Farquharson's Textbook of Operative Surgery

To
Margaret
and
Katharine

Farquharson's Textbook of Operative Surgery

Edited by

R. F. Rintoul
FRCS (Ed) FRCS
Consultant Surgeon, Nevill Hall Hospital, Abergavenny
Honorary Clinical Teacher, Welsh National School of Medicine
formerly
Clinical Tutor, University of Edinburgh
Senior Registrar, Royal Infirmary of Edinburgh
Surgical Tutor, Royal College of Surgeons

SEVENTH EDITION

CHURCHILL LIVINGSTONE
EDINBURGH LONDON MELBOURNE AND NEW YORK 1986

CHURCHILL LIVINGSTONE
Medical Division of Longman Group Limited

Distributed in the United States of America by
Churchill Livingstone Inc., 1560 Broadway, New York
N.Y. 10036, and by associated companies, branches
and representatives throughout the world.

First Edition 1954
Second Edition 1962
Third Edition 1966
Fourth Edition 1969
Fifth Edition 1972
Sixth Edition 1978
Seventh Edition 1986
International Student Edition of Seventh Edition 1986

ISBN 0-443-02572-X

British Library Cataloguing in Publication Data
Farquharson, Eric L.
    Farquharson's textbook of operative surgery. —
    7th ed.
    1. Surgery, Operative
    I. Title   II. Rintoul, R. F.
    617′.91   RD32

Library of Congress Cataloging in Publication Data
Farquharson, Eric L. (Eric Leslie)
    Farquharson's textbook of operative surgery.

    Includes bibliographies and index.
    1. Surgery, Operative. I. Rintoul, R. F. (Robert
Forbes) II. Title. III. Title: Textbook of operative
surgery. [DNLM: 1. Surgery, Operative. WO 500 F238t]
RD32.F32   1986   617′91   85-16661

Produced by Longman Group (FE) Ltd
Printed in Hong Kong

Preface to the Seventh Edition

When the First Edition of Mr Farquharson's Textbook was published in 1954, many surgeons were capable of practising a wide spectrum of general surgical operations and it was possible for a single author to provide comprehensive advice within a single textbook. Since then the widespread availability of synthetic materials for prosthetic implants and for atraumatic sutures has profoundly altered the surgical possibilities, with the additional benefit of smaller instruments, the operating microscope, and the fibreoptic bundle with its many and varied uses. Diagnostic methods are constantly changing; radiology is being increasingly replaced by ultrasound scanning, radioisotope scanning and, more recently, nuclear magnetic imaging. Many hospitals have the benefits of computerised axial tomography (CAT scanning) and some operations may be replaced by percutaneous surgery, or preceded by percutaneous biopsy by an 'interventional radiologist'. The surgeon of the 1980s can thus approach an operation with much more information about the patient than has hitherto been possible. However, the general surgeon of today must be aware of the basic techniques which are available and have a sound understanding of the reasons for applying these methods; it remains the objective of this textbook to provide this information in a single volume.

The publication of the Seventh Edition has been made possible only with the willing assistance of many colleagues in many hospitals throughout the UK. The whole text has been rewritten with the intention of providing guidance for the surgeon-in-training, particularly those preparing for the FRCS examinations. The book is also aimed at the surgeon practising in the smaller hospital at home or abroad, where more specialised advice is not otherwise available. For these, the simpler techniques have been described in a manner which will allow a surgeon of limited experience to operate with confidence and safety, should the situation demand that he proceed. References have been selected as a stimulus to further reading by supplying, where possible, details of an original article or of a more recent publication which covers the subject more comprehensively. The overall objective has been to maintain the continuity of style which Mr Farquharson introduced into his earliest teaching so as to provide an easily comprehensible and practical text.

The list of contributors follows, together with the list of artists who have painstakingly replaced the drawings. I am profoundly grateful to each of them for the skill and knowledge which they have contributed to the new edition and for their perseverance. As with the six previous editions, Mrs Farquharson has taken part in the preparation and her untiring enthusiasm and encouragement are acknowledged with gratitude.

With this edition, my wife has shared the enormous task of collecting, collating and checking the material from many sources. Without her help, it would never have appeared and she knows, I hope, how grateful I am.

Abergavenny, 1986   R. Forbes Rintoul

Preface to the First Edition

Most recently published works on operative surgery are the product of multiple authorship—the work of a number of eminent authorities, each writing on the specialty he has made his own. In support of such composite works, it is often stated that the progress of operative surgery in its many and varied branches has made the subject too vast to be covered adequately by a single author. It was with considerable diffidence, therefore, that I first approached such a task, but I believed that there was scope for a one-volume book written by a general surgeon and designed to present, as far as possible, the whole subject of operative surgery in balanced perspective from the viewpoint of the general surgeon in training.

With these aims in view, I have endeavoured to describe, in detail and with adequate illustrations, all the operations which the junior in general surgery is likely to undertake himself, and also the more commonly performed operations in which he may have to assist. In the specialised fields of surgery I have described in the same manner such operations as the general surgeon may at times be required to undertake when more expert help is not available. Most sections contain a short review of the surgical anatomy of the region; indications for operation, the choice of procedure, and pre-and postoperative treatment are discussed where pertinent.

Operations which are less frequently performed, and those which lie more strictly within the specialised fields, are described more briefly; the general scope and aims of the operation are discussed, but details of technique have as a rule been omitted. In this way it has been found possible to contain the work within a single volume of reasonable size.

Edinburgh, 1954   Eric L. Farquharson

Contributors

David C. Carter MD FRCS
St Mungo Professor of Surgery, University of Glasgow;
Honorary Consultant Surgeon, Glasgow Royal Infirmary

John Chalmers MD FRCS FRCS(Ed)
Consultant Orthopaedic Surgeon, Royal Infirmary of
Edinburgh; Senior Lecturer in Orthopaedic Surgery,
University of Edinburgh

James Christie FRCS(Ed)
Consultant Orthopaedic Surgeon,
Princess Margaret Rose Hospital
and Royal Infirmary of Edinburgh

Hugh A. F. Dudley ChM FRCS(Ed) FRCS FRACS
Professor of Surgery in London University, St Mary's
Hospital Medical School

Edward Hitchcock ChM FRCS FRCS(Ed)
Professor of Neurosurgery, Head of Department of
Neurosurgery, University of Birmingham

Geoffrey Hooper MMSc FRCS FRCS(Ed)
Senior Lecturer in Orthopaedic Surgery, University of
Edinburgh; Honorary Consultant Orthopaedic Surgeon,
Lothian Health Board

John Michael Stewart Johnstone FRCS(Ed)
Consultant General and Paediatric Surgeon, Leicestershire
District Health Authority

Jeremy Rae Braithwaite Livingstone FRCS(Ed)
FRCOG
Consultant Obstetrician and Gynaecologist, Royal Infirmary
of Edinburgh, Simpson Memorial Maternity Pavilion

D.B.L. McClelland BSc PhD(Leiden) FRCP(Ed)
Regional Director, Edinburgh and South-East Scotland Blood
Transfusion Service, Royal Infirmary of Edinburgh; Part-time
Senior Lecturer, Department of Clinical Pharmacology,
University of Edinburgh

Ian B. Macleod BSc FRCS(Ed)
Consultant Surgeon, Royal Infirmary of Edinburgh;
Honorary Senior Lecturer, Department of Clinical Surgery,
University of Edinburgh; Editor, Journal of the Royal
College of Surgeons of Edinburgh

Arnold G. D. Maran MD FRCS FACS
Head of Department of Otolaryngology, University of
Edinburgh; Consultant Otolaryngologist, Royal Infirmary and
City Hospitals, Edinburgh

J. E. Newsam MB FRCS(Ed)
Consultant Urological Surgeon, Western General Hospital,
Edinburgh; Honorary Senior Lecturer, University of
Edinburgh

R. F. Rintoul FRCS(Ed) FRCS
Consultant Surgeon, Nevill Hall Hospital, Abergavenny;
Honorary Clinical Teacher, Welsh National School of
Medicine

C. Vaughan Ruckley MB ChM FRCS(Ed)
Part-time Senior Lecturer, University of Edinburgh;
Consultant Surgeon, Royal Infirmary of Edinburgh

Michael N. Tempest MD ChM FRCS(Ed)
Consultant Plastic Surgeon, Welsh Regional Plastic Surgery
and Burns Centre, Chepstow; Consultant Plastic Surgeon,
University Hospital of Wales, Cardiff; Clinical Teacher in
Plastic Surgery, University of Wales College of Medicine;
Former Senior Lecturer in Plastic Surgery, University of
Ibadan, Nigeria

P. R. Walbaum FRCS
Consultant Cardiothoracic Surgeon, Royal Infirmary and City
Hospitals, Edinburgh

ARTISTS

Gillian Lee
Medical Artist, Buckhurst Hill, Essex

Ian Lennox
Senior Medical Artist, Edinburgh University Medical School

Eddy Lowe
Medical Artist, The Midland Centre for Neurosurgery,
Smethwick

Stephen McAllister
Senior Medical Illustrator, Tenovus Institute for Cancer
Research, Cardiff

Jean MacDonald
Senior Medical Artist, Department of Medical Illustration,
Glasgow Royal Infirmary

Anne McNeill
Medical Artist, Department of Clinical Surgery, Royal
Infirmary of Edinburgh

Contents

1 Operations on the skin and subcutaneous tissues   1
R. F. Rintoul & M. N. Tempest

2 Operations on muscles and tendons   16
J. Chalmers

3 Operations on blood vessels   26
D. B. L. McClelland, R. F. Rintoul & C. V. Ruckley

4 Operations on nerves   68
J. Chalmers & C. V. Ruckley

5 Operations on bones and joints   84
J. Chalmers

6 Operations on the hand and fingers   131
G. Hooper

7 Soft tissue injury   154
J. Christie

8 Amputations   163
J. Christie

9 Operations on the scalp, skull and brain   197
E. R. Hitchcock & A. G. D. Maran

10 Operations on the spine and spinal cord   213
E. R. Hitchcock

11 Operations on the face, mouth and jaws   220
A. G. D. Maran & M. N. Tempest

12 Operations on the neck and salivary glands   236
J. M. S. Johnstone, A. G. D. Maran & R. F. Rintoul

13 Operations on the breast   270
R. F. Rintoul

14 Operations on the thorax   283
J. M. S. Johnstone & P. R. Walbaum

15 Abdominal operations   309
J. M. S. Johnstone & R. F. Rintoul

16 Exploratory laparotomy   329
R. F. Rintoul

17 Operations on the stomach and duodenum   334
D. C. Carter & J. M. S. Johnstone

18 The spleen and portal hypertension   366
C. V. Ruckley

19 The liver and sub-phrenic space   374
I. B. Macleod

20 The gall-bladder, the bile ducts and the pancreas   381
J. M. S. Johnstone & I. B. Macleod

21 Operations on the appendix   408
R. F. Rintoul

22 Operations on the intestines   417
H. A. F. Dudley, J. M. S. Johnstone, I. B. Macleod & R. F. Rintoul

23 Operations on the rectum and anal canal   457
H. A. F. Dudley, J. M. S. Johnstone & R. F. Rintoul

24 Operations for hernia   480
J. M. S. Johnstone & R. F. Rintoul

25 Operations on the urinary tract   504
J. E. Newsam

26 The kidney, the adrenal glands and the ureters   528
J. E. Newsam & R. F. Rintoul

27 Operations on the bladder and prostate   574
J. E. Newsam

28 Operations on the male urethra and genital organs   607
J. M. S. Johnstone & J. E. Newsam

29 Gynaecological encounters in general surgery   636
J. R. B. Livingstone

Index   645

1
Operations on the skin and subcutaneous tissues

R. F. RINTOUL & M. N. TEMPEST

INCISIONS

All skin incisions should be carefully planned so as to give a good view of the deeper parts, and at the same time to avoid important structures. In general, when an incision has to be made in the neighbourhood of large vessels or nerves, it should be made parallel to, and not across, their long axis. For cosmetic reasons, however, incisions on the face or neck should be placed in a natural crease, for not only will the scar be less visible, but there will be less likelihood of keloid formation. Similar considerations arise in regard to incisions in the hand and fingers (p. 133).

A sharp knife should always be used, and the skin should be cut cleanly at one stroke throughout the distance required, the plane of the blade being held perpendicular to the skin surface (Fig.1.1). A fresh knife is used to incise the deeper layers so as to avoid contaminating them with organisms which may have been exposed by the skin incision.

An incision of adequate length should always be made. Short incisions may be appreciated by the patient, but they cannot be justified if they add unnecessary difficulties to the operation.

ARREST OF HAEMORRHAGE

All bleeding points should be secured with artery forceps. In order to minimise haemorrhage, any larger vessels which cross the line of incision should be identified and clamped between two pairs of forceps, before they are divided. Small superficial vessels are generally occluded by pressure alone, the forceps being left on for a minute or two, by *torsion* (twisting the forceps round several times), or by coagulation with the diathermy current. Larger vessels require to be ligatured or 'tied off' with fine thread or catgut. Every time this is done two foreign bodies are introduced—the ligature itself and strangulated tissue beyond it. Care should therefore be taken as far as possible to clamp the vessel alone, without taking up adjacent tissue; likewise the ligature should be of the finest material consistent with security, and the end should be cut as short as is practicable. When using diathermy, it is preferable to coagulate the vessel alone *without a mass of surrounding tissue* so as to ensure correct haemostasis and to avoid unnecessary tissue damage.

For the 'tying off' of bleeding points close co-operation between surgeon and assistant is required. The surgeon passes the ligature material around the forceps; the assistant holds the forceps, depressing the handle and elevating the point as much as possible, so that the tissue which is clamped becomes encircled by the ligature (Fig. 1.2). Just as the surgeon is tightening the first hitch of the knot the assistant *slowly* releases the forceps. If the forceps are released suddenly the tissue is liable to slip out of the grasp of the ligature.

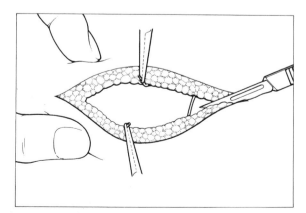

Fig. 1.1 Method of making skin incision and of arresting superficial haemorrhage.

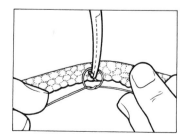

Fig. 1.2 Method of 'tying off' a bleeding point.

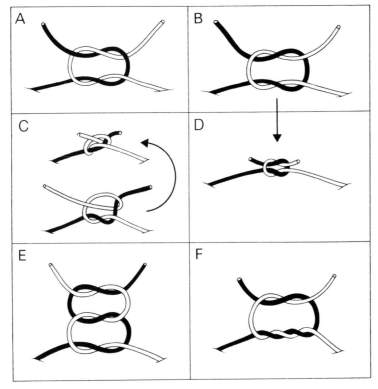

Fig. 1.3 Different varieties of knots: (A) *A 'granny' knot*. An unsafe knot, which should never be used. (B) *A reef knot*. Must be kept 'square' by tightening in the correct directions. (C) *A reef knot*—spoiled by careless tightening, so that an insecure knot results. The white strand has been pulled to the left. (D) The white strand has been correctly pulled to the right, the black to the left—see (B). (E) *Triple knot*. (F) *'Surgeon's knot'* with an extra turn to the first loop

KNOTS

Different types of knots

The simple and reliable *reef knot* is well known, and is universally advocated for surgical purposes. It is essential that it should be kept 'square' by being tightened in the correct directions, for an insecure slip-knot results if this precaution is not observed (Fig. 1.3). With slippery suture material such as catgut, nylon or other plastics, the ends should not be cut too short or the knot may slip. Multiple knots are required to provide a safe knot with monofilament nylon. The *triple knot* is a modification of the reef knot giving additional security, and allows the ends to be cut very short. The *surgeon's knot* is best suited to the ligation of large vessels and pedicles, when thicker ligature material is employed.

Tying knots with the left hand

This easily-learned accomplishment saves much time, especially in the tying of sutures, since there is then no need to lay down the needle, which is held throughout in the right hand. It is useful, both for the initial knot of a continuous suture, and for interrupted sutures so

that several of these can be obtained from the one length of material.

It is important to tie a reef knot, and to keep this 'square' by tightening it in the correct manner. A satisfactory technique is shown in Figures 1.4–1.9.

METHODS OF WOUND CLOSURE

After most operation wounds, except where sepsis or potential sepsis is encountered, the skin incision is closed by suture, in an attempt to obtain healing by first intention. One of the commonest causes of failure of such healing is imperfect haemostasis as the formation of a haematoma within the wound prevents accurate coaptation of the cut surfaces and predisposes to infection. All bleeding vessels must therefore be dealt with, and all dead space obliterated before skin stitches are inserted. Should it be impossible to do this, or should further bleeding be expected, the wound should be drained. Closed drainage by a fine tube to an evacuated bottle (*Redivac*) is now well established as a method of removing extravasated blood or serum and has done much to promote satisfactory healing of operation wounds.

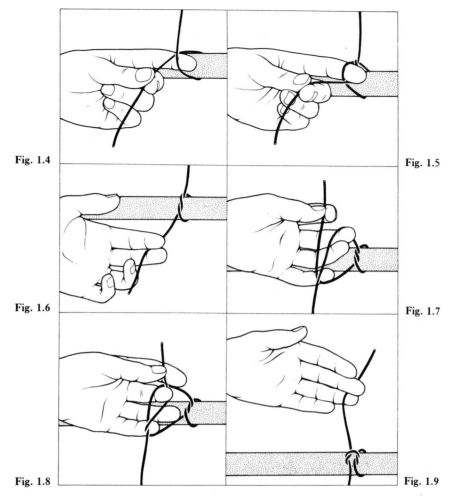

Figs. 1.4–1.9 Method of tying a reef knot with the left hand. Note how the knot is kept 'square' by tightening in the correct directions. (The end of suture material passing off the edge of each drawing is held in the right hand.)

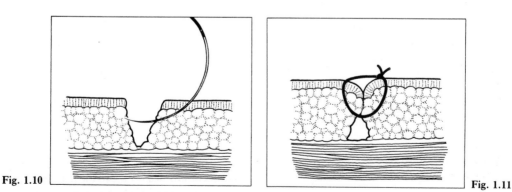

Figs. 1.10 & 1.11 Incorrect method of suturing which results in inversion of the skin edges so that dead space is left in the wound

Superficial stitches normally include only the skin and subcutaneous tissue. The needle should be made to pass perpendicularly through the skin in order that inversion of the edges may be avoided (Figs 1.12 and 1.13), and the stitches should be tied with only sufficient tightness to bring the skin edges together without constriction. Too tight stitches cause ischaemia of the tissue and result in delayed healing. In some situations, subcu-

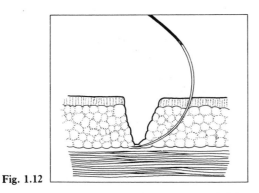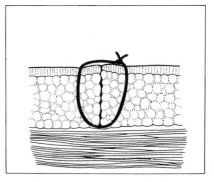

Figs 1.12 & 1.13 Correct method of suturing. The needle is introduced vertically through the skin, and traverses the entire thickness of subcutaneous tissue

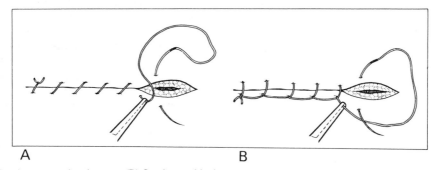

Fig. 1.14 (A) Continuous overhand suture. (B) Continuous blanket suture

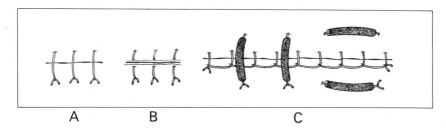

Fig. 1.15 (A) Ordinary interrupted sutures. (B) Eversion sutures. (C) Deep tension sutures threaded on rubber tubing showing simple type on the left and mattress on the right

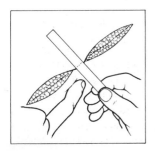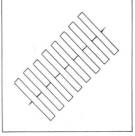

Figs. 1.16 & 1.17 Closure of skin wound by means of *Steri-strips*

ticular sutures may be used to approximate the dermal layer of the skin so that skin stitches are not required.

Deep stitches include, in addition, the deep fascia and one or more of the muscle layers and may be employed to obliterate any dead space in the depths of the wound. To prevent cutting of the skin, the parts of the sutures lying on the surface may be threaded on to short lengths of rubber tubing (Fig. 1.15).

Suture material Nonabsorbent material with a smooth surface should be employed for skin sutures. Silk, nylon, or a variety of different threads, specially treated to reduce absorbency, are in general use. When a neat scar

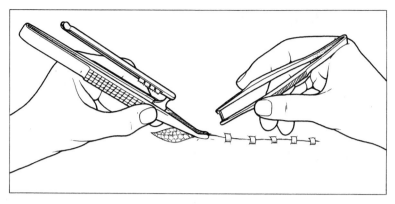

Fig. 1.18 Michel clips

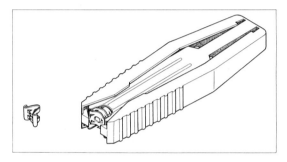

Fig. 1.19 Disposable skin clips and applicator

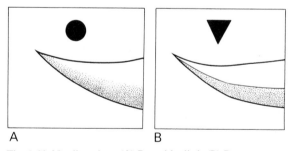

A   B

Fig. 1.20 Needle points: (A) Round bodied. (B) Reverse cutting

is particularly desired (e.g. in the head and neck), *Steri-strips* (Figs 1.16 and 1.17) or Michel or alternative clips (Fig. 1.19) may be used; they are removed after 3–4 days.

Needles

Except in certain situations, an ordinary round-bodied needle is not easily thrust through skin. Skin needles are usually triangular on cross-section, or have spear-shaped points. They may be straight or curved.

Types of suture

Various types of skin stitches in common use are shown in Figures 1.14 and 1.15. Superficial sutures may be either continuous or interrupted. Deep sutures are usually interrupted. Continuous suture saves much time in the closure of a long wound, but has the minor disadvantage that, should infection or haematoma formation occur, it is difficult to remove a part of the suture line for drainage without the rest becoming insecure. All knots are placed to lie at one side of the wound, so that they do not become buried in the scar.

SIMPLE TUMOURS AND CYSTS OF THE SUPERFICIAL TISSUES

Local anaesthesia

For minor operations on the skin and superficial structures a local anaesthetic has many advantages. It is the least toxic of all anaesthetics and has no after-effects, so that the patient can resume full activity immediately afterwards.

The drugs presently in most common use are the various proprietary forms of *procaine*, or of the longer-acting *lignocaine*—$\frac{1}{2}$ to 1% solution is commonly employed. A small quantity of adrenaline may with advantage be added to the solution. By its vasoconstrictor properties, it enhances the effect of the local anaesthetic and reduces bleeding. Proprietary solutions contain 1 part adrenaline in 200 000.

Infiltration anaesthesia aims at paralysing the nerve endings at the actual site of operation, the injection being made into the subcutaneous tissues immediately deep to the skin lesion and in the line of any incision that requires to be made. The infiltration of a small area can be carried out through one or two punctures with a fine hypodermic needle. Large needles, which are required for a wide infiltration, should not be introduced until the skin has been anaesthetised by injection through a fine needle. The best way of doing this is to raise a cutaneous wheal by the injection of a small quantity of anaesthetic solution

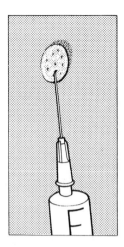

Fig. 1.21 The raising of a cutaneous wheal

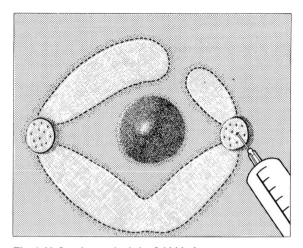

Fig. 1.23 Local anaesthesia by field block

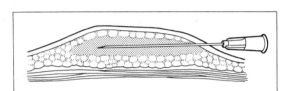

Fig. 1.22 Subcutaneous infiltration

within the layers of the skin. The needle is introduced in a direction almost parallel with the surface. As soon as its bevel disappears a few drops of solution are injected under pressure, so as to raise a round white wheal with a pitted surface (Fig. 1.21). This area is immediately insensitive. Further wheals are raised according to the extent of the infiltration required.

Field block
By this method the anaesthetic solution is injected into the tissues at some distance from the actual site of oper-ation, so that a zone of anaesthesia is created surrounding the operation area (Fig. 1.23). A fairly long needle is required for the injection, and a suitable number of skin wheals are raised for its insertion. It usually suffices to make the injection into the subcutaneous tissue alone, but in certain cases it may be advisable to infiltrate the muscle or other tissue lying deep to the lesion. Before any injection is made into the deeper tissues an aspiration test should be made, in order to ensure that the needle has not entered a blood vessel. The injection is then made while the needle is slowly withdrawn. Field block has advantages over infiltration anaesthesia in that the lesion is not obscured by local swelling.

Sebaceous cysts

For the removal of small cysts under healthy skin a linear incision is employed. If the cyst is markedly protuberant,

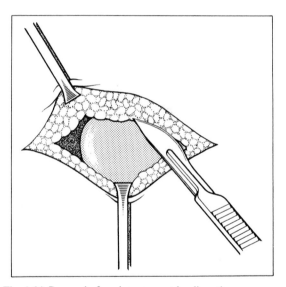

Fig. 1.24 Removal of a sebaceous cyst by dissection

or if the skin is thin and unhealthy, an elliptical segment of skin should be removed along with the cyst. The skin overlying the cyst is raised by careful dissection (Fig. 1.24); thereafter the cyst can be shelled out without difficulty using curved artery forceps to open the plane immediately adjacent to the cyst wall. An alternative method—that of *avulsion*—is particularly suited to the removal of sebaceous cysts on the scalp. A comparatively small incision is required, and the skin is raised for a short distance on one side only. The cyst is then delib-erately opened and the contents squeezed out. A pair of non-toothed dissecting forceps, with one blade outside the cyst and one blade within, is insinuated round the side of the cyst wall until this can be grasped at *its deepest part*, which is much tougher than the superficial part and will not tear easily. By traction on the forceps

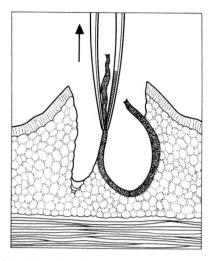

Fig. 1.25 Avulsion of a sebaceous cyst

(Fig. 1.25), the entire cyst wall can usually be avulsed with ease.

The wound is sutured, and a pressure dressing is applied to prevent haematoma formation in the cavity.

Infected sebaceous cysts
If any inflammation is present, removal of the cyst should always be deferred until this has subsided. If an abscess forms it should be incised and the contents evacuated; a cyst so treated seldom recurs.

Dermoid cysts
Superficial dermoid cysts occur as a rule in the face or scalp, the superciliary region being a common site. They are often firmly attached to the periosteum or bone, and may even have fibrous connections through bone diploë with dura mater, so that their removal may present some difficulty, and should be attempted only with the strictest aseptic precautions.

Implantation (dermoid) cysts occur on the hands and fingers. Their removal is described on page 152.

Papillomata
'Infective warts' which occur usually in crops may be treated successfully by local application (salicylic acid paint or the cryoprobe), or they may be destroyed by the diathermy current. Occasionally they require to be excised.

True papillomata should be excised if they are subject to pressure or friction, or if their removal is desired for cosmetic reasons. All excised skin lesions should be submitted to histological scrutiny since clinical examination does not always give a reliable guide to the future potential of the growth. If the wart has suddenly enlarged or has become ulcerated, malignant change must be suspected. The site of the lesion may arouse the suspicion of the surgeon especially on the sole of the foot where the so-called amelanotic melanoma can occur. This highly malignant tumour is not pigmented as its name implies. An elliptical incision around a suspicious wart should include an adequate margin of surrounding skin which will vary between 5 and 15 mm depending on the appearance of the wart and its situation.

Pigmented warts or naevi. The majority of these are benign, and remain so throughout life: occasionally they take on malignant characteristics, but this is rare before puberty. The excision should include a generous margin of surrounding skin (5–10 mm), since incomplete removal may stimulate the onset of malignant change.

Haemangiomata
These may take the form of a 'port-wine stain' (*capillary haemangioma*) or a definite tumour consisting of a spongy network of dilated blood spaces (*cavernous haemangioma*). *Port-wine stains* on the face are often flat and so extensive that instruction in cosmetic camouflage by an expert is the best form of advice that can be given. If the skin surface of the port-wine stain is irregular with numerous vascular excrescences, bleeding can be a serious nuisance and it may be justifiable to excise these lesions and apply a skin graft with the understanding that this will not eradicate the underlying lesion though it may improve the appearance and comfort the victim. Occasionally port-wine stains of the face may affect the deeper tissues extending into the brain (the Sturge-Kalischer-Weber syndrome) and be associated with fits and steady mental deterioration. Often calcification can be seen, on X-ray examination, in the brain. Recent work with *laser therapy* and *cryotherapy* suggests that these two techniques may offer some improvement in the appearance of the flat port-wine stain. Radiotherapy is useless.

Cavernous haemangiomata usually undergo dramatic spontaneous resolution within the first 2–3 years of life and a policy of 'wait and watch' is strongly advised. Surface ulceration will often speed up the process of resolution. Early excision is most unwise except possibly for the extensive lesions that may involve the eyelids where the question of retaining binocular vision is so important. If a major feeding vessel can be identified and palpated it is sensible to suggest ligating it. Various techniques to stimulate thrombosis in the lesions (such as injection of boiling water, saturated saline, intralesional diathermy, cryotherapy, even external pressure and steroids given systemically) have been recommended. Radiotherapy is absolutely contraindicated in the infant and young child and is probably unwise at any age.

Lipomata
Surgical removal offers no difficulty. Through an overlying skin incision, the tumour can usually be shelled out with ease from within its capsule, but care should be

taken that all extensions are removed. If the tumour is pedunculated, an elliptical incision is made around its base.

MALIGNANT TUMOURS OF THE SKIN

In all malignant tumours of the skin it is to be expected that permeation of the growth will have occurred, at least to some extent, into the tissue spaces at the periphery of the tumour, and in certain cases there will be evidence of spread to the regional lymph glands. Successful removal therefore necessitates the excision of a sufficiently wide margin of surrounding tissue along with the primary growth and involved regional glands also should be excised.

Squamous cell carcinoma (epithelioma)

This tumour is sensitive to radiotherapy, which may be used as an alternative or as an adjunct to operation. Radiotherapy, after histological confirmation, is preferable to operative removal in most anatomical sites. Excision of the growth should include at least 10–15 mm of healthy skin on all sides. Squamous cell carcinoma of the lip is discussed more fully on page 227.

Secondary deposits of squamous cell carcinoma in the regional lymphatic glands are generally less sensitive to radiotherapy than is the primary tumour. Block dissection of the regional glands should therefore be carried out when there is any suspicion that they are involved, either initially or during the patient's follow up. Radiotherapy alone may provide palliation when gland dissection is impracticable.

Basal cell carcinoma (**Rodent ulcer**) is slow growing; it

infiltrates deeply into the subcutaneous tissue, and even into bone, but seldom disseminates to the regional lymph glands. Again the choice in treatment lies between radiotherapy and excisional surgery. Application of the cryoprobe to a basal cell carcinoma allows tissue to be taken painlessly for histological examination and a small lesion may be destroyed by this procedure (Lloyd-Williams, 1978). If radiotherapy is not available, excision should include a margin of 5 mm on all aspects, including the deep surface. The resulting defect may require one of the plastic methods of repair for its closure (p. 9.).

Malignant melanoma

Variable degrees of pigmentation and nodularity should make the surgeon suspicious of malignant melanoma especially if there are adjacent satellite nodules. There seems to be little potential for a compound naevus to become malignant and excision is therefore carried out for diagnosis only. An established malignant melanoma, however, should be regarded as highly malignant until

it has been excised, when depth of penetration of the tumour into the dermis or subcutaneous tissues will give some guide to its aggressive potential. *Incision* biopsy is contraindicated except for a large lesion where major resection would result in unnecessary disfigurement in the event of the tumour being benign. In most cases, *excision* biopsy is necessary in order to establish a diagnosis of malignant melanoma and to plan any subsequent surgery. Since tumour thickness is a major determinant of survival (Meyer, 1985; Milton, 1980), the pathologist must report depth measurements of the melanoma and its level of invasion. Thus, a tumour which has not penetrated into the dermis may be cured by local excision while a thick tumour necessitates wider excision which will entail skin grafting or amputation.

The treatment of malignant melanoma is fraught therefore with difficulty and anxiety, and the surgeon carries an unusually heavy responsibility in the advice which he may offer. The following principles may be laid down for guidance:

1. The *minimal* treatment of *any* pigmented skin tumour is complete excision. Even for the most innocent-looking mole, a margin of 5 mm of healthy skin should be removed.

2. The excised tissue is examined histologically, either immediately by frozen section or within 48 hours. If the condition is shown to be a malignant melanoma—and even if the removal appears to have been complete—a wide excision of the previous wound and of the surrounding tissues should at once be carried out as described in the next paragraph.

3. A melanoma of 0.75 mm depth requires 1 cm clearance of normal skin, i.e. a further 5 mm should be removed in addition to the 5 mm already removed at the initial excision. A tumour of 1 mm depth requires 2–3 cm clearance and a tumour greater than 1.5 mm depth necessitates 5 cm clearance of normal skin. There is no evidence that excision of deep fascia or muscle provides any additional benefit.

4. (a) Melanomata under or near the nail of a finger or toe (*subungual*) should be treated by disarticulation of the digit at its base.

(b) Melanomata of the forefoot or of the posterior part of the foot may require a Syme amputation or a below knee amputation if there is extensive ulceration or bleeding.

(c) Melanomata of the anal canal are even more malignant than those in other situations and demand an abdominoperineal excision.

5. *Prophylactic* removal of regional lymph nodes (i.e. when they are not clinically involved by metastases) is not generally advised unless the primary lesion lies close to the lymph nodes. It may, however, be considered where the tumour is known to have been rapidly growing

and histological examination has shown invasion of the dermal lymphatics (Boulter, 1976). In all other cases, the patient is closely followed up for examination of the regional lymph nodes so that block dissection can be advised when there is clinical evidence of their involvement.

6. Radiotherapy appears to be of limited value in this relative radio-resistant tumour.

7. Intra-arterial perfusion with antimitotic drugs, systemic chemotherapy (Ghussen, 1985), endolymphatic infusion with radioisotopes (MRC Working Party 1979) and immunotherapy have all been used with some success, mainly for palliation in advanced cases.

SKIN GRAFTING

The highly specialized art of the plastic surgeon is invoked for the treatment of certain congenital lesions (cleft lip and palate: hypospadias: syndactyly), for the repair of complicated facial injuries, the treatment of major burns, the excision of certain malignant (or recurrent) tumours and reconstruction of the defects, quite apart from the treatment of conditions that could be regarded as aesthetic (scar revisions, rhinoplasty, breast reduction or augmentation). For this type of work special training and experience are required. To the general surgeon falls the humbler task of transplanting skin to cover raw areas or to replace scar tissue that is interfering with function.

It is now firmly established that skin is the best possible dressing for a raw surface. Skin grafting is, therefore, of special value in the treatment of burns, where, for several reasons, the normal process of epithelialisation may be unduly prolonged and healing may be complicated by infection, gross scarring and contractures. In certain full thickness burns immediate or early excision of the burn followed by immediate or delayed skin grafting may transform the situation and save weeks of suffering and disability. In deep dermal burns, too, tangential excision down to the zone of punctate bleeding with immediate cover using thin split skin grafts has been advocated by Janzekovic (1970) in Yugoslavia and this has revolutionised the treatment of this type of injury. Contracted scars in the neighbourhood of joints may need wide excision and intricate skin grafting manoeuvres that might well have been avoidable had the original wound been skin grafted.

Where there is actual loss of skin following trauma or the wide excision of malignant growths, immediate skin cover may be required. However, if this is impracticable for reasons such as difficulty in achieving haemostasis, uncertainty about the viability of the deeper tissues or the adequacy of clearance of a malignant lesion, it may be wiser to pack the cavity, dress the wound and close the defect later as a secondary procedure by one or more of the techniques to be described below.

Skin defects can be closed by one of three methods:

1. By local adjustment of the surrounding skin or by the advancement of skin flaps from the immediate neighbourhood. This method has obvious advantages in terms of colour match, texture and type of skin, but these flaps must be designed to lie in natural crease lines without tension and without producing additional unsightly scars in otherwise normal tissue.

2. By free skin transplants using either split-skin grafts of varying thickness or full-thickness skin grafts (*Wolfe grafts*). These grafts are completely detached from their origin and, to survive, must obtain adequate nourishment from the bed on which they are placed. As a general rule, the thinner the graft the more certain the 'take' but the final result may be often less satisfactory in appearance, function and durability.

3. By transfer of skin from another part of the body using a pedicled flap. Such a flap enables skin to be transferred along with the subcutaneous tissues which can provide the padding needed in the repair of complicated contour defects and the closure of heavily irradiated wounds. This type of repair requires several stages and careful planning. The introduction of microsurgical techniques has transformed the transfer of tissues from a distance and it is now possible to transfer a compound flap which includes not only skin and the subcutaneous tissues but also bone, muscle, tendons and nerves.

Adjustment of surrounding skin (local flaps)

The local tissues can be advanced, rotated or transposed to close the excisional defect or wound without tension using skin that is similar in texture and colour to the missing tissues. All incisions through the skin must be made cleanly with a sharp knife held at right angles to the surface. The tissues should be held with hooks or delicate forceps. Sharp needles and fine suture materials should be used and the sutures evenly spaced and tied without strangulating the tissues. Carefully placed subcuticular sutures will give an excellent scar.

Simple undercutting. Careful undermining of the adjacent tissues away from the edge of the wound may permit primary closure of quite a large defect without tension. The level at which this undermining should be carried out is important. In the face undercutting must be in the subcutaneous layer to avoid damaging the branches of the facial nerve (Fig. 1.27). In the limbs and over the trunk the most suitable plane lies on the deep fascia and the muscles themselves (Fig. 1.28); in the scalp, it is the layer between pericranium and the galea (Fig. 1.29). Carefully placed parallel incisions in the under surface of the galea may reduce tension on the suture line and give a little more advancement.

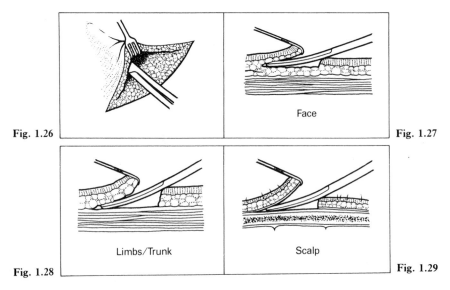

Fig. 1.26

Face

Fig. 1.27

Limbs/Trunk

Fig. 1.28

Scalp

Fig. 1.29

Figs. 1.26–1.29 Method of skin undermining (after McGregor, 1980)

V-Y advancement. This technique is more often seen in illustrations than in practice but it can be used in the repair of V-shaped lacerated wounds, the release of triangular-shaped scars, as a 'kite-flap' to close large circular defects and in the closure of certain finger tip injuries (the Kutler (Fisher, 1967; Kutler, 1949) or Kleinert (Atasoy, 1970) flap).

Rotation-advancement flaps are useful in the closure of defects, especially if the latter can be conveniently converted into a triangular shape. The ease with which these flaps can be used depends on the anatomical site of the defect and the laxity of the adjacent tissues. Almost every surgical textbook shows rotation flaps that are pitifully inadequate in size and with an axis of rotation that makes the illustrated result impossible. A very large flap is needed to close quite a small defect on the scalp (Fig. 9.4), on the face (Fig. 1.30) or a sacral bed sore. The flap must be raised in the appropriate tissue plane, (Figs 1.27–1.29) and if there is any serious difficulty in closing the secondary defect, this should be skin grafted.

Transposition flaps. Contracted linear scars commonly occur in the neck, the axillary fold or in the neighbourhood of joints where they may restrict or prevent movement. Simple excision of the scar combined with some plastic procedure to prevent recurrence of the contracture is required. Such a manoeuvre is the Z-plasty in which two interdigitating triangular flaps are transposed. The scar is excised (or incised along its crest) and from each extremity two incisions are made at an angle of 60°, so that the markings resemble the letter 'Z' (Fig. 1.32). The triangular flaps are then raised, transposed and sutured in their new position (Fig. 1.33). The effect of this manoeuvre is to lengthen the original axis of the scar and place a new axis across the contracture. It must be emphasised that it works best if the original scar is linear, with good quality skin on each side of the band. It is of no use in the release of broad thick contractures or in the closure of defects over convexities such as the skull. It is used widely as part of the treatment of Dupuytren's contracture in the hand and plastic surgeons regularly use it in the closure of difficult wounds. The permutations and combinations of this type of flap are superbly described by McGregor (1980).

Split skin grafts

These are the general purpose skin grafts most frequently used. They can be taken from any part of the body but the commonest donor sites are the anteromedial surface of the thigh and the inner aspect of the upper arm. The grafts may be cut at different depths. Thin grafts (*Thiersch grafts*) consist of epidermis only and are used mainly for covering granulating areas where the urgent need is to heal the wound quickly. The 'take' of these

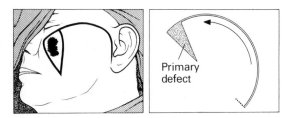

Primary defect

Fig. 1.30 Rotation flap to cover facial defect
Fig. 1.31 Advancement of the rotation flap. Dotted line shows 'back cut' to release tension

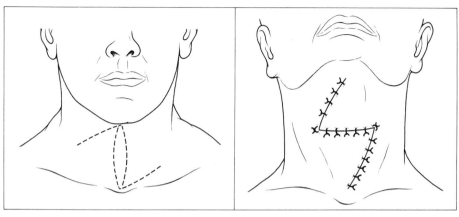

Fig. 1.32
Fig. 1.33

Fig. 1.32 Incisions for Z-plasty
Fig. 1.33 Completed Z-plasty

thin skin grafts is impressive even in the presence of infection but their inability to stand up to wear and tear and their tendency to contract relegates them to the category of temporary grafts that will need replacement later by thicker grafts or flaps. Thicker grafts (*split-skin grafts*) consist of epidermis, dermis and the superficial layers of the corium. They are far more durable and pleasing in appearance. Indeed the thicker split-skin grafts are almost indistinguishable from a full thickness graft. However, the surgeon must be cautious to select the least obtrusive donor site, since, the thicker the split-skin graft, the more unsatisfactory may be the healed donor surface.

Preparation of the recipient area
A clean 'tidy' freshly-made wound (by accident or deliberately by the surgeon's knife) presents no problems provided that complete haemostasis is secured by fine ligatures and careful use of the diathermy, preferably the bi-polar coagulator. The base of the wound should be as even as possible and any spaces between muscle bellies should be carefully obliterated by a few interrupted fine sutures. If these two criteria cannot be fulfilled it may be wiser to cut the skin graft and apply it some 36–48 hours later or to dress the wound and perform a definitive grafting operation 7–10 days later.

By contrast 'untidy' wounds and granulating areas may require careful preparation. Adherent sloughs must be excised and any crevices in the granulating area removed by cutting away the exuberant soft granulations. Frequent wet dressings with gauze soaked in saline, eusol or sodium hypochlorite (Milton) must be applied until a healthy, pink, painless flat granulating surface is produced. The fitness of the wound for grafting is probably best judged by the clinical appearances; information obtained by bacterial investigation is not always helpful and may be misleading. Complete sterility is usually unobtainable and is not essential. The presence of

B-haemolytic streptococci group A or coagulase positive staphylococci are contraindications to grafting but can be dealt with by systemic antibiotic therapy. Heavy pyocyaneus and proteus wound infections can interfere with graft 'take' and frequent wet dressings may be required to cleanse the wounds. However the indiscriminate local application of antibiotic powders, solutions and creams or various desloughing agents (enzymatic, chemical or hydrophilic) is an extremely expensive and largely worthless substitute for a good simple dressing technique.

In the operating theatre such a granulating area requires little extra preparation other than cleansing with povidone iodine or Hibitane followed by saline and rubbed down with a cotton gauze swab soaked in ether to remove any epithelial debris and greasy remnants from the tulle gras dressings that may have been used in the past. If some of the granulations are still exuberant and unhealthy in appearance, they should be scraped away to leave a yellow firm base. Bleeding is controlled by firm pressure with warm saline packs or packs soaked in hydrogen peroxide solution.

Cutting of the graft
The donor site, which should have been shaved if the surface was hairy, is prepared like any other operation site with povidone iodine, Hibitane, Cetavlon and spirit. The limb should be held firmly by the assistant whose hands give counter pressure from behind to present the surgeon with a flat surface from which the graft will be cut. The surgeon places a wooden board on the donor site just in front of the skin grafting knife. The blade of the knife and the edge of the wooden board are coated with liquid paraffin to allow a smooth gliding motion on the skin. The skin grafting knife is held firmly in the hand pressed firmly against the skin and with a steady to and fro sawing motion the knife and skin grafting board move steadily forwards (Fig. 1.35).

Although the blade in the knife may have been set at

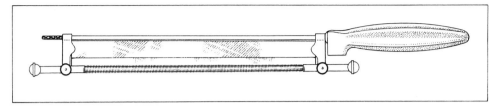

Fig. 1.34 Humby's skin-grafting knife (modified by Bodenham), with disposable wafer-type blades and with adjustable guard, allowing grafts of varying thickness to be cut

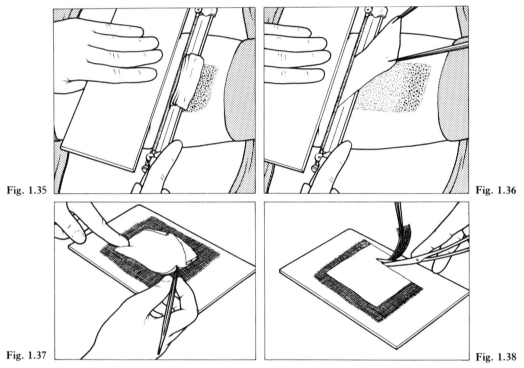

Fig. 1.35   Fig. 1.36

Fig. 1.37   Fig. 1.38

Figs. 1.35 & 1.36 A graft of varying thickness being cut
Fig. 1.37 The graft being spread out on tulle gras
Fig. 1.38 Strip being cut from the graft

a predetermined depth the surgeon must check the thickness of the graft. This can be judged by the translucency of the graft and the pattern of bleeding and appearance of the donor site. A very thin graft is translucent so that the knife blade will appear bluish grey in colour. A thicker graft will appear whiter in colour, the bleeding points on the donor surface will be few, far apart rather than closely packed and confluent as with the thinner grafts (Fig. 1.36). If the skin graft has been cut at too deep a level and subcutaneous fat appears in the wound, the surgeon has two choices: (a) to resuture the graft in place and take a thinner graft elsewhere or (b) to use the thick graft as a full-thickness graft and place a thin split-skin graft on the unintentionally deep donor site. The donor site should be dressed as soon as the grafts have been cut, using a layer of tulle gras, Gamgee tissue and a sterile crepe or elasticated cotton bandage carefully applied to exert even pressure, absorb any exudate and put the donor site at rest. An outer layer of Elastoplast or even plaster of Paris will give greater protection. The wound should be left undisturbed for 10–14 days and when the dressings are soaked off the donor site should be healed.

Preparation of the graft
The sheets of skin that have been cut are spread out, with their deeper surface uppermost, on a large sheet of tulle gras laid neatly and taut on a wooden board so that the squares of the tulle gras are lying correctly as squares. The skin is spread out evenly and, using a sharp scalpel

or pair of scissors, is trimmed so that the graft can be applied in sheets or strips (Fig. 1.38). When used as a single sheet the graft is cut to a suitable size and tacked to the edges of the defect by a few well-placed sutures that can be left long, if required, to help fix a tie-over dressing. When skin grafting a large area, the better sheets of skin should be reserved for the most important sites, namely across joints and flexion creases.

Strip grafting is useful in cases where, due to the state of the bed of the graft and the presence of infection, a complete 'take' cannot be guaranteed. In this case exudate or pus will not threaten a large sheet of skin and failure to take may be confined to only a few strips. A variant of this technique is to cut the strips into small squares about the size of postage stamps and apply these to the granulating surface leaving a small gap between each square. This is also one way of making a little skin go a long way but unfortunately the patchwork appearance of the final result is disfiguring and permanent.

Mesh grafting
The most efficient technique of making a split-skin graft go a long way is to pass the sheet of split skin through a meshing device that cuts the skin into a predetermined lattice pattern which allows the skin to be expanded by a factor of 4, 9 or 16. The final result may show a fine mesh-work pattern but this ultra-economical use of skin when donor sites are limited is a major advance in the life-saving skin cover of extensive burns.

Care of grafts: dressings or exposure
Failure of the split-skin graft to 'take' completely is due to:

1. A collection of serum or blood beneath the graft.
2. Infection and a collection of pus beneath the graft.
3. Accidental dislodgement of the graft, usually the result of a poor dressing technique or inadequate attention to fixation when the grafts are treated by exposure.

Pressure is certainly not essential for the take of a graft and it is debatable in any case how much pressure can be exerted by dressings and for how long it can be maintained. Nevertheless there is no doubt that a good firm dressing with evenly distributed pressure will keep the parts at rest during the early healing stages and protect the graft from unnecessary outside interference, both from the patient's, the nurses' and the surgeon's fingers. On a flat or evenly convex surface, firm crepe bandaging suffices over a layer of dry gauze or Gamgee tissue. A layer of Elastoplast or light plaster cast may be added for better protection. On a concave or irregular surface, fluffed-out gauze or pieces of polyurethane foam or cotton wool soaked in paraffin may be used to fill the cavity before bandaging as before. These dressings should be left undisturbed for at least 5–10 days and only removed earlier if there is pain, pyrexia or pus.

Full thickness grafts
These grafts which are composed of the full thickness of the skin are unsuitable for use on granulating areas but ideal for resurfacing clean surgical wounds produced by excision of scars or tumours. They are particularly useful where the texture and colour match of the skin are important and where durability of the skin cover is an advantage. For this reason they are widely used to correct facial deformities such as ectropion, scars and growths of the lips, nose and cheek and in the hand to correct hand deformities, burn contractures of the fingers, finger tip injuries and in the treatment of syndactyly.

The recipient site must be carefully prepared and absolute haemostasis achieved. An exact pattern is then made of the defect in metal foil or jaconet or paper. Any non-hairy part of the body can be chosen for the donor site, special preference being given to those sites where the donor site can be closed quickly and easily by primary suture. The postauricular sulcus (Fig. 1.39), the nasolabial fold, the supraclavicular and infraclavicular regions are good donor sites. So too, is the inframammary crease in the woman and the groin in both sexes, provided care is taken not to transplant hairy skin from the inguinal region. Flexion creases at the elbow or knee are best avoided as the resultant scars can be disfiguring. The pattern is laid on the donor site and the skin is cut at a superficial level, much as skin is raised in the dissecting room taking care not to button-hole the skin or raise too much subcutaneous fat in the process. Any excess fat must be trimmed away from the undersurface of the graft with sharp scissors. The donor defect is closed without tension after undermining the wound edges. The graft is then sewn into the surgically-created defect with fine sutures to give exact apposition at the graft-to-skin junction. Depending on the recipient site the graft may be left exposed or protected by a tie-over dressing.

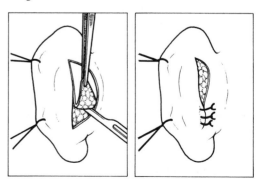

Fig. 1.39 Whole-thickness skin graft being cut from the post-auricular region
Fig. 1.40 Defect closed by suture

Pinch grafts

These grafts, originally described by Reverdin, are now no longer in favour. They are small cones of skin picked up with a sharp straight needle and cut through with a scalpel blade held flat against the skin surface. The graft, held on the needle, is then transferred to the granulating wound where it is pushed into the granulating surface. Several grafts are applied in rows to cover the surface leaving a gap of 0.5 cm between each cone. Its sole merit is that the grafts are hardy and can survive in the presence of sepsis. It may therefore have a place in chronic leg ulcers, tropical sores and bed sores.

The cosmetic appearance of the grafted area is exceedingly poor. The donor site disfigurement is appalling unless the pinch grafts are cut in a skin crease and the linear segment is then excised and closed itself by primary suture.

Pedicle flaps

In contrast to a free graft which is completely detached from its donor site and is transposed to the recipient site, a pedicle flap at all times maintains an intact circulation. This allows skin, subcutaneous tissue and/or fat to be transferred to resurface areas that are unsuitable for free split-skin grafts, that present a serious contour defect or sites at which further reconstructive work may be necessary such as tendon, nerve or bone graft repairs. Only when the flap is soundly inset into the recipient defect and has picked up a new blood supply can the pedicle be divided. There are two types of flap distinguished by their vascular anatomy.

Most of the traditional flaps in use belong to the category of 'random pattern' flaps in which the vascular distribution of the arteries and veins show little or no axial direction. For this reason the design of the flap must conform to some strict limitations in the length to breadth ratio which depends to a great extent on the elasticity of the tissues and the anatomical configuration of the donor and recipient sites. Good examples are the cross-finger flap and the cross-leg flap.

By contrast, an 'axial pattern flap' has a distinctly identifiable arteriovenous system in its long axis and long flaps can be raised with far fewer restrictions on their width. Good examples are:

1. The deltopectoral flap, based on the perforating intercostal arteries (Bakamjian, 1965).
2. The groin flap based on the superficial circumflex iliac artery (McGregor, 1972).
3. The hypogastric flap based on the superficial hypogastric vessels.

With all these flaps careful planning is needed. There must be no tension or torsion of the vascular pedicle and the maximum amount of the flap should be inset into the recipient area at the original operation. The closer the proximity between the donor and recipient areas, the more successful will be the result, though great care may be required in maintaining fixation of the limbs (Fig. 1.42).

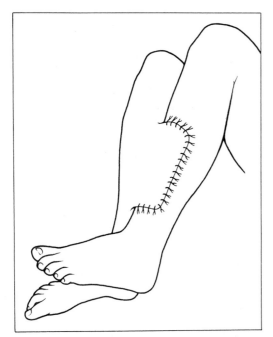

Fig. 1.41 Cross-leg flap

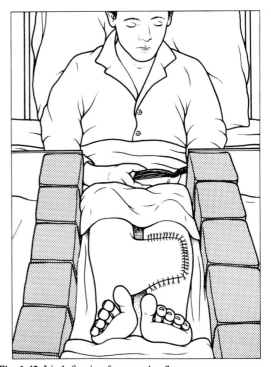

Fig. 1.42 Limb fixation for cross-leg flap

Interest in the vascular supply of other potential *axial pattern flaps* has encouraged a detailed re-examination and study of the blood supply not only to the skin and subcutaneous fat, but to the fascia, the underlying muscles, bones and nerves. Plastic surgeons now have at their disposal a very wide range of flaps, incorporating any number or all of these structures, that can be raised, transposed or rotated into local or distal defects. For example, the pectoralis major muscle with or without the overlying skin, can be raised on its vascular pedicle and transposed into the neck. The latissimus dorsi muscle can be transposed with or without some of its covering skin to reconstruct chest wall defects following mastectomy, defects in the neck or in the upper limb. Flaps containing skin and fascia (the tensor fasciae-latae flap) are invaluable in closing defects in the perineum, sacrum and ischial regions. Muscle flaps consisting of muscle only such as the gastrocnemius, soleus, gracilis and gluteus maximus flaps, can be used to cover difficult chronic wounds over the limbs and in the buttock region. Similarly in the lower limb below the knee, compound skin and fascial flaps have been proved to be far safer in closing difficult defects than simple skin flaps alone.

Many of these flaps, and others too, can be raised as free-flaps and transported to almost any site in the body provided there are suitable vessels at the recipient site to allow revascularization of the free flap by *microvascular anastomoses*. These compound flaps can be designed to include segments of bone and nerve which can themselves be revascularised at the same time.

The tube pedicle flap, associated so intimately with the names of Gillies (in the U.K.) and Filatov (in the Soviet Union) is a remarkably effective technique of transferring large or small quantities of skin and subcutaneous tissue to almost any part of the body in stages, either by 'waltzing' one end of the tube or attaching one end of the pedicle to an intermediate carrier such as the wrist or forearm (Fig. 1.43). Most of the pedicles raised in this way had a very large axial pattern component such as in the acromiothoracic pedicle or in the lower abdominal pedicle. Other tube pedicles had a far more random pattern of blood supply. Such operations required several stages, considerable skill in planning and execution by the surgeon and fortitude on the part of the patient. There is a tendency nowadays to relegate the technique to one of almost 'dinosaur status', but there is no doubt that it still has a place in certain complicated facial, trunk and limb reconstructions.

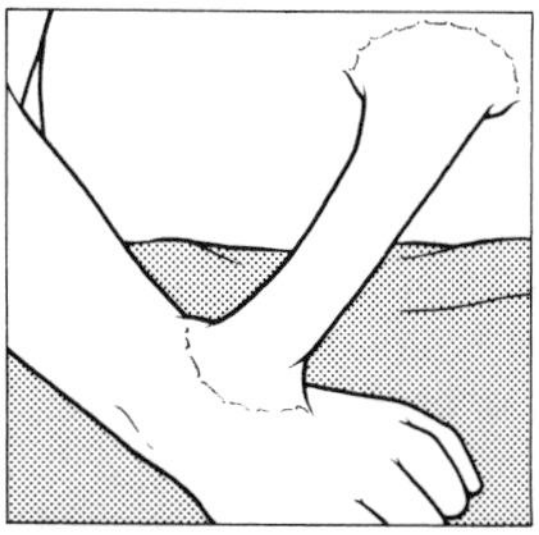
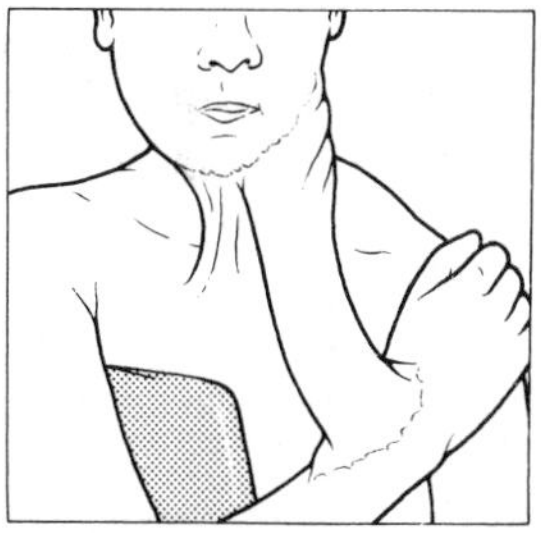

Fig. 1.43 Transfer of abdominal flap to wrist
Fig. 1.44 Pedicle flap carried on wrist to cover neck defect

REFERENCES

Atasoy E, Ioakimidis E, Kasdan M, Kutz J, Kleinert H E 1970 Reconstruction of the amputated finger tip with a triangular volar flap. Journal of Bone and Joint Surgery 52A: 921

Bakamjian V Y 1965 A two-stage method for pharyngo-oesophageal reconstruction with a primary pectoral flap. Plastic and Reconstructive Surgery 36: 173

Boulter P A 1976 Diagnosis and management of skin tumours. In: Hadfield J, Hobsley M (eds) Current surgical practice vol. 1. Arnold, London, p 246

Fisher R H 1967 The Kutler method of repair of finger tip amputations. Journal of Bone and Joint Surgery 49A: 317

Ghussen F, Nagel K, Groth W, Müller J M, Stützer H 1984 A prospective randomised study of regional extremity perfusion in patients with malignant melanoma. Annals of Surgery 200: 764

Janzekovic Z 1970 A new concept in the excision and immediate grafting of burns. Journal of Trauma 10: 1103

Kutler W 1949 A new method for finger tip amputations. Journal of the American Medical Association 133: 29

Lloyd-Williams K 1978 Cryosurgery and its applications. In: Hadfield J, Hobsley M (eds) Current surgical practice vol. 2. Arnold, London, ch 14, p 253

McGregor I A, Jackson I T 1972 The groin flap. British Journal of Plastic Surgery 25: 3

McGregor I A 1980 Fundamental techniques of plastic surgery and their surgical applications, 7th edn. Churchill Livingstone, Edinburgh. New Edition in preparation

Meyer K L, Childers S J 1985 The surgical approach to primary malignant melanoma. Surgery Gynaecology and Obstetrics 160: 379

MRC Working Party on Endolymphatic Therapy in Malignant Melanoma 1979 A clinical trial of endolymphatic therapy in malignant melanoma: Interim report of the progress of the Medical Research Council trial. British Journal of Surgery 66: 9

Milton G W, Shaw H M, Farago G A, McCarthy W H 1980 Tumour thickness and the site and time of recurrence in cutaneous malignant melanoma (Stage I). British Journal of Surgery 67: 543

FURTHER READING

Cason J A 1981 Treatment of burns. Chapman and Hall, London

Grabb W C, Smith J W 1979 Plastic surgery, 3rd edn. Little, Brown, Boston

Mathes S J, Nahai F 1979 Clinical atlas of musculo- and musculo-cutaneous flaps. Mosby, St. Louis

Mathes S J, Nahai F 1982 Clinical applications for muscle and musculo-cutaneous flaps. Mosby, St. Louis

Muir I F K, Barclay T L 1976 Burns and their treatment, 2nd edn. Lloyd-Luke, London. New Edition in preparation

O'Brien B McC 1977 Microvascular reconstructive surgery. Churchill Livingstone, Edinburgh

2

Operations on muscles and tendons

J. CHALMERS

AFFECTIONS OF MUSCLE

Disruption of muscle tendon unit

Disruption of a muscle tendon unit may occur at various points. The muscle may be detached from its bony origin or insertion; it may rupture through the belly, at the musculotendinous junction, in the tendinous portion itself, or through a sesamoid bone such as the patella (Fig. 2.1).

The site at which muscle or tendon rupture occurs is dependent upon a number of factors including the age of the patient and his general health. Disruption of the origin of a muscle may occur in the younger age groups, particularly where the origin or insertion is an epiphysis. Rupture within the belly of a muscle is most common in those indulging in vigorous athletic pursuits, such as rugby, as a result of indirect violence or from direct injury to the area while the muscle is contracting. Disruption at the musculotendinous junction is most commonly seen in early or advancing middle age. The sites at which this type of rupture are most common are in the tendo Achilles, the quadriceps and around the shoulder, both in the rotator cuff and in the long head of biceps. When such rupture occurs in these areas, surgical repair may be indicated, unless the patient's disability is small, or if he is elderly, when the condition is best treated conservatively.

The level at which injury occurs reflects the relative strengths of tissues at different periods of life. In injuries which are the result of intrinsic violence, the system gives way at the weakest point viz:-
   in children and adolescents, at an epiphysis
   in fit adults, through the belly of the muscle
   in middle age, through the tendon
   in elderly patients, through tendon or osteoporotic bone.
But there are many exceptions to these generalizations.

Muscle repair

Lacerations and ruptures through muscle bellies are difficult to repair, for sutures tend not to hold strongly in muscle tissue and can pull out when the muscle contracts. Small and incomplete ruptures are best left untreated for they cause no disability. They may, however, give rise to concern because a patient notices a 'tumour' proximal to the level of the injury when the muscle contracts. However, the innocent nature of the 'tumour' is apparent for it disappears completely when the muscle relaxes. Major muscle disruptions require to be sutured. Ragged muscle ends are trimmed and a series of mattress sutures are used to coapt the cut ends. The sutures should be placed, where possible, through tendinous tissue or fibrous muscle sheath. The suture line should be protected by splintage for about six weeks.

Muscle hernia

Muscle hernia results when the sheath of the muscle is torn or ruptured, so that the fibres bulge through the gap thus formed. Symptoms seldom warrant any operation but, if so, the defect in the sheath can be closed with a suture or a fascia lata graft. A quadriceps hernia is a common sequel to fascial transplant operations, in which

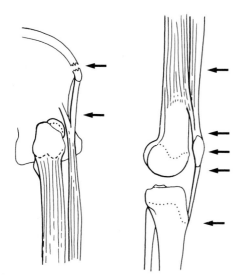

Fig. 2.1 Sites at which disruption of the quadriceps femoris muscle may occur

the defect in the fascia lata has not been sutured. The risk of such a hernia constitutes a definite disadvantage to the use of a fascial stripper.

Muscle abscesses (*pyomyositis tropicans*)

Abscesses in skeletal muscle are common in many tropical countries—the quadriceps, the pectorals and the glutei being most frequently affected. The aetiology is obscure, but the condition appears to arise as the result of repetitive trauma, when muscular haematomata become infected by blood borne organisms—usually *staphylococcus aureus*. Complete recovery after simple incision and drainage is the rule.

Traumatic ischaemia of the limb muscles

Traumatic ischaemia of the limb muscles is a complication of fractures, crushing injuries, gunshot wounds etc. The term *Volkmann's ischaemic contracture* is applied to the pathological changes which occur. Skeletal muscle in any situation may be affected, although it is most familiar when it occurs in the muscles of the flexor compartment of the forearm (Fig. 2.2). It is important to realize that the same changes can occur, both in the posterior aspect of the forearm and in the muscles below the knee where all the compartments are at risk, either singly or in combination. Early diagnosis is crucial. When it is diagnosed within a few hours of injury, treatment can be successful in preventing the established changes of Volkmann's contracture. If treatment is delayed for more than 4 or 6 hours, irreversible changes develop within the muscle.

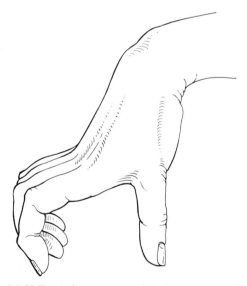

Fig. 2.2 Volkmann's contracture of the flexor muscles of the forearm leads to this disabling claw hand with flexion contractures of wrist and interphalangeal joints, and inability to grip

Extensive ischaemia resulting from the occlusion or division of a major artery or combination of smaller vessels does not usually present diagnostic difficulty. The cardinal signs of pain, pallor, paralysis and pulselessness are likely to be present. A much commoner and more insidious presentation is ischaemia, which is confined to a small area such as a closed osteofascial muscle compartment. In such a case, the periphery often has adequate circulation and peripheral pulses are present and yet, within the closed osteofascial compartment, muscles and nerves can suffer from ischaemia. The clinical features are: severe pain, which is aggravated when the muscle is put on a stretch; the affected muscles feel hard and tender; and loss of function may be demonstrated in nerves which pass through the compartment. If severe pain develops in an injured limb within 48 hours of injury, this complication must always be looked for and relieved if present.

Muscle ischaemia is the result of arterial insufficiency due to division of a main artery or to its occlusion by compression or intimal rupture with secondary thrombosis. Arterial spasm without structural damage to the vessel is now largely discredited, except in cases of wounding by high velocity missiles, which have traversed a limb in close proximity to the vessel. In general, time spent in attempting to relieve spasm by sympathetic blocks or other means merely delays the commencement of effective treatment. Compartment ischaemia is due to swelling within the compartment as a result of haematoma or post-traumatic oedema. The build up in pressure embarrasses venous drainage in the compartment, which in turn aggravates the swelling. If this vicious circle is not relieved, the arterial supply within the compartment is eventually cut off. If a severe degree of ischaemia persists for more than a few hours, the muscles undergo necrosis and, subsequently, replacement fibrosis with contracture. The nerves show a greater degree of resistance to ischaemia than muscle but again may suffer irreversible damage if treatment is delayed. Compartment ischaemia tends to be more common in crushing injuries or in association with fractures in which there has been a slight displacement for more severe injuries are likely to disrupt the compartments and so prevent the build up of pressure.

Treatment

As soon as traumatic muscle ischaemia is suspected, all constricting bandages and splints should be removed, the position of fractures or dislocations should be checked to ensure that they have been adequately reduced and in the particular case of supracondylar fractures of the humerus in children, an injury notoriously liable to be associated with Volkmann's ischaemia, the elbow should be gently extended. If these simple measures do not bring about relief, surgery should be carried out without

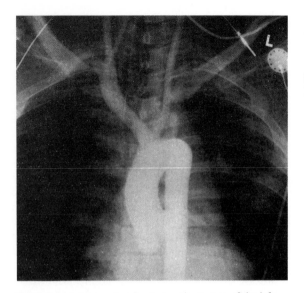

Fig. 2.3 Arteriogram showing traumatic rupture of the left subclavian artery which has sealed off spontaneously. Repair of the artery restored circulation to the arm

delay. An arteriogram may rarely be required to establish the site of arterial damage (Fig. 2.3). The major vessels are exposed proximal to the level of injury, where they may be readily controlled, and then traced to the site of injury, where external compressing agents are removed or the vessel damage repaired as described on page 35. If the vessel injury is associated with a fracture, it is frequently expedient to stabilize the limb by internal fixation of the fracture before the vessel repair is carried out.

Compartment compression is dealt with by division of skin and deep fascia throughout the length of the compartment. If more than one compartment is involved, it may be necessary to make two skin incisions to gain access, for example to all four compartments in the lower limb. Following division of the deep fascia, the swollen and congested muscles bulge through and rapidly resume a more normal colour, if the operation has been done in time. The condition of the main vessels and nerves within the compartment is then examined and, if necessary, they are repaired, although in general in compartment syndromes, decompression alone is sufficient to restore the circulation. No attempt should be made to close skin or fascia at this stage. A dressing is applied and the limb loosely bandaged. At four days, the wound is re-exposed under anaesthesia and delayed closure is carried out usually by means of skin graft or occasionally by skin suture, if the oedema has subsided sufficiently.

It is important to realize that where there has been ischaemia, the risks of infection, particularly anaerobic infection such as gas gangrene (p. 161), are consider-

ably increased. Antibiotic cover with penicillin in high dosage must be given and continued for 10 days. When ischaemia has complicated an open wound, such as a compound fracture, the risks of infection are increased further. It is extremely important that the most meticulous primary excision of the wound be carried out to minimize the risks of subsequent infection.

Late operations. The disability resulting from muscle ischaemia is due to contracture and shortening of the affected muscles. If the involved muscles retain some active function, the contracture may be overcome by either lengthening the tendons, for example the tendo Achilles in calf contracture, or by carrying out a muscle slide operation in which the origin of the affected muscles is mobilized from the bone and allowed to slide distally. This is an extensive procedure requiring a wide exposure and mobilization of the affected muscles and, if done inexpertly, can result in increased muscle ischaemia and nerve damage. Sometimes the infarct involves only part of the contents of the compartment producing localized fibrosis within part of one or more muscles. In this circumstance, it may be possible to excise the fibrosed tissue thus releasing the contractures and subsequently carry out tendon transfers to substitute for the missing muscles, as would be done in the case of paralytic disorder (p. 24).

Late operations should not be performed until at least 6 months have elapsed following injury in order to allow spontaneous recovery to take place.

REPAIR OF CUT TENDONS

Anatomy
A tendon is composed of longitudinal bundles of collagen fibres, loosely bound together. When it is cut or torn, the ends become frayed by separation of the collagen bundles, so that longitudinal sutures tend to cut out.

Where a tendon pulls round a curve or bend, it is enclosed within a synovial sheath, consisting of two layers continuous with one another through the medium of a narrow *mesotenon* (like the two-layered peritoneal reflection of the mesentery). This mesotenon, which is seen as a thin transparent membrane when a tendon is lifted from its bed, lies on the longitudinally convex side of the tendon, where it is away from friction; it carries the blood and lymph vessels which nourish the tendon itself.

Fibrous sheaths may be present in addition to synovial sheaths. They are necessary to prevent the tendons from slipping out of position as they pass round a bend. The fibrous sheaths of the fingers are described on page 144. The peroneal retinacula fulfil a similar function.

In the situations where a tendon pulls in a straight line, it has usually no synovial sheath; it is covered instead by a thin layer of *paratenon*, which is a specialized form of loose fat containing elastic fibres.

General considerations

When a tendon is severed in a synovial sheath, considerable retraction may occur—to a distance equal to the amplitude of movement of the tendon. Its ends become smoothly rounded over making no attempt to proliferate. Cut ends may remain loose within the sheath or they may become stuck down to the surrounding tissues, particularly if there has been any element of infection. When severed in paratenon, the tendon shows less retraction. New vascular connective tissue invades the gap between the tendon ends, which become linked by fibrous tissue. Initially the fibrous union has a loose and disorganized appearance but rapidly the fibres become orientated in the line of the tendon pull and the eventual scar closely resembles normal tendon. With subsequent use, the vascular adhesions associated with the repair break down and function is restored. This healing process will occur naturally in all situations except within the synovial sheath but, unless the tendon ends are approximated, either by surgical repair or external splintage, the tendon will heal with elongation and consequent impairment of function. Prognosis in tendon suture, therefore, depends on the type of tendon and the situation in which it has been divided; those in paratenon within the forearm or dorsum of hand being usually attended by a good result, while those in the synovial sheath depend to a much greater extent on the skill and experience of the surgeon. The poorest results of tendon repair are seen in the flexor tendons of the fingers, where they lie within the fibrous flexor sheath, where dense and permanent adhesions may form. Such adhesions may be minimized by atraumatic technique, the use of a nonirritant suture material and healing of the wound in conditions of absolute asepsis. Tendon suture, therefore, must not be regarded as a minor operation but should be carried out only in a fully equipped operating theatre with adequate assistance.

The preoperative clinical assessment is of great importance. Careful clinical examination should be carried out in order to establish with certainty which tendons (and nerves) have been divided, for the ends will have retracted from the site of injury and may be hard to find at operation unless the surgeon knows exactly which tendons he is seeking. Even in an unconscious or anaesthetized patient, however, the injured tendon may sometimes be deduced by the posture of the part (Fig. 2.4). General or regional anaesthesia may be used and a pneumatic tourniquet is essential. Primary tendon suture should be attempted only in incised wounds which are recent and afford good quality of soft tissue and cover, and in the case of divisions within the fibrous flexor sheath of the finger (p. 20), only if the surgeon has the necessary skilled experience. If any of these

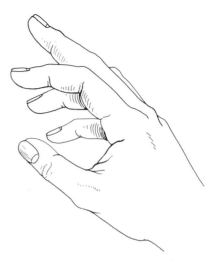

Fig. 2.4 In the unconscious patient posture of the fingers may indicate tendon damage. In this case the flexors of the long finger have been divided

conditions cannot be met, it is better that the wound be treated by simple excision and suture, and a secondary repair be carried out once skin healing has taken place.

Associated injuries. Fractures associated with tendon divisions are best stabilized by internal fixation. Nerves and important vessels divided at the level of the tendon injury can also be repaired at the same time.

Materials for tendon suture. These must be nonreactive in the tissues otherwise adhesions will form. Stainless steel wire, monofilament nylon, *Prolene* or *Mersilene* mounted on atraumatic needles are appropriate.

Techniques of tendon suture

The method of suturing employed should hold the cut ends of the tendon in firm apposition until healing is complete. It is necessary to obtain some sort of 'splicing' effect into the tendon ends, since simple longitudinal stitches will cut out between the fibres. To reduce the likelihood of adhesions to surrounding structures, the suture material should be buried as far as possible within the tendon.

Figure 2.5 illustrates two of the techniques which may be used to join tendon ends of equal size. The tendon ends, if ragged, are cut cleanly across and the suture material mounted on a fine, straight needle is passed through the tendon in a manner indicated in the diagrams.

Following tendon repair, it is necessary to protect the suture line from stress by appropriate splintage for 3 weeks in the case of upper limb tendons, and for 6 to 8 weeks in major weight-supporting tendons in the lower limbs. Gentle movements within the confines of the splintage may be allowed from an early date and once the

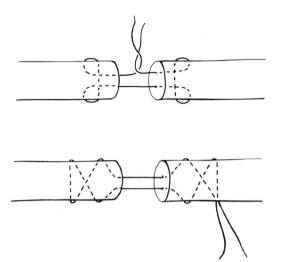

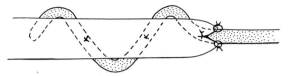

Fig. 2.6 The Pulvertaft suture for tendons of unequal size

Fig. 2.5 Two methods of suture of tendons of equal diameter.
Top the Kessler stitch
Bottom the Bunnell stitch

tendon to which it is being attached and therefore end to end suture is rarely possible and the technique illustrated in Figure 2.6 may be adopted.

In using a tendon graft, it is important to obtain correct tension otherwise the motor unit will not function properly. In the case of a finger flexor, the correct tension may be judged by comparison with the degree of flexion in the other fingers in the resting state.

splintage is removed, graduated active exercise is required to break down adhesions and regain movement.

Secondary tendon repair
The same techniques may be applied to secondary tendon repair but it is essential that the suture line should lie in healthy tissues. If the tendon is repaired in a scarred bed, it will become stuck down to the surrounding scar. Thus it may sometimes be necessary to carry out a plastic procedure in the overlying skin, or, if the deep tissues are scarred, it may be preferable to bypass the area by means of a tendon graft and thus avoid a suture line within the scar tissue.

Tendon grafting
The operation of tendon grafting is carried out when a gap exists between the tendon ends or where it is necessary to avoid a repair in scar tissue, or in the case of flexor tendon injuries in the finger within the fibrous flexor sheath, where a direct repair is likely to be associated with adhesion formation. The operation is almost invariably performed as a secondary procedure after skin healing. The tendons of palmaris longus and plantaris are most commonly used. A toe extensor may be used if other materials are not available. The palmaris tendon is best mobilized through a series of three or four short transverse incisions placed along the course of the tendon. Palmaris is sometimes absent—it is important to confirm its presence prior to anaesthesia. The plantaris, which gives an excellent length of strong, slender graft, is approached through a short incision in the medial aspect of the tendo Achilles near its insertion. The tendon is then removed using a tendon stripper. A tendon graft is usually of a smaller diameter than the

TENDON REPAIR IN SPECIAL SITUATIONS

Flexor tendon injuries in the hand
Tendon injuries occur most frequently in the hands because the hands are so exposed to risk of industrial or domestic injury. The particular problems of divisions within the fibrous flexor sheath have been referred to earlier and it is this structure which dictates the technique of repair (Fig. 2.7). Outside the fibrous flexor sheath, primary tendon repair may be carried out by one of the methods illustrated in Figure 2.5. It is sometimes

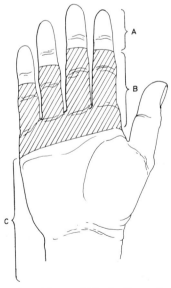

Fig. 2.7 Zones A and B are within the fibrous flexor sheath. Primary suture is permitted in Zone A, for a tenodesis at this level gives a good result.
Within Zone B tendon grafting is indicated, for adhesion at this level would lead to stiffness and poor function.
Within Zone C primary suture is satisfactory

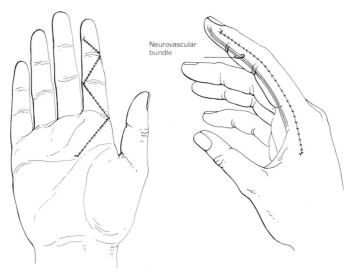

Fig. 2.8 Incisions which may be used for operations on the flexor tendons in the finger

prudent when all flexor structures are cut in front of the wrist, as in suicide attempts, to repair only the functionally most important tendons for, if all are repaired at the one level, they tend to fuse together. Thus it may be wise to repair flexor pollicis longus and flexor digitorum profundus only, resecting the sublimis tendon. Within the fibrous flexor sheath, if the superficial tendon alone is divided, the disability is negligible and it should not be repaired. If both tendons are divided, the sublimis is again sacrificed and the profundus repaired by means of a tendon graft, which bypasses the flexor sheath, done as a secondary procedure. Division of the profundus alone, distal to the superficialis tendon, may be repaired primarily even though it lies within the flexor sheath, for, although adhesions may form, a strong tenodesis at this level gives satisfactory function.

Flexor tendon graft in the finger

Incision. The incision must be placed so as to avoid cutting the flexor creases at a right angle, with a risk of scar contracture, and the neurovascular bundles must obviously be protected. Two incisions are widely used and are illustrated in Figure 2.8. The midlateral incision lies behind the neurovascular bundle, which is reflected forward in the volar skin flap, and must be carefully identified and preserved in the palmar extensions of this incision. The zigzag incision lies between the neurovascular bundles, the angles being placed at the flexor creases. This approach gives better access and is preferred by many. The fibrous flexor sheath is then excised leaving three intact pulleys to prevent bow stringing of the tendon graft. The superficial tendon is excised, if this has not already been done at the time of primary wound care, and the profundus is likewise

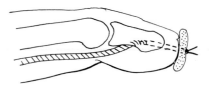

Fig. 2.9 Technique of attachment of the flexor tendon to the distal phalanx. The pullout stitch is fastened over a button at the finger tip and is withdrawn at 3 to 4 weeks when healing will have occurred. This technique can be adapted to attach tendon to bone in other situations

resected proximally to midpalm and distally to leave a short stump. The palmaris or plantaris graft is then attached to the proximal cut end of profundus by the technique illustrated in Figure 2.6, and is covered, if possible, with lumbrical muscle. The graft is then passed through the pulleys, which have been left, and is attached to the distal stump of profundus or to an osteo-periosteal flap elevated from the distal phalanx, using the pullout stitch shown in Figure 2.9. The tension of the graft should be adjusted to produce the same degree of resting flexion as is present in the adjacent fingers.

After the operation, the fingers are bandaged in semiflexion for 3 weeks. Thereafter active exercises are instituted, at first gently, and then with increasing vigour until maximum recovery is achieved, which may take several months.

Repair using silastic rod. An alternative technique has been developed in recent years, which utilizes a silastic rod to maintain the patency of the fibrous flexor sheath and to promote the formation of a new synovial sheath within it. This operation is done in two stages. At the first stage, the divided tendons are excised to midpalm and a rod of silastic of suitable calibre is placed within the flexor sheath, which is left intact except for a limited resection at the site of the original injury. The rod is anchored distally by means of a single stitch and the proximal end is cut obliquely in the midpalm. The cut ends of the flexor profundus and flexor superficialis are then sutured together in the midpalm. Postoperatively the finger is kept mobile by passive movement. Six weeks later a second operation is carried out at which the palmar and distal extremities of the old incision are reopened and a separate incision is made at the distal aspect of the forearm through which the superficialis tendon is identified and divided. It is mobilized carefully and brought out in the palmar wound. The suture line to profundus is freed from adhesions. The two ends of the silastic rod are then identified. The distal end of the superficialis graft is attached to the rod by suture and the rod is withdrawn at its distal end, drawing the tendon through the sheath. The tendon is then fixed as described above for the free tendon graft.

Repair of flexor pollicis longus
The simpler anatomy of the flexor of the thumb simplifies the surgical repair. Direct suture is often possible even within the fibrous flexor sheath, if this is excised widely from the site of suture. If there is much scarring, however, a tendon graft as for the finger flexors is preferable.

The results of surgical repair of the thumb flexor are usually superior to flexor tendon repair in the other digits which seldom achieves a full range of movement.

Extensor tendon repairs

Because the extensor tendons of the hand and wrist are surrounded by paratenon, their management is much easier and the end result generally more satisfactory than obtains with flexor tendon repairs. Primary suture is the treatment of choice and presents no particular problems apart from the particular injuries described below.

Mallet finger. This is caused by an acute flexion injury of the terminal segment, which either disrupts the extensor tendon or avulses it from its insertion with a fragment of bone. If the bony fragment is large, it should be reattached using a fine wire suture. If the tendon is disrupted, surgical repair is not necessary. Satisfactory healing can be obtained by immobilizing the terminal joint of the finger in full extension for 6 weeks. The splint is illustrated in Figure 2.10.

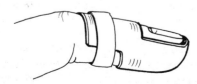

Fig. 2.10 Plastic finger splint used for mallet finger

Boutonnière deformity. This results from division or rupture of the central slip of the extensor expansion at the level of the proximal interphalangeal joint. It is very liable to be missed at the time of the initial injury since no immediate disability is apparent. With time, however, the two lateral slips of the extensor tendon slide forward around the sides of the joint and come to act as flexors leading to progressive flexion deformity of this joint with hyperextension of the distal interphalangeal joint. Splintage of the proximal interphalangeal joint in extension for 6 weeks using a splint such as is illustrated in Figure 2.11, is successful, if commenced early. Cases which present late may be left untreated if the disability or deformity are slight. Otherwise an attempt must be made to repair the central slip or reconstruct it by using one of the lateral bands.

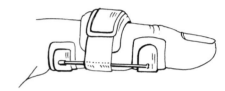

Fig. 2.11 Splint for boutonnière deformity

Rupture of the extensor pollicis longus tendon. This may occur at the level of the distal radius. It can be spontaneous as a result of repetitive activity or, more commonly, following an undisplaced fracture of the distal radius, which has led to irregularity of the groove in which the tendon lies. The rupture usually develops after an interval of some weeks. The rupture of this or indeed any of the extensor tendons of the fingers may complicate rheumatoid arthritis. The disability from rupture of the extensor pollicis longus tendon is not always great but, if it gives rise to handicap, surgical treatment is desirable. Direct suture is not possible because there is a large gap between the tendon ends and the most useful procedure is a tendon transplant using extensor indicis proprius as the motor tendon. This is divided through a short incision at the level of the neck of the second metacarpal—note that the extensor indicis proprius tendon lies towards the ulnar side of the extensor digitorum communis tendon of the index. Through a separate incision, it is joined to the distal part of the extensor pollicis longus tendon using the technique shown in Figure 2.13. The thumb is splinted in extension for three weeks and a uniformly satisfactory result is obtained.

Rupture of the tendo Achilles

This relatively common and disabling injury is frequently missed because, after the momentary acute pain of rupture, the patient experiences relatively little discomfort and may not seek medical advice. The presentation is very characteristic. The patient is usually a young adult engaging in athletic activity, who feels a sensation as if he had been kicked in the calf of his leg. Some plantar flexion is maintained through the action of the other long flexor muscles of the foot and toes but the patient is unable to stand on tiptoe and the loss of the normal tendon contour is apparent on clinical examination. Lateral calf compression fails to transmit a flexor action to the foot, as it does in the normal calf. As with other tendon ruptures in paratenon, spontaneous healing will take place but, unless this is carefully managed, the healing will take place with lengthening of the tendon and consequent loss of power in the calf muscle.

Conservative management
If the foot is placed in full equinus, the ruptured tendon ends are closely approximated and a plaster cast is applied in this position for 4 weeks. Because of the equinus attitude, the patient cannot usually weight-bear in such a plaster and must use crutches during this period. After 4 weeks, the plaster is replaced with one in 20 degrees of equinus in which weight-bearing is possible. This second plaster is kept on for a further 4 weeks. Thereafter the plaster is removed and for the next month the patient walks with a 1 centimetre raise to the heel of his shoe at all times. Normal athletic activity can be gradually resumed thereafter.

Surgical treatment
Many surgeons prefer surgical treatment. With the patient prone, an incision is made along the lateral border of the tendo Achilles. The paratenon is carefully incised and preserved along the length of the tendon. The ruptured tendon ends will be found to be frayed and have to be trimmed back. An end to end suture is then carried out with a nonabsorbable suture, using one of the techniques illustrated in Figure 2.5. A plaster cast is then applied with the foot in slight equinus, which is retained for 8 weeks. Weight-bearing is allowed. Thereafter the management is the same as in conservatively treated cases. The end result following both methods of treatment is similar.

Old ruptures of the tendo Achilles
If the degree of disability justifies surgical repair, a lateral incision is made, as for the acute rupture. The tendon ends will be found to be rounded off and widely separated so that direct suture is impossible. A central slip is mobilized from the proximal part of the tendon but left attached distally. The slip is then turned down and passed through the distal stump and sutured back upon itself with the foot in full equinus. The plantaris tendon, which is invariably intact, may be mobilized and woven across the gap to reinforce the repair. The foot is then

immobilized in an equinus plaster for 8 weeks, as for the acute injuries.

Other tendon injuries

Rupture of the quadriceps tendon
This usually takes place close to the patellar attachment. Immediate operative repair should be undertaken. A strong, non absorbable suture, such as stainless steel wire, is passed through a hole drilled transversely in the patella and the tendon is firmly anchored by a figure of 8 stitch to the bone. The knee is then immobilized in a plaster cylinder in extension for 6 weeks.

Similar techniques are used in the less common tendon avulsions in other situations, which include the patellar tendon, acute ruptures of the supraspinatus, the bicipital insertion, etc. The common rupture of the long head of biceps does not require repair.

TENOTOMY

Deliberate division of a tendon (*tenotomy*) is performed to lengthen a tendon which is causing deformity, or to weaken a muscle which is producing imbalance. Percutaneous tenotomy, using a tenotome, is often possible. Under anaesthesia, the tight tendon is placed on the stretch and the tenotome passed deeply to it and the tendon cut by displacing the tenotome towards the surface. The cut tendon ends then retract and, if healing occurs subsequently, it will do so with lengthening. This procedure is useful as part of the management of toe clawing and in the division of the adductor origins in adduction deformities of the hip. Division of the hamstrings in this way may be used to overcome flexion contractures of the knee in certain neurological disorders.

Subcutaneous tenotomy may be used, in the hands of the expert, to divide the lower end of sternomastoid in cases of torticollis but here, as in any other situation, the surgeon must be very aware of the other anatomical structures in the vicinity and open tenotomy in certain situations may be safer.

Lengthening of the tendo Achilles
The fibres of the tendo Achilles spiral through 90 degrees from origin to insertion. The rotation, when viewed from the back, is from medial to lateral. The technique for elongation of the tendo Achilles by a tenotomy, taking account of this rotation, is described.

A small incision is made on the medial aspect of the tendon near its insertion and the anterior two-thirds of the tendon is divided by means of a tenotome. A second short incision is made on the medial aspect of the tendon at its proximal end and the medial two-thirds are divided. Firm dorsiflexion of the foot then allows the tendon to

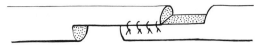

Fig. 2.12 Step cut lengthening of a tendon

elongate without loss of continuity. A walking plaster is then applied with the foot in neutral and is retained for 6 weeks.

Open tenotomy. Open lengthening or shortening of the tendon may be carried out by dividing the tendon in a stepcut fashion and resuturing it with adjustment in length, as shown in Figure 2.12.

TENDON TRANSFER

Tendon transfers are used either to restore active movement, where this has been lost as a result of neurological disease or damage to muscle and tendon, or to correct imbalance of muscle which might lead to deformity. In order for a tendon transfer to succeed, the following principles must be observed:

i. any fixed deformity must first be corrected either by soft tissue release or osteotomy;

ii. the muscle must be strong enough to perform the new task required of it—transfer of a tendon always weakens the muscle slightly;

iii. the muscle must have sufficient amplitude of motion to perform its new role;

iv. the transferred muscle should ideally have an allied or synergistic action to the muscle which it is replacing. Where its action is normally antagonistic, problems of retraining can be considerable, as, for example, when the below knee muscle normally acting in the stance phase of walking is transferred to the tendon of a swing phase muscle;

v. a straight line pull is desirable;

vi. it is of absolute importance that the transferred muscle can be spared from its original function.

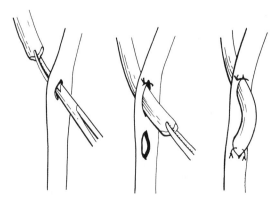

Fig. 2.13 Technique for linking two tendons

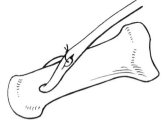

Fig. 2.14 Method for attaching a tendon to bone

Tendon transfers may be attached to an existing tendon or to bone (Figs. 2.13 and 2.14). Details of the very many tendon transfers available are to be found in more specialized texts. Examples of some of the more common procedures include:

Extensor indicis to extensor pollicis longus, which is described on page 22, and transfer of the tibialis posterior tendon to the dorsum of the foot for paralytic foot drop deformity.

Triple transplantation for radial nerve paralysis. In this condition there is drop-wrist together with loss of extension in the fingers and thumb. The following tendon transplantations may be carried out:

i. pronator teres to extensor carpi radialis brevis

ii. flexor carpi ulnaris to the extensors of the fingers

iii. palmaris longus to extensor pollicis longus.

STENOSING TENOSYNOVITIS

In the condition of stenosing tenosynovitis there is some obstruction to the free movement of a tendon within its sheath, due either to a thickening of the tendon or to fibrosis and constriction in the sheath.

De Quervain's syndrome. This is the most common example of this condition and affects the extensor pollicis brevis and abductor pollicis longus tendons as they lie on the radial styloid. The patient experiences localized pain at this site during movement of the thumb with local tenderness and usually a nodular swelling at the site of the lesion. Injection of hydrocortisone 25 mg into the tendon sheath may relieve a significant proportion of cases and is always worth a trial in the first instance. If this fails, surgical decompression is invariably successful.

A *transverse incision* is made over the lesion with great care being taken to preserve the cutaneous branches of the radial nerve which cross this incision and which, if injured, may cause as much discomfort as the primary disease. The thickened tendon sheath is then incised longitudinally and a strip of sheath is removed (Fig. 2.15). It is important to note that the abductor pollicis longus may have more than one tendon and careful search must be made to ensure that each has been decompressed.

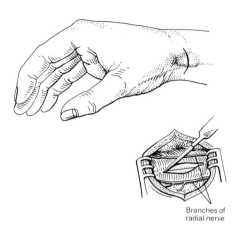

Branches of
radial nerve

Fig. 2.15 Operation to release a De Quervain's lesion—note the proximity of the terminal branches of the radial nerve

Trigger finger. This is due to stenosing tenosynovitis affecting the flexor tendons at the level of the metacarpophalangeal joint. The lesion consists of a swelling of the flexor tendons at this point together with narrowing and thickening of the proximal margin of the fibrous flexor sheath. The powerful flexors can pull the thickened tendon proximal to the area of stenosis but the less powerful extensors are less able to straighten the finger, which may lock in a position of acute flexion or release with a sudden jerk. A thickened and tender nodule can be palpated in the tendon during finger movement. Surgical decompression is indicated and is carried out through a short *transverse incision* overlying the nodule. Care is taken to identify and protect the digital nerves—this is particularly important in the case of trigger thumb in which the radial digital nerve crosses the lesion and is particularly vulnerable. The constricted segment of the fibrous sheath is then incised longitudinally.

FURTHER READING

Lamb D W, Kuczynski K 1981 The practice of hand surgery. Blackwell Scientific Publications, Edinburgh

Nistor L 1981 Surgical and non-surgical treatment of Achilles tendon rupture. Journal of Bone and Joint Surgery 63A: 394

Seddon H J 1956 Volkmann's contracture: Treatment by excision of the infarct. Journal of Bone and Joint Surgery 38B: 152

Sheridan G W, Matsen F A 1976 Fasciotomy in the treatment of the acute compartment syndrome. Journal of Bone and Joint Surgery 58A: 112

3
Operations on blood vessels

D. B. L. McCLELLAND, R. F. RINTOUL & C. V. RUCKLEY

Anatomy

An artery consists of three coats. The outer coat or *tunica adventitia* is composed of fibrous and elastic tissue, and contains the periarterial sympathetic nerves; it is attached only loosely to the middle coat, and can be stripped from it without difficulty. The middle coat or *tunica media* constitutes the main thickness of the arterial wall; it is composed of plain muscle with a proportion of elastic tissue, this proportion being greater in the large vessels. The inner coat or *tunica intima* lines the lumen of the vessel. It consists of a layer of endothelial cells, supported on a basement membrane of elastic tissue.

When an artery is completely divided, its cut ends contract *and retract* to a very marked degree, as the result of spasm of the muscular coat. In this way spontaneous arrest of haemorrhage may be brought about. The tunica adventitia, which has less power of contraction, and which may also be loosely attached to surrounding tissues, remains projecting beyond the other coats at the cut ends, and requires to be trimmed away before end to end repair of the vessel can be effected.

A vein has a structure very similar to that of an artery, except that all coats (especially the tunica media) are much thinner. A characteristic feature of veins is the presence of valves designed to prevent reflux of blood. If, for any reason, a vein becomes dilated, or the seat of inflammatory changes, its valves may be rendered incompetent. Valves are absent from the venae cavae, from the pulmonary veins, and from the veins of the portal system.

The concept of *collateral circulation*, important in all areas of surgery, is particularly relevant to vascular operations. The surgeon should be constantly aware of the alternative channels by which blood can bypass vessels obliterated by disease, by trauma or by the surgeon. Branches which can provide collateral circulation should, if possible, be preserved during dissection.

BASIC TECHNIQUES IN ARTERIAL SURGERY

The exposure of specific arteries is dealt with in later sections; there are however certain principles common to all vascular operations, attention to which should enable the inexperienced surgeon to avoid serious trouble.

The dissection and control of arteries

When exposing an artery it is important to mobilize enough of the vessel and its branches to ensure complete proximal and distal control. The inexperienced surgeon is advised to place slings of plastic, rubber or umbilical tape around a vessel to aid dissection and give control of a vessel which has been opened. However vascular surgeons often dispense with slings in order to simplify and expedite the operation. Once an artery has been exposed the best plane of dissection for mobilization and control is deep to the adventitia. This does not apply to veins. Vessels should always be handled gently, since trauma to the wall commonly leads to thrombosis, and in particular they should never be grasped or clamped with an instrument likely to cause damage. Remember that the soft elastic intima can easily be split without visible damage to the adventitia. Any clamp should be applied with the minimal compression required to control flow.

Modern vacular clamps have relatively atraumatic jaws. Particularly good in this respect is the Fogarty hydragrip vascular clamp with its compressible disposable plastic inserts which clip into the jaws of the instrument (Fig. 3.1A). There is no clamp that will avoid causing damage if it is applied to a heavily calcified vessel, in which case a soft area of wall should be sought before a clamp is applied or a sling drawn tight. If vascular clamps are not available in the emergency situation, a serviceable substitute can be made by sheathing a non crushing gastro-intestinal clamp with cloth or rubber tube. Better still a sling of tape or fine silastic tube can be passed through a length of stiff plastic tube to act as a 'snub' as shown in Figure 3.1E.

As a general rule, and particularly in the case of aneurysms, the distal clamps should be applied before the proximal ones and before the vessels are mobilized in order to minimize distal embolism.

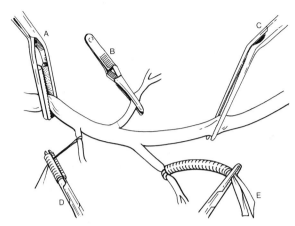

Fig. 3.1 Methods of controlling blood vessels. (A) Fogarty soft jaw clamp. (B) Bull dog clamp. (C) Atraumatic metal jawed vascular clamp. (D) Double ligature sling. (E) Sling with snub

Haemorrhage
Bleeding can usually be controlled by direct compression at the bleeding point while the vessel is exposed and controlled above and below. Where this is not practicable, as in the case for example of ruptured aortic aneurysm, the aorta can be compressed by the assistant just above the neck of the aneurysm or above the pancreas through an opening in the lesser sac while the neck is identified and clamped. If there is difficulty finding the neck or if there is serious bleeding a quick method is for the aneurysm to be opened and the surgeon's index finger inserted into the neck of the sac to give immediate control of bleeding and provide a guide to the positioning of a clamp. An excellent method of controlling aortic bleeding from within is by means of a Foley catheter, while Fogarty embolectomy catheters (p. 45) can be used for the same purpose in smaller arteries.

Arteriotomy (incision into an artery)
This should, as a general rule, be made longitudinally, allowing one to see a greater area of the inside of the vessel; it can readily be extended and it gives access to the orifices of branches, advantages which outweigh the only benefit of a transverse incision which is that it can be closed with less tendency to narrow the lumen. However, in vessels of 4 mm or less, especially if made simply for the purpose of embolectomy, a transverse incision may be preferable and unlike an arteriotomy in a large vessel should be closed with interrupted sutures. A longitudinal incision in an artery smaller in diameter than the common femoral generally requires to be closed with a small patch of vein, taken usually from the long saphenous.

Suturing and suture materials
Nonabsorbable sutures must be used. Silk has largely been discarded because of its irritant qualities and a tendency to be associated with late aneurysm formation. Teflon coated braided dacron is a satisfactory material but the best, especially for small vessels is soft, pliant, monofilament polypropylene. A useful standard size of suture for femoral and popliteal arteries and others of equivalent size is 5/0. Finer sutures are used for smaller vessels while as large as 3/0 may be used on the aorta.

Needles should be round bodied or, in the case of dense graft material or heavily diseased arterial wall, tapercut.

Before opening an artery, any loose adventitia should be removed since it is thought to be thrombogenic if it encroaches on the suture line or is carried inward with a stitch inserted from outside. During closure special care must be taken to include the intima in every stitch (unless of course an endarterectomy has been performed) since the dissection of an intimal flap is probably the commonest cause of early thrombosis after reconstruction. When closing an arteriotomy a continuous suture is used, seeking to obtain slight eversion of the cut edges. As one approaches the end of the closure it may be difficult to see the end of the arteriotomy and to ensure that all layers are included in the stitch. It is therefore advised that a separate end stitch should be placed at the opposite end of the incision, as shown in Figure 3.2. Accurate suturing is more important in vascular surgery than in most other areas and in dealing with medium to small vessels (as distinct from microvascular surgery) the use of magnification ($\times$ 2–4) by means of a loop or spectacles fitted with binocular lenses is often advisable.

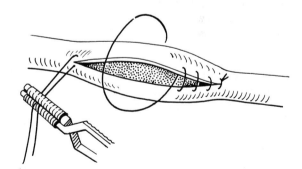

Fig. 3.2 Closure of arteriotomy

Vascular anastomoses
There are many different techniques for joining blood vessels to each other or to synthetic grafts. In constructing an end to end anastomosis care must be taken to avoid narrowing the lumen and it may be preferable, especially when dealing with small vessels, to bevel the ends as shown in Figure 3.11. It is usually more convenient to use continuous sutures but interrupted sutures may be preferred when dealing with an unusually

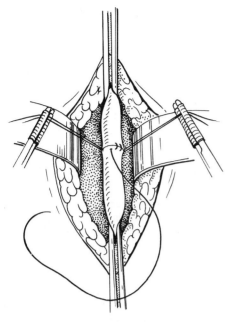

Fig. 3.3 Standard end to end anastomosis. Note the stay sutures and the continuous suture which slightly everts the edges

difficult part of an anastomosis especially if the artery is friable or when joining vessels of very small diameter.

Broadly, there are two main techniques for either end to end or end to side anastomosis. The first is to place anchoring sutures at the beginning as shown in Figure 3.3. This has the advantage of stabilizing the vessels and grafts but may limit access. The second, which is preferred by the author, is to take advantage of the remarkable frictionless qualities of the newer polypropylene monofilament suture materials. With the cut ends some distance apart a posterior row of continuous sutures is placed and then drawn tight, concertina fashion, to approximate the vessels (Fig. 3.11). The anterior layer is then easily completed. A similar principle can be applied to end to side anastomosis (Fig. 3.13).

EXPOSURE OF THE MAIN VESSELS OF THE NECK AND LIMBS

The commonest indication for exposure of a main artery is elective reconstruction for chronic obliterative disease. Emergency exploration may be undertaken in acute occlusion or when arterial injury is suspected. Reconstruction is seldom attempted in veins owing to the liability to thrombosis but may be needed in a case of severe trauma to ensure limb survival. Venous thrombectomy is rarely performed but venous interruption has a place in the management of thrombo-embolism.

The carotid arteries

Endarterectomy for the prevention of stroke is perhaps the most frequent vascular operation in the neck. Others include excision of carotid body tumour, carotid sinus denervation, ligation for cerebral haemorrhage from aneurysm and exploration in cases of trauma.

Anatomy

The common carotid artery begins its course in the neck behind the sternoclavicular joint. Thence it passes upwards in a line towards the lobule of the ear, but ends opposite the upper border of the thyroid cartilage by dividing into external and internal carotid arteries. It is enclosed along with the internal jugular vein and the vagus nerve in the carotid sheath of deep cervical fascia; the vein is lateral to it, and the nerve lies in the groove behind the two vessels.

Superficial relations. These are sternomastoid, sternohyoid, sternothyroid and omohyoid—this last muscle crossing it obliquely at the level of the cricoid cartilage; at this level also, the ansa hypoglossi and the superior and middle thyroid veins lie in front of the artery. It is overlapped to a variable extent by the lobe of the thyroid gland.

The external carotid artery

This begins at the bifurcation of the common carotid artery, at the upper border of the thyroid cartilage, and runs upwards to end behind the neck of the mandible, by dividing into maxillary and superficial temporal arteries. It leaves the carotid triangle by passing under cover of the posterior belly of the digastric, and its upper part occupies a groove on the deep surface of the parotid gland.

The internal carotid artery

This begins at the bifurcation of the common carotid artery, and ascends to enter the skull through the carotid canal, which lies opposite the lower border of the external auditory meatus. It is at first posterolateral to the external carotid artery, and then deep to it. It is enclosed in the carotid sheath, with the internal jugular vein posterolaterally, and with the vagus nerve deep to the interval between them. Sternomastoid overlaps it laterally. *It has no branches in the neck.*

Superficial relations. These, in the carotid triangle, are the cervical branch of the facial nerve, the hypoglossal nerve, and the common facial and lingual veins, as these pass backwards to join the jugular.

Exposure

For exposure of the carotid arteries the head is turned to the opposite side and slightly extended. A sand bag is placed between the shoulder blades. The ideal incision from the cosmetic point of view is placed in the skin

Care must also be taken to avoid damage to the vagus nerve and the internal jugular vein which can be retracted gently on slings.

The exposure of the common carotid artery and internal jugular vein in the lower part of the neck is essentially similar. A skin crease incision is made at the level of the cricoid cartilage. The carotid sheath is exposed above the omohyoid which can be retracted downwards. The internal jugular vein, the descendens hypoglossi and the vagus nerves should be identified and separated before any attempt is made to pass a sling round the artery.

Subclavian and axillary arteries
Exposure may be necessary for the arrest of haemorrhage, the treatment of aneurysms (generally associated with a cervical rib) or for atheromatous occlusion.

Anatomy
The subclavian artery crosses the front of the cervical pleura at the root of the neck. It arches from the sterno-clavicular joint to the outer border of the first rib, where it becomes the axillary artery. It rises to a level 1–2 cm above the clavicle, when the shoulder is depressed. Scalenus anterior crosses the artery, dividing it into three parts. The subclavian vein lies in front of scalenus anterior, at a lower level than the artery, and behind the clavicle.

Superficial relations of third part. Skin, superficial fascia, platysma, supraclavicular nerves, deep fascia; external jugular vein and its tributaries (transverse cervical, suprascapular and anterior jugular veins); supra-scapular artery; nerve to subclavius.

The axillary artery runs downwards and laterally behind the clavicle to become the brachial artery. Its second part lies deep to the pectoralis minor with the axillary vein just below and medial to it throughout its course.

Superficial relations of axillary artery. These, encountered after fascial layers, are pectoral muscles and nerves; acromiothoracic vessels; termination of cephalic vein.

Exposure
The third part of the subclavian artery is the most accessible and may be exposed in the first instance. The arm is placed at the side and is drawn downwards in order to depress the shoulder; the head is turned to the opposite side. An incision is made 1–2 cm above the clavicle from sternal head of sternomastoid to anterior border of trapezius. Superficial fascia and platysma are incised in the same line and the deep fascia is divided. The external jugular vein may cross the field and have to be divided between ligatures. Omohyoid is retracted upwards, and the third part of the subclavian artery is now exposed, with the scalenus anterior muscle medially,

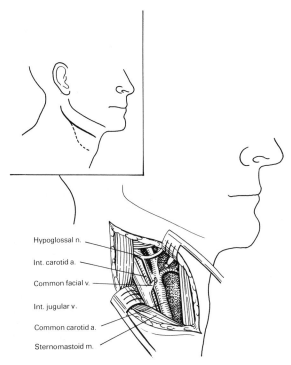

Fig. 3.4 Exposure of the great vessels on the right side of the neck

Hypoglossal n.
Int. carotid a.
Common facial v.
Int. jugular v.
Common carotid a.
Sternomastoid m.

crease, and there are few neck operations for which adequate exposure cannot be thus obtained, but if greater longitudinal exposure is required, an 's' shaped incision may be preferred (Fig. 3.4). In order to avoid damage to the cervical branch of the facial nerve the upper end of the incision should not approach nearer than 1.5 cm to the angle of the mandible. Platysma and deep fascia are divided in the line of the incision and the flaps are dissected a little way upwards and downwards. The anterior border of sternomastoid is freed and the muscle retracted posteriorly. The common facial vein crosses the field and must be divided between ligatures. The internal jugular vein is displaced backwards to expose the carotid arteries. The descendens hypoglossi nerve on the anterior surface of the carotid sheath is preserved. Fluctuations in blood pressure due to disturbance of baroreceptors can be avoided by infiltration of the tissues in the carotid bifurcation with 0.5 cc of 1% Xylocaine. In the case of carotid endarterectomy there is a danger that mobilization of the arteries will release thrombus into the cerebral circulation. Extreme gentleness should therefore be used in dissection.

Care must be taken to avoid damaging the hypoglossal nerve, which can be mobilized by division and ligation of the small vessels which tether it posteriorly before it crosses the carotid arteries. To extend the access superiorly the posterior belly of the digastric can be divided.

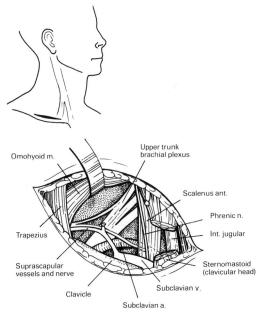

Omohyoid m.

Upper trunk
brachial plexus

Scalenus ant.

Phrenic n.

Int. jugular

Trapezius

Suprascapular
vessels and nerve

Sternomastoid
(clavicular head)

Clavicle

Subclavian v.

Subclavian a.

Fig. 3.5 Exposure of the right subclavian artery

and with the upper and middle trunks of the brachial plexus to its lateral side. The transverse cervical artery, lying under cover of omohyoid, and the suprascapular artery, crossing the subclavian, are preserved.

Exposure of the *second and third parts* of the subclavian artery and the *axillary artery* is normally required for aneurysms and atheromatous occlusion. The upper limb is abducted and is supported on an arm board or on a small table (Fig. 3.5). A long incision is made, beginning at the anterior edge of the sternomastoid and continuing in the line of the vessels to the anterior axillary fold. The first stage of the dissection has already been described. Division of the sternomastoid and scalenus muscles, with care to avoid damage to the phrenic nerve, brings the second part of the subclavian artery into view. If necessary the middle third of the clavicle may be resected and pectoral muscles divided in the line of the incision to complete the exposure of the arteries.

The root of the neck is a hazardous area for the inexperienced surgeon. The subclavian artery is relatively thin walled and bleeding from it or one of the great veins is very difficult to control. In emergency situations to gain rapid control of the third part of the subclavian and the first part of the axillary artery there should be no hesitation in resecting the middle third of the clavicle. To gain control of the proximal subclavian or the brachiocephalic trunk a sternal split is necessary with a lateral extension through the second intercostal space.

Brachial artery

The brachial artery may be exposed easily anywhere in its course. Exploration is most likely to be required for

embolism or iatrogenic trauma inflicted in the course of cardiological investigations. Exposure may also be necessary to investigate possible damage associated with fractures of the humerus.

Anatomy
The brachial artery begins as a continuation of the axillary artery at the level of the lower border of teres major. It runs downwards and slightly laterally, at first medial to the humerus and then in front of it. It ends in the cubital fossa, at the level of the neck of the radius, by dividing into radial and ulnar arteries. The artery is accompanied by venae comites in its lower part and by the basilic vein in the upper part.

Relations in the upper arm. The artery lies successively on the long and medial heads of triceps, the insertion of coracobrachialis, and brachialis. The biceps overlaps it on the lateral side. The median nerve, at first lateral, crosses in front of the artery in its middle third, and then runs along its medial side. The ulnar nerve is on the medial side of the artery in its upper half but diverges from its lower half. The medial cutaneous nerve of the forearm also lies to its medial side in the upper half of the arm.

Relations at the bend of the elbow. The brachial artery enters the cubital fossa, with the tendon of biceps on its lateral side, and the median nerve on its medial side. These structures lie on the brachialis muscle, which forms the upper part of the floor of the fossa. They are roofed over by deep fascia containing the bicipital aponeurosis, which stretches from the tendon of biceps to blend with the fascia over the medial side of the forearm. The superficial fascia overlying the fossa contains the median cubital and other veins.

Branches. The branches of the artery are the profunda, which arises near its commencement and accompanies the radial nerve spirally round the humerus; the ulnar collateral artery, which arises in the middle of the arm, and accompanies the ulnar nerve to the back of the medial epicondyle; the supratrochlear artery arises just above the elbow and runs also to the medial epicondyle.

Exposure in the upper arm
The upper limb is abducted and rotated laterally and is supported with the forearm resting on a small table (Fig 3.6). The upper arm should be entirely free; if it is supported in any way, displacement of the muscles will render the approach more difficult. An incision is made along the medial edge of the biceps, and the deep fascia is divided in the same line. Care is taken to avoid the basilic vein which pierces the deep fascia in this situation. The biceps is mobilized and drawn laterally to expose the artery with its venae comites and the median nerve in close relationship (see anatomical description above).

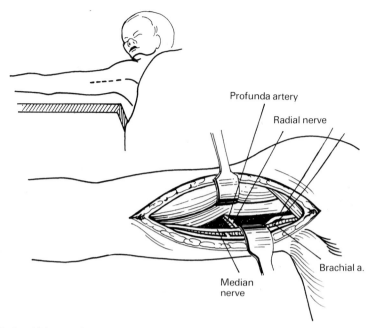

Fig. 3.6 Exposure of the brachial artery in the upper arm

Exposure at the bend of the elbow

The arm is abducted and supported on a table in the position of lateral rotation. An incision is made in the antecubital region along the medial border of the biceps tendon. The deep fascia, including the bicipital aponeurosis, is incised vertically, and the biceps tendon is retracted to the lateral side to display the contents of the fossa. (This is accomplished more easily if the elbow is flexed slightly to allow relaxation of the muscle). The brachial artery lies in the centre of the fossa, between the tendon of biceps and the median nerve (Fig. 3.7).

Iliac arteries

Exposure of the three iliac arteries is most often required for atheromatous occlusion. Temporary or permanent control of the external iliac may be required for high wounds of the femoral artery or septic wounds in the upper thigh, and ligature of the internal iliac artery may be indicated for secondary haemorrhage after hysterectomy.

Anatomy

The external iliac artery begins at the pelvic brim as a terminal branch of the common iliac artery, and runs downwards to pass deep to the midinguinal point, where it becomes the femoral artery.

Relations in the inguinal region. The artery lies on psoas, with its vein to the medial side. The femoral nerve is 1–2 cm lateral, with the small genitofemoral nerve in between. Anteriorly, it is in contact with the peritoneum; below the peritoneal reflection it is related to the muscles

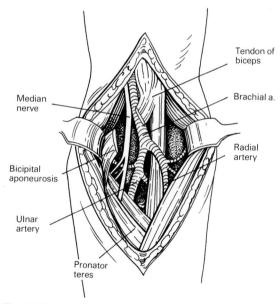

Fig. 3.7 Exposure of the brachial artery and its terminal branches in the cubital fossa. (For the sake of clarity the veins have been omitted)

of the abdominal wall immediately above the inguinal ligament—transversus, internal oblique, and external oblique from within outwards.

Branches. These branches are the inferior epigastric which runs upwards into the rectus sheath, and the deep circumflex iliac which courses laterally along the back of the inguinal ligament.

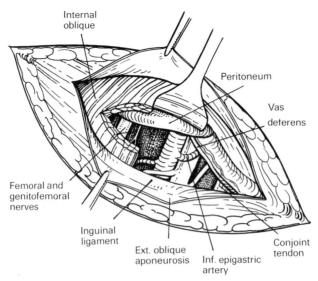

Fig. 3.8 Extraperitoneal exposure of the external iliac vessels at the groin

Exposure

Exposure by the extraperitoneal route is the method of choice where the lesion is unilateral. The common, external and internal iliac arteries can be exposed in their whole length by an oblique muscle cutting incision in the lower abdomen, displacing the peritoneum and its contents forwards and medially out of the iliac fossa.

For extraperitoneal exposure of the external iliac artery alone, the patient is placed in a moderate Trendelenburg position and an incision is made 1–2 cm above and parallel to the middle of the inguinal ligament. The inguinal canal is opened and the muscular fibres of internal oblique are divided just above the inguinal ligament. Transversalis fascia is incised and the spermatic cord is retracted medially and upwards. The inferior epigastric artery should, if possible, be preserved as the peritoneum is gently raised to display the external iliac artery and vein (Fig 3.8).

Intraperitoneal exposure

This is required where the lesion is bilateral or involves the bifurcation of the aorta. The small intestine is packed off within the peritoneal cavity or, if that is not possible, it is wrapped in moist towels or exenterated into a polythene bag over the right side of the wound. The aorta and right iliac vessels are exposed by division of the overlying peritoneum followed by blunt dissection. The right ureter must be seen and mobilized out of the way. The left iliac arteries are exposed by dividing the peritoneum lateral to the pelvic mesocolon.

Femoral artery

The common femoral artery is most frequently exposed during embolectomy or reconstruction. Wounds of the femoral artery are among the most common vascular lesions encountered. Exposure of the artery, in order that its condition may be investigated, is an integral part of the exploration of most penetrating wounds of the thigh.

Anatomy

The femoral artery, beginning as a continuation of the external iliac at the midinguinal point, runs obliquely downwards through the femoral triangle and subsartorial canal. Surgeons refer to the proximal portion, above the origin of the profunda, as the common femoral and the distal as the superficial femoral artery. It ends at the junction of the middle and lower thirds of the thigh by passing through the opening in adductor magnus, to become the popliteal artery. Its position is indicated by the upper two-thirds of a line drawn from the midinguinal point to the adductor tubercle, the thigh being slightly flexed and rotated laterally.

Relations in the femoral triangle. The femoral vein is on its medial side; the femoral nerve is 1–2 cm lateral. Four small branches arise near its origin—the superficial epigastric, the superficial circumflex iliac, and the superficial and deep external pudendal. The profunda femoris artery arises from the lateral side of the femoral artery 3–4 cm below the inguinal ligament; it runs medially behind the femoral artery to disappear between the adductor muscles.

Relations in subsartorial canal. The canal is formed by adductor longus and magnus posteriorly, vastus medialis anterolaterally, and the fibrous roof and sartorius anteromedially. Within the canal the femoral vein is posterolateral, the saphenous nerve is anteromedial, and the nerve to vastus medialis is lateral.

Exposure in the upper two-thirds of the thigh

An incision of adequate length is made in the line of the artery. The long saphenous vein, lying in the superficial fascia, is preserved, in case it may be required for reconstruction. The deep fascia is incised, and the sartorius muscle is mobilized. To expose the upper part of the femoral vessels, and the profunda vessels, sartorius is retracted laterally. To expose the femoral vessels in their lower part, sartorius is retracted medially, and the underlying bridge of fibrous tissue which roofs over the subsartorial canal is divided. In this way the femoral vessels may be exposed in their entire length.

Exposure at the femoropopliteal junction

The limb is flexed slightly at hip and knee joints, and is rotated laterally. The operator may find it more convenient to stand at the opposite side of the table, so that he faces the field of operation. An incision is made extending upwards from the adductor tubercle for 20 cm in the line of the artery and downwards along the posterior border of the tibia for 10 cm. The long saphenous vein is identified and held aside. The sartorius is mobilized and retracted backwards. The underlying fascia is divided in the line of the incision, to open up the subsartorial canal. The femoral vessels are now exposed, the vein lying posterolateral to the artery. The saphenous nerve and a branch of the artery, the descending genicular, are seen and preserved. The proximal part of the popliteal artery may be exposed by retracting or dividing the tendon of adductor magnus. The popliteal fascia is then incised and dissection is carried out through the popliteal fat, keeping close to the popliteal surface of the femur so as to avoid disturbing the popliteal vein. To expose the artery distally, the origin of the medial head of gastrocnemius is divided and retracted backwards.

Popliteal artery

Exposure of this artery may be indicated as part of an exploratory operation in wounds of the popliteal fossa, or for the treatment of aneurysms.

Anatomy

The popliteal artery begins as the continuation of the femoral at the opening in adductor magnus. It runs downwards in the popliteal fossa to end at the lower border of popliteus by dividing into anterior tibial and the tibial peroneal trunk which in turn divides into posterior tibial and peroneal branches. It gives off small branches to the knee joint and to the surrounding muscles.

Relations. The popliteal vein is medial to the artery in its lower part, but crosses it posteriorly to lie posterolateral to it in its upper part. The medial popliteal nerve crosses the vessels posteriorly from lateral side above to medial side below.

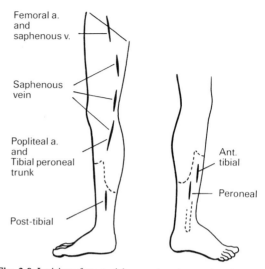

Fig. 3.9 Incisions for arterial reconstructions and saphenous vein removal in the leg. Note that the incisions avoid potential flaps for amputation

Exposure

The popliteal artery can be approached through a longitudinal posterior incision directly over the line of the vessel, with the patient lying prone. An alternative approach to the distal popliteal and the tibial peroneal trunk is a lateral one with excision of the upper end of the fibula. The best approach however in the majority of cases is through a medial incision which, as well as giving access to the popliteal artery and tibial peroneal trunk, also facilitates removal of the saphenous vein which is commonly required for reconstruction or repair.

With the patient supine, the thigh is externally rotated and the knee is flexed 30 to 60 degrees. A longitudinal incision is made beginning 1 cm posterior to the medial condyle and carried down parallel to and 1 cm behind the posteromedial border of the tibia (Fig. 3.10). Care must be taken to avoid damage to the saphenous vein which is close to the skin at this level. The crural fascia is divided to expose the tendons of semitendinosus, gracilis and semimembranosus. These may be retracted

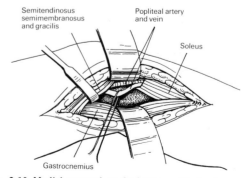

Fig. 3.10 Medial approach to the lower popliteal artery

anteriorly, or divided to give access to the popliteal space. The medial head of gastrocnemius is retracted and the fat gently separated to expose the neurovascular bundle covered with a thick layer of fascia which is incised longitudinally. The popliteal vein is retracted posteriorly and must be separated with great care since venous bleeding in the popliteal fossa can be difficult to control and damage to the vein is likely to lead to thrombosis. The artery is then separated from the tibial nerve and encircled with a sling. For exposure of the origins of the tibial arteries the anterior tibial vein which crosses the artery must be divided and the soleus muscle incised at its origin from the posterior surface of the tibia.

Distal reconstruction

If the popliteal artery is obstructed it may sometimes be feasible to take a vein or synthetic graft down to a tibial or peroneal artery in mid or lower calf. If this is to be successful there should be an intact arterial arch in the foot. Appropriate incisions are illustrated in Figure 3.9.

WOUNDS OF ARTERIES

Control of bleeding

As a first aid measure profuse bleeding from a limb should be controlled by pressure pad and bandage rather than by tourniquet, a potentially dangerous implement. No attempt should be made to apply artery forceps within a wound that is bleeding profusely since it is impossible to identify the damaged vessel with any accuracy, and there is a serious risk of injuring neighbouring structures.

The patient should be prepared for a definitive operation, carried out with adequate lighting and with all necessary facilities. If the bleeding has been temporarily arrested by packing or by local pressure, it may be possible, after gently removing the dressings, to explore the wound in a relatively bloodless field. If, however, there is still profuse bleeding, it will be necessary to apply a tourniquet, or to expose the main artery at a proximal level, where it can be occluded, either by a temporary ligature or by an arterial clamp.

Permanent ligature

In the case of the larger vessels of the limb—axillary, brachial, femoral and popliteal, permanent ligature should be avoided if possible, because of the risks of subsequent ischaemia, if not of actual gangrene. (The subclavian artery constitutes an exception to this general rule; because of an abundant collateral circulation, it can usually be ligatured with safety in necessitous cases).

Reconstruction is usually possible and reversed saphenous vein is preferred to synthetic materials, especially if there is wound contamination. Where there

is associated bone damage fractures should, if possible, be stabilized prior to reconstruction of the vessels (the two being done at the same operation); but if this means delay, temporary cannulae can be used to connect the vessels and maintain viability of the limb until definitive reconstruction is performed. The smaller arteries—i.e. those below the elbow and knee—normally have an adequate collateral circulation, so that reconstructive measures, which are very difficult because of the small size of the vessel, do not usually require to be considered. If both vessels of the forearm or lower leg are injured, an attempt should be made to reconstruct the larger.

Arterial haematoma

This may occur in cases of arterial injury where the extravasated blood cannot escape to the surface—either because there is no external wound, or because the external wound is too small. The resulting haematoma may be either circumscribed or diffuse, depending upon the resistance offered by the tissues. If the vessel wound is small it may become sealed off and the haematoma gradually absorbed. A large haematoma, by exerting pressure on the smaller vessels, may cause obstruction to the collateral circulation. When the haematoma is not absorbed its outer layers become organized, and the central part forms a cavity constantly distended by the circulating blood; it shows expansile pulsation, and may now be described as a *traumatic arterial aneurysm*.

If the haematoma is increasing in size, or if the circulation of the limb is embarrassed, immediate operation should be undertaken. If practicable, a tourniquet is applied; if not, it may be necessary to expose the main vessel at a proximal level, and to apply a clamp or temporary ligature. The haematoma is then explored through an adequate incision. All clots are removed, so that the bleeding point can be identified. If necessary, the tourniquet or clamp can be cautiously released after the vessel has been exposed.

In the case of arteries above the elbow or knee, an attempt should usually be made to repair or to reconstruct the damaged vessel. If the operator lacks the necessary experience or facilities, he may perforce have to be content with simple ligation of the vessel, as close to the injury as possible. Although this entails some risk of ischaemia of the limb, such risks will have been lessened if the operation has been successful in arresting the bleeding, and in evacuating the haematoma which may have been embarrassing the collateral circulation. Vessels below the elbow or knee can usually be ligatured with impunity although many surgeons believe that these too should be repaired wherever possible.

When there is no obvious increase in the size of the haematoma, and when the circulation of the limb remains satisfactory, it is best to postpone operation, in order to allow the establishment of a collateral circulation, or possibly to permit the patient being transferred to a centre where vascular surgery is undertaken.

A contracted and empty artery

This may result from the pressure of bone fragments after fracture, from crushing injuries without fracture, or from the disruptive force of a high velocity missile traversing the tissues in close proximity.

It was formerly believed that the condition of the vessel was due to a state of spasm, which involved also the distal ramifications of the artery, and, by reflex action, vessels forming the collateral circulation. It is now thought that simple contusion of the artery is the most important factor; this leads to rupture of the intima, localized contusion of the media, thrombosis and occlusion. Spasm may play a part in producing ischaemia, especially in the smaller vessels, but it should never be assumed to be solely responsible if signs of circulatory deficiency persist in the distal part of the limb for more than 2 to 3 hours after the injury. Failure to explore the artery and relieve underlying damage within 4 hours of the onset may result in permanent ischaemic muscle damage.

Operation

This is the only effective treatment, and, in the absence of spontaneous recovery, should not be delayed. The vessel is exposed by an adequate incision, enlarged until a normally pulsating length of vessel is seen above the pulseless segment. If there is doubt as to what part spasm may be playing this segment may then be covered with a warm 2% solution of papavarine sulphate (a smooth muscle relaxant) and left for a few minutes. Alternatively, an attempt may be made to inject the solution directly into the lumen of the artery, this method being used also to test the patency of the vessel. The damaged segment is the proximal end of the contracted part of the artery. It should be excised and a reconstructive operation performed.

TECHNIQUES IN ARTERIAL REPAIR

Following the great advances in vascular surgery during the past 25 years, it is now known that repair of torn arteries, even in the face of considerable technical difficulties, is successful in a gratifying proportion of cases, and such treatment is now urged wherever it is anatomically possible. When direct repair is impracticable, reconstructive methods, employing either an autogenous vein graft or a woven plastic prosthesis, are advised. Even if the artery becomes occluded later, it may remain open long enough to ensure wound healing and a viable limb.

The successful repair of vascular injuries demands a meticulously careful technique, which includes gentleness in handling, absolute asepsis, and scrupulous care in the placing of sutures.

Before any attempt is made to repair a damaged artery, attention must be paid to the toilet of the wound in the soft parts, and all bruised and devitalized tissue should be excised. The damaged vessel is exposed, and is mobilized sufficiently to allow temporary ligatures or special arterial clamps to be applied above and below the site of injury. Any fracture is dealt with by some form of internal fixation prior to arterial reconstruction. If there is delay and the viability of the limb is at risk, a temporary cannula or shunt can be inserted. Treatment of the arterial wound depends essentially on the degree of damage to the vessel wall. Clean cut wounds without bruising are uncommon; if they are placed longitudinally or have caused only partial division of the vessel, they may be closed by direct suture; a cleanly severed vessel may be repaired by immediate end to end anastomosis. More frequently, however, there is bruising or destruction of a segment of the vessel wall, with or without complete severance of continuity. If there is the slightest doubt about arterial damage, for example if there is any diminution of pulse volume distal to a contused area, an arteriotomy must be made in order that the intima can be examined. A contused segment should be excised, so that cleancut ends can be approximated for suture. The resultant gap does not necessarily preclude end to end anastomosis, since it can often be bridged with surprisingly little difficulty, by mobilization of the vessel above and below. Monofilament or fine teflon coated braided dacron are suitable suture materials. Carrel's method of everting sutures, which bring intima into contact with intima, is generally advocated, although a simple over and over suture may be equally effective. A combination of the two may also be used.

End to end anastomosis

The two segments are milked free of blood clot, and a few ml of heparin solution (10 units per ml of saline) are irrigated into each: some of the same solution may also be injected into the vessel on the far side of each clamp. The cut ends are then approximated by two stay sutures inserted at equidistant points. These sutures, held on forceps, are used to steady the vessel and to rotate it as required, while the anastomosis is completed around the entire circumference (Fig 3.3). Stitches, which may be horizontal mattress to evert the edges or over and over, are placed about 2 mm apart and 2 mm from the cut edge. Heparin solution is used to irrigate the vessel which is flushed out by temporary release of clamps before the arteriotomy is closed. After the suture has been completed, the distal clamp is released first. The resulting retrograde flow is at a relatively low pressure: any obvious leaks are at once recognized, and are closed

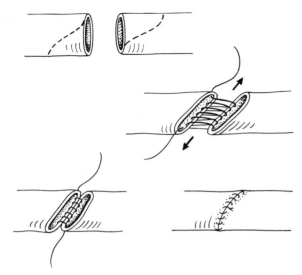

Fig. 3.11 An alternative technique for end to end anastomosis. The ends are bevelled to reduce the risk of constriction. A running posterior monofilament suture draws the ends together and is continued around the front of the vessel

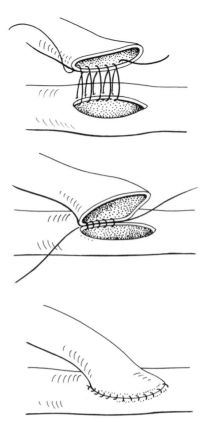

Fig. 3.13 An alternative technique for end to side anastomosis using a monofilament pursestring to approximate the posterior layer

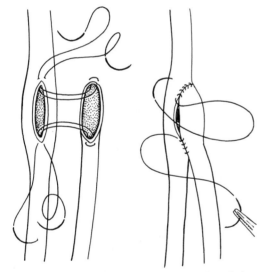

Fig. 3.12 Vascular anastomosis by the end to side technique

by additional sutures. The proximal clamp is then gradually released, light gauze pressure being maintained on the outside of the anastomosis throughout. Oozing generally ceases spontaneously within a few minutes, but one or two further sutures may be required.

ARTERIAL RECONSTRUCTION

Most restorative operations on arteries take one of two forms—disobliteration or graft. The remarkable expan-

sion of vascular surgery in recent years can largely be attributed to the development of a variety of synthetic grafts which provide admirable substitutes for arteries.

Indications for arterial reconstruction
The strongest indications arise in the case of congenital abnormalities, such as coarctation of the aorta (although this is often dealt with by direct anastomosis) and in arterial injuries which include aneurysms and arteriovenous fistulae of traumatic origin. In obliterative vascular disease the indications are less clearcut since this is usually a widespread and progressive condition. Patients carry particular risk of complications due to obliterative disease in vessels supplying vital organs—particularly brain, kidneys and heart; myocardial infarction being the commonest cause of death in patients who undergo surgery for atherosclerosis. As a general rule the more localised the occlusion and the larger the vessel affected the better the outlook for reconstruction.

Autogenous vein
This is the material of choice for the reconstruction of small and medium sized arteries. As a rule a suitable vein

is readily available, and will often survive in the presence of mild infection. A successful vein graft eventually becomes thickened to take on many of the characters of an artery. The long saphenous vein (when normal) is the ideal substitute for an artery of comparable size. It may be used either to bridge a gap resulting from the excision of an injured segment or to bypass a diseased segment. The vein is exposed throughout its length by single or multiple incisions. Its branches should be tied with fine silk 2–3 mm from the main vessel to avoid 'crimping' the adventia. It is removed, its distal end cannulated and gently distended with heparinized blood to check for haemostasis. It is reversed (because of the valves) and sutured end to end in the case of trauma or end to side in the case of bypass for obliterative disease by the methods of suture already described. The vein should be sutured under a moderate degree of tension, otherwise it stretches when arterial blood is admitted and may become tortuous and liable to thrombose.

Synthetic prostheses

Tubes of woven or knitted dacron (Terylene) in various shapes and sizes have become available to replace segments of arteries. They are now accepted as the ideal grafting material *for arteries the size of the external iliac or larger*. For smaller arteries vein should be preferred since this carries higher patency rates and lower risk of infection. Alternatives if vein is not available, include expanded polytetrafluoroethylene (Goretex) and the Dardik biograft which is terylene reinforced gluteraldehyde-treated human umbilicial vein. A graft will thrombose unless there are also patent distal vessels to ensure good run-off flow, and this is especially true of reconstruction of small calibre arteries.

Fate of plastic prostheses

It has been shown that dacron is an effective arterial substitute, and that the grafts can remain patent and function well for many years. Grafts removed many years after implantation have shown a smooth glistening luminal surface, consisting mainly of collagen bundles and compressed fibrin and a surface layer of flattened epithelial cells. The plastic fibres of the prosthesis remain unchanged as an intermediate layer, but are permeated by cells growing from the adventitia to form a densely adherent covering or sheath of fibrous tissue. Muscle and elastic fibres appear to be absent, or are present only in very small quantities.

Thrombo-endarterectomy

This is an alternative method of restoring flow through a thrombosed artery, provided that the affected segment is short, and the cases are carefully selected. The artery is opened longitudinally, and the thrombus, together with the diseased intima and its atheromatous plaques,

is removed through a plane of cleavage *in the media*, the adventitia and the outer layer of the media being left behind. The incision in the artery may be closed by a patch graft of vein or of dacron if direct suture appears to narrow the lumen (Fig. 3.15).

Bypass grafting

This term denotes the insertion of a graft or synthetic prosthesis, by end to side anastomosis, to short-circuit an obstructed segment of artery—usually the femoral (Fig. 3.14). Certain advantages are claimed for the method. (1) Exact matching of the calibre is unnecessary. (2) There is less narrowing of the vessel than occurs at the points of end to end anastomosis of a replacement graft, since, owing to the oblique cutting of the bypass graft, the suture line represents the widest part of the union. (3) There is less interference with the collateral circulation and the operation imposes less strain on the patient, since the vessel requires to be exposed only through a small incision above and below the obstructed segment, the graft being passed through a subfascial

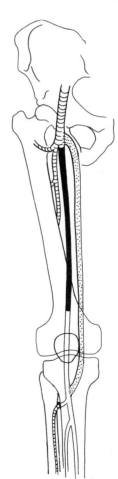

Fig. 3.14 Bypass graft for blocked femoral artery

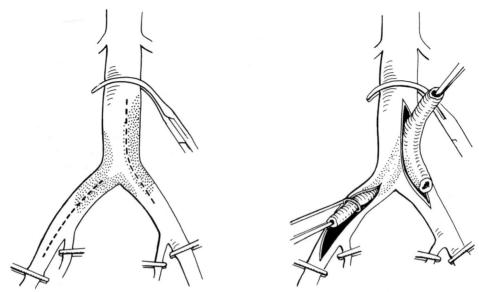

Fig. 3.15 Thrombo-endarterectomy of the aorta and iliac arteries. The thrombus and atheromatous material are removed through a plane of cleavage in the media, the adventitia and the outer layer of the media being left in situ

tunnel. As noted earlier autogenous vein is the graft material of choice in limb vessels. When vein is not available, alternatives which may be considered include gluteraldehyde stabilized, dacron-reinforced human umbilical vein graft (Dardik) or expanded polytetrafluoroethylene (PTFE). These materials, like vein, can if necessary be used to bypass diseased arteries right down to the level of the ankle provided that there is adequate run off in the form of a patent arterial arcade in the foot.

Profundaplasty
This operation, first described in 1972, may help to preserve an ischaemic limb if the popliteal vessel is unsuitable to receive a bypass graft from the femoral artery. It can be combined with a graft from a higher level. Biplane arteriography is usually required to demonstrate profunda origin stenosis. The arteriotomy in the common femoral artery is extended into the profunda femoris, and closed with a vein patch or with the distal toe of a dacron graft.

Arterial dilatation
A recent innovation in the management of obliterative arterial disease is the development of transluminal angioplasty, the dilatation of a stenosed segment, under local anaesthesia and radiological control, by means of a balloon (Gruntzig) catheter. In large arteries, e.g. the iliacs, the early results are most encouraging (Youkey, 1983).

Microvascular surgery
Advances in operating microscopes, in miniature instruments, suture materials and in surgical techniques have led to the development of the new specialty of microvascular surgery. Opportunities to apply these techniques are not numerous but may arise in several different fields including nerve and vessel repair, digit or limb reimplantation, hand surgery, free grafts in plastic surgery, organ transplantation and extracranial-intracranial bypass. The practical details of microvascular surgery are beyond the scope of this text (O'Brien, 1977). Training courses are now available in a number of centres.

ANTICOAGULANT THERAPY

Anticoagulant therapy is indicated in all conditions where it is considered desirable to reduce the normal clotting power of the blood—i.e. in most thromboembolic states. These include coronary thrombosis, pulmonary embolism, cavernous sinus thrombosis, mesenteric embolism and thrombosis, peripheral arterial embolism and peripheral phlebothrombosis. In treatment of these conditions, anticoagulant therapy is employed in order to prevent extension of the thrombosis and to encourage retraction and shrinkage of the clot; prophylactically, it serves to prevent further thrombotic episodes.

Contraindications
Contraindications to anticoagulant therapy are the presence of an actual or potential bleeding surface (as may occur for the first 2 or 3 days after operation) and blood dyscrasias involving impairment of the normal mech-

anism for the prevention of bleeding. Old and frail patients, and those with severe liver or kidney damage, should be given the drugs in much reduced dosage. It is frequently necessary, however, to weigh the risks in these conditions against those of pulmonary embolism; as a rule the latter consideration will over-ride the former. If operation is intended on a patient who is being maintained on an oral anticoagulant the latter should be replaced by heparin several days before the operation. Heparin can be quickly reversed by protamine sulphate if perioperative bleeding is a problem.

Heparin

Heparin has at least two modes of action on the coagulation system and three main clinical uses. In combination with heparin cofactor it inhibits Factor Xa. This is thought to be the mechanism of action of low dose subcutaneous heparin, a proven prophylactic against postoperative pulmonary embolism. In a dose of 5000 units twice or thrice daily it is given by deep subcutaneous injection into the fat of the abdominal wall. The first dose is given approximately 1 hour before operation and it is continued postoperatively until the patient is mobile. Such doses do not alter the clotting time.

In large dosage heparin also blocks the thrombinfibrinogen reaction. Large doses of heparin, e.g. 5–15 000 units intravenously, are used to prevent thrombosis during arterial operations and may be reversed at the end of the procedure. Similarly large doses are used for the initial treatment of acute thrombotic or thrombo-embolic episodes. Heparin is excreted rapidly by the kidneys, and when used in 'therapeutic' doses is controlled by estimation of the clotting time, which should be maintained at between 15 and 20 minutes, or at 2 or 3 times that existing before therapy. Such prolongation of the clotting time indicates adequate heparinization. Continuous intravenous infusion is the method of choice and 1–2000 international units can be administered each hour by means of a saline drip or ideally by low volume infusion pump. Deep subcutaneous injection into the fat of the abdominal wall may be used to replace intravenous administration after the first day, an injection of 15–25 000 units being given twice daily. In severe forms of thrombosis such as extensive venous thrombosis heparin should be continued for a week to 10 days before converting to oral anticoagulant. During conversion the two should be overlapped by 4 or 5 days.

Antidote

Withdrawal of the heparin is followed by restoration within a few hours of the normal clotting time. If, however, severe haemorrhage should occur, or should operation become urgently necessary, intravenous injection of 5 to 10 ml of a 1% solution of *protamine sulphate* will immediately restore normal clotting.

Oral anticoagulants

These drugs owe their anticoagulant action, partly to their ability to reduce the blood prothrombin by inhibiting its formation in the liver, and partly by lowering the concentration of *Factor VII*, which is essential to the formation of thromboplastin. They differ from heparin in three important respects. Firstly, they can be given by mouth; secondly, their action is not fully developed for 24 hours or more; thirdly, since they are metabolized slowly and have a cumulative action, there is some danger of haemorrhage. Because of this, the dosage must be carefully controlled by regular estimation of the prothrombin time, which should be maintained at $1\frac{1}{2}$ to $2\frac{1}{2}$ times that of normal plasma. In this country, warfarin sodium is at present the preparation of choice.

Dosage

Warfarin should be started in two doses of not more than 15 mg at 24 hour intervals. Thereafter, doses must be carefully controlled by estimation of prothrombin time, carried out at first daily and then at increasing intervals of time until the desired prolongation of prothrombin is established. The usual maintenance dose of warfarin is 5–10 mg daily. It is clear that these drugs should not be used unless laboratory facilities of a high order are available—a disadvantage which offsets to some extent their low cost as compared with heparin—but blood samples for the estimation of prothrombin time can now be sent by post to most laboratories.

Antidote

Since 48 hours may elapse after withdrawal of the drug before the prothrombin time returns to normal, a specific antidote is more necessary than in the case of heparin, should severe haemorrhage occur or an emergency operation be required. Such an antidote is found in *Vitamin K1 (phytomenadione)*, 15 to 25 mg of which can be administered either by mouth or by intravenous injection.

Thrombolytic therapy

Although streptokinase and urokinase have been widely available for many years their therapeutic roles are not well defined. Both achieve their effect by activating circulating plasminogen. Urokinase is derived from human urine. Streptokinase is derived from streptococcal cultures. These agents are relatively expensive. In acute arterial occlusion, especially in the case of embolism, surgery is preferred as a more dependable means of restoring the circulation. In deep vein thrombosis streptokinase may be considered in major iliofemoral thrombosis if it is of recent onset i.e. within 4 to 5 days and there is no potential source of bleeding such as a peptic ulcer, recent operation or fracture.

Many clinicians believe that lytic therapy is indicated in massive pulmonary embolism. The co-operative study of the National Heart and Lung Institute in the U.S.A. (1970) showed that urokinase in comparison with heparin significantly accelerated the resolution of pulmonary thrombo-emboli at 24 hours as demonstrated by pulmonary arteriogram, lung scans and right heart pressures. However, no significant difference in 2 week mortality was noted (a larger trial would have been required), moreover bleeding occurred in 45% of patients receiving urokinase in contrast to 27% of those receiving heparin alone. In subsequent trials no difference in therapeutic effect was observed between urokinase and streptokinase. These agents should not be used without expert haematological advice.

ARTERIOGRAPHY

Outlining of an entire arterial system can be obtained by radiography after the injection of an opaque medium into the parent trunk. This method of investigation may give valuable information in cases of arterial injury or disease. It may demonstrate the site of any narrowing or constriction, or aneurysm or of arteriovenous fistula. It may indicate the extent of occlusive vascular disease, and the state of any collateral circulation. The opaque media commonly used at the present time are organic iodine compounds in which the pharmacological action of iodine is suppressed. They are radioinactive and are not retained in the body; they have some irritant action and may cause inflammation or even thrombosis in veins. This latter hazard can be avoided by dilution of the medium or by the use of one of the newer nonionic contrast media.

Aortography

This is used to investigate the circulation, not only in the aorta and its main branches, but also in the arteries of both lower limbs. It is of special value in demonstrating occlusive lesions at the aortic bifurcation or in the iliac arteries, and in outlining the renal blood vessels and parenchyma in cases of suspected tumour or essential hypertension. It is also being used extensively in the diagnosis of many other abdominal conditions. Three methods are in use.

Translumbar aortography

This term implies the injection of contrast medium into the aorta by percutaneous puncture in the lumbar region. With the patient in the prone position and under general anaesthesia a needle, 15 cm in length and 1–3 mm in external diameter, is entered immediately below the 12th rib on the left side, 4 finger breadths from the midline. It is directed forwards and medially until it strikes the

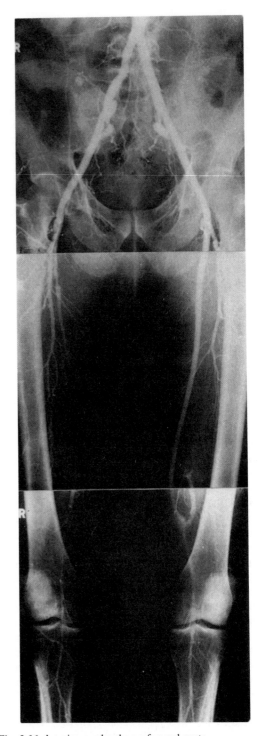

Fig. 3.16 Arteriogram by the perfemoral route

body of the 2nd lumber vertebra; it is then withdrawn slightly and realigned so that it slips forward past the side of the vertebral body, to enter the aorta which is lying immediately in front. Successful entry into the lumen of the vessel is suggested by a sensation similar to that obtained from puncture of the spinal theca, and is confirmed by the escape of blood in rhythmic jets. 40 to 60 ml of solution, warmed to body temperature (in order to prevent spasm of the vessels) is injected under pressure as rapidly as possible, and three or four exposures are made in quick succession, as fast as the films can be changed. Possible complications, which are fortunately very rare, include (1) separation of a calcified intimal plaque which may become an embolus, (2) the initiation of a dissecting aneurysm as a result of the injection having been made intramurally, and (3) thrombosis of mesenteric or peripheral arteries.

Transfemoral catheterization method
By percutaneous puncture of one or other femoral artery, and by the introduction of a fine polythene catheter in a cardiac direction, an aortogram can be taken at any desired level without difficulty. This is the most frequently used method, since it is generally regarded as being both easier and safer than translumbar aortography. The use of appropriately shaped catheters allows the selective catherization of aortic branches—including mesenteric and renal vessels and the branches from the aortic arch to the head and upper limbs.

Transbrachial or transaxillary aortography
This method, whereby a catheter is introduced proximally into the brachial or axillary artery, percutaneously or by open operation, is used to outline the aortic arch and its branches and the descending thoracic aorta when the transfemoral route is not available.

Peripheral arteriography
For investigation of the distal circulation in the lower limb, 10 to 15 ml of contrast medium may be injected into the femoral artery, by percutaneous puncture just below the inguinal ligament, either general or local anaesthesia being employed. If there is any difficulty in entering the artery by percutaneous puncture or the operator lacks the necessary experience, the artery can be exposed through a small incision.

Renal arteriography is described on page 506.

ARTERIAL ANEURYSMS

Traumatic aneurysms may follow penetrating wounds of arteries, or they may occur as a late result of simple contusion when the injured segment of vessel subsequently gives way. Non-traumatic aneurysms are usually associated with generalized arterial degeneration.

In the early stages of development of a traumatic aneurysm—when the condition is better described as an *arterial haematoma* (p. 34)—conservative treatment should be employed, unless there is a progressive increase in the swelling or acute circulatory failure due to compression of the collateral vessels. Should these conditions be present, immediate operation is indicated. After evacuation of the haematoma, continuity of the artery is restored if at all possible, either by simple repair, or by one of the reconstructive methods which have been described—except in the case of vessels below the elbow or knee, where simple ligation is the procedure of choice.

In most cases, however, it is desirable to postpone operation until the primary wound has soundly healed, and an adequate collateral circulation has developed. The optimum time for intervention will vary with each case. If the condition is progressive, operation may be demanded within a few days; if it is relatively quiescent, operation may be delayed for several months.

Choice of operation
This depends very largely upon the size of the artery concerned, and on the possibility of an adequate collateral circulation. Except in the case of the smaller vessels, simple ligation alone is now discarded, since it has been shown to have two great disadvantages. If the collateral circulation is adequate for nutrition of the limb, it also maintains blood flow through the aneurysm which therefore fails to close; if the collateral circulation is inadequate, the risk of gangrene is considerable.

Ligature with obliteration of the sac
This is an appropriate procedure in the case of vessels below the elbow or knee. It is best carried out from *within* the aneurysmal sac, and the term 'obliterative endo-aneurysmorrhaphy' (Matas, 1888) is applicable. The method is as a rule effective in preventing recurrence; in addition it combines simplicity and safety, since surrounding structures are not disturbed and possible interference with the collateral circulation is reduced to a minimum. The steps in the operation are shown in Figure 3.17.

Ligature with excision of the sac
This is a more certain method of preventing recurrence, but, owing to the extent of the dissection required, damage may be inflicted upon the collateral circulation on which the nutrition of the part depends.

Reconstructive procedures
Advances in the reconstructive surgery of arteries (pp. 36 & 37) have revolutionized the treatment of aneurysms. This applies particularly to aneurysms of the aorta. Most aortic aneurysms prove fatal within a limited time, either by rupture, by embolism or by pressure on surrounding structures, and there is no medical treatment which will influence the natural course of the disease.

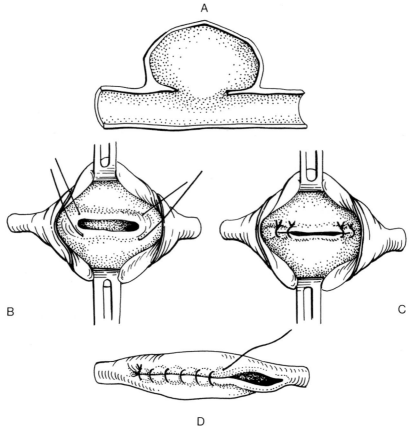

Fig. 3.17 Obliterative endo-aneurysmorrhaphy
(A) Cross section of artery with false sac
(B) Sutures placed to close the arterial openings within the sac
(C) Sutures tied
(D) Closure of the sac

Aneurysms of the aorta and large arteries
The surgical treatment of these aneurysms has advanced rapidly in recent years so that it is impossible to do more than lay down certain general principles for guidance.

Arch of aorta
Aneurysms of the arch (especially of the central part) carry the problem of maintaining an adequate cerebral circulation during the reconstructive procedure. A temporary bypass may be constructed—usually to the innominate artery. In the case of dissecting aneurysms treatment using hypotensive agents may be the first choice in the hope of effecting intramural thrombosis failing which the condition is dealt with either by division and suture of the aorta (thus effecting closure of the dissection) or by replacement of the affected segment with a prosthesis. These procedures may have to be combined with reconstruction of the aortic valve.

Descending thoracic aorta
The risks of temporarily clamping this vessel concern, not the brain, but the spinal cord and kidneys. This may be avoided by the construction of a temporary bypass. When there is associated coarctation, much less risk arises, for a collateral circulation has already been established.

Abdominal aorta
Fortunately aneurysms of the abdominal aorta seldom develop above the level of the renal arteries, so that these vessels, together with the coeliac and superior mesenteric, are usually unaffected. The inferior mesenteric artery is usually found to be occluded at its origin. The standard treatment is replacement with a plastic prosthesis, either a simple tube or more commonly a bifurcation graft. No attempt should be made to excise the posterior part of the aneurysmal sac. After exposure through a long midline or transverse abdominal incision, by the intraperitoneal route described on page 32, the

aorta above the sac and the iliac arteries distally are controlled with suitable clamps. Most surgeons give 5–10 000 units of heparin intravenously in elective cases prior to cross clamping. At the end of the procedure, if there is any sign of bleeding, the heparin is reversed with protamine. If a variety of graft is to be used which requires preclotting, such as knitted dacron, then this must be done before the heparin is given. The sac is opened in the midline and the contents evacuated. The mouths of any bleeding lumbar arteries are closed with stitch ligatures. The prosthesis is laid in the sac and sutured as an inlay or end to end to the aortic or iliac stumps (Fig. 3.18). The passage of Fogarty embolectomy catheters down both limbs prior to completion of the distal anastomoses is a recommended precaution

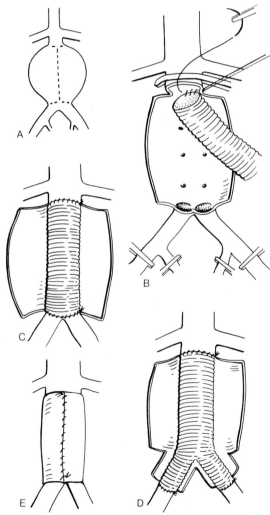

Fig. 3.18 Graft replacement for aneurysm of the abdominal aorta. The graft, which may be simple tube or bifurcation, is laid within the aneurysmal sac. The sac and peritoneum are closed over the graft

against postoperative ischaemia, especially if systemic heparin has not been used. The sac is loosely sutured around the graft in order to give it a supportive covering. Care should be taken to separate the graft and particularly the suture lines from overlying bowel, if necessary by interposing a pedicle of omentum, because of the danger of later fistula. The 5-year survival rate of electively treated abdominal aneurysms is about 60% as compared with 10% for untreated cases. Most centres advise early operation since rupture of an aortic aneurysm is an emergency which requires urgent operation and carries a mortality of around 50%.

Iliac, femoral and popliteal aneurysms
A restorative operation, with either replacement or bypass, is the ideal treatment. The indications for replacement are increasing size, distal embolism or acute occlusion. If gangrene has developed by the time the patient seeks treatment, amputation will of course be required.

Innominate, subclavian and axillary aneurysms
The subclavian artery can usually be ligatured with safety, provided that this is done beyond the first part, the branches of which provide an adequate collateral circulation. For aneurysms of the innominate and axillary arteries, a reconstructive operation should if possible be attempted.

Arteriovenous aneurysms (fistulae)
Fistulous communication between an artery and a vein is rarely met within civilian life, but is a common sequel to the penetrating wound of warfare. Depending on the presence or absence of an aneurysmal sac between the communicating vessels, the terms *varicose aneurysm* or *aneurysmal varix* may be employed, but the distinction is a somewhat arbitrary one.

Natural cure is most unlikely—indeed the condition is usually progressive. When the fistula involves the main vessels of a limb, signs of defective circulation develop in the distal part of the limb. In carotidojugular fistulae, cerebral and occular effects may predominate. The effects on the general circulation may be even more serious. The diversion of blood from the normal arterial bed results in a marked fall in the diastolic pressure, with a corresponding rise in pulse pressure. Increased venous return to the heart gives rise to progressive left ventricular enlargement. The larger the fistula, and the nearer it is to the heart, the more serious will be its effects. Operation is indicated before cardiac decompensation has become established.

Quadruple ligature
This is a suitable method for the smaller vessels. The artery and vein are exposed above and below the fistula,

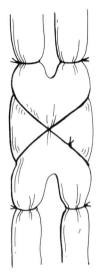

Fig. 3.19 Arteriovenous fistula; quadruple ligation and obliteration

and each vessel is ligatured in both situations. Ligatures are applied also to any other vessels communicating with the sac. Thereafter the sac may be obliterated with further ligatures (Fig. 3.19). Every effort is made to avoid damage to important collateral vessels, on which the circulation of the limb depends.

Reconstructive operations

These are indicated in the case of the larger vessels. Direct repair may be possible especially in the early stages using a vein or dacron patch on the artery if necessary (Fig. 3.20). Later, it is advisable to excise the affected segment of the artery and to replace it, if direct repair is not possible, with an autogenous vein graft.

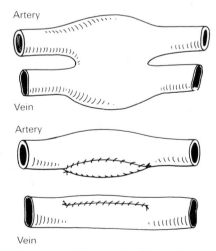

Fig. 3.20 A reconstructive operation for arteriovenous fistula

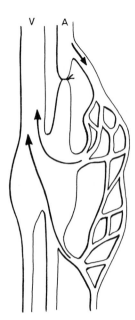

Fig. 3.21 Ligature of the artery alone, in arteriovenous fistula, is likely to cause gangrene

Simple ligature of the artery alone, proximal to the fistula, is contraindicated in the case of the main vessel of a limb, for it will almost invariably be followed by gangrene. The reason for this is that the collateral circulation lacks the force to drive it into the capillary bed distal to the fistula; it takes instead the course of least resistance through the fistula back to the heart (Fig. 3.21).

ACUTE ARTERIAL OCCLUSION

Despite the advent of thrombolytic therapy acute arterial occlusion remains a surgical condition. Thrombosis can usually be distinguished by an antecedent history of claudication and is often precipitated by a hypotensive episode. If it is quite clear that an episode of acute ischaemia is due to thrombosis rather than embolism then emergency thrombectomy should not be attempted unless the surgeon is prepared and equipped to go on to an arterial reconstruction in the likely event of failure to clear the thrombus. Sometimes however exploration may be the only means of distinguishing between the two.

Arterial embolism is usually secondary to severe heart disease, especially auricular fibrillation, the embolus lodging at major arterial bifurcations—the aortic, the common iliac, the femoral or the popliteal. It occurs often in elderly and unfit patients, so that the mortality is high, and the major surgical procedures are contraindicated.

Following lodgement of the embolus, there is propagation of thrombosis both proximal and distal to the site of embolism. The main object of anticoagulant therapy (intravenous heparin) is to obviate this progressive clotting, but it is the modern view that all emboli in major arteries should be removed, even if the limb is viable and the circulation appears to be adequate. Anticoagulant therapy is invaluable, however, if there is to be some delay while the patient is being transferred to a centre where vascular surgery is undertaken. A successful embolectomy prevents propagation of the clot, and may obviate irreversible ischaemic changes in the limbs. No arbitrary time limit can be set, but once infarction has occurred in the calf muscles, evidenced by tenderness and fixed plantar flexion, salvage is unlikely (Gregg, 1983).

Embolectomy catheters
The slender balloon catheter, devised by Fogarty (1963, 1971) has been a most significant advance in vascular surgery, and is now an indispensible instrument for embolectomy. This catheter is 80 cm long and is available in sizes 4 to 7F. It has a delicate inflatable balloon close to its tip, the balloon being of varying sizes. The catheter is threaded into the artery to a level beyond which no clots are thought to be present. The balloon is then inflated with sterile water or air until slight resistance is felt, and the catheter is withdrawn with the balloon in its inflated state, bringing with it any clots present within the lumen. The inflation should be gradually increased to match the widening calibre if the catheter is being withdrawn proximally and vice versa.

Aortic and iliac embolectomy
Effective removal of aortic and iliac emboli has in the past been accomplished by direct exposure of these vessels; in addition bilateral inguinal incisions are required for the removal of more distal thrombi. Such an approach is a very formidable procedure in a critically ill patient.

By means of the embolectomy catheter
Aortic bifurcation and iliac emboli, together with any distal thrombi, can now be removed *via* the femoral arteries, which are approached below the inguinal ligament, and the procedure can be carried out very expeditiously under local anaesthesia. The entire abdomen should, however, be prepared and draped, since, if extraction of the clot by the embolectomy catheter is unsuccessful, it may be necessary to expose the aortic bifurcation by laparotomy. Through incisions below the inguinal ligaments, the femoral arteries are exposed; they are elevated with tapes passed above and below the origin of the profundae, and these branches are controlled in the same way. An incision 1–1.5 cm in length is made

into the femoral artery just above the origin of the profunda. Attention should first be paid to removal of thrombi in the distal arterial tree i.e. both from the distal part of the femoral artery and from the profunda. After the catheter has been passed as far distally as possible, the balloon is inflated until mild resistance is felt, and is then withdrawn, additional fluid or air being injected gradually as the calibre of the vessel increases. Ideally the clearance of the distal arterial tree should be checked by peroperative arteriography. It can be misleading to rely on good backflow alone. Arteriography can be done simply by positioning a cassette, draped in a sterile towel, under the limb and the hand injection of 10–20 ml of contrast fluid through a cannula into the distal lumen. After all thrombi have been removed, a solution of heparin (10 units per ml of saline) is injected into the distal vessels, which are then occluded by atraumatic arterial clamps. A larger size balloon catheter is now introduced into the main trunk, and is passed upwards into the aorta to a level well above the embolus. The balloon is then inflated with the appropriate amount of fluid, and is extracted as previously described, bringing the clot, or a considerable part of it, with it. The catheter should be passed repeatedly until no further clots can be delivered, and until a forceful blood flow is obtained. After one side has been cleared (Fig. 3.22), the procedure should be repeated from the opposite femoral artery. If the embolus has been a saddle-shaped one at the bifurcation of the aorta, about half of it can be expected to be removed through each femoral artery. Finally the arteriotomy incision is sutured. Anticoagulant therapy is continued after operation, not only to prevent further embolisation, but also to prevent venous thrombosis, which is a frequent sequel to arterial embolisation.

Peripheral arterial embolism
The common femoral artery is the most frequent site for peripheral embolism (40% of all cases), the clot lodging at the point where the profunda artery branches off. Localized bulging, with pulsation above the embolus and a state of immobile constriction below, may be seen but this sign is by no means always present. The circulation is controlled by means of slings applied to the artery above and below; a longitudinal incision is made in the arterial wall, when, if the diagnosis is correct, clot will be present in the lumen. From the groin the Fogarty catheter can be passed down the profunda to the lower thigh and down the superficial femoral artery as far as the ankle. Thrombus is removed as described above.

Pulmonary embolectomy and venous thrombectomy
These are discussed in the section on venous thrombosis (p. 52).

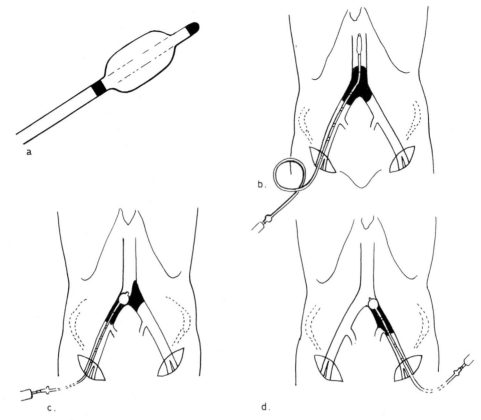

Fig. 3.22 Balloon catheter embolectomy
a Tip of Fogarty catheter showing inflatable balloon
b Catheter tip above embolus after introduction through right femoral artery
c Clot being dislodged by withdrawal of inflated balloon
d Residual clot being removed through left femoral artery

VARICOSE VEINS

Anatomy

The superficial veins of the lower limb are collected into two main trunks—the long saphenous vein, which extends the whole length of the limb and the short saphenous vein, which extends upwards only as far as the knee.

The long saphenous vein

This is formed by the union of veins on the medial side of the foot. It passes in front of the medial malleolus, and ascends to the medial side of the knee, lying just behind the femoral condyle. In the thigh it inclines laterally and forwards towards the saphenous opening, which lies 3–4 cm below and lateral to the pubic tubercle. It pierces the cribiform fascia, and passes deeply through the saphenous opening to join the femoral vein.

Tributaries. The more important of these, together with their usual anatomical arrangement, are shown in Figure 3.23. Considerable variations however exist; a high medial or lateral superficial femoral vein may be mistaken for the main trunk, and very occasionally this latter is double. Special note should be made of the tributary (J in Fig. 3.23) which ascends along the medial side of the calf, behind and parallel to the main trunk, and joining this just below knee level. This vessel has important communications with the deep veins, through 'perforators' (usually three in number) which traverse the deep fascia at fairly constant levels. It is in relation to this tributary, rather than to the main trunk of the long saphenous vein, that varicosities and ulcers in the lower leg commonly develop.

The short saphenous vein

This is formed by the union of veins on the lateral side of the foot. It crosses behind the lateral malleolus, and then ascends obliquely backwards towards the middle of the popliteal fossa, where, after receiving several small tributaries, it pierces deep fascia to enter the popliteal vein. It frequently communicates with the deep veins

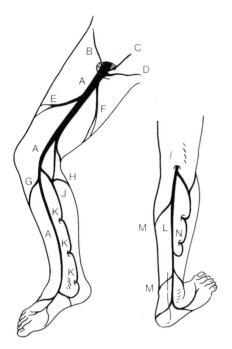

Fig. 3.23 Anatomy of long and short saphenous veins
A = Long saphenous vein, main trunk; B = Superficial
external iliac vein; C = Superficial epigastric vein;
D = Superficial external pudendal vein; E = Lateral
superficial femoral vein; F = Medial superficial femoral vein;
G = Anterior vein winding round tibia below knee;
H = Posterior vein, joining (or occasionally replacing) short
saphenous vein; J = Posteromedial vein, which lies parallel to
and behind main trunk of long saphenous vein, and anastomoses
with arches arising from; K = perforating veins—usually three
in number and constant in position; L = Short saphenous vein,
with M = medial tributaries which may communicate with
medial perforators; N = connection with lateral perforating
vein, a handsbreadth above malleolus

Assessment

The first and most important thing is for the surgeon to
learn to recognize the patterns of varicosities which are
characteristic of particular sites of incompetence. For
example, if there are varicosities on the medial side of
the thigh it can usually be assumed, even if it is not
immediately obvious, that there is saphenofemoral
incompetence. Indeed one of the commonest mistakes in
varicose vein surgery is failure properly to deal with
incompetence at this level. Prominent varicosities in the
lower half of the medial side of the calf are usually associated with incompetent perforators, especially if there
are associated skin changes of pigmentation, eczema or
ulceration. The presence of a retromalleolar venous flare
extending down on to the foot is a clear sign of the existence of an incompetent perforator at its apex. Varicosities on the lateral side of the calf may stem from
short saphenopopliteal incompetence or from connections with an incompetent long saphenous vein. Careful examination will distinguish the two, provided
that the surgeon bears in mind the variations which
may occur in the termination of the short saphenous
vein.

Before the operation, with the patient standing, the
main venous channels are palpated, percussed and
marked with an indelible marker. The simplest and most
widely used test (*Trendelenburg*) depends on observation
of the filling of varicosities before and after systematic
removal of rubber tourniquets (the most distal first)
which have been applied with the leg elevated. *Doppler
ultrasound* is a valuable noninvasive tool, simple in application, which can be used to demonstrate saphenofemoral or saphenopopliteal reflux, perforator incompetence
and patency of deep veins.

When there is a history of deep vein thrombosis phlebography is the most reliable method of confirming
patency of deep veins. If however there is no oedema,
venous claudication or severe skin changes it can be
assumed that there is not a deep vein occlusion sufficient
to preclude varicose vein surgery. Ascending phlebography is performed by injection of contrast medium
into a foot vein. The medium is directed into the deep
veins by tourniquet above the ankle. *Phlebography* can
be used to locate perforating veins but is seldom justified for this indication, physical examination being
preferred.

Injection therapy, which came back into favour in the
1960's as a result of the work of Fegan (1963), is not
necessarily an alternative to operation. It has a useful
place for the abolition of minor varices unrelated to
saphenous incompetence and is particularly effective in
dealing with residual or recurrent varices postoperatively. If saphenofemoral or saphenopopliteal incompetence is present the sclerosis of distal varicosities offers
no prospect of long term benefit.

through a 'perforator' a handsbreadth above the lateral
malleolus (Fig. 3.23).

Variations from the normal arrangement frequently
occur. The vein may pierce the deep fascia in the upper
part of the calf, or occasionally it may remain superficial
throughout, joining the long saphenous vein as one of its
medial tributaries near the knee. Before any treatment
of varicose veins can be planned, it is essential to determine by careful examination whether the varicosities
involve the long or short saphenous system, and to what
extent they have developed in relation to communicating
or *perforating* veins which pass through fascia and muscle
to connect with the deep veins of the limb.

Special tests have been designed in order to determine
the choice of treatment. They fall into three main groups:
(1) tests for valvular incompetence at the saphenofemoral
and saphenopopliteal junctions; (2) tests for incompetent
perforating veins; (3) tests for patency of the deep veins.

Choice of operation

The various components of varicose vein surgery are saphenofemoral ligation (Trendelenburg), saphenopopliteal ligation, multiple ligations, stripping and the ligation of perforators superficial or deep to the deep fascia.

Crucial to the correct choice of operation is careful physical examination, as described above, with the aim of detecting the points at which there is reflux from the deep to the superficial system. When varicosities stem from saphenofemoral incompetence, as is the case in the great majority of both primary and secondary varicose veins, the Trendelenburg operation is indicated. Since saphenofemoral reflux and perforator incompetence frequently coexist it is usually necessary to add multiple incisions through which the major tributaries of the saphenous systems are interrupted and perforators ligated. As an alternative to multiple incisions some surgeons prefer to deal with high incompetence and to follow this with avulsions through multiple tiny stab incisions. The long term benefits of these methods are unproven and they will not be discussed further. The stripping of the long saphenous vein is less popular than hitherto owing to the importance of that vein as arterial replacement. If points of incompetence are carefully located and dealt with, stripping can, with advantage, be omitted. If stripping is performed without incompetent perforators being ligated the varicose condition will, in the long run be worse rather than better. If stripping is performed it should be carried out only from knee to groin. Stripping of the long saphenous vein in the calf serves no proven additional benefit, gives rise to postoperative discomfort, and carries a high probability of damage to the saphenous nerve.

Sclerotherapy

Many different solutions have been employed during the past 50 years. The common objective is to induce endothelial damage and so initiate a chemical phlebitis. The injected vein eventually shrinks and becomes organized into fibrous tissue so that complete obliteration of the vein results. Two satisfactory solutions are ethanolamine and sodium tetradecyl sulphate (STD). In the technique of compression sclerotherapy (Fegan) the sites of incompetent perforators are located as accurately as possible.

Up to eight 2 ml syringes are each loaded with 0.5 ml of sclerosing solution. The patient sits vertically on a waist high couch with the legs horizontal. In this position the vein contains sufficient blood for venepuncture. The lowest injection site is selected first. The needle is inserted, the leg is elevated to empty the vein and the sclerosant injected while the vein is compressed with the fingers above and below the needle. Compression is then applied by means of elastocrepe bandage over Sorbo rubber pad or cotton wool ball. The procedure is repeated at several sites, working proximally. A full length two way stretch elastic stocking is fitted over the completely injected and bandaged leg.

The importance of walking for 1 hour immediately and 3 miles each day is emphasized. Provided that the patient remains relatively comfortable and the bandages firm they are not disturbed for 3 weeks.

Trendelenburg operation

This operation is considered to be an essential part of any surgical treatment for varicosities involving the long saphenous system. It implies the removal of a segment of the proximal end of the long saphenous vein, together with the ligature of all tributaries entering this segment. For many years it was employed as the sole method of operative treatment for such varicosities, but at the present time it is usually combined with other procedures, such as stripping and multiple ligatures. The operation may be performed on an outpatient, but it is not one which an inexperienced house surgeon should undertake. If the upper end of the long saphenous vein is visible or palpable when the patient stands up, its position should be indicated by skin marking before the operation is commenced.

An incision 5 to 8 cm in length is made below and parallel to the medial half of the inguinal ligament, at the level of the saphenous opening which is 3 cm below and lateral to the pubic tubercle—just medial to the femoral pulsation. As soon as a small cut has been made in the deep fascia, the fat can be separated by blunt dissection in the line of the saphenous vein. The vein is then cleared to a level of 7 to 8 cm below the opening.

The saphenous trunk is divided between clamps applied about the middle of the exposed part. Using the clamp as a convenient tractor, the upper segment of vein is raised from its bed; its three named tributaries in this part—the superficial external iliac, the superficial epigastric and the superficial external pudendal—and any others discovered, are clamped and divided. The superior margin of the saphenous opening is retracted upwards, so that the vein can be cleared right up to its junction with the femoral.

Although traction with a haemostat on the proximal stump of the long saphenous vein is very helpful for dissection, care must be taken when it comes to ligation not to tent up and thus constrict the common femoral vein. A nonabsorbable transfixion suture is used for the proximal ligation (Fig. 3.24). The cut ends of the tributary veins are ligated.

Attention is then turned to the distal stump. An important step is ligation of the medial superficial femoral tributary (F in Fig. 3.23). This can usually be reached by retraction on the lower margin of the wound with the knee flexed. Sometimes a separate incision is

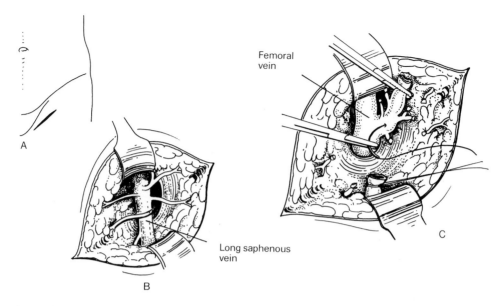

Fig. 3.24 Saphenofemoral ligation (Trendelenberg)
(A) The incision is centred on a point 3–4 cm below and lateral to the public tubercle.
(B) All the tributaries of the upper end of the long saphenous vein are exposed, ligated and divided.
(C) The proximal stump of the long saphenous vein is transfixed and ligated

required. The lower stump is then ligated unless stripping is intended.

The groin wound is closed with interrupted subcutaneous catgut and nonabsorbable skin sutures. If a stripper is present it is led out of the lateral end of the wound and the adjacent skin suture left untied until the leg has been bandaged (vide infra).

Difficulties and complications
Difficulty in finding the saphenous vein is overcome by enlarging the incison. A high medial or lateral superficial femoral tributary may be mistaken for the main trunk. If the main trunk of the saphenous vein is double, both divisions should be ligatured. Mistaken identification of the main vein, or any anatomical variations from the normal will at once become apparent as the vein is traced upwards towards the saphenous opening. Tearing of the femoral vein or slipping of the ligature on the saphenous stump causes alarming haemorrhage. The greatest danger is that the surgeon, in his natural anxiety to arrest haemorrhage, may apply forceps blindly in the depths of the wound, and by so doing may cause irreparable damage to the femoral artery or vein. All that is required is to pack gauze firmly into the wound, and to lower the head of the table. *The gauze is left in situ for at least 5 minutes*: when it is removed the haemorrhage will be reduced to a mere trickle. If the ligature has slipped, the stump of the saphenous vein can then be picked up without difficulty.

A tear in the femoral vein should be sutured with fine nonabsorbable material on a round bodied needle. This is best achieved by using a fine nozzle suction close to the tear to clear blood from the field unless bleeding can be controlled by finger compression of the vein above and below the wound.

Vein stripping
Mayo's original 'ring' stripper which was passed outside the vein, has now been replaced by the intraluminal variety. This consists of wire or plastic 85–90 cm in length with an olivary tip on one end and acorn-shaped head on the other. Modern disposable strippers have detachable acorns of various sizes (Fig. 3.25).

Technique
For stripping of the upper half of the long saphenous vein, it is advised that a Trendelenburg operation should first be carried out at the groin i.e. the vein is exposed and all tributaries entering its upper segment are divided. The vein is then transfixed and ligated at its junction with the femoral and is divided below the ligature. The distal end is temporarily controlled with a loosely tied ligature held in a haemostat (Fig. 3.26). The long saphenous vein is now exposed through a skin crease incision three finger breadths below the knee joint; the stripper is introduced (Fig. 3.26B) and is passed upwards until it emerges through the upper end of the vein in the groin incision, the loosely tied ligature allowing it to do this (Fig. 3.26 A). The stripper is drawn upwards until arrested by the acorn-head, which is of course too large to enter the vein.

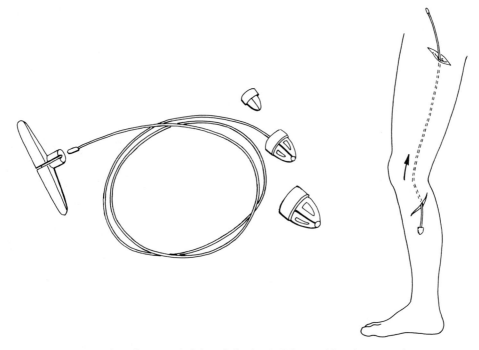

Fig. 3.25 The plastic disposable stripper has a range of sizes of olive heads. It is passed from knee to groin

A ligature of strong silk is now tied firmly around the vein containing the stripper, so that the vessel is anchored against the acorn-head (Fig. 3.26 C). The vein is then divided below the ligature and the lower cut end is tied off. The vein is not stripped out at this stage. It will usually be necessary for further incisions to be made in the leg to ligate large tributaries and perforating veins. All wounds are closed with non-absorbable sutures. In the groin incision the suture alongside the stripper is left untied, the loose ends being controlled by haemostats. Wounds are dressed and the leg elevated and bandaged. An excellent way of ensuring that compression is effectively maintained postoperatively and the bandages kept in place is to apply an elastic *graduated* stocking on top of the bandage—but untapered tubular elastic bandage is potentially harmful and must be avoided. Finally traction is applied to the stipper to avulse the vein and the last suture is tied, sterility being maintained by using the haemostats to tie the knot. If this procedure is followed, and if during the Trendelenburg operation the medial superficial femoral vein has been dealt with as described above, there should be no haematoma formation—a common cause of postoperative discomfort after stripping.

Ligature of the short saphenous vein
This is indicated when varicosities involve this vein or its tributaries. A transverse incision is made across the lower part of the politeal fossa at the level of the head of the fibula. (A vertical incision is liable to heal with keloid formation). The short saphenous vein is identified, and is ligatured and divided at the level where it pierces deep fascia to join the popliteal vein. The surgeon must be aware of the anatomical variations which commonly occur. Other superficial veins of the region, entering either the short saphenous or the popliteal vein, are dealt with in the same way (Dodd, 1965).

Vein ligatures
In most operations for varicose veins it is not sufficient simply to carry out saphenous ligations with or without stripping. It is necessary also to ligate varicose tributaries at their junctions with the saphenous veins and to ligate perforating veins at the point at which they traverse the deep fascia. If it is intended to follow high ligation with a course of sclerotherapy then the need for multiple ligations may be less.

Incisions near to joints should be made transversely; all other incisions should be longitudinal otherwise the scope for dissecting out veins is severely restricted. Where perforators are suspected, for example at the medial border of soleus, the incision should be carried straight down to the level of the deep fascia. Superficial veins crossing the line of the incision should be ligated but in the lower calf the circulation to the skin should not be jeopardized by extensive superficial dissection. At the level of the deep fascia wound flaps can be raised by gently separating subcutaneous fat from deep fascia. This

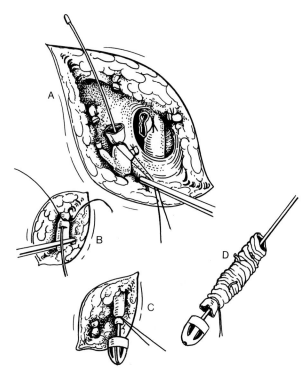

Fig. 3.26 Stripping operation for varicose veins
(A) Trendelenberg operation. Long saphenous vein ligatured and divided at junction with femoral. Tributaries divided between ligatures
(B) Long saphenous vein exposed just below knee. A ligature is placed around the vein and the stripper inserted
(C) Ligature tied to anchor vein against acorn head of stripper and vein divided
(D) The complete vein after avulsion telescoped against the head of the stripper

plane of dissection can be extended over quite a wide area to reveal the presence of perforators which can be then ligated. Where the changes of chronic venous insufficiency are present: induration, eczema and ulceration, the ligation of perforators is best achieved at subfascial level as described in the following section.

After-treatment following operations on veins
Patients who have undergone minor operations, such as a few ligatures, can usually remain completely ambulant, since exercise obviates stasis in the deep veins, and reduces the risk of thrombosis. For the same reasons, however, they should avoid standing for any length of time for the first few days after operations, and, when seated, should keep the limb elevated. When more extensive procedures, involving multiple ligations of varices, stripping, skin grafting etc. have been employed, a more restful convalescence is usually advised, and a firm supporting bandage should be worn until healing is complete. It is the author's policy to prescribe graduated compression hose to be worn for at least 3 months after operation.

VENOUS ULCERS

The majority of patients with ulcers in the lower leg have other causative or aggravating disorders of which the more important are arterial insufficiency, obesity, arthropathy at the knee or ankle, rheumatoid vasculitis, hypertension, neurological deficit, chronic skin disorders and diabetes.

Nevertheless, stasis and hypertension in the superficial veins is undoubtedly an important factor in the majority of ulcers in the lower third of the calf—the so-called 'ulcer-bearing area'. Such ulcers are most commonly located on the medial side in relation to the main perforating veins. When the valves of these perforating veins become incompetent the rise in deep venous pressure caused by each calf contraction is transmitted outwards to the overlying superficial veins. Occlusion of the deep veins by thrombus aggravates the problem. Incompetence of valves in deep veins, an alternative sequel to deep vein thrombosis, results in excessive pressure being transmitted to the superficial veins not only during exercise but also at rest while standing or sitting.

Chronic hypertension in the venous side of the capillary circulation results in the skin changes characteristic of venous insufficiency: pigmentation, eczema, induration and ulceration. Contact dermatitis commonly supervenes as a result of sensitivity to antibiotics or other locally applied medicaments. These changes are the consequence of increased capillary permeability with escape of blood constituents into subcutaneous tissue. Lysis of red cells and haemosiderin deposition leads to pigmentation. Protein is deposited around each capillary, forming a fibrin wall which interferes with tissue oxygenation and nutrition.

The basis of all *conservative treatment* is to abolish venous congestion by elevation of the part if the patient can be kept at rest, or by means of firm compression by bandages or elastic stockings if he or she is ambulant. The importance of correctly applied high quality elastic bandage or properly fitting hosiery cannot be overemphasized. The patient will rapidly discard items which are uncomfortable or ill fitting. Elastic bandages seldom provide sustained compression for more than a few hours and they must be regularly reapplied. Such bandages must always include the forefoot and extend to the knee. Compression should be maximal in the lower calf and diminish as the bandage ascends. The same is true of stockings of which the most generally useful types are of knee length.

A full account of the management of leg ulcers is beyond the scope of this book. However, it may be said that provided that the associated conditions are treated and the venous hypertension counteracted by physical measures the nature of the ulcer dressings are of secondary importance. Paste-impregnated bandages are the most generally useful dressing. Agents which tend to cause allergy, especially local antibiotics, should be avoided. *Operation* is usually advocated without undue delay for the younger patient, but a preliminary period of conservative treatment is advisable, in order to reduce oedema and to obtain complete or partial healing of the ulcer before surgical intervention. In the case of older patients, operation may be reserved for those in whom conservative treatment is unsuccessful. It should not, however, be postponed for too long, for the results are less favourable when the ulcer is of long standing; in such cases, where irreversible changes may have occurred, skin grafting is likely to be an essential part of the treatment.

If dilatation or varicosity is present in the superficial venous system, this should be treated by one of the methods already described. It is usually advised that such treatment should include ligation or injection of perforating veins in the vicinity of the ulcer.

Where there is advanced skin change with inflammation or induration perforators should be ligated under the deep fascia. This is most conveniently performed under tourniquet. In such cases it is the author's policy to deal with venous incompetence at high levels by the conventional methods already described. Wounds are then closed and dressed, the leg elevated and exsanguinated by means of an Esmarch rubber bandage and a thigh tourniquet. The lower leg is redraped. A generous straight incision is made behind the medial margin of the tibia in the lower half of the leg. If there is an ulcer in the line of incision, it should be excised. Any large veins in the subcutaneous tissue should be ligated but undercutting of the skin flaps should be avoided as far as possible. The incision is carried down to and through the deep fascia. The latter is easily separated from underlying muscle to reveal perforators at the medial border of soleus where they are ligated. Suspected perforators on the lateral side are sought at the lateral border of soleus, if necessary, through a separate incision. Where both lateral and medial perforators require to be dealt with both may be reached through a posterior median incision. Such an incision should deviate to one or other side of the Achilles tendon at its lower end. The patient should be warned before operation that the wound may be slow to heal. He or she should be kept in bed with elevation, for 3 to 4 days. The wound is then inspected and mobilization commenced if healing is progressing satisfactorily. If an ulcer has been excised, the raw area is covered with tulle gras, and is grafted 4 or 5 days later. Firm supporting bandages are worn until healing is complete.

VENOUS THROMBOSIS AND EMBOLISM

The effective management of this condition depends very much on accurate diagnosis; the unreliability of clinical diagnosis is well known. For the detection of venous thrombosis Doppler ultrasound, the radio-iodine uptake tests and various types of plethysmography all have their place but if active treatment, especially thrombolytic therapy or surgery is planned, phlebography is still the most important investigation. Similarly, lung scanning or pulmonary angiography are of prime importance if pulmonary embolism is suspected. The opportunities for successful pulmonary embolectomy are, however, rare.

The majority of patients with venous thrombosis and/or pulmonary embolism can be satisfactorily treated with a week to 10 days of intravenous heparin overlapped with and followed by oral anticoagulants. Life threatening pulmonary embolism or major deep vein thrombosis of recent onset (within 4 days) which carries the risk of lethal embolism or post-thrombotic problems should be treated with Streptokinase, provided that there is no obvious bleeding risk such as an active peptic ulcer or a fracture or major operation within the last 10 days. There are two possible surgical approaches to venous thrombosis: venous thrombectomy and venous interruption.

Venous thrombectomy
This operation is seldom performed today although some authors still recommend it for phlegmasia caerulea dolens. While it is not technically difficult to remove thrombus from an occluded vein, especially since the advent of the Fogarty catheter, there is a high frequency of rethrombosis, despite anticoagulation, and follow up studies have shown the majority of results to be disappointing. Furthermore, the patients in whom thrombectomy carries the best chance of success, those with newly formed iliofemoral deep vein thrombosis (DVT), are those who are most likely to respond to thrombolytic therapy with streptokinase.

Venous interruption
The prime indication for venous interruption is pulmonary embolism which has occurred despite properly controlled anticoagulation. It should also be considered where there is phlebographically demonstrated recent thrombus in a patient in whom thrombolytic therapy or anticoagulation is contraindicated. Any patient who requires abdominal surgery and who has a well documented history of thrombo-embolism should be considered for caval plication at the same operation. Venous interruption carries the theoretical risk of precipitating a post-thrombotic syndrome but in fact, in the majority of cases, collateral veins ensure that the patient remains without troublesome symptoms.

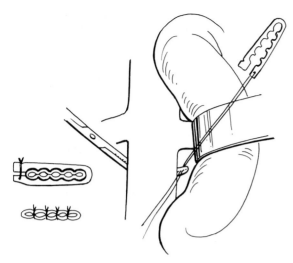

Fig. 3.27 Caval plication. Clip and suture plication are shown in cross-section. The Miles serrated clip is placed around the inferior vena cava just below the renal veins, with the help of a silk ligature

Femoral vein ligation

Ligation of the superficial femoral vein may be indicated where bilateral phlebography has shown the DVT to be confined to one limb below the level of the profundafemoral junction. The common femoral vein is exposed through a vertical incision 1 cm medial to the pulsation of the common femoral artery. The long saphenous vein provides a ready guide to the common femoral vein

which is followed down to the confluence of deep and superficial tributaries. The latter is ligated with silk flush with the lower border of the profunda. The superficial femoral vein can be safely ligated without causing symptoms of venous obstruction in the limb, on account of the generous connections between calf veins and the profunda system.

Caval interruption

The simplest way of preventing thrombus from ascending to the lungs is to ligate the inferior vena cava below the renal veins. This method has frequently been adopted in the past but it is liable to cause oedema of the lower limbs and to be followed later by the development of collaterals large enough to transmit major emboli. Preferred alternatives involve the conversion of the lumen of the cava to a series of smaller channels. This can be achieved at open operation by suture plication or by the application of a serrated clip (Miles, 1964) or indirectly by the transluminal insertion of a filter such as the Greenfield filter (1973, 1983).

For direct plication the inferior vena cava is best exposed through a right paramedian incision although it can readily be reached through a midline or transverse incision. The peritoneum at the lateral border of the second part of the duodenum is incised and the duodenum reflected medially. The cava is then exposed by blunt dissection, teasing away loose areolar tissue. The right renal vein is identified first, the left usually joining the cava at the same level although the left kidney

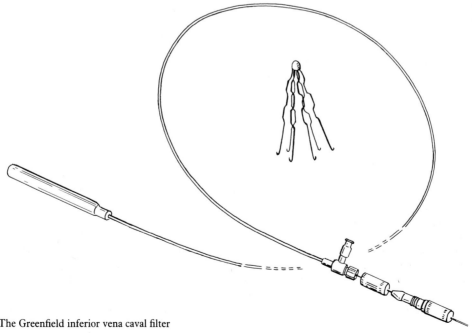

Fig. 3.28 The Greenfield inferior vena caval filter

lies higher than the right. A sling is passed around the cava below the renal veins, great care being taken to avoid damage to lumbar veins. A serrated Miles clip is placed across the cava and tied in place with a silk ligature (Fig. 3.27). The alternative method of suture plication consists of the insertion of three or four nonabsorbable sutures through the anterior and posterior walls thus converting the lumen to a series of small channels.

Transluminal filters

Several varieties of filter have been devised for insertion by way of a peripheral vein. The Greenfield (Fig. 3.28) and Mobin-Uddin are both suitable for insertion under radiological control via the right internal jugular vein. An intravenous pyelogram is first performed to check the position of the kidneys. The operation is carried out under local anaesthesia, a considerable advantage in a patient suffering from pulmonary embolism. A transverse incision 3 cm above the medial end of the clavicle is centred over the lateral edge of sternomastoid. The latter is partly divided to give access to the internal jugular vein which is mobilized with care, the most difficult part being the posterior wall which is adherent to fascia of the carotid sheath. A sling is placed around the vein for distal control, and a vascular clamp applied to the upper end. At an earlier stage the filter, which consists of a fenestrated 28 mm diameter disc of silastic mounted on six stainless steel alloy sharpened spokes, has been screwed on to a threaded stylet and loaded into a catheter mounted applicator capsule. This is now inserted via a venotomy in the internal jugular vein and advanced under fluoroscopic control to the level of the disc between the third and fourth lumbar vertebra where it is ejected from the capsule. After the filter has been impacted by upward traction the stylet is unscrewed to release it. The catheter is removed and the venotomy closed. Intravenous heparin is restarted after 12 hours, maintained for 7 to 10 days and followed by oral anticoagulant for a minimum of 3 months. The Greenfield system includes a filter carrier which allows the insertion to be made from the perfemoral approach in appropriate cases. Approximately 50% of these patients thrombose their inferior vena cavas below the filter but in only about 5% does this give rise to chronic swelling. Other reported complications include misplacement of the filter in a renal or iliac vein and proximal migration of the filter. These complications are exceedingly rare particularly with experienced operators. Provided that the stringent indications are adhered to the lifesaving potential of the procedure more than justifies the complication rate.

After any type of caval interruption, elevation, ankle exercises, elastic support and early ambulation are vigorously promoted postoperatively.

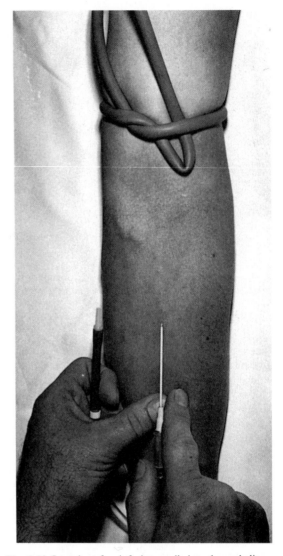

Fig. 3.29 Insertion of an infusion needle into the cephalic vein in the forearm. The tubing, emptied of air, is ready to be attached.

INTRAVENOUS INFUSION

Choice of vein

Cannulation of the venous system may be required for the intravenous infusion of fluids, for transfusion of blood products, for the administration of drugs or for parenteral feeding when alternative routes are unsuitable. Access is also required for measurement of the central venous pressure (p. 310). The choice of vein thus depends on the individual requirements for each patient, and on the patency of the veins. In general, it

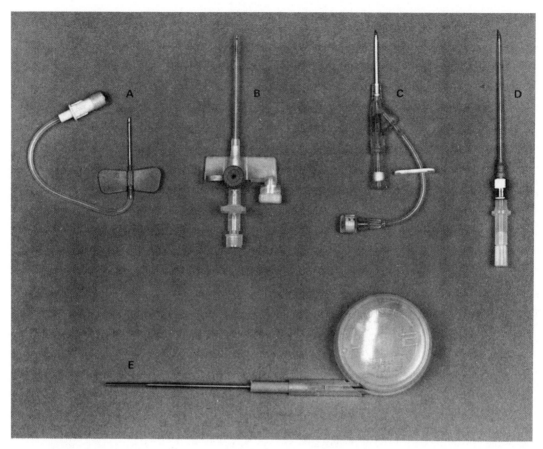

Fig. 3.30 Types of intravenous needle cannulae for percutaneous use: The Butterfly (A) and the Venflon (B) needles incorporate side plates to allow rigid fixation. Each can be used for intermittent drug administration (through a syringe) or for 'drip' infusion; the Venflon needle allows for both functions. The Y-can (C) is also dual purpose. Cannulae (B), (C) and (D) (Jelco) consist of a fine needle within a plastic cannula. After it has been confirmed, by aspiration of blood, that the vein has been entered, the needle is withdrawn, and the infusion tubing is connected to the cannula. The 'drum cartridge catheter' (E) is advanced by rotation of the drum after the attached needle has been used to puncture the vein

is an advantage to use veins on the dorsum of the hand or on the forearm for isotonic fluids and central veins for irritant solutions. The cephalic vein on the radial side of the forearm (Fig. 3.29) can usually be identified even when the veins generally are collapsed and it is of convenient size. Since it lies between the wrist and elbow joints, the cannula is less likely to be disturbed by movement, and there is no need for splintage. In an emergency, veins of the cubital fossa are easily identified, but it is best to insert a long cannula which will not obstruct when the elbow is flexed. Splinting of the elbow should be avoided since the necessary bandaging may interfere with the smooth flow of the infusion. Three sites are available for rapid infusion (p. 357) or for the placement of a cannula within the right heart, namely the basilic, subclavian and jugular veins. Use of the cephalic vein in the upper arm or of the long saphenous vein anterior to

the medial malleolus is not recommended because of the tendency of these veins to become thrombosed and because of the immobility imposed by an infusion in the leg. A careful aseptic technique is essential in all cases, especially for the insertion of a 'central venous line' where colonization of the catheter tip by bacteria can lead to septicaemia or thrombosis of the great veins.

Percutaneous puncture of vein
Simple puncture by a needle has obvious advantages in expediency, but the maintenance of an infusion through a needle alone is somewhat precarious. Several types of needle cannulae are now available; by their use a plastic cannula can, in association with a special needle, be introduced into a vein by percutaneous puncture. These are illustrated in Figure 3.30. This method of infusion is usually possible except in shocked patients, in whom

the veins may be very collapsed. No attempt will be made to describe the technique of entering a vein with a needle; this will usually be learned by demonstration and perfected by practice. Confirmation that the vein has been entered should be obtained by aspirating blood into a syringe before the infusion is connected up; otherwise it may extravasate into the tissues around the vein. The needle or cannula should be secured by strapping, so that it will not be pulled out of the vein by minor strains or jerks on the tubing.

In the technique for central venous catheterization, the appropriate vein is punctured, an intravenous catheter is advanced towards the heart and both the needle and stilette are withdrawn. Some indication of the position of the catheter tip is obtained by comparing the length of the stilette with the length of catheter which is visible outside the vein. However, radiographic confirmation of the catheter position should be obtained whenever possible. Access through the basilic vein is obtained either by direct puncture at the medial border of the biceps muscle or through the median cubital vein. The subclavian vein is more commonly entered below rather than above the clavicle and requires experience for its safe usage (Ross, 1980). With the patient's head rotated to the opposite side and tilted head downwards, the needle is introduced below the midpoint of the clavicle and advanced towards the back of the sternoclavicular joint keeping close to the clavicle. The internal jugular vein is punctured deep to the sternomastoid, aiming in the direction of the vein at the sternal end of the clavicle. A short cannula in the external jugular vein is a suitable alternative.

Cannulization by exposure of vein ('cut down')

This allows the cannula to be inserted with greater accuracy into the vein, and to be firmly secured with an encircling ligature. A larger cannula can be employed, so that a more rapid infusion can be given if desired, and, since there is less tendency both to thrombosis and to leakage into the tissues, the flow can be maintained more evenly and for longer periods. Various proprietary brands of intravenous catheter, made of nylon or other plastic, are now widely used. They can be inserted for a considerable distance into the vein and are therefore less likely to become dislodged. This ensures the efficiency of the 'drip' and also allows for measurement of the central venous pressure (p. 310) if the catheter is passed so that its tip lies in the superior vena cava. A catheter incorporating a radio-opaque marker can be placed with accuracy in the central veins since its position is readily seen on a routine chest X–ray. When the need for rapid blood transfusion can be anticipated, it is preferable to use a short wide diameter cannula or even the obliquely trimmed end of the transfusion set (Dudley, 1973).

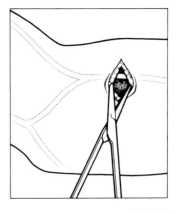

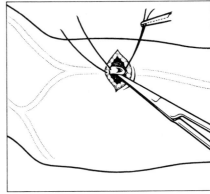

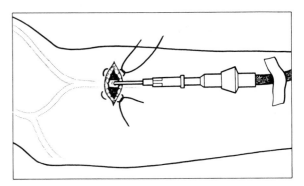

Fig. 3.31 Method of exposing a vein in the forearm and of tying in a cannula

In a conscious patient a little local anaesthetic solution is infiltrated intradermally in a line transversely across the vein, and a small incision is made. The superficial fascia is cleared by inserting the points of sharp scissors, and opening them on each side of the line of the vein (Fig. 3.31). When the vein has been isolated in this way two ligatures are passed around it; the distal one is tied and held in forceps, the proximal one is half tied in readiness to receive the cannula and its ends are left loose. With sharp pointed scissors a nick is made in the vein between the ligatures, the distal one being used as a retractor. The cannula, which should have been filled with the infusion solution in order to exclude air bubbles, is quickly inserted, and the proximal ligature is tied to enclose it. At this point, it is convenient to pass a stitch through the skin and to tie it round the base of the cannula, in order to prevent it from being pulled out of the vein before the tubing can be fixed with strapping. The skin wound is closed with two mattress sutures.

BLOOD TRANSFUSION AND BLOOD PRODUCTS

Transfusion of blood has been a well established part of clinical practice since early in the present century. The crucial first development in safe transfusion was Landsteiner's discovery in 1901 of the major human blood group system (the ABO system). In recent years, transfusion has become an increasingly powerful and specialized form of therapy; safe transfusion requires access to specialist facilities for the collection, testing and processing of blood and for the necessary tests on the patient. In the absence of these facilities, transfusion of blood is potentially very hazardous and should only be considered in life threatening emergencies. Medical staff who are likely to face such situations should obtain some basic training in the necessary techniques from an established transfusion department.

Collection and storage of blood

All blood for standard transfusion is collected into a citrate anticoagulant solution which also contains dextrose to preserve the viability of red cells during storage. The simplest solution is acid citrate dextrose (ACD). This may be supplemented with phosphate (CPD)and adenine (CPD-adenine) to further prolong red cell viability.

Normally 400–450 ml of blood is withdrawn into 70–100 ml of anticoagulant mixture. Blood must be collected into suitable containers: ideally, plastic blood collection packs should be used. These are supplied by several manufacturers, sterile and ready for use with an integral tube and needle for blood collection. They can be safely stored for long periods, but must be used within their labelled shelf life. Detailed instructions for use are supplied with the packs.

Glass bottles with a suitable connecting tube and vents are used for blood collection in some countries. These bottles and tube systems must be specially prepared using pyrogen free materials and sterilized before use. (Further practical details on blood collection are given at the end of this section.) Plastic blood collection packs are simpler and safer to use for both collection and transfusion of blood, and greatly facilitate the preparation of blood components.

Blood must be stored at 2–6°C in properly controlled refrigerators. During storage many physiologically important changes occur. These are summarized in Table 3.1. The maximum permissable storage period is 21 days for ACD blood, 28 days for CPD blood and 35 days for blood in CPD-adenine, as the viability of red cells declines sharply thereafter. However, many other important changes occur more rapidly, in particular the loss of functional platelets and coagulation factors V and VIII.

Table 3.1 Some changes in blood collected into ACD and stored at 4°C

		Days of storage			
		0	7	14	21
Red cell viability	%	95	90	85	75
Platelet viability	%	95	0	0	0
Coagulation factors V VIII	%	95	30	30	30
Potassium (mmol)		3.5	10	25	30

Essential transfusion immunology

Transfusion immunology is now a complex and specialized field. An understanding of certain aspects is essential to all clinicians involved in using transfusion therapy.

Red cell antigens and antibodies

The ABO system. By far the most important red cell antigens are those of the ABO blood group system. This is because most normal individuals have *naturally occurring* antibodies to red cell antigens of the ABO system in their plasma (see Table 3.2). These antibodies can cause rapid intravascular destruction of transfused red cells which are ABO-incompatible, frequently leading to a fatal haemolytic transfusion reaction. From Table 3.2 it is clear that Group O patients, since they have antibodies to both A and B red cells, are at the greatest risk. Since half the population is of Group O, the risk of ABO incompatibility is ever present.

The Rhesus (Rh) system. Although there are five different antigens within the Rhesus System, designated C D E, c̄, ē, the most important is the Rh(D) antigen, since this is the most immunogenic and most often associated with clinical problems. For this reason Rhesus typing is routinely restricted to Rh(D) typing, and individuals are designated as Rh(D) positive or negative. The reasons for the importance of the Rh system are as follows:

i. Individuals who are Rh(D) negative can be easily stimulated to produce antibodies to Rh(D) by transfusion of Rh(D) positive red cells. These antibodies can produce severe transfusion reactions.

ii. Anti Rh(D) antibodies in a pregnant women cause haemolytic disease in an Rh(D) positive fetus. It is there-

Table 3.2 The ABO blood group system—antigens and antibodies

Blood group	Frequency in the population*	Red cell antigens	Antibodies in serum
0	50	None	Anti A and Anti B
A	35	A	Anti B
B	10	B	Anti A
AB	5	A and B	None

*The proportions vary greatly in different populations. These percentages are for a UK caucasian population.

fore *essential* to avoid transfusion of Rh(D) positive blood to Rh(D) negative women of child bearing age.

iii. Patients with anti Rh(D) antibodies must be transfused with Rh(D) negative blood. Owing to the low incidence of Rh(D) negative individuals, this can cause serious problems for a blood bank.

Other red cell antigens There are numerous other red cell antigen systems which may cause transfusion problems. Although these are quantitatively less important than the ABO and Rh systems, they can be involved in serious transfusion reactions. Safe transfusion therefore requires that any patient should be tested for the presence of unexpected antibodies against all antigens on the red cells to be transfused. If the patient is known to have a red cell antibody, donations which do not contain the relevant antigen must be found.

Leucocyte and platelet antigens and antibodies
Leucocytes and platelets also have very complex antigen systems and patients can develop antibodies against these. Leucocyte antibodies are a common cause of transfusion reactions, although these are not normally severe. The development of platelet antibodies may make patients clinically resistant to platelet transfusion and require the use of increased doses of random donor platelets or the provision of HL-A typed platelets.

The investigation and management of these problems require specialized advice and facilities.

The provision of compatible blood
It cannot be overemphasized that the testing required to supply compatible blood is a specialized task which should be done by trained staff using appropriate techniques, reagents and equipment. The details of the compatibility testing method will depend on local practices and also on the urgency with which the blood is required. It should only very rarely be necessary to transfuse blood without some form of compatibility test.

Transfusion of uncrossmatched blood
In massive, exsanguinating bleeding, it is justifiable to start transfusion with Group O blood. However, Group O should no longer be considered as a 'universal donor' for several reasons:
    i. If Group O Rh(D) positive blood is used, the Rh(D)

negative patient is likely to be immunized, leading to the risk of future transfusion problems and haemolytic disease of the newborn.

ii. Group O Rh(D) negative blood can be used, but its widespread use in this way will seriously reduce the ability of a blood bank to supply Group O Rh(D) negative blood to patients, such as women of child-bearing age, who *must* receive it.

iii. Transfusion of uncrossmatched Group O blood carries the risk of adverse reactions due to a patient having antibodies against red cell antigens other than those of the ABO system.

iv. Group O blood may contain high levels of antibody to Group A and B red cells which can haemolyze the recipient's red cells.

v. The transfusion of Group O blood to a patient of Group A or B causes difficulties in subsequent compatibility testing because the patient's blood following transfusion contains a mixed population of red cells.

Group specific transfusion
An alternative to the use of Group O blood is to determine the patient's ABO and Rh type and transfuse blood of the same ABO and Rh type. This carries the major hazard that any error in typing or in the subsequent identification of the patient with the donor's blood can lead to a fatal ABO incompatible transfusion.

'Group and antibody screen' In some clinical situations it is possible, in a planned transfusion system, to test the patient's blood in advance, to determine the ABO and Rh group and to test for the presence of any unexpected red cell antibodies. The procedure is known as a 'Group and Antibody Screen'. When this information is available and up to date in the blood bank, it is possible in an extreme emergency to issue safely blood of the correct ABO and Rh type, but again, extreme care must be taken to ensure correct identification of the patient and the blood to be transfused, and the blood bank should recheck the ABO groups of patient and blood units and perform a rapid compatibility test while the blood is being transported.

Compatibility testing
Clinical staff with access to a blood bank do not require detailed knowledge of laboratory procedures but should

be aware of certain organisational aspects of the cross-matching laboratory to obtain the safest and most effective service from the blood bank.

Identification procedures. The aim of compatibility testing is to ensure that blood of the correct type is transfused to the patient. The main cause of serious transfusion accidents are CLERICAL MISTAKES LEADING TO WRONG IDENTIFICATION OF THE PATIENT, BLOOD SAMPLE OR BLOOD TO BE TRANSFUSED. The doctor who takes a blood sample for compatibility testing is responsible for making sure that the sample tube is fully labelled with the patient's full identification, that the request form is fully completed and the correct blood sample and request form are sent together to the blood bank.

The ward staff who set up a blood transfusion are responsible for checking that the blood which is supplied for a named patient is transfused to the correctly identified patient. The patient's name and blood group should be recorded on a label on each unit of blood supplied, and this should be checked with the appropriate information on the patient's identity band.

Response time of the blood bank. It is essential to find out from the blood bank the speed with which it can respond to urgent and less urgent requests for blood and to communicate clearly to the blood bank the urgency with which blood is needed for any patient. This will allow the blood bank to select the safest form of compartibility testing which can be carried out in the time available. Local arrangements differ widely and transport delays may be a major limiting factor in the urgent supply of blood.

Information required by the blood bank. It is essential to inform the blood bank about any clinical features of the patient which may indicate that transfusion problems are likely. In particular, patients who have had pregnancies, or have given birth to infants with haemolytic disease, patients with a history of previous transfusions or transfusion reactions will all alert the blood bank to look for antibodies causing problems in the supply of compatible blood.

Samples required by the blood bank. The blood bank must have a sufficient volume of the patient's blood to carry out compatibility testing. Normally 10 ml of clotted blood should be submitted, or a minimum of 1 ml of blood for each unit of blood required.

If no blood bank is available, clinical staff must be trained and equipped to undertake the simplest form of compatibility testing which can provide reasonable safety in an emergency situation.

Clinical considerations in the use of blood and blood products

In recent years a large range of potent therapeutic products derived from whole blood have become available.

The purpose of these products is firstly to provide in a safe and highly concentrated form replacement for deficiencies of particular blood components and secondly to make the most efficient possible use of each blood donation by ensuring that patients receive only that part of the donation which they require. The correct use of blood component therapy therefore improves the care of patients and makes the best use of donated blood. Table 3.3 lists the major blood products and some indications for their clinical use.

Transfusion in acute blood and fluid loss

The aim of replacement therapy should be to maintain the patients' circulatory volume and oxygen delivering capacity at an optimal level by the use of an appropriate combination of red cell containing preparations and other fluids. It is no longer considered desirable to replace blood loss ml for ml as this may not be the most effective regime and may expose the patient unneccessarily to the complications of transfusion.

The average healthy adult can lose 500 ml of blood rapidly with no ill effects (the equivalent of a routine blood donation) and, given adequate fluid replacement with crystalloid or colloid solutions, a loss of one to two litres can be sustained without irreversible hypotension. Children, the elderly and patients with cardiac or pulmonary disease are less resistant to blood loss (and more susceptible to the risks of over-transfusion) and so require a more exacting approach to transfusion.

Having made a clinical assessment of blood loss the following points should be considered:

Does the patient need *blood* or can some *safer fluid* be used?

Oxygenation must be maintained; in the fit patient, a haematocrit of 30% with the associated reduction in blood viscosity provides optimal capillary flow and adequate tissue oxygenation. Low plasma viscosity will be better maintained by fibrinogen-free crystalloid or colloid solutions than by plasma. *Coagulation factor levels* must be maintained at an adequate level. In patients who have no liver disease or congenital deficiency of clotting factors and who are not receiving anticoagulant therapy, there is a large reserve capacity for resynthesis of clotting factors. Since a defect of greater than 50% in levels of coagulation factors is compatible with normal blood clotting, replacement in the bleeding patient is not required. In patients receiving more than 10 units of blood however a falling platelet count may be associated with a bleeding tendency and administration of platelet concentrates may be indicated.

A general replacement policy for the acutely bleeding patient should be based on a planned sequence of crystalloid solutions, colloid solutions and whole blood or red cell concentrates.

Transfusion of the anaemic surgical patient

Although there are no standards for the desirable haemoglobin level in surgical patients, it is often accepted in clinical practice that patients should not be subjected to anaesthesia or major surgery with a haemoglobin of less than 10 g. However, in some situations, patients may be intentionally haemodiluted with the aim of increasing capillary blood flow and tissue oxygenation and patients who are well adapted to low haemoglobin levels (for example patients on chronic haemodialysis) tolerate surgery at low levels of haemoglobin. In such cases it is essential that transfusion support is immediately available. If preoperative transfusion is required, red cell concentrates should be used in preference to whole blood.

Blood components

Many blood transfusion services make a major effort to obtain fresh plasma from as many blood donations as possible for the preparation of blood products (Table 3.3). This policy requires the informed co-operation of clinicans to make use of the resulting red cell concentrates in place of whole blood in the many situations in which this is clinically appropriate.

Whole blood

This should be reserved for the actively bleeding patient who requires a substantial transfusion. Ideally, whole blood should be used within a transfusion policy in which the initial replacement of red cells is in the form of red cell concentrates.

Fresh whole blood (less than 6 hours old)

Table 3.1 indicates the rapid decline in platelets and clotting factors V and VIII in stored whole blood. In situations where whole blood is the only available product, patients requiring large volume transfusions (10 units or more) should if possible receive fresh blood, especially if there is evidence of bleeding due to thrombocytopaenia. However, if platelet concentrates and coagulation factor replacement are available, there should be no need for fresh blood and specific replacement should be given.

Red cell concentrates, plasma depleted blood, packed red cells

In each of these products, a proportion of the plasma has been removed from the blood donation to give a red cell preparation with a haematocrit of 60–90%, depending on the local product. These preparations should be used for non urgent transfusion to correct anaemia. When used for rapid transfusion, the flow rate is slow because of high viscosity and the concentrated red cells should be diluted with sterile physiological saline infusion solution before transfusion. This can conveniently be done using an infusion set with a 'Y' piece which allows simultaneous collection of the pack of concentrated red cells and a

Table 3.3 Blood components

Product	Indications	Special precautions	Shelf life
Whole blood	Massive haemorrhage	Must be ABO + Rh compatible	21 Days (ACD) 28 Days (CPD) 35 Days (CPD-Adenine)
Red blood cells (Red cell concentrate)	Most routine transfusions and for massive replacement as part of planned programme	Must be ABO + Rh compatible	As above
Leucocyte-depleted red cells	Patients with transfusion reactions or risk of sensitisation to leucocyte antigens	Must be ABO + Rh compatible	Depends on method of preparation
Platelet concentrates	Bleeding due to thrombocytopaenia	Should be ABO compatible	24–72 hours
Fresh frozen plasma	Bleeding due to uncharacterized coagulation factor deficiency or coumarin overdose	Must be ABO compatible	1 year at −40°C
Cryoprecipitate of factor VIII & fibrinogen	Bleeding with fibrinogen depletion	Must be ABO compatible	1 year at −40°C
Albumin 5% 15–20%	Acute volume expansion Symptomatic hypoproteinaemia		4 years 4 years
Factor VIII	Haemophilia A		2 years
Factor IX	Haemophilia B Coumarin anticoagulant reversal		2 years
Immunoglobulins	Prophylaxis of various interactions (see text)		4 years

container of saline for infusion. Red cells should *not* be diluted with calcium containing solutions such as Ringer lactate or with solutions containing dextrose.

Leucocyte depleted red cells
Red cell suspensions with a high proportion of leucocytes and platelets removed are prepared by several methods and are of value in the patient who has experienced transfusion reactions due to leucocyte antibodies or who is likely to require repeated transfusions.

Platelet concentrates
Platelet concentrates are prepared from fresh blood donations by centrifugation. About 60% of the platelets from the donation are suspended in 20–30 ml of plasma and can be stored under proper conditions for 24–72 hours. Their use is required when patients with a bleeding tendency due to thrombocytopaenia require surgery and occasionally in the massively transfused patient who develops a bleeding tendency due to dilutional thrombocytopaenia. An adult patient commonly requires a dose of 6 platelet concentrates (pooled from 6 donors) to provide haemostasis. These should be given immediately before surgery and infused quickly. Platelets should be stored at 18–22°C, not at 4°C. An alternative source is the use of platelet-rich plasma but the large volumes (150–180 ml per donation) limit the dose of platelets which can be given.

Fresh frozen plasma
This is prepared by separating the plasma from fresh blood and freezing as rapidly as possible at –30 to –40°C. Fresh plasma is a useful source of all coagulation factors and is of use in the patient with a bleeding tendency due to an uncharacterized lack of clotting factors or in the absence of products to permit more specific factor replacement. Fresh plasma is of particular value in patients bleeding due to liver failure or overdosage of anticoagulants. In these cases, volumes of 500–1000 ml may be required to achieve adequate haemostasis. Note that this product requires 30 to 60 minutes to thaw before use.

Fresh dried plasma
This is a freeze dried equivalent of fresh frozen plasma and the indications for its use are similar.

Freeze dried plasma (outdated)
Plasma obtained from outdated donations of blood is pooled to prepare this product which contains albumin, fibrinogen and the non labile clotting factors. It is a valuable colloid fluid for volume replacement and as a source of plasma proteins in the burned patient but if alternative albumin containing solutions are available, these are equally effective as volume replacement, more

convenient, and are free from the risk of transmitting hapetitis.

Albumin solutions
These preparations have the major disadvantage of high cost. Stable Purified Protein Solution (SPPS) or Plasma Protein Fraction (PPF) contain 4–5% albumin, 85–95% of the total protein being albumin, with a sodium concentration of 140 mmol/1. Purer albumin solutions with a low sodium content (salt poor albumin) are usually supplied as 10% or 25% solutions and are substantially more costly than SPPS. All these preparations are pasteurized to remove the risk of hepatitis virus transmission.

The indications for use of albumin solutions include the following:

Volume replacement in shock or hypovolaemia. Large volumes of crystalloid solutions (Ringer's lactate) have been used successfully to replace massive extra and intravascular fluid losses, but excessive volumes may lead to pulmonary oedema. Initial volume replacement should therefore employ crystalloid solutions ($\frac{1}{2}$–2 litres, depending on the size, age and fitness of the patient). Thereafter, a colloid should be used before transfusion of blood. Albumin solutions are satisfactory but costly for this phase of resuscitation and for most patients synthetic volume expanders such as dextrans or hydroxyethyl starch may be used. Initial resuscitation with albumin solutions should be avoided since there is evidence that this may increase pulmonary complications in some groups of patients. In patients who are likely to develop hypoalbuminaemia, it is logical to use albumin solutions in preference to other colloids.

Burns. Albumin solutions may be used to replace the protein loss in burned patients, although it is not certain whether plasma may be superior since it contains many other proteins which may be important to the burned patient.

Hypoproteinaemia. Concentrated (15 or 25%) salt poor albumin solutions are valuable in the treatment of hypoalbuminaemia when this is severe enough to cause clinical complications such as oedema. Albumin solutions should not be used to correct hypoproteinaemia in chronic conditions such as liver failure, and are not effective in correcting nutritional hypoproteinaemia since the aminoacids of albumin are poorly metabolized and the infused albumin increases the catabolism of endogenous albumin.

Specific coagulation factors
Fibrinogen. Although concentrated freeze dried fibrinogen is available, it carries a high risk of transmitting hepatitis and is rarely used. Fibrinogen replacement should only be required in bleeding patients whose plasma fibrinogen is less than 1 g per 100 ml. The simplest and safest source is cryoprecipitate. This is prepared by

freezing fresh plasma and thawing under controlled conditions. A precipitate forms which contains fibrinogen and Factor VIII. Each donation of cryoprecipitate contains 150–300 mg of fibrinogen and 6–12 donations usually produce haemostatic levels in an adult patient. An alternative is to infuse 500–1000 ml of fresh plasma rapidly. In patients who may not tolerate this volume, a diuretic must be given.

Factor VIII concentrates. Factor VIII concentrates are used in the treatment of haemophilia A. There are two main preparations—cryoprecipitate (see above) and freeze dried preparations of intermediate or high purity. The surgical management of haemophiliac patients may require large quantities of these products and requires specialist clinical and laboratory support.

Factor IX concentrates. Although developed for the treatment of Haemophilia B, these products have a role in the correction of severe coagulation factor deficiencies due to liver failure or coumarin anticoagulant. These products carry a significant risk of transmitting hepatitis and are potentially thrombogenic in certain patients.

Immunoglobulins
Preparations of immunoglobulin G (IgG) are prepared from pooled donor plasma (Human Normal Immunoglobulin (HNI)) or from donors with particular specific antibodies (Human Specific Immunoglobulin (HSI)). All these products are administered by intramuscular injection.

Human normal immunoglobulin (HNI). This provides effective prophylaxis against hepatitis A for 2 to 4 months when given in a dose of 750 mg (adult dose) and is effective in prophylaxis of measles in exposed children. HNI is also used as maintenance for replacement therapy in patients with immunoglobulin deficiency. In the treatment of severe bacterial infections in surgical patients, large doses of special preparations of HNI, modified for intravenous use, have been given. The efficacy of this treatment remains to be demonstrated.

Human specific immunoglobulin. A range of preparations exists, including the following:

Anti Rh(D). This is used in the prevention of sensitization of Rh(D) negative mothers who give birth to Rh(D) positive infants. It may also be used to prevent immunization following the accidental or unavoidable administration of Rh(D) positive blood products to an Rh(D) negative patient.

Anti hepatitis B surface antigen (anti HBsAg). Administered within a short period of a proven parenteral innoculation with hepatitis B positive blood, this product confers a degree of protection against hepatitis B infection.

Anti tetanus. In a dose of 250 iu, human antitetanus immunoglobulin is a safe and effective part of tetanus prophylaxis and should be given, in addition to the other normal measures, to all patients who have not had appropriate immunization in the past 5 years and who have a contaminated wound in which adequate surgical toilet has been delayed. This product, being a human immunoglobulin, has none of the risks of allergic reactions associated with the horse anti tetanus globulins previously employed.

Side effects and hazards of blood transfusion
The relative risks and benefits of transfusion therapy must be assessed by the clinician in each case before taking the decision to transfuse. The main risks are as follows:

Haemolytic transfusion reactions
These occur when there is an incompatibility of donor red cells and recipient plasma, usually because a clerical mistake leads to ABO incompatibility. In a severe case, the reaction will begin after a very small volume of blood has been transfused and will be characterized by shock, chills, fever, dyspnoea, back pain, pain at the infusion site and headache. This may be followed by haemorrhage (due to disseminated intravascular coagulation, haemoglobinuria, oliguria, renal failure and jaundice). The essential steps in the management of an acute haemolytic transfusion reaction are shown in Table 3.4.

Febrile reactions
These occur in about 1% of transfusions, often due to sensitisation to leucocyte or platelet antigens. The reactions are usually minor. Transfusion should be stopped, 100 mg of hydrocortisone and an antihistamine should be given and transfusion restarted. Some patients with severe repeated reactions of this type require to receive a leucocyte and platelet depleted preparation of red cells.

Allergic reactions
Urticaria, occasionally with chills or fever, occurs in up to 3% of blood recipients. Premedication with antihistamine may prevent or reduce the symptoms. Occasional severe anaphylactic reactions occur in rare patients who are deficient in immunoglobulin A (IgA) and who have anti IgA antibodies. These must be managed as any severe anaphylactic reaction, with adrenalin, hydrocortisone and oxygen.

Bacterial contamination of blood
This is a rare hazard, with modern transfusion methods, but the risk is always present, especially if blood is not stored constantly at 4°C and if plastic blood bags are carelessly handled. A heavily contaminated blood donation may appear almost black in colour and if it has been allowed to separate, there may be a layer of haemolytic staining above the red cell layer. Transfusion will cause a rapid, severe and potentially fatal collapse due to endotoxic shock. The transfusion must be stopped immediately and intensive therapy for septicaemic shock

Table 3.4 Management of acute haemolytic transfusion reaction

Investigation	Treatment

1. Check all documentation for errors. Return blood to blood bank and request urgent investigation
2. Take blood for
  Blood bank (10 ml)
  Blood urea and electrolytes (10 ml)
  Coagulation tests (10 ml)
3. Do an ECG—look for evidence of hyperkalaemia
4. Repeat biochemical and coagulation screens 2–4 hourly until patient is stable.
	1. Stop transfusion immediately
	2. Hydrocortisone 100 mg i.v.
	3. Insert bladder catheter, drain bladder and monitor urine output.
	4. Mannitol 20% 100 ml i.v. and 100 ml physiological saline
	5. Frusemide 150 mg i.v.
	6. Wait 2 hours: if urine output is still below 100 ml/hour repeat mannitol 20%, 100 ml
	7. Wait 2 hours. If urine output still below 100 ml/hour, start treatment for acute renal failure
	8. If evidence of hyperkalaemia start insulin-glucose, or resonium therapy
	9. If evidence of disseminated intravascular coagulation seek advice on blood product replacement and/or heparinization

initiated, including high doses of antibiotics active against gram positive and gram negative organisms.

Fluid overload
In anaemic, elderly, the very young, or patients with cardiopulmonary disease, careful observation, the use of red cell concentrates and diuretics are required to avoid this complication.

Transmission of disease
The transmission of Hepatitis B by transfusion has been largely prevented in many countries by introducing costly donor screening programmes. In some communities where the prevalence of Hepatitis B is very high, this may not be practicable.

Hepatitis due to other viruses (non-A, non-B hepatitis) cannot be prevented by donor screening and may occur in 2% or more of recipients. All donations are tested for syphilis and this, together with storage at 4°C, effectively removes the risk. Malaria, Brucellosis, toxoplasmosis, Chaga's Disease, cytomegalovirus, EB virus, may all be transmitted by transfusion.

Emergency collection of blood
A plastic blood collection set with integral needle should be used. If this is not available, blood for immediate retransfusion may be collected into a sterile glass container, containing a 3.8% sterile solution of trisodium citrate (50 ml for 450 ml of blood). If a glass container is used it *must* be vented to avoid the build up of air pressure which can lead to fatal air embolism in the donor. The donor should lie horizontal. A sphygmomanometer is placed on the forearm, inflated to 60 mmHg and the large antecubital vein located. The skin should be prepared with a disinfectant such as alcohol. Once the cannula is inserted, blood should flow freely into the collecting container and must be mixed gently with the anticoagulant during collection. The donor should clench and unclench his 'fist to promote venous flow. A

maximum of 450 ml should be withdrawn from an adult donor. The donor should rest lying down for at least 10 minutes after completing donation.

Provision of compatible blood in an emergency
It is essential to transfuse blood which is either of *Group O or of the same ABO group as the recipient*. To ensure this, the ABO group of the recipient and of all potential donors must be determined with no possibility of error. Compatible donors must be selected and a final check for compatibility of donor and recipient should be done before transfusion. The materials required for this testing are shown in Table 3.5.

Table 3.5 Materials required for blood typing and compatibility check in an emergency.

For method 1 (Appendix 1)

Syringes and needles for venepuncture
plain sample tubes—5–10 ml, no anticoagulant
clean small test tubes and rack
centrifuge to separate blood samples
felt pen or wax pencil
pasteur pipettes and teats
physiological saline
microscope with low power lens

Blood typing antisera: Anti A
                          Anti B
                          Anti A + B
Must be stored and used according to manufactures instructions

For method 2 (Appendix 2)

Syringes and needles for venepuncture
tubes to take anticoagulated blood samples
clean microscope slides
felt pen or wax pencil
pasteur pipettes and teats
microscope with low power lens

Blood typing sera   Anti A
                     Anti B

The key to safe ABO typing is to use potent typing sera. These must be obtained from commercial suppliers or blood transfusion organizations. They must be stored according to instructions, used only within their shelf life and used according to the instructions supplied with them.

Two procedures for emergency compatibility testing are described. The first (Appendix 1) should be used if a centrifuge is available. The second procedure (Appendix 2) should be used only if no centrifuge is available, since this procedure is considerably less effective in detecting incompatibilities.

APPENDIX I

Procedure for emergency compatibility testing when a centrifuge is available to separate the blood sample.

First
Determine the patient's ABO blood group
1. Obtain and label a 10 ml sample of blood from the patient. Allow this to clot fully
2. Centrifuge to separate red cells and serum
3. Using clean test tubes, label tubes and place in test tube rack as shown below

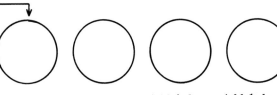

To this tube add 10 drops of saline solution. Then add one drop of patients red cells

Add 1 drop of Anti A   Add 1 drop of Anti B   Add 1 drop of Anti A + B

Then to each of these tubes add 1 drop of the patient's cell suspension

4. Centrifuge gently
5. Examine each tube for agglutination: this will be shown by tight clumping together of the red cells, which cannot be dispersed by gentle shaking.
6. The blood group is determined as follows

Blood Group

Typing Serum	A	B	O	AB
Anti A	+	−	−	+
Anti B	−	+	−	+
Anti A + B	+	+	−	+

+ = agglutination
− = no agglutination

Second

Determine the blood group of each potential donor
1. Obtain and label a 10 ml sample of blood from each potential donor and allow to clot fully
2. Repeat for each donor the procedure described for grouping the patient

Third

Select donors of compatible ABO group. If possible select donors of the same group as the patient. If insufficient donors of the patient's group are available select donors of group O.

Fourth

Test for compatibility between the patient and the selected donors.
1. Take the cell suspension tubes for each selected donor and place in a test tube rack as shown
2. Add two drops of the *patient's* serum to the second row of test tubes as shown

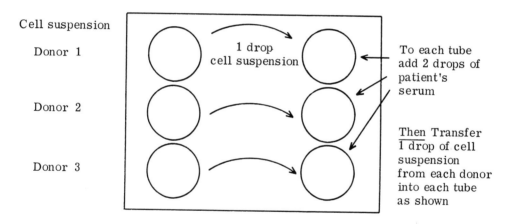

Cell suspension

Donor 1   1 drop
             cell suspension   To each tube
                                                 add 2 drops of
                                                 patient's
                                                 serum

Donor 2

                                                 Then Transfer
                                                 1 drop of cell
Donor 3   suspension
                                                 from each donor
                                                 into each tube
                                                 as shown

3. Centrifuge gently and examine for agglutination or haemolysis
4. Examine all negative results under low power lens of the microscope
5. Select as compatible those donors who show no evidence of agglutination by naked eye or microscopic examination

Note This procedure is insensitive and will not detect all incompatibilities due to irregular antibodies.

APPENDIX 2

Blood typing procedure for use in emergency if no certrifuge is available

1. Microscope slides are labelled as shown for the patient and for each donor
2. One drop of each standard typing sera (Anti A and Anti B) is added to each slide
3. One drop of anticoagulated blood from the patient is added to the first slide as shown

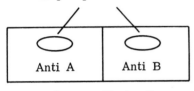

1 drop of patient's blood

Typing Sera   Typing Sera
Anti A   Anti B

Determine Patient's Group

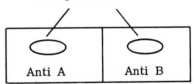

1 drop of donor blood.

Typing Sera   Typing Sera
Anti A   Anti B

Determine Potential Donor's Group

Repeat for each potential donor

4. The slide is gently rocked to mix cells and serum for the period recommended in the instructions with the typing serum for the slide technique
5. A positive result is shown by agglutination (clumping of the cells) with one or other typing sera. This can be seen easily with the naked eye. A negative result is shown by the cells remaining free in suspension. If possible, this should be confirmed under a low power microscope when the cells can clearly be seen to be floating free from each other
6. The same procedure is used to group each donor
7. Blood groups are determined as follows:

| | Blood Group | | | |
Typing Serum	A	B	O	AB
Anti A	+	−	−	+
Anti B	−	+	−	+
Anti A + B	+	+	−	+

+ = agglutination
− = no agglutination

8. Donors of the same blood group as the patient are selected. If insufficient donors of the patient's blood group are available, group O blood may be used to transfuse patients of groups A, B, and AB

Compatibility test for use in emergencies if no centrifuge is available

Procedure
a. Mark out a microscope slide for each donor as shown
b. Add drop of the patient's anticoagulated blood
c. To the slide for donor number 1 add 1 drop of anti-coagulated blood from donor 1

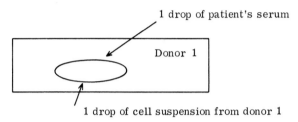

1 drop of patient's serum

Donor 1

1 drop of cell suspension from donor 1

d. Gently rock the slide to mix
e. After 5 minutes, examine the slide for the presence of agglutination (see Appendix 2, para. 5).
f. Repeat the procedure for each donor.

Note This procedure is insensitive and will only detect gross incompatibilities. Clinically important incompatibilities can be missed; the procedure must only be used in emergency situations where no laboratory support is available.

REFERENCES

Dodd H 1965 The varicose tributaries of the popliteal vein. British Journal of Surgery 52: 350.
Dudley H A F 1973 Some aspects of modern battle surgery. Journal of the Royal College of Surgeons of Edinburgh 18:67
Fegan W G 1963 Continuous compression technique of injecting varicose veins. Lancet 2: 109
Fogarty T J, Cranley J J, Krause R J, Strasser E S, Hafner C D 1963 A method for extraction of arterial emboli and thrombi. Surgery Gynaecology and Obstetrics 116: 241
Fogarty T J, Daily P O, Shumway N E et al 1971 Experience with balloon catheter technic for arterial embolectomy. American Journal of Surgery 122: 231
Greenfield L J, McCurdy J R, Brown P P, Elkins R C 1973 A new intracaval filter permitting continued flow and resolution of emboli. Surgery 73: 599
Greenfield L J, Stewart J R, Crute S 1983 Improved technique for insertion of Greenfield vena caval filter. Surgery Gynaecology and Obstetrics 156: 217

Gregg R O, Chamberlain B E, Myers J K, Tyler D B 1983 Embolectomy or Heparin therapy for arterial emboli? Surgery 93: 377
Matas R 1888 Traumatic aneurism of the left brachial artery. Medical News of Philadelphia 53: 462
Miles R M, Chappell F, Rennor O 1964 A partially occluding caval clip for prevention of pulmonary embolism. American Surgeon 30: 40
National Heart and Lung Institute, Bethesda, USA 1970 Urokinase pulmonary embolism trial. Phase 1 Results. Journal of the American Medical Association 214: 2163
O'Brien B McC 1977 Microvascular reconstructive surgery. Churchill Livingstone, Edinburgh and New York
Ross A H M, Anderson J R, Walls A D F 1980 Central venous catheterisation. Annals of the Royal College of Surgeons of England 62: 454
Youkey J R et al 1983 Percutaneous transluminal balloon angioplasty of the iliac artery for contralateral ischaemia. Surgery 94: 100

FURTHER READING

American association of blood banks technical manual 1981 8th edn. American Association of Blood Banks, Washington D.C., U.S.A.
This manual describes the full range of technical procedures.
Mollison P L 1979 Blood transfusion in clinical medicine. Blackwell, London
A comprehensive text dealing with the theoretical basis of transfusion

National Transfusion Organisations have procedure manuals. These should be available to any medical staff who may have to carry out emergency transfusion.
Petz L D, Swisher S N 1981 Clinical practice of blood transfusion. Churchill Livingstone, Edinburgh
A clinically orientated text which comprehensively describes all aspects of modern transfusion therapy.

4

Operations on nerves

J. CHALMERS & C. V. RUCKLEY

Anatomy of the nerve trunk and mechanism of regeneration

Structure of a peripheral nerve

A major peripheral nerve is made up of a large number of fibres—there may be as many as 50 000 in the median nerve of the forearm. Each fibre consists of an *axon* and its cellular coverings. The axon is the process of a nerve cell lying within the central nervous system or a ganglion of the autonomic nervous system and links this cell with an appropriate end-plate, the structural unit being called a *neurone*. The peripheral nerves carry, to a varying degree, fibres concerned with motor, sensory and sympathetic functions. Two main fibre types occur—the *myelinated* and *unmyelinated*. In the former, the Schwann cell sheath, which invests all peripheral nerve fibres, is wrapped around the axon in many layers, which contain the myelin, a complex lipo-protein (Fig. 4.1). At intervals along its length, the myelin sheath is interrupted at the nodes of Ranvier. In unmyelinated fibres, the Schwann cell layer contains no myelin.

Myelinated fibres conduct more rapidly than unmyelinated fibres and transmit the efferent impulses to skeletal muscle and the afferent impulses from some sensory endings concerned with pain and light touch. The majority of sensory fibres are, however, unmyelinated as are those of the sympathetic nervous system.

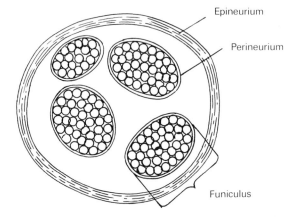

Fig. 4.2 Diagramatic cross section of a peripheral nerve

Groups of nerve fibres are aggregated into bundles or fascicles which are surrounded by a thin, but well organized layer of connective tissue, the *perineurium*. The fibrous layer, which binds the fascicles together to form the peripheral nerve, is called the *epineurium* (Fig. 4.2). Fascicles tend to branch and regroup along the length of the nerve forming as it were an intraneural plexus so that the cross-section arrangement of bundles varies from point to point along the course of the nerve.

The investing membranes of a peripheral nerve are surprisingly strong so that it is not uncommon to find the major nerves as the only intact structures in a severely injured limb. The peripheral nerves are supplied by many small nutrient arteries which communicate freely within the nerve. It is possible, therefore, to mobilize quite long lengths of nerve without damaging the blood supply.

CLASSIFICATION OF NERVE INJURIES

Nerve injuries may be divided into three degrees of severity. In first degree nerve injuries (*neurapraxia*), axons are not disrupted but nerve conductivity is temporarily

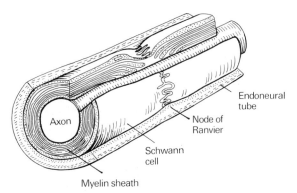

Fig. 4.1 Details of myelinated nerve

lost, probably as a result of local dispersal of the myelin sheath. Many pressure palsies are of this type. In second degree nerve injuries (*axonotmesis*), greater violence produces disruption of the axons but the supporting connective tissues of the nerve remain in continuity. In third degree injuries (*neurotmesis*), the nerve is completely divided.

Nerve injuries may also be classified as *degenerative* and *non-degenerative* lesions. In the former there is degeneration of the axon distal to the site of injury and proximally as far as the first node of Ranvier, while chromatolysis takes place in the parent cell (Wallerian degeneration). Second and third degree injuries are of this type, while non-degenerative lesions are of the first degree.

Following division of a nerve, elastic traction causes the ends to separate and spontaneous recovery never takes place. At the proximal stump a traumatic neuroma forms which consists of numerous fibrils sprouting from the cut end of the severed axons together with proliferation of the supporting tissues within the nerve. In the distal stump a bulbous end forms consisting of the supporting elements only.

Recovery following nerve injury

In first and second degree nerve injuries, being lesions in continuity, complete and perfect recovery may be anticipated. In first degree injuries, this may take place within hours or days of the injury. In second degree injuries, the recovery time depends on the distance between the level of injury and the end organ supplied by the nerve, axonal regeneration occurring at the rate of about 1 mm per day. In third degree nerve injuries, recovery does not take place unless surgical repair of the divided nerve is carried out. Even then, recovery is usually imperfect for it depends on the success with which axons reconnect with distal Schwann cell sheaths (which will guide them to the periphery) and also on the element of chance, which seems to govern whether motor axons reach motor end-plates and sensory axons reach sensory end organs.

Factors which influence recovery include age of the patient, the younger having the better prognosis; the level of the lesion, the more proximal having poorer prognosis; the violence which produces the original injury, the more severe the violence the poorer the prognosis. Mixed nerves, which carry both motor and sensory functions, such as the median or ulnar nerve, have a poorer prognosis than for example the radial nerve, which is largely a motor nerve and usually recovers well. A large gap between the nerve ends at the time of repair militates against recovery for repair involves either extensive mobilization of the nerve with damage to its blood supply, or a nerve graft, which seldom succeeds as well as a direct suture.

Clinical features

Whatever the degree of nerve injury, the presentation may initially be similar with loss of all functions carried by the nerve. Thus there will be flaccid paralysis, sensory impairment and loss of sympathetic function, notably sweating and vasomotor control. These last observations can be very important for they enable a peripheral nerve injury to be diagnosed even in an unconscious patient, the lack of sweating being easily detected clinically by simply stroking a finger over the injured limb; denervated skin feels more slippery than the normally sweating skin.

As a working rule, closed injuries of nerves are usually of the first or second degree whereas injuries associated with open wounds are usually of the third degree and in any event with open wounds, it is possible to establish the nature of the nerve injury with certainty during the course of the wound excision. In practice, then, nerve injuries associated with closed wounds are treated conservatively until a reasonable period has elapsed to allow for spontaneous recovery and the nerve is explored surgically only if the anticipated recovery does not take place. A reasonable recovery interval may be estimated from the fact that axonal regeneration takes place at about 1 mm a day. By measuring the distance from the site of injury to the first muscle or area of skin supplied by the nerve, an estimate of the likely rate of recovery can be calculated.

An advancing Tinel sign, that is a point of sensitivity on the course of the injured nerve, is also a useful guide to the progress of recovery and gives an indication that at least part of the nerve is in continuity. Difficulties in the assessment of nerve injuries can arise when several degrees of nerve injury are present at the same time. Thus in traction injuries of the brachial plexus, it is not uncommon to have all three degrees of nerve injury involving different nerve roots. In such circumstances surgical exploration may be necessary to establish the severity of injury and plan treatment.

Electrophysiological assessment of nerve injuries. Changes in the conductivity of nerves and in the electrical activity of muscles may occur following nerve injury and can be used to aid clinical diagnosis and give an objective measure of recovery.

Nerve conductivity. Peripheral nerves may be stimulated by surface electrodes placed along their course and the resultant response in a peripheral muscle is picked up by electrodes placed over the muscle. Likewise afferent sensory potentials may be detected in a nerve in response to peripheral sensory stimulation within the nerve territory. Both motor and sensory conduction tests give an indication of the integrity of the nerve and the conduction velocity can be assessed by measuring the distance between stimulus and recording electrode and the time taken for the stimulus to reach that point. Conduction velocity is frequently delayed in first degree nerve injuries and is particularly characteristic of compression lesions of peripheral nerves. The level of injury may be localized by identifying a segment of the nerve in which maximum delay occurs. In second or third degree nerve injuries no conductivity takes place after Wallerian degeneration is established (i.e. by the end of the second week). The return of measurable conductivity may precede the clinical signs of recovery.

Electromyography. When a needle electrode is placed in a normally innervated resting muscle no electrical activity is detected, whereas in denervated muscle small 'fibrillation' potentials can be detected firing at irregular intervals. In first degree nerve injuries fibrillation potentials do not occur.

MANAGEMENT OF NERVE INJURIES

Whatever the degree of nerve injury, it is important that the tissues supplied by the nerve should be maintained in healthy condition pending recovery. The patient must be advised of the need to protect anaesthetic skin from accidental injury and he must be shown how to retain by passive movement the mobility of joints whose muscles are paralysed. It may be necessary to provide some form of splintage to maintain function during the recovery period. Thus a drop-foot splint is required for a lateral popliteal nerve injury and a wrist and finger extension splint in radial nerve injuries.

Surgical repair of divided nerves

Whether nerves should be repaired at the time of the primary wound treatment or as the delayed secondary procedure, is a subject for debate. The argument in favour of a primary repair is that it spares the patient the need of a further operation. However, if the wound is extensive and the result of considerable violence, definitive nerve repair is best done as a delayed procedure, because it would add considerably to the length of the initial wound treatment, also because it is difficult to identify the extent of nerve damage and therefore the amount of nerve which must be resected. Furthermore the delicate epineurium does not hold sutures well. Primary nerve repair is probably best restricted to clean, incised wounds of limited extent where the surgeon has the necessary experience, instruments and time at his disposal. In all other circumstances at the time of primary wound treatment, the cut ends of the divided nerve should be identified and approximated with two or three sutures carefully placed so that the correct rotation of the nerve is maintained. It is often easier to match the cut ends of the nerve at this stage than at a secondary procedure. Isolating the site of nerve division with a silastic tube is useful in preventing adhesion of the nerve to the surrounding muscles or tendons, which may also have been damaged at the same level.

Secondary nerve repair

Secondary nerve repair is carried out after an interval of several weeks when associated muscle and tendon injuries have healed and the possibility of infection has been eliminated. The incision should be long enough so that the nerve may be identified in healthy tissues proximal and distal to the level of injury and it is then easy to dissect to the injured site. It is difficult and unwise to try and identify the nerve within scar tissue at the site of injury. Having identified the point of division, the neuroma is resected with a fresh scalpel blade or razor beyond the limit of scar tissue, which can be recognized when the nerve bundles pout separately from the cut surface (Fig. 4.3). The epineurium at this stage has proliferated and is easy to suture. The suture material should be fine and nonreactive, 6/0–8/0 nylon or prolene are suitable. Two lateral sutures are first placed in the epineurium joining the nerve ends in their correct orientation, which is of paramount importance. This will have been facilitated by the correct placement of sutures at the time of the primary approximation and can be helped by matching small blood vessels or nerve bundles. It is obvious that the quality of recovery in a mixed nerve will depend largely on the correct matching of the nerve ends. Using the two lateral sutures as stay sutures, the nerve may be rotated to allow further sutures to be

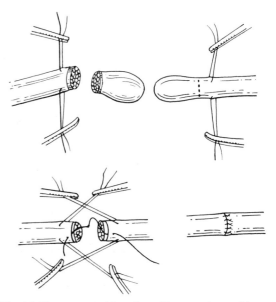

Fig. 4.3 Nerve suture. Note the guide suture inserted into the epineurium at corresponding points on the circumference and held with dissimilar pair of forceps. These help to maintain correct orientation of the nerve ends throughout the repair

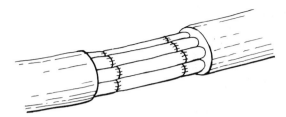

Fig. 4.4 Cable grafting. Multiple lengths of a smaller expendable nerve may be used to bridge a gap in a larger nerve. Shows sutures between epineurium of the graft and perineurium of the fascicles (by microsurgical techniques)

placed around the periphery on the superficial and deep aspects of the nerve (Fig. 4.3). It is important that the suture line should not be under tension, which means that gaps greater than 2 or 3 cm cannot be repaired by direct suture unless length can be gained by some device such as anterior transposition of the ulnar nerve at the elbow or by flexing joints over which the nerve passes. Larger defects can only be repaired by means of a nerve graft. A nerve, which can be spared, such as the sural or saphenous, is used and a sufficient length is obtained to allow enough segments to match the diameter of the nerve which is being bridged. The epineurium of each graft is then sutured to the perineurium of fascicles of the recipient nerve using the operating microscope and microsurgical technique (Fig. 4.4). Recovery following nerve grafting is always imperfect and the quality of the result reflects the skill and experience of the operator.

Partial nerve division
Partial nerve division presents particular problems of management for attempts at repair may result in damage to the intact portion of the nerve. If the partial division represents a small proportion of the nerve, primary repair coupled with wrapping the nerve in silastic sheeting

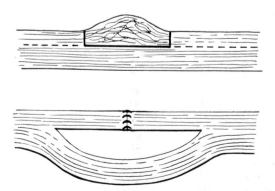

Fig. 4.5 Loop suture used to repair partial division of a nerve. The intact and damaged fascicles are carefully separated and the damaged portion resected and repaired as shown

may achieve a good recovery. If this fails and significant disability persists, the nerve may be repaired by loop suture as illustrated in Figure 4.5, in which the damaged portion of the nerve is carefully dissected from the intact portion and a formal secondary repair of the injured part of the nerve carried out. This can only be done if the gap is very small; for larger defects an inlaid cable graft is required.

Postsurgical management
Following surgical repair by any of the foregoing techniques, it is necessary to protect the suture line from tension for three weeks. This requires immobilizing the limb, usually with the joints over which the nerve passes in a position of flexion, by means of a plaster cast which is removed at the end of three weeks and gentle mobilization of the limb commenced. If acute flexion of any joint has been necessary in order to overcome shortening of a nerve, then mobilization of the joint must be gradual and may be achieved by either serial changes of the plaster cast producing progressively lesser flexion or else by means of a turnbuckle plaster, in which a hinge with a series of graduated stops allows gradual extension of the limb over a period of three or four weeks.

OPERATIONS ON INDIVIDUAL NERVES

The brachial plexus
The commonest injuries to the brachial plexus are the result of traction. This may occur at birth but in adult life it is frequently the result of motor cycle injuries, the head and shoulder being forced apart by the violence resulting from contact with the ground.

Anatomy
The brachial plexus lies partly in the antero-inferior corner of the posterior triangle of the neck, partly behind the clavicle, and partly in the axilla. It consists of trunks, divisions, cords and branches. The *upper trunk* arises from the anterior rami of C5 and 6; the *middle trunk* from C7; and the *lower trunk* from C8 and T1. Behind the clavicle the trunks divide into anterior and posterior divisions. The upper two anterior divisions unite to form the *lateral cord*; the lower anterior division forms the *medial cord*; all three posterior divisions unite to form the *posterior cord*.

Main branches of the cords. The *median nerve* is formed by the union of a branch of the lateral cord and a branch of the medial cord. The *ulnar nerve* is the main continuation of the medial cord; the *radial nerve*, of the posterior cord. Other branches are the *musculo-cutaneous* (lateral cord); the *medial cutaneous nerves of arm and forearm* (medial cord); the *circumflex nerve*, and the *nerve to latissimus dorsi* (posterior cord).

Traction lesions

Traction lesions of the brachial plexus are of three types—*upper*, when roots C4, 5 and 6 are involved; *lower*, when roots C7, 8 and T1 are involved; or *total*, when the entire arm is rendered flaccid and anaesthetic. In management of traction lesions in adult life it is important that a clear prognosis be established at an early stage. The injury to the brachial plexus may be non-degenerative when recovery will occur and satisfactory functional recovery will be achieved in the hand. Where a lesion is degenerative and in continuity, proximal recovery may occur but the prognosis for the hand is poor. Where a complete avulsion of the roots has taken place, the prognosis for that particular level is hopeless and no recovery can be expected.

Prognostic indicators. Injuries of the upper roots of the plexus tend to do better than complete injuries or injuries of the lower roots.

Supraclavicular lesions have a worse prognosis than infraclavicular. Severe pain lasting for more than six months carries a poor prognosis. Horner's syndrome is associated with a poor prognosis for lesions of the lower roots.

Nerve root avulsions from the cord do not recover and are irreparable. These can be recognized on myelography by the presence of a traction meningocele at the level of avulsion.

Management

In the management of traction injuries of the brachial plexus, as in all other forms of peripheral nerve injury, meticulous attention must be paid to the prevention of contractures by ensuring that all joints are kept mobile by being put through a full passive range of movements regularly. The anaesthetic skin should also be protected and care taken to avoid pressure sores etc.

In lesions with good prognostic indications treatment is conservative and recovery is anticipated. In those with poor prognostic features early surgical exploration is advocated in some centres with a view to establishing the prognosis and, if possible, to carrying out surgical repair. Direct repair of the plexus is rarely possible and repair can only be effected by means of cable grafts using the sural or saphenous nerve. These operations require a high degree of skill and experience and should be performed only in specialized centres. Even in the best hands, the recovery rate following surgery is poor.

If at a year following a brachial plexus injury, the arm remains totally flail and anaesthetic, the patient may choose to have a shoulder arthrodesis and a forearm amputation followed by the fitting of a prosthesis. Others may prefer to retain the useless limb. Only a few highly motivated patients achieve functional use of their prosthesis. Amputation of the limb does not relieve painful symptoms.

Median nerve

The median nerve is the most frequently injured of all the peripheral nerves because of its exposed situation on the flexor aspect of the forearm and hand where incised wounds are common. It is also very vulnerable to compression within the tight confines of the carpal tunnel.

Anatomy

The median nerve originates in two roots arising from the medial and lateral cords of the brachial plexus. In the upper arm it descends first along the lateral side of the brachial artery, then crosses it anteriorly to run on its medial side into the cubital fossa. It leaves the fossa between the heads of pronator teres, and descends in the forearm between flexor sublimis and flexor profundus. In the lower third of the forearm it becomes more superficial by emerging at the lateral side of flexor sublimis. It comes to lie 2.5 cm above the wrist in front of the sublimis tendons, to the medial side of flexor carpi radialis, between it and palmaris longus (which may, however, be superficial). It then enters the palm of the hand, passing deep to the flexor retinaculum.

Motor distribution. The median nerve supplies all the muscles on the front of the forearm (except flexor carpi ulnaris and the ulnar part of the flexor digitorum profundus). In the palm it supplies the short muscles of the thumb (except the adductor) and the lateral two lumbricals.

Sensory distribution. The skin of the thumb and of the lateral two and a half fingers (except on the dorsum of their proximal segments) is supplied by digital branches of the median nerve. The greater part of the palm is supplied by the palmar branch. The sensory distribution of the median nerve is one of the most important tactile areas of the body and has been aptly called the eyes of the hand.

Median nerve injury

The possibility of a median nerve injury at or above the elbow can be investigated most simply by asking the patient to clench his fist. If the nerve is injured above elbow level, this movement is impossible, since the thumb and the lateral two fingers have no power of flexion. Flexion of the medial two fingers by flexor profundus is preserved. In the case of wounds about the wrist, the clinical diagnosis of median nerve injury is less easy, since the branches to the long flexor muscles will usually be intact. Paralysis of the thenar muscles will, however, be present, and can be detected from the patient's inability to bring the thumb into opposition. Anaesthesia will be found in the area of sensory distribution of the nerve. When dealing with the common incised wounds on the flexor aspect of the forearm, it is of great importance to make a careful clinical assessment of the

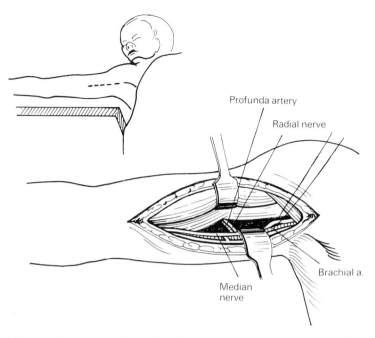

Fig. 4.6 Exposure of median nerve in upper arm. Note that the nerve crosses the brachial vessels from lateral to medial side as it passes distally

extent of the tendon and nerve injury prior to surgery for the divided ends of these tissues may retract and be difficult to find at the time of the wound excision, unless the surgeon knows precisely which structures he is to look for.

Considering that the median is a mixed nerve, the degree of recovery after suture is better than might be expected. Some 60% of patients regain adequate motor and sensory function.

Exposure of the median nerve in the upper arm and cubital fossa is closely related to the brachial artery (Fig. 4.6) and the operation is similar to that described

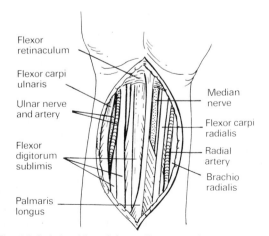

Fig. 4.7 Relationships of the median nerve above the wrist

for exposure of the artery (p. 30). Just above wrist level (where injuries are common), the nerve lies medial to flexor carpi radialis tendon, either lateral or superficial to the sublimis tendons (Fig. 4.7). Owing to its flattened shape it is easily mistaken for a tendon.

Postoperatively, following repair of the median nerve, the suture line should be protected by immobilization of the arm in an appropriate position. Where the nerve has been injured above the elbow or around the elbow, flexion of the elbow will often allow the nerve to be sutured without tension. Where the injury is more distal in the forearm, there is often a temptation to flex the wrist in order to allow closure of the gap but this should be resisted as the nerve will inevitably become adherent to the site of the injury and a traction lesion will result as the flexed wrist is subsequently straightened. Even although the nerve is injured distally in the forearm, any tension at the repair should be relieved by flexion of the elbow.

Carpal tunnel syndrome
The median nerve, in common with most other peripheral nerves, may be subject to compression where it passes through the confined anatomical tunnels. Carpal tunnel syndrome is by far the most common of these 'entrapment' neuropathies. It affects usually women around the time of the menopause, who are regularly awakened with pain centred on the median distribution but often radiating diffusely to involve the whole hand and forearm. The patient has to exercise the hand in

order to promote venous return and allow the symptoms to subside. During the day, the discomfort may return during activities involving repeated gripping movements with the wrist flexed. Objective neurological changes persist within the median nerve territory only after the syndrome has been present for many weeks or months. The syndrome has many variations and may less commonly affect men and adults of any age. Commonly some space-occupying condition, such as oedema or synovitis within the carpal tunnel, is the precipitating factor. Delay in electrical conductivity of the median nerve across the wrist may confirm the diagnosis in cases of doubt.

In mild cases of short duration, conservative measures may be tried. These include the provision of a night splint, which immobilizes the wrist in a neutral position, or an injection of hydrocortisone 25 mg into the carpal tunnel, the site of injection being placed just medial to the palmaris longus tendon, which lies comfortably between the median and ulnar nerves (Fig. 4.8). If symptoms persist, surgical decompression is necessary. The operation can be satisfactorily done with Bier's regional anaesthesia. The incision curves gently from the ulnar border of the tendon of palmaris longus where it crosses the distal wrist crease and extends to the midpalm (Fig. 4.9). The palmar fascia is incised to expose the transverse carpal ligament, which is then divided vertically at its midpoint (normally medial to the median nerve) but care must be taken to avoid injury to the nerve, which may be adherent to the under surface of the

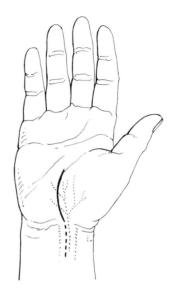

Fig. 4.9 Incision for carpal tunnel decompression is placed slightly towards the ulnar side of the midline to avoid the palmar cutaneous branches of the median nerve

ligament. It is wise therefore when the first opening is made in the ligament to pass a dissector underneath it to protect the deeper structures from injury. The ligament must be completely divided, the median nerve inspected and a neurolysis carried out if it is found adherent to the surrounding tissues. The skin only is closed and early mobility of the hand encouraged.

Ulnar nerve

Whereas injuries to the median nerve are particularly important because of the sensory loss which ensues, with ulnar nerve lesions the motor loss of the intrinsic muscles of the hand which control fine skilled finger movements is the main complaint, the ulnar sensory distribution being less critical than that of the median nerve. The ulnar nerve is subject to compression at two sites: on the medial aspect of the elbow and at the wrist where it passes through tight anatomical tunnels.

Anatomy

The ulnar nerve originates as the main continuation of the medial cord of the brachial plexus. In the upper arm it descends along the medial side of the brachial artery in its proximal half; it then deviates medially, accompanied by the ulnar collateral artery, and pierces the medial intermuscular septum to enter the back of the arm, where it runs down under cover of the medial border of triceps. At the elbow it is closely applied to the back of the medial epicondyle, from which it passes on to the medial ligament of the joint. It enters the forearm deep to the aponeurosis joining the humeral and ulnar heads of flexor carpi ulnaris and runs down under cover

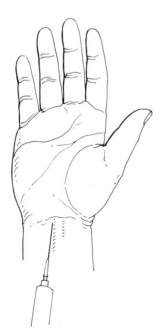

Fig. 4.8 Site of injection into the carpal tunnel to the medial side of palmaris longus tendon

of this muscle, lying on flexor digitorum profundus. Approaching the wrist the nerve becomes superficial between flexor carpi ulnaris and flexor digitorum sublimis. It then pierces deep fascia and enters the palm by passing superficial to the flexor retinaculum within Guyon's canal. In the lower third of the forearm, and at the wrist, the nerve is closely related to the ulnar artery which lies on its lateral side.

Motor distribution. In the forearm the ulnar nerve supplies only flexor carpi ulnaris, and the medial half of flexor digitorum profundus. In the hand it supplies most of the short muscles—the hypothenar muscles, all the interossei, the medial two lumbricals, and the adductor pollicis.

Sensory distribution. The medial 1½ fingers and the medial border of the palm are supplied by the ulnar nerve.

Ulnar nerve compression

At the elbow the cubital tunnel is bounded superficially by the aponeurosis which joins the two heads of origin of flexor carpi ulnaris and on its deep surface the medial ligament at the elbow joint. This tunnel becomes progressively narrowed as the elbow is flexed. Any encroachment on the tunnel from pathology in the elbow joint, such as chronic arthritis, may compress the ulnar nerve. Tardy ulnar neuritis may occur many years after an elbow fracture, commonly after an injury of the lateral condyle, causing a valgus deformity. At the wrist, the nerve is closely tethered as it passes through Guyon's canal and again is vulnerable at this site to any space-occupying lesion, such as a ganglion. Unlike median nerve compression, ulnar nerve compression is usually painless but presents a slow and insidious loss of sensation and motor power within its territory. The level of compression can be identified by careful neurological examination—thus, if the sensory impairment involves the dorsal aspect of the hand, the lesion is probably at the elbow for the dorsal cutaneous branch of the ulnar nerve separates from the main trunk above the wrist. If the dorsal sensation is preserved, then the lesion lies probably at the wrist. If all sensation is intact but the ulnar innervated intrinsic muscles are paralyzed, then the compression must involve the deep palmar branch of the ulnar nerve after it has separated from the main trunk as it passes deeply into the palm at the level of the piso-hamate ligament. Surgical exploration of the nerve at the site indicated by the clinical examination will then identify the compressing agent and allow the nerve to be released.

Exposure in the upper arm is by an approach similar to that described for the brachial artery (p. 30). The ulnar nerve is identified to the medial side of the vessels in the upper half of the arm. It is then traced downwards as it diverges from the vessels and pierces the medial intermuscular septum, to enter the posterior compartment of the arm.

Exposure at the elbow. A curved incision is made in the line of the nerve, and with its centre just behind the medial epicondyle. By division of the deep fascia the nerve is exposed as it lies in the postcondylar groove. In the distal part of the wound the nerve passes out of sight between the two heads of flexor carpi ulnaris; it is exposed by longitudinal separation of the fibres of the muscle. As the nerve is elevated from its bed, five branches may be encountered. An articular twig to the elbow joint can be divided; the other branches are muscular (two to flexor carpi ulnaris, and two to flexor digitorum profundus), and these should be preserved.

Anterior transposition

After any operative treatment (neurolysis or nerve suture) at the level of the elbow, *the nerve should never be replaced in its original bed behind the medial epicondyle*, but should be transposed to the front of the elbow, so that it may pursue a shorter course, where it will be less subject to stretching and friction. This procedure, which can overcome up to 7–8 cm of shortening, greatly facilitates any form of nerve repair which involves trimming or resection. The operation of anterior transposition (Fig. 4.10) is specific for the conditions of traumatic neuritis and of recurrent dislocation of the nerve. After the nerve has been exposed and freed, its displacement may at first be prevented by the muscular branches; these may be elongated by separating them gently in a proximal direction from the parent trunk. When this has been done, the nerve can usually be brought without difficulty to the front of the medial epicondyle. In the upper part of the wound, the medial intermuscular septum is resected as its presence can result in continuing pressure on the nerve. The common flexor origin is now divided 1 cm distal to the medial epicondyle and the ulnar nerve displaced anteriorly to lie deep to the flexor muscles on the anterior capsule of the elbow joint. The common flexor origin is re-attached by suture and the elbow is subsequently immobilised at 90 degrees of flexion in a plaster splint for three weeks to allow the muscles to heal. Subcutaneous transposition of the ulnar nerve leads to recurring ulnar neuritis and should not be done.

Exposure at the wrist requires no special description. The nerve lies between flexor carpi ulnaris and flexor digitorum sublimis, and enters the palm by passing superficial to the flexor retinaculum. The ulnar artery is closely applied to its lateral side.

Post-operative position. When the nerve has been injured near the wrist, flexion of the wrist should be avoided for the reasons stated above in relation to the median nerve. Any shortage of tissue should be made up by anterior transposition (see above).

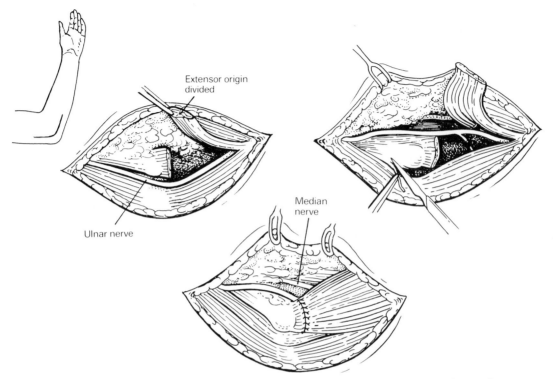

Fig. 4.10 Anterior transposition of the ulnar nerve. The nerve is brought to lie in front of the elbow deep to the extensor muscles and in the same plane as the median nerve

Figures 4.1, 4.8, 4.9, 4.10 are adapted from illustrations in Lamb D W & Kuczynski K (eds) 1981 The practice of hand surgery. Blackwell, Edinburgh

Radial nerve

Because of its close relationship to the humerus the radial nerve may be injured in fractures of this bone or may be involved in callus formation. The important posterior interosseous branch of the radial nerve may be injured in fractures of the upper third of the radius, to which it is closely related and is subject to compression during its course through supinator.

Anatomy

The radial nerve begins as the direct continuation of the posterior cord of the brachial plexus, and descends behind the axillary artery. In the upper part of the arm it passes backwards between the long and medial heads of triceps, and then winds round the humerus, under cover of the lateral head and between it and the medial head. In the lower third of the arm it pierces the lateral intermuscular septum, and runs down to the front of the lateral condyle, lying in the cleft between brachialis and brachio-radialis. The profunda artery and veins accompany the nerve in its course around the humerus. At the level of the epicondyle the radial nerve gives off its posterior interosseous branch, and then crosses the capsule of the elbow joint to enter the forearm, where

it runs distally under cover of brachio-radialis. In the lower third of the forearm it emerges at the posterior border of brachio-radialis and descends over the abductor and extensor tendons of the thumb to supply the skin of the lateral two-thirds of the dorsum of the hand, and part of the dorsum of corresponding digits.

The *posterior interosseous nerve* (which is entirely motor) passes to the back of the forearm by winding round the lateral side of the upper third of the radius, through the substance of the supinator muscle. It then descends between the superficial and deep muscles, and breaks up into branches supplying them.

Motor distribution. The radial nerve, from its main trunk, supplies triceps, brachio-radialis, extensor carpi radialis longus, anconeus, and part of brachialis. Through its posterior interosseous branch it supplies all remaining muscles on the back and radial side of the forearm; these include the dorsiflexors of the wrist (except extensor carpi radialis longus), the extensors of the fingers and thumb, and the long abductor of the thumb.

Sensory distribution is unimportant, since there is considerable overlap from adjacent nerves—the lateral cutaneous of forearm (from musculocutaneous), and the posterior cutaneous (from ulnar).

Radial nerve injury

Injury to the radial nerve occurs most commonly in the distal part of the upper arm, so that its branches to triceps are intact. All other muscles supplied by it (see above) are likely to be weakened or paralyzed, and a characteristic *drop wrist* deformity is present. The inability of the patient to extend his thumb may be the first sign. Sensory loss is restricted to a small area on the dorsal aspect of the first web. Lesions of the posterior interosseus nerve are characterized by dropping of the fingers alone for the radial wrist extensors are usually preserved and there is no sensory loss.

Since the radial nerve is mainly motor, repair is more successful than is the case with any other important nerve trunk. Full functional recovery may be expected in 70 to 80% of cases, but, if the lesion has been at a high level, it may not be complete until well over a year from the time of operation.

Infra-axillary exposure. The radial nerve at first lies posterior to the proximal part of the brachial artery, and the approach to this part is similar to that described for the artery (p. 30).

Exposure in the middle third of the arm. Here, the nerve passes obliquely round the posterior surface of the humerus, lying in the musculospiral groove. An incision is made on the back of the arm in the line of the nerve. The interval between the long and lateral heads of triceps is opened up, and further distally the lateral head is divided in the line of the nerve. The fascial roof of the groove is incised to expose the nerve, which, accompanied by the profunda vessels, lies partly on the bone and partly on the upper fibres of the medial head (Fig. 4.11). Branches of the nerve to the triceps muscle should be carefully preserved.

Exposure in the lower third of the arm is obtained by downward prolongation of the above incision, and by opening up the cleft between the brachialis and brachioradialis muscles.

Exposure of the posterior interosseous branch. Repair of this nerve is unlikely to be practicable but the nerve may require to be exposed in operations on the upper part of the radius or in compression lesions of this nerve within the supinator muscle. Its origin from the radial nerve on the front of the lateral epicondyle should first be identified. From there it is traced down to the point where it enters the substance of the supinator deep to the arcade of Frose. By division of the superficial fibres of this muscle, the nerve is completely displayed.

Sciatic nerve

Injuries of the sciatic nerve are common in warfare but are seldom encountered in civilian practice except as a complication of fracture dislocations of the hip. In cases where there is a complete lesion of the nerve, all the muscles of the lower leg and foot are paralyzed, and, if the injury is in the buttock, the hamstrings also are involved. There is complete anaesthesia of the sole of the foot. When the lateral popliteal part of the nerve is injured, paralysis is confined to the muscles of the anterior and lateral compartments of the leg, and the foot adopts an attitude of *equinovarus*; sensation in the sole is preserved.

The results of operative repair are uncertain usually because the lesions result from extreme violence such as gunshot wounds and also because of the distance between the level of injury and the peripheral end organ so that, even after a satisfactory repair, irreversible muscle atrophy may have taken place before axonal regen-

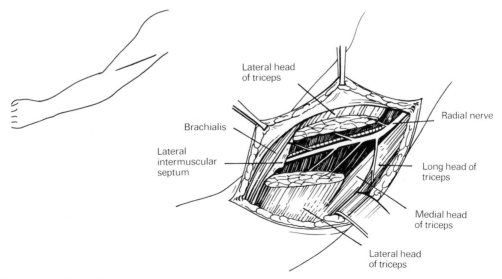

Fig. 4.11 Exposure of the radial nerve on the posterior aspect of the upper arm

eration. More peripheral lesions of the lateral popliteal nerve have a better outlook.

Anatomy

The sciatic nerve arises as a terminal branch of the sacral plexus (L4 and 5; S1, 2 and 3). It leaves the pelvis through the greater sciatic foramen below piriformis. It descends through the gluteal region, and ends about the middle of the back of the thigh by dividing into medial and lateral popliteal nerves. The *medial popliteal nerve* continues down the middle of the back of the thigh to the popliteal fossa. The *lateral popliteal nerve* deviates laterally, and runs down under cover of biceps to the posterior surface of the head of the fibula, where it can be readily compressed against the bone.

In the buttock the nerve is covered posteriorly by gluteus maximus; anteriorly it lies successively on the ischium, on the obturator internus with the gemelli, and on the quadratus femoris. The inferior gluteal vessels are medial to it.

In the thigh it is crossed superficially by the long head of biceps, and is overlapped by semimembranosus. Anteriorly, it lies on adductor magnus.

Distribution. The sciatic nerve innervates the hamstrings, part of adductor magnus, and all muscles below the knee. It provides the sensory supply of the limb below the knee, with the exception of those areas supplied by the saphenous branch of the femoral nerve— the medial aspect of the leg, and the medial border of the foot as far as its middle.

Exposure in the buttock. With the patient prone, and with the knee pillowed to hyper-extend the hip, a curvilinear incision is made as shown in Figure 4.12. In the lower vertical part of the incision, the deep fascia and the iliotibial tract are divided lateral to the posterior cutaneous nerve of the thigh, which can be seen shining through. Above this, gluteus maximus is split in the line of its fibres between the middle and lower third. The lower portion is retracted medially to expose piriformis with the sciatic nerve appearing at its lower border. Piriformis may be divided or retracted to expose the nerve within the sciatic notch.

Exposure in the thigh. An incision is made vertically down the back of the thigh. The posterior cutaneous nerve is sought for and safeguarded. The long head of biceps, which crosses the nerve from medial to lateral

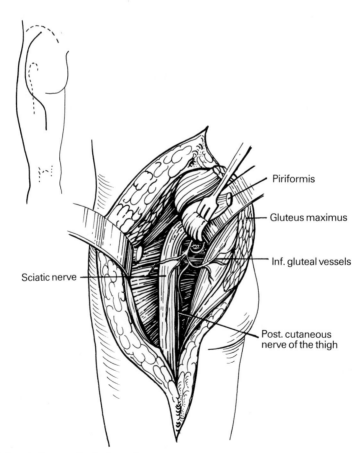

Sciatic nerve

Piriformis

Gluteus maximus

Inf. gluteal vessels

Post. cutaneous nerve of the thigh

Fig. 4.12 Exposure of the sciatic nerve in the buttock

side, is mobilized and retracted laterally. The nerve, or its terminal branches, can now be found embedded in fat on the surface of adductor magnus.

Facial nerve

Direct suture of the facial nerve is rarely possible but the nerve lends itself ideally to nerve grafting for its function is exclusively motor and the nerve consists of a single fascicle, which is readily bridged by a single segment of the long saphenous nerve or great auricular nerve (p. 266).

Where nerve repair is not possible, dynamic muscle transfers may succeed. These are designed to achieve (a) acceptable balance of the face at rest, (b) active closure of the eye, and (c) some voluntary control of lips and cheek.

A segment of temporalis muscle is transferred to the eyelids; a segment of the same muscle or of masseter is utilized to raise the corner of the mouth, and the anterior belly of digastric, to lower it. In order to impart adequate length to these muscular slips, 'tendons' manufactured from fascia lata, are added to them.

Other nerves

Compression lesions

Compression lesions can affect all the major peripheral nerves of the body and detailed description of each is not possible. Common lesions of the median and ulnar nerves have been described above on pages 72 and 75; the same principles of management apply to other nerves. The lesions are recognized by spontaneous loss of function or the development of paraesthesiae within the territory of a specific nerve. The site of compression can usually be deduced from a knowledge of the anatomy of the nerve. If recovery does not take place within a reasonable time, exploration at the site of compression is indicated. Other common examples include the lateral cutaneous nerve of the thigh as it passes beneath or through the outer end of the inguinal ligament (meralgia paraesthetica), and the lateral popliteal nerve at the neck of the fibula.

Morton's neuroma

A curious form of nerve entrapment involves the plantar digital nerve running to the cleft between the third and fourth toes. At this site, the nerve becomes compressed between the metatarsal heads and develops a thickening, sometimes fibrotic and sometimes cystic, within its substance. The patient experiences attacks of sudden severe pain, which shoot between these toes at irregular and unexpected intervals when walking, especially on uneven ground. Local tenderness can be elicited at the site of the neuroma. If the condition is persistent and fails to respond to a metatarsal insole, the lesion should be

surgically explored through a plantar incision centred on the neuroma, which can be readily identified and resected. The level of resection should be 2 or 3 cm proximal to the metatarsal heads so that the neuroma, which will inevitably form on the cut stump will not be subjected to pressure.

OPERATIONS ON THE SYMPATHETIC NERVOUS SYSTEM

General considerations

The operation of sympathectomy may be carried out (1) to improve the circulation in the limbs by the abolition of vasoconstrictor tone; (2) for the relief of visceral and causalgic pains; and (3) as a cure for hyperhidrosis.

Circulatory disorders of the limbs

It is in these conditions that sympathectomy finds its greatest field of usefulness. All sympathetic fibres to the upper limb emerge from the spinal cord between the 2nd and 8th thoracic segments, and thereafter pass through the upper three thoracic ganglia. Fibres to the lower limb, emerging from the cord between T.9 and L.2, pass through the lumbar ganglia. Removal of the lumbar 2 and 3 ganglia will thus cut off the entire sympathetic supply to the limb concerned. Importance has in the past been attached to the fact that a lumbar ganglionectomy is essentially a preganglionic operation as regards the innervation of vessels below the knee, for the fibres supplying these vessels have their cells in the sacral ganglia which remain undisturbed, whereas in the corresponding operation for the upper limb both pre- and postganglionic fibres are divided. It was to these differences that the apparently better results of lumbar ganglionectomy were ascribed, and the operation of *preganglionic rami-section* came to be recommended in place of ganglionectomy for denervation of the upper limb. It has been established, however, that the vessels behave in the same way after ganglionectomy as after preganglionic section, and most surgeons now prefer to remove the second and third, and the lower third of the first thoracic ganglion for upper limb denervation. Removal of the whole 'stellate' ganglion (the fused inferior cervical and 1st thoracic ganglia) interferes with the sympathetic supply to the head and neck and causes Horner's syndrome.

Causalgia

This term is used to designate the persistent and intense pain which may follow minor amputations, or partial injury to a mixed nerve. The aetiology of the pain is obscure, but complete relief can often be obtained by sympathectomy (Baker, 1969).

Hyperhidrosis of the limbs can be completely abolished by sympathectomy. When sweating is sufficiently profuse to cause serious mental distress, the operation should be advised.

Peripheral vascular disease—selection of cases
The sympathetic nerves control the tone of all arteries which have a considerable amount of smooth muscle in their walls. For practical purposes this means the medium sized and small arteries and arterioles of the limbs and the arteriovenous anastomoses. Sympathectomy may be indicated to obtain vasodilatation where the peripheral vessels show an excessive response to cold or emotion or where there is already obstruction of the main artery and dilatation of the resultant collateral circulation is desirable.

Raynaud's syndrome, acrocyanosis and erythrocyanosis
These are conditions where the vasoconstrictor response is excessive. Sympathectomy is rarely required in true Primary Raynaud's in young women, but may provide symptomatic relief should the attacks continue and become more frequent or prolonged. Improvement may also follow cervicodorsal sympathectomy in Secondary Raynaud's syndrome, but is liable to be temporary and be followed by relapse. Removal of the second and third lumbar ganglia improves the circulation in the cold, blue leg syndromes of young women and in neurological disorders where muscular paralysis may be associated with vasoconstriction and low blood flow to the distal part of the limb.

Thrombo-angeitis obliterans
This involves the arteries distal to the knee and the elbow, but sympathectomy may help to delay the progress of the disease in the early stages and to lead to more limited amputations when these become necessary.

In *atherosclerosis*, there is slow and often widespread occlusion of the main vessels to the limb. In cases where direct reconstructive surgery is not possible, sympathectomy may be done with the intention of dilating the collateral circulation. This often makes the foot warmer, brings temporary relief of pain, or improves ulceration.

Tests for vasomotor release
The potential response to sympathectomy can be tested by inducing reflex vasodilatation, by spinal anaesthesia or by paravertebral block. However, these tests are not always reliable and are seldom thought to be a necessary preliminary to sympathectomy today.

Paravertebral block
This implies the interruption of sympathetic pathways by injection into paravertebral trunks of ganglia. It is employed not only as a discriminative test, but also as a method of treatment. A single injection of local anaesthetic may give immediate (albeit temporary) relief of causalgic pain; it may abolish vasospasm in a limb for a sufficiently long time to tide the patient over some circulatory crisis. The injection of alcohol or phenol (Reid, 1970) may confer lasting benefit, and may be employed as an alternative to operation.

Cervicothoracic block
Long slender needles of the type used for lumbar puncture are employed. The patient should be placed in the lateral position with his spine fully flexed. The head is supported on a pillow to prevent lateral bending of the cervical spine. Three wheals are raised 4 cm lateral to the spinous processes of C.7, T.1 and T.2. A long needle is introduced through each wheal perpendicular to the skin surface until it makes contact with the neck of the rib (usually the one below). It is then manipulated so that it passes below the rib, and is inclined medially at an angle of 25 degrees towards the sagittal plane, so that it impinges on the side of the vertebral body. This contact should be obtained at a depth of not more than 3 cm beyond the rib; in the absence of contact within this limit of penetration, the needle should be directed more medially. A rubber marker transfixed by the needle is a useful way of ensuring that the safe depth of penetration is not exceeded. After an aspiration test to ensure that the needle has not entered a blood vessel, 5 ml of 1% procaine is injected slowly. It is an advantage to insert all three needles before any injection is made, since the direction of the first needle, if correctly placed, serves as a useful guide to the insertion of the remaining two needles. After a successful injection the upper limb and the face and neck on the affected side should become hot and dry; in addition there should be enophthalmos and constriction of the pupil (*Horner's syndrome*).

Lumbar block
This procedure is best carried out in a department of Radiology so that the position of the needle can be checked by screening. The injection of a small volume of radiological contrast material helps to confirm the appropriate site for injection.

The patient lies in the lateral position with the spine fully flexed and the waist supported by a pillow; wheals of local anaesthetic are raised 7–10 cm lateral to the upper extremities of the spinous processes of L.2 and 3. A 19 gauge needle 12–18 cm in length is introduced perpendicularly through each wheal until it makes contact with the transverse process. It is then partially withdrawn and re-inserted in a more upward direction so that it passes above the transverse process. At a depth of 2 to 3 cm beyond the process its point should be felt to scrape against the side of the vertebral body; if such contact is not obtained the needle is directed more medially. Local anaesthetic is infiltrated at each stage. A rubber marker should be used for the correct measurement of penetration. Any sharp pain indicates that the needle has struck a lumbar nerve, and its direction should at once be changed. After the needles have been placed and aspiration tests carried out 5 ml of 1% procaine (temporary block), or 4 ml of 8% phenol in Urografin (permanent block) is injected through each. If the injection has been correctly placed, there should be immediate cessation of sweating in the lower limb on the affected side; the degree of improvement in the circulation will depend upon the capacity of the vessels to dilate.

Cervicothoracic sympathectomy

This implies the removal at least of the 2nd and 3rd thoracic ganglia, which contain the cells of most of the post-ganglionic fibres supplying the upper limb. Preganglionic fibres are believed to reach these ganglia by one or two routes. They may travel by white rami communicantes from the 2nd and 3rd thoracic nerves (the sympathetic outflow from T.1 being distributed mainly to the head and neck). If they are derived from spinal roots lower than T.3, and enter corresponding ganglia of the sympathetic chain, they must thereafter ascend in the chain in order to synapse with post-ganglionic fibres supplying the upper limb. For complete denervation of the upper limb, it may be thought advisable to remove the small lower part of the stellate ganglion (the part representing the 1st thoracic ganglion), the division being made below the level where the rami communicantes from the 1st thoracic nerve join the ganglion, so that a Horner's syndrome is avoided. For hyperhidrosis affecting the head and neck, it is necessary to remove the whole stellate ganglion (or at least to divide the rami from T.1) and thus to accept a Horner's syndrome. For axillary hyperhidrosis or for anginal pain, the upper four or five thoracic ganglia should be removed.

Anterior approach

This method involves a somewhat difficult dissection but produces less post-operative pain than the alternative approaches. Both sides can be done at the one sitting, and convalescence is rapid. The ganglia may be approached above or below the arch of the subclavian artery. The former is preferred. The first part of the operation is similar to that described for exposure of the third part of the subclavian artery (p. 29) except that the clavicular head of sternomastoid is divided to expose scalenus anterior and the phrenic nerve. Thereafter (the phrenic nerve being safeguarded) scalenus anterior is divided at its insertion into the 1st rib. The subclavian artery, which is now exposed in the greater part of its length, is gently mobilised (Fig. 4.13) and retracted downwards. The thyrocervical artery is seen and ligated with silk. The vertebral artery does not appear at all in the field, and the internal mammary artery remains medially. The suprapleural membrane is detached from the inner border of the 1st rib, and the pleura is displaced downwards and laterally to expose the bodies of the upper three thoracic vertebrae and the posterior ends of the corresponding ribs. The sympathetic trunk is identified crossing the necks of the ribs (the 'stellate' ganglion lying on the 1st rib) and is divided just below the 3rd thoracic ganglion. The upper segment is drawn upwards and laterally, and the rami passing to and from the 2nd and 3rd ganglia are divided, after which these

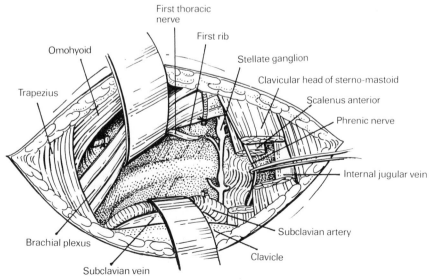

Fig. 4.13 Cervicothoracic sympathectomy by the anterior route above the arch of the subclavian artery

ganglia are removed. The lower third of the stellate ganglion is also removed.

Axillary approach

This method was described by Hedley Atkins and the bilateral procedure is advocated by Campbell (1982). It gives easy and direct access to the upper thoracic ganglia, but is a less convenient approach to the stellate ganglion. An incision 10–12 cm in length is made in the medial wall of the axilla along the line of the 2nd intercostal space, and is deepened through the fibres of serratus anterior until the space is reached. The only structure of importance to be avoided here is the nerve to serratus anterior, but this is usually behind the posterior end of the wound, and is therefore not seen. The pleural cavity is entered after division of the intercostal muscles. A rib spreader is introduced, and the intercostal space is forcibly enlarged to an extent of 5–6 cm. This must be done very slowly to obviate postoperative pain. By means of a gauze roll and a suitable retractor, the lung is drawn downwards. The sympathetic chain should now be seen through the parietal pleura (Fig. 4.14), and the various ganglia are identified—the stellate, from its position on the neck of the first rib. The overlying pleura is then incised, and the sympathetic chain is divided below the 3rd thoracic ganglion (or, when indicated, below the 4th or 5th). The ganglia above the level of section are now mobilised and turned upwards, care being taken to avoid damage to the delicate intercostal veins, and the rami communicantes attached to these ganglia are divided. The chain is finally divided above the 2nd ganglion, or through the lower part of the stellate ganglion if desired. Any bleeding from intercostal vessels is carefully arrested. An intercostal drain is inserted. After inflation of the lung, the wound is closed.

Posterior approach
This method, which entails resection of part of the 3rd rib posteriorly, may cause a certain amount of after-pain so that convalescence is more prolonged. It is therefore not recommended.

Lumbar ganglionectomy

Preganglionic fibres for the lower limb leave the spinal cord in the lower four or five thoracic and upper two lumbar nerves. They enter corresponding ganglia of the sympathetic chain, and descend in the chain to synapse around postganglionic cells in the lower lumbar ganglia and in the sacral ganglia. Removal of the 2nd and 3rd ganglia denervates the limb from the middle of the thigh distally: removal of the 1st ganglion denervates the groin and the upper half of the thigh. It should be noted that, in regard to the sympathetic innervation of vessels below the knee (i.e. in the sciatic distribution) this is a preganglionic operation, for the fibres supplying these vessels have their cell stations in the sacral ganglia, which are not disturbed. In a bilateral operation, the 1st lumbar ganglion on at least one side should be left, since removal of both ganglia may cause sterility, due to paralysis of the ejaculatory mechanism.

The extraperitoneal approach is now accepted as the standard method, since it entails no intra-peritoneal disturbance. Both sides can be done at the one sitting without adding materially to the operative risk. The patient lies partly on his side and a transverse or oblique incision is made in the loin extending from the anterior axillary line to the lateral border of the rectus. The muscles are divided in the same line, and the peritoneum is displaced medially and forwards off the posterior abdominal wall, the genital vessels and the ureter being raised with it. The sympathetic chain is found lying in the groove between the vertebral bodies and the psoas mus-

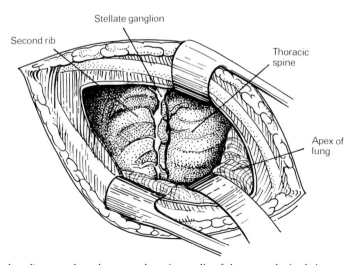

Fig. 4.14 Axillary (transpleural) approach to the upper thoracic ganglia of the sympathetic chain

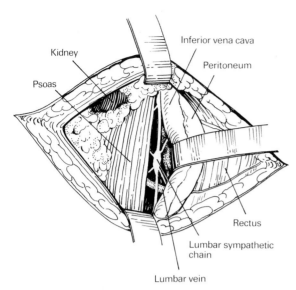

Kidney

Psoas

Inferior vena cava

Peritoneum

Rectus

Lumbar sympathetic chain

Lumbar vein

Fig. 4.15 Right-sided lumbar ganglionectomy by the extraperitoneal route

cle. On the right side it is behind the inferior vena cava (Fig. 4.15); on the left side it is overlapped by the aorta. The first lumbar ganglion must be sought for high up under cover of the crus of the diaphragm; the 4th ganglion may be obscured by the common iliac vessels. *The intraperitoneal approach* may be employed when the abdomen has to be opened on account of some other condition. With the patient in the Trendelenburg position the peritoneal cavity is opened by a lower midline or paramedian incision, and the intestines are packed off into the upper abdomen. For exposure of the left sympathetic chain, the peritoneum is incised along the lateral side of the descending colon, which is then raised from the posterior wall and retracted medially. For exposure of the right sympathetic chain the caecum and ascending colon may be mobilized in a similar manner, or a more direct approach may be made by incising the overlying peritoneum lateral to the inferior vena cava.

REFERENCES

Baker A G, Winegarner F G 1969 Causalgia. A review of twenty-eight treated cases. American Journal of Surgery 117: 690

Campbell W B, Cooper M J, Sponsel W E, Baird R N, Peacock J H 1982 Transaxillary sympathectomy—is a one stage bilateral procedure safe? British Journal of Surgery 69: Supplement, p S 29

Reid W, Watt J K, Gray T G 1970 Phenol injection of the sympathetic chain. British Journal of Surgery 57: 45

FURTHER READING

Seddon H 1975 Surgical disorders of the peripheral nerves, 2nd edn. Churchill Livingstone, Edinburgh

Spinner M 1978 Injuries to the major branches of the peripheral nerves. W B Saunders Co, Philadelphia

Sunderland S 1978 Nerves and nerve injuries, 2nd edn. Churchill Livingstone, Edinburgh

5

Operations on bones and joints

J. CHALMERS

The introduction of infection at a bone or joint operation leads to consequences which may well be disastrous. Meticulous attention must, therefore, be paid to the aseptic ritual. Elective operations should not be performed in the presence of any systemic infection or of septic skin conditions, even although these are well removed from the site of operation. Preparation of the skin should be especially thorough, but the ritual of shaving and enclosing the limb in sterile drapes for 24 hours prior to surgery is no longer practised. There is now much evidence to show that shaving the skin at an interval before surgery is undertaken increases the risk of infection by creating small nicks or abrasions, which may harbour organisms. Shaving, if required, should be carried out immediately before operation and be limited to the operation site. The only preoperative skin preparation which is necessary is thorough cleansing with soap and water.

'No-touch' technique

This technique was at one time used by many orthopaedic surgeons. It requires that the gloved hand should be regarded as potentially contaminated, since sweating of the hands within the gloves carries to the surface organisms from the deeper layers of the skin, and gloves frequently become perforated at operation. The theatre sister should not touch any instruments or swabs by hand, but only with sterile forceps. Needles are threaded with forceps, and are passed to the surgeon in a needle holder. The skin incision is made through surgical adhesive film and the knife is discarded. The surgeon must not introduce his fingers into the wound, and should avoid touching the business end of the instruments. Needles are held in holders, and forceps are used throughout for swabbing and for the tying of ligatures and sutures; blood on the glove is evidence of failure of the technique. Few surgeons now adhere to the full discipline since the fingers, used carefully and judiciously, provide the most delicate and sensitive surgical instruments. The use of double gloves in high risk situations overcomes most of the potential hazards of perforated gloves. Nevertheless, tradition dies hard and most orthopaedic surgeons still practise a modified technique, which might be described as 'not much touch'.

Identifying the operation site

In orthopaedic surgery there is frequently no external evidence of disease of a joint once the patient is anaesthetised and accidents have occurred in which the wrong limb has been operated upon. To avoid such disasters the surgeon should personally confirm the site of surgery prior to anaesthesia and mark the operation site with a skin pencil.

Tourniquets

Tourniquets are used where possible in limb surgery except in cases of peripheral vascular disease. Properly used they limit blood loss and provide a dry operative field. Improperly used, they can cause damage to nerve or vessel. If applied too tightly, or too loose, they may increase bleeding by impeding venous return without occluding the arterial circulation. Only pneumatic tourniquets with a pressure gauge should be used. The cuff should be applied to the upper arm, the proximal thigh or mid calf where muscle bulk will protect the nerves. Before inflating the tourniquet the limb should be exsanguinated by elevation for a few minutes or by applying an Esmarch bandage from the periphery proximally. Elevation is sufficient in most circumstances and has the advantage of leaving a small amount of blood in the limb which helps to identify the vessels and allow their control during the operation. The tourniquet should be inflated to 50 mmHg above the arterial pressure. The safe duration of tourniquet time varies with the age of the patient and the health of his blood vessels. In experimental animals tourniquets have been retained for three hours without lasting ill effect but in practice an hour and a half is probably a wise limit. Tourniquets are not a substitute for haemostasis and it is important that all cut vessels should be ligated or coagulated. In major wounds particularly around vascular areas, such as the elbow or knee, it is wise to release the tourniquet before wound closure to confirm that satisfactory haemostasis has been secured, for a wound haematoma creates an environment favourable to infection and may cause wound breakdown.

In addition to careful haemostasis, wound drainage for one or two days is indicated in most orthopaedic operations. Suction drainage is most effective and represents one of the major advances in operative technique in recent years.

Antibiotic cover

With the introduction of major joint replacement surgery there has been a new incentive to control operative infection which is a major hazard in this type of surgery. Among the various measures which have been tried are the use of ultra clean air enclosures which have proved of value but are expensive additions to operating rooms and are not generally available. The use of appropriate antibiotic cover during and after operation has proved almost as valuable and has reduced the incidence of sepsis to less than 1% in some series. For maximal effect the antibiotic should reach high circulating blood levels during surgery and is best given intravenously at the time of anaesthetic induction. Wide spectrum antibiotics such as Cefuroxime have been most widely used and a suggested routine is 750 mg intravenously at induction and repeated intramuscularly or intravenously at six and twelve hours after surgery. None of these measures however is a substitute for gentle, careful surgical technique with good haemostasis and excision of any traumatised or devitalised tissues at the completion of the operation.

Aspiration of joints

Joint aspiration is frequently required for diagnostic or therapeutic purposes. As the synovial cavity is a continuous one, aspiration may be carried out on any aspect of a joint. The site should be selected therefore so as to avoid important anatomical structures and cause least discomfort to the patient. The tissues at the chosen site are infiltrated with local anaesthetic such as 1% lignocaine using a fine bore needle; the skin and joint capsule are the most sensitive structures. The infiltrating needle is left in situ for two minutes to mark the track while the anaesthetic is taking effect. With thin serous effusions the fine infiltrating needle may be adequate to allow diagnostic aspiration, but for thicker effusions such as blood or pus a wider bore needle is selected and introduced along the anaesthetised track.

Osteotomy

Osteotomy is the surgical division of bone. It may be performed to correct deformity of a bone or joint and to relieve pain in osteoarthritis. Common indications are metatarsal osteotomy to correct hallux valgus or to relieve pressure on a prominent metatarsal head, upper tibial osteotomy for osteoarthritis of the knee, supracondylar osteotomy for deformities resulting from polio-myelitis, intertrochanteric osteotomy for osteoarthritis of the hip, spinal osteotomy for kyphotic deformity in ankylosing spondylitis and osteotomy of any bone to correct congenital deformities or malunited fractures. Many of these procedures will be considered in the subsequent sections, but a few general principles may be considered here.

Osteotomies are in general precise operations designed to produce a specific realignment of a bone. It is necessary therefore to study the patient and the X-rays before operation and plan the exact level of bone section or the amount of bone removal required before surgery. The bone section should be done with minimal trauma so as to avoid bone necrosis. Thus it is best to avoid power saws, which may generate heat, and use sharp osteotomes or hand operated drills or saws. When the osteotomy has been completed internal fixation is usually applied to hold the correction.

A useful technique which has application particularly in children is the two stage procedure of 'osteotomy-osteoclasis'. In this procedure which is most widely used for supracondylar osteotomies of the femur, an appropriate wedge is removed leaving a small part of the cortex intact. The wedge is then broken into chips which are reinserted into the defect and a plaster cast is applied. Two weeks later under anaesthesia the plaster is wedged to complete the osteotomy and to produce the desired correction. No internal fixation is required.

OPERATIONS ON THE UPPER ARM AND SHOULDER

Exposure of humerus

Anterior approach to upper half
The patient lies on his back with the shoulder slightly raised by a flat sandbag placed beneath the lower part of the scapula. An incision is made as shown in Figure 5.1. For a full exposure it begins *behind* the highest point of the shoulder over the spine of the scapula, crosses the shoulder anteriorly to the coracoid, and then descends in the line of the medial border of the deltoid as far as the insertion of this muscle. The cephalic vein is identified lying in the delto-pectoral sulcus. Injury to the vein is avoided by deepening the incision through the medial fibres of deltoid, thus leaving a narrow strand of muscle protecting the vein. To obtain full exposure of the upper end of the humerus, the anterior part of deltoid should be mobilized at its origin from the anterior border of the lateral third of the clavicle. Henry (1973) advises that a sliver of bone comprising this border should be severed with a chisel, and swung laterally with the muscle fibres attached 'like a curtain on a rod'. This procedure allows very full exposure of the upper half of

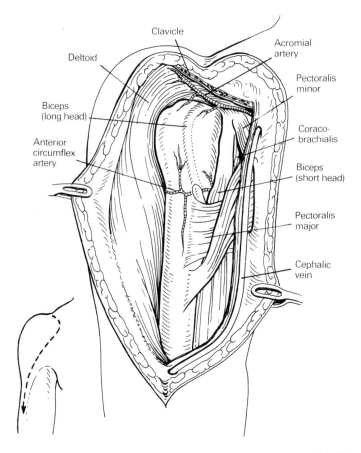

Fig. 5.1 Anterior exposure of shoulder and proximal humerus. The approach passes between deltoid and pectoralis major using the cephalic vein as a guide; the deltoid may be detached from the clavicle

the humerus and of the shoulder joint (Fig. 5.1). At the close of the operation, the strip of bone bearing the deltoid origin is easily reattached with a single stitch.

Anterior approach to the lower half
The incision lies just lateral to the sulcus marking the lateral border of biceps, and so avoids the cephalic vein which lies in the sulcus (Fig. 5.2). The biceps is mobilized and retracted medially to expose the brachialis. The fibres of this muscle are then split by means of a blunt dissector, which is directed towards the front of the humerus in the midline. In this way the lateral strip of brachialis acts as a buffer protecting the radial nerve, while the medial strip protects the musculocutaneous nerve and, farther away, the main neurovascular bundle (Fig. 5.2). The split in brachialis may be carried down to within 2.5 cm of the epicondyles without opening the elbow joint. Flexion of the joint relaxes the muscles, and allows them to be retracted to give wide exposure of the bone.

Exposure of the shoulder joint

Anterior approach
The anterior approach utilizes the upper part of the Henry exposure of the upper part of the humerus. It is not always necessary to detach the anterior fibres of the deltoid from the clavicle but, having retracted the deltoid laterally, the front of the shoulder is still obscured by the coracoid process and its attached muscles. These may be mobilized either by dividing the muscles (coracobrachialis, the short head of biceps and pectoralis minor) 1 cm below their origins, or, preferably, by dividing the tip of the coracoid with an osteotome and displacing it medially with its muscles still attached. It simplifies reattachment at a later stage if the coracoid is first drilled and tapped with a screw, which is then removed before osteotomy and used to reattach the coracoid on completion of the operation. The front of the shoulder joint now lies exposed, covered only by the subscapularis muscle.

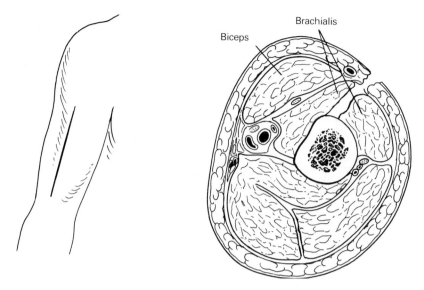

Fig. 5.2 Anterior exposure of distal humerus. The approach is made lateral to biceps and splits brachialis

Posterior approach to the shoulder joint

The patient lies on his side with the affected arm uppermost. The arm is freely draped to allow an assistant to change the position as required. The skin incision follows the spine of the scapula, extending laterally to the tip of the acromion. The deltoid muscle is mobilized from the spine of the scapula and from the acromion and is reflected distally and laterally (Fig. 5.3), care being taken to avoid damage to the axillary nerve, which emerges through the quadrilateral space distal to the teres minor. The shoulder joint is now hidden by the tendons of teres minor and infraspinatus and is exposed by separating these muscles or, if need be, by dividing the tendons 1 cm from their insertion and reflecting them medially, care being taken to avoid injury to the suprascapular nerve, which enters infraspinatus at the base of the acromion.

Posterior approach to the humerus

The posterior approach is more widely used than the anterior approach, being more appropriate for the reduction and internal fixation of fractures. In this ap-

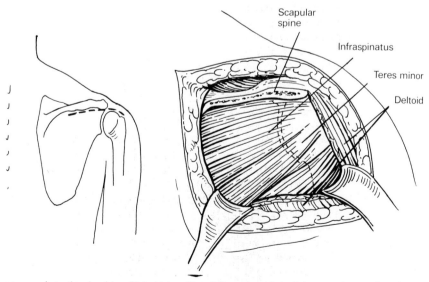

Fig. 5.3 Posterior approach to the shoulder. Deltoid is reflected from the spine of the scapula exposing the posterior muscles of the rotator cuff

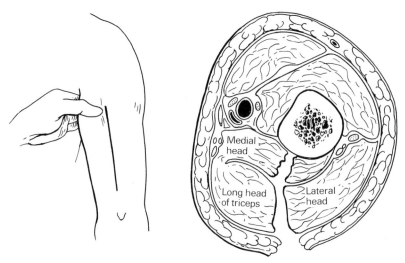

Fig. 5.4 Posterior approach to humerus

proach, the radial nerve is at risk and its course must be constantly borne in mind. It crosses the middle third of the humerus obliquely from the medial to lateral side, lying deep to the long and lateral heads of triceps and lateral to the medial head of triceps. It enters the anterior compartment by passing through the lateral intermuscular septum to enter brachialis in the distal third of the upper arm. Both the nerve and its branches to the triceps must be carefully preserved.

The patient lies in the lateral position. The incision extends vertically down the middle of the posterior surface of the upper arm. The deep fascia is divided and the long head of triceps is identified in the proximal part of the wound by virtue of its mobility when compared with the lateral head and deltoid. The plane between the long and lateral heads is developed and the radial nerve and profunda artery are identified deep to these heads and carefully protected. As these muscle bodies become fused in the lower part of the wound, they have to be separated by sharp dissection. This then exposes the medial head of triceps, lying more deeply, and this muscle is split vertically in the mid-line to expose the posterior shaft of the humerus (Fig. 5.4).

Transacromial approach to the shoulder
This approach gives good access for surgery to the rotator cuff and fixation of fractures of the greater tuberosity. The skin incision is made in the coronal plane centred over the most prominent lateral point of the acromion and extending 5 cm both proximally and distally. The trapezius and deltoid muscles are split in the line of their fibres up to the acromion. Short flaps of conjoint aponeurosis, periosteum and bone are raised with an osteotome, as shown in Figure 5.5, and the acromion is then split with an oscillating saw and separated with a self-retaining retractor, exposing the

subdeltoid bursa and the underlying rotator cuff. Rotation of the arm allows access to the whole of the rotator cuff. When closing the wound, the acromium is repaired by suture of the overlying aponeurotic and periosteal flaps.

Recurrent dislocation of the shoulder
In the great majority of cases, the dislocation is anterior and is due either to stretching of the anterior capsule, or more commonly, to separation of the glenoid labrum from its bony attachment. Although recurrent posterior dislocation is very rare, accounting for only 2% of shoulder dislocations, it is nevertheless important to recognize that it can occur, for the operative treatment of the two types is, of course, entirely different.

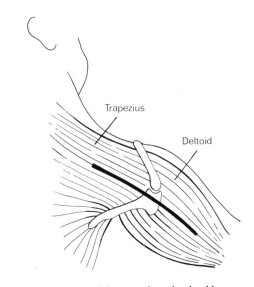

Fig. 5.5 Transacromial approach to the shoulder

In *recurrent anterior dislocation* a wedge-shaped defect may arise in the posterior part of the head of the humerus as a result of its repeated contact with the anterior margin of the glenoid and this notch, when present, facilitates redislocation. The surgical correction of recurrent anterior dislocation involves the repair or reinforcement of the anterior capsular structures and also limits external rotation and so prevents the humeral notch from engaging with the anterior margin of the glenoid.

The standard anterior approach to the shoulder is used (p. 86). The subscapularis tendon is divided 2 cm medial to its insertion. Before the division is completed, a holding suture is placed in the proximal part of the muscle, for otherwise it will retract and be difficult to recover. Ideally the tendon should be divided separately from the underlying capsule, but this can be difficult for the two structures are frequently fused at this level. The anterior capsule is then incised and the nature and extent of the capsular damage inspected by external rotation of the arm. The periosteum overlying the front of the neck of the scapula is elevated and the underlying bone is roughened with an osteotome so as to allow subsequent adhesion of the soft tissues. The distal stump of the subscapularis tendon and the underlying capsule are then sutured to the periosteum or labrum at the front of the neck of the scapula by means of three strong, but absorbable, mattress sutures which are all placed in position with the arm externally rotated and tied with the arm internally rotated. The medial capsular flap is brought to overlap the subscapularis tendon and sutured under moderate tension; the medial cut end of the subscapularis is brought as a separate layer to overlap the capsule and is in turn sutured to the soft tissues in the region of the lesser tuberosity. There are thus four overlapping layers reinforcing the front of the shoulder joint and limiting external rotation (Fig. 5.6). The coracoid process is then reattached and the wound closed. The arm is thereafter bandaged in internal rotation for three weeks, following which gentle, progressive mobilisation of the shoulder is begun.

The above operation is known as the *Putti-Platt procedure* after the two eminent surgeons, who independently described it. It remains the most widely used operation for it combines simplicity with a high success rate.

Alternative procedures include the *Bankhart operation* in which the detached labrum is reattached to the glenoid margin by sutures passed through drill holes in the margin of the glenoid made with a right-angled dental drill. This is usually combined with a double breasting of the subscapularis as in the Putti-Platt procedure. Anterior bone blocks may also be used, utilizing the tip of the detached coracoid process, which is screwed to the anterior surface of the neck of the scapula or a free bone

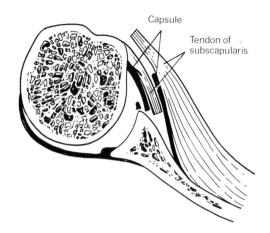

Fig. 5.6 The Putti-Platt repair of recurrent dislocation of the shoulder. The anterior capsule and subscapularis tendon are overlapped

graft is taken from the iliac crest and placed intracapsularly. The latter is secured by tucking it into the pocket which lies in front of the neck of the scapula, or it may be placed anterior to the capsule and fixed to the neck of the scapula by means of a screw.

Recurrent posterior dislocation of the shoulder
The standard posterior approach is used. The infraspinatus tendon is divided 2 cm from its insertion and the posterior capsule incised. The pathology is usually a detachment of the posterior labrum from the glenoid and repair is effected by means of a bone block, which can be tucked into the space beneath the detached labrum and left projecting 1 cm. Alternatively it may be placed outside the capsule and secured in position by screwing it to the neck of the scapula, as in the anterior bone block procedure.

Operations on the rotator cuff
These may be required for ruptures or avulsion of the rotator cuff, for calcium deposits in the cuff or for supraspinatus tendonitis. Acute ruptures or avulsions are recognized by inability to initiate abduction of the shoulder, although passive abduction is free and active abduction can be sustained above 90 degrees. The transacromial approach to the shoulder is used and the tear in the rotator cuff is then identified by rotating the arm to bring it into view. The retracted proximal ends of the torn tendons are mobilized, brought laterally and sutured under an osteoperiosteal flap, the sutures passing through drill holes in bone at the point of attachment. The arm may be supported by the side in a sling following this operation and passive movements commenced within a few days. Active movements are delayed for three weeks.

Supraspinatus calcification occasionally requires surgery, either because of intense local pain, which has failed to respond to injections of local anaesthetic and hydrocortisone (which should always be attempted in the first place), or because the size of the calcified mass may be so great as to produce an actual block to abduction by engaging against the undersurface of the acromion. These lesions may be approached through a short coronal incision placed over the lesion distal to the acromion process. The deltoid fibres are split in the line of the incision and the chalky, inflamed area of the rotator cuff is then immediately identified. The calcified mass is incised and the chalk-like material curetted. No postoperative immobilization is required.

Acromioclavicular joint lesions
Subluxation of the acromioclavicular joint is a minor displacement limited by the integrity of the conoid and trapezoid ligaments. It causes few symptoms and requires no surgical repair. If these ligaments are completely disrupted, the outer end of the clavicle displaces upwards and backwards producing an ugly shoulder contour, but little disability. There is no conservative treatment. Many surgical procedures have been described, including insertion of a lag screw through the clavicle into the coracoid process, or transfixation of the reduced acromioclavicular joint by means of a Rush pin or stout Kirschner wire, the latter being bent over at its lateral extremity to prevent medial migration. The screw, or wire, should be removed after eight weeks to allow restoration of the normal movement which takes place between the clavicle and the scapula.

Arthrodesis of the shoulder
This operation is rarely performed but may be indicated in chronic arthritis or to stabilize the shoulder in certain paralytic disorders such as poliomyelitis or brachial plexus injuries.

It is essential that the shoulder be fixed in the optimum position for the patient's needs. In general this is in 40 degrees of abduction, 20 degrees of flexion and 25 degrees of internal rotation, i.e. a position in which the hand may readily be brought to the mouth. Many techniques of shoulder fusion are described. A simple and effective method consists simply of denuding the joint surfaces of articular cartilage and transfixing them in the desired position with a trifin nail or compression screw, with or without a bone graft fashioned from the fibula or the spine of the scapula. An anterior approach is used with a proximal extension to the incision to allow detachment of the deltoid from the acromion. The subscapularis and anterior capsule are then divided and the cartilage removed from the joint surfaces with gouges and osteotomes. A guide wire is then inserted through the lateral aspect of the upper end of the humerus to reach the centre of the glenoid and over this a cannulated trifin nail or cannulated screw is inserted, the length having been judged by X-ray. Following wound closure, the arm is immobilized in a shoulder spica. It greatly facilitates the application of the spica if the body part of the jacket is applied to the conscious patient prior to surgery. The spica is retained for at least eight weeks, or until there is radiological evidence of union.

OPERATIONS ON THE ELBOW AND FOREARM

Exposure of the elbow joint
The *lateral approach* gives wide access to the elbow joint with minimum damage to the soft parts. It is performed with the patient's arm across his chest. The incision is centred on the lateral epicondyle and extends 5 cm proximally and distally. The lateral intermuscular septum is identified above the epicondyle, and, using it as a guide, the anterior muscles, brachioradialis and the common extensor origin are separated from the posterior muscles, triceps and anconeus (Fig. 5.7). The incision is deepened to bone and to the capsule of the elbow between these muscles. If the operation is to be limited to the front of the elbow as for removal of a loose body, an incision is made in the anterior capsule. Conversely, if access is required to the posterior part of the joint, the capsule is opened behind the epicondyle. Very wide exposure of the entire elbow may be obtained by dividing the lateral ligament and hinging the elbow open. Postoperatively a sling is worn for ten days.

The posterior approach
This approach is particularly useful if a very wide exposure of the elbow is required for reconstruction of comminuted fractures involving the elbow joint or for elbow arthroplasties. With the arm supported on a rest across the trunk, an incision is made, starting in the

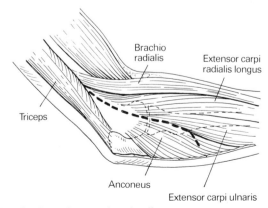

Fig. 5.7 Lateral approach to the elbow

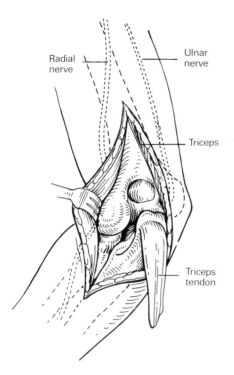

Fig. 5.8 Posterior approach to the elbow

midline, 8 cm proximal to the olecranon and passing close to the lateral margin of the olecranon and distally for a further 5 cm along the posterior aspect of the ulna. The skin flap is retracted medially to allow exposure of the ulnar nerve behind the medial epicondyle and the position of the nerve is kept constantly in mind throughout the operative procedure. A tongue-like flap of triceps tendon is turned down to its insertion into the olecranon and the triceps incised in the midline down to bone. The capsule and muscular attachments to the epicondyles are then elevated as widely as may be required by the operative procedure, great care being exercised to protect the ulnar nerve (Fig. 5.8).

Arthrodesis of the elbow
This operation is rarely performed and the indications and individual requirements of the patient are so varied that there is no standard technique. The optimal functional position must be established before operation by trial fixation in plaster casts.

Through the posterior approach, the joint surfaces are denuded of cartilage and transfixed in the predetermined position by means of a screw or strong Kirschner wires. Circumstances may require the head of the radius to be excised.

Arthroplasty of the elbow is still undergoing development. Many different models are being used at the present time and many difficulties have been encountered.

Until time has established the worth of these various procedures they are best left in the hands of their innovators.

Exposure of the radius
The best approach to the shaft and lower end of the radius is through an incision overlying the medial border of the brachioradialis (Fig. 5.9). Distally, the incision should reach the radial styloid; proximally, it is carried up as far as is thought necessary. The cephalic vein, which crosses the line of incision in the middle third of the forearm, is divided between ligatures. The three long muscles which form the radial border of the forearm: brachioradialis, extensor carpi radialis longus and extensor carpi radialis brevis, and the radial nerve which lies on the deep aspect of brachioradialis, are mobilised and retracted laterally to expose the lateral surface of the shaft of the radius. The insertion of pronator teres to the middle of this surface, and the muscles arising from the anterior and posterior surfaces, are detached subperiosteally. The radial artery is displaced medially with the anterior muscles, and is carefully safeguarded. If the hand is now turned into full pronation, the lower two-thirds of the radius is widely exposed.

For *exposure of the upper third of the radius*, the incision, which still overlies the medial border of brachioradialis, is carried up into the upper arm to a point 8 cm above the elbow. The cleft between brachioradialis and

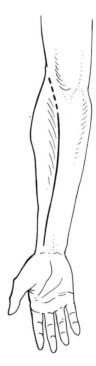

Fig. 5.9 Incision for exposure of the radius

the tendon of biceps is opened up, the radial recurrent vessels being divided between ligatures. The radius is exposed by a longitudinal incision made upon its anterior surface, through the most anterior fibres of supinator, the knife being kept immediately lateral to the biceps tendon. A rougine is now worked laterally around the bone to detach the fibres of supinator inserted into its anterior, lateral and posterior surfaces. In order to avoid the possibility of injury to the posterior interosseous nerve, which winds around the bone in the substance of supinator, it is essential that the instrument should be kept close to the bone throughout. If only the head and neck of the radius require to be exposed, and if wide access is not essential, a better approach is through an incision made directly over the posterior surface of the upper end of the bone.

Exposure of the ulna

The ulna is subcutaneous in its entire length, and can be exposed by an incision made along or adjacent to its posterior border.

OPERATIONS ON THE WRIST

The most commonly performed operations about the wrist are those on nerves and tendons described on pages 18 & 73. The wrist may be exposed from any aspect, according to the needs of the particular procedure. The *dorsal approach* gives widest access and is most suitable for arthrodesis. A longitudinal dorsal incision is made curving obliquely across the wrist. The extensor retinaculum is detached from its ulnar extremity and mobilized towards the radial side. The wrist is exposed by separating the digital extensors towards the ulnar side, and the extensor pollicis longus tendon (which is freed from its groove on the dorsal aspect of the radius) and the radial wrist extensors towards the radial side. The capsule is then incised and reflected as required to expose the carpus.

Removal of ganglia

The term ganglion, apart from its use in reference to nerve tissue, is employed to denote a tense cystic swelling containing gelatinous material, which may develop in relation to joints and tendon sheaths. Although it may occur about any of the joints of the extremities, by far the commonest site is the dorsal surface of the wrist. It is therefore convenient to consider it here.

Ganglia frequently disappear spontaneously as a result of rupture and it is always worthwhile attempting this procedure therapeutically. The ganglion and its surroundings are injected with local anaesthesia and its contents dispersed either by manual pressure or by insertion of a wide bore needle. Many ganglia are painless and are best left alone, if they do not respond to this simple treatment. Where a ganglion continues to recur, and produces symptoms such as pressure on adjacent nerves or justified cosmetic concern, excision is indicated, but the patient should be warned that recurrence is possible.

The excision of a ganglion can sometimes be a difficult and time-consuming operation, which must always be carried out under a tourniquet and with full awareness of the anatomical relations in the vicinity. Bier's regional anaesthesia is ideal. A transverse incision is usually made so that the underlying cutaneous nerves can be easily identified and avoided. The investing fascia is incised longitudinally and the adjacent tendons are mobilized. Resection of the ganglion is then proceeded with, great care being taken to try and identify its communication with a synovial cavity. Not infrequently a ganglion can migrate some distance from its point of origin and if its connecting neck is not identified and excised, it may recur.

Arthrodesis of the wrist

This may be indicated to treat a painful wrist which has been disorganized by chronic arthritis or by trauma. The extent of the arthrodesis is determined by the extent of the disease. Thus in traumatic arthritis resulting from fractures of the distal radius, it may be necessary only to fuse the radius to the proximal bone of the carpus, which leaves a small amount of wrist movement from the remaining carpal joints. If the arthritis is more widespread, the arthrodesis may have to be extended to include the metacarpals and it may be necessary also to excise the lower end of the ulna. So long as forearm rotation is maintained, a stiff and painless wrist causes very little disability.

The dorsal approach, as described above, is used and by flexing the wrist the residual articular cartilage is removed from the carpal joint surfaces, using gouges, osteotomes and sharp curette. Chips of cancellous bone obtained from the iliac crest are then packed into the residual gaps and crevices, with the wrist in flexion. The wrist is brought into the ideal position of 20 degrees of extension, thus compacting the bone grafts. The joint capsule is repaired as far as possible and the extensor retinaculum, which has been carefully preserved, is placed deep to the extensor tendons and resutured at its ulnar attachment. The wrist is immobilized in plaster for eight weeks.

Many prefer to elaborate the above procedure by the addition of an onlay bone graft. This is obtained from the outer aspect of the wing of the ilium at a site selected to give the correct curvature required by the operation site. A bed is prepared for the graft from the distal radius to the bases of the middle three metacarpals and the graft is cut and shaped to match (Fig. 5.10) If it fits well, no internal fixation is required. If it appears un-

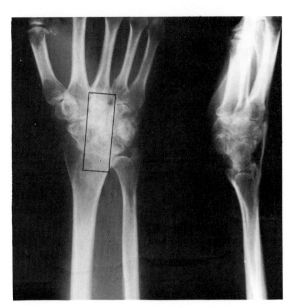

Fig. 5.10 X-ray showing the position of the posterior onlay graft for wrist fusion

stable, it may be temporarily transfixed by Kirschner wires, which are removed when the plaster is changed at two weeks.

OPERATIONS ON THE HIP AND THIGH

Aspiration of the hip joint
The needle may be inserted perpendicular to the skin at a point 2.5 cm below and lateral to the midinguinal point. The femoral artery, which lies deep to this point, should be safeguarded by palpation.

An alternative method is to introduce the needle just above the tip of the greater trochanter, and to pass it upwards and medially in the line of the femoral neck, following the bone until the joint is reached.

Exposures of the hip joint

The anterior approach
This gives excellent exposure with minimal muscle damage, and is widely used. The incision passes from just below the middle of the iliac crest to the anterior superior spine, and then extends vertically downwards for 10 to 12 cm (Fig. 5.11). Superficial and deep fascia are divided in the line of the incision. Gluteus medius and tensor fasciae latae are detached sub-periosteally from the iliac crest and are reflected downwards. The dissection is continued distally in the thigh in the interval between tensor fasciae latae laterally, and the sartorius and rectus femoris medially, care being taken to preserve the lateral cutaneous nerve of the thigh. The joint capsule is now exposed and is incised or excised according to the needs of the operation.

The anterolateral exposure of the hip
This approach gives more generous access to the hip joint than the anterior and is widely used for arthroplasty procedures. The operation can be done with the patient supine, a sandbag being placed under the buttock on the side of operation, or it may conveniently be done with the patient on the orthopaedic table, which

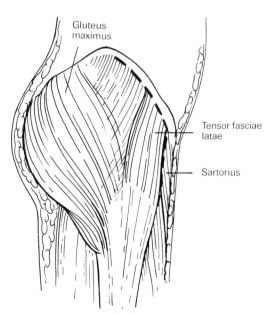
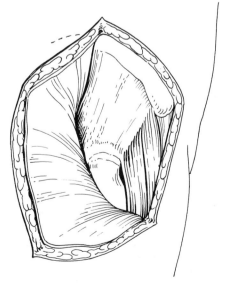

Fig. 5.11 Anterior approach to the hip

allows greater freedom of manipulation of the leg by an unsterile assistant at the foot of the table, if required. The incision commences just below the iliac crest at a point 2.5 cm posterior to the anterior superior spine. It passes to the midpoint of the greater trochanter and then distally along the line of the femur for 5 cm. The fascia lata is then incised in the lower part of the wound just posterior to the insertion of tensor fasciae latae. Continuing the dissection upwards in the line of the skin incision, the plane between the muscle bellies of tensor fasciae latae anteriorly and gluteus medius and minimus posteriorly is then defined and the overlying fascia divided up to the iliac crest. The plane between these muscles is developed down to the side wall of the pelvis securing a number of vessels which cross the line of dissection. The nerve to tensor fascia femoris also crosses between the muscle groups and may be preserved if a limited operation is being carried out, but usually has to be sacrificed, if a major arthroplasty is being undertaken. No disability appears to result from denervation of this muscle. At the proximal end of the wound, the origins of the glutei and tensor are fused together and have to be separated by sharp dissection. If need be the exposure can be increased by stripping the glutei posteriorly off the iliac crest. The capsule of the hip joint is concealed at first by a very constant fat pad. When this is removed, the entire anterior and superior capsule of the hip joint is exposed and may be incised or excised as widely as the operation requires. The reflected head of rectus femoris may be removed but it is rarely necessary to detach the direct head.

The posterolateral approach

There are a number of variations of this approach but the most widely used is the 'Southern' approach of Austin Moore. The patient is supported in a true lateral position with the lower leg flexed to 90 degrees at the hip and knee. The incision (Fig. 5.12a) starts in front of the posterior superior iliac spine and extends to the midpoint of the greater trochanter and then distally in the line of the femur for a similar distance. The fascia lata and the gluteal insertion to it are divided in the line of the lower part of the incision and the split is extended proximally separating the fibres of gluteus maximus in the line of the proximal part of the skin incision. The split gluteus maximus is then held apart by a self-retaining retractor exposing the short external rotator muscles covering the posterior surface of the hip joint. These are from above downwards: piriformis, the obturator internus with the gemelli and quadratus femoris. The sciatic nerve which emerges below piriformis to lie on the posterior surface of the other rotators midway between the greater trochanter and the ischium should be identified and protected throughout the operation (Fig. 5.12b). By internally rotating the hip, the short rotator muscles

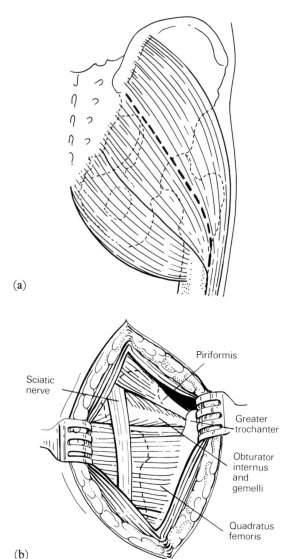

(a)

(b)

Fig. 5.12(a) Incision for posterior approach to the hip. (b) Structures on posterior aspect of the hip exposed by splitting the fibres of the gluteus maximus

become better defined and are divided close to their insertion, the proximal ends having first been secured by stay sutures. It is not always necessary to divide the piriformis or the quadratus femoris, nor it is necessary to detach gluteus medius and minimus from the greater trochanter. Having divided the external rotator muscles, the capsule of the hip joint is exposed and is incised as necessary for the procedure. If hip dislocation is required, it is achieved by internal rotation of the leg which must be carried out gently in osteoporotic elderly patients. If there is resistance to dislocation, it is best to divide the neck with the head in situ and remove it piecemeal thereafter.

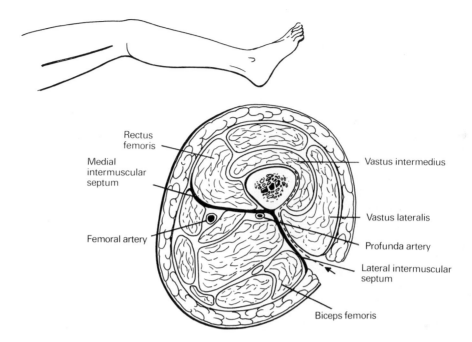

Rectus femoris

Medial intermuscular septum

Femoral artery

Vastus intermedius

Vastus lateralis

Profunda artery

Lateral intermuscular septum

Biceps femoris

Fig. 5.13 Posterolateral approach to the shaft of femur

Exposure of the shaft of the femur

The posterolateral approach causes minimal damage to the quadriceps and therefore is least likely to cause knee stiffness. It is now the standard approach to the femur and supersedes Henry's anterior approach. The patient lies on his side and a skin incision is made along the axis of the femur just behind the midlateral line of the thigh and is extended as far as may be required to give access to the objective of the operation (Fig. 5.13). The fascia lata is incised along the length of the skin incision just posterior to the iliotibial band. This exposes the vastus lateralis which is separated by blunt dissection from the lateral intermuscular septum as far as its origin from the linea aspera. The muscle is detached from its origin by an incision made about 0.5 cm lateral to the linea aspera since this allows the perforating vessels to be secured as they are encountered. If the muscle is detached from the linea itself the cut vessels may retract out of sight and be more difficult to find. The vastus lateralis and the remaining quadriceps muscles can then be mobilized from the lateral aspect and front of the femur by bone levers giving good access to the bone.

At wound closure only the fascia lata and skin require to be sutured. A conventional tourniquet can only be used for lesions of the distal femur, but it is possible to secure a tourniquet at a high level by passing a Steinmann pin into the lateral aspect of the femur in the upper thigh and placing the cuff of the tourniquet above it.

Total prosthetic replacement of the hip joint

One of the greatest advances in orthopaedic surgery in recent years has been the development of prosthetic joint replacements. The hip joint was the first to be developed and has remained the most successful of all joint replacements with a success rate exceeding 90% in many large series. The most widely used model is that developed by Charnley (1979) (Fig. 5.14). The two components of the prosthesis are secured to bone with methylmethacrylate cement. Although highly successful in properly selected cases, the prosthesis can fail mechanically either by breakage of the femoral component or more commonly loosening of the cement/bone bond. The other important cause of failure is infection, which, if it becomes established, requires a major revision operation with a much reduced success rate. The consequences of these complications are so serious that it follows that this operation should only be carried out where the clinical indications are unequivocal and where the surgeon is confident in the sterility of his theatre environment. The operation is indicated for severe pain or disability in the hip joint of an elderly patient despite conservative treatment. The common underlying pathological conditions are osteoarthritis, rheumatoid arthritis, avascular necrosis of the head of the femur or failure of primary treatment of a fractured neck of femur. The operation should not be carried out for chronic arthritis due to an infectious cause unless the infection has been eradicated. Occasionally the operation may be-

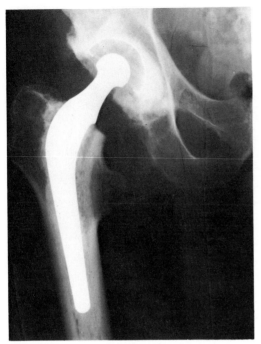

Fig. 5.14 The Charnley hip prosthesis as seen on X-ray. The acetabular component is made of high density polyethylene and the femoral of stainless steel

come necessary in a younger patient who suffers from bilateral hip joint disease, for example rheumatoid arthritis or ankylosing spondylitis, but in these circumstances the patient should always be advised that the procedure may not last indefinitely because of wear or loosening.

The operation is normally carried out under antibiotic cover (p. 85). The incision used depends on the surgeon's preference; both the anterolateral and posterior approaches are suitable. Charnley recommends the true lateral approach with division of the greater trochanter, which allows very generous exposure both of the acetabulum and of the shaft of the femur and is of particular value in a difficult case but has the disadvantage that the trochanter has to be firmly secured at the end of the operation which adds to the operative time and to the possible complications. This approach is not widely adopted for routine use. Nevertheless the inexperienced surgeon may well find this the easiest and safest approach and would do well to read Charnley's description. Having dislocated the hip, the head is removed with an osteotome or Gigli saw. The acetabulum is prepared by removal of all soft tissue, sclerotic bone and residual cartilage down to the level of the acetabular fossa, using cranked gouges. Two or three holes are made in the roof of the acetabulum and in the ischium to provide additional anchoring points for the cement. The blood and bony fragments are washed out of the acetabulum, using an antibiotic solution, and the acetabulum thoroughly dried. An acetabular cup of appropriate size is then selected. A mix of methylmethacrylate cement is firmly pressed into the exposed cancellous bone of the acetabulum and into the anchorage holes and the acetabular component is inserted using the appropriate guide to ensure correct placement, which should be at an angle of 45 degrees from the longitudinal axis of the body. A common fault is to have the cup facing too laterally. Excess cement should be removed before it hardens. The femoral shaft is then reamed with the appropriate reamers and again thoroughly irrigated with antibiotic solution. A trial reduction of the femoral component is carried out without use of the cement to ensure correct fit. Stability is best achieved by a fairly tight reduction and a range of prostheses with different femoral neck lengths is available as required. Cement is inserted into the femoral canal either by a cement syringe or by digital pressure. During the insertion process the shaft is vented by a plastic catheter which is removed when the filling is complete. The femoral component is inserted with the neck pointing medially to the normal axis of the femur. Once the cement is hardened, the hip is reduced and the wound closed in layers over a suction drain. The patient mobilizes quickly and is allowed to walk after two days and may leave hospital in ten or twelve days when the wound has healed. Prolonged physiotherapy is not usually required.

Arthrodesis of the hip
Arthrodesis of the hip is now rarely performed as arthroplasty is in general a more acceptable solution to a chronic hip problem. Nevertheless, there remain some indications for this procedure, notably severe post-traumatic arthritis in a young and active person in whom an arthroplasty would be unlikely to last long. A satisfactory arthrodesis of the hip allows a comfortable, painless gait but an awkward sitting posture and, as with arthrodesis of any joint, it throws greater stress on neighbouring joints. Thus the spine and knee of the same leg tend to develop degenerative changes over a period of years. However, it is now possible to convert an arthrodesed or ankylosed hip to replacement arthroplasty when a patient reaches an appropriate age and the arthrodesis may then be regarded as an interim procedure, which will carry a patient through his most active working years.

Many techniques of arthrodesis are described, the one to be described here has the merit of simplicity and safety.

Ischiofemoral or V-arthrodesis
With the patient supine upon the orthopaedic table, the hip joint is carefully positioned to lie in 20 degrees of flexion, 5 degrees of external rotation and no abduction or adduction. If contraction of the hip joint prevents this position from being achieved, then an osteotomy must

be carried out as described later. A midlateral incision is made extending from the greater trochanter distally for 10 cm. The lateral aspect of the upper femur is exposed subperiosteally and a guidewire is inserted under X-ray control as described in the internal fixation of fractures of the neck of femur (p. 123). The guidewire is aimed to cross the hip joint and enter the thick bone in the roof of the acetabulum just above the pelvic rim, and is advanced towards the sacro-iliac joint for about 6 cm. The length of nail is measured from the guidewire and a triflanged nail is driven across the hip joint into the pelvis, thus stabilizing the hip in its optimal position. A lateral incision is then made over the fibula of the same leg and the bone is exposed between the lateral and posterior muscle groups. The midportion is stripped of soft tissues and an 8 cm length is removed for use as a graft. The bone should be cut with a Gigli saw or oscillating power saw since it tends to splinter if divided with an osteotome or bone cutters. The fibular wound is closed and the patient turned to the prone position and retowelled. The hip wound is then extended as for the conventional posterior approach to the hip joint (p. 94). The gluteus maximus is split in the line of its fibres and the posterior aspect of the hip joint covered by the external rotators is exposed. The sciatic nerve is identified as it emerges from the lower border of piriformis and a tape is passed round it. A guidewire is in-

serted from the lateral aspect of the femur, 1 cm below the point of entry of the nail. The wire is advanced medially, proximally and posteriorly aimed towards the thick part of the ischium just below the hip joint, which is identified by finger palpation. Cannulated drills are advanced over the guidewire, across the femur and into the ischium, the largest drill being slightly less then the diameter of the fibular graft. The graft, which has been pointed by means of a file at one end, is then punched through the hole in the femur into the ischium for a distance of 3 cm. In order to prevent a fracture occuring at the site of the hole in the femur, it is prudent to attach a short plate to the triflange nail as in the fixation of an intertrochanteric fracture. The V formed by the graft and nail both traversing the femur and penetrating the pelvis give great stability to the arthrodesis and no additional immobilization is required. The patient may get up on crutches soon after the operation and protected weight-bearing is allowed with the help of crutches. Full weight-bearing should be possible in six weeks. Fusion takes place progressively through the fibular graft which hypertrophies and ultimately the hip joint itself fuses (Fig. 5.15).

The purpose of turning the patient from supine to prone position during the course of the operation is to enable the identification and protection of the sciatic nerve, which can be damaged if the graft is inserted blindly. The operator will be impressed by the close relationship between the graft and the sciatic nerve.

Arthrodesis combined with osteotomy

If the ideal position of the hip joint cannot be obtained (because of uncorrectable deformity) the above procedure should be carried out with the hip joint in its deformed position and a corrective subtrochanteric osteotomy is performed with the patient supine on the orthopaedic table, as a secondary procedure two weeks later—the osteotomy site being secured by a seven hole plate. Some surgeons prefer to combine the arthrodesis and osteotomy as a one stage procedure but it can be difficult to get the ideal position by this means and the two stage procedure described above is safer and simpler.

Intertrochanteric osteotomy

Division of a bone in the vicinity of an osteoarthritic joint with correction of deformity may relieve pain in a high proportion of cases and in many instances produce an improved radiological appearance, at least for a number of years. This well tried procedure can be a useful interim procedure in patients too young for arthroplasty, but who have failed to respond to conservative measures. Intertrochanteric osteotomy for osteoarthritis of the hip and upper tibial osteotomy for osteoarthritis of the knee, (p. 105) are the most com-

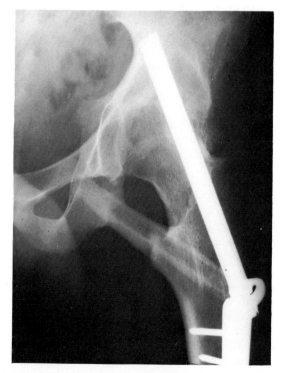

Fig. 5.15 X-ray showing V-arthrodesis of the hip. Note the hypertrophy of the fibular graft

mon procedures of this kind. The ideal indications for this procedure are severe pain with preservation of at least 50% of movement in the affected joint.

The patient is placed on the orthopaedic table and two-plane X-ray control is established as for pinning a fractured neck of femur (p. 123). A midlateral incision is made extending distally to the greater trochanter for about 10 cm and the shaft of the femur is exposed as for internal fixation of an intertrochanteric fracture (p. 124). It is useful to place the anterior bone lever just above the lesser trochanter, to serve as a guide for the osteotomy. A guidewire is inserted into the centre of the neck of the femur under X-ray control, and a second guidewire is passed across the femur to confirm the level of the osteotomy, which should lie just above the level of the lesser trochanter. A flanged nail is driven into the neck of the femur, the length being measured to stop short of the articular surface by 2 cm to ensure that no penetration of the joint takes place. The osteotomy is carried out at the selected level either by using a Gigli saw or by perforating the bone with a series of drill holes, completing the osteotomy with an osteotome. The use of a power saw tends to produce some heat necrosis at the site of osteotomy which may delay healing.

In the past it has been the practice to displace the shaft of the femur medially at the osteotomy site by at least half the diameter of the bone; however there is no evidence which supports the need for this displacement and subsequent replacement arthroplasty, if required, is made more difficult if the osteotomy site has been displaced. It is therefore customary now simply to correct any pre-existing deformity at the osteotomy site, and achieve stabilization by the attachment of seven hole plate to the nail. Other techniques of fixation may be used, such as compression plate or fixed angle nail plate, according to the preference and experience of the surgeon.

Early mobilization is allowed, the patient taking part-weight for the first six weeks and full-weight thereafter.

Excision arthroplasty of the hip (Girdlestone pseudarthrosis)

Excision of the head and neck of the femur is an operation originally developed for the management of septic arthritis of the hip. It may appear of historic interest only in these days of artificial hip joints. Nevertheless, in many parts of the world where the facilities for hip joint replacement are lacking and where social customs, particularly the need to adopt the squatting posture, demand a very full range of hip movement, excision arthroplasty may still have a place in the management of a severely disorganized hip joint resulting from infection or chronic arthritis. The operation may be performed through the anterolateral or posterior approach. The head and neck of the femur are cleanly removed to leave

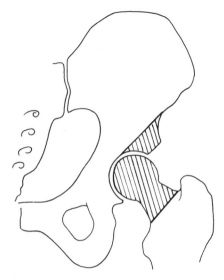

Fig. 5.16 Extent of bone resection in a Girdlestone pseudarthrosis

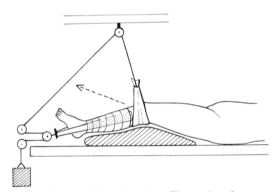

Fig. 5.17 Hamilton Russell traction. The resulant force shown by the arrow corresponds to the axis of the femur

a smooth intertrochanteric surface. The superior margin of the acetabulum is likewise resected to leave a smooth lateral surface to the pelvis (Fig. 5.16). The limb is then supported postoperatively in Hamilton Russell traction (Fig. 5.17). This form of traction maintains length and correct rotation of the limb and is applied for four to six weeks until a fibrous scar has formed at the operation site, so as to limit subsequent telescoping. The patient mobilizes, at first non-weight-bearing and gradually taking increased weight. Inevitably the limb will shorten and an appropriate shoe raise will subsequently be required. The patient will usually need the support of a walking stick in his opposite hand.

Congenital dislocation of the hip

Congenital dislocation of the hip is theoretically a preventable condition and in an ideal world surgical procedures should rarely be required. Potentially unstable hips may be recognized at birth by Barlow's modification of Ortolani's test, and if the hips are splinted in a position of abduction, flexion and lateral rotation for eight to twelve weeks, they will usually stabilize in the reduced position. If they escape detection at birth, subluxation or dislocation is then not usually recognized until the child begins to walk at a year. Even at this stage conservative treatment with gentle traction and progressive abduction may achieve reduction. Forceful attempts at manipulative reduction cause avascular necrosis of the upper femoral epiphysis with disastrous results. The older the child at diagnosis the higher the incidence of imperfect reduction because of soft tissue obstruction within the acetabulum, usually an inturned fibrocartilaginous labrum or limbus. Operative reduction is then required. Excessive anteversion of the femoral neck may have developed which must also be corrected by lateral rotation osteotomy of the femur, otherwise recurrent subluxation is likely. If concentric reduction and correction of anteversion is achieved before the age of three by either conservative or surgical means, there is good prospect that the acetabulum will develop normally and give good containment of the femoral head. If perfect reduction has not been obtained by this age, the acetabular roof is unlikely to develop fully and an innominate osteotomy may be required to stabilize the joint.

Open reduction of congenital dislocation of the hip
This operation is normally performed between one and three years in infants in whom conservative reduction has failed. A preoperative arthrogram will confirm the displacement and indicate the nature of the obstruction. The anterior approach (p. 93) is used. A transverse skin incision below the anterior superior spine may be used to leave a less conspicuous scar. The anterior capsule is exposed and opened through an H incision. Careful probing or digital palpation will confirm the nature and extent of the soft tissue obstruction which is then excised. An inturned limbus may be identified and lifted up with a blunt hook. At operation it is possible to assess the degree of anteversion by flexing the knee and hip to 90 degrees and measuring the angle between the neck and the axis of the tibia. When the head of the femur has been reduced the position of maximal stability is assessed, usually abduction with some flexion and internal rotation, and a plaster cast is applied to hold the legs symmetrically in this position for four weeks. At the end of this period, if excessive anteversion is present, a lateral rotation osteotomy is carried out through the upper femur. A lateral approach (p. 95) is made to the upper end of the femur which is exposed subperiosteally. Two guide wires are inserted, above and below the osteotomy site, at an angle to each other which corresponds to the desired amount of correction. An osteo-

tomy is then carried out between the wires at a level about 2 cm below the lesser trochanter using a sharp osteotome and the bone is derotated until the two wires are parallel. A four hole plate is used to stabilize the osteotomy site, and a hip spica is applied for four weeks. Some surgeons add an element of varus at the osteotomy site by bending the plate a few degrees believing that this gives greater containment of the femoral head and in older children a small segment of the femur may be removed to produce some femoral shortening and so reduce the tension of the soft tissues at the hip joint.

Iliac osteotomy
Many techniques of pelvic osteotomy have been described. The most widely adopted is that of Salter (1961) (Fig. 5.18) which may be combined with open reduction of the dislocation. The hip is exposed through the anterior incision which is extended backwards to the mid point of the iliac crest. The iliac apophysis is split along the line of the crest and the lateral half with the periosteum of the external surface of the ilium is stripped as far as the sciatic notch and the acetabulum and the medial half with the periosteum of the inner aspect is stripped for a similar extent. After open reduction of the hip joint and lengthening of the adductors and iliopsoas if required, an osteotomy is performed from the anterior superior spine to the sciatic notch using a Gigli saw or thin osteotomes, great care being taken to protect the sciatic nerve and superior gluteal vessels as they pass through the sciatic notch. The distal fragment is tilted outwards and forwards and wedged open in this position by means of a suitably shaped graft cut from the iliac crest. Stability is further ensured by placing a Kirschner wire across the osteotomy site through the graft. The split iliac apophysis is then sutured together and after wound closure a single hip spica is applied with the hip in slight abduction flexion and medial rotation. The plaster is removed after six weeks and mobilization commenced.

OPERATIONS ON THE KNEE

Aspiration of the knee
Effusion occurs more commonly in the knee than any other joint. Aspiration is required to relieve discomfort of a large effusion or for diagnostic purposes. The knee joint cavity extends at least 3 cm proximal to the upper pole of the patella and aspiration is most comfortably and easily carried out in this suprapatellar pouch by the technique described on page 85.

Arthroscopic surgery of the knee
In recent years, techniques of arthroscopic surgery have been developed for such procedures as the removal of

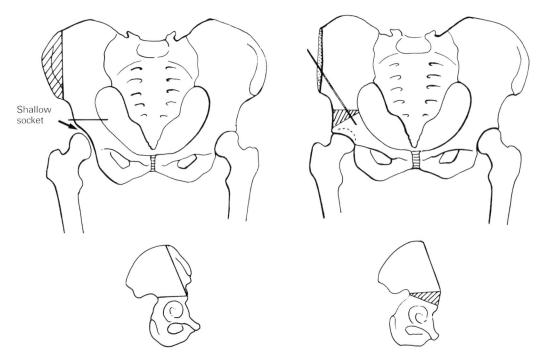

Shallow
socket

Fig. 5.18 Diagram of the Salter innominate osteotomy

torn cartilages, loose bodies and joint biopsies. These endoscopic procedures may be performed as day case surgery and the patient experiences less discomfort and speedier convalescence.

Arthroscopic surgery is a rapidly expanding field at the present time and its use is being extended to a wider range of joints and to more varied pathology. The techniques, however, are difficult and are best acquired by apprenticeship and experience.

Exposure of the knee joint

The knee joint is so superficial and accessible surgically that the possible surgical approaches are infinite. The one approach which may be regarded as standard is the anteromedial approach, which allows wide access and is appropriate for such procedures as synovectomy and replacement arthroplasty of the joint. The incision commences in the midline, 8 cm proximal to the patella and curves distally about 1 cm medial to its medial border, ending near·the tibial tubercle. The vastus medialis and joint capsule are divided in the line of the skin incision and the synovial membrane is incised throughout its length. The patella may then be everted and dislocated laterally to expose the entire anterior aspect of the knee joint (Fig. 5.19). Flexing the knee increases exposure of the intercondyle area and the lateral recesses. Sometimes it is necessary to detach the medial third of the patellar tendon from the tibial tubercle in order to displace the patella fully.

Replacement arthroplasty of the knee joint

In contrast to the hip, for which one basic design of arthroplasty and one basic technique of insertion with minor variations has been widely accepted, the state of knee arthroplasty at the present time is less well established. More than 100 designs of artificial knee joint are currently available—few have been subjected to prolonged clinical trials. The general experience, however, seems to suggest that they are less reliable and enduring than the hip arthroplasty. It is not possible therefore to recommend a standard textbook procedure at present. Ideally the surgeon who wishes to embark on knee arthroplasty should acquire first-hand experience of one of the many techniques available at the hands of an expert and concentrate on the perfection of one technique. Until experience has clearly indicated which of the many options is most reliable, it is probably wise for the occasional operator to avoid knee arthroplasty altogether. As for all types of replacement arthroplasty, these operations are best restricted to the elderly and severely disabled. They are not procedures for the young and active.

Synovectomy of the knee

Synovectomy may be useful in patients suffering from rheumatoid arthritis who experience severe pain in association with marked synovial reaction, persistent effusion, in whom good joint movement is retained and in whom the X-rays show good preservation of the joint

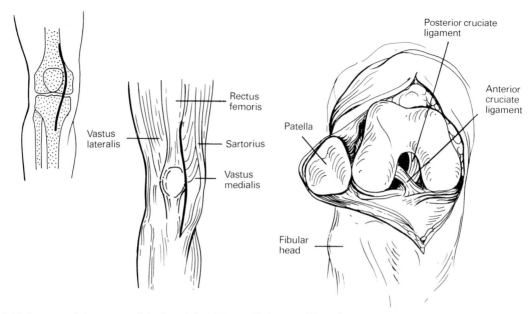

Fig. 5.19 Anteromedial exposure of the knee joint. The patella is rotated laterally

surface. It also has an established place in the management of haemophilic arthropathy (in patients who experience frequent bleeds) before advanced joint disorganization has occurred. The anteromedial approach (p. 100) is used. All accessible synovial membrane is stripped from the undersurface of the capsule and from the underlying bone, commencing with the suprapatellar pouch and extending to the lateral recesses and to the intercondylar area as far as can be reached. Through this approach about three-quarters of the synovial lining of· the knee can be removed. Bone nibblers are useful for clearing the synovium in the more remote recesses of the joint. In rheumatoid arthritis a clear plane of separation is easily developed between the synovium and the underlying tissues. In haemophilic patients this plane tends to be obliterated.

Post-operative management is important. The knee must be splinted for the first few days until the quadriceps has regained control and thereafter knee mobilization is pursued with active physiotherapy. Manipulation under anaesthesia may be required in two weeks, if 90 degrees of flexion has not been achieved by then.

Removal of the medial meniscus
The menisci of the knee perform a valuable weight distributing function. Following their removal, the weight transmitted across the knee joint is concentrated at much smaller areas of contact of the incongruous articular surfaces and degenerative arthritis will usually develop after an interval of some years. For this reason menisci must be conserved if at all possible. Meniscectomy should only be undertaken when the meniscus

is so damaged that it no longer performs its useful function. Clinical diagnosis of a torn meniscus can be difficult and in one large series was accurate in only 60% of cases. Arthrography or arthroscopy greatly increase the diagnostic accuracy and should be used whenever the diagnosis is in doubt. In recent years, it has also been recognized that degeneration of the meniscus is a common accompaniment of ageing and that in most cases it is not a source of lasting symptoms. The finding of degenerative changes therefore in a meniscus is not per se an indication for meniscectomy. Meniscectomy is indicated when the cartilage tear produces mechanical instability or locking of the knee or gives rise to persistent localized pain and tenderness.

Preoperative treatment
The patient should be taught how to carry out quadriceps exercises before operation. These exercises, which are essential to prevent wasting of the muscles, are difficult to learn after operation when the knee is painful and heavily bandaged.

Operation
A pneumatic tourniquet should be used. The knee is flexed over the end of the operating table. The surgeon sits facing it with the foot resting in his lap. An anteromedial incision is made, which may be vertical or oblique (Fig. 5.20), the latter having the advantage of avoiding the infrapatellar branch of the saphenous nerve which if injured can cause postoperative discomfort. The capsule is divided in the line of the skin incision. The synovial membrane is picked up most eas-

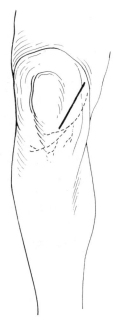

Fig. 5.20 Incision for removal of medial meniscus. The oblique incision avoids the infrapatellar branch of the saphenous nerve

ily at the proximal end of the incision over the femoral condyle and is incised in its turn. The margins of the wound are retracted and the meniscus inspected. A bucket handle tear may be found displaced into the intercondylar area or a longitudinal split may be identified in the undisplaced cartilage. The anterior horn of the cartilage is hooked forward with a blunt hook and this may disclose marginal or parrot beak tears or a posterior peripheral tear. If no pathology is identified, the diagnosis is incorrect and the cartilage should be left in situ. The knee must then be carefully inspected for other abnormality which might have caused the patient's symptoms.

If the damage is a bucket handle tear, only the displaced portion need be removed and this is done by dividing its two points of attachment. This simple, atraumatic procedure leaves a rim of healthy meniscus which may still perform a useful function. If total meniscectomy is required, the anterior horn is hooked upwards with a blunt hook, a knife is passed beneath the meniscus sweeping laterally and upwards into the intercondylar area to detach the anterior horn. This is then grasped with a Kocher's or similar forceps and the meniscus firmly drawn forwards. The peripheral attachments are divided with a sharp knife. This is easily accomplished for the anterior half because it is under direct vision but the posterior half of the meniscus is largely out of sight and is much more difficult to mobilize. Powerful retraction and the use of Smillie knives

with an end-cutting surface are useful here. The cartilage should be pulled onto the cutting edge of the knife by means of the Kocher's forceps and gradually mobilized and pulled into the intercondylar area. Once this displacement has been achieved, the posterior attachment is easily divided. If a substantial part of the posterior horn breaks away and is left behind, a separate posteromedial incision may be required. The site for this incision is identified by passing a curved artery forceps through the anterior wound so that its point can be felt at the joint line on the postero-medial aspect. A short, vertical incision is then made centered on the point of the forceps. The fragment of posterior horn is seen and removed under vision. The synovium, capsule and skin are closed with absorbable sutures, a compression bandage is applied and the knee splinted in extension with a plaster slab or a canvas splint. The splint and bandage are retained for ten days, during which time the patient practises quadriceps exercises. He may take weight on the limb or use crutches according to his inclination and can be discharged from hospital the day after operation. Following removal of the plaster, a short period of supervised physiotherapy will speed his recovery.

Removal of the lateral meniscus
Injuries of the lateral meniscus are less common but can occur and cystic change within the meniscus may also necessitate meniscectomy.

Operation
This is similar to that described for the removal of the medial meniscus. The central portion of the lateral meniscus is free of capsular attachment and therefore peripheral dissection may be slightly easier. The lateral geniculate artery should be looked for and cauterised as it can cause troublesome bleeding after the tourniquet is removed.

Removal of loose bodies from the knee
The knee is a large and complex joint and only a small part of it can be inspected through any one incision. It is important therefore that a loose body be located either by the patient or by X-ray prior to surgery. A blind exploration of the knee to find a loose body is likely to be unsuccessful. When the loose body has been located, a short incision is made directly over it and the loose body removed. In the case of non-radio opaque loose bodies, these should be located prior to surgery and securely transfixed with a needle before the joint is opened.

Operation for osteochondritis dissecans
Osteochondritis dissecans usually involves the intercondylar aspect of the medial femoral condyle. The fragment, if not separated in young children, may go on to spontaneous healing following a period of immobiliz-

OPERATIONS ON BONES AND JOINTS   103

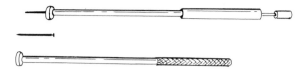

Fig. 5.21 Instruments used for the insertion of the Smillie pin. (See also Fig. 5.42)

ation of the joint. Surgical treatment is not required. If, in the adolescent, the fragment is clearly mobile and causing symptoms it should be removed, or if very large, repositioned and secured by Smillie pins. The incision is the same as that for medial meniscectomy. The softened and mobile area of cartilage, if not detached, can be easily identified by palpation with a blunt dissector. An incision is made through the margin of the loose fragment, which is then removed. If very large, the fibrotic, sclerotic bed is curetted and drilled at a number of points to improve vascularity. The fragment is then repositioned and pinned, using Smillie pins and the appropriate introducer (Fig. 5.21). If the fragment has been separated from its bed for some time, it will no longer fit the bed from which it came and no attempt should then be made to reposition it. Following removal of an osteochondritic fragment, the defect heals remarkably well with fibrocartilage in time. Fortunately the lesion usually occupies a non-weight bearing area. The postoperative management is as described for meniscectomy.

Patellectomy
Patellectomy is indicated for comminuted fractures and occasionally in severe cases of chondromalacia patellae and when osteoarthritic change is concentrated in the patellofemoral joint. A transverse incision is made over the patella and the vertical incision is made in the retinacular fibres which cover the bone. Using sharp dissection with a scalpel, the patella is carefully shelled out of its tendinous attachments, preserving them as far as possible. The aponeurotic flaps are overlapped with mattress sutures, a compression bandage is applied and the knee supported in a plaster splint until the quadriceps have recovered their activity. Mobilization can be commenced usually at the end of two or three weeks, except in traumatic cases in which the lateral expansions of the quadriceps mechanism have also been injured, in which case they must be splinted for six weeks to allow healing of the extensor mechanism.

Recurrent dislocation of the patella
This occurs most commonly in young girls in whom there is some minor congenital abnormality such as excessive genu valgum, poor development of the lateral femoral condyle, small and high patella or joint laxity. As many of these minor anomalies are inherited, it may

be familial and is often bilateral. Recurrence may also follow traumatic dislocation of the patella which has not been protected sufficiently after the first incident to allow the capsule to heal.

Many operations are described for the treatment of this disorder and the selected procedure must take account of the underlying pathology: for example, in the presence of severe genu valgum, a supracondylar osteotomy would be appropriate. An operation widely practised in the past has been the distal and medial displacement of the insertion of the patellar tendon into the tibial tubercle, which may be appropriate where the patella is high and laterally displaced (*Hauser's operation*). However, it is becoming increasingly recognized that re-routing of the patella in this way leads to later degenerative arthritis in the patellofemoral joint and this procedure must now be rarely indicated. It must never be carried out in a growing child for it would damage the upper tibial growth plate causing tibial recurvatum.

A less traumatic procedure consists of the formation of a check ligament from the lateral third of the patellar tendon—the *Roux-Goldthwait procedure*. This was originally developed for the younger child but it works well at all ages.

Operation
A midline incision is made from the lower pole of the patella to the tibial tuberosity. A release incision is made in the lateral capsule, the patellar tendon is identified and a vertical split is made separating the lateral third from the medial two-thirds. The lateral portion is detached from the tibial tuberosity and passed underneath the tendon to be sutured to an osteoperiosteal flap on the anteromedial aspect of the upper tibia (Fig. 5.22). The knee is immobilized in a plaster cylinder for six weeks, quadriceps exercises being maintained throughout and continued during the post-plaster mobilization period.

Popliteal cyst (Semimembranosus bursa)
This appears as a tense cystic swelling in the popliteal fossa to the medial side of the midline. It is the result of a one-way valvular mechanism which allows the escape of synovial fluid from the knee into the normal semimembranosus bursa. The condition is usually painless and tends to resolve with time and rarely requires treatment. Very large and painful cysts may be excised through a transverse incision. It is important to identify and close the communication with the knee joint.

Arthrodesis of the knee
This operation is occasionally indicated in a joint destroyed by infective arthritis or by degenerative arthritis in a young person who is unsuited for replacement arthroplasty.

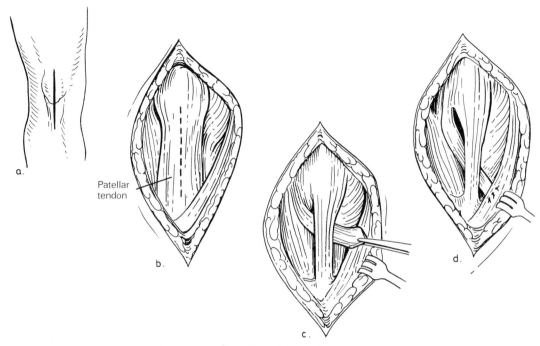

Patellar tendon

Fig. 5.22 Roux-Goldthwait procedure for recurrent dislocation of the patella

The most satisfactory and consistently effective technique is the compression arthrodesis as described by Charnley.

Operation
With the patient supine, a transverse or S-shaped incision is made at the level of the middle of the patella. The incision is deepened through the joint capsule at both sides and the infrapatellar tendon is divided. The knee is then flexed to expose the collateral and cruciate liga-

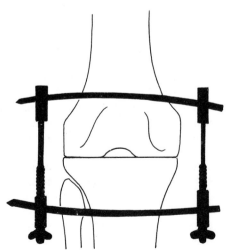

Fig. 5.23 Arthrodesis of the knee using the Charnley compression apparatus

ments which are divided, allowing the tibia to be displaced forward in relation to the femur. The joint surfaces are then resected with a tenon saw removing as little bone as possible. The cut surfaces should be flat and so shaped that, when co-apted, the limb is in normal alignment with regard to abduction and adduction and in about 15 degrees of flexion. Steinmann pins are inserted transversely through the distal femur and upper tibia at their mid points about 5 cm from the bone ends. The compression apparatus (Fig. 5.23) is applied to the ends of the pins and the wing nuts tightened to produce moderate bowing of the Steinmann pins; this will produce rigid stability at the site of arthrodesis. The wound is closed and a plaster cylinder applied. At four weeks, the compression apparatus is removed and a new plaster reapplied for a further four weeks, by which time the arthrodesis should be consolidated.

Muscular imbalance of the knee
Isolated paralysis of the quadriceps does not give rise to great disability for the knee may be stabilized in extension through the action of gluteus maximus in extending the femur when the foot is securely balanced on the ground. Even slight flexion contracture at the knee may render this mechanism incompetent however and a supracondylar osteotomy to correct the flexion deformity may then be required. When gluteus maximus is also paralysed and the foot muscles are incompetent, a caliper is necessary to stabilize the knee.

A persistent tendency to flexion deformity at the knee due to imbalance between overacting hamstrings and weak quadriceps—characteristic of spastic paralysis—can be corrected by *Egger's operation*, in which the hamstring muscles are detached from the tibia and re-attached to the distal femur, where they reinforce hip extension rather than knee flexion.

Flexion deformities in the knee may also develop in chronically sick and elderly patients, who are bed- or chair-bound and neglected. If their deformities cannot be corrected by continuous traction, tenotomy of the hamstring tendons may be required, and if this proves inadequate, the origin of the two heads of gastrocnemius and the proximal attachment of the posterior capsule of the knee joint are erased from the bone and allowed to slide distally.

Supracondylar osteotomy

Severe genu valgum or varum and knee flexion deformity may be corrected by supracondylar osteotomy. The technique of osteotomy—osteoclasis described on page 85 may be used. Alternatively, in older children or adults, a complete osteotomy may be carried out with the removal of an appropriate wedge of bone to allow correction of the deformity and the osteotomy site is then stabilized by internal fixation, either with metal staples or a short plate. A plaster cast is applied and maintained for five or six weeks until there is radiological evidence of union.

Quadricepsplasty

Occasionally following fractures of the distal femur, adhesions may develop between the quadriceps mechanism and the underlying bone, which limit knee flexion. If this gives rise to significant disability, the operation of quadricepsplasty is indicated. This operation is a major undertaking and should only be carried out in patients who are well-motivated to co-operate with the extensive and often painful postoperative physiotherapy which is required.

Operation. A midline vertical incision is made in the front of the distal thigh continuing into the anteromedial incision of the knee (p. 100). The knee joint is first opened and any adhesions, which may be present within the knee joint itself, are divided. Sometimes these constitute the main source of contracture and no further dissection is required. However, usually it is necessary then to isolate the rectus femoris from the remaining components of the quadriceps and adhesions between the quadriceps and the bone are separated, as they are identified. After operation the knee is immobilized in a plaster splint in 90 degrees of flexion. The splint is removed at intervals throughout the day to allow the knee to be extended but the flexed position is retained throughout the night. Splintage is discarded when the

patient has regained active control of the range of movement gained during the operation. Physiotherapy may have to be continued for several months.

High tibial osteotomy

High tibial osteotomy is carried out for osteoarthritis of the knee in patients with varus or valgus deformity. It is particularly successful in cases in which the arthritis is largely confined to one compartment of the knee. The osteotomy is carried out just above the patellar tendon insertion about 2 cm below the tibial articular surface. A wedge of bone is excised to restore the normal alignment of the limb. It is essential, before the operation is undertaken, to measure precisely the amount of correction required so that the correct thickness of wedge is removed. X-ray control is required during the operation.

The operation of lateral wedge osteotomy will be described as this is more commonly performed. The exposure for medial wedge osteotomy is easier because of the absence of the fibula, but otherwise is similar.

Lateral wedge osteotomy. A transverse incision is made over the upper tibia extending from the head of the fibula to the tibial tuberosity. It is prudent to identify the common peroneal nerve on the lateral aspect of the neck of the fibula and mobilize it so that it can be kept out of harms way during the rest of the operation.

The lateral surface of the upper tibia is exposed subperiosteally as far as the patellar tendon and the lateral ligament and biceps tendon are detached carefully from the head of the fibula preserving the continuity of their attachment to the fascia on the lateral aspect of the upper fibula. The proximal 1.5 cm of the head of the fibula is then removed with an osteotome. This allows access to the posterior surface of the tibia. A guidewire is inserted at the level of the proposed osteotomy 2 cm below the articular surface and passed medially to emerge from the medial cortex at the same level. Its position is confirmed by X-ray. Bone spikes are then placed in front of the tibia deep to the patellar tendon and posteriorly passing it in contact with the bone while the knee is flexed. This ensures that the popliteal vessels and nerves are held out of the way. While an assistant holds the soft tissues away from the bone with these spikes, the surgeon, with broad osteotomes, carefully cuts a wedge of predetermined thickness, using the guidewire to mark the proximal surface of the wedge. This avoids the risk of drifting too close to the articular surface. When the wedge removal is completed the guidewire is withdrawn. The osteotomy is held closed by the assistant and is secured by two offset staples (Fig. 5.24). The soft tissues are repaired and a compression bandage and plaster backslab applied.

Early weight-bearing is allowed and knee mobilization is commenced at two weeks, but a protective plaster slab

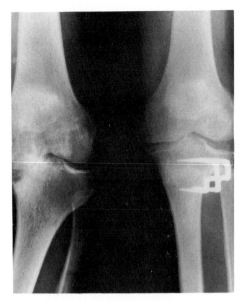

Fig. 5.24 X-ray showing upper tibial osteotomy for medial compartment osteoarthritis with genu varum

is retained while weight-bearing for a further two weeks. Thereafter unprotected weight-bearing is allowed.

OPERATIONS ON THE ANKLE

Exposure of the ankle joint

The anterolateral approach gives excellent exposure of the ankle and tarsal joints, and causes minimal disturbance to the soft parts. The incision, shown in Figure 5.25, begins in front of the fibula 5 cm above the joint, and is carried downwards between the lateral malleolus and peroneus tertius, to end over the base of the fourth metatarsal. The superior and inferior extensor retinacula are divided as far as is necessary to expose the capsule of the ankle joint.

Arthroplasty of the ankle

At the present time, replacement arthroplasties of the ankle are being developed and undergoing trial. The value of these procedures is not yet established.

Arthrodesis of the ankle

This may be required for post-traumatic arthritis following intra-articular fractures involving the ankle joint and occasionally in chronic arthritis of inflammatory origin.

Many techniques for ankle arthrodesis are described. Charnley has developed a compression technique similar to that which is now standard for the knee. His approach to the ankle joint is through the transverse anterior incision, dividing all the extensor tendons and the anterior joint capsule and lateral ligaments, which allows the ankle to be opened widely. The joint surfaces are then resected and Steinmann pins passed through the distal tibia and the talus and the compression apparatus attached as in the knee arthrodesis. The extensor tendons are repaired and the wound closed. Charnley states that this very radical approach does not give rise to any lasting disability. A compression arthrodesis can, how-

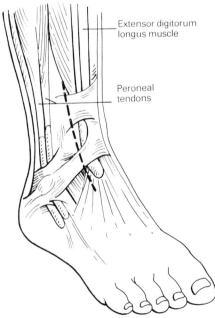

Extensor digitorum longus muscle

Peroneal tendons

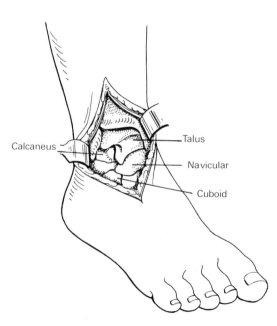

Calcaneus

Talus

Navicular

Cuboid

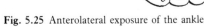

Fig. 5.25 Anterolateral exposure of the ankle

ever, be satisfactorily performed through two lateral incisions with preservation of all tendons, although the more limited access undoubtedly makes the resection of the bone ends more difficult. A simpler, non compression method works well in most instances.

Technique

The ankle joint is exposed through the anterolateral approach. The ankle joint is opened and the articular surface is excised from the distal tibia and from the talus. The dissection is carried down on the medial side removing the articular cartilage from the medial malleolus and from the medial surface of the talus. The lateral surface of the talus is dealt with similarly but it is not usually possible nor necessary to excise so much on the lateral side as on the medial side. Cancellous chips are removed from the anterior iliac crest. With the foot in full plantar flexion the cancellous chips are packed into the resultant gap and the foot is then brought up to neutral or a position of 5 degrees of plantar flexion if there is some shortening. The foot and ankle are immobilized in a below knee plaster for eight weeks or until arthrodesis is sound. Weight-bearing is allowed after two weeks.

OPERATIONS ON THE HINDFOOT

Calcaneal osteotomy

Inversion of the calcaneus may exist as an isolated deformity or be part of a residual club foot deformity in which case it may be associated with a short tendo-Achilles. Correction of the deformity is obtained by eversion osteotomy of the calcaneum.

Operation

The patient lies prone. The incision extends obliquely across the medial aspect of the heel and proximally along the medial border of the tendo-Achilles for 3 cm. The tendo-Achilles is divided in a stepcut manner. The neurovascular bundle behind the medial malleolus is identified and preserved and the calcaneum is exposed subperiosteally on its superior and medial aspect. An osteotomy is carried out as shown in Figure 5.26. A wedge of cortical bone obtained either from the tibia or from the bone bank is driven into the osteotomy site from the medial aspect, holding it open in the desired position. The tendo-Achilles is repaired, if necessary with lengthening, and a knee plaster is applied and weight-bearing allowed after two weeks. The plaster is retained for eight weeks.

In pes cavus deformities associated with heel inversion, where the os calcis is of normal length, it is better to obtain correction by removing a wedge from the lat-

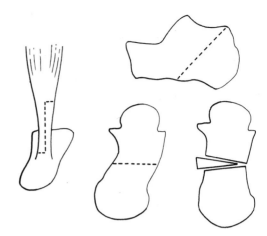

Fig. 5.26 Correction of heel inversion by an opening wedge osteotomy of the calcaneum

eral aspect of the os calcis, producing slight shortening of the bone and relaxation of the plantar soft tissues.

Triple fusion

In this operation arthrodesis of the subtalar and midtarsal joints is carried out. The operation is designed to produce a well shaped and stable foot and is indicated in a wide range of deformities and paralytic disorders of the foot. The operation should not be carried out until skeletal growth has ceased. The incision is shown in Figure 5.27 and is deepened to expose the lateral and dorsal aspects of the tarsus, care being taken to preserve

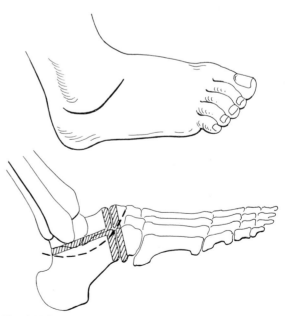

Fig. 5.27 Incision and extent of bone resection in the operation of triple fusion

the extensor tendons. The soft tissues are mobilized as close to the bone as possible until the subtalar and midtarsal joints are fully exposed. Using thin osteotomes, the joint surfaces are resected in parallel to each other, exposure of the medial parts of the joints being obtained by an assistant forcibly inverting the foot. Appropriate wedges may be removed to correct any deformity. Sometimes a short medial incision over the talonavicular joint is necessary to allow complete clearance of the joint surfaces. If the joint excision has been accurately performed the bone surfaces should then be closely opposed with correction of deformity. The three joints are stabilized by transfixion with Kirschner wires or by use of small staples. Any residual gaps between the bone surfaces should be packed with cancellous bone graft. A below knee plaster is applied over a padded dressing and this is changed to a close fitting plaster at two weeks when the Kirschner wires can be withdrawn. Weight-bearing is allowed at four weeks; the plaster cast is removed at eight to ten weeks, when there is radiological evidence of union.

Pes Planus

Mobile flat foot does not require surgical correction. Spasmodic flat foot due to a congenital tarsal coalition may be cured before the age of fourteen by excision of the anomalous bar. In older children, if the symptoms warrant it, a triple fusion may be required.

Pes Cavus

Most cases of pes cavus cause little disability and do not require surgical treatment. There is no entirely satisfactory surgical correction for this deformity. *Steindler's operation*, which involves division of the shortened structures of the sole at their attachment to the calcaneum, produces temporary benefit only. Correction of heel inversion (p. 107), if present, may improve the posture of the foot as a whole and likewise correction of the associated toe clawing may also improve foot function. Occasionally a triple fusion or wedge resection of the midtarsal joint may be required, but the results of this procedure in pes cavus are disappointing.

Congenital talipes equinovarus

Club foot, which does not respond readily to conservative manipulation and corrective strapping, should be released surgically at an early stage, ideally between two to four months. If the deformity is allowed to exist for a longer period, adaptive changes occur in the bony skeleton, which makes full correction thereafter difficult and triple fusion may become necessary at a later stage. Early soft tissue release is therefore ideal.

The incision is made from the medial border of the tendo-Achilles to below the medial malleolus and forward to the medial border of the foot. The tibialis pos-

terior, flexor digitorum longus, the neurovascular bundle and the flexor hallucis longus are identified behind the medial malleolus in that order from front to back. The neurovascular bundle is traced to its terminal branching in the sole of the foot and carefully preserved throughout the subsequent operation. The tendo-Achilles is then lengthened in a stepcut manner. The tibialis posterior, flexor digitorum longus and flexor hallucis longus tendons are lengthened in the same way. The capsule and ligaments on the medial and inferior aspects of the talonavicular joint are widely opened to allow correction of the talonavicular subluxation, which is a feature of the club foot deformity, and the ligaments on the medial aspect of the subtalar joint are similarly divided. Finally division of the capsular ligaments on the plantar aspect of the midtarsal joint are divided and it is now possible to manipulate the foot into full correction of its varus and inversion deformities. The stepcut tendons are now repaired with appropriate lengthening. The foot is immobilized in the correct position in a well padded plaster cast. The corrective plaster is maintained for at least ten weeks.

Paralytic drop foot deformity

Paralytic drop foot may result from poliomyelitis or injury to the lateral popliteal nerve. The deformity can be controlled by one of the many varieties of drop foot splint but, if the patient finds this unacceptable, surgical correction is possible. If the tibialis posterior muscle is acting normally, triple arthrodesis may be carried out,

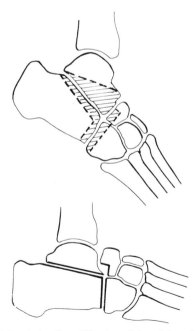

Fig. 5.28 Lambrinudi modification of the triple arthrodesis to correct paralytic drop foot deformity

the tendon tibialis posterior being then transferred through the interosseous membrane to be attached to the dorsum of the foot where it will act as a dorsiflexor. If this muscle is paralysed, a Lambrinudi variation of the triple arthrodesis is carried out in which a wedge of bone is removed from the plantar aspect of the talus, as shown in Figure 5.28 and the triple fusion is carried out with the talus in full equinus and the rest of the foot in dorsiflexion.

OPERATIONS ON THE FOREFOOT

Ingrowing toenail

Persistent ingrowing toenail is best treated by wedge resection as illustrated in Figure 5.29. In carrying out this procedure, care must be taken to remove the entire nail fold and the germinal zone related to the piece of nail which is being removed. This fans out laterally at the base of the nail and meticulous dissection must be carried out to ensure that an irregular spike of nail does not recur.

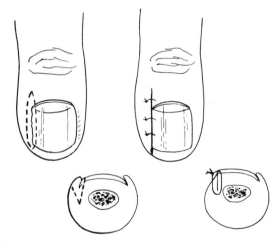

Fig. 5.29 Wedge resection for ingrowing toenail

Radical excision of the nail bed (Zadek's operation)

This is indicated for more general deformities of the nail such as onychogryphosis. The nail is first avulsed. The flap of skin overlying the base of the nail is elevated proximally and the sub-adjacent germinal layer of the nail bed is excised, paying particular attention to the lateral extensions, which are loosely attached to the bony expansion at the base of the terminal phalanx. The flap of skin is then sutured back to the base of the nail bed. If the skin underlying the nail is metaplastic and unhealthy, it is better to excise this entirely and to cover the residual defect with a skin graft.

Claw toes

Clawing of the toes is usually a feature of pes cavus but can occur independently. The common cause is a muscle imbalance resulting from weakness in the intrinsic muscles of the foot. If the clawing is severe and giving rise to symptoms, surgical correction is possible. If the toes can be corrected passively, the operation of choice is a flexor to extensor transfer whereas, if the deformity is fixed, interphalangeal fusion is preferred.

Flexor to extensor transfer in toes—Girdlestone's operation
Through separate dorsolateral incisions at the base of each toe, the fibrous flexor sheath is exposed and incised. The flexor tendons are divided as far distally as possible and the long flexor alone is brought to the dorsal aspect of the toe. It is passed through the extensor expansion and sutured to it with fine, non-absorbable suture. Thereafter the flexor tendon will act in the manner of the intrinsics, i.e. it will flex the metatarsophalangeal joint and extend the interphalangeal joints. Following the operation, the toes are held in the correct position by means of a plaster cast which extends forward to the tip of the toes. The plaster cast is retained for four weeks.

Interphalangeal fusion
Through mid-dorsal incisions in each toe, the extensor tendon is split longitudinally, the dorsal capsule of each joint is incised and the articular surface of the bone ends resected. Small, sharp chisels and gouges are useful here. When the two joints have been cleared in each toe, a Kirschner wire is used to transfix them. This is first inserted into the proximal surface of the middle phalanx and guided through the distal phalanx to emerge at the tip of the toe. It is then driven retrogradely across the proximal interphalangeal joint. The wire is removed after four weeks, during which time the patient may walk in an open-toed sandal.

Hammer toe

This term is applied to a flexion deformity at the proximal interphalangeal joint of the toe, usually the second. The condition is best treated by arthrodesis of the affected joint using a peg in socket procedure, which has the additional advantage of shortening the toe slightly, for a hammer toe is usually excessively long.

The first step in the operation consists in subcutaneous tenotomy of the extensor tendon in order to correct the dorsiflexion deformity of the first phalanx. The dorsal corn is excised by a longitudinal elliptical incision and the extensor tendon and dorsal capsule are incised. The head of the proximal phalanx is cleared and, with small bone shears and an osteotome, is shaped into a peg which should include the dorsal cortex to give increased strength. Then using a suitably sized drill or burr, a hole is bored into the base of the middle phalanx. This phalanx is now impacted on to the peg and no additional fixation should be required, although it is prudent to support the toe with a collodion splint for the first week or two. Weight-bearing in an open-toed sandal is allowed immediately.

Mallet toe

This is a flexion deformity of the terminal joint. The bones are too small at this level to allow a spike arthrodesis and it is sufficient simply to resect the joint surfaces and stabilize them with a short Kirschner wire, as in the Lambrinudi procedure.

Hallux valgus

Hallux valgus is exceedingly common, particularly among women in the Western world. Only a minority of cases produce significant symptoms and operative treatment should therefore be very selectively used. There is no point in carrying out any operative procedure for this condition, unless the patient agrees thereafter to wear shoes designed for function rather than fashion, for unsuitable footwear with high heels and narrow toes is undoubtedly a constant aggravating factor in the production of this deformity. Once the toe begins to deviate from its normal alignment, the condition tends to get progressively worse because the long tendons now bowstring to the lateral side and the mechanical advantage of the adductor is increased whereas that of the abductor is diminished. Any operative correction of hallux valgus must take these factors into account.

Many operations have been described to correct this deformity and the choice of procedure depends to some extent on the age and sex of the patient and on the degree of the deformity. Correction of the alignment by metatarsal osteotomy is indicated in young people in whom the joint remains relatively healthy. In older women, a Keller's arthroplasty is the operation of choice; while in men and when faced with a very gross deformity, arthrodesis is likely to produce the most satisfactory result.

Metatarsal osteotomy

There are many ways of carrying out this procedure; some exceedingly complex. The *Wilson osteotomy* has the virtue of simplicity and in a recent review proved to be as satisfactory as any. A dorsomedial incision is made over the distal half of the first metatarsal, which is then exposed subperiosteally. An oblique osteotomy is then carried out through the neck of the metatarsal, as illustrated in Figure 5.30. The osteotomy can be performed with an oscillating saw or by multiple drilling completed with an osteotome. The hallux and the metatarsal head are then rotated into normal alignment and the meta-

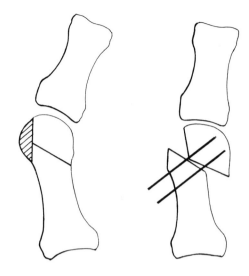

Fig. 5.30 Diagram of Wilson's osteotomy

tarsal head is displaced laterally in relation to the metatarsal shaft where it may be stabilized by two Kirschner wires. It is important that no dorsal angulation should take place at the osteotomy site. The medial bony projection from the stump of the metatarsal is removed and after wound closure a plaster is applied with the hallux held in slight overcorrection. A new weight-bearing plaster is applied in two weeks and retained for a further two weeks and thereafter the patient may walk in an orthopaedic sandal. At eight weeks the osteotomy is united and the Kirschner wires are removed.

In older patients hallux valgus deformity is usually part of a more widespread disorganisation of the forefoot, characterized by collapse of the transverse arch with excessive pressure and pain under the metatarsal heads and frequently dorsal and lateral subluxation of the metatarsal phalangeal joints of one or more of the small toes with consequently poor toe function, which again puts excessive pressure on the metatarsal heads. The hallux valgus deformity may be so severe that the hallux comes to lie over or under the neighbouring toes. In such a foot, surgery confined to the hallux valgus deformity alone would relieve only one component of the patient's discomfort and additional procedures, such as metatarsal osteotomies and excision of the dislocated proximal phalanges may also be required. No operative procedures, however, are going to restore such a foot to its pristine condition, and the patient must be made fully aware of this before surgery is undertaken.

Keller's arthroplasty

A dorsomedial incision is made over the base of the proximal phalanx and the metatarsal head and neck. The soft tissues are stripped from the bones by sharp

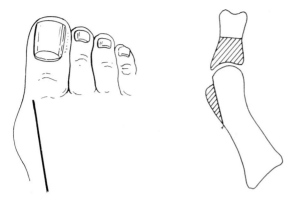

Fig. 5.31 Incision and extent of bone removal in Keller's arthroplasty

dissection. The structures which must be mobilized include the joint capsule and the four short muscles, which are attached to the base of the proximal phalanx. The medial prominence of the metatarsal head is trimmed as shown in Figure 5.31 and at least half of the proximal phalanx is removed. The skin only requires closure. The toe is then bandaged in slight overcorrection and the patient may walk in a wooden soled sandal within a few days. The patient should when possible maintain the foot in elevation until the postoperative swelling has subsided. Intrinsic exercises should be maintained postoperatively until maximal toe function is restored. It is sometimes useful to keep a small silicone rubber wedge between the first and second toes for some months after operation, if there is any tendency towards recurrence.

Hallux rigidus

Stiffness of the metatarsophalangeal joint may occur during adolescence when the common pathology is osteochondritis dissecans of the metatarsal head. At this age it is rarely painful and no treatment is usually required, although, if the patient finds the condition limiting, removal of a dorsal wedge at the base of the proximal phalanx may give a more useful arc of movement by allowing increased dorsiflexion.

In older people hallux rigidus is caused by osteoarthritis. It is extremely common and only a minority of people have symptoms sufficiently troublesome to warrant surgery. In some, discomfort is due simply to pressure on the marginal osteophytes which develop around the osteoarthritic joint, and simple removal of the osteophytes will bring sufficient relief. When the pain arises from the joint itself, Keller's arthroplasty or arthrodesis is carried out. Arthrodesis is probably the better procedure in the working man but should only be performed when some dorsiflexion is possible at the interphalangeal joint. Keller's arthroplasty is more suitable in women, who in general prefer to retain some

movement in the metatarsophalangeal joint to allow them to wear varying heights of heel.

Arthrodesis of metatarsophalangeal joint

The joint is exposed as in the Keller's operation. Marginal osteophytes are removed and the articular surfaces are denuded of cartilage and then shaped to form close contact. The arthrodesis is stabilized by means of a transfixion screw with 5 or 10 degrees of dorsiflexion in men and rather more in women. Slight valgus should also be allowed in women to facilitate subsequent shoe fitting. A below knee walking plaster extended forward to support the toe is worn for six to eight weeks.

Clawing of the hallux

Flexion deformity of the interphalangeal joint of the big toe may develop following tibialis anterior paralysis, or more commonly as part of the generalized clawing associated with pes cavus resulting from weakness of the intrinsic muscles. The first metatarsal is abnormally flexed and painful callosities tend to develop under the metatarsal head and over the dorsum of the clawed toe. *Jones' operation* is designed to correct both aspects of the deformity by interphalangeal fusion and tendon transfer of extensor hallucis longus tendon to the neck of the first metatarsal. A transverse incision is made on the dorsal aspect of the interphalangeal joint and the joint surfaces are resected using sharp chisels. The joint is stabilized in a straight position by two crossing Kirschner wires. The extensor hallucis longus tendon is divided as distally as possible and a hole is drilled through the neck of the first metatarsal large enough to allow the tendon to be passed through and sutured back on itself in moderate tension. A below knee walking plaster is retained for five weeks. The Kirschner wires are removed at eight weeks when the arthrodesis is solid.

Overlapping fifth toe

This is a common congenital deformity in which the fifth toe overlies the fourth and is subject to pressure from shoe wear. It is best corrected by the *Butler operation*. The skin incision starts in the dorsal aspect of the foot at the base of the fifth toe and passes distally to encircle the toe near its base. Care must be taken to ensure that the digital nerves and vessels are preserved. The incision then extends on to the plantar pad at the base of the toe, where a small circle of skin is removed to match the diameter of the toe. Through the dorsal incision, the extensor digitorum longus tendon and dorsal capsule of the metatarsophalangeal joint are divided. This allows the toe to be displaced into its correct position, where it is anchored by suturing the skin of the toe to the margin of the circular skin defect. This leaves a small deficiency of skin on the dorsal aspect of the toe but the skin in this region is loose and readily closed.

Metatarsal head resection or forefoot arthroplasty

Patients with rheumatoid arthritis frequently develop disabling metatarsalgia due to loss of toe function, dislocation of the metatarsophalangeal joints and excessive weight borne by the metatarsal heads. Excision of all the metatarsal heads may produce marked relief of pain. Such an operation does not, however, improve the function of the forefoot and it must be reserved for people with rheumatoid arthritis, who generally have multiple joint problems and restricted walking ability. The operation is not suitable for forefoot disorganization in non-rheumatic cases, nor is it suitable for patients when there is any doubt about the peripheral circulation as delay in wound healing is a feature of this procedure.

Technique

Three longitudinal incisions are made in the dorsal aspect of the foot at the level of the metatarsophalangeal joints. One is placed on the dorso-medial aspect of the big toe, as for Keller's arthroplasty, and the other two between the remaining toes. Through these incisions, the bases of the proximal phalanges of the toes, which are usually dislocated dorsally, are exposed and at least half of the proximal phalanx of each toe is excised. The metatarsal heads are exposed and excised with an oblique cut, as shown in Figure 5.32. The trimmed metatarsal necks should then present a smooth and uniform curve. If one projects beyond this alignment, it will certainly give rise to pain subsequently. Finally, an ellipse of skin, transversely orientated, is removed from the sole of the foot just behind the weight-bearing pad, which in this deformity has been drawn forwards to face anteriorly rather than plantarwards. When this elliptical plantar wound is closed, the weight-bearing pad is drawn back to its proper position and the now rather floppy toes fall into better alignment. A light compres-

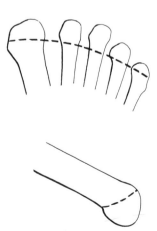

Fig. 5.32 Metatarsal head resection showing the amount of bone to be removed

sion bandage is applied to hold the toes in this position and when the wounds are healed a below knee walking plaster is applied for three weeks. Physiotherapy is directed towards strengthening the foot and toe muscles during the period of immobilization and subsequently to restore a moderate degree of toe function.

Not infrequently, some toes are more severely affected than others and the surgeon may in this event be tempted to carry out a metatarsal head resection only in the more troublesome toes. This, however, is invariably unwise for the remaining toes then become painful in turn.

In the non-rheumatic foot, in which only one or two metatarsal heads are displaced into the sole, a dorsal displacement osteotomy of the affected metatarsal may give relief. This operation is frequently indicated in conjunction with Keller's arthroplasty where one or more of the adjacent metatarsophalangeal joints may be affected in this way. Through a short incision the dorsal aspect of the neck of the affected metatarsal is divided obliquely. No fixation is required and immediate weight-bearing is allowed. The osteotomy will unite with dorsal displacement thus relieving pressure on the offending metatarsal head.

OPERATIONS FOR OSTEOMYELITIS

Improved social conditions and more effective treatment of primary foci of infection have greatly reduced the frequency and severity of osteomyelitis in developed countries. Elsewhere it continues to be a major problem. If infection is allowed to become established in bone it tends to cause extensive bone necrosis as a result of toxaemia and by interruption of the local blood supply. This is caused by pressure exerted by the inflammatory products together with periosteal stripping produced by the abscess when it escapes from bone under pressure. When large areas of bone death occur the organisms can linger there safe from the natural defences of the body and from antibiotics which cannot penetrate in the absence of a good blood supply. A state of chronic osteomyelitis is then established which may last for a lifetime. Other serious complications include damage to the adjacent growth plate and involvement of neighbouring joints.

Typically acute osteomyelitis is a disease of childhood and the common sites of involvement are the metaphyses frequently of the femur and upper tibia, but no bone is immune. In the adult the haemopoietic bones of the spine and pelvis are the most common locations. The infection usually reaches bone by the blood stream from a focus elsewhere such as a boil or infected wound or a urinary tract infection. The organism is the staphylococcus aureus in over 90% of cases but the rest are due to a wide range of organisms and the pattern may vary in different countries. Salmonella infections, for example, are common in countries with a high incidence of sickle cell disease.

Treatment is directed towards aborting the infection before it has a chance to become entrenched and involves both conservative and surgical measures. The first step is to try to identify the organism by blood culture, swabbing any obvious superficial source of infection or by local aspiration of the infected site. Antibiotic therapy is commenced immediately thereafter, before the bacterial confirmation is available. The antibiotic selected must be effective against staphylococcus aureus which may be assumed to be penicillin resistant, but should also cover the less common organisms including the coliforms which may occasionally be responsible. They must be administered intravenously and in high concentration initially. Developments in chemotherapy are so rapid that it is difficult to recommend in a textbook a drug regime that can be guaranteed to endure to the next edition, however at the time of writing, cloxacillin coupled with gentamycin or one of the injectable cephalosporins would be appropriate. Once the organism is identified and its sensitivity known the antibiotics can be varied accordingly. Chloramphenicol is of value if salmonella typhi is suspected. Once the acute illness has subsided the drugs may be administered orally and must be continued for at least three weeks after the symptoms and signs have settled. Surgery is indicated if an abscess is detectable when the child is first seen or if the antibiotic therapy has not produced a dramatic improvement in the patient's condition within 24 hours. The operation consists of a surgical incision down to bone at the level of maximal swelling and tenderness. Any subperiosteal abscess is evacuated and several drill holes are made in the metaphysis to allow the release of an intraosseus abscess. The wound is irrigated with an antibiotic solution and then closed over a vacuum drain. The limb should be splinted in a plaster cast to relieve pain and prevent pathological fracture, but the site of infection must be windowed to allow observation.

Osteomyelitis may also arise from infection introduced through compound wounds or during the course of surgery. This should be preventable by good surgical technique and by meticulous wound excision (p. 156).

Chronic osteomyelitis
Once chronic osteomyelitis is established, chemotherapy will do no more than control the recurrent exacerbations of infection. The key to management is surgical removal of sequestra and the eradication of abscess cavities and dead space by saucerisation and filling the resulting defect with viable soft tissue such as a muscle flap. Sometimes the chronic infection takes the form of diffuse sclerosis with multiple sinus tracks but no large cavities

or sequestra. In such cases surgical excision of the entire area of infected bone offers the only prospect of cure. This may be possible if the bone is expendable such as the clavicle or fibula but is obviously more difficult in the major weight-bearing bones, although the development of microsurgical techniques, which enable the transplant of a living fibula with attachment of it's blood supply, now offers the prospect of repairing large defects in any long bone following excision for chronic infection or tumour. Operations for chronic osteomyelitis have therefore to be varied according to circumstance. It is useful at the outset to inject the sinus track with a dye such as methylene blue. The incision should excise the sinus and the surrounding scar and follow the sinus to the bone which is exposed subperiosteally as widely as may be necessary. X-ray can help to identify the site of the sequestrum or cavity during the operation. Once this has been located, the cavity is saucerised—that is completely deroofed, using osteotomes and gouges and the margins bevelled as extensively as may be required to produce a crater whose opening is wider than its base. Sequestra, which are usually easily identified by their white and crenated appearance, are lifted out and the wall of the cavity closely examined for other loculi or communicating sinuses. A local flap of muscle is then mobilized with care to preserve its blood supply and this is used to fill the cavity. If no muscle is available the wound should be dressed and left open. A few days later, when clean and granulating, a split skin graft may be used to line the cavity. At a later date when all signs of infection have subsided, the cavity may be filled by cancellous bone.

It must be recognized that many cases of chronic osteomyelitis will recur, despite such radical surgery.

OPERATIONS FOR BONE TUMOURS AND CYSTS

Bone tumours are exceedingly varied in their histogenesis and in their behaviour. Table 5.1 lists the more common of these tumours and gives some indication of their frequency. Malignant primary bone tumours are exceedingly rare, and with advances in endoprosthetic replacement and in chemotherapy, it is desirable that these should be managed in specialized units if available.

Benign tumours and cysts are much more common and easier to manage. Many show a tendency to spontaneous healing; these include most fibrous cortical defects, some chondroblastomas, aneurysmal bone cysts and simple cysts. Others are symptomless and therefore require no treatment except perhaps bone biopsy if their nature is uncertain.

Surgery is required for those which cause significant

Table 5.1 Classifications of primary bone tumours

Histological type	Benign	Frequency	Malignant	Frequency
Haemopoietic			myeloma	XX
			reticulum cell sarcoma	X
Chondrogenic	osteochondroma	XXXX	primary chondrosarcoma	X
	chondroma	XXXX	secondary chondrosarcoma	X
	chondroblastoma	X		
	chondromyxoid fibroma	X		
Osteogenic	osteoid osteoma	X	osteosarcoma	X
	benign osteoblastoma	X	parosteal osteosarcoma	X
Unknown	giant cell tumour	X	malignant giant cell tumour	X
			Ewing's tumour	X
			adamantinoma	X
			malignant fibrous histiocytoma	X
Fibrogenic	fibroma	XX	fibrosarcoma	X
	fibrous cortical defect	XXXX		
Notochordal			chordoma	X
Vascular	haemangioma	X	haemangioendothelioma	X
	aneurysmal bone cyst	X		

The number of X's gives an approximate indication of frequency; X implying rarity and XXXX common occurrence.

symptoms such as pain, pathological fracture or swelling sufficient to be disfiguring or to cause mechanical effects on other tissues. Surgery consists of simple excision or curettage with, if necessary, the repair of a residual defect with bone grafts. If a pathological fracture due to a benign tumour or cyst has occured, it is often wiser to delay surgical treatment until the fracture has healed. Some illustrative examples:

Osteochondromas

These cartilaginous capped exostoses arising at the metaphyses may be solitary lesions or multiple in the condition of diaphyseal aclasis. Only large and troublesome tumours (Fig. 5.33) require treatment and these are simply excised by dividing their origin from bone; as a rule they are devoid of soft tissue attachment. Growth of an osteochondroma in adult life suggests the possibility of malignant transformation to chondrosarcoma and a wider local resection is then indicated.

Chondromas

These cartilaginous tumours may be left if they are asymptomatic. Otherwise they are treated by curettage and bone graft replacement if large. The small chondromas which occur so commonly in the phalanges will heal following curettage without the need of bone graft.

Osteoid osteomas

These are small and intensely painful tumours of osteoblastic derivation. Frequently they may be overlooked on routine X-ray because of their minute size, but a bone scan will always reveal them as a 'hot spot'. Local excision is indicated and is invariably curative provided that the osteogenic nidus is removed.

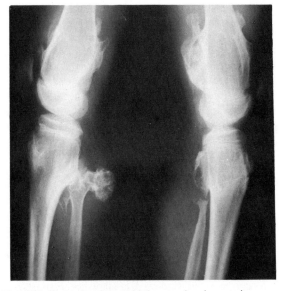

Fig. 5.33 X-ray showing multiple osteochondromata in diaphyseal aclasis. Note that some are sessile and others pedunculated

Giant cell tumour

This often gives rise to problems of management because of its common subarticular location in major joints. Although it responds to radiotherapy, there have been so many reports of irradiation induced sarcoma following this treatment that it is no longer recommended. Although most giant cell tumours behave in a benign fashion, a minority assume malignant characteristics and this raises a further difficulty in treatment. If the tumour occurs in a bone which may be resected without loss of function, such as the distal ulna or proximal fibula, then local resection is the treatment of choice. When the tumour occurs in an epiphysis around the knee or hip and major fracture has not occurred, then curettage and packing with bone grafts should be tried in the first instance (Fig. 5.34). The success rate with this simple procedure can be high but it depends on the thoroughness with which the curettage is done. It is important to obtain the bone graft (if autogenous graft is used) with separate instruments and gloves to avoid the possibility of tumour transfer to the donor site. If the tumour presents with a major fracture or if it recurs following local surgery, then wide local resection with major bone graft or endoprosthetic replacement is required (Fig. 5.35).

Malignant bone tumours

Malignant bone tumours tend to present with pain, swelling or pathological fractures—symptoms which are common to many other benign orthopaedic conditions such as osteomyelitis or stress fracture. It is of absolute importance therefore that a biopsy be obtained before radical treatment is undertaken. It is wise also to make a routine of sending biopsy specimens for both histological and bacteriological examination. Ewing's tumour and osteomyelitis, for example, may present in an identical fashion with pain, fever, raised ESR and similar X-ray appearance, and the diagnosis may be missed if biopsy is sent to the inappropriate laboratory.

The biopsy wound should be small, and so situated that it may be excised during subsequent surgery.

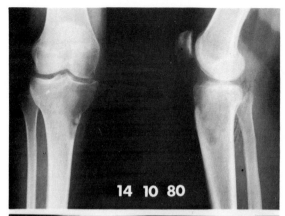

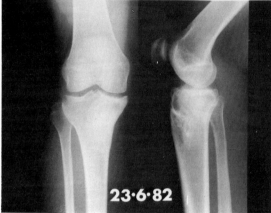

Fig. 5.34 X-rays showing giant cell tumour of upper tibia treated by curettage and bone graft

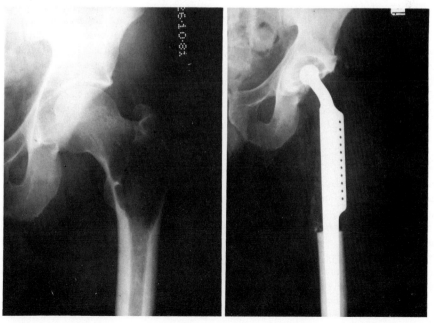

Fig. 5.35 X-rays showing giant cell tumour of proximal femur treated by endoprosthetic replacement

Ideally several specimens should be obtained from the tumour, for bone tumours frequently vary in their histological characteristics from place to place. Trephine needle biopsies are of value in situations such as the vertebral bodies where open biopsy would involve a major operation.

The management of these rare tumours has altered greatly in recent years. Amputation is no longer regarded as the only surgical procedure available and chemotherapy in conjunction with surgery or radiotherapy has significantly improved the prognosis of osteosarcoma and Ewing's tumour in particular. Historically patients suffering from these tumours had a survival rate of less than 20%, whereas recent series with survival rates at five years in excess of 50% are being reported.

Radical local surgery without amputation for malignant bone tumours should be undertaken only if it is possible to remove the tumour with a wide margin of normal tissue and yet leave enough useful function in the limb to make it better than a prosthesis. Limbs should not be preserved at a risk to the patient's life unless metastatic spread has already occurred.

To assess resectability of a tumour, it is desirable to have preoperative arteriography and CT scans of the limb in order to establish the tumour extent, and an endoprosthesis must be constructed to replace the resected bone or joint. Frozen sections at the time of surgery are useful to confirm that the limits of resection are tumour free. Chondrosarcomas, which in general are more slowly growing and less invasive than osteosarcomas, are most suitable for this type of surgery, but some osteosarcomas, fibrosarcomas and aggressive giant cell tumours may also be treated in this way. If the criteria for local resectability cannot be met then amputation well above the level of tumour must be performed. Chemotherapy, usually involving a combination of drugs including Adriamycin, Methotrexate, Vincristine and Cisplatin, is now given additionally in most cases of bone sarcoma. The optimal therapeutic regime has still not been established and many different courses of treatment are being evaluated. It is best that such treatment be supervised by an oncologist.

Metastatic bone tumours

These are much more frequent than primary malignant tumours. Breast, bronchus, prostate, thyroid and kidney are the common primary sites, although most malignant tumours will occasionally involve bone.

The treatment of these lesions is inevitably only palliative and depends on the nature of the primary tumour. Breast and prostatic secondaries, for example, may be controlled by hormonal therapy and by local radiotherapy. If pathological fractures occur or appear inevitable, it is often possible to stabilise the bone by curetting the local tumour and packing the resulting

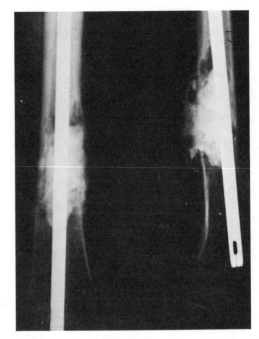

Fig. 5.36 X-ray of pathological fracture through a metastatic deposit stabilized by intramedullary nail and methylmethacrylate cement

defect with methylmethacrylate cement incorporating an internal fixation device such as shown in Figure 5.36.

Bone cysts

Simple bone cysts and aneurysmal bone cysts both may undergo spontaneous healing with time and symptomless lesions do not necessarily require treatment. If large, painful and a source of repeated pathological fracture, they should be treated by curettage and bone grafting, although a high recurrence rate may be anticipated and the operation may have to be repeated.

Recent reports suggest that simple bone cysts may be cured by the injection into the cyst of Methylprednisolone in doses ranging from 40–200 mg. Two needles are introduced into the cyst, one to allow fluid to escape and the other for the introduction of the steroid. The healing response may not be apparent for several months and repeat injections may be necessary.

OPERATIONS ON FRACTURES

Surgeons tend to polarise into two groups with regard to fracture management—the conservative school take pride in the closed treatment of fractures, while others regard most fractures as a surgical challenge. Both approaches require skilled management. Both can lead to good functional results and each has its range of complications. Conservative management avoids the risk of introducing infection to the fracture site but it involves more prolonged immobilization of the limb or patient with complications of stiffness or osteoporosis, sometimes referred to as 'plaster disease' by the surgically disposed. Surgical treatment often permits earlier mobilization and more accurate reduction of a fracture but at the risk of introducing infection and devitalizing bone as a result of the soft tissue stripping required.

There are some broad areas of agreement, however, which may be used as guidelines. Most fractures in children heal readily and can be well managed conservatively. Minor malalignments will, in general, remodel with growth. Fractures which cannot be reduced or maintained in reduction because of soft tissue interposition or muscle forces are best openly reduced and internally fixed—examples are certain fractures of the olecranon, patella, radius and ulna and fractures involving weight-bearing joints where perfect reduction is desirable if subsequent degenerative arthritis is to be avoided. Fractures in the elderly which, if treated conservatively, would involve prolonged immobilization in bed, are best treated by surgical means, if this will permit earlier mobilization. A hospital bed is a dangerous environment for the elderly and infirm. In patients with multiple injuries, particularly those with severe head or spinal injuries, internal fixation of limb fractures may facilitate nursing care. Pathological fractures due to malignant disease should, where possible, be treated by internal fixation for natural healing rarely occurs. In most other instances, the choice of treatment will reflect the training and experience of the surgeon and the environment in which he works. Ideally the surgeon should be familiar with both methods and be prepared to select the technique most appropriate to the individual patient.

A bewildering wide range of internal fixation devices is now available, many incompatible with each other in the type of metal used and in the calibre and type of screws and bolts and each requires its own range of instrumentation. It is desirable therefore that each surgeon should decide on one compatible system and become thoroughly familiar with its use. It need hardly be said that an atraumatic and aseptic technique is essential. With composite implants, such as plates and screws, it is important that all components be of the same metal, otherwise electrolytic reaction may occur. Titanium, chromium cobolt alloys and certain standards of stainless steel are acceptable.

Compound fractures
The principles governing the management of compound fractures are the same as those which obtain for any wound. Surgical excision of dead or severely damaged tissue and the removal of foreign material is essential, if infection is to be avoided. Infection of bone is in gen-

eral much more intractable than infection of soft tissue and fracture healing is likely to be delayed or to fail altogether in the presence of infection. If possible, a tourniquet is used in the initial stages of the operation. The injured part is thoroughly cleansed with a mild antiseptic solution, such as hibitane or cetavlon, and the wound irrigated with saline. The wound is extended, if necessary, to allow adequate inspection and excision of the deeper layers. Failure to enlarge the wound is the most common fault in the management of a compound fracture. Not infrequently a sharp spike of bone may have caught up fragments of clothing, earth or other highly contaminated materials which are then drawn back into the tissues when the limb is straightened. Small wounds associated with fractures are the tip of the iceberg and should alert the surgeon to the larger area of potential trouble beneath the surface.

Following wound extension, each layer is then carefully excised, removing the contaminated and damaged tissues, but respecting the major nerves and vessels. The fractured bone ends must be delivered to view and any completely detached fragments of bone be removed. Soiled bone must be curetted or nibbled away and the wound again irrigated with saline. At this stage, the tourniquet should be released and the vitality of the tissues confirmed—healthy muscle should contract when lightly pinched with forceps.

Wound closure should only be carried out in wounds of limited extent, which can be closed without tension, otherwise the wound should be simply dressed and left open for delayed primary closure or skin grafting after an interval of about four days, as discussed in the management of wounds in general on page 155.

Wide spectrum topical antibiotics applied by spray or in irrigation fluid are of value at the completion of the wound excision but systemic antibiotics are not essential in well excised wounds of limited extent. It is prudent, however, to give penicillin specifically to counter tetanus or gas gangrene in extensive wounds where the adequacy of the excision is in doubt.

It is tempting to carry out internal fixation when the fracture is exposed to view, but, in general, this is best avoided for the introduction of foreign material seems to inhibit the natural defences of the body against any residual bacteria, which may remain after even the most careful wound excision. There are, however, some circumstances which justify the risks of internal fixation of compound fractures. For example, if a major vessel has been damaged and requires repair or grafting, an unstable fracture may subsequently compromise the vascular repair and internal fixation is then justified. External fixation, using skeletal pins mounted to a rigid external scaffold, as shown in Figure 5.37, may be of great value in the management of severe injuries with extensive soft tissue loss, requiring multiple dressings and skin graft-

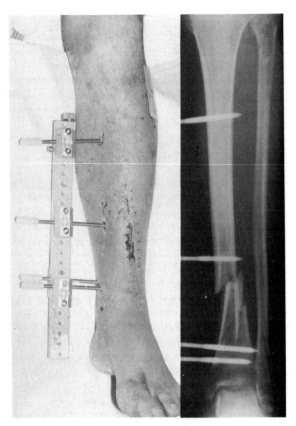

Fig. 5.37 External fixator used to stabilize a compound tibial fracture

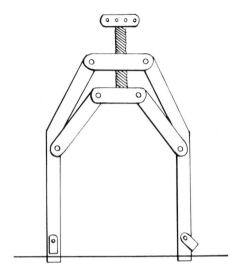

Fig. 5.38 Tensioning device used to apply traction to a Kirschner wire

ing procedures. This technique maintains the fracture in good position while allowing free access to the wound.

In most other circumstances, the compound fracture is immobilized by a wellpadded plaster cast or Thomas splint as for a closed fracture.

Skeletal traction

Skeletal traction may be used as an alternative to skin traction as a means of maintaining length and alignment and rotation of a fracture. It is commonly used for fractures of the femoral shaft, but has occasional applications elsewhere.

The traction is applied by a metal pin passing through bone. The *Steinmann pin*—a sharpened pin, 3 mm in diameter—or the *Denham pin*, are used. The latter is similar to the Steinmann but has a central threaded segment which, when screwed into cortical bone, resists lateral movement and hence reduces the risk of infection.

The usual site for the application of skeletal traction is through the upper end of the tibia. Under general anaesthesia, the pin is inserted by hand using the T shaped introducer through the cortical bone just below

the tibial tubercle. It is important that the pin is placed at right angles to the axis of the shaft of the tibia, otherwise asymmetric traction may result in undue stress on the ligaments on one side of the knee. The points of emergence of the pin through the skin should be left exposed but may be protected with a mild antiseptic, such as betadine cream. A metal stirrup or U-loop, to which the traction cord is attached, is fixed to the pin. Figure 5.38 illustrates one method of use. The traction should not exceed 10 kg except for short intervals and should never be so great as to cause distraction of the fracture—usually 5–8 kg is sufficient. It is important that the stirrup rotates freely about the pin so that the pin itself is not turned with every movement, otherwise pin tract infection will develop.

Other sites which are occasionally used for skeletal traction include the olecranon, the supracondylar region of the femur and the calcaneum. In these sites the finer Kirschner wire, which has its own telescopic introducer and stirrup attachment, may be preferred.

TECHNIQUES OF INTERNAL FIXATION

Having decided that internal fixation is required, the surgeon must then decide when the operation should be performed and which technique should be used. In general, surgery need not be delayed if the patient's general condition is satisfactory unless there is gross local swelling or local infection. Superficial skin abrasions and blisters are likely to become more infected with time and indicate early, rather then delayed, surgery.

A case can be made for delaying surgery in fractures of major long bones and in multiple injuries in which the risk of fat embolism is high, not because internal fixation increases the chance of fat embolism, but because it may be more difficult to diagnose following a major operation. The risk will have passed by three days and surgery is then safer. There is evidence that delaying surgery for up to two weeks has no adverse effect on subsequent fracture healing and it has even been suggested that healing may be enhanced by this period of delay.

Choice of technique

Ideally internal fixation should not only hold the fracture reduced, but it should be strong enough to support the fracture and allow early mobilization of the part and of the patient without need of additional splintage. The methods available include Kirschner wire transfixation (suitable for fractures of small bones or for small intra-articular fragments) screws and bolts (suitable for larger fragments as in comminuted fractures of the tibial plateau) metal plates and screws, with or without compression and intramedullary nails and rods which are

useful for long bone fixation and for fractures of the neck of the femur. Most of these techniques are illustrated in the subsequent sections on individual fractures. Figure 5.39 illustrates some of these devices.

Note on screw fixation

Various types of screws are available for different purposes and it is important that the surgeon should understand the principles of their use. There are two basic types—self-tapping and those which require the hole to be pre-tapped. A self-tapping screw has a point designed to cut its own thread in bone. The bone is pre-drilled with a drill which is smaller than the diameter of the screw so that the thread of the screw will engage in the bone. Thus a standard screw of 4 mm diameter requires a 3 mm drill. A self-tapping screw should be long enough to allow the point to emerge from the distal bone surface, otherwise bone may grow into the cutting grooves of the point and make subsequent removal difficult. A non-self-tapping screw requires that the bone be pre-drilled and then pre-threaded with a tapping cutter. It is claimed that this latter method gives better fixation but in practice both types are satisfactory. Cortical bone screws have a shallow thread and cancellous bone screws a deeper thread and it is obviously essential that the correct tap be used for each.

When joining two pieces of bone together by means of screws, it is essential to overdrill the proximal fragment with a drill wider than the thread of the screw so that the two fragments can be impacted together (Fig. 5.40). If the screw thread engages in each fragment, tightening the screw cannot approximate them.

Compression fixation

Compression has been shown to promote bone healing in arthrodesis of the knee, (p. 104) and it is suggested that it is of value in the management of fractures also. Whether this is due to any effect on the biology of fracture healing, or simply to secure fixation and close coaptation which results from compression, is a matter of debate. An accurately reduced, compressed fracture will heal with minimal external callus but it has the disadvantage that bone being so firmly splinted becomes locally osteoporotic from lack of stress so that refracture may occur following the removal of the fixation device. Nevertheless, compression techniques are acquiring in-

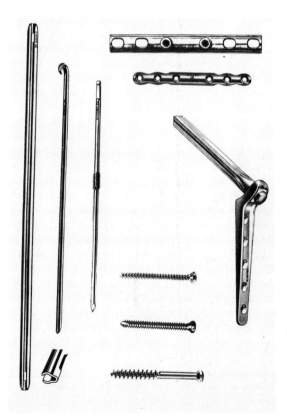

Fig. 5.39 Various internal fixation devices referred to in text: From *left* to *right*: Küntscher nail, Rush pin, Denham pin, compression plate (oval holes), standard plate, trifin nail and adjustable angle plate; Screws: *top* cortical; *middle* cortical self tapping; *bottom* cancellous

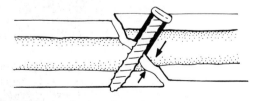

Fig. 5.40 Screw fixation of a cortical bone fracture (see text)

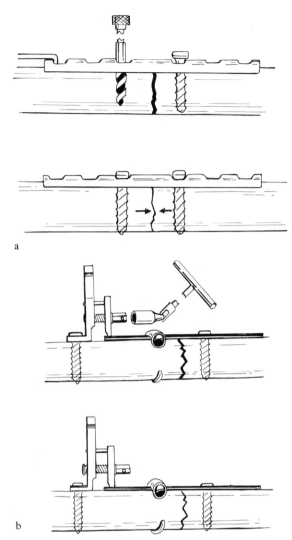

Fig. 5.41a & b Two techniques of compression plating.
a. Uses a self-compression plate with oval slots for the screws. The first two screws are inserted in the end of the slot away from the fracture. As the sloping shoulder of the screw is tightened against the plate, the fracture is compressed.
b. A conventional plate with round screw holes is attached to one side of the fracture with a single screw. The tensioning device is then fixed to the bone as shown and tightened to apply the desired pressure at the fracture site. The remaining screws are then inserted and the tensioning device is removed

creasing popularity. Two methods of compression plating are illustrated in Figure 5.41.

Illustrative examples of internal fixation of fractures

Intra-articular osteochondral fractures
These fractures may occur in the elbow, where they usually involve the capitellum or the radial head, and in the knee, where the lateral condyle of the femur or the undersurface of the patella are the common sites, usually complicating dislocation of the patella. They can be overlooked on X-ray, because the bone component may be a small inconspicuous flake while the larger cartilage component is, of course, invisible on X-ray. If neglected, they form loose bodies in the joint and the residual crater in the joint surface may lead to later osteoarthritis. Operative treatment is therefore necessary. The joint is opened at the site of injury, the loose fragment, if small, is removed and, if large, restored and fixed by Smillie's pins or Kirschner wires, which are driven through the fragment into the subadjacent bone, the head of the pin being buried below the cartilage surface (Fig. 5.42).

Fractures of the lateral condyle of the humerus, even in children, usually fail to unite and, unless internally fixed by means of a screw or Kirschner wire, cubitus valgus will develop and tardy ulnar palsy is likely to ensue. When using Kirschner wires to fix small fragments or small bones it helps to insert them with a power drill, rather than with the hand introducer, for the force required by the latter may displace the fragments.

Olecranon fractures
In fractures of the olecranon, the proximal fragment is pulled away by the action of triceps and healing by bone will not occur. Fibrous union may suffice for an elderly person but, if strong extension power is to be restored, internal fixation is necessary.

Through a curved lateral incision, the fracture site is exposed, the proximal fragment is drawn proximally with a bone hook and the fracture surfaces curetted of loose fragments or blood clot. The fracture is then accurately reduced and held by two towel clips. The bone fragments are stabilized by means of an oblique screw. The screw must be directed obliquely to engage the opposite cortex of the ulna (Fig. 5.43).

An alternative method, known as tension band wiring is illustrated in Figure 5.44. Having reduced the fracture, the surgeon inserts two Kirschner wires across the fracture site and bends the projecting ends over to prevent their migration down the shaft. A small hole is then drilled transversely through the posterior cortex of the ulna about 2 cm distal to the fracture site. A wire is passed through the hole and round the projecting Kirschner wires in a figure-of-eight fashion and tightened with tension. Early mobilization is encouraged for elbow movement increases the compression across the fracture.

Fractures of the radial head
Severely communited fractures of the radial head should be excised. The posterolateral approach minimizes risk of injury to the posterior interosseous nerve. An incision

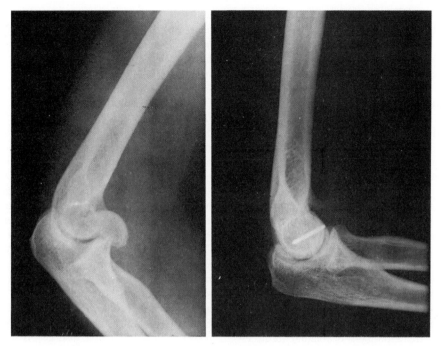

Fig. 5.42 X-ray of elbow showing fixation of intra-articular fracture by a Smillie pin. (See also Fig. 5.21)

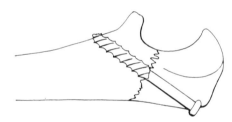

Fig. 5.43 Screw fixation of olecranon fracture

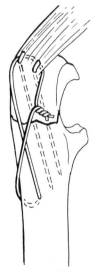

Fig. 5.44 Tension band wiring of olecranon fracture

is made from the tip of the lateral epicondyle, in the direction of the subcutaneous border of the ulna, about 4 cm from the tip of the olecranon. The interval between the anconeus muscle and the common extensor origin is identified and developed. Deep to this lies the capsule of the elbow joint. On opening the capsule, the radial head is readily visualised and can be removed. Displacement of the upper radial epiphyses occurs in children. If manipulative reduction fails the upper end of the radius is exposed and the displaced head of the bone is pressed into position. The radial head should never be removed during the growing period for this will result in relative overgrowth of the ulna with disorganization of the inferior radio-ulnar joint. Less severe fractures of the radial head can be treated conservatively, although loose displaced marginal fragments may be excised, or if large, internally fixed by small screws.

Fractures of the radius and ulna
These fractures are difficult to manage conservatively because of the opposing muscle forces, which act on the radius at different levels. In adults, internal fixation is usually required, for near perfect reduction must be achieved if forearm rotation is to be maintained. The bones are approached separately, otherwise cross union may occur. The fractures are then manipulated into reduction with bone forceps and stabilized by six-hole plates and screws. Compression plating may give sufficient stability to allow external fixation to be dispensed

with. In other circumstances a full arm plaster should be used for at least five weeks.

Fracture of the ulna with dislocation of the radial head (Monteggia fracture)

This fracture has a bad reputation because of the common complication of persistent dislocation of the head of the radius. The key to management lies in perfect reduction of the ulnar fracture coupled with repair or reconstruction of the annular ligament of the radial head, if this remains unstable. Postoperative fixation in plaster is required for five weeks.

Plaster fixation for forearm fractures

It is sometimes stated that in order to obtain or maintain reduction of forearm fractures, it may be necessary to immobilize the forearm in full supination or pronation. These extreme positions are dangerous, for, if the arm should stiffen in either of these positions, severe functional disability will result. Forearm plasters should therefore always immobilize the arm in a mid-position of rotation where subsequent stiffening will be less of a handicap. If extreme positions of rotation are necessary in order to maintain reduction of any fracture, then internal fixation is undoubtedly a preferable method of treatment.

Fractures of the upper end of the femur

Fractures of the upper end of the femur occur most commonly in elderly women, usually as a result of a relatively minor injury, such as a simple stumble. Most are pathological fractures, the common underlying abnormality being osteoporosis but sometimes with a component of osteomalacia. A high proportion of the affected patients have associated illnesses which add to their infirmity and complicate the management of their fracture.

Less frequently these fractures occur in younger individuals, usually as a result of considerable violence.

These fractures may be classified as *transcervical* (intracapsular) or *trochanteric* (extracapsular). With intracapsular fractures many of the nutrient vessels which run proximally to the head from the base of the neck are disrupted leaving only a small variable contribution from the artery of the ligamentum teres. As a result, delayed healing of this fracture is common and avascular necrosis of the femoral head a frequent complication. Fractures of the trochanteric region, on the other hand, maintain a good blood supply on both sides of the fracture line and healing is rarely a problem.

Transcervical fractures may be further classified according to Garden's classification: (I) incomplete fracture, in this the inferior cortex remains intact while the superior cortex is impacted; (II) complete fracture without displacement; (III) complete fracture with partial displacement; (IV) complete fracture with full displacement. The prognosis worsens and the complication rate increases through stages I to IV and this classification therefore is a useful guide to management and treatment.

Transcervical fractures

There is no satisfactory conservative treatment for these injuries. Garden grade I fractures may sometimes heal spontaneously but a proportion of them come unstuck in the first two or three weeks and it is therefore prudent to internally fix them all. As transcervical fractures occur generally in the elderly and debilitated in whom the consequences of prolonged bed rest and immobilization are most damaging, surgical treatment, which will allow early mobilization, is almost routinely performed. The timing of operation is important. Many of these patients arrive in hospital dehydrated and hypothermic, having been lying helpless on the floor for some hours before being discovered. Others may have cardiac failure, respiratory infection, recent stroke, etc. and a day or two spent in assessing the patient thoroughly and in treating any remediable disorder, is time well spent. The mortality in this group of patients is high but can be reduced by careful preoperative preparation.

Choice of operation

Two types of procedure are available:
1. internal fixation with an intramedullary device and;
2. excision of the head of femur with prosthetic replacement

The high failure rate of internal fixation both in terms of union and in the complication of avascular necrosis, has popularised prosthetic replacement, but this also has its range of complications: the acetabulum may fail to stand up to the unyielding pressure of a metallic femoral head and infection and dislocation may occur in this elderly and unfit group of patients. In general internal fixation is preferred for younger and fitter patients and for fractures in the Garden grades I and II. A replacement may be preferred for the very elderly and unfit and for grades III and IV, particularly in those patients with severe osteoporosis in whom the bone is too weak to support internal fixation devices.

Internal fixation

Many techniques of internal fixation are described, which is a sure indication that none is entirely satisfactory. A single Smith Peterson pin is usually inadequate and some form of multiple fixation is preferable (Fig. 5.45). No form of fixation will, however, succeed unless an accurate reduction of the fracture is obtained.

To achieve reduction of an intracapsular fracture the patient is anaesthetized and placed on an orthopaedic table. The affected limb is put on gentle traction and

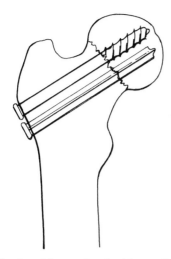

Fig. 5.45 Fixation of fractured neck of femur. Two flanged nails or one nail and a cannulated screw, as shown, give better fixation than a single device

slight internal rotation. Anteroposterior and lateral X-rays are taken and the position assessed. If reduction has not been achieved, adjustment of the position of the leg can be simply made using the controls of the orthopaedic table. Forceful manipulative reduction of these fractures can be harmful by further jeopardising the blood supply.

In a small percentage of cases in which a satisfactory reduction is not achieved by such simple manoeuvres, open reduction may be required.

Method of internal fixation. With the patient on the orthopaedic table and the fracture reduced, X-ray tubes or the image intensifier are positioned to allow AP and lateral projections of the hip. A straight lateral incision is made over the upper end of the femur from the tip of the greater trochanter distally some six to ten centimetres depending on the obesity of the patient. The tensor fasciae latae and the fascia lata itself are split in the line of the skin incision, the vastus lateralis muscle is split longitudinally or reflected forwards from its origin and the lateral aspect of the shaft of the femur is thus exposed. Two guidewires are inserted into the femoral neck from the lateral aspect of the femur across the fracture site and into the head of the femur under X-ray control. The two wires should be separated sufficiently to allow the two internal fixation devices to be inserted and should diverge slightly. The placing of the guidewires becomes easier with increasing experience. When the cortical bone is hard, pre-drilling of the lateral cortex with a 4 mm drill simplifies the insertion of the guidewire and any subsequent adjustments that may be necessary. Two flanged nails or a flanged nail and a cannulated screw of a length carefully measured from the guidewires to give maximal fixation in the head are then

driven into position, checking at frequent intervals during their insertion that the guidewire is not advancing with the nail, which may sometimes happen if the pin becomes slightly off line. When the nails or nail and screw are inserted, the guidewires are removed and the wound closed. Rapid mobilization is allowed and the patient encouraged to walk with assistance within 48 hours.

Femoral head replacement

If this procedure is selected, either the antero-lateral or posterior approaches (pp. 93 & 94) may be used according to the preference of the surgeon. The posterior approach gives better access to the femoral shaft in stocky, obese patients. The joint capsule is opened, the femoral head removed and the neck of femur trimmed, if required, with bone cutters or reciprocating saw, to present a flat, smooth surface angled to match the flange of the prosthesis and allowing slight anteversion. It is of paramount importance that the prosthesis selected should match as closely as possible the size of the original head, otherwise high points of pressure will develop within the acetabulum, which will lead to early acetabular erosion. The correct size is measured by means of graded templates. The femoral shaft is then reamed using a notched broach corresponding to the stem of the prosthesis. No force should be used for it is easy to penetrate the shaft in these elderly patients with fragile bones. If difficulty in passing the broach is experienced, the usual cause is inadequate removal of the superior cortex of the neck. With the Moore's prosthesis, particularly, it is necessary to excise the superior cortex of the stump of the neck as far as the face of the trochanter. The prosthesis is then inserted into the shaft of the femur and gently reduced into the acetabulum. Excessive force on the shaft of the femur during this manoeuvre may cause it to fracture. Tissue forceps are first placed on the cut margins of the capsule so that it can be held out of the way and, using the appropriate plastic punch, pressure is placed on the prosthetic head in the direction of the acetabulum, while gentle traction is maintained by the assistant on the femur. The femur is rotated to follow the head into the acetabulum rather than being used as a lever to rotate it in. The Moore's prosthesis (Fig. 5.46) is used without cement; the Thomson prosthesis may be used with or without cement. If it is to be cemented, a preliminary trial reduction should be carried out to ensure the correctness of the fit. With the posterior approach particularly, dislocation may occur in the early postoperative period if the hip is allowed to flex acutely as when sitting in a low chair or on a low toilet seat and this is therefore to be avoided for the first few days. Walking, however, is perfectly safe and should be encouraged when the patient's condition allows.

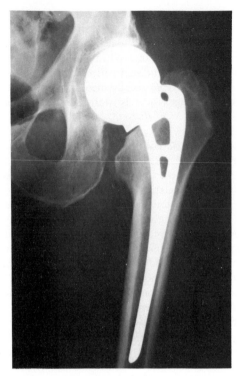

Fig. 5.46 X-ray of Moore's prosthesis

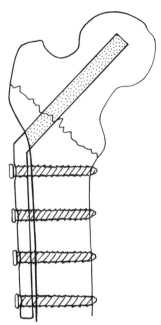

Fig. 5.47 Method of fixation of a trochanteric fracture

Trochanteric fractures

Although these fractures have a good blood supply and healing is rarely a problem, stabilization can present technical difficulties, particularly if there is much comminution involving the medial cortex. Reduction is carried out on the orthopaedic table and usually presents no problems. If there is any difficulty, it is easy to expose the fracture site and obtain reduction under direct vision. The approach is similar to that for internal fixation of the femoral neck fractures but requires to be extended distally down the shaft of the femur for 15 cm or more according to the length of plate selected. The most commonly used fixation device consists of a nail inserted into the femoral neck attached to a plate which is screwed to the shaft of the femur (Fig. 5.47). Protected weight bearing may be started early but full weight-bearing is avoided in the unstable fractures for at least six weeks.

Complications of fractures of the upper end of the femur

Avascular necrosis

Some degree of avascular necrosis develops in all displaced fractures of the femoral neck. In about 30% of those who survive long enough, the necrosis is sufficiently extensive to allow segmental collapse of the femoral head to take place. This complication does not always give rise to distressing symptoms or require treatment but, for those patients who have persistent and severe pain and progressive disability, total replacement arthroplasty of the hip joint is the appropriate solution.

Non-union

A certain percentage of displaced fractures of the femoral neck will not unite even with what appears to be adequate internal fixation. In this event the pins may cut out of the head and the fracture displaces once more. If the acetabulum remains healthy, a femoral head replacement is appropriate. If a penetrating nail has damaged the acetabulum, a total hip replacement arthroplasty is preferred. If non-union occurs in a young patient without gross displacement, a subtrochanteric osteotomy may allow healing to take place.

Penetration of the acetabulum by a fixation device

With both intracapsular and extracapsular fractures, settling at the fracture site may result in the fixation device penetrating through the femoral head into the acetabulum. This complication can be reduced if the nail is left 0.5 to 1 cm short of the joint surface at the initial fixation or by using a sliding nail. If penetration occurs while the fracture remains ununited, the fixation device should be left in situ unless pain is severe. When the fracture has united, the fixation device can then be removed.

Subtrochanteric femoral fractures

Transverse fractures occurring just below the lesser trochanter are particularly characteristic of Paget's disease and osteomalacia but may occur in normal bone when subjected to sufficient trauma. The proximal fragment tends to flex, abduct and externally rotate due to the unopposed action of iliopsoas and the hip abductors. Conservative management is consequently difficult. Internal fixation with pin and plate is therefore usually indicated. The plate must be long enough to allow at least six screws to be attached to the distal fragment and if there is much comminution or if the bone is pathologically soft, it is wise to support the limb on Hamilton Russell traction (see Fig. 5.17) for the first few weeks.

Midshaft femoral fractures
With fractures through the middle third of the femur the surgeon has the option of conservative treatment, for example using skeletal or skin traction with the limb supported on a Thomas splint, or internal fixation. Internal fixation may be achieved by one or more strong plates and screws or by an intramedullary nail. The former requires extensive exposure of the bone with consequent damage to blood supply, but confers stability to resist all forces including rotation. Intramedullary fixation may be achieved with minimal or no exposure of the fracture site but may not always control rotational forces if there is much comminution.

In simple fractures in adults intramedullary fixation with a Küntscher nail is now the most widely adopted procedure.

Intramedullary nailing of femoral shaft fractures
Before embarking on intramedullary fixation of any bone the surgeon must ensure that he has available all the instruments necessary for insertion *and the removal* of a nail in the event of the nail becoming jammed. It is useful also to know the length of the nail required by taking an X-ray of the intact opposite limb bone with a measuring rod taped on the skin surface at the same level as the bone. Closed intramedullary nailing can be done successfully in practiced hands, but requires an orthopaedic table which allows intraoperative skeletal traction with patient in the lateral position, image intensification and extensive instrumentation including flexible power drive cannulated reamers. Any surgeon embarking on this procedure should read a full description beforehand (King & Rush, 1981).

Open intramedullary nailing of the femur is more widely practiced. The patient is placed on his side with the fractured leg uppermost. The fracture site is then exposed through a posterolateral approach (p. 95) and the bone ends immobilized and cleared of loose fragments. The proximal fragment is then reamed retrogradely from the fractured surface using a hand or power driven reamer, starting with the smallest that will comfortably fit and increasing up to 14 or 15 mm for an adult. The reamers should be advanced to penetrate through the greater trochanter. The distal fragment is reamed to the same diameter, care being taken not to penetrate the knee joint. The nail is selected of the same diameter as the largest reamer used and of a length which will reach to the level of the upper pole of the patella and proximally to emerge 2 cm above the greater trochanter.

The nail is then inserted into the proximal fragment

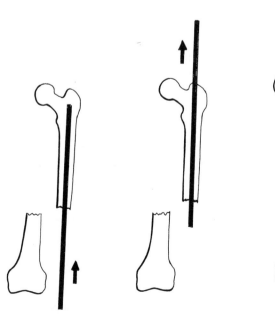
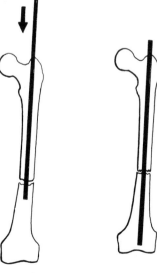

Fig. 5.48 Open method of insertion of intramedullary nail

and driven proximally until it can be felt to reach the subcutaneous tissues of the buttock; this is facilitated by flexing and adducting the hip joint. The nail is exposed in the buttock through a small stab wound and is withdrawn until the end reaches the level of the fracture. The fracture is then reduced and stabilized by a bone clamp while the nail is driven distally until only 2 cm are left emerging above the greater trochanter (Fig. 5.48). If the nail is allowed to project further from the bone it causes discomfort and damage to the gluteal muscles, while burying the nail too deeply will make its removal difficult if this should subsequently become necessary.

Force should never be used when driving a nail, for a jammed nail can be very difficult to extract. If the nail is not passing easily it should be withdrawn and replaced with one 1 mm narrower. A check X-ray should be taken before wound closure to confirm the correct length and location of the nail. While the fracture site is still exposed the stability of the fracture should be tested, particularly with regard to rotation. If rotational stability is not secured, the limb should be supported on Hamilton Russell traction for a few weeks, otherwise early mobilization and weight-bearing is allowed.

Supracondylar fractures of the femur may be managed conservatively but can prove troublesome because of the tendency of the distal fragment to flex due to the pull of the gastrocnemius. Internal fixation is consequently often preferred and the condylar blade plate illustrated in Figure 5.49 is suitable.

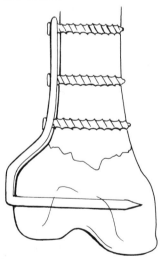

Fig. 5.49 Supracondylar fracture of femur stabilized by a condylar blade plate

Fractures of the patella

A similar principle may be used in transverse fractures of the patella (Fig. 5.50), but comminuted displaced fractures of the patella must be excised (p. 103).

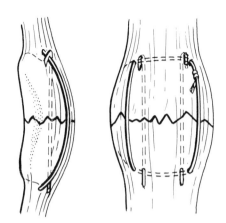

Fig. 5.50 Tension band wiring of patella

Tibial fractures

Fractures of the tibial plateau
These are common injuries particularly among pedestrians struck by a car. The fractures are often associated with ligamentous injury and both knees may be involved. Treatment depends on the severity of the injury and on the age and activity of the patient.

Ideally, as with all fractures involving the joint surface, perfect reduction should be the objective but severe comminution makes this difficult to achieve and in the old and inactive surprisingly good results can be obtained by a conservative routine of early mobilization. In younger patients in whom degenerative arthritis has more opportunity to develop, an attempt should be made to restore the joint surface and stabilize major fragments. Depressed segments of articular surface should be elevated to their normal situation and supported there by packing bone graft beneath. Major fragments are secured with cancellous screws or a bar bolt (Fig. 5.51). Major ligamentous injuries should be repaired at the same operation.

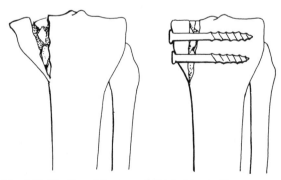

Fig. 5.51 Fixation of fracture of tibial plateau with cancellous screws

Tibial shaft fractures

More controversy surrounds the management of these fractures than any other and large series of successful results are reported by advocates of both the conservative and the surgical schools. Clearly both can work and the arguments outlined on page 117 should guide the decision. Improved plaster techniques allowing early knee movement (Sarmiento, 1981) have overcome many of the criticisms of plaster fixation.

If internal fixation is used there is a choice as with most long bones between plate and screws, and intramedullary nailing which can be done as a closed procedure with greater facility than with the femur, although still requiring modifications to the operating table and a range of specialized instruments (for a full account read Adams, 1985).

Plate or screw fixation has the disadvantage of requiring an open operation on a superficial bone with the possibility of skin breakdown and infection. This risk, however, can be largely avoided if the skin incision is curved over the anterior muscle compartment where any difficulties in closure or subsequent breakdown will expose muscle rather than fracture and skin graft, if required, will have a receptive bed.

The deep facia is incised in the line of the skin incision and is reflected medially to the periosteum which is incised along the lateral surface of the tibia and mobilised to expose the fracture site. A six-hole heavy duty plate is then applied to the lateral surface, preferably with compression by the technique illustrated on page 119. The lateral surface is chosen when possible because it avoids a subcutaneous situation but all aspects of the tibia are accessible to fixation if the circumstances of the fracture dictate.

Oblique fractures of the tibia lend themselves to accurate fixation by means of transfixation screws as illustrated in Figure 5.52. It is important when applying these techniques to obtain perfect reduction and to overdrill the proximal fragment so that the screw thread will not engage, see Figure 5.40. Obviously screw fixation alone will not allow unprotected weight-bearing but it is a useful and relatively minor adjunct to conservative management when reduction is difficult to maintain. Plate fixation also is not secure enough to allow unprotected weight-bearing for several weeks.

Ankle fractures

Ankle fractures are exceedingly common, second only in frequency to the Colles fracture of the wrist. They may involve the medial or lateral malleoli alone or together, and in severe displacements, the posterior margin of the tibial articular surface. These fractures may be associated with ligamentous disruption. In general an ankle injury becomes unstable only if two or more of the stabilising components are broken, i.e. a malleolus plus

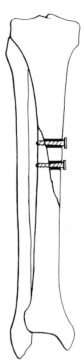

Fig. 5.52 Screw fixation of oblique tibial fracture

a major ligament or two malleoli, and by the same token stability may be restored even if one of these structures is left unrepaired.

Unstable ankle injuries should be treated routinely by internal fixation for perfect reduction is required, as in all weight-bearing joints, and this is difficult to maintain by plaster alone. Isolated displaced medial malleolar fractures require fixation otherwise non union is common because of the pull of the powerful deltoid ligament which holds the bone fragments apart. Isolated fractures of the lateral malleolus on the other hand without demonstrable joint instability under anaesthesia may be managed conservatively by a below knee walking plaster.

Medial malleolar fractures are treated by screw fixation as in Figure 5.53, or, if the fragment is too small, two Kirschner wires inserted from different angles may be used.

Lateral malleolar fractures may be fixed by screw or plate or intramedullary rod such as the Rush pin according to the fracture pattern.

Diastasis of the inferior tibiofibular joint should be stabilized by a transverse tibiofibular screw as shown in Figure 5.54 but it is important to remove this screw when the plaster is removed at eight weeks for normal ankle motion requires a mobile inferior tibiofibular joint in order to accommodate to the variable width of the talar articular surface during flexion and extension.

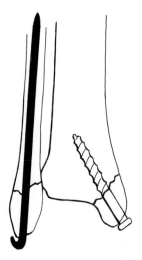

Fig. 5.53 Methods of stabilising malleolar fractures

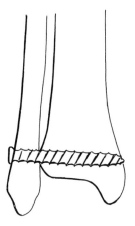

Fig. 5.54 Screw fixation of tibiofibular diastasis

Posterior marginal fragments of the tibial articular surface if small may be ignored but if large, i.e. representing more than a quarter of the tibial articular surface, they should be accurately reduced and internally fixed. The fragment is usually posterolateral and is therefore exposed through a vertical incision between the tendo-Achilles and the fibula. The flexor hallucis muscle obscures the fracture and is retracted proximally, the fracture surfaces are then cleared and accurate reduction is obtained under vision. Two cancellous screws are used to secure fixation.

Treatment of non-union

Non-union of a fracture is usually the result of infection, poor blood supply, inadequate fixation, soft tissue interposition or unrecognized bone pathology. Non-union is easy to recognize when the bone ends become sclerosed and a pseudo joint develops, but this may not occur for many months or even years and for practical purposes it is better to define non-union as failure of healing within a reasonable arbitrary period of eight weeks for an upper limb fracture or 12 to 16 weeks for a lower limb fracture. It is recognized that some ununited fractures at this stage may be examples of delayed union which if immobilized for a further period might go on to spontaneous healing, but the distinction between delayed and non-union at this stage is impossible and in order to ensure healing with minimal further delay, all fractures at this stage which are unhealed should be considered for further treatment.

Non-unions of the femoral neck have been considered on page 124.

Other common sites of non-union are the tibial shaft, the humerus especially in obese elderly individuals, the forearm bones if the initial fixation was inadequate and the scaphoid, but no fracture is immune from this complication. Treatment consists of rectifying the causal factor and promoting union by the addition of cancellous bone graft. It is not possible to describe the infinite variety of procedures which may be required but the treatment of the common tibial non-union will serve as an illustration.

The fracture site is exposed by the curved incision described on page 127. If infection is encountered, all dead and unhealthy tissue is excised, the wound irrigated with an antibiotic solution and methylmethacrylate beads containing Gentamicin are placed in the infected area and the wound closed. Once the organism has been identified systemic antibiotics are given and further surgery delayed for two weeks. By that stage the infection should be under control. The wound is opened, the antibiotic beads removed and cancellous strip grafts applied. Systemic antibiotics are continued until union occurs. If at the first operation no infection is encountered cancellous strip grafts (p. 129) are applied as a primary procedure without disturbing the fracture site if it is in good position and well stabilised by fibrous scar (Fig. 5.55). If the position requires adjustment or if the fracture is grossly unstable, internal fixation is used together with cancellous strip grafting. Unless the internal fixation is absolutely secure, external plaster fixation is also used until the fracture is healed, usually within 8 to 12 weeks. During this time weight-bearing is encouraged within the plaster.

Principles of bone grafting

Microscopic areas of bone death occur constantly throughout the skeleton as a result of minor trauma or focal vascular occlusion. These necrotic areas are continually repaired by a process of revascularisation, resorption of the dead bone and its replacement by new living bone which subsequently undergoes remodelling to restore the normal architecture of the part. In this way a constant process of skeletal renewal goes on

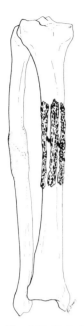
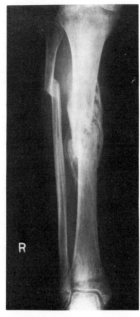

Fig. 5.55 Techniques of cancellous strip grafting for non-union

throughout life. Larger areas of bone death resulting from more extensive vascular insult such as occurs in Perthes disease or as a result of fracture, is dealt with in the same way, although the larger the fragment the slower its eventual replacement. There is then a fundamental biological reaction to dead bone which attempts to replace it with living bone. This property is made use of in the operation of bone grafting. Bone taken from one situation and transplanted to another inevitably dies and is consequently replaced by living bone. By appropriately shaping and locating the graft it is possible for the surgeon to create new bone formation where he wishes. Thus cavities in bone may be induced to heal and defects in bone resulting from trauma or disease may be repaired. Bone may be used to bridge joints to create arthrodesis and in the case of ununited fracture, where the natural healing process has for some reason lost its impetus, bone may be conducted across the fracture site through the medium of the graft to restore bony union.

Although allografts of bone produce the same immunological reactions as the allografts of other tissues, this is of little consequence as all free grafts of bone, whether from the same individual or another, die and

are treated in the same way. Thus allografts of bone, and bone which has been preserved by freezing or freeze drying, can be used surgically without regard to immunological reaction.

In bone grafting operations the following points are of importance: small grafts are more rapidly replaced than large and the least possible amount of bone should be used. Cancellous bone is more readily revascularised and offers less volume of bone to be resorbed than cortical and should be used unless there is some over-riding mechanical requirement which demands cortical bone.

Bone grafts are at their weakest during the process of resorption and replacement by immature living bone and they must be supported by splintage until remodelling occurs.

Cancellous strip grafting

This is the standard operation for an ununited fracture. The iliac crest is used as the donor site. An incision is made parallel to and just below the crest extending from the anterior superior spine posteriorly as far as required. The lateral surface of the ilium is exposed subperiosteally, the crest with its attached muscles is detached with an osteotome and reflected medially, care being taken to leave the anterior superior spine undisturbed. The medial aspect of the ilium is exposed subperiosteally. Using a sharp chisel rather than an osteotome, thin slivers of cancellous bone are cut from the exposed margin of the ilium, five or six slivers, 6–10 cm in length being sufficient for most fractures. The detached crest is then carefully sutured back to the periosteum and muscles on the outer face of the ilium over a vacuum drain and the wound closed.

The fracture site is then exposed subperiosteally on all its aspects and the cancellous slivers are placed around it like barrel staves (see Fig. 5.55). Thin slivers long enough to reach healthy living bone on either side of the fracture site are ideal and will form a guide and stimulus to conduct the new bone across the fracture site. The scar tissue between the bone ends should be left undisturbed unless it is necessary to alter the position of the fracture for this confers some stability to the fracture site and does not act as a barrier to healing. If the position requires alteration, internal fixation should be used together with bone grafting.

It is important to obtain the graft before exposing the fracture site, otherwise unrecognized infection at the latter might contaminate the donor area.

REFERENCES

Charnley J 1979 Low friction arthroplasty of the hip, theory and practice. Springer, Verlag, Berlin

Henry A K 1973 Extensile exposure, 2nd edn. Churchill Livingstone, Edinburgh

King K F, Rush J 1981 Closed intramedullary nailing of femoral shaft fractures. A review of 112 cases treated by the Kuntscher technique. Journal of Bone and Joint Surgery 63A: 1319

Salter R B 1961 Innominate osteotomy in the treatment of
congenital dislocation and subluxation of the hip. Journal
of Bone and Joint Surgery 43B: 518
Sarmiento A, Latta C L 1981 Closed functional treatment of
fractures. Springer Verlag, Berlin

FURTHER READING

Adams J C 1985 Standard orthopaedic operations, 3rd edn.
Churchill Livingstone, Edinburgh
Apley A G, Murphy W 1981 Where do we stand in the
treatment of fractures? In: Hadfield J, Hobsley M (eds)
Current surgical practice. Vol 3. Arnold, London, ch 13
Barlow T G 1962 Early diagnosis and treatment of congenital
dislocation of the hip. Journal of Bone and Joint Surgery
44B: 292
Burrows H J, Wilson J N, Scales J T 1975 Excision of
tumours of humerus and femur with restoration by
internal prostheses. Journal of Bone and Joint Surgery
57B: 148

Campbell's Operative orthopaedics 1980, 6th edn. Edmonson
A S, Crenshaw A H (eds) C V Mosby Co, London
Freeman M A R 1981 Reconstructive surgery in arthritis, In:
Hadfield J, Hobsley M, (eds) Current surgical practice,
Vol 3. Arnold, London, ch 14
Hooper G 1984 A colour atlas of common operations on the
foot. Wolfe Medical Publications Ltd, London
Hooper G 1985 A colour atlas of minor operations of the hand.
Wolfe Medical Publications Ltd, London
Hoppenfeld S, de Boer P 1984 Surgical exposures in
orthopaedics—the anatomic approach. J B Lippincott Co,
London
Hughes S P F 1983 Second generation joint replacements.
British Journal of Hospital Medicine, Vol 30, p 234
Muller M E, Allgower M, Schneider R, Willenegger H 1979
Manual of internal fixation, 2nd edn. Springer Verlag,
Berlin
Rockwood C A, Green D P (eds) 1984 Fractures in adults, 2nd
edn. J B Lippincott Co, London
Sweetnam R 1983 Limb preservation in the treatment of
bone tumours. Annals of the Royal College of Surgeons of
England 65: 3

6
Operations on the hand and fingers

G. HOOPER

GENERAL CONSIDERATIONS

Anaesthesia

Adequate anaesthesia is essential for operations on the hand. The method of obtaining anaesthesia should be compatible with use of the tourniquet (see below).

General anaesthesia or a brachial plexus block are indicated for major and prolonged operations. Bier's block is very suitable for minor operations (such as carpal tunnel release, removal of a ganglion, or decompression of tendon sheaths) but the tourniquet becomes uncomfortable after a while and the technique is unsuitable for procedures lasting more than about 15 minutes.

Local anaesthetic infiltration is not recommended for routine use in hand surgery; although anaesthesia may be adequate the local anatomy tends to be obscured by oedematous tissue. A digital nerve block is acceptable for operations on the distal part of the finger; 3–4 ml of 1% lignocaine *without adrenalin* is injected into the web spaces on either side of the finger around the dorsal and palmar digital nerves (Fig. 6.1). Subcutaneous infiltration of local anaesthetic in a tense ring around the base of the finger should be avoided as there is a small but real risk of causing mechanical embarrassment to the circulation.

Tourniquet

A tourniquet should be used whenever possible. A bloodless field is a great aid to precise identification and handling of tissue in the hand.

A finger tourniquet has a limited place, in operations on the distal part of the finger. The traditional type of finger tourniquet applied by clipping rubber tubing around the base of the finger is not recommended as the pressure exerted is very variable and it is not possible to exsanguinate the finger; a much more effective device is the finger of a rubber glove (Figs. 6.2 & 6.3). If a finger tourniquet is used it should be applied after the digital nerve block has been inserted.

For most operations an inflatable tourniquet is used. Before inflation the limb is emptied of blood by applying a rubber bandage firmly from the fingertips to the upper

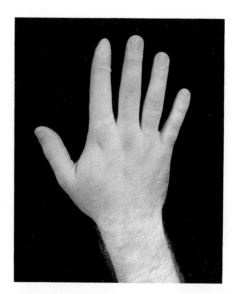

Fig. 6.2 Finger tourniquet. The finger of a rubber glove is placed over the finger

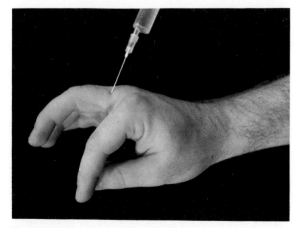

Fig. 6.1 Digital nerve block anaesthesia

131

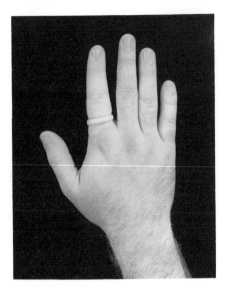

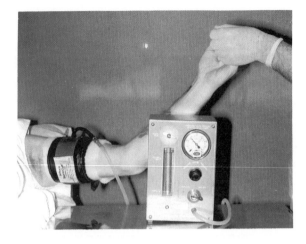

Fig. 6.5 Pneumatic tourniquet. The tourniquet is inflated and the rubber bandage removed

Fig. 6.3 Finger tourniquet. After cutting the end of the finger of the rubber glove it is rolled to the base of the finger

arm (Figs. 6.4 & 6.5). The inflation pressure of the tourniquet is 50 mm of mercury above systolic pressure; it is essential that the pressure is checked regularly during the operation. The tourniquet may be left in place for up to 1½ hours in a fit young patient. Tourniquets should be checked and calibrated regularly during routine theatre maintenance and unreliable or suspect equipment taken out of service immediately. If these simple rules of use are not kept then problems will certainly arise (Fletcher & Healy, 1983)

The preliminary bandaging must be omitted if the hand is infected as there is a theoretical risk of promoting spread of infection proximally. In these

circumstances the arm is elevated for several minutes before the pneumatic tourniquet is inflated in the usual way.

Skin preparation

The hand is painted with an antiseptic such as Betadine, using two sponges in holders; one supports the hand while the other is used for painting (Fig. 6.6). When there is an open wound on the hand, skin preparation is slightly modified (p. 136).

Position of the hand

The hand should rest on a small table and the surgeon and any assistants should be seated comfortably. A lead hand (Fig. 6.7) can be used to support the hand in position during the operation if so desired.

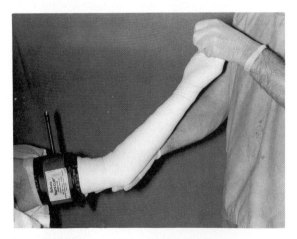

Fig. 6.4 Pneumatic tourniquet. After applying the tourniquet around the upper arm, the arm is exsanguinated by wrapping a rubber bandage around it

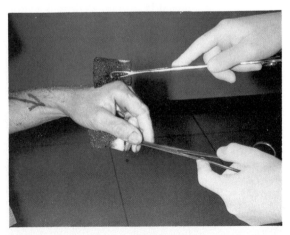

Fig. 6.6 Skin preparation. Note the use of two sponges in holders, one to support the hand and one to paint it

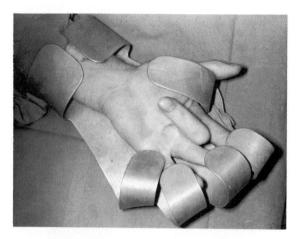

Fig. 6.7 A lead hand in use

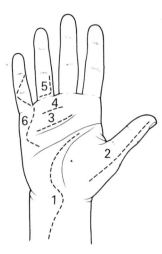

Fig. 6.9 Acceptable incisions on the palmar aspect of the hand:
1. An incision should not cross the wrist at right angles.
2. The 'mid-lateral' incision must lie dorsal to the ends of the flexor creases in the digits.
3. A transverse skin crease incision.
4. A transverse palmar incision.
5. Transverse incisions may be made in the flexor creases of the digits and may be extended by mid-lateral incisions.
6. The useful volar zig-zag incision. The apices of the skin flaps must lie at the end of the flexor skin creases

Elaborate and specialized instruments are rarely needed in hand surgery but the surgical instruments that are used (scissors, forceps, needle-holders, skin hooks and other retractors) should be of a size appropriate to the delicacy of the procedure and in excellent repair.

Magnification is a useful aid. For most purposes suitable magnification is provided by ×2 or ×3 loupes (Fig. 6.8). If higher magnification is needed the operating microscope is used.

Incisions

Incisions in the hand should be planned with care as wrongly placed incisions can damage important structures, or may contract on healing. To avoid scar contractures incisions in the hand should not cross skin creases at a right angle; they should be placed to avoid the crease if possible.

Short incisions in a finger should be placed transversely and on the palmar surface they should, if poss-

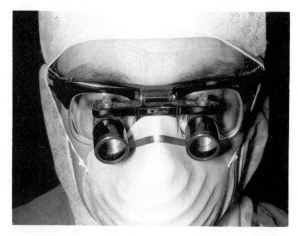

Fig. 6.8 Magnifying loupes

ible, lie in a flexion crease. A longer exposure can be made through a 'mid-lateral' incision, well behind the digital vessels and nerves; unless the incision lies posterior to the ends of the flexor creases it is prone to migrate to the flexor aspect of the finger and heal with contraction. A volar zig-zag incision (Fig. 6.9) avoids this problem.

In the palm, transverse incisions in the flexion creases should be used whenever possible. Zig-zag incisions meeting the flexion creases at 45° are acceptable alternatives (Fig. 6.9). At the wrist, incisions should lie transversely or meet the flexor crease at 45° (Fig. 6.9). For wide exposure at the wrist a transverse incision can be extended by proximal and distal extensions at either end (Fig. 6.10).

In circumstances where a longitudinal incision has been made at right angles across a skin crease the incision can usually be broken up by Z-plasties (p. 10) to avoid scar contractures. Many surgeons favour this technique for dealing with Dupuytren's contracture in the hand (p. 148).

Position of immobilization

If it is necessary to immobilize the hand for any time after surgery or injury, care must be taken to avoid secondary contractures of the interphalangeal (IP) and metacarpophalangeal (MCP) joints. Anatomical studies (Kuczynski, 1968) have shown that the relevant capsular

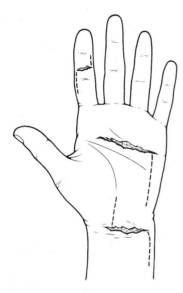

Fig. 6.10 Extending a transverse incision or traumatic wound. Incisions should never cross skin creases at right angles

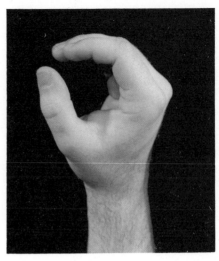

Fig. 6.12 Position of function. If the hand becomes stiff in this position it will still be of some functional use. For reasons discussed in the text, it is *not* the correct position for immobilization of the hand

structures are at their maximum length when the IP joints are extended, the MCP joints are flexed to 90° and the thumb is fully abducted from the palm (Fig. 6.11). It is necessary to hold the wrist in about 15° of dorsiflexion to maintain this position with comfort. This is the 'position of immobilization' and it differs from the 'position of function' described by Kanavel (1939) (Fig. 6.12). The 'position of function' is the posture in which a stiff hand will be of most functional use; the

'position of immobilization' is the position which will prevent or minimize stiffness.

The position of immobilization can be maintained by a correctly applied boxing glove dressing, reinforced with a plaster back slab to prevent flexion of the wrist (Fig. 6.13). If it is necessary to splint only part of the hand, for example a broken finger, the joints of the part should be placed in the position described above. The thumb must always be immobilized in abduction in

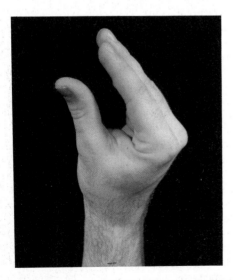

Fig. 6.11 Position of immobilization. The wrist is slightly dorsiflexed, the interphalangeal joints are extended and the metacarpophalangeal joints are flexed. The thumb lies parallel to the fingers

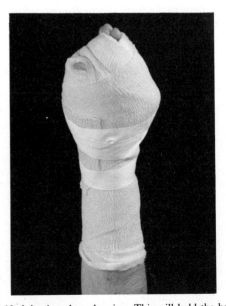

Fig. 6.13 A boxing glove dressing. This will hold the hand in the position of immobilization. A plaster back slab should be applied to keep the wrist dorsiflexed

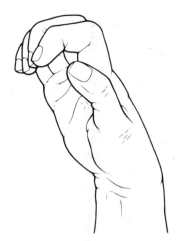

Fig. 6.14 A hand with multiple contractures. This type of crippling hand deformity is still, unfortunately, most often the result of failure to splint the hand in the correct position, to elevate the swollen hand or to supervise the rehabilitation of the patient

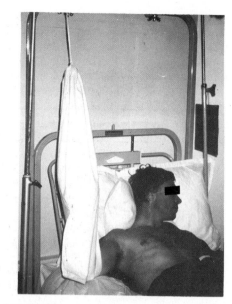

Fig. 6.15 Elevation of the hand

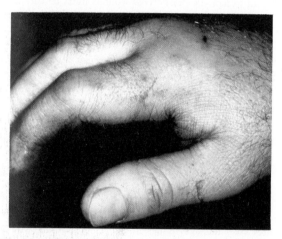

Fig. 6.16 When the hand is even slightly swollen it assumes an undesirable position. The metacarpophalangeal joints are extended, the interphalangeal joints are flexed and the thumb is adducted. Unless the swelling is reduced by elevation and the hand is splinted in the correct position (Fig. 6.11), secondary contractures will occur (Fig. 6.14)

relation to the palm, to prevent a contracture of the first web space. A thumb that lies in the plane of the palm is useless because it cannot be opposed to the fingers (Fig. 6.14).

It cannot be too strongly emphasized that one of the most common causes of hand dysfunction after surgery or injury, and one that is entirely preventable, is incorrect splintage.

Avoidance of swelling

Oedema is an inevitable accompaniment of trauma and infection but its devastating effects on the hand can be prevented by simple measures. Swelling is prevented, and treated, by elevating the hand and encouraging the patient to exercise the hand if the primary condition allows. Swelling of any severity is an indication for admission to hospital—it cannot be controlled by outpatient supervision. The hand is elevated in a roller towel (Fig. 6.15); this should be done as a routine after every operation on the hand, and the hand must be kept elevated until the patient is able to demonstrate that he is able to walk about with the hand held up and exercise it (if it is not splinted). Broad arm slings encourage dependency of the hand and are never needed after surgery or injury. The patient should be warned against their use.

When the hand is swollen the MCP joints tend to straighten, the IP joints to flex and the thumb to adduct—in other words the hand is held in the very position in which secondary joint contractures are most likely to occur (Fig. 6.16). It is therefore imperative that the swollen hand, in addition to being elevated, is splinted in the position of immobilization until the swelling is under control.

Rehabilitation

The hand does not get better by itself after surgery or injury. All patients, and some more than others, need supervision and instruction in appropriate use of the hand. In most patients who have had minor operations this will consist of reassurance that no damage can be done by putting the hand through a full range of movements, and ensuring that exercises are being done regularly. At the other extreme a few patients will need prolonged inpatient and outpatient treatment by physiotherapy and occupational therapy to restore mobility and function after severe injury or extensive reconstructive surgery. This type of supervision is a vital part of the overall management of the patient undergoing hand surgery and must never be neglected.

INJURIES OF THE HAND

It is the *initial* assessment and treatment of hand injuries which determines the final result. A trivial injury that is mismanaged can result in permanent disability— disability that might never have occurred had the patient not sought medical attention. It follows that:

1. New patients should be dealt with by a surgeon who has some training and experience in the management of hand injuries.
2. Full surgical technique (i.e. aseptic precautions in a properly equipped operating theatre) is essential in managing wounds.
3. Appropriate anaesthesia must be provided.
4. All except the most trivial wounds must be carefully explored so that all foreign matter may be removed and the full extent of the injury determined. A tourniquet is essential.
5. Primary closure of the skin and repair of other structures is carried out *only if conditions permit*.

Management of wounds

Skin preparation
Dirt should be removed from the skin of the hand using an appropriate preparation; soap and water is usually suitable but a solvent may be needed for greasy dirt. Skin preparation is completed by painting around the wound with an antiseptic. It is most important that antiseptic solutions are not allowed to enter the wound as they may damage tissues in the hand, but the wound should be irrigated with normal saline solution.

Wound excision
All wounds are contaminated with bacteria to a varying degree. Bacterial proliferation will cause clinical infection, and must be prevented by removing contaminated and dead tissue. Any ragged, devitalized or grossly contaminated skin edges are excised to leave the wound edges as healthy as possible. It is better to accept a slight deficiency of skin rather than leave doubtful skin that is almost certain to become infected. Subcutaneous fatty tissue which often prolapses through the skin on the palmar surface should also be excised.

The wound is thoroughly explored to ensure the removal of any foreign material and all devitalized tissue, and to identify possible damage to the deeper structures. If the wound must be enlarged any incision used for this purpose should conform with the principles given on page 133. Thorough irrigation using normal saline in a syringe will clear blood clot and superficial debris from the wound and allow more precise exploration.

Bleeding points should be coagulated with diathermy.

Wound closure
Primary suture is permissible if:
1. The wound is recent—not more than 4–6 hours old.
2. Contamination has been minimal.
3. The skin edges can be brought together without tension.

If these conditions do not pertain *the skin should not be sutured*. There are three main options if a wound has not been primarily sutured:

1. Adequate closure can often be obtained by pressure of dressing alone, any parts which remain unclosed being allowed to heal by granulation. With such treatment healing of small wounds may be expected to occur without infection and with the formation of a supple scar, a result far superior to that obtained when primary suture has been followed by even a mild degree of sepsis.

2. A wound with skin loss may be left open and the hand splinted and elevated. After 2–3 days the wound is inspected in the operating theatre and the wound is closed by some form of skin grafting, or a decision is made to allow the wound to close by granulation. This form of management has relatively little place in the care of hand wounds and is definitely not indicated if tendons, bones and joints are exposed, when treatment should be as in (3) below.

3. The wound is covered by an appropriate form of skin graft at the time of the original excision.

The indications for these various methods are best illustrated by discussing the management of some common types of wound of the hand.

Linear cuts and lacerations
The wound should be carefully explored but excision of tissue is seldom needed. Recent wounds may be closed primarily.

Bursting injuries
These are the result of severe compression such as may occur when the hand is trapped in rollers. The skin may literally burst open, exposing tendons, bones and joints. Because of the swelling it is impossible, and in any case it is undesirable, to close the wound primarily. All dead and contaminated tissue is carefully removed. A few loose stitches may be necessary to secure a covering for exposed tendon and bone. The hand is splinted in the position of immobilization and elevated. Further inspection is carried out 48 hours later when the swelling will be much less. Wounds with edges lying in contact may

be left to heal; gaping wounds or areas of skin loss should be closed by an appropriate skin grafting procedure.

Wounds with raised skin flaps

The displaced skin is thoroughly cleaned with saline; ragged edges and obviously devitalized parts are excised. The viability of the flap can be assessed by deflating the tourniquet cuff and examining the flap for return of colour and arterial bleeding. If the flap is considered viable it is secured in position with a few stitches without tension, and the hand is splinted and elevated. Firm dressings prevent the accumulation of blood under the flap. It is seldom that such a flap is found to have an intact circulation and as a general rule the skin flap with a distal base is always suspect. It is advisable to remove doubtfully viable skin during the initial surgical procedure rather than take a chance and be presented with an area of necrotic skin and surrounding infection at a subsequent wound inspection. The gliding structures of the hand underlying such a flap may be irrevocably damaged.

If partial or complete excision of a flap has been decided upon the skin defect is dealt with as described in the next section.

Wounds with skin loss

All loss of skin in the hands and fingers should be made good by skin grafting as soon as practicable. This not only hastens healing, but by preventing infection it avoids fibrosis and contracture, and preserves the function of deep tissue that would otherwise be exposed.

Partial thickness grafts as a method of skin replacement in the hand are less satisfactory on the palmar than on the dorsal surface because the grafted skin is relatively easily traumatised. Full thickness grafts of some variety are generally indicated when there has been loss of skin from the palmar surface of the hand. Free full thickness grafts have good wearing characteristics, but have the disadvantage of lack of sensation and inability to take over exposed tendon and bone.

A pedicle flap is necessary to cover tendon and bone. Such flaps should be planned and executed by a surgeon with special training in the techniques of plastic surgery; an ill-designed flap can create more problems than it solves. General guidance on the types of flap available are given on page 14. Suffice it to say here that, depending on the defect, it may be possible to use locally based pedicle grafts from the hand or it may be necessary to raise a flap from more distant sites such as the groin or deltopectoral areas. Wherever the flap is obtained it is of the utmost importance that, in so far as is possible, swelling of the hand due to dependency is avoided and secondary stiffness due to joint contracture is prevented.

Occasionally the skin of an injured finger that must be amputated can be preserved with its blood supply intact and used to cover a defect in the hand.

One special type of injury associated with skin loss that should be mentioned is the *ring avulsion*. In this injury, fortunately uncommon, the patient's ring is accidentally torn from the finger, removing the skin as a distally based sleeve of tissue. The injury often occurs when, in jumping from the back of a truck, the ring is caught on some projection on the tailboard. Tempting though it is to replace the skin on the finger this should not be done as the digital vessels are almost always either avulsed or thrombosed and death of the skin is inevitable. Immediate amputation is indicated unless circulation is definitely present in the skin.

Finger tip injuries

A *subungual haematoma* is usually caused by a crushing injury to the finger tip. A collection of blood forms under tension below the nail. The blood is easily evacuated by drilling the nail with an unwound paper clip that has been brought to red heat in a flame.

Traumatic amputations of the finger tip are exceedingly common injuries. If soft tissue alone has been lost the wound will usually close rapidly if protected by dressings. If bone is exposed it should be trimmed back to allow primary closure of the skin, using local advancement flaps if necessary (p. 9). Finger length should not be conserved if the result is a tight tender scar adherent to bone. There is little place for partial or full thickness free grafts in finger tip injuries; the former lacks stability to hard use and the latter lacks sensation: the result of using either type of graft is often a finger that is overprotected by its owner.

Injuries involving the nail bed require extremely careful repair if abnormal nail growth is to be avoided (Kleinert, 1967).

Wounds with division of nerves

The principles of management of nerve injuries are dealt with on pages 70–71, and specific features of injuries to the median, ulnar and radial nerves are described on pages 72–77. It need only be emphasized here that when there is a wound overlying a nerve it is mandatory to test the appropriate motor and sensory functions and if there is any doubt whatsoever about nerve function the wound should be explored in circumstances that will allow primary repair if indicated.

Severed digital nerves should be repaired primarily if possible. The cut ends of the nerve are opposed using three sutures of 8/0 Prolene. Splintage of the digit should be maintained for three weeks thereafter. Recovery of the nerve is usually good as it is of course a pure sensory nerve.

138   FARQUHARSON'S TEXTBOOK OF OPERATIVE SURGERY

Wounds with division of tendons

The techniques of tendon repair and the management of specific tendon problems in the hand have been dealt with on pages 19–22. Once again it must be emphasized that careful clinical examination of the injured hand is essential to exclude such injuries, and if there is any doubt about the action of the tendons the wound must be explored in circumstances that will allow the appropriate repair or reconstruction to be carried out.

As noted on page 19, when flexor tendons are cut in the fibrous flexor sheath healing occurs with adhesions around the tendon resulting in limitation of movement. For this reason primary repair should not be attempted, except under circumstances discussed below. The safe procedure is to close the skin wound and carry out delayed tendon grafting.

In the last decade there has been a return to the practice of primary flexor tendon repair in 'no man's land' (the previously prohibited area of the fibrous flexor sheath) by many experienced hand surgeons, with results that are equal to those obtained by delayed tendon grafting (Lister, 1977). The technique is demanding on both patient and surgeon (as indeed is flexor tendon grafting) and is totally contraindicated if the patient is likely to be unco-operative, or in any tendon injury other than a straightforward clean cut. The flexor tendons are repaired using buried wire or nylon sutures and a running 6/0 Prolene suture is inserted around the circumference of the tendon junction. The flexor sheath is repaired and the skin is closed. Elastic band traction is attached to the finger nail (Figs. 6.17 & 6.18), allowing active extension of the finger but only passive flexion; with this arrangement there is no stress across the tendon repair. Passive movement of the tendon within the sheath lessens the tethering effect of the inevitable adhesions that form around the healing

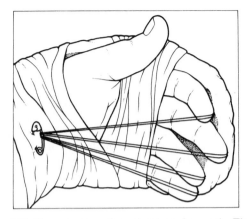

Fig. 6.18 Finger traction after primary tendon repair. The patient is encouraged to extend the fingers actively, against the tension in the elastic bands. Passive overdistraction of the tendon repair is prevented by the back slab which keeps the wrist and metacarpophalangeal joints flexed by about 30°

tendon. The traction is maintained for a minimum of four weeks and requires daily supervison.

Bites

All wounds sustained from contact with teeth are potentially serious, because of the risk of infection. Except in countries where rabies is endemic, human bites are much more dangerous than dog bites because of the virulence of the organisms involved (Chuinard & D'Ambrosia, 1977).

Bites of all descriptions, and any wound sustained from an adversary's teeth, should be treated with great respect. Exploration and excision should be particularly thorough and should be carried out with adequate anaesthesia. *It is safer if no stitches are inserted in the wound.* Often a tooth will penetrate a metacarphophalangeal joint when the fist is clenched; when the MCP joint is extended the puncture wound becomes sealed by the extensor hood. The patient some days after the incident may present with an early septic arthritis of the MCP joint. The joint should be explored, thoroughly irrigated with saline and the wound left open. The hand is immobilized in the optimum position. Pending identification of the bacteria involved a broad spectrum antibiotic is prescribed. Careful supervision of the patient is essential if stiffness is to be avoided.

Foreign bodies in the hand

Unless the foreign body can be identified easily by palpation its removal is likely to be much more difficult than would appear. Many inert foreign bodies can be left *in situ*. If exploration is indicated it must be performed under adequate anaesthesia with tourniquet control. A radio-opaque body should be identified on radiographs taken in two planes immediately before

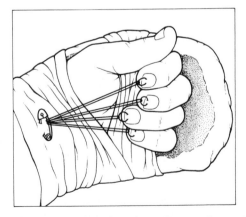

Fig. 6.17 Finger traction after primary flexor tendon repair. Elastic bands are attached to sutures passed through the nails of the involved fingers and keep the fingers passively flexed

operation. To assist in location a paper clip may be taped to the skin and after taking the radiograph a corresponding mark is made on the skin surface. If a needle or similar elongated object is being sought the incision should be made across the long axis, provided this does not conflict with the principles laid down on page 133.

Wooden foreign bodies may be contaminated, so the wound should not be stitched after their removal.

Splinter below the nail. As a rule, attempts have already been made to extract the splinter which has become broken off well below the nail bed. Under a local anaesthetic, a V-shaped portion of nail overlying the splinter is removed with scissors. This allows the splinter to be lifted out and provides drainage should infection supervene (Fig. 6.19).

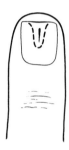

Fig. 6.19 Removal of a splinter below the nail

Injection injuries. Material may be injected under very high pressure from industrial grease guns and paint sprays. The usual history is that the nozzle blocked and then cleared suddenly as the user was testing it against his finger. The entry wound may be a quite innocent-looking puncture but the injected material has often penetrated for a considerable distance into the hand. If left, the extensive tissue damage becomes manifest over a few days and amputation is usually necessary. Treatment consists of early recognition of the severity of the injury and immediate exploration, which may be extensive. As much as possible of the injected material is removed, together with all obviously devitalized tissue.

Traumatic amputation of the hand
Crushing or mangling injuries of the hand must be treated by adequate excision of dead and contaminated tissue according to the principles outlined already. All viable tissue must be conserved for use in any secondary reconstructive procedure, and skin loss should be made good as soon as possible.

Replantation
When part of the hand has been amputated by a clean cut without severe crushing, surgical replantation using microsurgical techniques may be feasible. The indications for replantation vary somewhat among surgeons, but the following are general guidelines:

Unsuitable: Patient with significant medical or psychological problems.
Heavily contaminated, crushed or improperly preserved parts.
Single fingers.
Amputations at or distal to the interphalangeal joint.

Suitable: Thumb amputations.
Multiple amputations of fingers (not all parts are necessarily replanted).
Transmetacarpal, transcarpal and distal forearm amputations.

Preservation of parts. The amputated part is placed in a sterile polythene bag which is sealed and placed *on* ice. Ice, saline, antiseptics and preservatives should *not* be placed in the bag with the part. An occlusive dressing is placed on the stump and the patient and the part are transferred to a centre where microsurgical skills are available, and where a final decision can be made about the feasibility of replantation. Because of the limited amount of soft tissue in the hand, and especially in the fingers, replantation may be a possibility for up to 24 hours after injury.

Technique of replantation. Two surgical teams are initially needed, one to identify structures in the amputated part and the other to identify structures in the stump. Because of the length of the operation further surgical help may be needed during the procedure; replantation is a team effort, not a 'one-man show'.

The part is reattached by internal fixation of the bones, after first shortening them. Unless skeletal shortening is carried out the microvascular repair will be under tension and will surely fail. In the fingers the sequence of repair is:
1. Repair tendons.
2. Repair vessels under the microscope using 10/0 sutures; as a general rule at least two veins must be repaired for each artery. Vein grafts are often needed to reconstruct the vessels.
3. Finally the digital nerves are repaired.
Obviously this sequence may require some modification when amputations at other levels are dealt with.

After operation a close watch must be kept on the circulation, and reoperation to inspect the anastamoses may be necessary if there is suspicion of thrombosis. Reconstruction using vein grafts is usually needed if a segment of thrombosed vessel has to be removed.

Fractures in the hand
Fractures of the metacarpal bones and phalanges are extremely common. Like all injuries in the hand, they can cause long term disability if mismanaged. Many fractures need little or no treatment beyond encourage-

ment in normal use of the hand; and overtreatment, in the form of unnecessary splints and plasters, must be avoided. Other fractures, particularly displaced fractures, those involving joint surfaces or those associated with soft tissue damage may require very careful attention.

The main factor governing management is the stability of the fracture. Stability can usually be gauged from the clinical and radiographic appearance of the injury. Some common patterns are:

Stable. Isolated fractures of the metacarpal bones, undisplaced fractures of the phalanges.

Unstable. Multiple fractures of the metacarpal bones, fractures of the base of the thumb metacarpal involving the trapezio-metacarpal joint (Bennett's fracture), transverse and oblique fractures of the phalanges with displacement, fractures involving the condyles of the phalanges.

Stable undisplaced fractures do not need to be immobilized. Active use of the hand is advised. Taping an injured finger to an adjacent one (Fig. 6.20) will often give the patient some confidence in using the hand.

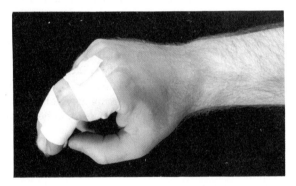

Fig. 6.20 Garter strapping for stable fractures of the phalanges. The interphalangeal joints must be left free. Some absorbent material should be placed between the fingers to prevent pressure sores over bony prominences

Unstable fractures must be reduced and held in position. If there are several fractures in the hand the whole hand should be splinted in the position of immobilization using a boxing glove dressing supported by a plaster slab. The hand must be elevated to control oedema. If there is only one fracture of a phalanx it can be splinted with a strip of metal covered with foam rubber (Fig. 6.21); uninjured digits are left free of splintage. The splint keeps the metacarpophalangeal joint flexed to a right angle and the interphalangeal joints straight. The surface marking of the MCP joint, and hence the position for placing the bend in the splint, is the distal palmar skin crease. Particular care should be taken to avoid rotational deformities in fractures of the proximal phalanges by ensuring that the palmar part of

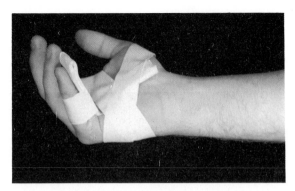

Fig. 6.21 Splintage for unstable fractures of the phalanges. Note that:
1. The splint is well covered with tape to prevent scratching from the edges of the metal.
2. The bend in the splint lies at the distal palmar skin crease.
3. The palmar part of the splint points to the tuberosity of the scaphoid, to prevent malrotation of the finger.
4. It is unnecessary for the splint to extend proximal to the wrist

the splint points to the tuberosity of the scaphoid at the base of the thenar eminence.

Some fractures cannot be stabilised easily by external splintage and internal fixation should be considered for them. Common examples are Bennett's fracture, fractures involving the condyles of the proximal phalanges and multiple displaced fractures of the hand. Internal fixation should also be considered in displaced open fractures with significant soft tissue damage (see below).

Adequate internal fixation of most fractures can be

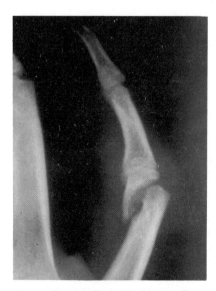

Fig. 6.22 X-ray of a typical unstable fracture. Fractures of the condyles of the proximal phalanges are often displaced, resulting in significant deformity of the finger

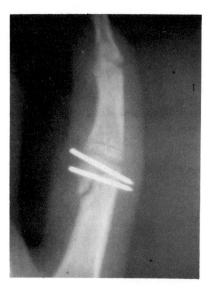

Fig. 6.23 Internal fixation of an unstable fracture. When the fracture has been reduced it is often possible to insert the Kirschner wires percutaneously on a power drill

obtained by the use of fine (0.035″ or 0.045″) Kirschner wires driven by a power drill. It is usually possible to reduce the fracture closed and then introduce the wire percutaneously (Figs. 6.22 & 6.23). A check radiograph is then obtained. (It is not good practice to introduce the wire under image intensifier screening as the surgeon's hands may be exposed to an unacceptable level of radiation over the course of several such procedures.) Open reduction is sometimes needed if the fracture cannot be reduced accurately. Wires can be cut short or left protruding through the skin according to choice: there is no firm evidence that protruding wires are associated with a higher incidence of infection and the wire is of course easier to remove; however the exposed wire can injure adjacent fingers and may be inadvertently withdrawn if the end catches on some object such as clothing. Wires may be removed from bone about three weeks after injury as the fracture is usually stable by this time. It should be mentioned that fractures of the phalanges remain visible for many weeks on radiographs, so that assessment of healing is made clinically, not radiographically.

Compound fractures
Open fractures of the fingers pose special problems, because the combination of a fracture and damage to the gliding tissues such as tendons can result in a stiff, largely useless digit which interferes with the function of the other fingers. This problem is likely to arise when either the proximal or intermediate phalanges have been broken, since the tendons pass over them. Treatment of compound fractures of the terminal phalanges is

directed towards obtaining a stable finger tip that will stand up to heavy work and, since bone healing is seldom a problem, appropriate management of the wound is the priority.

In all open fractures careful débridement is necessary; damage to soft tissue structures should be identified and a decision made about primary reconstruction. Associated damage to tendons, vessels or nerves is an indication for internal fixation with Kirschner wires to allow accurate repair of the soft tissues. Extensor tendons should be repaired with fine nonabsorbable mattress sutures. Primary repair of flexor tendons is not indicated when there is an open fracture at the same level but it must be realized that if a decision is taken to conserve the finger and carry out secondary flexor tendon grafting when the fracture has healed, the patient and surgeon are committed to a programme of management lasting several months with a very uncertain outcome. Primary amputation should be considered when an open fracture of a single finger is associated with considerable damage to soft parts. There is little point in 'saving' a finger if the result is a stiff, painful and useless part. This is particularly so in the case of the manual worker to whom an early return to work and settlement of any compensation claim are of great economic importance.

Multiple open fractures in the hand should be stabilized with multiple Kirschner wires for 3–4 weeks, until soft tissue healing allows mobilization of the hand. In this type of injury some degree of functional impairment is almost inevitable but it should be minimized by treatment. A minimum of Kirschner wire should be used, placed so that the hand can be brought into the position of immobilization. If at all possible the wires should avoid transfixing tendons.

Primary arthrodesis of an interphalangeal joint (p. 149) is indicated when an open intra-articular fracture is complicated by damage to tendons, but circulation and sensation in the finger are unimpaired. An arthrodesis of a metacarpophalangeal joint of a finger should never be done, as function of the other, normal, fingers may be impaired. Fusion of the MCP joint of the thumb is permissible.

INFECTIONS OF THE HAND AND FINGERS

Severe infections of the hand are fortunately less common than formerly. This is no doubt attributable to better treatment of wounds and antibiotic treatment of early infections. Nevertheless, when severe infections do occur they can rapidly cripple a hand unless managed correctly. A false sense of security can be engendered by treatment with antibiotics which may suppress but not eradicate infection.

The general principles of management of hand infections are quite straightforward and comprise:
1. Rest in the position of immobilization.
2. Elevation to minimize oedema.
3. Appropriate antibiotic treatment.
4. Surgical drainage of localized pus.
5. Rehabilitation when the infection is under control.

Antibiotics
Most infections are due to pencillin-resistant staphylococci. Until the organism has been cultured and identified it is appropriate to treat the patient with a broad-spectrum antibiotic that is active against penicillinase-producing organisms. Antibiotic treatment should be continued until after the patient begins to regain active, pain-free hand movements.

Surgical treatment
If there is a localized abscess it must be drained surgically by the most direct route. Adequate anaesthesia and a bloodless field are both essential for any drainage operation. Without them adequate exploration of the abscess cavity is impossible and there is a distinct risk of overlooking a 'collar stud' extension of the abscess.

Subcuticular infections

Septic blisters
These are common on the palmar surface of the fingers and in the finger webs. The epidermis becomes elevated by a collection of pus within the layers of the skin. The raised epidermis may be shaved off with a scalpel. A careful search must be made for any track leading to a deeper abscess which must be explored and laid open.

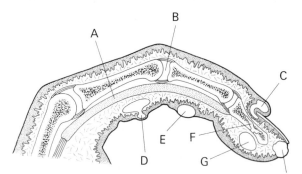

Fig. 6.24 Infections that may affect a digit:
A. Tendon sheath infection
B. Septic arthritis
C. Paronychia
D. Subcuticular abscess with subcutaneous 'collar stud' extension
E. Subcuticular abscess
F. Osteomyelitis
G. Pulp space infection
H. Apical pulp space infection

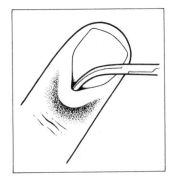

Fig. 6.25 Paronychia. Pus is drained by separating the nail fold from the nail with artery forceps

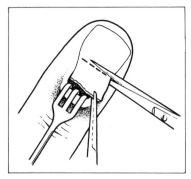

Fig. 6.26 Paronychia. If infection has extended beneath the nail, part of it must be removed to ensure free drainage

Paronychia
This is an infection of the nail fold (Fig. 6.24). Mild cases can be aborted by antibiotic treatment; if this is unsuccessful or too late, pus will collect deep to the nail or spread around it in a horseshoe fashion. Pus under the nail is drained by removing an appropriate amount of the proximal part of the nail (Figs. 6.25 & 6.26). Part of the nail fold must be lifted as a flap to gain access.

Carbuncles in the hand
Like carbuncles elsewhere, these result from a staphylococcal infection of hair follicles and therefore occur on the dorsum of the hand or the proximal segments of the fingers. They respond well to antibiotic treatment and surgical intervention should be restricted to the removal of any sloughing tissue.

Subcutaneous infections

Pulp space infections
The three pulp spaces on the flexor aspect of the fingers are separated by the flexor creases where the skin is attached to the underlying fibrous flexor sheath. The fatty tissue in the terminal space is subdivided into

15–20 compartments by fibrous septa between the skin and the periosteum of the terminal phalanx. Infection in the terminal pulp space therefore does not spread down the finger, but causes a rapid build up of pressure which may be associated with sloughing of the overlying skin and osteomyelitis of the terminal phalanx. Necrosis of the terminal phalanx is not unusual and is probably secondary to bone infection, although thrombosis of vessels due to pressure or bacterial toxins may be involved.

In the early acute phase antibiotic treatment is often successful. If localization of pus occurs, indicated by persistent pain, localized tenderness and perhaps subcuticular pointing of pus, then it should be drained by the shortest route. An 0.5 cm incision is made over the most tender point (Fig. 6.27) and deepened until pus is encountered. Extensive incisions are unnecessary but the original incision may have to be extended to allow thorough exploration and drainage of the cavity. Sloughing tissue may be excised but only obviously dead, sequestrated bone fragments should be removed.

An apical abscess is a special type of pulp infection. Infection is localized to the area under the free margin of the nail, just dorsal to the tip of the phalanx (see Fig. 6.24). Treatment consists of evacuating the pus through a small incision over the most tender point. If there is much pus under the nail a triangular segment should be removed, as in the treatment of a retained splinter beneath the nail (p. 139).

Infection in the middle and proximal pulp spaces is less common than in the terminal space. The spaces are bounded, but not entirely closed, by attachments of the skin creases to the fibrous flexor sheaths and laterally by fascial attachments between the skin and the phalanges; they are not subdivided by fibrous septa. Localized pus, which can track to the web spaces, should be drained by a longitudinal incision over the point of maximum tenderness, or where there is visible pointing.

Web space infections

The space between the bases of the fingers communicates with the dorsum of the hand and proximal pulp spaces of the fingers via loose connective tissue at the side of the fingers. Infection in these areas can spread to the web spaces, or the spaces may become infected directly from an abrasion on the overlying skin.

In the early stages the infection is in the nature of a diffuse cellulitis which may resolve with antibiotic therapy. Later the adjacent fingers are separated by the swollen web, which bulges out both palmwards and dorsally, and adjacent web spaces may become involved.

Any drainage operation should be delayed until the infection is localized, and then the abscess should be drained by the most direct route, usually a short transverse incision on the palmar surface about 1 cm proximal to the web margin (Fig. 6.28). If the incision is kept short it is most unlikely that the digital nerves and vessels will be injured.

Tendon sheath infection

The synovial sheath of the flexor tendons is usually infected by direct puncture wounds, particularly where the skin is in close contact with the sheath at the skin creases, but infection may also spread into it from adjacent lesions.

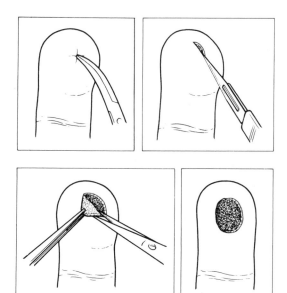

Fig. 6.27 Terminal pulp space infection. The point of maximum tenderness is found by clinical examination. An incision is made at this point. The wound may be enlarged by removal of skin to ensure that there is a cavity that can drain freely

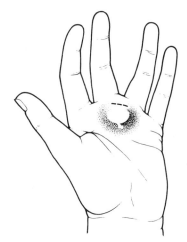

Fig. 6.28 Drainage of a web space infection

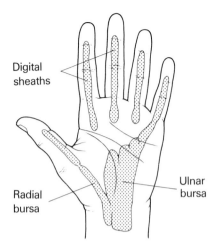

Fig. 6.29 The synovial sheaths in the hand

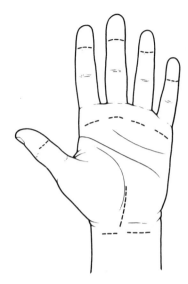

Fig. 6.30 Incisions for drainage of synovial sheaths in the hand

Each digit has a fibrous and synovial sheath. The synovial sheaths surround the flexor tendons; those of the index, middle and ring fingers end proximally at about the level of the metacarpophalangeal joints, but the sheath of the thumb is continuous with the radial bursa, and that of the little finger with the ulnar bursa (Fig. 6.29). The ulnar bursa is the name given to the synovial sheath that surrounds all the tendons passing to the fingers in the palms; it extends about 2.5 cm proximal to the wrist joint. There is usually a communication between the radial and ulnar bursae, deep to the flexor retinaculum. Spread of infection from the little finger into the ulnar bursa is uncommon, but spread of infection from the thumb sheath to the radial bursa is not infrequent.

In an established, untreated tendon sheath infection there is severe, throbbing pain and swelling of the finger which takes up a slightly flexed position. Passive movements cause severe pain. This clinical presentation is considerably modified by antibiotic treatment: swelling is not marked and limited passive and active flexion may be possible without pain. However there is usually localized tenderness along the sheath and passive *extension* of the proximal interphalangeal joint causes pain.

When the ulnar bursa is infected there is swelling of the whole hand, and swelling often extends above the wrist. The fingers are characteristically held in a semi-flexed position and passive extension causes severe pain. Compression of the median nerve in the carpal tunnel also contributes to the pain. Infection of the thumb and radial bursa causes swelling of the thumb and thenar eminence, and the thumb is held slightly flexed.

Surgical exploration is indicated for any tendon sheath infection that has not settled completely after 48 hours of adequate antibiotic treatment. The fibrous sheath is exposed through volar incisions placed at the entrance of the sheath and the distal skin crease of the finger

(Fig. 6.30). A 1 mm diameter catheter is threaded up the sheath from the proximal incision and the sheath is thoroughly irrigated with normal saline. The hand is splinted in the position of immobilization in a boxing glove dressing, the irrigation is continued and antibiotics are given systemically. If the ulnar bursa is infected it should be explored through a longitudinal incision on the volar aspect of the wrist, care being taken not to cross the wrist at a right angle (Fig. 6.30). The flexor retinaculum is divided, carefully protecting the median nerve, to expose the ulnar bursa which should be opened and irrigated.

The radial bursa is approached through an incision on the ulnar border of the tendon of flexor carpi radialis, with careful identification and retraction of the median nerve. The distended radial bursa is identified, opened and an irrigation catheter passed into it.

It is rare now to encounter extensive sloughing of the flexor tendons due to delay in treatment. When it occurs amputation of the finger should be considered because permanent stiffness is inevitable and may well compromise the function of other fingers.

Septic arthritis in the hand

Infection of interphalangeal and metacarpophalangeal joints may be due to extension of infection from surrounding soft tissues, or follow penetrating injuries of the joint (p. 138). Wounds of the knuckle sustained by contact with an adversary's teeth are particularly dangerous.

In the early stages infection is confined to the synovial membrane and splintage, elevation and antibiotic treatment may be sufficient to control it. However, infections are seldom encountered at this early stage and it is safer to recommend exploration of all penetrating injuries under antibiotic cover. The extensor tendon is retracted or, if it has been partially divided, the wound is extended to allow a clear view of the joint. Any fragment of bone and cartilage is lifted out and the joint is thoroughly irrigated with normal saline. The wound is left open and the hand is splinted until the infection has settled. Thereafter active movements are commenced.

Infections of the palmar spaces

The *palmar subaponeurotic space* (or superficial middle palmar space) lies deep to the palmar aponeurosis and superficial to the flexor tendons (Fig. 6.31). It contains the superficial palmar arch and the digital branches of the median and ulnar nerves.

The *ulnar and radial bursae* have already been described.

The *midpalmar space* extends between the little and ring finger metacarpal bones and lies between the interossei and the ulnar bursa (Fig. 6.31). The tendon sheaths of the middle and ring fingers project into the space and prolongations of the space (the lumbrical canals) extend towards the web spaces between the digits (Fig. 6.32). Proximally the space is in continuity beneath the flexor retinaculum with the space of Parona above the wrist.

The *thenar space* lies deep to the thenar muscles and superficial to adductor pollicis (Fig. 6.31). It is separated from the mid-palmar space by a septum which extends from the long finger metacarpal bone. A lumbrical canal extends from the space towards the radial

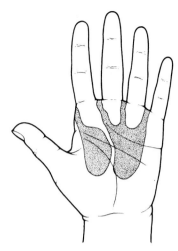

Fig. 6.32 The thenar and middle palmar spaces are extended to the web spaces by the lumbrical canals

border of the index finger (Fig. 6.32). The tendon sheath of the index finger communicates with the space.

Infection of the palmar subaponeurotic space is not uncommon and is usually secondary to an abrasion or penetrating wound of the palm. When pus is localized in the palm it must be drained and a careful search made for any connection with another, deeper collection since 'collar stud' abscesses are often found in this region (Fig. 6.31). It is now extremely uncommon to encounter infections of the deep palmar spaces. They are usually secondary to spread of infection from appropriate tendon sheaths, or a web space infection tracking down a lumbrical canal. The characteristic sign of deep infection is loss of the normal concavity of the palm, together with swelling of the dorsum of the hand. Passive movements of the fingers are limited and extremely painful. Localization of pus usually becomes evident by tracking to the surface of the palm or one of the webs. The mid-palmar space is drained through one of the appropriate lumbrical canals (Fig. 6.33) and the thenar space via the lumbrical canal on the radial border of the index finger; if pus points elsewhere it may be drained directly.

Other infections

Cellulitis and lymphangitis. These are usually due to streptococcal infection and are spreading infections that usually do not localize. As there is no local collection of pus, drainage is not needed. Indeed, surgical interference is positively dangerous and may cause further spread of infection. Treatment is by rest, elevation and antibiotics.

Pyogenic granuloma. This lesion is the result of an abnormal response to a minor penetrating injury. An infected mass of granulation tissue appears at the site of the injury (Fig. 6.34). It is painful and bleeds easily.

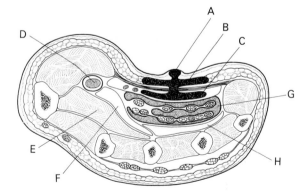

Fig. 6.31 A transverse section through the proximal part of palm:
A. Subcuticular palmar abscess
B. Subcutaneous palmar abscess
C. Subaponeurotic palmar abscess
D. Flexor pollicis longus tendon in radial bursa
E. Adductor pollicis
F. Thenar space
G. Ulnar bursa
H. Deep palmar space

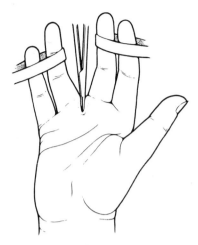

Fig. 6.33 Draining the middle palmar space along a lumbrical canal

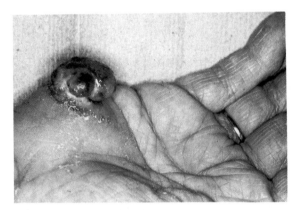

Fig. 6.34 Pyogenic granuloma

Much of the granulation tissue lies below the skin; careful exploration and removal of all involved tissue is necessary.

CONGENITAL ANOMALIES OF THE HAND

Malformations of the hand are not particularly uncommon, occurring in about 1 per 1000 live births. Many different types of anomalies are seen and, rather than attempting to be comprehensive, this section will deal with the principles of their management; the role of surgical treatment, rather than details of surgical operations, will be described.

Classification
Deformities may be:
1. Isolated, affecting only the hand and upper limb.
2. Associated with other congenital anomalies, perhaps together recognized as a malformation syndrome.

3. Associated with a generalized skeletal dysplasia.

It is most important for the parents to have advice from a clinical geneticist on the pattern of inheritance, if any, of the congenital deformity affecting the child. Many deformities have no genetic basis (e.g. those associated with thalidomide ingestion during pregnancy) but others have a very clear cut inheritance.

In describing the deformity it is best to keep to a very simple overall classification of types. One such, used by many hand surgeons, is given in Table 6.1, together with examples of some of the many anomalies.

Table 6.1 Classification of congenital anomalies of the hand

Type	Example
Failure of formation of parts	
i. Transverse	Congenital absence of forearm and hand
ii. Longitudinal	Absence of radius and thumb ('Radial club hand')
Failure of separation of parts	Syndactyly (fused fingers)
Duplication	Polydactyly (extra digits)
Overgrowth	Macrodactyly (isolated overgrowth of a digit)
Congenital constriction band syndrome	Partial amputation or annular grooves
Associated with skeletal dysplasias	Multiple enchondromatosis (Ollier's disease) often affects the hands
	The hand is abnormally shaped in many skeletal disorders, e.g. Marfan's syndrome, achondroplasia
Miscellaneous (Conditions not classifiable elsewhere)	Camptodactyly (contractures of the IP joints)
	Clinodactyly (congenital lateral curvature of the little finger)

Principles of management
Because of the relative rarity of individual anomalies it is important that children with these conditions are seen by a surgeon with appropriate special experience, preferably soon after birth. Many congenital anomalies of the hand do not require, or are not amenable to, any form of surgical treatment and in any case the need for surgery is seldom pressing; however it is important to establish an early relationship with the parents and to advise them on the likely programme of management for their child.

The aim of surgical treatment is to improve hand function; surgery to improve appearance is undertaken only if there will be no deterioration in function. The goal of reconstruction is a hand that has active pinch and grasp; good skin sensation is fundamental to this. Prolonged, careful observation of the use the child makes of his limb is necessary before any decision about surgery can be made, and here the help of an occupational therapist with special interest and experience in this field can be invaluable. Children are able to develop extremely useful patterns of function even in the presence of severe anomalies.

Timing of surgery

Soft tissue procedures, such as removing a useless floating extra digit, can be done at an early age but sometimes more complicated soft tissue operations (such as separating a syndactyly) are best left until the hand is larger as this makes any surgery much easier. Bone and joint procedures and tendon transfers (which may be required for example in providing a thumb) should be delayed for the same reason; however, if the proposed surgery is likely to alter the pattern of prehension it should not be long delayed as it is more difficult for the older child to develop a new pattern of prehension. Generally speaking, it is desirable to have all major procedures completed before the child is due to go to school for the first time as by then he has established a pattern of use of the hand and disruption of education should be kept to a minimum.

DUPUYTREN'S CONTRACTURE

Dupuytren's disease affects the palmar and digital fascia in the hand, and occasionally the plantar fascia in the foot. It is extremely common in middle-aged and elderly people in Britain and many other countries where the population is of mainly European origin, but rarely affects Chinese, Indian or African people. A fairly strong autosomal dominant pattern of inheritance has been demonstrated in a proportion of patients in several studies. There is probably an association with some other disorders, notably epilepsy, alcoholic cirrhosis and diabetes, but the link is not clear. The disease is equally common in manual and non-manual workers, but injury may occasionally cause progression of the disease in someone who is prone to develop it. Women are affected less often than men in the middle years and there is some evidence that the disease is less severe in women.

The characteristic early lesion is a collection of fibroblasts and contractile myofibroblasts in the longitudinal fibres of the fascia, or between the fascia and the skin, forming a nodule. Nodules coalesce to form cords of fibrous tissue extending into the fingers. Shortening of these cords causes contractures of the fingers.

Clinical features

The ulnar part of the hand is most often affected, al-

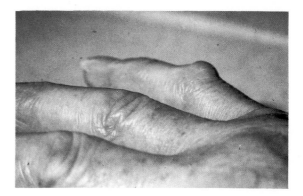

Fig. 6.35 A knuckle pad (Garrod's pad) on the dorsum of the proximal interphalangeal joint of the little finger

though thumb involvement is not rare. Early nodules are often uncomfortable and their removal may be requested for this reason. However surgical removal is often followed by rapid recurrence and progression to contracture and it is preferable to inject the lesion with a long-acting corticosteroid preparation, which often relieves the discomfort. The same management is recommended for the fibrofatty pads (Garrod's pads, Fig. 6.35) sometimes seen on the dorsum of the proximal interphalangeal joints in young patients who have a strong likelihood of developing Dupuytren's disease in later life.

If cords of affected fascia are confined to the palm, finger contractures do not occur. It is only when they pass into the fingers that shortening of the cords is likely to pull the fingers into flexion. If the metacarpophalangeal joint is pulled into flexion (Fig. 6.36) a secondary joint contracture is very unlikely to develop, since the tethering band still allows further active flexion, thus bringing the capsular ligaments of the MCP joint to their full length (see 'Position of Immobilization', p. 133). In

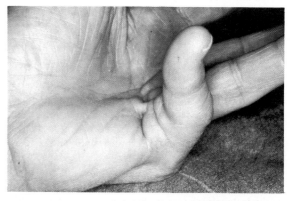

Fig. 6.36 Dupuytren's contracture. There is a 90° flexion contracture of the metacarpophalangeal joint of the little finger

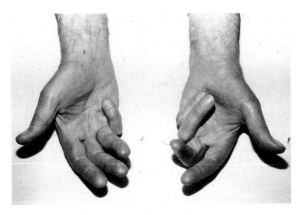

Fig. 6.37 Dupuytren's contracture. Severe contractures of the proximal interphalangeal joints of fingers in both hands

contrast if the proximal interphalangeal joints are pulled into flexion by their tethering cords (Fig. 6.37) secondary joint contractures rapidly occur, for the cord prevents the PIP joint being put in full extension, the position in which the capsular ligaments are at full length. These points are of great importance in predicting the likely results of fasciectomy.

Treatment

The treatment of established Dupuytren's contracture is surgical. The type of operation, and its timing, should be decided on an individual basis.

Timing

The rate of increase of contractures is very variable; in some patients they remain static for many years and in others become severe within a few months. Surgery should be carried out before secondary joint contractures have developed; thus there is no urgency when the MCP joint alone is affected, since secondary contractures do not occur and a good correction can always be obtained, but if the PIP joint is involved surgery should not be long delayed for secondary joint contractures may result in a permanent flexion contracture, even after removal of the involved fascia.

Types of operation

Local fasciectomy is the treatment of choice. Recovery is rapid after this procedure, in which only the affected, abnormal fascia is removed. *Radical fasciectomy*, i.e. removal of all fascia, normal and abnormal, is no longer practised; it is followed by severe swelling and stiffness of the hand and the overall results are poor. *Subcutaneous fasciotomy* is seldom done although it has a small place in the management of elderly unfit patients with a single longitudinal cord causing flexion of the MCP joint. The cord is cut with a tenotomy knife in the palmar region; it is risky to cut the cord in the finger be-

cause of the close relationship of the digital nerves and vessels to it.

Incisions. Local fasciectomy is carried out in a bloodless field with adequate anaesthesia.

Many incisions have been described and each surgeon has his own particular favourites. The main points to bear in mind are:

1. The cords of abnormal tissue must be adequately exposed.
2. The principles of siting scars on the hand described on page 133 must be observed.
3. There is no single method of dealing with Dupuytren's contracture because the extent and severity vary so much between patients.
4. Skin flaps must be made as thick as possible, but one should be aware of the fact that the digital nerves and vessels may lie superficial to affected fascia in the finger. Therefore a direct cut down on to the fascia must be avoided and the flaps must be raised from it with due care.

The most frequently used incisions are illustrated in Figure 6.38. A single cord may be dissected out through a longitudinal incision from the palm to the finger, which is closed with Z-plasties. A good, simple exposure is the volar zig-zag exposure of Bruner. Mid-lateral incisions in the fingers are preferred by some, but the exposure is not so good. If a wider exposure of the palmar fascia is needed a transverse incision is placed in the distal palmar crease, and this can be combined with incisions entering the fingers. At the end of the procedure

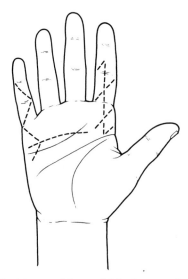

Fig. 6.38 Incisions used for partial fasciectomy. A volar zig-zag incision provides good exposure and may be combined with a transverse palmar incision when a wider exposure of the palmar fascia is needed. Many surgeons use a longitudinal incision to expose the abnormal fascia and then break up the incision with multiple Z-plasties

the transverse palmar wound is left open, thus allowing any haematoma to drain freely; recovery is rapid and painfree. The transverse wound closes in quickly, leaving a fine scar (McCash, 1964).

Following excision of the involved tissue, with careful identification and preservation of the digital vessels and nerves, the tourniquet can be released to allow identification and coagulation of any small bleeding vessels. Many surgeons do not release the tourniquet at this point, but rely on careful identification and coagulation of vessels during dissection to ensure haemostasis. The results of both techniques are probably equally good.

Postoperative management

The hand is placed in a boxing glove dressing with a dorsal back slab and kept elevated to minimize swelling. After a few days the dressings are removed and mobilization is started under the supervision of a physiotherapist. A night splint to keep the MCP joints and IP joints extended is worn for several weeks.

Recurrence. This is not uncommon, particularly in young patients with a strong diathesis. It is usually apparent within 2 years of operation. Treatment is by further fasciectomy and, if the skin is involved, excision of the affected skin and replacement with a full thickness free skin graft taken from the inner aspect of the upper arm.

Recurrence should be distinguished from extension, which is development of the disease elsewhere in the hand.

Amputation. Amputation of a finger is rarely indicated as a primary treatment but is sometimes requested by a patient who has had several operations for recurrent disease in a finger. Dorsal skin from an amputated finger can be used to replace involved skin in the palm; there is some evidence that recurrence is uncommon beneath such a graft.

SURGERY OF THE ARTHRITIC HAND

The hand can be affected by many types of arthritis, the most frequently encountered being osteoarthritis, rheumatoid arthritis and psoriatic arthropathy.

Osteoarthritis

In the hand this typically affects the distal interphalangeal joints and the trapeziometacarpal joint at the base of the thumb.

Distal interphalangeal joints

Osteoarthritic lipping of the distal interphalangeal joints is manifested as Herberden's nodes. Pain is often slight despite advanced arthritic changes on radiographs

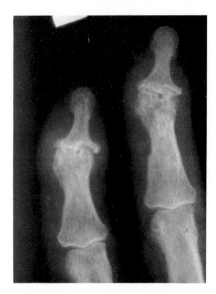

Fig. 6.39 X-ray of osteoarthritis affecting the distal interphalangeal joints

(Fig. 6.39). If pain is a problem arthrodesis of the affected joint is indicated (see below).

Occasionally a ganglion (or 'mucous cyst') arises from the dorsum of an osteoarthritic interphalangeal joint, and typically lies to one or other side of the extensor tendon. Successful removal is by no means easy and operation is only indicated if the ganglion is very large or otherwise troublesome. The neck of the ganglion must be dissected down to the joint and removed. Abnormally thin skin over the lesion should be excised and a local rotation flap used to close the defect (Kleinert et al, 1972) (Fig. 6.40). Unless these precautions are taken recurrence or a synovial fistula may occur, and arthrodesis of the joint may be necessary.

Arthrodesis of an IP joint. The technique described by Lister (1978) is recommended for arthrodesis of the IP

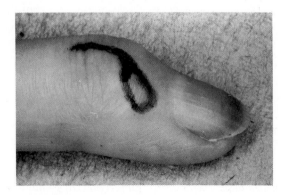

Fig. 6.40 Removal of a mucous cyst. Abnormal skin over the cyst should be removed and the defect closed by advancing a flap of normal skin

joints and the MCP joints of the thumb. (As noted previously, arthrodesis of the MCP joints of fingers is very disabling and should not be done.)

The distal IP joint is approached through an H-shaped incision on the dorsum of the finger, the proximal IP joint through a curved dorsal skin incision with reflection of the extensor tendon. Collateral ligaments are divided to allow complete dislocation of the joints and careful removal of all articular cartilage; the normal configuration of the joint surfaces should be maintained to allow contact of cancellous bone. Using a 0.035″ Kirschner wire on a power drill, two parallel holes are drilled 0.5 cm either side of the joint. A loop of No. 0 (BS Gauge 26) monofilament stainless steel wire is passed through the holes. A 0.035″ diameter Kirschner wire is then driven retrograde from the joint and then, whilst holding the bones in contact at the desired angle, back across the joint. The wire loop is then tightened and its twisted end buried in soft tissue. Very stable fixation is obtained with this technique (Fig. 6.41). The longitudinal wire should remain in place for about 6 weeks.

Recommended angles for arthrodesis are shown in Table 6.2.

Trapeziometacarpal joint of thumb (Fig. 6.42)
This most often affects middle-aged women, causing pain and sometimes a progressive adduction deformity

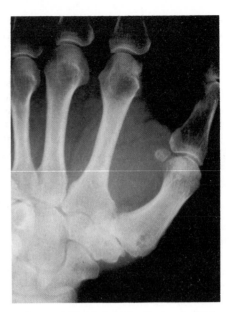

Fig. 6.42 Osteoarthritis of the trapeziometacarpal joint of the thumb

of the metacarpal bone of the thumb. Surgical treatment is indicated only if conservative treatment, in the form of anti-inflammatory analgesics, local steroid injections, or rest in plaster, have been unsuccessful. Several different operations are available:

Arthrodesis. The joint is approached through the anatomical snuff box, the remains of the cartilage removed, and the surfaces apposed and stabilized with Kirschner wires, with the thumb in an abducted position. It is by no means easy to obtain a solid arthrodesis; care must be taken to place the cancellous surfaces in close apposition and a scaphoid-type plaster is worn for 6 weeks.

Osteotomy. This is a very simple procedure. A dorsally based wedge of bone is removed from the metacarpal bone about 1 cm from the joint. The osteotomy is closed and held with an intraosseous loop of wire (Fig. 6.43) (Wilson & Bossley, 1983).

Arthroplasty. Excision arthroplasty is performed by removing the trapezium. It is surprisingly difficult to remove all the bone but important that this be done. Pain relief is good, but the thumb tends to be weak in gripping.

The trapezium may be replaced by a silicone rubber spacer; this is a form of interposition arthroplasty (Swanson, 1972). Total replacement of the trapeziometacarpal joint with a miniature artificial ball and socket joint has been described but is still under evaluation.

Rheumatoid arthritis (Figs. 6.44–6.47)
The surgery of the hand affected by rheumatoid arthritis is a highly specialized field which is more properly covered in detailed texts to which the reader is referred

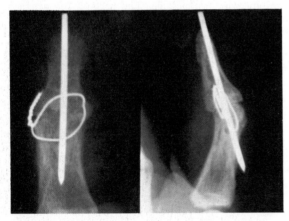

Fig. 6.41 X-ray showing arthrodesis of an interphalangeal joint. Intraosseous wiring is a very reliable method

Table 6.2 Recommended angles for arthrodesis

Thumb	MCPJ	20°	IPJ	10–20°
Index finger	PIPJ	20°	DIPJ	10°
Middle finger	PIPJ	30°	DIPJ	10–20°
Ring finger	PIPJ	40°	DIPJ	15–30°
Little finger	PIPJ	50°	DIPJ	20–40°

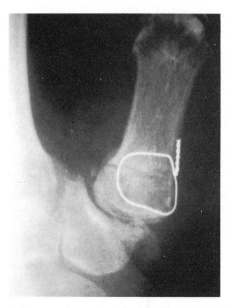

Fig. 6.43 Metacarpal osteotomy for trapeziometacarpal osteoarthritis of the thumb

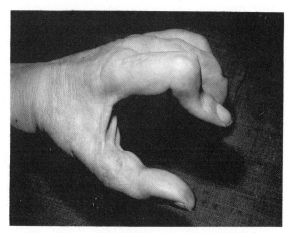

Fig. 6.45 Rheumatoid arthritis. Boutonnière deformity caused by rupture of the central slip of the extensor apparatus over the proximal interphalangeal joint

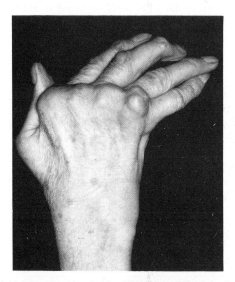

Fig. 6.44 Rheumatoid arthritis. Ulnar deviation of the fingers and subluxation of the metacarpophalangeal joints. (Reproduced with permission from Lamb & Hooper, 1985)

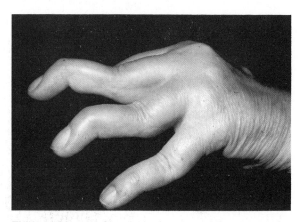

Fig. 6.46 Rheumatoid arthritis. Swan-neck deformity of several fingers

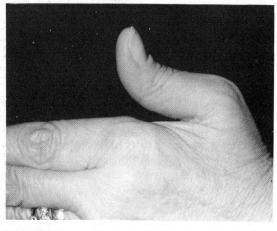

Fig. 6.47 Rheumatoid arthritis. Z-deformity of the thumb. (Reproduced with permission from Lamb & Hooper, 1985)

(Green, 1982; Flatt, 1983). However, because the condition is so common, some general principles of surgical management are given here.

The aim of surgical treatment of the hand affected by rheumatoid arthritis is to relieve pain and improve function. A deformed hand is not in itself an indication for operation. As with congenital hand anomalies, careful assessment of the patient's capabilities by an occupational therapist with particular experience of the

Table 6.3 Surgical treatment of rheumatoid arthritis in the hand

Problem	Operation
Wrist	
Synovial proliferation beneath extensor retinaculum	Synovectomy or decompression of extensor compartment
Subluxation of head of ulna	Excision of head of ulna
Rupture of extensor tendons	Reconstruction by tendon transfer, grafting or suture to adjacent tendons
Painful unstable wrist	Arthrodesis
Carpal tunnel syndrome	Decompression of carpal tunnel
Flexor synovitis	Synovectomy
Metacarpophalangeal joints	
Instability and ulnar deviation (Fig. 6.44)	Arthroplasty and realignment of extensor apparatus
Fingers	
Flexor synovitis	Flexor synovectomy
Boutonnière deformity (Fig. 6.45) Swan neck deformity (Fig. 6.46)	Various procedures, depending on types and mobility of deformity
Unstable PIP joint	Arthrodesis
Thumb	
Rupture of extensor pollicis longus tendon	Tendon transfer using extensor indicis proprius
'Z' deformity (Fig. 6.47) Adduction deformity	Various procedures, depending on type and mobility of deformity

condition is always necessary before embarking on reconstructive surgery. Provision of simple aids for everyday activities may achieve far more than any surgical operation.

The common problems associated with the rheumatoid hand and their surgical treatments are listed in Table 6.3. Several procedures may be needed in the same hand and careful planning is necessary. It is preferable to carry out several small procedures, rather than combine them as one major hand reconstruction. If multiple operations are needed they should commence with simple, usually highly successful procedures, rather than complex ones requiring a lot of effort and determination on the part of the patient in the rehabilitation period. Souter (1979) has recommended the following sequence:
1. Dorsal wrist surgery.
2. Flexor tendon surgery.
3. Metacarpophalangeal joint surgery.
4. Proximal interphalangeal joint surgery and correction of other finger deformities.

5. Realignment of the thumb in the most useful position relative to the reconstructed fingers.

TUMOURS IN THE HAND

Many of the common tumours found in the hand are not neoplastic in nature.

Ganglia
The pathogenesis of ganglia is unclear but they may be due to herniation of synovial tissue from joints.

Common sites are the wrist on the dorsomedial and occasionally volar aspects. In the fingers pea-sized ganglia may be found attached to the proximal part of the fibrous flexor sheath. Surgical treatment is recommended only if the lesion is large and unsightly or if its nature is uncertain, since about 50% will disappear spontaneously. Ganglia should be excised in a bloodless field with adequate anaesthesia. The incision should be large enough to allow good exposure of the ganglion; cutaneous nerves must be protected when the skin is cut. It is important to trace the connection of the ganglion down to the wrist joint, to excise it and to leave the joint capsule open (Angelides & Wallace, 1976). Failure to remove the communication with the joint is followed by rapid recurrence.

Pigmented villonodular synovitis
This lesion, also known as 'giant cell tumour of the tendon sheath' is usually found in the middle-aged. It usually presents as a painless swelling on the flexor aspect of the finger or on the dorsum, arising from the distal interphalangeal joint (Fig. 6.48). Sometimes erosion of the bone is seen on radiographs. Treatment is by excision which should be complete to prevent local recurrence.

Implantation dermoid
This lesion is the result of implantation of skin into sub-

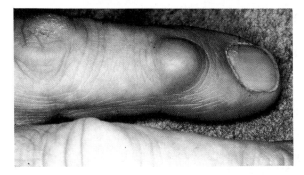

Fig. 6.48 Villonodular synovitis arising from the distal interphalangeal joint

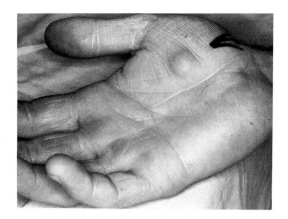

Fig. 6.49 Implantation dermoid

cutaneous tissue by minor trauma, and is common on the flexor aspects of the hand or fingers (Fig. 6.49). The removal of an implantation dermoid through a suitably placed incision presents no difficulty.

Glomus tumour
This tumour arises from the glomus body. It is usually a well encapsulated tumour less than 1 cm in diameter, most often found in the terminal segment of a finger. The patient complains of pain, tenderness and cold sensitivity, leading to protection of the finger. If examination of the finger is permitted the tumour may be palpable, or visible as a purplish lesion under the nail bed. Exploration and complete excision is necessary. If the tumour is subungual, part of the nail must be removed.

Squamous carcinoma
The back of the hand is not an uncommon site for this tumour, especially in those exposed to sunlight or industrial irritants. Management is discussed on page 8.

Malignant melanoma
The hand is a relatively rare site for this tumour but when it does occur the thumb is most often involved and the lesion is usually subungual. It may fungate around the nail fold and then be mistaken for a chronic nail bed infection and be treated inappropriately. The management is discussed on page 8.

Other conditions in the hand

Nerve compression lesions
See page 73.

Tenosynovitis
See page 24.

REFERENCES

Angelides A C, Wallace P F 1976 The dorsal ganglion of the wrist: Its pathogenesis, gross and microscopical anatomy, and surgical treatment. Journal of Hand Surgery 1: 228

Chuinard R G, D'Ambrosia R D 1977 Human bite infections of the hand. Journal of Bone and Joint Surgery 59A: 416

Fletcher I R, Healy T E J 1983 The arterial tourniquet. Annals of the Royal College of Surgeons of England 65: 409

Kanavel A B 1939 Infections of the hand, 7th edn. Ballière, Tindall and Cox, London

Kleinert H E, Putcha S M, Ashbell T S, Kutz J E 1967 The deformed finger nail, a frequent result of failure to repair nail bed injuries. Journal of Trauma 7: 177

Kleinert H E, Kutz J E, Fishman J H, McCraw L H 1972 Etiology and treatment of the so-called mucous cyst of the finger. Journal of Bone and Joint Surgery 54A: 1455

Kuczynski K 1968 The proximal interphalangeal joint. Anatomy and causes of stiffness in the fingers. Journal of Bone and Joint Surgery 50B: 656

Lamb D W, Hooper G 1985 Colour Aids to Hand Conditions. Churchill Livingstone, Edinburgh

Lister G 1978 Intraosseous wiring of the digital skeleton. Journal of Hand Surgery 3: 427

Lister G D, Kleinert H E, Kutz J E, Atasoy E 1977 Primary flexor tendon repair followed by immediate controlled mobilization. Journal of Hand Surgery 2: 441

McCash C R 1964 The open palm technique in Dupuytren's contracture. British Journal of Plastic Surgery 17: 271

Souter W A 1979 Planning treatment of the rheumatoid hand. Hand 11: 3

Swanson A B 1972 Disabling arthritis of the base of the thumb. Treatment by resection of trapezium and flexible (silicone) implant arthroplasty. Journal of Bone and Joint Surgery 54A: 456

Wilson J N, Bossley C J 1983 Osteotomy in the treatment of osteoarthritis of the first metacarpophalangeal joint. Journal of Bone and Joint Surgery 65B: 179

FURTHER READING

Flatt A E 1977 The care of congenital hand anomalies. C V Mosby, St. Louis

Flatt A E 1983 Care of the arthritic hand, 4th edn. C V Mosby, St. Louis

Green D P 1982 Operative hand surgery. Churchill Livingstone, New York

Hueston J T, Tubiana R 1974 Dupuytren's disease. Churchill Livingstone, Edinburgh

Lamb D W, Kuczynski K 1981 The practice of hand surgery. Blackwell, Oxford

Lister G 1984 The hand. Diagnosis and indications, 2nd edn. Churchill Livingstone, Edinburgh

7

Soft tissue injury

J. CHRISTIE

Tissue devitalization contamination and infection

Whenever a wound is inflicted, some devitalization of tissue (cellular damage) is inevitable. When the wound is made with a sharp knife the damage is comparatively slight and interferes little with healing. The majority of accidental wounds, however, are inflicted by contact with some blunt or ragged object, or by crushing, and in these wounds tissue devitalization may be extensive. All wounds which are not made under the aseptic conditions of an operating theatre are potentially infected and most accidental open injuries, whether civilian or military, cause contaminated foreign material to enter the tissues. Organisms lie on the surface of the wound for a period of time and multiply in that situation. During this period of 12 or 24 hours there will be no local evidence of infection and there is unlikely to be any constitutional disturbance that might suggest sepsis. A certain number of wounds however will develop evidence of infection after this period if left untreated. Organisms will flourish locally, enter the lymphatics and the characteristic signs of local inflammation will appear along with signs of a general systemic disturbance.

Many variables determine whether wound infection supervenes. It is well known for instance that organisms can be cultured from the surface of some 25% of apparently clean surgical wounds, but that this contamination is not inevitably followed by infection. Infection is more likely to supervene when there is devitalized or injured tissue present, when foreign material is left behind or when highly virulent organisms are involved. The resistance of the patient is also critical and it is known that in conditions of immunodeficiency, or when there is vascular disease or diabetes present, infection is more likely to occur. The wound should be treated as soon as practicable, as delay also leads to an increasing incidence of infection.

TYPES OF WOUNDS

Wounds caused by sharp instruments

Frequently sharp instruments, knives, cut glass, or ragged pieces of metal, will cause an incised wound with comparatively little tissue destruction. It must be remembered though that this kind of wound may penetrate deeply causing sharp injury to important structures, making careful and critical examination essential. By and large however there does not tend to be the kind of massive tissue destruction that is caused by blunt injury.

Wounds caused by blunt force

Many wounds are caused by bludgeoning force so that the skin and underlying tissues are opened, usually by shearing stress, and tearing injury may occur as a result of the considerable violence involved. As a general rule, the amount of tissue damage that occurs relates to the degree of violence involved. When this type of blunt wound has occurred, shearing and devitalization of the skin, as well as of underlying fat and muscle, should be suspected and treatment should take account of this. The accompanying table shows energy levels in open fractures from different mechanisms (Chapman quoted by Gustilo, 1982) and gives an idea of the severity of violence that is to be expected.

	Joules
Fall from a pavement	135
Skiing injury	400–700
High velocity gun shot wound	3 000
Bumper injury at 20 mph	135,000

Gunshot wounds

Shotgun injuries

Injuries caused by a shotgun vary very much in their severity. For the first few feet after discharge from the barrel of a shotgun the pellets will travel in a 'shot-cloud' and are closely followed by the wadding. A patient struck by the discharge at this close range will sustain severe penetrating injury at the point of impact and the pellets will spread rapidly through the soft tissue causing widespread damage. The wadding will also enter the wound but usually remains fairly discrete within the soft tissues.

After shotgun injury it is usually fruitless to attempt to remove more than a small proportion of the retained pellets. It is however of great importance to remove the wadding if this has been injected into the wound, as the material from which it is made is usually irritating; also the central entrance wound should be laid widely open.

Low velocity gunshot wounds
Many pistols and rifles discharge bullets which have a relatively low velocity (< 360 m (1200 feet) per second). Unless these are soft nosed or hollow bullets which break up and cause widespread injury, relatively little damage may occur within the tissues, though of course major and vital structures can be damaged. A low velocity bullet passing through the soft tissues will tend to leave a track which is not surrounded by much tissue necrosis. There may be small entrance and exit wounds though a larger exit wound may occur if the bullet breaks up. The bullet is sometimes retained within the tissues.

The form of surgical treatment required will depend upon whether major structures have been damaged. In general, though, a low velocity injury through soft tissue, with small entrance and exit wounds, does not need to be laid open unless some underlying vital structure is involved. The entrance and exit wounds should be adequately débrided and cleaned with iodine, and it is wise for the patient to be given an antibiotic. Removal of a retained bullet is not essential.

High velocity gunshot wounds
High velocity missiles, with a speed of greater than 900 m (3000 feet) per second, may cause considerable tissue destruction. The higher velocity bullet carries a great deal of kinetic energy which may be imparted into the tissues. Furthermore the faster bullet tends to wobble as it passes through soft tissue and resistance to its passage is increased; thus a greater proportion of its kinetic energy is transferred causing increased damage.

As the bullet passes through flesh, a phenomenon occurs (first reported by Woodruff in 1898) known as *cavitation*. The tissues are accelerated away from the bullet during its passage, and a momentary cavity forms filled with water vapour, immediately behind the travelling missile (Fig. 7.1). The tissues become stretched and sheared from their blood supply. The cavity, if deep, will close rapidly but not before air and debris have been sucked in through the bullet track. Tissues sheared from their blood supply become necrotic for up to several centimetres around the bullet track. These bullet tracks must be laid open and excision of necrotic tissue undertaken.

Usually a high velocity bullet causes a small entrance wound and when it passes through flesh over a large distance, it may cause a relatively small exit wound, but cavitation will have occurred within the tissues. When

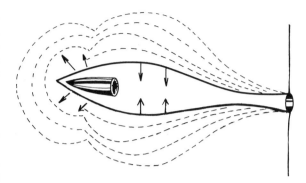

Fig. 7.1 Illustrating the passage of a high velocity missile through soft tissue

the bullet passes through a relatively short track, as through a limb, the site of exit may coincide with the site of maximum energy transfer, causing a large exit wound.

A large exit wound also occurs when the bullet shatters bone, and multiple fragments exit along with the metal.

Lawnmower injuries
Injuries caused by lawnmowers are becoming relatively common in most Western communities. The blades usually revolve in a circular fashion on a vertical axis and cause fairly extensive injury, commonly of the feet. There are a number of virulent bacteria particularly gram negative organisms, which may be injected into the tissues, so that these wounds are probably best left open primarily.

Injuries caused by teeth
Injuries caused by biting (particularly human tooth wounds) are also rife with relatively aggressive organisms. Here again it is wise to leave the wound open in the first instance, secondary suture being carried out later.

TREATMENT OF WOUNDS

The primary and most important aspect of the treatment of all recent accidental civilian and war wounds is careful and expert surgery. Appreciation of the severity and extent of tissue damage is critical, and the surgical procedure must always take account of this.

Surgical wound excision is the treatment of choice for all significant wounds in both civilian and military practice, whenever practicable.

Surgical débridement is a procedure originally described during the Napoleonic wars, and is not so formal nor so extensive as excision of the wound.

It cannot be stressed enough that wound excision is the single most important step in preventing wound infection. The operation is exacting and consists of careful excision of the wound edges, fat, fascia and underlying muscle to the furthest depth and cavity of the wound.

Débridement on the other hand refers to the excision, in a looser way, of necrotic and unhealthy looking tissue. There are situations in which débridement is more appropriate than wound excision, particularly after a lengthy period of time has elapsed between wounding and surgery, for the treatment of wounds of the face, or in the management of wound infection.

The retention of dead tissue or inanimate foreign material within the wound poses the greatest single threat to uncomplicated healing. Wound excision will undoubtedly remove a relatively small number of healthy cells but its primary intent is to remove dead or inanimate matter, also abraded and potentially infected surfaces. Only viable and healthy tissue should be left behind except in exceptional circumstances.

Many high energy shearing, or bullet wounds, will leave dead tissue behind, and it is important to appreciate the potential consequences of injury; only a high index of suspicion will frequently allow the surgeon to make an adequate exploration and excision of all the injured areas.

Antibiotics are now established as having an important role to play (Gustilo, 1982) in the prevention of wound infection. By and large they should be given in high doses intravenously, as soon as possible after injury, and should be continued over the period of surgery. High doses of intravenous cephalosporins in particular have been shown to diminish the risk of infection following injury. These should be started almost as soon as the patient is admitted and should be continued for at least 3 days.

Wound excision

This is a carefully planned operation designed to remove all devitalized and contaminated tissues which might predispose to the development and spread of infection. It involves therefore, the excision, not only of the skin edges, but of all tissues lining the wound cavity. Primary excision is the treatment of choice in all significant recent wounds whether military or civilian. It is important to remember that shearing injuries may have caused devitalization of skin and underlying muscle which will require adequate exposure and excision. High velocity bomb or bullet wounds should also be laid open, and the dead and necrotic tissue underneath carefully excised.

The operation should be attempted only if it can be performed during the first 18 hours or so after injury. Beyond that time it is probably wiser to revert to the less extensive procedure of wound débridement. After 12 hours or so considerable judgement may be required in deciding which of the two operations is most appropriate.

Operation

Except after hand injury where a bloodless field is particularly desirable, the use of a tourniquet is not usually advised. The tourniquet tends to obscure potential bleeding points and makes the recognition of devitalised tissue somewhat difficult; theoretically also it may reduce the resistance of the part to infection.

Skin preparation is carried out over a wide area around the wound. Soap and water is the best agent for preliminary cleansing, and is usually effective in removing ingrained dirt and grease; subsequently an iodine preparation or Cetavlon wash may be used with advantage. Care should be taken to prevent washings from the surrounding skin entering into the wound by light gauze packing if necessary. After cleansing, the skin is dried with spirit and is prepared with one of the commonly used antiseptics.

The edges of the wound are now excised with a sharp knife (Fig. 7.2). Where the skin is only lightly injured it is adequate to excise a strip some 2 mm or 3 mm wide. Where there is more extensive abrasion and injury a wider margin of skin must be removed. Once the skin has been excised subcutaneous tissues are similarly carefully excised with the knife. The skin wound is enlarged,

Fig. 7.2–7.5 *Stages in the operation of primary wound excision*

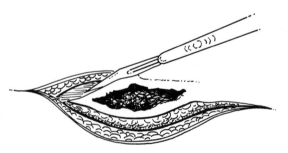

Fig. 7.2 Excision of the skin edges

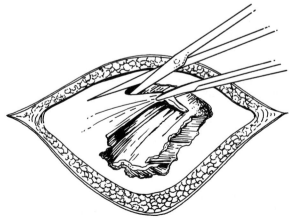

Fig. 7.3 Excision of wound in deep fascia

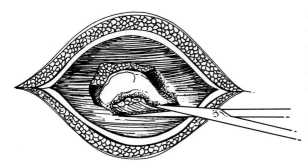

Fig. 7.4 Removal of the devitalized muscle

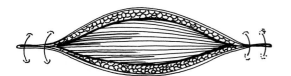

Fig. 7.5 Wound partially sutured

should this prove to be necessary, by further incisions which should usually be made in the long axis of a limb. Deep fascia is excised in a similar way, and muscle is trimmed back also using a knife or scissors. Devitalized muscle tissue carries the greatest danger of infection, and the colour, contractile response and the bleeding capacity of the muscle will determine how much should be excised. Bruised and ischaemic muscle fibres are usually darker than normal, do not contract when cut, and do not bleed. All devitalized fibres are excised with scissors. Successive snips are made in a direction away from the damaged area until healthy fibres are encountered; these are recognized by brisk response to the stimulus of cutting, and by oozing of blood from the cut ends. When wide retraction of severed muscles has occurred, it may be necessary to enlarge the wounds considerably through skin and deep fascia in order to obtain access to all damaged tissues. Foreign bodies are removed along with small detached fragments of bone. Bone fragments with a periosteal or muscular attachment should be left behind. Larger bone fragments that contribute to stability should also be retained. The treatment of arterial or nerve injuries has been discussed in previous chapters. Careful arrest of haemorrhage is most important. Bleeding points are clipped as they appear, and are ligatured with fine sutures, or are coagulated with diathermy. On completion of the excision the wound should have only viable tissues left behind. During the procedure, the tissues should be copiously washed with saline, and should be handled delicately.

Wound débridement (surgical toilet)

This operation consists of the removal of foreign bodies and debris from the wound, together with the excision of any devitalized skin tags and of obviously necrotic tissue. Many surgeons use the term débridement to describe the operation undertaken primarily after injury. It should be stressed that wound excision is nearly always to be preferred in the early period after injury and that the simpler removal of foreign material and debris from the wound, along with excision of devitalized tissue is a procedure that is appropriate when significant time has elapsed before the patient can be taken to surgery, or in special circumstances such as wounding of the face. The preparation of the skin around the wound is similar to that described for wound excision, and the operation is different only in that formal excison of the wound edges is not undertaken. The more obviously abraded or injured tissues are removed along with foreign material and dirt. Healthy tissues are not disturbed.

Wound closure

After wound excision or débridement has been carried out, the surgeon has to decide whether the wound should be completely sutured, partially sutured or left widely open and packed with gauze. The decision is one which requires considerable judgement. It is frequently tempting to suture the wound throughout its length in an attempt to obtain healing by first intention. Successful primary healing is pleasing to the patient and surgeon alike, but the risk of infection is always greater after primary wound closure. Infection may be disastrous particularly when there is an underlying fracture.

Extensive wounds of any kind after severe violence, particularly when there is impregnation of foreign material with extensive tissue necrosis, should probably be left open after wound excision has been completed. Similarly wounds that are more than 18 hours old and that have been dealt with by débridement should also be left open, as should high velocity bullet injuries whose track has been laid wide open in order to excise necrotic tissue. Experience in the Second World war, also more recently in the Korean war and Vietnam conflicts, has again established that many wounds are best treated open after appropriate excision (Dudley, 1973).

After the first 5 days of being left open, wounds develop a remarkable resistance to infection and many may be closed relatively safely. It is also striking that wounds left open and allowed to discharge freely *ab initio* rarely become infected.

Primary suture

Many cleanly incised wounds may be closed by primary suture after excision. It is unwise however to close a wound that has been untreated for about 18 hours since injury. When a wound is closed by primary suture there should be no large underlying cavity and the tissues within the wound should be entirely healthy. When there is a large cavity which cannot be obliterated it is usually wiser to leave the wound open, or to use a system of closed irrigation for some days. Interrupted nonabsorbable sutures may be used to close a cleanly incised wound.

No wound should be closed under tension. Tension is liable to occur whenever there is significant swelling after injury, particularly after crushing injury of a limb or when there is an underlying fracture. When a medium suture breaks before drawing the wound edges together, skin tension is likely to be too great to allow safe closure. In these circumstances the wound is best left open. It is also wise to leave wounds caused by lawnmowers, or by human or animal bites, open for a period of days before formal secondary suture.

Partial primary suture

The centre of the wound may, on occasion, be left open. This is safer than wholly closing the wound and allows many extensive injuries, also those that have had to be extended in order to gain adequate access, to be closed up to the point that skin tension develops. The central part of the wound or indeed one of its ends may be left open, and is usually covered by a light gauze dressing. Alternatively a small drain may be left in the depths of the wound. This is a wise precaution when a cavity remains in the wound, as it will prevent the retention of blood, serum or other exudate. It is rare that a wound which is allowed adequate drainage in this way becomes infected. Retention of infected exudate and bacterial toxins are the most potent factors allowing further spread of infection.

Gauze packing

Gauze packing of an open wound may be necessary when there has been heavy contamination or much devitalization of tissue. It is also necessary when, due to tissue loss, a large cavity is left behind. Usually only light packing is used so as to hold the wound open. Tullegras, or Sofratulle gauze is laid on the tissues and the packing is laid into the dressing. It is important that the cavity is only lightly packed and that free drainage is allowed from the wound. When a wound is packed open, secondary suture or some plastic procedure such as skin grafting, may be required at a later date.

Delayed primary suture

Delayed primary suture is the optimum treatment for a wound which has been left open and packed with gauze in the first instance. This is not always possible and some wounds, particularly those with skin loss, may require skin grafting procedures or transposition flaps.

Delayed primary suture is usually undertaken some 5 days after the original procedure. The wound should be free from infection on clinical inspection and culture, and the surfaces of the wound should be clean. When there is a copious discharge present or obvious dead tissue and slough, the procedure should be delayed.

The technique is similar to that described for primary suture. When there is a large cavity and dead space cannot be obliterated, it is wiser not to close the entire wound but to allow drainage from the area of the cavity. Alternatively the wound may be closed over the cavity but irrigation should be used. The wound should only be closed secondarily if tension can be avoided.

Immobilization

All severe soft tissue wounds should be immobilized after initial treatment. Rest encourages healing by preventing movement and muscle spasm. Immobilization is particularly useful when it is necessary to transport the patient after initial treatment, and will considerably diminish mortality. Usually a plaster cast is employed to achieve immobilization, and is frequently split after application to avoid the risk of compression as the injured area swells. The joints above and below the wound are usually also included in the cast, in a suitable position of function. The Thomas splint is often more appropriate when treating injuries of the thigh.

When a compound fracture is present, other forms of immobilization such as an external fixation device, or formal traction within a splint may be more appropriate.

When a plaster cast is used, certain rules should be stringently observed:

1. When considerable swelling of the limb is anticipated the plaster cast should be split throughout its length. If the cast is not split initially, the surgeon should ensure that there will be regular observation of the limb during the period in which the swelling may be anticipated, and the cast should be split whenever there is the remotest suspicion of ischaemia.

2. Encircling dressings, bandages or wool are liable to become saturated with hardened and dried blood, and thus become rigid. When a plaster cast is split, the underlying dressings must also be divided so that skin is visible throughout the length of the split. The plaster must be split from end to end.

3. A window may be cut in the plaster so that regular inspection can be carried out (Fig. 7.6). It is important that the plaster window is retained and that, after inspection of the wound is completed, the plaster window is replaced and held in place with firm compression bandaging (Fig. 7.7), otherwise oedema will occur locally.

4. A wound which has been left completely open, and packed with gauze, may safely be enclosed in plaster without a window (closed plaster method). The wound is usually exposed after 5 days in these circumstances so

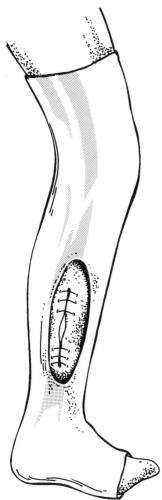

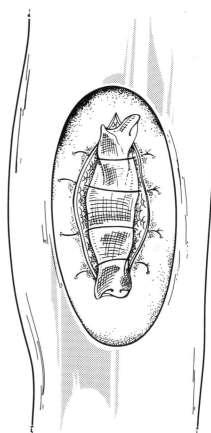

Fig. 7.6 Soft tissue wound of the leg, treated by immobilization in plaster. A window in the cast over the full extent of the wound allows periodic inspection and dressing.

Fig. 7.7 Delayed primary suture of leg wound as seen through plaster window. The wound has been left open and a swab held in place by suture

that secondary suture may be undertaken or whatever other procedure appears to be appropriate. Winnet Orr used the closed plaster technique extensively during the First World war when faced with massive evacuations of injured troops. Their wounds were treated by early excision, left open and a closed plaster was applied. This treatment met with considerable success.

TREATMENT OF INFECTED WOUNDS

65 to 70% of accidental wounds yield potentially pathogenic organisms when cultures are taken on admission to hospital (Patzakis, 1974). The vast majority of these

wounds will not develop infection if appropriately treated. Those wounds that are not associated with severe tissue destruction, flap elevation or avulsion, and which have only a minimal to moderate crushing component, should be associated with an infection rate of less than 2%. More severe injuries with extensive damage to the soft tissues, including muscle, skin and neurovascular structures particularly when accompanied by fracture, will probably have an infection rate of anywhere between 10% and 40%.

Wound infection does not usually appear for 2 or 3 days after injury. Initially when there is cellulitis, and bacteriological cultures reveal a pyogenic organism, strict rest and the administration of high dose antibiotic therapy are appropriate. A certain number of these wounds will not however respond rapidly to this treatment, and other wounds will present late with already established infection.

The management of established infection requires considerable judgement. When it is clear that there is pus present within the wound, early surgical débridement is advisable. Surgery is also indicated when it is suspected that necrotic tissue or slough is retained within the wound, or when there is retained foreign material or debris, though again considerable judgement is required and a vain search should not be made for shotgun pellets, pieces of shrapnel or multiple fragments that are widely dispersed in the tissues. By and large, however, there is an increasing tendency towards early exploration and drainage of the wound and radical débridement of necrotic tissues, particularly when there is established infection after a compound fracture. In these circumstances bone is treated rather like soft tissue and necrotic or grossly infected bone tends to be excised leaving only healthy tissue behind.

It should be emphasized that the decision to proceed to early radical débridement of an infected wound should be carefully thought out, should not be undertaken overhastily, and is not usually appropriate during the early phase of cellulitis. When there is a fracture present wound débridement is generally more pressing so as to prevent intractable osteomyelitis; in general, simple soft tissue infection tends to be more benign in its behaviour when there is no underlying fracture and there is less urgency in proceeding to early débridement.

When early débridement of a wound is undertaken, the tissues should be packed open and free drainage allowed to occur. The wound is left undisturbed for 24 hours before being inspected and subsequently having regular dressing procedures.

As soon as appropriate cultures and sensitivities have been reported, high dose antibiotic therapy is commenced. The wound should be immobilized, and the patient observes a regime of strict rest. When there is an underlying fracture, it is usually stabilized with a plaster cast or with an external fixation device.

Following débridement of the infected wound, treatment will depend upon the subsequent course of the infection. Usually wound discharge will rapidly diminish as will the surrounding oedema and inflammation. Normally the wound will look clean and relatively uninfected after some 5 days and secondary suture may be contemplated at that time. The wound may however retain slough or necrotic material and this may require excision. It may prove impossible to close the skin and in these circumstances split skin grafting may be necessary after healthy granulation tissue has developed. It is sometimes appropriate to close the wound over irrigation when there is a large cavity and dead space

cannot be obliterated. Irrigation should not be used for more than 3 to 5 days.

Débridement of an infected wound
This is the procedure used when it is judged that an established infection will be most appropriately managed by surgical intervention. The wound is opened up usually throughout its length. When there are sinuses present it may not be necessary to open up the entire wound, but the sinus tracks should be exposed, and the sinuses entirely excised including surrounding scar tissue if practicable. Fresher wounds are opened throughout their length and are explored to their depths. Pus is gently swabbed out and any loculi or cavities are opened. Necrotic tissue is identified and is excised with scissors until the wound edges appear to be healthy. The wound should not be swabbed too vigorously or considerable bleeding will occur. When bone is involved necrotic or infected looking bone is usually excised. The wound is then packed widely open.

Secondary suture
This may be carried out as soon as the infection has been overcome, but is only suitable in a certain number of patients. Appropriate antibiotic cover should be available. The skin edges should be healthy and there should be early ingrowth of epithelium. There should be no residual adherent slough and no infected crevices within the wound. Granulation tissue should look healthy, firm and reddish in colour. Residual discharge should be minimal and nonpurulent.

Techniques
Skin flaps are mobilized by under cutting, with or without excision of the wound margins, and are approximated over the granulating area with interrupted sutures. Tension must be avoided and it is always better to leave part of the wound open than to force it closed with tight stitches. When secondary closure is possible, a drain should be left in the wound to allow any further discharge to escape freely.

Closed irrigation
This is used when an infected wound is closed over dead space, or when considerable bleeding is anticipated. Two tubular surgical drains are placed in the wound through adjacent skin. Saline, or saline containing antibiotics, is run into the wound through a drip giving set and through one of the tubular drains. As the wound is closed the other drain will start to drain first blood and then irrigation fluid. If this does not occur a syringe may be used to suck the irrigation out through the drain. Subsequently this drain is connected to a collecting bag. It is important to run the irrigation through briskly so that

blood clots do not occur as these will block the irrigation system. As the effluent irrigation becomes clear the rate of irrigation system may be reduced. Usually this kind of closed irrigation system is retained for no longer than 5 days.

Secondary haemorrhage

Secondary haemorrhage usually occurs as the result of wound sepsis. A small premonitory haemorrhage may occur and suggests that the patient should be kept under careful observation. A significant increase in bleeding requires that the wound is gently opened and the bleeding vessel, normally an artery, is sought and tied off. If no single large vessel can be identified gauze packing may be used alone, and is removed some 3 to 4 days later in the operating theatre.

Severe haemorrhage which threatens to exsanguinate the patient and which cannot be controlled by gauze packing must be treated by proximal ligation. Very occasionally it is necessary to ligature the main vessel of the limb, but this should be undertaken only in exceptional circumstances as it will involve the risk of distal gangrene, especially so in the lower limb. When the procedure is used in order to save life the risk is sometimes justified.

OPERATIVE TREATMENT IN GAS GANGRENE

Prophylaxis

The anaerobic organisms producing gas gangrene infection are saprophytes which flourish in devitalized or necrotic tissue, especially fleshy muscle. Early wound excision is therefore the best preventative measure. If this is contraindicated or is impracticable, débridement should be as thorough as possible. Antibiotics should also be used in high doses from the moment the patient is admitted to hospital, and should be continued intravenously for at least 3 days. It should be stressed however that when conditions are ripe for the development of gas gangrene in the wound, antibiotics will not prevent this dangerous disorder. When there is considered to be a serious risk of gas gangrene, the wound should always be left widely open. Injudicious primary suture of a contaminated wound may well be a determining factor in the development of the disease. A wound which is left open and packed rarely becomes infected. Other factors which predispose to the condition include delay in adequate primary treatment, also any interference with the blood supply to the part, e.g. injury to the main vessel of the limb, tourniquets, tight plasters and compartment syndromes.

Hitchcock has shown that frank necrosis of tissue or muscle is not necessary for gas gangrene to develop. It is sufficient that relative local hypoxia occurs in order that the clostridial spores may be converted to vegetative forms with rapid multiplication.

Gas gangrene is seen most commonly after trauma, and almost half of the patients who present will have an open wound. Some 30% of the patients however will develop gas gangrene after routine surgical operations and a small proportion will have primary gas gangrene without open injury to the skin (Hitchcock, 1982).

Operative diagnosis

Early diagnosis is a matter of life and death, and no hesitation should be felt in exploring the wound at the first suspicion of anaerobic infection. Stitches are removed and the wound margins are retracted. In assessing the nature of the infection a distinction should be drawn between *true gas gangrene* (clostridium myositis) and *anaerobic cellulitis*. True gangrene is essentially an infection of fleshy muscle; it involves previously healthy fibres, and spreads longitudinally within the sheaths, so that a muscle or group of muscles may be involved throughout its entire length. In anaerobic cellulitis the infection is confined to cellular connective tissue within the wound, and to muscle which is already necrotic from trauma or vascular damage. In both conditions collections of malodourous gas may be found in the depths of the wound, or raising blebs on the skin surface, and small areas of necrosis will be found throughout the tissues.

The wound, having been opened up, is enlarged if necessary to permit a thorough examination. A search is made for areas of discolouration, and for gas bubbles in the subcutaneous tissue and in the depths of the wound. Muscle sheaths are opened and the fibres are inspected. In the early stages of anaerobic infection the affected fibres are paler than normal, a lustreless pinkish grey shade being described; later they become deeply congested, slate blue or frankly gangrenous, and bubbles of gas may be seen between them.

Conservative operation

'In the established case of gas gangrene, bold surgery, blood transfusion, and Penicillin are essentials' (Stammers, 1948). The use of antitoxin is somewhat controversial and in a recent review Hitchcock does not believe that its administration affects the course of the disease. If antitoxin is to be given 200 000 units should be given together with a blood transfusion which is repeated as necessary.

The affected region is exposed by a long skin incision which is placed in the long axis of the limb, and has the wound at its centre. The sheaths of the affected muscles are opened up by longitudinal incision until healthy fibres are exposed. All fibres which show even a suspicion of infection are ruthlessly excised until healthy muscle, which bleeds and contracts on section, is revealed. Adjacent muscles are examined and, if necessary, are treated in the same way. Owing to the longitudinal spread of the infection an entire muscle or group of muscles may require to be removed. Any discoloured areas of skin or fascia are excised too. The wound is dusted liberally with Penicillin powder and is kept widely open by means of gauze packing. Penicillin therapy is continued in high dosage by intravenous administration.

In *anaerobic cellulitis* the infection is confined to cellular connective tissue within the wound, and to necrotic muscle fibres. Such tissues alone require to be removed. The excision is therefore much less radical than that required for true gas gangrene.

Hyperbaric oxygen therapy can be used as an adjunct to surgery and may assist to the extent that a more distal amputation can be undertaken when ablative surgery is required (Darke, 1977).

Amputation

The fact that gas gangrene tends to be confined to indi-

vidual muscles or groups of muscle saves many limbs from amputation. Except when there is *massive gangrene*, the wound should always be explored before amputation is considered, in the hope that the infection can be eradicated by conservative operation. Indications for amputation are:

1. Massive gangrene, where the infection involves most of the muscles in the injured segment of the limb; here amputation is the only possible lifesaving measure;
2. The coexistence of a compound fracture, and extensive disease.
3. Serious impairment of blood supply as will occur when the main artery of the limb is damaged.

The amputation must be sufficiently high to allow all infected muscle to be removed but it need not necessarily be above the level of subcutaneous spread. The wound is left widely open and is packed with gauze.

REFERENCES

Darke S G, King A M, Slack W K 1977 Gas gangrene and related infection: classification, clinical features and aetiology, management and mortality. A report of 88 cases. British Journal of Surgery 64: 104
Dudley H A F 1973 Some aspects of modern battle surgery. Journal of the Royal College of Surgeons of Edinburgh 18: 67
Gustilo R B 1982 The management of open fractures and their complications W B Saunders, New York
Hitchcock C R 1982 Gas gangrene in the injured extremity. In: Gustilo R B (ed) The management of open fractures and their complications, W B Saunders, New York, p 183

Patzakis M, Harvey J I P, Ivler D 1974 The role of antibiotics in the management of open fractures. Journal of Bone and Joint Surgery 56A: 532
Stammers F A R 1948 War supplement, British Journal of Surgery 2: 274

FURTHER READING

Owen-Smith M S 1981. High velocity missile wounds. Arnold, London

8

Amputations

J. CHRISTIE

INDICATIONS FOR AMPUTATIONS

Amputation of a limb or part of a limb is required when the vitality of the part is destroyed by injury or disease or when the life of the patient is threatened by the spread of a local condition. Amputation may also be desirable in patients with deformity or paralysis, where it is considered that the patient would be better served by an artificial limb. The decision to proceed to amputation is usually taken after careful consideration. Other alternatives may be available and many factors must be taken together in determining the most suitable management for the individual patient. Assessment on an inpatient basis is often helpful and the opinion of a specialist in some other field of endeavour may be invaluable. In considering the indications for amputation it is necessary to make a clear distinction between the upper and lower extremities. It is important to preserve stability and length in the lower limb and if these cannot be restored, the patient may well be better off with an artificial limb. Stability is not essential to useful function of the upper limb and even a grossly deformed or shortened arm may be preferable to a replacement prosthesis (Figs. 8.1–8.3).

The majority of patients who come to amputation in Britain have vascular disease and of these some 20% have diabetes. Some 10% of patients lose a limb as a result of some other cause, most commonly injury. The majority require amputation of the lower extremity; a small and important group have loss of the upper extremity, occasionally bilateral. The amputation rate is 1 to 1.5 per 10 000 of population; 75% of the patients are aged 60 years or more.

Wounds and injuries

Amputation surgery is sometimes required after injury to a limb. This is usually only considered after the most serious kind of crushing force or when there is traumatic amputation with irretrievable damage to the blood vessels or to the nerve supply of the extremity. Occasionally massive loss of soft tissues or a combination of injury to bone and soft tissue may preclude limb salvage. Techniques of vessel and nerve repair in combination with planned reconstructive surgery to the bone and soft tissues allows the extremity to be saved except after the most mutilating of injuries. Reattachment of the totally severed limb is now possible and should be practised when it is probable that the outcome will be superior to that offered by an artificial limb. In general, when there is sharp traumatic amputation, reattachment may be an entirely worthwhile procedure. This is particularly true in the upper extremity when amputation has occurred through the forearm or hand. Traumatic avulsion of a limb usually causes extensive soft tissue injury and reattachment is likely to be unrewarding.

Microsurgical techniques are also available: these allow small distal vessels to be anastomosed enabling the digits to be reattached after traumatic amputation. When there is significant crushing this is not likely to be successful but it is frequently well worth attempting to resuture the thumb or one or more of the fingers after sharp traumatic amputation particularly at a proximal level.

There are of course certain risks in attempting to preserve a severely mangled limb, particularly of infection—occasionally gas gangrene. Antibiotics given prophylactically will diminish the danger, although when devitalized tissue is present serious infection may still occur. Immunization against the anaerobic organisms is essential in these circumstances.

Vascular disease

The majority of patients who require amputation in Northern Europe and America have vascular disease. Many of these have widespread disease of the vascular tree with major vessel involvement. A relatively small number of patients, particularly those with diabetes, have peripheral arteriolar disease and consequently relatively localized peripheral ischaemic changes. In these circumstances it is often possible to contemplate one of the more conservative amputations.

Infections

Acute infection
Certain acute infections such as gas angrene can some-

Figs. 8.1–8.3 Showing that the first metacarpal and little finger may allow a competent grip. This man returned to work as a miner after amputation during the First World War. Note the hypertrophy of the little finger. (Redrawn from a patient of Mr James A Ross)

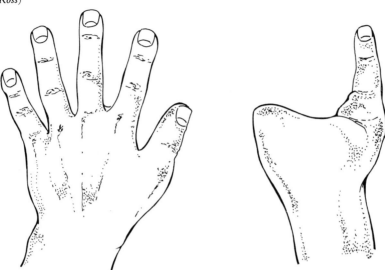

Fig. 8.1 Both hands for comparison following recovery from extensive injury on the right

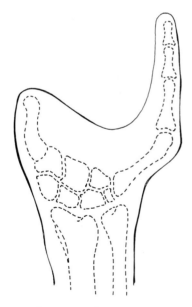

Fig. 8.2 Drawing from X-ray of right hand

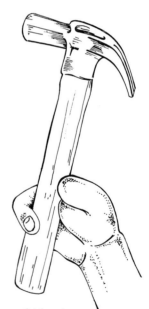

Fig. 8.3 Showing useful function

times lead to the need for amputation surgery. Gas gangrene may occur after serious injury or compound fracture particularly when there has been severe crushing and devitalization of the soft tissues. Gas gangrene also occurs occasionally after surgery to a limb that is severely affected by vascular disease.

Other fulminating infections, for instance severe infection in the finger, may occasionally cause extensive damage and require amputation of the digit.

Chronic infection
Chronic infection particularly of bone and joints may lead to amputation, especially if there is progressive deterioration in the general health or a threat of amyloid, both of which may occur as the result of prolonged suppuration. In the lower limbs the loss of function resulting from osteomyelitis or septic arthritis may be such that the patient would be better served by an artificial limb.

Malignant tumours

Certain tumours of the extremities may be treated most suitably by amputation in an attempt to achieve cure or in an attempt to relieve severe local symptoms. Carcinoma arising in the soft parts of the limb may sometimes necessitate amputation, especially if it has infiltrated so as to involve bone. The decision to amputate in the presence of malignant disease should be carefully taken and other available alternatives such as prosthetic skeletal replacement should be considered. (Some tumours such as osteosarcoma may sometimes be managed with reconstructive surgery, rather than by amputation. There is evidence now that the results of irradiation and chemotherapy in the management of Ewing's sarcoma may produce results that are not worse than those achieved after amputation surgery, irradiation and chemotherapy p. 116.)

Deformity

Deformity may be congenital or acquired. Acquired deformity is frequently the result of some underlying neurological disease such as cerebral palsy, myelomeningocele or infantile paralysis. Reconstructive surgery can achieve surprisingly good results in many conditions of this nature which were formally treated by amputation. Shortened bones may be lengthened, malalignment corrected and flail joints stabilized. Amputation is however appropriate if the patient is likely to be better served by an artificial limb. This is seldom true in congenital deformity of the upper extremity where reconstructive surgery is almost always preferable but in the lower limb amputation may be entirely appropriate when deformity is severe.

Congenital limb deficiency

Congenital absence of a limb or part of a limb may lead to the need for amputation or corrective surgery and prosthetic fitting. Congenital absence of the forearm and hand is the commonest deficiency of the upper limb requiring the provision of an artificial limb. Congenital amputation through the upper arm is less common and bilateral absence of the upper extremities is rare now that *Thalidomide* is no longer prescribed.

The focal femoral deficiencies, congenital absence of the fibula and more rarely absence of the tibia may lead to the need for amputation surgery in the lower limb. Congenital ring constriction also occurs and sometimes requires amputation.

Gangrene

Gangrene occurs usually as the result of ischaemic disease of a limb or of serious infection. Massive gangrene is, of course, an absolute indication for amputation. In *dry gangrene*, which is usually the result of vascular disease, amputation may with advantage be delayed until a line of demarcation has formed. It may be found that the extent of gangrene is less than was suggested by the area of skin involvement, and by skin grafting methods it may be possible to conserve a little extra length of stump. In *moist gangrene*, which is usually infective in nature, especially the serious type known as gas gangrene, amputation is often a matter of considerable urgency (p. 162).

OPTIMUM LEVELS FOR AMPUTATION

The level at which an amputation should be carried out does not entirely depend upon the extent of the injury or disease. Consideration must be given also to the function desired in the remaining stump. This differs very markedly in the upper and in the lower limb. Even the most fragmentary portion of a hand is of much greater value to the patient than the best prosthesis, and every effort must be made to conserve as much tissue as possible. On the other hand, zealous attempts to preserve a seriously diseased foot may be misguided and amputation at an appropriate level is often to be preferred.

The great majority of patients who suffer amputation above the level of the wrist or ankle joint will eventually be fitted with an artificial limb, and their future activity and wellbeing depends largely upon the efficiency with which that limb can function. It is necessary therefore for the surgeon to work in close co-operation with the prosthetist in fashioning a stump to which the best possible prosthetic socket can be fitted. Many patients who come to amputation are old and will require amputation of the lower limb. It is important when possible to preserve the knee joint as very much less energy expenditure is required to walk with a below knee prosthesis than with amputation at the above knee level.

Up to a certain point a longer stump is preferable but too long a stump may be an encumbrance leaving a bony tip that is poorly protected by soft tissues. The prosthetist may also find it difficult to accommodate the longer stump and, in the lower limb, length discrepancy may be impossible to avoid. An amputation at the appropriate level on the other hand will provide a stump that is suitable for patient and prosthetist alike.

Certain optimum levels shown in Table 8.1 have been advocated though these should not be accepted too rigidly. Amputations at other levels may be appropriate and when necessary prosthetic design can be varied to accommodate most levels of amputation. A golden rule is that too low a level of amputation can be remedied; too high removal of a limb is beyond repair. Sometimes in older patients who have no prospect of walking a higher amputation usually at the above knee level is chosen to achieve rapid healing and an early return to the wheelchair. Amputation surgery may also be modified

Table 8.1 Guidelines

Forearm	Optimum length of stump is 20 cm as measured from tip of olecranon. An 8 cm stump is the minimum for useful function. Between these levels as much bone as possible should be saved.
Upper arm	Optimum length of stump is 20 cm as measured from acromion. Above this level as much bone as possible should be saved.
Lower leg	*Syme's amputation.* The tibia and fibula are divided at or immediately above the level of the ankle joint.
	Site of election. Length of tibial stump is 14 cm. An 8 cm stump is the minimum for useful function (see p. 187). Between these levels as much bone as possible should be saved.
Thigh	Optimum length of stump is 25–30 cm, as measured from tip of trochanter. Above this level as much bone as possible should be saved.

in underdeveloped countries to adapt to local circumstances, where only the most simple type of prosthesis is likely to be available.

Choice of level in vascular disease and diabetes

Vascular disease
The mortality rate after amputation for peripheral vascular disease is between 10 and 25%, and is higher with advancing age. One third of these patients will be dead after two years and two thirds will have died after five years (Warren & Kilm, 1968). About 10% of the patients surviving after amputation will lose the remaining limb each year, slightly more during the first year after amputation. Of below knee amputees, 60% will make good use of their artificial limb compared with 40% of patients who have amputation at the above knee level. Walking metabolic expenditure after above knee amputation is some two times greater than that of a normal individual (Peizer, Wright & Mason, 1969). This compares with an increase in walking metabolic expenditure of about 20% after below knee amputation. It is hence abundantly clear that, wherever possible, below knee amputation is preferable to the above knee level. Ghormley in 1947 described below knee amputation using a long posterior flap. This has become popular recently and, partly because of its success, there has been an increasing tendency to attempt below knee amputation wherever possible. Some 75% of patients who come to amputation for vascular disease now have successful surgery at the below knee level.

Arteriography, thermography, Doppler instrumentation and dye attentuation studies as well as clinical examination can be helpful in determining the level at which amputation will be successful.

Diabetes
Patients with diabetic gangrene of the lower limb or intractable infection frequently do not have extensive major vessel disease and a relatively conservative excision may be possible. A diabetic ulcer with underlying osteomyelitis may require local resection only. Amputation of one or more toes or ray resection in the fore part of the foot may be sufficient. When there is more extensive involvement transmetatarsal amputation or amputation of the toes may be indicated. Amputation through the midfoot level or Syme's amputation may also be appropriate.

When there is absence of peripheral pulses in diabetes, reconstructive vascular surgery may prevent the need for a more radical amputation, or may precede a relatively conservative operation in the foot.

Clinical examination of the peripheral pulses, skin viability, tissue turgor, nail growth, hair growth and distal sensation are all important in determining the level at which amputation will succeed in diabetes.

Choice of level in neoplastic disease
Occasionally a benign tumour causing great deformity may require amputation surgery. Large lymphatic malformations or angiomatous tumours fall into this category. When malignant disease is suspected, biopsy should be carefully interpreted before embarking upon definitive surgery. It is usually better to wait for paraffin sections than to rely on frozen section particularly when bone is involved.

Low grade tumours may require local ablation or block resection. Aggressive tumours such as osteosarcomata may require more radical removal. Advice from an oncologist may be useful. Secondary deposits can be effectively sought using isotope studies and CT scans.

Choice of level in children
Children usually require amputation as a result of trauma, malignant disease, congenital abnormalities or limb shortening. Growth of a limb after amputation in the child will be affected. After above knee amputation the major growing epiphysis of the femur is removed and very little increase in length will occur. It is therefore essential that as much length as possible is preserved, and if at all possible a through knee amputation is to be preferred. Growth in length of the stump is also diminished after below knee amputation as the proximal tibial epiphysis fails to contribute the expected amount of growth. It is therefore essential that 13 cm of tibia should be preserved if at all possible and the tibia may easily be shortened later if necessary. Proportionate amputation is therefore not appropriate in the child.

Bony overgrowth also occurs in the immature stump, such as the appositional new growth beyond the site of section of the tibia, fibula or femur. This bony overgrowth does not increase stump length significantly but periosteal spikes of new bone form beneath the tip of the stump and cause discomfort. Overgrowth is more common in the younger patient and frequently requires revisional surgery.

Syme's amputation is preferable to below knee amputation in children as the distal growing epiphysis of the tibia is preserved.

Site of amputation in the presence of skin loss

Occasionally there is extensive skin loss or degloving of skin after a severe crushing injury. It is important to realize that full thickness skin cover is not necessary over the entire stump area, and length may be preserved, even though it is necessary to contemplate skin grafting over some of the stump. This may be undertaken as a secondary procedure. Such a stump may prove to be remarkably durable despite fairly large areas of split skin graft cover.

Choice of level in the presence of sensory deficiency

Sensory deficiency of the foot frequently leads to indolent penetrating ulcers and metatarsal osteomyelitis. When intractable lesions of this nature are present amputation may be necessary. Syme's amputation may prove to be very successful despite sensory deficiency of the heel (Srinavasan, 1973). Stump care must however be meticulous. Midfoot amputation may also succeed in these circumstances provided that the heel skin is good and stump care is appropriate.

METHODS AND TECHNIQUE OF AMPUTATION

The stump

The optimum length for amputation stumps in different situations has already been discussed. The stump should be firm and smoothly rounded, and it should be conical in shape, tapering distally. Opposing groups of muscles should be fixed together over the end of the sectioned bone so that vascularity and muscular control of the stump may be maintained. Suture of the muscles over the divided bone in this way is known as *myoplasty* (Fig. 8.4). The opposing muscle groups may also be anchored to the divided bone by sutures passed through their substance and fixed through drill holes into the bone end (*myodesis*). Any muscle placed over the bone end is converted into fibrous tissue, but this serves as an effective cushion which protects the skin from pressure against the bone. The joint proximal to the amputation should have a full range of movement and contractures should be avoided if at all possible. The skin should be neatly cut and sutured without too much

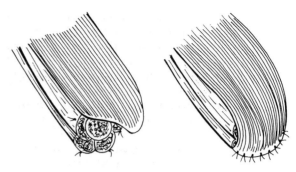

Fig. 8.4 Showing above knee myoplasty before and after suture

tension; there should be no folds or puckering and 'dog-ears' should be avoided. Skin should be freely moveable both on the bone and on the subcutaneous tissue. A terminal scar is satisfactory in the upper limb. It is less desirable in the lower limb though does not cause the patient much discomfort in a well manufactured socket.

Bone should be sectioned carefully and rounded off so that there are no sharp edges. A bone file should be used for this purpose. The tip of the sectioned bone should be covered with a periosteal or osteoperiosteal flap to enhance the vascularity and weight bearing properties of the stump.

Methods of amputating

All amputations (except the guillotine method) are designed to provide the bone stump with an adequate covering of skin and soft tissues.

Guillotine amputation

This is the most primitive type of amputation. All tissues of the limb are divided at the same level, and the bone end is left exposed on the cut surface. This method is useful when the distal part of the limb is trapped (as by machinery or in mining accidents), and an amputation has to be carried out on the spot. It may be employed also in the presence of gross sepsis. As a rule reamputation must be performed at a higher level in order that the bone end may be covered with soft parts. The operation is now generally regarded as unsatisfactory, because, unless special precautions are taken (Fig. 8.16), considerable retraction of the soft parts occurs and the exposed bone is very liable to secondary infection.

Circular amputation

This should not be confused with the guillotine method. The skin and muscles are divided circularly, but at a lower level than the bone, so that they provide a covering for the bone stump. The proposed level of bone section is first determined and the circular skin incision is made at a distance below this equal to the diameter of the limb. When skin and subcutaneous tissues have been incised they are allowed to retract upwards, and then at the new level of the skin edge the muscles are divided down to the bone. A large scalpel or amputation knife is employed for division of the soft parts; it should be used with a sweeping circular motion, the blade being kept perpendicular to the surface of the bone. Retraction of the cut muscles then takes place, and is assisted by stripping the bone with an elevator until the level for section is exposed. The circular method is most suited to a cylindrical segment of a limb, e.g. the upper arm.

Elliptical or oval amputation

The advantage of this over the circular method is that it does not leave a terminal scar. It is very similar to the method of amputating by a single flap. The upper end of the ellipse is placed at the level of bone section; the lower end should lie at a distance below this equal to the diameter of the limb. The bone is exposed by raising the flap of skin and muscle in the manner described for the flap operation.

Amputation using a racquet incision

In this method a straight incision is carried proximally from a circular or elliptical incision. The method is used especially for disarticulation at the metacarpo or metatarsophalangeal joint, and is applicable also to a disarticulation at the shoulder and hip.

Amputation using flaps

This is the most widely used method of amputation. Either two flaps cut from opposite sides of the limb or a single flap may be used. In order that the bone may be adequately covered it is essential that the combined length of the two flaps, or the total length of a single flap, should be equal to one and a half times the diameter of the limb at the level of bone section. Each flap should be cut to a semicircular rather than a rectangular shape, since a conical and not a cylindrical stump is desired. Amputation at the below knee level in vascular disease is most suitably undertaken with a single long posterior flap. This has a better blood supply than an anterior flap and its use appears to offer improved wound healing. When there is normal vascularity equal anterior and posterior flaps may be used or a long posterior flap to avoid terminal scarring.

When unequal flaps are used the shorter flap should be rather broader than the longer flap so that the skin edges to be sutured are of equal length. A good blood supply to the flaps must be assured particularly when a single long flap is employed. When the flaps have been marked out by the skin incision, they are dissected upwards until the level of bone section is reached. The distal part of the flap should consist of skin and deep fascia alone, but the proximal part should contain sufficient muscle to cover the bone end. As the flap is dissected upwards, the knife is gradually made to cut more deeply until at the level of bone section all muscles have been divided. It is better to cut the flaps over generously (and to trim off redundant skin later if required) than to end up short.

Choice of method

In succeeding sections of the chapter certain classical amputations are described, and the method which is most suited to each is detailed. These operations, however, are not universally applicable, and in a number of patients the operation is modified by the extent of injury or disease.

The most appropriate operation may be one which will allow as much as possible of the limb to be saved. This is particularly true when the injury or disease extends up to or beyond the optimum level for amputation (see Table 8.1). Difficulty always arises when there has been crushing injury with marked destruction of the soft parts. Enough bone should be removed to allow the bony stump to be adequately covered, but length should be preserved by using whatever viable tissue is available from whatever aspect of the limb. It is sometimes reasonable to cover the bone end with muscle and to contemplate split skin grafting at a later date in order to preserve length, though extensive areas of skin grafting should probably best be avoided. When there is extensive mangling, the skin on one side of the limb may be uninjured, and the use of this as a single flap will avoid unnecessary sacrifice of bone (Figs. 8.5–8.7). If the skin is destroyed up to the same level around the greater part of the limb circumference the circular method of amputation may be most appropriate.

Management of the soft tissues

Skin

The skin should be handled carefully during amputation surgery. Skin flaps should be neatly cut; although dog-ears will disappear, a poorly formed stump will delay limb fitting often for some weeks after amputation. On the rare occasions when a guillotine amputation is used, elastoplast traction to the leg may be applied in order to draw the skin and tissues distally. When there has been a severe crushing injury the limb must be carefully inspected for degloving. When this occurs the skin is sheared from its blood and nerve supply and will become necrotic. This is best appreciated by pinching the cuticle between the thumb and index finger. The fact that the skin has sheared off from the underlying tissues can usually be easily felt. The availability of skin flaps is frequently determined by the injury and in certain circumstances it may be necessary to consider skin grafting.

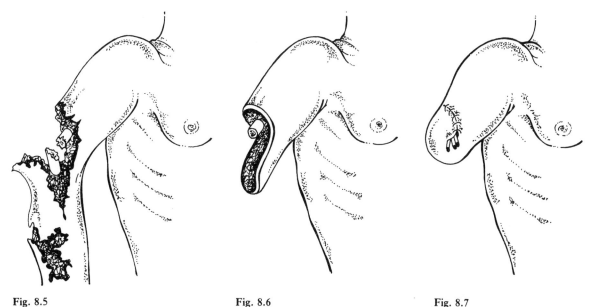

Fig. 8.5   Fig. 8.6   Fig. 8.7

Figs. 8.5–8.7 Injury often dictates the most appropriate skin closure. In order to preserve length, a single medial flap has been used

Muscle

Some form of myoplasty should be performed as a routine. Diederich described careful closure of opposing muscle groups over the bone end. Younger patients should also have the muscles anchored to the bony stump by sutures passed through drill holes. Opposing muscle groups are then closed over the bone end.

Patients with peripheral vascular disease normally have the Diederich type of myoplasty (1963) though a few surgeons also anchor the muscles to the bony tip in ischaemic disease. It is important to judge the amount of muscle that is to be left behind fairly accurately and to avoid too floppy a stump on the one hand and too bony a stump on the other. When there is vascular disease present, skin and muscle should be raised as one flap in an attempt to preserve blood supply.

Nerves

The major nerves are usually divided cleanly with a knife. The nerve is pulled down before division and allowed to retract into the soft tissues. The sciatic nerve is ligatured first to prevent bleeding. A fine suture is used.

Tingling and phantom feeling is commonplace after amputation, and this is more prominent after loss of an upper extremity. A feeling of parasthesia in the absent foot or arm is almost invariable but this is frequently a relatively minor symptom. More severe phantom discomfort and pain can occur, particularly when there has been delay in wound healing or after severe traction injury, and may be difficult to treat.

Bone division

After division of the bone during amputation, all sharp edges and prominences should be carefully rounded off with a bone file (Fig. 8.8). Various authors including Loon (1962), Ertl (1949) and Mondray (1952) have described techniques of osteoplasty. In the younger and more active patient it is usually wise to raise up a sleeve of periosteum before the bone is divided. This is closed over the bony stump and is said to provide a more comfortable stump. During below knee amputation in the younger patient it may be helpful to create a bony bridge between the divided tibia and fibula. To do this osteoperiosteal flaps are raised from the tibia (before it is divided) using a small osteotome. Periosteum is lifted off

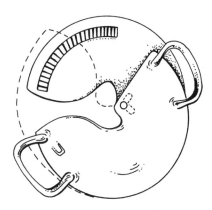

Fig. 8.8 Retractor for use in thigh amputation. It protects the tissues while bone is being sawn

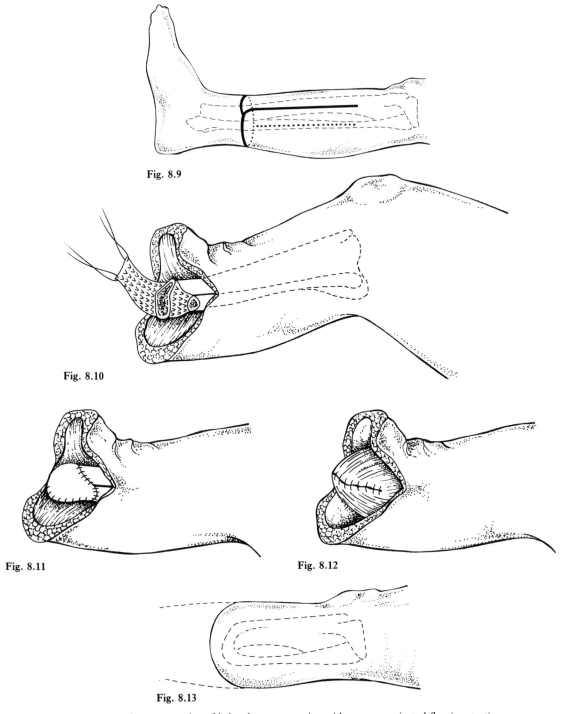

Fig. 8.9

Fig. 8.10

Fig. 8.11   Fig. 8.12

Fig. 8.13

Figs. 8.9–8.13 Diagrammatic representation of below knee amputation with an osteoperiosteal flap (see text)

with flakes of cortical bone. After division of the tibia and fibula at approximately the same level the periosteal flaps are swung across to be sutured to the periosteum on the fibula (Figs. 8.9–8.13). With time a bony bridge should form between the two bones. The advantage of this technique is that a more stable and non-compressible below knee stump is formed.

Swanson (1964) in America has developed silastic implants in the shape of a champagne cork to plug the end of the bony stump. The technique is not widely used in Britain but is likely to be an area in which there will be further research.

Postoperative management

Immediate postoperative fitting

Berlamont of Berkplage was probably the first to introduce immediate postoperative fitting. Normally a plaster is applied to the stump and a prosthetic extension is fixed to the plaster in order to allow partial weight bearing immediately after surgery (Fig. 8.14). In a prospective study, Mooney (1971) found that there were less complications of wound healing if plaster over a soft dressing only was applied. The addition of weight-bearing through a prosthetic extension increased healing complications considerably. In their series the use of a simple elastocrepe bandage was associated with highest incidence of problems.

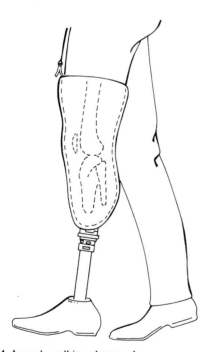

Fig. 8.14 An early walking plaster pylon

Immediate postoperative fitting is not used extensively in Britain at present and the provision of a prosthetic device is usually delayed until the wound appears to be healing, though not necessarily healed.

Controlled environment

Controlled environment treatment is a form of post-surgical dressing applied to the stump (Redhead & Snowdon, 1978). A polyvinyl chloride sleeve is placed over the amputation stump and seals proximally. A consul is attached distally to the sleeve and pumps sterile air into the sleeve at constant pressure and humidity. This dressing may be used for some days after amputation and intermittent positive pressure can be applied. It is unlikely to be adopted as routine management in the postamputation period in most centres and will be reserved for specialized problems.

Postoperative dressing

The author's practise is to use a fluffed gauze and wool dressing after below knee amputation, after which the leg is encased in a plaster cylinder (see Fig. 8.48). This is retained for 10 days unless there appears to be an indication for inspecting the wound in which case the plaster is cut off. After above knee amputation some surgeons prefer to use a plaster cast though many still use an elastocrepe bandage.

It is usually the surgeon's intention to provide the patient with an artificial limb as soon as the wound appears to be healing favourably. The wound need not be entirely healed though should in other respects be reasonably stable. It is often perfectly appropriate to commence limb fitting and walking training some nine or ten days after the amputation. A simple temporary device such as the Little pneumatic walking aid, or a plaster with prosthetic extension, may be used to commence walking training; alternatively an artificial limb may be made up, the socket normally being manufactured from a cast of the amputation stump. After surgery every effort should be made to keep the patient mobile and to prevent flexion contractures occurring in the joints.

AMPUTATION IN THE PRESENCE OF SEPSIS

Amputation in the presence of sepsis presents two main problems. It is necessary to decide at which level amputation is likely to succeed and also which method of surgery is most appropriate.

There is always a risk of infection occurring at the site of amputation and the wound should usually be left open. It is sometimes justifiable to close the wound primarily in the presence of distal infection but in these circumstances free drainage should be allowed from the wound through a drain site, or irrigation may be used. It is to be stressed however that in the presence of severe infection the wound should only be closed in exceptional circumstances.

Sometimes the surgeon may prefer to plan the amputation in two stages. The first stage then represents a preliminary amputation to remove the infected part. Subsequently a secondary procedure is planned in order to provide a satisfactory stump.

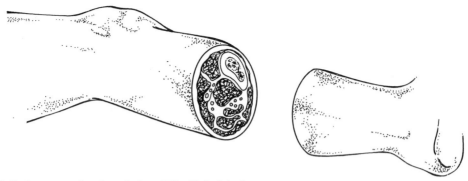

Fig. 8.15 Guillotine amputation through the middle third of the leg

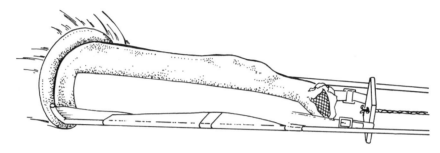

Fig. 8.16 A method of applying traction after a guillotine amputation in order to prevent retraction of the soft parts

Method of amputating

There are various techniques available to the surgeon when frank infection is present in a limb that requires amputation. Frequently the leg is amputated at its definitive level and flaps are raised in the usual manner but at the end of the operation the wound is left open and the flaps are closed gently over gauze packing. This may be removed after five days and the flaps closed in the normal way. Alternatively the surgeon may decide simply to excise the distal infected part, using a guillotine type of amputation (Figs. 8.15 & 8.16) if necessary, and proceeding to definitive amputation at the site of election when it is clear that the infection has settled.

Level of amputation

When a first stage of provisional amputation is undertaken this should usually be as low as possible in order to preserve enough tissue to allow a satisfactory definitive amputation at some later stage. The procedure should of course be carried out through viable tissues but need not necessarily be above the level of infection provided that free drainage is ensured. In this way maximum length can be conserved. Even when it is hoped that the amputation will be definitive it should if possible be carried out below the optimum level in case further bone resection is required later.

AMPUTATIONS IN THE FINGERS AND HAND

Anatomy

For the performance of amputations in the hand, the surgeon should know the exact position of the various joints and the arrangement of the tendons to the different digits.

Surface marking of joints (Fig. 8.17)
The distal interphalangeal joint is at a level 6 mm distal to the crease on the palmar surface: on the dorsum it is 3 mm distal to the knuckle prominence when the finger is flexed. *The proximal interphalangeal joint* is opposite the distal of the two creases which are seen close together on the palmar surface; on the dorsum it is 6 mm distal to the knuckle prominence. *The metacarpophalangeal joint*: the level of this joint is 18 mm proximal to the crease at the finger web; on the dorsum the joint level is 12 mm distal to the knuckle. *The wrist joint* is opposite the proximal of the two main creases on the anterior surface of the wrist.

Tendons
Each digit has at least four tendons, or sets of tendons; those required for the movements of flexion, extension, abduction and adduction.

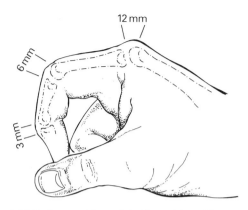

Fig. 8.17 Surface markings of the finger joints. The measurements given indicate the distance of each joint distal to the angle of the knuckle

In the fingers flexor profundus is inserted into the base of the terminal phalanx, and the flexor sublimis by slips into the middle phalanx. The extensor tendon, by means of its tripartite expansion, is inserted into both middle and distal phalanges. The interossei are inserted into the extensor hood; each of the four lumbrical muscles, arising from the tendons of flexor profundus in the palm, passes on the radial side of the metacarpophalangeal joint, also to join the extensor expansion on the dorsum of the proximal phalanx.

In the thumb the long flexor and the long extensor tendons insert into the base of the distal phalanx. The remaining tendons insert into the base of the proximal phalanx, except abductor pollicis longus, which extends only as far as the base of the metacarpal.

Structures of metacarpophalangeal and interphalangeal joints
The capsule of these joints is greatly strengthened in front by the tough *rotor plate*, which has a firm distal attachment to the base of the phalanx.

Posteriorly, the capsule merges with the expanded extensor tendon. The joints are opened from the dorsum, therefore, when this tendon has been divided.

Arteries
The four *palmar digital arteries* arise from the superficial palmar arch. The three medial ones run towards the webs, and each divides into two branches which supply contiguous sides of the fingers; the fourth runs to the ulnar side of the 5th finger. The *radialis indicis* runs along the lateral side of the index finger, and the *princeps pollicis* supplies a branch to each side of the thumb; both of these arise directly from the radial artery.

Indications
Amputations in the fingers and hand are required most commonly after injury. Amputation of a finger may be required also when there is serious infection, to prevent spread of the infection to the palm, or because a stiff or deformed finger has resulted. Occasionally amputation may be required for neoplastic disease.

Principles of amputation
The surgeon should usually conserve as much tissue as possible though certain principles will act as a guide in establishing the optimum level for amputation, particularly in the fingers. The extent and nature of injury will determine the availability of skin and soft tissues, and will allow the surgeon to judge the most suitable method of closure. Skin closure should not be under tension and soft tissue cover over the bony stump is desirable, otherwise an adherent and painful scar will result. It is of course preferable to cover the bony stump with volar skin and soft tissue though this is not always practicable. Where possible amputation through the middle or distal phalanx is preferable to disarticulation at the interphalangeal joint since the attachment of flexor and extensor tendons is thereby preserved. At a level proximal to the insertion of the tendons to the middle phalanx, some surgeons prefer to preserve a stump of the proximal phalanx which will be actively flexed by residual intrinsic attachment, and to some extent will assist the power grip. Disarticulation of the long or ring fingers at the metacarpophalangeal joint has the disadvantage of allowing coins and small objects to pass through the hand and is less popular than section through the proximal phalanx. When the index or little finger requires shortening proximal to the sublimis insertion, the surgeon must decide whether a stump of the proximal phalanx should be left. A few surgeons argue that a proximal phalangeal stump may be useful to the manual worker as it enhances power grip and preserves the width of the hand and metacarpal arch. The long finger however largely takes over the function of the index finger in these circumstances and is used for pinch grip and fine work. Disarticulation of the index or little finger at the metacarpophalangeal joint leaves a somewhat ugly hand, and most surgeons prefer to remove the finger through the metacarpal head by oblique section. This will produce a more acceptable cosmetic result and in the index should be distal enough to preserve the attachments of the deep transverse ligament of the palm.

Formal amputations are rarely possible after injury and flaps should be obtained from residual undamaged skin. Removal of bone is reduced to the minimum which is compatible with adequate cover of the stump. It is important to provide adequate skin cover over the bone as any tension will leave a tender and adherent scar. The scar should be placed dorsally if possible using a longer volar flap.

It is sometimes possible to devise a skin flap from a

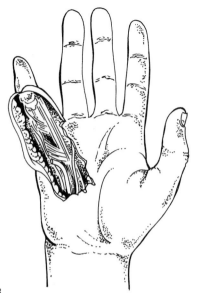

Fig. 8.18

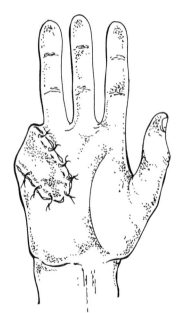

Fig. 8.19

Figs. 8.18 & 8.19 Skin from a finger used to replace a defect in the palm

seriously injured finger in order to cover a skin defect in the palm of the hand. The finger is split longitudinally and the bones and nail bed are removed. The skin is then opened out and sutured into the defect in the palm after being trimmed as required (Figs. 8.18 & 8.19).

The digital nerves should be drawn out and sectioned carefully and should be allowed to retract into the soft tissues. There is evidence that cauterization of the nerve trunk using diathermy may prevent at least to some ex-

tent the occurrence of painful digital neuromata which are not uncommon after digital amputation and which may be extremely troublesome.

Amputation of the terminal phalanx of a finger

Most traumatic amputations occur at the tip of the digit. It is important that good quality skin should be used to cover the bone and this should not be allowed to become adherent. As elsewhere in the hand volar flaps are most suitable. An effort should be made to preserve the base of the phalanx in order to preserve the tendon insertions to the stump. When this is not possible amputation through the middle phalanx may be preferred.

It is sometimes possible to preserve the tip of the finger by using local advancement flaps as described by Kutler (see p. 10). In general, split skin cover over the tip of a digit is unsatisfactory since it lacks sensation and often becomes adherent in the region of the bony stump. In small children there are remarkable powers of tissue regeneration and simple cleaning and dressing of the digit may be all that is required. Skin grafts should not be considered.

Formal amputation of the terminal phalanx (Fig. 8.20)

When the situation allows, a formal procedure should be undertaken. A transverse incision is made on the dorsal surface of the digit about 6 mm distal to the knuckle; it is continued as far as the lateral border of the finger on each side and is deepened down to the base of the phalanx. A long palmar flap is then cut; this should extend almost to the tip of the finger and must be rectangular and not pointed in shape. It is carefully dissected, the knife being kept close to the phalanx. The bone is then divided with bone shears close to its base, after which the flap is folded back and secured with three or four interrupted sutures. As a rule there are no vessels which require ligature.

The incision for *disarticulation* through the terminal joint is made a little more proximally and the joint is opened by division of the flattened extensor tendon. The volar flap is then carefully fashioned, the terminal phalanx removed along with the nail bed, and the flap is sutured over the intermediate phalanx.

Many surgeons prefer amputation through the distal third of the intermediate phalanx rather than disarticulation at the interphalangeal joint, since the latter may leave a somewhat expanded or drumstick appearance.

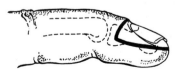

Fig. 8.20 Incision for formal amputation of terminal phalanx of finger

Alternatively, the condyles of the intermediate phalanx may be trimmed.

Amputation through the middle or proximal phalanx
Unequal anteroposterior flaps (the longer being on the palmar side), or a single long palmar flap, are employed. The digital vessels may require to be ligatured. As much as possible of the 2nd phalanx should be preserved for the sake of its tendon insertions. If these can not be preserved amputation through the proximal phalanx, at the base of the finger or obliquely through the meta-carpal head, is preferable.

In the index or fifth fingers, unless half of the middle phalanx can be preserved, most surgeons feel that the finger should be shortened obliquely through the meta-carpal head. The middle finger will then acquire the important functions of the index. A few surgeons prefer to preserve a stump of the proximal phalanx (Fig. 8.21) and believe that this contributes to power grip, particularly in manual workers. The long and ring fingers are probably best shortened through the proximal phalanx unless the tendons inserted into the middle phalanx can be preserved (Fig. 8.22).

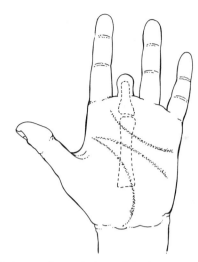

Fig. 8.22 Amputation at the base of the long or ring fingers should preserve a stump of the proximal phalanx

avoided in infection and this helps to limit spread of disease.

The *operation* is very simply performed. Two lateral flaps are cut by an incision which begins over the dorsum of the metacarpophalangeal joint and passes round each side of the finger a little distal to the web (Fig. 8.23). The digital arteries are secured and the flexor and extensor tendons are divided. The proximal phalanx is then cleared as far as its base, which is divided cleanly with an osteotome or bone shears. The skin flaps fall naturally together and are secured by two or three stitches. The retention of the base of the phalanx causes no undue projection.

Disarticulation at the metacarpophalangeal joint
This classical operation is less often employed than pre-

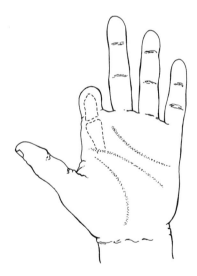

Fig. 8.21 A stump of the index or little finger proximal phalanx should rarely be left

Amputation through the base of the proximal phalanx
Amputation of the long or ring fingers may be best undertaken through the base of the proximal phalanx. The attachment of the interosseous muscles to the proximal phalanx are preserved and the palmar ligaments supporting the metacarpal arch are also retained. Scarring in the web is kept to a minimum and there is no fear of injuring the lumbricals and interossei to the adjacent fingers. The need for dissection towards the palm is

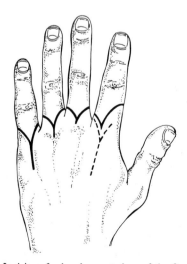

Fig. 8.23 Incisions for basal amputations of the fingers

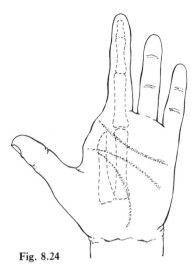

Fig. 8.24

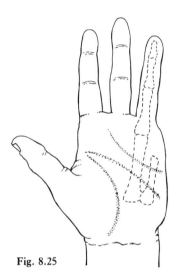

Fig. 8.25

Figs. 8.24 & 8.25 Amputation at the base of the index or little finger should normally be through the metacarpal head by oblique section

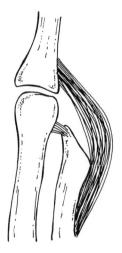

Fig. 8.26 Showing use of the first dorsal interosseous muscle to cover the stump

collateral ligaments with the interosseous tendons are then cut and the disarticulation is completed by division of the expanded extensor tendon. No attempt should be made to anchor the tendons in any way. When it is the index or 5th finger that requires to be removed it is an advantage to make a longer flap on the marginal side so that the scar falls towards the midline of the hand and is less subject to pressure.

Removal of a metacarpal head?
The deformity resulting from disarticulation of the index or little finger through the metacarpophalangeal joint is somewhat conspicuous. The hand has a very much better cosmetic appearance if the metacarpal head is sectioned obliquely, preserving the attachment of the metacarpal ligament, and the metacarpal arch. After oblique removal of the metacarpal head the stump of the metacarpal should be covered by interosseous muscle (Figs. 8.24–8.26).

Amputations in the thumb
Every effort must be made to preserve as much of the thumb as circumstances will allow, as it is of pre-eminent importance in the hand. Reconstructive procedures should be employed whenever practicable in order to avoid loss of length. Replantation surgery may also be used in certain circumstances. Even a stump composed of the metacarpal alone or of part of the metacarpal is of great value. No formal amputations need to be described. Flaps are obtained from available skin, and the minimum amount of bone is removed.

    When there is skin avulsion from the thumb leaving part of a phalanx exposed, it may be possible to achieve skin cover using grafting procedures so as to avoid sac-

viously as it has certain disadvantages as already outlined. Disarticulation of the index or little fingers leaves a somewhat ugly hand; disarticulation of the long or ring finger allows small coins to drop through and it is preferable to leave the base of the proximal phalanx.

    The *incision* is similar to that described for amputation through the base of the proximal phalanx, except that it begins more proximally over the metacarpal neck and so becomes racquet shaped. The flexor tendon is first divided, and the dissection is carried proximally until the joint is exposed. The digital arteries are secured. Disarticulation is most easily performed from the palmar aspect, the strong palmar ligament being divided. The

rificing the segment of bone which could not otherwise be covered.

Amputations in the hand
No formal amputations require to be described, for it is essential that as much of the hand as possible should be saved. When fingers and metacarpal heads are lost, the remaining parts of the metacarpals form a most useful pad against which the thumb can be opposed. Even a stump composed of the carpal bones alone is of value especially if the thumb or part of the thumb can be saved also.

DISARTICULATION AT THE WRIST JOINT

This operation is rarely practicable, owing to the difficulty of obtaining flaps sufficiently long to cover the expanded ends of the forearm bones. Preservation of the inferior radio-ulnar joint allows the power of pronation and supination to be retained but these movements cannot be transmitted to an artificial hand. The circumference of the forearm changes in rotation, and the artificial socket is either too tight to permit the change of shape or too loose to secure a firm hold on the stump. The operation has, therefore, little to commend it, and an amputation through the lower third of the forearm is usually to be preferred.

AMPUTATION THROUGH THE FOREARM

Anatomy

Muscles
Anterior surface. The superifical muscles are pronator teres, flexor carpi radialis, palmaris longus, flexor digitorum sublimis and flexor carpi ulnaris. Pronator teres passes obliquely laterally to gain insertion into the middle of the lateral surface of the radius. The other muscles run down to the wrist keeping the above relationship from lateral to medial side, although flexor sublimis is on a somewhat deeper plane. The deep muscles are flexor digitorum profundus, which clothes the anterior and medial surfaces of the ulna in its upper three-fourths, flexor pollicis longus which covers the anterior surface of the radius to a similar extent, and pronator quadratus which covers the anterior surface of both bones in the lower fourth.
Lateral border and dorsum. The superficial muscles are brachioradialis, extensor carpi radialis longus, extensor carpi radialis brevis, extensor digitorum communis, extensor digiti minimi and extensor carpi ulnaris. The deep muscles are abductor pollicis longus, extensor pol-

licis brevis, extensor pollicis longus and extensor indicis; these all become superficial in the lower third of the forearm, the three tendons of the thumb crossing to the radial side.

Vessels
The radial artery in the upper two-thirds of the forearm is overlapped by brachioradialis; in the lower third it lies superficially between brachioradialis and flexor carpi radialis. *The ulnar artery* runs a deeper course lying on the surface of flexor profundus; it becomes superficial towards the wrist and passes anterior to the flexor retinaculum. *The anterior interosseous artery* runs down on the front of the interosseous membrane; *the posterior interosseous artery* is found between the superficial and deep muscles of the dorsum.

Nerves
The median nerve is at first deep to flexor sublimis, but appears on its radial side just above the wrist. *The ulnar nerve* lies on flexor profundus on the medial side of the ulnar artery; with the artery it becomes superficial at the wrist. *The radial nerve* accompanies the radial artery in the middle third of its course in the forearm; it then turns dorsally and breaks up into its terminal sensory branches. Its more important *posterior interosseous* branch runs a deep course among the dorsal muscles, breaking up into branches which supply them.

Operation
For the fitting of an artificial hand the optimum length of the forearm stump is 16–20 cm measured from the olecranon. A stump measuring less than 8 cm is useless for transmitting movement to an artificial elbow joint, so that, if this amount of bone cannot be conserved, an amputation through the upper arm may be preferred. Between these levels as much of the limb as possible should, of course, be saved.

The circular method of amputation is applicable to the lower third of the forearm which is roughly cylindrical, while the flap method is best in the upper two-thirds. In cases of injury, however, flaps will be obtained from whatever skin is available. Vessels and nerves are identified during the division of the muscles and are dealt with in the usual manner (p. 169). When the muscles have been divided the knife is entered between the two bones in order to divide the interosseous membrane and the muscular fibres arising from it. Both bones are then cleared for a short distance with an elevator, so as to expose bare bone to the saw. The radius being the more movable bone is divided first. Muscles which have a humeral attachment should be sutured over the bone ends, so that all possible mobility of the elbow joint may be retained.

Krukenberg amputation

The Krukenberg amputation is used infrequently in patients with bilateral loss of the arms through the forearm. The operation separates radius and ulna, so allowing pincer function and providing relatively crude grasp. Usually the operation is used on one side only, though bilateral Krukenberg procedures have been discussed. Those requiring more detailed information are referred to a recent article by Mathur et al (1981).

DISARTICULATION AT THE ELBOW JOINT

Disarticulation at the elbow is not a popular operation. The stump is club-shaped and unsightly, and the artificial limb cannot be fitted with a mechanical elbow joint at the correct level. In cases of injury there are unlikely to be sufficient soft parts available to cover the expanded end of the humerus. The one advantage of the operation is that the artificial limb, which must be fitted by means of a lacing leather, or a plastic, socket secures a very firm hold on the stump and does not tend to rotate.

Technique

For a formal operation all the various methods of amputating have been individually recommended: circular, elliptical, racquet, and flap methods. The choice will depend upon the conditions present. It should be noted that voluminous flaps are required, owing to the relatively large size of the lower end of the humerus.

Muscles and tendons are divided just below the joint level. *The brachial artery* is identified in the middle of the cubital fossa on the medial side of the biceps tendon, and *the median nerve* lies just medial to the artery. *The ulnar nerve* is found between the medial epicondyle and the olecranon, in company with branches of the ulnar collateral and supratrochlear arteries. *The radial nerve* runs in front of the radio-humeral joint, and is accompanied by the profunda artery. These vessels and nerves are dealt with in the usual manner. It is recommended that the disarticulation should be commenced from the lateral side, the knife being entered between the head of the radius and the capitellum.

AMPUTATION THROUGH THE UPPER ARM

Anatomy

Muscles

Biceps lies superficially on the anteromedial aspect of the arm and is easily identified. *Coracobrachialis*, which is posteromedial to biceps, extends only as far as the middle of the humerus. *Brachialis* is closely applied to the

front of the humerus in its lower two-thirds. *Triceps* forms the muscular mass on the posterior aspect.

Vessels

The brachial artery runs a fairly superficial course, being overlapped by the medial border of biceps. Its main branches are the *profunda* which accompanies the radial nerve, and the *ulnar collateral* which accompanies the ulnar nerve. *The cephalic vein* ascends in the superficial fascia at the lateral border of biceps.

Nerves

The median nerve is at first lateral to the brachial artery, but crosses anteriorly in the middle of the arm to reach its medial side. *The ulnar nerve* deviates medially from the artery, and passes posteriorly through the medial intermuscular septum to reach the back of the medial epicondyle. *The radial nerve* runs a spiral course round the back of the humerus under cover of triceps. It pierces the lateral intermuscular septum to reach the front of the lateral condyle, where it lies between the brachioradialis and brachialis. *The musculocutaneous nerve* pierces coracobrachialis and runs down between biceps and brachialis. It pierces deep fascia a little above the elbow to become the lateral cutaneous nerve of the forearm. *The medial cutaneous nerve* of the forearm pierces deep fascia in the middle of the arm and runs superficially over the medial side of the elbow.

Operation

Amputation should not be carried out through the lower 7–8 cm of the humerus since the stump is then too long to allow the fitting of a mechanical elbow joint at the correct level. A stump measuring 20 cm from the acromion is regarded by prosthetists as ideal. Above this level as much of the limb as possible should be conserved. It should be noted that a stump which is much shorter than this is incapable of transmitting movement to an artificial limb, but is of the greatest value in preserving the normal contour of the shoulder (Fig. 8.28).

Either the circular, the elliptical or the flap method is employed, the choice depending upon the conditions present. If the flap method is favoured, the flaps should be made lateral and medial rather than anterior and posterior. The vessels and nerves are identified during division of the muscles and are dealt with in the customary manner.

AMPUTATION AT THE SHOULDER

Anatomy

Muscles related to the shoulder joint

On three sides the joint is strongly supported by mus-

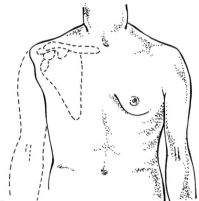

Fig. 8.27

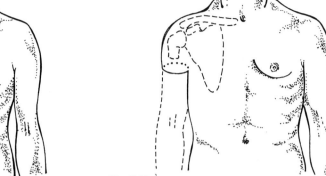

Fig. 8.28

Figs. 8.27 & 8.28 Disarticulation through the shoulder joint results in unsightly angular deformity. Amputation through the upper end of the humerus preserves the contours of the shoulder, although the stump is useless

cles, the insertions of which are fused with the capsule: *anteriorly*, subscapularis; *superiorly*, supraspinatus and infraspinatus; *posteriorly*, teres minor. *Inferiorly*, the joint is related to the long head of triceps, but this is in contact with the capsule only when the arm is abducted. The long head of biceps passes through the joint cavity over the head of the humerus. More remote relations are: *anteriorly*, short head of biceps and coracobrachialis, which lie on subscapularis and are in turn covered by pectoralis major and by the anterior fibres of deltoid; *superiorly*, the main part of deltoid arising from the acromion arch; *posteriorly*, the posterior fibres of deltoid.

Vessels
The axillary artery lies anteromedial to the joint, separated from it by subcapularis. When the arm is abducted to a right angle its course is indicated by a straight line drawn from the mid point of the clavicle to the junction of the arm with the posterior axillary fold; when the arm is by the side this line is curved. Its *posterior humeral circumflex* branch, which may be encountered in amputations at the shoulder, runs round the surgical neck of the humerus under cover of deltoid. *The axillary vein* is on the medial side of the artery. *The cephalic vein* ascends in the groove between pectoralis major and deltoid.

Nerves
At the level of the shoulder joint the brachial plexus has evolved into the main nerve trunks of the limb. These lie grouped around the axillary artery. The *medial and musculocutaneous nerves* are lateral, the *ulnar nerve* is medial, the *medial cutaneous nerve of the forearm* is anterior, and the *radial* and *circumflex nerves* are posterior. *The median cutaneous nerve of the arm* lies on the medial side of the vein.

In amputations at the shoulder the head and tuber-

osities of the humerus should always if possible be preserved. If a disarticulation through the joint is performed the acromion process alone remains to form the prominence of the shoulder; the normal rounded contour is lost, and an angular and unsightly shoulder results (Fig. 8.27). Disarticulation may, however, be necessitated by certain injuries, or be considered advisable in cases of malignant disease of the humerus.

Disarticulation at the shoulder joint
The classical method of carrying out this operation was first described by Spence in 1856, and, with no more than slight modifications, it is still employed at the present time.

The approach to the joint is by the racquet method. With the arm held slightly abducted and rotated laterally the incision is made as shown in Figure 8.29. It begins just lateral to the tip of the coracoid process and extends downwards in the line of the humerus; at the level of the axillary folds it splits to encircle the limb. The vertical part of the incision is deepened, and the clavicular fibres of the deltoid and the pectoralis major tendon are divided. The knife is now swept round the lateral and posterior sides of the incision, and is made to cut deeply to the bone, so that the deltoid muscle is divided cleanly a little above its insertion. The large lateral flap containing the deltoid is turned upwards, care being taken to avoid injury to the posterior humeral circumflex which enters its deep surface. The tuberosities of the humerus and the shoulder joint are now exposed. By cutting against the superior and anterior surfaces of the anatomical neck of humerus the capsule of the joint, together with the capsular muscles and the long head of biceps are divided. The limb is rotated first medially and then laterally to allow this part of the operation to be carried out. The head of the humerus is then dislocated forwards, and the disarticulation is completed. The

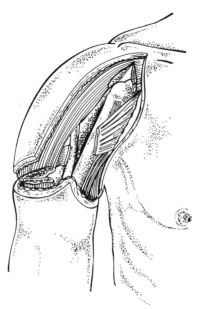

Fig. 8.29 Spence's method of disarticulation at the shoulder joint

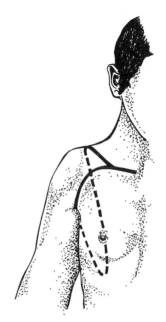

Fig. 8.30 Incision for inter-scapulo-thoracic amputation

knife is now inserted between the humerus and the soft parts on the medial side and is made to cut downwards to the bone. The remaining muscles, together with the brachial vessels and the nerve trunks, are divided above the lower level of the skin incision on the medial side. In Spence's original technique, division of the medial flap was completed in one sweep by bringing the knife sharply through the tissues from within outwards into the skin incision already made. It was the duty of the assistant to grasp the partially formed flap, following the track of the knife, and to secure the vessels by pressure between the finger and thumb. After the flap had been divided the vessels were picked up and ligatured. In modern practice it is customary to identify and ligature the vessels before the division is carried out. The flaps are trimmed if necessary and are sutured. Drainage of the wound for 24 to 48 hours is advisable.

Amputation through the upper end of the humerus
In cases where it is found possible to conserve the upper end of the humerus, the first stages of the operation are very similar to those described for disarticulation. The deltoid flap is not reflected so far upwards, and the capsular muscles are not, of course, divided. For section of the bone an electric or Gigli saw is recommended. Longer flaps may be required, depending upon the amount of humerus which it is possible to retain.

INTER-SCAPULO-THORACIC AMPUTATION

This operation is sometimes necessary for malignant growths involving the scapula or the upper end of the humerus. It consists in removal of the upper limb altogether with the scapula and the lateral two-thirds of the clavicle. The incision is shown in Fig. 8.30. Its horizontal part is used to expose the clavicle which is cleared and divided with a Gigli saw near its medial end. The lateral or main part of the bone is elevated, and its middle third is removed. Through the access thus afforded the subclavian vessels are divided between ligatures, and the trunks of the brachial plexus are treated by simple section at a higher level. In the anterior part of the racquet incision pectoralis major and minor are divided close to the chest wall. From the posterior part of the incision the medial flap is raised as far as the vertebral border of the scapula. Removal of the forequarter is then completed by division of the muscles which attach the scapula to the trunk—trapezius, levator scapulae, the rhomboids, serratus anterior and latissimus dorsi. All haemorrhage is arrested, and the flaps are sutured with drainage.

AMPUTATION OF THE TOES

Anatomy

Metatarsophalangeal and interphalangeal joints
The metatarsophalangeal joints are situated 2.5 cm proximal to the free border of the web. In the lateral four toes, the proximal and distal interphalangeal joints are respectively 6 mm and 3 mm distal to the joint prominence on the dorsum. In the great toe the inter-

phalangeal joint is at a level midway between the base of the nail fold and the joint prominence.

The capsule of these joints is greatly strengthened below by the tough *plantar ligament*, which is firmly attached to the base of the phalanx. In the first metatarsophalangeal joint this ligament is replaced by the two sesamoid bones. Dorsally the capsule is deficient, its place taken by the expanded extensor tendon.

The toes

Each toe, provided that it is not deformed, takes at least a proportion of the weight borne by the forefoot; it relieves the pressure on the head of its metatarsal, and contributes largely to the normally resilient gait. The little toe is of less value than the others in this respect, but its removal leaves the head of the 5th metatarsal forming a prominence on the side of the foot, over which a painful corn is very liable to develop. Amputation of any toe, therefore, should not be undertaken lightly, nor should it be performed for conditions such as hammer toe, which can be corrected by other measures (p. 109). It is necessitated as a rule by crushing injuries, or for deformities which are incapable of correction.

The great toe has, of course, much greater functional importance than all the others, and should be conserved whenever possible, If partial amputation is unavoidable every effort should be made to obtain a stump which will be mobile and capable of weight-bearing.

Partial amputation of the great toe

Amputation of the terminal phalanx

If a functionally useful stump is to be obtained, it is essential to preserve the base of the terminal phalanx, into which the long flexor and extensor tendons are inserted. In cases of injury, flaps are obtained from whatever skin is available. Preference should, if possible, be given to a longer flap on the plantar aspect, so that the scar will not be subjected to pressure. The incision for a formal amputation is shown in Figure 8.31. The long plantar flap is reflected back, the knife being kept close to the bone, in order to avoid injury to the plantar digital arteries which provide the blood supply to the flap.

The bone is divided with bone shears or with a sharp osteotome just distal to its base. If a *disarticulation* is necessary the joint is best opened from the plantar surface. The flap is folded over the end of the stump and is secured with a few interrupted sutures.

Amputation through the proximal phalanx

A stump comprising less than one complete phalanx is of little or no value for weight-bearing; it tends to become dorsiflexed and in the way. No more than the base of the phalanx should therefore be preserved.

Amputation of the great toe at its base

The base of the proximal phalanx should always if possible be retained, for thereby the insertions of the short muscles of the toe remain intact. These muscles are of value in giving support to the head of the metatarsal and ensure a better stump.

The formal operation is carried out by the racquet method. The incision is shown in Figure 8.32. It should be noted that the handle of the racquet is placed well to the lateral side of the dorsum, in order that pressure on the scar will be avoided; it extends proximally as far as the head of the metatarsal. The blade of the racquet encircles the toe obliquely so that the medial flap extends almost as far distally as the interphalangeal joint. The flaps are dissected back and the digital arteries are secured and ligatured. The long tendons are divided. The first phalanx is cleared and divided with an osteotome just distal to its base. The flaps fall naturally together and are opposed with a few interrupted sutures.

Disarticulation at the metatarsophalangeal joint

The incision is similar to that described above, except that the straight part extends proximally as far as the neck of the metatarsal, and a shorter flap on the medial side will suffice. The flaps are reflected back to expose the joint, and the digital arteries are secured. The long

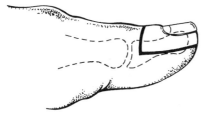

Fig. 8.31 Incision for amputation of terminal phalanx of great toe

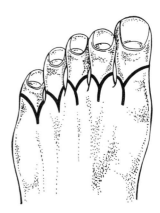

Fig. 8.32 Incisions for basal amputations in the toes

tendons are divided. The joint is opened from the plantar surface, the insertions of the short muscles being divided along with the capsule against the base of the proximal phalanx, so that the sesamoid bones are preserved. When the disarticulation has been completed the capsular structures are sutured together over the exposed metatarsal head in order to support it and to prevent retraction of the short muscles.

Partial amputation in the lateral four toes

Such amputations are frequently condemned as being unsatisfactory, as the stump is usually useless for weight-bearing, and tends to become dorsiflexed and in the way. This cannot be accepted, however, as a general rule. The stump of a toe may have no weight-bearing value, but if it consists of one phalanx or more it acts as a useful spreader to keep the adjacent toes in normal alignment. The second toe is particularly valuable in this respect, and its loss predisposes to hallux valgus. Dorsiflexion of the stump can usually be prevented by tenotomy of the extensor tendon (p. 23) at the time of amputation, and by exercises afterwards. Amputation through the base of the proximal phalanx is preferable to disarticulation at the metatarsophalangeal joint, since it entails less interference with the important metatarsal arch.

Amputations through the base of the middle or terminal phalanx are again preferable to a disarticulation, since the tendon insertions are preserved. The technique is similar to that described for partial amputation in the great toe.

Disarticulation of the lateral four toes

Disarticulation at the metatarsophalangeal joint should be carried out in cases of injury where the base of the phalanx cannot be preserved. It is indicated also in the relatively common deformity in which one toe has become displaced backwards on the others, and is pressed upon by the shoe; such a toe is useless, both for weight-bearing and as a spreader to the other toes.

As in the case of the great toe the racquet approach is employed. The incisions for the different toes are shown in Figure 8.32, and the operation follows the lines already described. The inexperienced operator should note that the metatarsophalangeal joints are situated much further proximally than would be anticipated.

Amputation of all of the toes

Amputation of all of the toes is usually indicated where there is fixed clawing or dislocation of the metatarsophalangeal joints leading to gross deformity. This frequently occurs in rheumatoid arthritis, and amputation of the toes may sometimes be preferred to forefoot arthroplasty.

Flint and Sweetnam reported their experience of the procedure in 1960, and Green discussed the technique in 1985. Dorsal and volar incisions run across the toes sweeping into the web spaces as they pass across the foot. The toes are disarticulated at the metatarsophalangeal joint, the arteries are secured, and the long tendons and nerves are divided and allowed to retract.

AMPUTATIONS IN THE FOOT

Amputations through the foot, particularly through its midpart, have had a relatively poor reputation over many years. Warren (1968) and Pederson (1954) described the use of the transmetatarsal amputation which now has an established place in surgical practise particularly in patients with diabetes and relatively localised peripheral vascular disease of the toes.

Recently there has been increasing interest in amputations more proximally in the foot. Amputation through the metatarsal bases or disarticulation at the tarsometatarsal joints (described by William Hey of Leeds, 1810 and by Lisfranc, 1815) may be extremely useful after trauma, particularly crushing injuries of the forefoot. This type of amputation may also be used in the diabetic foot.

Chopart's amputation or disarticulation through the midtarsal joints (the talonavicular joint on the medial side of the foot and the calcaneocuboid joint on the lateral side of the foot) has generally been considered to be an unsatisfactory procedure. Recently, Bingham writing in Murdoch's Textbook (1970) stated that with suitable tibialis anterior transplant a satisfactory stump may be achieved. This is particularly so after injury but the procedure has yet to establish its place in the diabetic foot. It is particularly important to note that unless a satisfactory tibialis anterior transfer to the neck of the talus can be achieved the procedure is likely to fail.

In undertaking amputation through the foot a long volar flap should be used when at all possible. When a junctional scar, that is a scar between volar and dorsal skin, is placed in a weight-bearing area considerable discomfort is likely to ensue. One of the conspicuous advantages of amputation through the foot is that an ordinary shoe or surgically made boot may be adequate footwear and a formal artificial limb is usually not necessary.

Transmetatarsal amputation

There are several series which have been published to show that transmetatarsal amputation, performed for peripheral vascular disease, particularly in diabetes, is attended by a large percentage of successful results. The absence of palpable pulsation below the femoral artery is not an absolute contra-indication to the operation provided that the skin on the dorsum of the foot is warm and well nourished and there is no spreading infection.

Technique

The amputation is effected by the use of a long plantar flap, which extends to a level just proximal to the flexion crease at the base of the toes; the dorsal part of the incision crosses the necks of the metatarsals, at which level these bones are divided. Since primary healing is always in some doubt, the flaps must be handled with great gentleness and not held with dissecting forceps; they should be trimmed as required and sutured accurately, so that the skin is neither redundant nor under tension (Figs. 8.33 & 8.34). It is advised that the stitches should be left in place for fourteen days.

Tarsometatarsal amputation

A long volar flap is used if possible. The foot is shortened through the bases of the metatarsals or by disarticulation at the tarsometatarsal joint. The long toe flexors and extensors should be anchored to the soft tissues of the foot. After closure of the wound a padded dressing is applied.

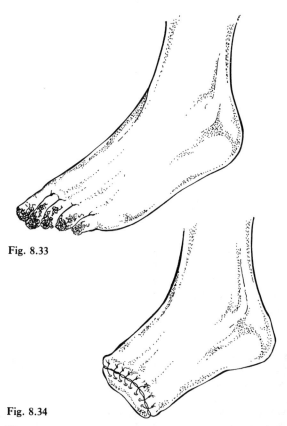

Fig. 8.33

Fig. 8.34

Figs. 8.33 & 8.34 Transmetatarsal amputation for dry gangrene of the toes. A long plantar flap is employed, and the metatarsals are divided at the levels of their necks

Midtarsal or Chopart's amputation

A long volar flap and a shorter dorsal flap are raised from the skeleton of the foot provided suitable skin is available. The midtarsal joints are exposed and disarticulation of the foot is completed through the talonavicular joint on the medial side of the foot and through the calcaneocuboid joint on the lateral side. The tibialis anterior is identified and is sutured into a drill hole through the neck of the talus. The remaining long extensor muscles and long flexors are anchored to soft tissues particularly to the remains of the midtarsal capsule. The long volar flap is swung over the divided foot and sutured on the dorsum. A padded dressing and a below knee plaster are applied in order to maintain the ankle in the neutral position. The plaster should be retained for six weeks in order to allow the tibialis anterior muscle to anchor in the neck of the talus.

SYME'S AMPUTATION

Anatomy

Structure of the ankle joint

The capsule is attached on all sides to the margins of the articular surfaces, and is arbitrarily divided into *anterior, posterior, medial and lateral ligaments*. The medial (*deltoid*) ligament is fanshaped and very strong. Its apex is attached to the malleolus; its base to bony points over a wide area on the medial side of the foot.

Anterior relations of ankle joint

The following structures are in contact with the anterior ligament, from medial to lateral side: tibialis anterior, extensor hallucis longus, anterior tibial vessels, anterior tibial nerve, extensor digitorum longus and peroneus tertius. In the superficial fascia, the long saphenous vein is found anterior to the medial malloelus, and terminal branches of the musculocutaneous nerve lie lateral to the midline.

Structures between medial malleolus and heel

The following structures enter the sole of the foot behind and below the medial malleolus and are bound down by the flexor retinaculum: tibialis posterior, flexor digitorum longus, posterior tibial vessels, posterior tibial nerve and flexor hallucis longus. They lie in that order in the line between the malleolus and the heel. At this level the posterior tibial artery and nerve both divide into medial and lateral plantar branches.

Structures between lateral malleolus and heel

Peroneus longus and brevis lie in contact with the lateral ligaments of the ankle joint. The short saphenous vein lies in the superficial fascia behind the malleolus.

Posterior relations of the ankle joint

The joint is separated from the tendocalcanei by a wide interval filled with fat. The posterior tibial vessels and nerves and the flexor group of tendons are in contact with the medial part of the posterior ligament before they pass below the medial malleolus. The peroneal artery and the peroneal tendons lie behind the lateral part of the ligament.

Aims of Syme's operation

This operation, first described by Syme in 1842, is the classical amputation in the region of the ankle. The tibia and fibula are divided at or immediately above the level of the joint, and their ends are covered with a single flap obtained from the skin of the heel. The end of the stump is at a height of about 6–8 cm from the ground.

Syme's amputation has established itself as a procedure that will provide a durable stump which may be entirely satisfactory. Some 50% of patients are able to walk on the stump without a prosthesis (which may prove to be useful at night), and many become involved in strenuous work. It is difficult to provide a woman with an attractive prosthesis and occasionally the Syme's stump tends to migrate sideways. This amputation is particularly suitable in young men who have a crushing injury of the foot, but the unsightliness of the prosthesis is a drawback in the female although it does not entirely preclude the operation.

Recently the Syme's amputation has been used in patients with diabetes and Wagner (1977) has presented a large series of successful Syme's procedures in diabetic patients using a somewhat modified technique. Srinavasan (1973) has shown that the amputation may be used successfully in the sensory deficient foot. There can be no question that Syme's amputation is of special value to patients who do not have access to modern artificial limbs, for they can be fitted with a simple appliance known as the 'Elephant boot'. This is inexpensive to manufacture and gives lasting service (Fig. 8.35).

Technique

The surgeon stands at the end of the table facing the foot, which either overhangs the table or is raised by a sandbag placed under the lower third of the leg. The incision is shown in Figure 8.36. The knife is entered below the tip of the lateral malleolus and is carried with a backward inclination across the sole to a point 2 cm below the medial malleolus. (It was formerly taught that the incision should be carried to a point below *and behind* the medial malleolus, but this entails some risk of dividing the posterior tibial artery before it has given off its important calcanean branches, on which the nutrition of the heel flap depends). The two ends of the incision are then joined by the shortest route across the front of the ankle joint. Throughout the incision all structures

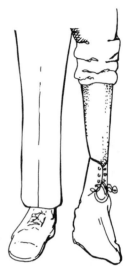

Fig. 8.35 Primitive 'elephant boot' prosthesis that can be used after Syme's amputation

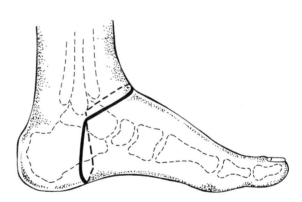

Fig. 8.36 Incision for Syme's amputation

are divided down to bone. On the anterior surface these include the extensor group of tendons and the anterior tibial vessels and nerve. On the medial side, below the malleolus, the incision divides the flexor group of tendons and the plantar vessels and nerves. Laterally, the peroneal tendons are cut. The ankle joint is then opened by division of its anterior ligament; the lateral ligaments are cut from within outwards, and the foot is dislocated in a plantar direction to expose the back of the joint.

The next part of the operation is the most important and the most difficult. It consists in the division of the posterior ligaments of the joint, the detachment of the insertion of the tendocalcaneus and the dissection of the calcaneum out of the heel flap. During these stages of the operation the plantar dislocation of the foot is steadily increased (Figs. 8.37–8.41). There is great danger of wounding the posterior tibial and peroneal arteries when the posterior ligament is cut, for both arteries are

Figs. 8.37–8.41 *Stages in a Syme's amputation*

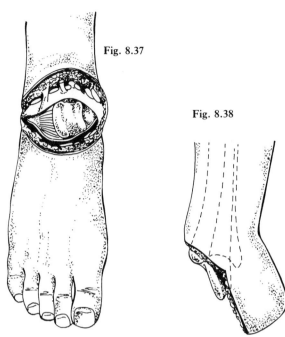

Fig. 8.37

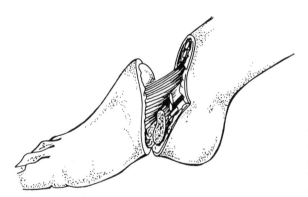

Fig. 8.38

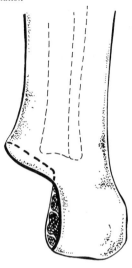

Fig. 8.40 Showing the heel flap prior to closure

Fig. 8.37 Division of the anterior structures and opening of the ankle joint

Fig. 8.38 Division of medial and posterior ligaments of ankle joint, prior to dissection of the calcaneum out of the heel flap

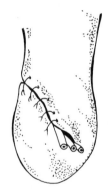

Fig. 8.41 Operation completed

Fig. 8.39 Bones about to be divided

closely applied to the back of the ligament. Their branches which supply the skin of the heel are also in danger when the calcaneum is being dissected out of the flap. To avoid such accidents, which may result in sloughing of the flap, *the knife is kept closely applied to the bone throughout these stages of the operation.*

In the original technique the heel flap was dissected off the calcaneum and the Achilles tendon was divided as the first stage of the operation. This alternative method is entirely satisfactory.

The anterior tibial artery, the medial and lateral plan-

tar arteries, and the two saphenous veins are the main vessels which require ligature. As the stump is to be an end-bearing one, particular attention should be paid to the shortening of nerve trunks, so that these do not become involved in scar tissue at the end of the stump. Anterior tibial and musculocutaneous nerves are identified, and cut short. The medial and lateral plantar nerves should be dissected upwards out of the heel flap to their point of origin from the posterior tibial nerve; this trunk is then divided well above the ankle region.

If the articular surface of the tibia and fibula are healthy, the malleoli alone are removed. Otherwise the bones are divided immediately above the level of the ankle joint. The saw is applied exactly at right angles to the axis of the leg. The heel flap is folded over the bone ends, and after being trimmed as required is sutured in position. Drainage may be provided by a strip of corrugated plastic brought out at one corner of the wound; this is removed within 48 hours.

Syme's amputation in diabetes

When Syme's amputation is undertaken in the diabetic patient several modifications must be considered. In the first place it is probably wise to cut the heel flap slightly larger. The incision usually starts about 1 cm in front of the medial malleolus and passes across the front of the ankle joint to 1 cm in front of the lateral malleolus and then by the shortest route across the sole of the foot.

Wagner (1977) prefers a two-stage amputation. During the first stage the heel is enucleated in the usual way but the medial and lateral malleoli are not removed. The wound is closed and when it is soundly healed some five or six weeks later, the malleoli are removed through small incisions at a second stage procedure. Some surgeons however prefer to remove the malleoli during the first operation but most leave the distal articular surface of the tibia and do not section the tibia as previously described.

When there is significant infection in the foot as is often the case in diabetes it may be wise to close the Syme's amputation over irrigation. Two tubular drains may be left in the cavity of the stump. Saline, containing an appropriate antibiotic, runs into the cavity through one of the drains, and escapes into a urinary bag through the other. The irrigations may be run fast enough to keep the effluent fluid relatively clear. The drains may be retained for up to 10 days.

OTHER AMPUTATIONS AT THE ANKLE

Modified Syme's amputation

Many modifications of Syme's original amputation have been described, with variations of the incision and of soft tissue and bony procedures. In general the original technique has outlived all of these variations. Figure 8.42

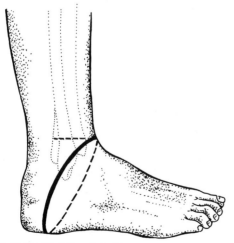

Fig. 8.42 Modified Syme's incision

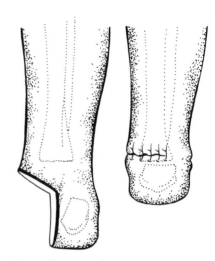

Fig. 8.43 Pirogoff's amputation

shows Syme's amputation using an elliptical incision and with division of the tibia and fibula slightly higher than usual. It is doubtful whether this operation has anything to commend it and it has not won widespread approval.

Pirogoff's amputation (Fig. 8.43)

This is similar to Syme's amputation except that the posterior part of the calcaneum is retained in the heel flap, and is opposed to the sawn surface of the tibia by sutures which take up the periosteum or are passed through drill holes in the bones. It provides a longer stump than does Syme's amputation, and one which is even better suited to end-bearing, but in view of the difficulty of fitting an artificial foot with an ankle joint at the correct level, it is seldom employed nowadays except in underdeveloped countries.

AMPUTATION THROUGH THE LEG AT THE BELOW KNEE LEVEL

Anatomy

Muscles

Anterior group. Tibialis anterior lies immediately lateral to the tibia in the upper two-thirds of the leg. Extensor digitorum longus is lateral to tibialis anterior and in front of the fibula. Extensor hallucis longus lies between tibialis anterior and extensor digitorum, and partly hidden by them. In the lower third these muscles pass on to the front of the tibia, where they are joined by peroneus tertius.

Lateral group. Peroneous longus and brevis cover the lateral surface of the fibula, brevis being anterior and on a deeper plane. In the lower third both muscles incline backwards to pass behind the lateral malleolus.

Posterior group. The muscular mass of the calf is composed of gastrocnemius superficially and soleus which is immediately deep to it. These muscles (together with the unimportant plantaris tendon) combine to form the tendo calcaneus. The deep muscles are popliteus (which does not extend below the upper third of the leg), flexor digitorum longus, flexor hallucis longus and tibialis posterior. Flexor digitorum longus is closely applied to the back of the tibia, and flexor hallucis longus to the back of the fibula. Tibialis posterior lies between them on the interosseus membrane, and is on a still deeper plane.

Vessels and nerves
The anterior tibial artery enters the anterior compartment of the leg by piercing the upper part of the interosseous membrane. In the upper two-thirds it runs a deep course on the anterior surface of the membrane; in the lower third it lies on the front of the tibia. *The posterior tibial artery* runs for the greater part of its course between soleus and the fascia covering tibialis posterior; distally it is directly behind the ankle joint. The *posterior tibial nerve* accompanies the artery on its lateral side. The *peroneal artery* is found on the back of the interosseous membrane, close to the fibula. *The long saphenous vein* ascends in the superficial fascia on the medial surface of the leg; *the short saphenous vein* on the posterior surface.

Objectives of amputation
Amputation at the below knee level through the middle third of the leg is the operation of choice when it is not possible to preserve the foot or the heel. The ideal length of tibial stump is 14 cm. A stump that is shorter than 8 cm tends to slip out of the socket of an artificial limb and is very difficult to accommodate comfortably and effectively in the patellar tendon bearing prosthesis. When it is not possible to save at least 8 cm of the tibia the patient may be better served by knee disarticulation or amputation through the thigh.

A distinction should be made between those amputations that are undertaken as a direct result or consequences of peripheral vascular disease and amputations in which vascular disease is not a problem. Ghormley described below knee amputation using a long posterior flap in 1947. Burgess (1981) has been largely responsible for popularising this technique and it is probably now the most commonly used method of below knee amputation in patients with vascular impairment. Recently amputation at the below knee level using a long posteromedial flap using an elliptical incision has been described, but only the conventional long posterior flap technique will be described here.

Patients who do not have ischaemic disease in the limb, particularly younger patients, are probably better served by amputation at the below knee level with careful myoplasty and osteoplasty. In these patients equal or unequal skin flaps may be used. Unequal flaps have the advantage that the scar is not terminal and may be placed away from the sectioned tibia, though this is not particularly important if the patient is to be provided with a patellar tendon bearing prosthesis.

Myoplasty is designed to anchor the opposing muscle groups firmly around and over the sectioned bone. When osteoplasty is used a periosteal sleeve may either be closed over the sectioned bone (and is thought to provide a more comfortable stump) or periosteal strips raised from the tibia are sutured across to the fibula in the hope that bony union between the sectioned tibia and sectioned fibula may occur. This provides the patient with a firmer stump.

Conventional below knee amputation
The proposed level of bone section is marked by a scratch on the skin, and the flaps are marked out. The combined length of the two flaps should be equal to $1\frac{1}{2}$ times the diameter of the limb at the level of bone section. The skin is incised and the long saphenous vein will be encountered at the medial corner of the anterior flap, and the short saphenous vein at the middle of the posterior flap. The flaps are dissected back in the usual way. The periosteum covering the subcutaneous surface of the tibia should be raised (in lieu of deep fascia in this area) along with the anterior flap; the posterior flap may contain some muscle at its base. Division of the muscles is completed at the level of bone section. The posterior tibial vessels and nerve are encountered between the soleus and tibialis posterior in or near the midline. The knife is introduced between the bones, and the interosseous membrane along with any remaining muscle fibres is divided. The anterior tibial vessels and nerve and the peroneal vessels lie on opposite sides of the membrane, the latter being close to the fibula. Vessels and nerves are dealt with in the usual manner.

The fibula is divided first—a little higher than the tibia, so that its end will not press on the skin; it is an additional advantage if the saw cut is made obliquely. The tibial stump is bevelled anteriorly, also to avoid pressure on the skin by the bone edge (see Fig. 8.46); this is conveniently done before the main saw cut. The posterior muscles are sutured across the bone end to the periosteum that has been raised with the anterior flap. If haemostasis is assured and dead space avoided, drainage is probably unnecessary but does no harm, provided that the drain is removed within 48 hours.

In patients where less than 14 cm of tibia can be preserved, flaps should be cut in any manner which will entail least sacrifice of bone. Removal of the fibula in these patients may allow the use of flaps which would otherwise be too small.

Amputation with a periosteal bridge
Whatever form of amputation is used at the below knee

level, myoplasty (suture of the opposing muscle groups over the end of the tibia) should be used. Many surgeons prefer a slightly more complex procedure in those patients not affected by vascular disease. The operation is designed to fashion a secure myoplasty, and also fashion a periosteal bridge between the tibia and the fibula which will ultimately form a bony bar between the two bones (see Fig. 8.10). The technique described here is derived from descriptions by Loon (1962), Ertl (1949) and Mondray (1952), and has been recommended by Murdoch (1968).

Anterolateral and posteromedial vertical incisions are made on the leg from a point about 2.5 cm above the proposed level of bone section. These incisions are taken distally so as to allow 8 to 10 cm of the tibia to be exposed beyond the proposed level of section. The incisions are then joined circularly around the leg. The anteromedial and posterolateral skin flaps formed in this way are dissected proximally from the deep fascia. The anterior group of muscles including the extensors and the peroneals are now divided transversely at the same level as the distal skin incision. The entire group of muscles is raised from its bed on the tibia and the fibula, leaving periosteum undamaged. The posterior group of muscles is dealt with in the same way being raised from the posterior aspect of the tibia and fibula, once again leaving periosteum and interosseus membrane undamaged.

The fibula is divided at the level of proposed tibial

section and is removed with the interosseous membrane. Two osteoperiosteal flaps are now raised from the intact tibia, one on its medial aspect and one on its lateral aspect. Periosteum is raised with an osteotome and small flakes of cortical bone are also lifted from the tibia. When both osteoperiosteal flaps are completed to the level of proposed tibial section, the tibia is divided and prepared. The lateral osteoperiosteal flap is now sutured to the deep surface of the fibula and the medial tibial osteoperiosteal flap is drawn across the divided end of the tibia and is sutured to the lateral side of the fibula, thus creating a bridge between the two bones (see Fig. 8.11).

The major vessels are isolated and ligatured, and the posterior tibial nerve is divided and allowed to retract. The muscle groups are sutured under light tension over the tibia and fibula after suitable tailoring. Usually most of the soleus and deep posterior muscles must be removed. It is necessary to secure both groups of muscles by anchoring sutures to the periosteum of the tibia at the base of the osteoperiosteal bridge to prevent lateral dislocation of the muscle groups.

The skin flaps are now tailored and sutured over a Redivac drain.

Below knee amputation is vascular disease (Figs. 8.44–8.47)
Below knee amputation in the presence of vascular disease is undertaken normally without a tourniquet. The

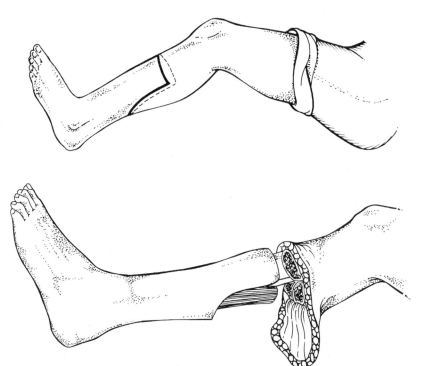

Fig. 8.44

Fig. 8.45

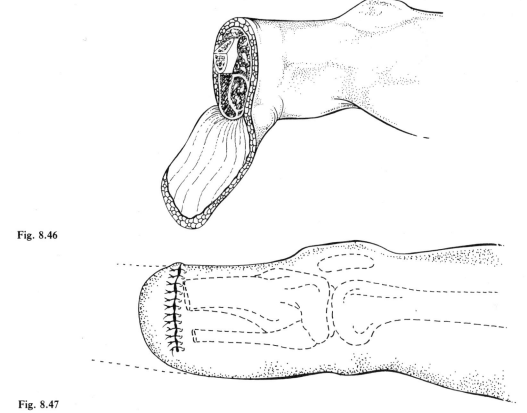

Fig. 8.46

Fig. 8.47

Figs. 8.44–8.47 Below knee amputation using a long posterior flap

below knee stump should not be shorter than 8 cm but is frequently cut slightly shorter than when the tissues are otherwise healthy. A short anterior flap is marked out and will cross the leg transversely no more than 1 cm distal to the proposed site of tibial section. A long and somewhat square posterior flap is marked out and will be almost 1½ times the diameter of the leg in length, or approximately 12 cm. The anterior or transverse incision is made through skin and deep fascia and divides the anterolateral group of muscles transversely. The tibia is exposed on its subcutaneous and lateral surfaces. The short anterior flap fashioned in this way is raised from the tibia proximally for approximately 1 cm. The antero-lateral muscles are also raised from the interosseous membrane and the fibula. The anterior tibial vessels are ligatured and the nerve is divided and allowed to retract. The tibia is now divided, most conveniently with a Gigli saw. The peroneal muscles and musculocutaneous nerve are divided over the fibula which is sectioned with large bone cutters or a Gigli saw, 0.5 cm proximal to the site of tibial section.

Attention is now turned to the posterior flap. Skin is incised and the posterior muscle groups are divided

obliquely from the tibia to the skin incision. This is conveniently done using an amputation knife. The posterior tibial nerve is divided and allowed to retract and the posterior tibial vessels are divided and ligatured.

The posterior mass of muscles including the gastroc-nemius, the soleus and the deep posterior muscles should be tailored carefully so that the posterior flap is not too bulky. Virtually all of the deep posterior muscles will require to be removed and much of the soleus will also be removed. The gastrocnemius is tapered to the tip of the flap. Bone ends are prepared in the usual way and carefully rounded off. The wound is closed, sutur-ing the posterior muscles to the periosteum overlying the tibia and to the deep fascia overlying the anterior group of muscles. The skin is closed over a suction drain.

Postoperative management after below knee amputation
Whatever technique of below knee amputation is used it is probably wise to apply a padded wool and gauze dressing which is encased in plaster of Paris to the midthigh level. A window may be cut over the patella for inspection (Fig. 8.48). The immediate postoperative

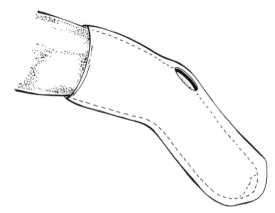

Fig. 8.48 Plaster of Paris dressing after below knee amputation. A wool and gauze dressing is applied to the stump before the plaster is wrapped. A window is cut over the patella to allow inspection

fitting of a prosthetic extension is popular with some surgeons but is not widely used.

AMPUTATION THROUGH THE LEG IN THE UPPER THIRD

It has already been stated that, in patients to whom modern artificial limbs are available, this is not a good amputation, and that if at least 8 cm of tibia cannot be conserved, it may be preferable to amputate at or above the knee.

Rarely however and in communities in which modern artificial limbs are not available this can prove to be an excellent amputation as it adapts to the simplest type of artificial limb: the historical 'peg-leg'. On this the patient *kneels*, and the weight is borne, therefore, on a surface which is well accustomed to pressure. With such an appliance a 5 cm stump of tibia is ideal, and a longer stump is only an encumbrance (Fig. 8.49). Flaps should be fashioned so that the scar does not lie on the kneeling surface. It should be emphasized, however, that this amputation is rarely used now.

DISARTICULATION AT THE KNEE JOINT

Through knee amputation provides a stump with some inherent advantages. The femoral condyles are expanded and allow for satisfactory suspension of an artificial limb. There is a large end bearing surface which is extremely comfortable within the socket of an artificial limb. There are however certain disadvantages: the stump is long and it is difficult to level the knee centre of a prosthetic extension with that of the natural knee of the normal leg. The knee therefore looks ugly. The

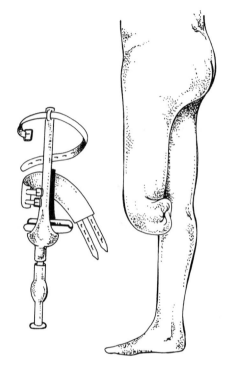

Fig. 8.49 The 'peg-leg' amputation. Seldom used now

amputation is very suitable for young and active men but tends to be less popular in young women with unilateral loss of a leg. It has been recommended for use in vascular disease but is no substitute for below the knee amputation when this is possible. Some patients who require through knee amputation in ischaemic disease develop discomfort over the lateral femoral condyle because of ischaemic changes in the skin at that site. For this reason it is not an amputation that can be wholeheartedly recommended in vascular disease and the author's preference is for above knee amputation when there are significant ischaemic changes in the leg, when the below knee level is not likely to succeed. Through knee amputation is always to be preferred to above knee amputation in the child as it preserves the distal growing epiphysis of the femur.

Technique
The operation is carried out with the patient lying on his face. Unequal anterior and posterior flaps may be used or medial and lateral flaps as described by Smith in 1852. If a long anterior flap is used this will extend to a level 2.5 cm below the tibial tubercle and is completed after flexing the knee. The shorter posterior flap should be about half the length of the anterior flap. Equal anterior and posterior flaps, or a circular incision are infrequently used. When medial and lateral flaps are used, the lateral flap is marked out from 2.5 cm below

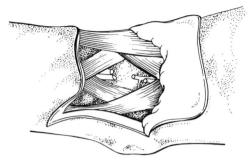

Fig. 8.50 Posterior approach to the knee in disarticulation

the tip of the patella vertically downwards to the upper border of the tibial tubercle and then curves laterally to the midline of the posterior popliteal crease at the back 2.5 cm above the joint line. The lateral flap should extend to at least 2.5 cm beneath the upper border of the tibial tubercle and should be approximately half of the AP diameter of the leg in length. The medial flap should be approximately 4 cm longer than the outer flap in order to provide ample skin over the stump. Once the skin flaps have been prepared the popliteal fossa is opened and its contents defined. The popliteal vessels are divided between ligatures, below any branches that might supply the flaps (Fig. 8.50). The popliteal nerves are sectioned cleanly at the upper limit of the fossa. All muscles bounding the fossa, together with the posterior capsule lining its floor, are divided and the joint cavity is laid open. The knee is now flexed to a right angle, the capsule of the knee joint is exposed and the ligamentum patellae is divided at the front, and is turned upwards. The capsule of the knee joint is divided, the menisci removed and the cruciate ligaments are also divided. The patella is left in situ and the ligamentum patellae is sutured to the cruciate ligaments and the remains of the posterior capsule of the joint. The skin flaps are closed after trimming and a suction drain is left in the knee joint. The scar will lie either posteriorly when a long anterior flap is used or in the intercondylar area when medial and lateral flaps are used.

After through knee amputation there is frequently a synovial discharge from the wound for some days, but this resolves spontaneously.

AMPUTATION THROUGH THE THIGH

Anatomy

Muscles

The anterolateral group consists of sartorius and quadriceps femoris. Sartorius runs obliquely down the thigh from lateral to medial side. The quadriceps is formed by rectus femoris and the three vasti, which combine to form the patellar tendon. The vasti clothe the shaft of the femur on its lateral, anterior and medial surfaces.

The medial group consists of gracilis and the three adductors. Gracilis runs down superficially. Adductor magnus, by far the bulkiest muscle of the group, extends down as far as the adductor tubercle. Adductors longus and brevis have high insertions into the femur, and are encountered only in amputations above the middle of the bone.

Posterior group ('hamstrings') are biceps, semi-tendinosus and semi-membranosus. Biceps is inserted into the head of the fibula. The other two muscles both pass to the medial side of the upper end of the tibia.

Vessels

The femoral artery lies along the upper two-thirds of a line drawn from the midinguinal point to the adductor tubercle (when the thigh is slightly flexed, abducted and rotated laterally). In the upper third of the thigh the artery is medial to sartorius; in the subsartorial canal in the middle third, it is posterolateral. At the junctions of middle and lower thirds it passes through the opening in adductor magnus to become the *popliteal artery*, which is closely applied to the femur. *The femoral vein* in its lower part is posterior or posteromedial to its artery; in its upper part it is medial. *The profunda vessels* lie deeply on the anterior surface of adductor magnus. *The long saphenous vein* ascends in the superficial fascia on the medial side.

Nerves

The femoral nerve breaks up into branches immediately below the inguinal ligament; the only one requiring to be recognized in an amputation is the saphenous nerve, which accompanies the femoral artery as far as the opening in adductor magnus.

The sciatic nerve divides at a varying level in the thigh into *medial* and *lateral popliteal nerves*; these nerves lie on the posterior surface of adductor magnus, the lateral popliteal nerve passing under cover of biceps.

Objectives of amputation

The patient with amputation through the lower or middle-third of the thigh is fitted with an artificial limb which is usually in total contact with the stump and which will allow at least some weight to be taken by the ischial tuberosity against the upper and posterior rim of the socket. The femoral stump acts as a lever and moves the artificial limb. Its ideal length is 25–30 cm as measured from the tip of the trochanter or some 70% the length of the femur. The bone should be divided 8–10 cm above the knee joint. When the amputation is at the above knee level in children as much length as possible should be preserved as the distal growing epiphysis of the femur is lost.

The through knee level in children is used if at all possible in order to preserve this epiphysis. When no more than 15 cm of the femur can be preserved in the adult, the thigh tends to slip out of the socket of the artificial limb and is not efficient as a lever. When disease or injury is so severe that no more than 10 cm of the femur can be preserved, disarticulation through the hip joint is probably preferable so that a Canadian No 1 prosthesis may be fitted. A tourniquet may be used during above knee amputation but must be applied on the thigh. It has the advantage of returning to the body blood which could otherwise have been lost with the discarded limb.

When through thigh amputation is used, opposing muscle groups are sutured together over the bone end so that muscle action on the stump remains balanced. Otherwise unopposed flexors of the hip and adductors of the thigh will tend to pull the stump into flexion and adduction.

Amputation through the lower third of the thigh

An appropriate method of amputating at this level is by unequal anteroposterior flaps, the longer flap being placed anteriorly. The extremity of the anterior flap is in the neighbourhood of the proximal border of the pa-

tella; the posterior flap is half the length of the anterior. The quadriceps tendon is divided at the level of the anterior incision, and is raised in the flap (Figs. 8.51 & 8.52). The hamstrings are cut at the level of the posterior incision. The femoral vessels are identified as they pass through the opening in adductor magnus. The medial and lateral popliteal nerves are found on the back of this muscle, the latter under cover of biceps. The lower tendinous fibres of the adductor are divided, and the vessels and nerves are dealt with in the usual way. The femur is sawn transversely, 8–12 cm above its lower end. The quadriceps tendon is turned back over the bone stump, and is sutured to the hamstrings. The flaps are approximated and sutured. Drainage for 48 hours may be advisable as a precautionary measure, but if all bleeding points are ligatured it is not necessary, since the section is made through tendinous muscle, and oozing is minimal.

Myoplasty

Younger and more active patients who do not have vascular disease are probably better served by a technique of myoplasty with myodesis that anchors the vastus lateralis, adductors and hamstrings to the femur by sutures passed through drill holes in the bone. Murdoch

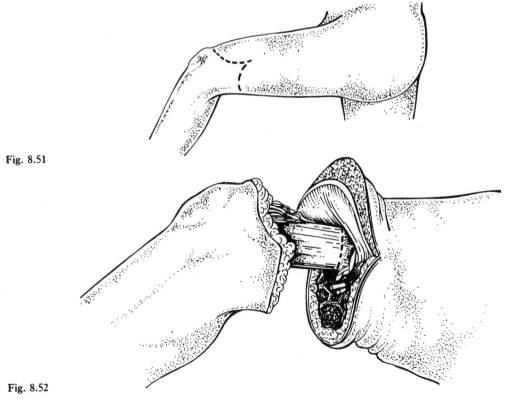

Fig. 8.51

Fig. 8.52

Figs. 8.51 & 8.52 Amputation through the lower third of the thigh

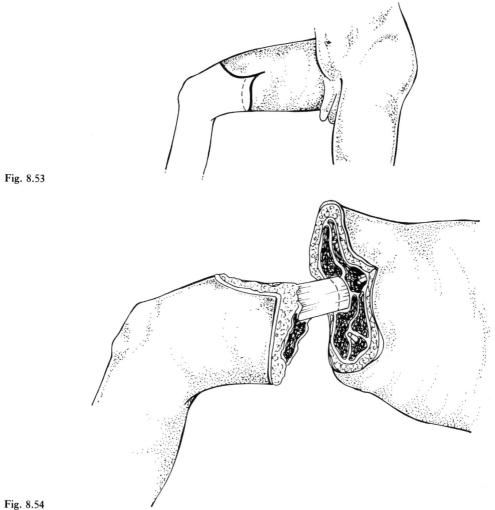

Fig. 8.53

Fig. 8.54

Figs. 8.53 & 8.54 Amputation through the middle third of the thigh

(1968) has recommended that these muscles are divided at the level of bony section, and that the quadriceps expansion is left long, is drawn over the end of the divided bone and sutured to the anchored hamstrings posteriorly (see Fig. 8.4).

Amputation through the middle third (Figs. 8.53 & 8.54)

At this level the flaps may be placed *anterolaterally* and *posteromedially*, to avoid the risk of splitting the femoral artery longitudinally, but their exact position will, of course, depend upon the amount of bone which can be preserved. The flaps are reflected proximally, the knife being made to cut more and more deeply, so that at the level of bone section all muscles have been divided. The femoral and profunda arteries, and the medial and lateral popliteal nerves (or the sciatic nerve) are dealt with in the usual manner. The flaps are trimmed as required, and are sutured. Drainage for 48 hours is essential, owing to the large area of cut muscle from which considerable oozing may occur.

Amputation through the upper third

When more than 10 cm of the femur, measured from the tip of the greater trochanter, cannot be preserved disarticulation through the hip joint is probably appropriate. When 10 cm of the stump or more can be retained the skin flaps will be fashioned as available and muscle will be trimmed as required. It is usually possible to provide a patient with a short stump of this nature with some form of suitable artificial limb.

Supracondylar amputations

Supracondylar amputations are mentioned simply to dismiss them as being of little value to the patient. There is little purpose in performing the Gritti-Stokes amputation in which the patella is anchored to the divided femur after its articular surface has been removed. This procedure risks non-union between the patella and the femur.

Amputation through the distal femur does not allow the prosthetist enough room to place a prosthetic knee device beneath the socket is such a way that the prosthetic knee centre will level with that of the remaining normal knee. It is suggested therefore that these amputations should no longer be used.

AMPUTATION AT THE HIP

Anatomy

Muscles related to the hip joint
On all sides the joint is covered with muscle which is partly fused with the capsule. *Anteriorly* there are rectus femoris, iliopsoas and pectineus, in that order from lateral to medial side; more remote anterior relations are sartorius and tensor fasciae latae. *Posteriorly* lie piriformis, obturator internus (with the gemelli) and quadratus femoris; covering these is gluteus maximus. *Inferiorly*—obturator externus.

Vessels and nerves
The femoral artery enters the thigh behind the mid-inguinal point, lying on the psoas muscle. *The femoral vein* is on its medial side, and the *femoral nerve* lies laterally. The *sciatic nerve* lies on the posterior surface of obturator internus and quadratus femoris, under cover of gluteus maximus.

When more than 10 cm of the femur, measured from the tip of the greater trochanter, cannot be preserved, disarticulation through the hip joint is the amputation of choice and allows the patient to be fitted with the Canadian No 1 prosthesis (Fig. 8.55). This has a large socket which encloses the amputation stump and encircles the patient at his waist. It is a comfortable socket which allows the patient remarkably good function. Disarticulation is usually required after certain injuries or in some patients with sarcoma involving the upper part of the femur.

Disarticulation at the hip joint
Two classical methods have been described: the method of the anterior racquet, and that of the single posterior flap. The second method is to be preferred from the point of view of limb fitting, as it yields a firmer and more compact stump, but the choice will necessarily depend upon the conditions present. The incisions for the two methods are shown in Figure 8.56. The handle of

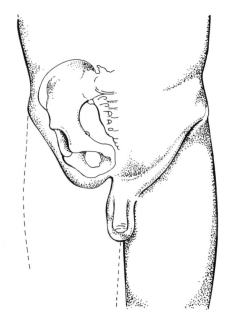

Fig. 8.55 Disarticulation of the hip joint. The proximal femur should be removed entirely

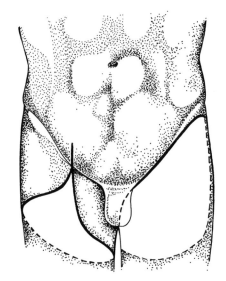

Fig. 8.56 Incisions that may be used for amputation at the hip

the racquet is placed in the line of the femoral vessels, and the medial flap is the longer, so that the scar will fall away from the perineum. In the alternative method the original length of the single posterior flap should be $1\frac{1}{2}$ times the anteroposterior diameter of the limb at the level of the hip joint; the anterior part of the incision is 2.5 cm below and parallel to the inguinal ligament. In each method the first part of the operation consists in exposure and ligation of the femoral vessels. The anterior muscles are divided in the line of the incision, and the joint is opened from the front. The adductors, the hamstrings and gluteus maximus are cut so that portions of them remain in the flaps. The sciatic nerve is found lying deep to gluteus maximus, and is cut short. Disarticulation is completed by division of the capsule and of the remaining short muscles which are inserted into the trochanteric area. The flaps and muscle stumps are trimmed as required to prevent flabbiness of the stump. (In the method of the single posterior flap, all muscles are cut close to the pelvis, with the exception of those required to give reasonable bulk to the flap.)

INTER-INNOMINO-ABDOMINAL AMPUTATION

This operation may be undertaken for the removal of malignant growths of the pelvic bones or upper end of femur, or of the related soft tissues. Gordon-Taylor published in 1959 a personal series of 108 cases, with no deaths in the last 50. He urged that this amputation should always be preceded by a biopsy, since metastases in the pelvic bones from an unsuspected renal carcinoma may present an X-ray picture very suggestive of primary sarcoma.

Technique
An elliptical incision is advocated, its lateral part overlying the iliac crest and its medial part crossing the medial side of the limb a little below the perineum, but this may be varied according to the situation and extent of the tumour. The abdominal muscles attached to the iliac crest are divided close to the bone, and the peritoneum is stripped medially. The common iliac vessels are ligatured in continuity. The inguinal ligament is divided at each end; the conjoined tendon and rectus muscle are severed close to the pubis, and the spermatic cord is displaced medially. The pubic bone is cleared on its anterior and posterior surfaces, and the symphysis is divided with a strong knife or with a chisel. The posterior part of the ilium is cleared, the greater sciatic notch is identified, and with the aid of curved forceps of Gigli saw is passed through its apex. The ilium is then divided upwards and outwards towards the back of the iliac crest.

The innominate bone, together with the lower limb, can now be drawn away to expose the lumbosacral trunk, and the first and second sacral and obturator nerves; these are injected with local anaesthetic and are divided. The external iliac, obturator, gluteal and pudendal vessels are divided, but should be ligatured first, since, although the common iliac vessels have already been tied, fairly brisk bleeding may still occur. Separation of the hindquarter is completed by the division of psoas, piriformis and levator ani, and by the detachment of ischiocavernosus and the crus penis from the ischiopubic ramus. The stumps of muscles are sutured together to give as much support as possible to the peritoneum.

Recently there have been minor modifications to Gordon-Taylor's technique. Sir Gordon-Taylor himself later replaced ligature of the common iliac artery by individual ligations of the external iliac artery, and internal iliac artery beyond the origin of the superior gluteal vessel. This safeguards the blood supply to the large posterior flap.

REFERENCES

Burgess E M, Matsen F A 1981 Determining amputation levels in peripheral vascular disease. Journal of Bone and Joint Surgery 63A: 1493

Dederich R 1963 Plastic treatment of the muscles and bone in amputation surgery. Journal of Bone and Joint Surgery 45B: 60

Ertl J 1949 Amputations stumpf. Chirurgie 20: 218

Flint M, Sweetnam R 1960 Amputation of all toes. Journal of Bone and Joint Surgery 42B: 90

Ghormley R K 1947 Amputation in occlusion vascular disease in peripheral vascular disease. W H Saunders & Co., Philadelphia

Green R M, Rob C G 1985 Amputation of all the toes. In: Dudley H, Carter D C eds. Rob and Smith's Operative Surgery 4th edn. Butterworths, London, p 402

Hey W 1810 Practical observations in surgery, 2nd edn. Cader and Davies, London

Lisfranc J 1815 Nouvelle méthode operation pour l'amputation patient du pied dans son articulation tarso metatarsiennei. Gabon, Paris

Loon H E 1962 Below knee osteomyoplasty. Artificial Limbs 6(2): 86

Mathur B P, Nardang I C, Piplani C L, Majid M A 1981 Rehabilitation of the bilateral elbow amputee by the Krukenberg procedure. The Journal of the International Society for Prosthetics and Orthotics Vol. 5: No. 3

Mondray F 1952 Der muskepkrafige oberations. Unfterschenketstumpf. Chirurgie 23: 517

Mooney V, Harvey J P, McBride E, Snelson R 1971 Comparison of postoperative stump management: plaster vs. soft dressings. Journal of Bone and Joint Surgery 53A: 241

Murdoch G 1968 Myoplastic techniques. Bulletin of Prosthetic Research 10–9: 4

Murdoch G (ed) 1970 Prosthetic and orthotic practice. Arnold, London, p 141

Pederson H E, Day A J 1954 The transmetatarsal amputation in peripheral vascular disease. Journal of Bone and Joint Surgery 36A: 119

Peizer E, Wright D W, Mason C 1969 Human locomotion. Bulletin Prosthetic Research 10: 12

Redhead R G, Snowdon C 1978 A new approach to the management of wounds of the extremities—controlled environment treatment and its derivatives. Prosthetic and Orthotic International 2: 148

Srinavasan J 1973 Syme's amputation in insensitive feet. Journal of Bone and Joint Surgery 55A: 558
Swanson A B 1964 The Krukenberg procedure in the juvenile amputee. Journal of Bone and Joint Surgery 46A: 1540
Wagner F W Jr 1977 Amputations of the foot and ankle: lumbar status. Clinical Orthopaedics 122: 62
Warren R, Kilm R B 1968 A survey of lower extremity amputations for arterial insufficiency. J and A Churchill Ltd., London

9

Operations on the scalp, skull and brain

E. R. HITCHCOCK & A. G. D. MARAN

OPERATIONS ON THE SCALP

Anatomy
The various layers of the scalp are shown diagramatically in Figure 9.1.

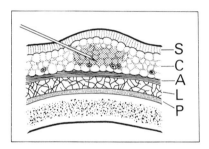

Fig. 9.1 Drawing to show the layers of the scalp and the depth at which local anaesthetic should be injected

Skin is thick and dense, and contains many sebaceous glands.

Connective tissue binds down the skin to the galea aponeurotica, so that these three layers of the scalp move as one. It consists of a dense network of fibrous tissue containing only small lobules of fat, and forms the main thickness of the scalp; within it lie the vessels and nerves.

Aponeurosis. The *galea aponeurotica* is a thin but dense aponeurosis, into which are inserted the frontal and occipital muscles. Its lateral margins blend with the strong temporal fascia.

Loose areolar tissue occupies the space between the galea and the pericranium. This space is limited by the origins of the frontal and occipital muscles, and on each side by the attachment of the galea to the temporal fascia. It is traversed by emissary veins which connect the dural sinuses with veins of the scalp. It constitutes the 'dangerous layer' of the scalp, since within this space blood or pus may collect, and may spread over the entire dome of the skull. Infection within the space may extend via the emissary veins to the dural sinuses.

Pericranium may be regarded as the periosteum on the external surface of the skull. It is continuous with the outer layer of the dura at the foramen magnum, and is attached to it at the sutures. Unlike periosteum elsewhere, it is easily stripped off the bone, and has little share in providing its blood supply.

Local anaesthesia in the scalp
Lignocaine 2% is commonly used with adrenaline 1:200 000. For injections of amounts greater than 20 ml it is usual to dilute the adrenalin to 1:400 000 but lignocaine without adrenalin can be used. Approximately 10 ml of fluid should be injected for each 3 cm of incision. It is important to avoid subgaleal injections because the nerves lie in the connective tissue layer into which the anaesthetic solution should be injected. Because the layer is dense injection into it requires considerable pressure. If there is little resistance it implies that the solution is diffusing into the subaponeurotic space and satisfactory anaesthesia will not be obtained.

Arrest of haemorrhage in the scalp
Whenever possible operative incisions should be made vertically in line with the main vessels. When long incisions are required they should be made in short sections whilst the cut edges are compressed against the skull by the assistant's finger tips (Fig. 9.2). Before the pressure is relaxed curved artery forceps are applied to the cut edge of the galea at 1 cm intervals and then pulled back so that the galea is drawn over the cut surface, stretching and occluding the bleeding vessels. A more efficient method is by the application of Raney clamps over skin and galea. These methods are necessary because the scalp vessels are enmeshed in the fibrofatty layer and cannot be picked up· with forceps in the customary manner.

Wounds of the scalp
The smallest scalp wound is potentially serious because infection may result in a troublesome and prolonged cellulitis of the scalp. It is particularly dangerous if the wound overlies a depressed fracture, below which the

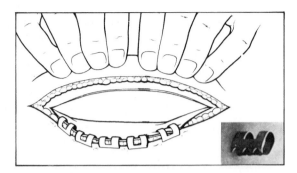

Fig. 9.2 Method of arresting haemorrhage in an operative incision in the scalp—first by pressure with the assistant's finger tips, and later by drawing the cut edge of the aponeurosis over the wound margins. Inset shows a Raney clip used in neurosurgical practice

dura may be torn, because then there is the risk of the development of a cerebral abscess. The extent and severity of the wound is determined by careful examination and by skull radiographs. This preliminary procedure may suggest that, after simple first-aid treatment, the patient should be transferred to a neurosurgical centre.

Shaving of the hair. In simple scalp wounds without gross contamination it is usually sufficient to shave the hair for a distance of 5 cm around the wound. Before doing so the selected area should be cut as short as possible with scissors and then thoroughly washed with soap and water. A safety razor has advantages over a 'cut-throat' since a supply of new blades can be made readily available although the 'cut-throat' razor does not clog so readily.

Débridement. In simple cases débridement (as contrasted with complete excision of the wound) is adequate and where necessary a local anaesthetic is infiltrated *through clean undamaged skin* in order to avoid the spread of infection. Under a good light the scalp edges are retracted and the wound is carefully examined, bleeding being temporarily arrested by gauze packing and scalp compression. Tags of devitalized tissue (skin, galea or pericranium) and any foreign material are removed and the wound is thoroughly washed out with saline. If the wound is grossly contaminated antibiotic solution can be applied locally.

Excision of the wound is essential when gross contamination is present, or if an underlying fracture has been detected. Local or general anaesthesia will be required depending on the extent of the damage and the age of the patient and a large area of the surrounding scalp (the whole scalp in large wounds) should be shaved. The wound edges and all devitalized tissue are meticulously excised but excision should be limited to only a few millimetres since there is a considerable risk of producing

a scalp defect which will require special procedures to close.

Methods of suturing the scalp
In simple scalp wounds, where excision has not been necessary, the cut edges are brought together loosely but accurately with a minimum number of interrupted sutures. A two layer closure should always be done in wounds more than 3 or 4 cm in length (Fig. 9.3).

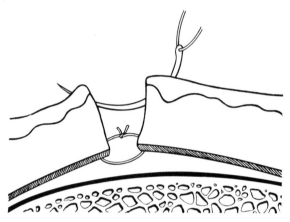

Fig. 9.3 Scalp suture in two layers—the deeper suture has not yet been tightened

Operative incisions and traumatic wounds *after excision* should always be repaired in two layers. First, the galea is approximated by interrupted sutures of fine silk, or preferably absorbable material, placed about 1 cm apart which take the main strain of the suture line and ensures sound healing. The skin edges are then brought accurately together by a further layer of interrupted sutures. Rarely bleeding from a scalp vessel continues after wound suture but can be controlled by pressure or additional skin sutures. Very large lacerations, especially if there are flaps permitting collections of blood, should whenever possible be drained by suction for 24 hours but if this is not available it is safer to leave the wound undrained.

Repair of defects. Every effort should be made to bring the scalp edges together. Because of the excellent blood supply, some wound tension is permissible although healing is then very dependent upon complete absence of infection and, despite the additional loss of tissue, careful débridement and wound excision should be performed. By undercutting, the scalp edges can usually be approximated by one of the plastic procedures illustrated (Figs. 9.4 & 9.5) a two layer closure always being performed. These are not minor procedures, however, and should not be attempted by the inexperienced.

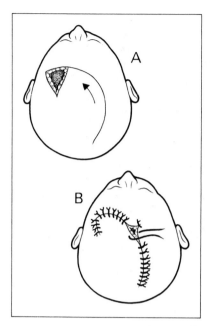

Fig. 9.4 Repair of scalp defect by a single rotational flap

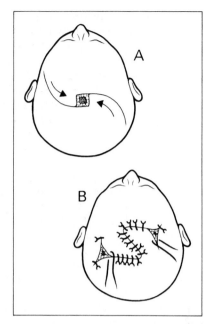

Fig. 9.5 Repair of scalp defect by double rotational flaps

OPEN WOUNDS OF THE SKULL AND BRAIN

Transfer to a neurosurgical centre

There is no reason why patients requiring neurosurgical treatment should not be transferred to a specialist hospital equipped for neurosurgical work but before considering this it is very important to ensure that there are no other injuries such as rupture of the abdominal viscera which may require treatment in situ. Occasionally a neurosurgical team will travel to the hospital in such cases but in general the need for the neurosurgical team to be available for the reception of casualties from a wide area implies that the neurosurgeon is reluctant to move from his base for a single case. Doubts as to the best procedure can usually be resolved by telephone consultation with the neurosurgical centre.

Whenever possible, skull X–rays should be carried out on the patient's admission to hospital since these may reveal an unsuspected fracture or one more extensive than first diagnosed, thus altering the entire plan of treatment. Patients with head injuries, however, are very often extremely restless and X–rays of good quality cannot be obtained. In these situations it is often better to defer further radiographs until the patient's condition has stablised or simply to proceed as a matter of urgency in dealing with the fractures already shown. If the scalp wound is found in association with an underlying skull or brain injury and when transfer to a neurosurgical centre has been decided upon, the initial treatment should be confined to simple first-aid measures. The scalp should not be shaved for fear of introducing further infection and the wound should not be disturbed or probed. Gauze dressing with crepe bandage should be applied although if there is brisk bleeding from the scalp it is permissible to control this with loose sutures.

A general surgeon is unwise to operate on any scalp wound until he has excluded a fracture by radiography. 'Probing' the wound by finger or instrument to detect fractures is unreliable and quite unacceptable. Nevertheless there is an undeniable need for the general surgeon to be able to deal with head injured patients for whom it may be impossible in the circumstances which exist to obtain more expert care. Most of the surgery of head injuries is not beyond the scope of one well grounded in general surgery.

Treatment of a large scalp wound

To reduce the risks of infection and facilitate the operation, the entire scalp should be shaved. A local anaesthetic is usually quite satisfactory, the solution being injected into the scalp a few centimetres from the wound margin on each side. This enables all operative procedures to be carried out painlessly since the skull and brain are insensitive and the dura contains few nerves. In a restless and unco-operative patient and with extensive scalp laceration a general anaesthetic is recommended. It has the additional advantage that a clear airway is assured and the anaesthetist becomes a valuable member of the team keeping constant watch on the patient's respiratory state, attending to resuscitive measures. A meticulous excision of the wound is performed but wide removal of healthy tissue should be avoided so as to leave as little denuded skull as possible. When the wound is a small one it is frequently necessary to obtain better access—either for the purpose of thorough excision or in order to deal effectively with an underlying fracture. In the latter case general anaesthesia is preferable to procedures under local anaesthetic. The wound may be enlarged by extending the extremities into an 's' shaped wound. Alternatively a small laceration can be excised and sutured and then a '∩' shaped flap of scalp (which includes the sutured wound) is cut and reflected, haemorrhage being controlled by the methods described earlier.

Treatment of underlying fractures

If the fracture is a clean linear one, without displacement, then no special treatment is required and the scalp wound, after excision, is carefully sutured. When a fracture is comminuted all small bone fragments should be removed but larger fragments, especially in cosmetic areas, can be washed in antibiotic solution and replaced.

Depressed fractures

Having exposed the whole extent of the depression, a small burr hole is made through undamaged bone at the periphery of the depression through which an elevator is introduced and used as a lever to raise the depressed fragments (Fig. 9.6). Only the most minor depressions

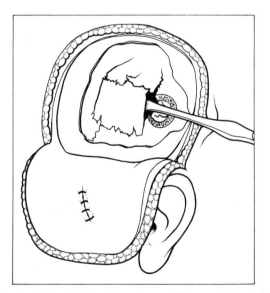

Fig. 9.6 Method of elevating a depressed fracture of the skull through an opening made with burr or trephine in undamaged bone adjoining the defect. In compound fractures all bone fragments which are contaminated should be removed

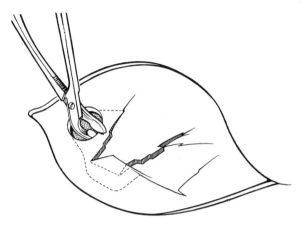

Fig. 9.7 Rongeur of depressed and comminuted fragment

can be dealt with in this way and it may be safer for the inexperienced operator to refer this procedure to a neurosurgical centre as he may do more harm than good. Grossly depressed and comminuted fragments should not be dealt with in this way but the bone edges rongeured away to allow the loose fragments to be carefully removed (Fig. 9.7). Fragments in the region of a venous sinus should not be elevated by a general surgeon. Any resultant defect in the skull is unlikely to cause symptoms but if necessary can easily be repaired at a later date by means of one of the rapidly hardening acrylic plastics.

Treatment of the dura

The dura is often intact in compound fractures and in such cases should never be opened unless from its bulging and plum coloured appearance there is strong reason to suspect a subdural haematoma. When a dural tear is present its whole extent should be exposed by removal of bone as required. Small pieces of felt with attached thread (patties) should be placed beneath the tear to protect the usually swollen underlying brain. Ragged dural edges should be sparingly excised but the tear should not be enlarged unless the underlying brain requires inspection. The dural tear should be carefully sutured with interrupted sutures of fine absorbable material, but if, as is often the case, the dura has retracted, then small tears may be covered with gelfoam and larger defects covered with a transplant of pericranium or fascia lata. If the patient's condition does not permit this a large sheet of gelfoam is applied over the surface of the brain and dural repair left for a later operation. No attempt should be made to close the dura if there is swollen brain.

Arrest of haemorrhage from dural vessels

All dural vessels are best sealed by the coagulating diathermy current (Fig. 9.8), the vessels being grasped with sharp-pointed dissecting forceps which are then

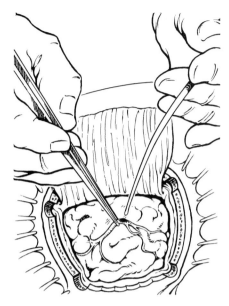

Fig. 9.8 Coagulation of dural vessels

touched with the electrode. This is usually adequate for most vessels and silver clips are rarely necessary. Bleeding from the surface of the dura can be controlled by the application of muscle grafts taken from the temporalis muscle; when hammered or crushed to a thin sheet they adhere firmly to any tissue against which they are pressed. Gelatine haemostatic foam is also effective.

Tearing of dural sinus
Repair is best left to the expert but haemorrhage may be controlled by elevating the patient's head and applying a muscle graft or gelatine foam. Very large tears may be closed by a running silk ligature over which a muscle stamp or gelatine foam is pressed until bleeding ceases. If the tear cannot be repaired then the sinus must be under-run with a ligature or plugged with a muscle graft accepting the very considerable risk that the interruption of major venous drainage from the brain may well result in severe cerebral oedema.

Treatment of brain injury
Penetrating wounds of the brain are usually due to indriven fragments of bone but it is common for these to be embedded at any depth within the brain. Operation is designed to remove all devitalized cerebral tissue, extravasated blood, bone fragments and any accessible foreign bodies; in addition all haemorrhage must be arrested. A complete débridement of this nature is dependent upon adequate exposure and direct vision. It is usually necessary, therefore, to perform a small craniotomy or enlarge the opening of the skull with rongeur forceps. Penetrating wounds of the brain are best dealt with by neurosurgeons.

Removal of damaged brain tissue
Damaged cerebral tissue can be removed by irrigation and suction. A gentle jet of warm saline is directed into the wound from a syringe and weak suction (25–30 cm Hg) through a finebore nozzle (3 mm lumen) is used to remove all devitalized brain matter and blood clot but leaving healthy brain matter alone. Suction is continued until the cavity is surrounded by healthy, undamaged brain tissue during which procedure any indriven bone fragments are discovered and removed with forceps. The utmost gentleness must be observed since any kind of rough handling will lead to destruction of valuable brain tissue or to interference with blood supply. The most meticulous attention must be paid to the arrest of haemorrhage for otherwise a postoperative clot is likely to form and to compress the brain. Bleeding points are controlled by diathermy coagulation.

Gunshot wounds of the brain
The wound of entry is often small and may be overlooked or treated as a simple scalp wound. The inner table is invariably more extensively fractured than the outer table and indrawn bone fragments are usually present. The missile may still be within the brain. Operative treatment is carried out as described above and the wound track in the brain followed and cleared of all damaged tissue. In the case of through-and-through wounds both entrance and exit wounds should be similarly treated. The question of whether a missile or other foreign body embedded in the brain should be removed depends upon its accessibility. When it lies within the track of brain destruction it will naturally be removed as part of the débridement. When it lies very deep in the brain the last portion of its track is often invisible. Attempts to follow and extract it can result only in further damage to healthy brain tissue. A deeply embedded foreign body may cause no symptoms when left in situ provided the area of more gross destruction in the superficial part of its track has received adequate attention. Attempts to remove deeply embedded foreign bodies are best left to neurosurgeons. The treatment described is effective for gunshot wounds due to low velocity missiles but many modern high velocity missiles unfortunately produce considerable brain pulping at a distance from the track.

Fractures involving the paranasal air sinuses.
Frontal fractures or those involving the thin floor of the anterior fossa often extend into the frontal or ethmoidal air sinuses and constitute a potential danger of pneumatocele, meningitis or brain abscess. The diagnosis is made from the radiograph or from the observation of cerebrospinal fluid rhinorrhoea but alternatively the condition may be found during wound exploration. If, during the exploration of an open wound, a fracture is found to extend into an air sinus, most commonly the

frontal, dural tears in the vicinity should be carefully repaired. If there is a large defect in the sinus wall then it is usual to remove the mucous lining on the grounds that the risk of infection is reduced and a muscle graft should be placed in the sinus.

Cerebrospinal fluid rhinorrhoea
Provided adequate antibiotic treatment is continued for several weeks the risk of meningitis or brain abscess is small but if there is a profuse CSF rhinorrhoea or if a pneumatocele develops a dural graft should be applied as soon as the patient's condition permits.

EXTRADURAL AND SUBDURAL HAEMORRHAGE

Extradural haemorrhage is due most commonly to traumatic rupture of the middle meningeal vessels and occasionally tears of the dural veins or sinuses. Subdural haemorrhage may result from rupture of veins passing to the superior longitudinal sinus or the lateral sinuses and also from cerebral laceration. It is unnecessary to know the detailed course of the middle meningeal artery other than to appreciate that it enters the scalp through the foramen spinosum in the temporal fossa and then divides into an anterior and posterior branch embedded in the outer layer of dura.

Extradural or subdural haemorrhage although uncommon are very important closed head injuries since active surgical intervention is necessary and the results of energetic intervention are most gratifying. A massive haemorrhage not only produces local compression of the brain but also dangerous displacements which block cerebrospinal fluid pathways producing a rapid rise in intracranial pressure. Surgery consists of the evacuation of the clot and arrest of bleeding.

Operation is justified on the *suspicion* of extradural or subdural haemorrhage but if practicable the patient should be referred to a neurosurgical centre or if doubt exists advice by telephone should be sought. If, however, such facilities are not available the operation, which is, or can be, a relatively simple one, is well within the scope of a general surgeon and should not be withheld merely because expert aid is not available. The mortality after such operations is high but is rarely due to the operative trauma. Death is frequently attributed to concurrent brain injury but failure of diagnosis or hesitancy to operate in the early stages of clot formation is certainly a factor of equal importance. Exploration through a burr hole in the skull is a simple matter to determine whether a surface haemorrhage has occurred. Performed under local anaesthesia it entails so little risk yet is more than justified, even when negative findings are obtained. If an

extradural or subdural haemorrhage is present simple enlargement of the exploratory opening is often all that is required to provide the access necessary for treatment of the condition.

Diagnosis
Extradural haemorrhage is relatively uncommon, forming about 2% of all head injuries. The classical picture of a latent or 'lucid' interval following the injury, lasting for a few minutes to several hours, is the exception rather than the rule. Where it does occur it is followed by headache, giddiness and drowsiness, deepening into a coma but extradural haemorrhage should always be suspected when after some degree of recovery from the initial concussion the patient's condition deteriorates. As restlessness and drowsiness develop the pulse rate falls and blood pressure rises. Minor pupillary inequalities are not generally helpful and it is the *trend* of the changes in the signs which is so important in the diagnosis. A fixed, dilated pupil almost invariably means raised intracranial pressure—usually on the same side, although it can be due to cerebral oedema or intracerebral haematoma. A late sign of grave prognostic import, it usually indicates downward displacement of the midbrain and compression of the cerebral peduncle on the opposite side against the tentorial rim, with stretching of the third nerve.

Subdural haemorrhage is more common than extradural haemorrhage and because it is usually associated with major brain injury, a true 'lucid interval' is rare and the clinical picture is therefore much less characteristic. In the *acute* form deterioration in consciousness may appear within a few hours of injury but in the *subacute* form several days may elapse before deterioration is evident. A *chronic* form may not manifest itself for several weeks or months. *Acute* subdural haematomas are usually accompaniments of severe brain laceration and oedema, and are rarely compressive.

Localising signs
These are of great assistance in diagnosis especially in extradural haemorrhage where the bleeding is relatively confined. As the clot increases in size there is weakness of the opposite side of the body which may become bilateral, and unilateral or bilateral spasticity. Decortication or decerebration are signs of further deterioration and appear first on the side of the injury. A deterioration in the conscious level invariably precedes all other signs. Localization of the site of the lesion is obtained by finding ipsilateral pupillary dilatation and contralateral motor signs such as paralysis. Usually the haematoma is on the same side as the pupil which is the more dilated. Radiological evidence of the fracture line crossing the middle meningeal groove is of value both in confirming and in localizing an extradural haemorrhage.

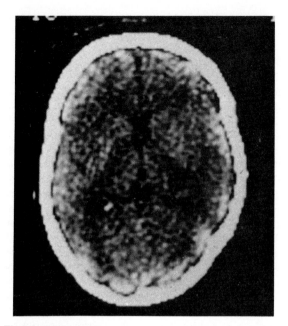

Fig.9.9 CAT scan

Special investigations
Echo-encephalography has been displaced by the use of
computerized axial tomography (Fig. 9.9) but if the
latter is not available (and in general it is restricted to
major centres) an echo-encephalogram may reveal
midline displacement. Computerized axial tomograms,
however, although not essential in the management of
head injuries are extremely valuable in permitting accurate diagnosis and delineation of haemorrhage and
oedema. X–rays are passed through the head as a gener-
ator rotates around it and the rays are detected, stored
and computed to produce images of the skull and brain
in different horizontal planes. Extracerebral haematomas
are demonstrated as high density shadows producing
ventricular distortion. Until this expensive apparatus
becomes generally available the majority of head injured
patients will be evaluated largely on clinical grounds.

Burr hole exploration
Extradural bleeding will usually have occurred below the
external evidence of injury manifested in the form of an
abrasion or bruising or a boggy swelling of the scalp.
Urgent exploration is best performed at the site of the
external injury and it must be recognized that this may
indicate the beginning of a fracture running into the
temporal region. If in doubt the burr hole should be
made in the temporal region, just above the zygoma. If
a fracture is seen on the X–ray to cross an arterial groove
at another site then the burr hole can be made at this
site. If no haematoma is found at the initial exploration
similar exploration should be carried out on the opposite
side at once.

Preparation and position of patient
For an urgent procedure preparation may be minimal but
whenever possible the entire scalp should be shaved since
both sides may require exploration. A special head rest
is not essential and the head can be placed on a soft sand
bag or pillow. The head is elevated and turned to the
opposite side, the surgeon and assistant standing at either
side of the patient's head. Towels are applied to shut off
the operation area (if possible over an overhead table)
leaving an area beneath which the anaesthetist will have
free access to the nose and mouth.

Anaesthesia
Either local or general anaesthesia may be employed.
Endotracheal intubation ensures a good airway and
prevents straining and increase of intracranial pressure.
Light anaesthesia is sufficient if the line of the incision
is infiltrated with local anaesthesia and the anaesthetist
may prefer to control ventilation by giving a muscle relaxant.

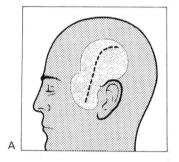

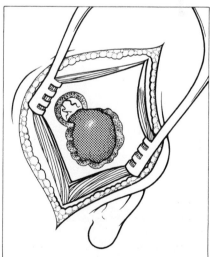

Fig. 9.10 Operation for extradural haemorrhage. (A) shows
area to be infiltrated with local anaesthetic and the incision
employed. (B) the initial opening in the skull is made with a
burr or trephine, and is then enlarged with rongeur forceps to
allow adequate access to the clot

Incision

The incision begins at the lower border of the zygoma halfway between the eyebrow and meatus and runs upwards and slightly backwards for about 5 cm (Fig. 9.10). Haemorrhage is controlled by digital pressure and a self-retaining retractor placed in the superficial part of the wound. The superficial temporal artery is often severed and should be controlled by diathermy coagulation. In the lower part of the wound the temporalis muscle, covered by fascia, is incised and the muscle split down to the bone. A strong self-retaining retractor is placed in the split down to the bone to hold the muscle fibres apart. The burr hole is made immediately above the midpoint of the zygomatic arch, using a perforator on a Hudson's brace (Fig. 9.11). The perforator should be turned rapidly to prevent sudden perforation of the bone and when the inner table is penetrated a characteristic rocking sensation is produced. The perforator should then be replaced with a burr and the hole enlarged. Because the burr tapers and cuts a funnel-shaped hole it is very safe to use but the surgeon should still be careful, especially in the thin bone of the temporal fossa. If an extradural haemorrhage has occurred the clot will now be seen presenting in the burr hole, or alternatively, the dura may be plum coloured and bulging due to the presence of subdural haemorrhage. In either case the burr hole should be enlarged by the rongeur. If the dura appears normal in colour (pinkish white shade) but is tense it is probable that cerebral oedema is present but

if the dura is slack the exploration should be regarded as negative.

Treatment of extradural haematoma

The first essential is to enlarge the wound of access, for not only must the blood clot be removed but, if possible, the site of the bleeding should be identified and secured. The skin incision is extended upwards and backwards and the split in the temporalis muscle also extended. If necessary the temporal fascia is incised transversely along the temporal line and the muscle fibres on each side of the split scraped from their origin. By strong retraction a much wider skull exposure can now be obtained. The burr hole is then enlarged in the direction indicated by the situation of the clot, usually towards the skull base. The clot is evacuated by suction and displacement with a smooth instrument or blunt probe and washed away with a stream of saline. As the clot is removed the ruptured meningeal vessel may come into view but its identification may be difficult on account of continued haemorrhage. A clear field in the depths of the wound can be obtained by irrigating with warm saline but the essential feature is to have good suction. Haemostasis is achieved by diathermy coagulation or the application of a silver clip. If the artery is ruptured at the base of the skull at the foramen spinosum, and diathermy coagulation fails to control the haemorrhage a small plug of cotton wool or bone wax may be inserted.

Frequently the site of the haemorrhage is not visible

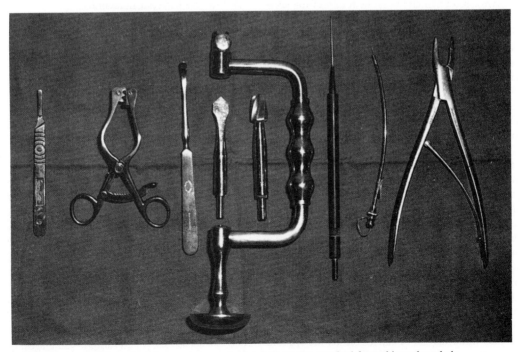

Fig. 9.11 Hudson's brace with skull perforator, burrs and other instruments required for making a burr hole

and it is unnecessary to search for it. The wound should be drained, ideally by vacuum drainage, the end of the drain being placed in the extradural space. If the clot is extensive and passes posteriorly the skin incision may be extended into a ∩-shaped flap and either a formal craniotomy performed or further bone removed by rongeur. Dural haemorrhage may be difficult to control after the vessels have been stripped off from the deep surface of the skull. It is helpful in these circumstances to put small pieces of gelfoam or muscle between the dura and undersurface of the bone and to stitch the dura to the pericranium over the bone edges (Fig. 9.12).

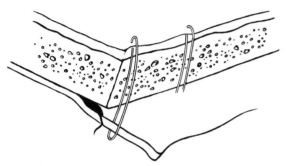

Fig. 9.12 Hitch stitches for control of an extradural blood vessel

Treatment of subdural haemorrhage

Such haemorrhages are usually due to rupture of the cortical veins, most commonly in the region of the lesser wing of the sphenoid, i.e., on the inferior surface of the frontal lobe or around the temporal pole. It may, however, gravitate to other situations such as the parietal region. As soon as subdural haemorrhage is suspected exploration should be carried out by means of burr holes. The first is made in the temporal region, as in the case of exploration for extradural haemorrhage, and the diagnosis is at once confirmed if the dura is dark in colour and bulging. The dura should be carefully incised and the incision extended in a semilunar or cruciate manner, whilst the underlying brain is protected by a retractor or small felt patty. The haematoma is now aspirated as completely as possible by suction, aided by flushing with warm saline. If bleeding continues the burr hole and dural incision can be enlarged in the direction from which the haemorrhage appears to come, so that the bleeding vessel can be located and sealed by diathermy coagulation. If the surgeon is satisfied that all bleeding has been arrested the wound may be closed, but otherwise it should be drained. If no subdural blood is found at the temporal burr hole a second burr hole is made in the frontal region, and if the finding here is also negative a third burr hole may be made in the parietal region. This is a procedure that may require to be repeated on

the opposite side. If on the first exploration the underlying brain is slack then it is unlikely that there is any large increase of intracranial pressure and further explorations are unnecessary. On the other hand if the brain is tight but no subdural blood found, although the commonest cause is cerebral oedema, a search must be made on the opposite side to exclude a subdural haematoma. Subdural haematomas are commonly associated with severe cerebral laceration and haemorrhage and to deal with this a large area of brain must be exposed and devitalized brain tissue and intracerebral clot removed by a combination of irrigation and suction.

The wound is closed by approximating the split temporalis muscle with two or three interrupted sutures and the scalp sutured in two layers.

Cerebral oedema is commonly associated with extra- and subdural haemorrhage. Treatment is by the intravenous administration of hypertonic solutions such as mannitol, which by its osmotic action causes fluid to be withdrawn from the swollen brain into the general circulation. One gram per kilogram body weight is given rapidly and thereafter continued as a 25% solution at the rate of approximately 100 ml per hour. Levels above 300 osmoles per litre of serum osmolality should be avoided.

The response of the brain to steroids is a controversial topic. If they are to be given, the dosage should be high, such as 50 to 100 mg of Dexamethasone, followed by 4 to 8 mg every 3 hours. Ventilation may be necessary to maintain arterial oxygenation to reduce $PaCO_2$ but the value of controlled hyperventilation is questionable, except for these special situations.

SIMPLE DEPRESSED FRACTURES

These fractures are frequently unassociated with brain damage, and in the absence of neurological signs it is often unnecessary and may indeed be dangerous to elevate them. If, however, the fragment is depressed for more than the whole thickness of the skull, or if it is lying end-on, or is obviously spiculated, operation is generally advocated. The depressed area of bone is exposed by turning down a '∩' shaped scalp flap and the fracture is elevated by the method described on p. 200. The dura should not be opened unless it is already torn or there is evidence of underlying injury and unattached bone fragments should not be removed for they will readily consolidate as healing occurs.

Indentation of the skull, without true fracture, may occur in infants. When the depression is sharply incurved, operation is indicated. Through a curved incision a small opening is made at the margin of the depression and a smooth periosteal elevator inserted and used to elevate the depressed area of bone.

OPERATIONS FOR ACUTE MASTOIDITIS

Because of the availability of chemotherapy for the primary condition infection of the tympanic (mastoid) antrum as a complication of acute otitis media is now rarely found in any serious form—at least in the acute stage of the condition. When infection does occur it is usually well controlled by chemotherapy whilst pus tends to track superficially to form a subperiosteal abscess requiring only simple drainage and therefore the risk of intracranial complications is small. The classical operation of Schwartze for drainage is therefore now seldom required. It is sometimes indicated, however, in more chronic stages of otitis media when profuse purulent otorrhoea, pulsating and increasing in amount, together with pyrexia and mastoid tenderness persist after adequate antibiotic treatment or when headache or drowsiness suggest intracranial suppuration. If chemotherapy is not available or is ineffective, operation may be necessary in the acute stage. In established mastoiditis, there is a risk of facial nerve paralysis, labyrinthitis, sigmoid sinus thrombosis, meningitis, otitic hydrocephalus and brain abscess. If any of these occur or threaten to occur, the mastoid must be decompressed.

Mastoidectomy

With the patient's head turned to the side on a sandbag, a postauricular incision is made 2 cm from the post aural crease right on to the bone of the mastoid. It should extend the length of the ear. The periosteum of the mastoid is elevated until the anterior edge of the mastoid is seen and, superiorly, the elevator should demonstrate the superior wall of the external meatus. Imaginary tangents are drawn from these surfaces and they are found to intersect on the mastoid. The triangle bounded by these tangents and the edge of the external meatus is called Macewen's triangle and is the surface marking of the antrum (Fig. 9.13). Entry into the mastoid should be at this point in order to keep the operator clear of the facial nerve and dura. Once the mastoid antrum is found, the rest of the mastoid air cells can be drilled out (or chiselled if no drill is available). The dura is protected by smooth bone as is the sigmoid sinus. The middle fossa dura of the transverse sinus may be exposed in the depth of the cavity and should be approached with great care.

If *extradural infection* is present the exposed dura is thickened and oedematous with granulations and in such cases all the affected bone should be removed until healthy dura is exposed. The lateral sinus should not be opened. The wound is then irrigated with antibiotic solution and the upper part of the wound closed with interrupted sutures. A small thin rubber drain is stitched into the lower part of the wound and pus removed from the external ear into which a small pack is inserted. A dry gauze dressing is applied over the wound which is left undisturbed for 5 days.

If a general surgeon is performing this surgery, it is an emergency situation and the above procedure should suffice. After this the patient should be referred on to an otolaryngologist for specific management of the ear condition. It is probably dangerous for an inexperienced operator to proceed further than merely draining the mastoid abscess. The facial nerve may well be transected and if the dura is inadvertently opened in the presence of infection the resulting complications may be serious.

SPECIAL DIAGNOSTIC PROCEDURES

Cerebral isotope scanning (Fig 9.14)
This is a well established and harmless diagnostic pro-

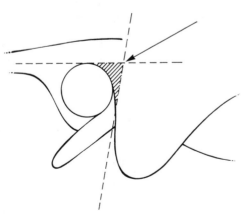

Fig. 9.13 Site for drilling in mastoid infection (Macewen's triangle). Triangle marked by two tangents and margin of auditory meatus

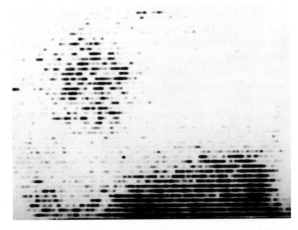

Fig. 9.14 Cerebral isotope scan showing increased uptake in the high posterior parietal region caused by a meningioma

cedure. A short life radioactive isotope is injected intravenously and the radioactive emission from the head measured by a special scanning Geiger counter, which produces a picture of the radioactive densities within the skull. Vascular lesions such as tumours and abscess appear as areas of increased density.

Angiography

Angiography aids in the diagnosis of cerebral tumours and because of the characteristic features of blood supply to different tumours it may indicate the nature of the tumour as well as its site (Fig. 9.15). Its particular application, however, is in the revelation of abnormalities of the cerebral vessels such as aneurysms or angiomata. A number of contrast media are available (*Conray* or *Urographin* are generally used).

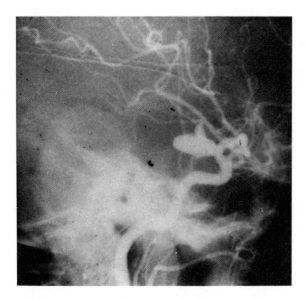

Fig. 9.15 Carotid angiogram showing aneurysm of the intracranial carotid artery

The operation is carried out in the X-ray department, usually under general anaesthesia and the injection is made, in the first instance, on the side believed to be affected. Common carotid injection is the simplest of direct puncture procedures. The patient lies on his back with the neck slightly extended and local anaesthetic is injected, about one finger's breadth above the clavicle, in front of the sternomastoid and behind the carotid. This tends to elevate and steady the artery. An 18 gauge needle is inserted through the carotid and then withdrawn until arterial blood spurts out. A large syringe with a contrast medium is attached to the needle and approximately 8 ml of contrast medium injected rapidly under pressure. An immediate exposure (*arteriogram*) is made followed by a quick change of film and a second

exposure (*phlebogram*) 2 to 3 seconds later. The lateral radiograph is usually taken first and the same procedure followed to obtain an anteroposterior view. No more than 50 ml of contrast medium should be injected for bilateral carotid angiography.

Ventriculography (Fig. 9.16)

This is much less commonly done than previously. The procedure is performed under local anaesthesia and past methods of biparietal burr holes have been superseded by frontal burr holes made immediately in front of the coronal suture in the midpupillary line. In this situation a ventricular cannula is introduced through the burr hole, diametrically, until the frontal horn is penetrated, first on the normal side. Successful entry into the ventricle is shown by the escape of cerebrospinal fluid from the cannula when the stylet is removed. A similar procedure is done on the, supposedly, abnormal side and cerebrospinal fluid is withdrawn 5 to 10 ml at a time and replaced by a slightly smaller quantity of air. It is also possible to perform ventriculography through a single burr hole. Instead of air, water soluble contrast media, such as *Conray*, may be introduced, to give better visualization. The interpretation of ventriculograms depends on abnormalities or inequalities in the size of the ventricles, on displacements and on filling defects.

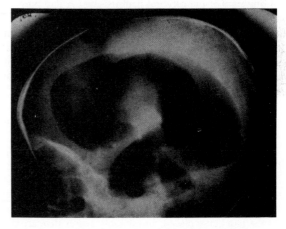

Fig. 9.16 Air ventriculogram showing gross hydrocephalus

Lumbar air encephalography

This is rarely performed but has value in the demonstration of suprasella masses. It is dangerous to perform in patients with increased intracranial pressure.

Computerized axial tomography (Fig. 9.17)

This expensive device has largely replaced ventriculography and to some extent angiography in the case of tumours. It is possible, by injecting intravenous contrast media, to reveal areas of increased vascularity.

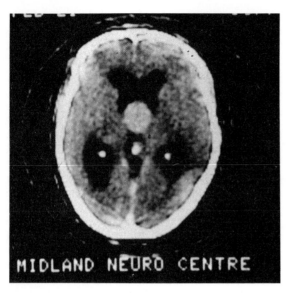

Fig. 9.17 CAT scan showing choroid cyst of the third ventricle

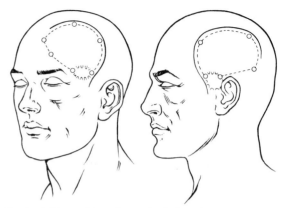

Fig. 9.18 The position of osteoplastic flaps for exposure in the frontoparietal and parietal areas. Dotted lines are shown between burr holes

METHODS OF ACCESS IN BRAIN OPERATIONS

The osteoplastic flap

This method is now universally adopted for the exposure of any part of the cerebral hemispheres. A flap may be made in the frontoparietal, parietal or parieto-occipital regions of the skull, according to the estimated position of the cerebral lesion and must be of sufficient size to give the access which is required. The increasing use of the microscope in neurosurgery has encouraged the use of much smaller exposures than formerly.

The true osteoplastic flap (Fig. 9.18), where the bone flap is cut and turned down with the scalp adherent to it, is rarely, if ever, performed nowadays.

The scalp incision is '∩'-shaped, the base of the flap being sufficiently broad for an adequate blood supply and scalp haemorrhage arrested by the methods described on p. 197. Four or five burr holes are made along the periphery of the exposed skull, the two holes at the base of the flap being placed considerably nearer than are the ends of the scalp incisions so that the narrow base can be rongeured more easily. The hand operated Hudson's brace, used in conjunction with a burr, is used for making the burr holes. The dura is separated from the skull with a curved dissector insinuated through the burr holes. By means of a special guide a Gigli saw is passed between adjacent holes and the intervening bone is divided—with an outward bevel so that the freed portion of skull, when replaced, will not sink below its normal level. Haemorrhage from the diploë of the skull is arrested by rubbing in bone wax, and meningeal haemorrhage by diathermy coagulation. Bleeding from the dural

sinus may be controlled by applying a muscle graft.

Incision of the dura (Fig. 9.19)
It is usual to employ a 'U' shaped incision with its base towards the saggital sinus. If the dura appears tense it is advisable to carry out a ventricular puncture and aspiration of cerebrospinal fluid before opening the dura widely, as otherwise serious herniation of the brain may occur.

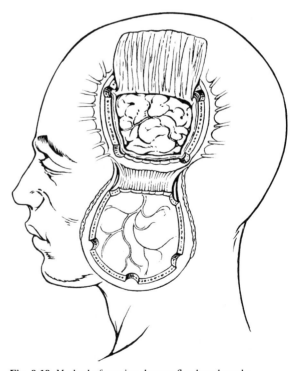

Fig. 9.19 Method of turning down a flap based on the temporalis muscle. The skin flap has been reflected along with the skull flap and the dura opened as a U-shaped flap

Replacement of the flap

At the end of the operation, after suture of the dura, the portion of skull is replaced in position and the scalp repaired in two layers.

Posterior fossa approaches

The operation is done with the patient in the three-quarter prone, or ENT position, the head firmly held in a head holder. The prone position, with the neck flexed, is easier to achieve but great care should be taken to avoid pressure on the abdomen and chest by the interposition of appropriately placed sand bags.

A skin incision (Fig. 9.20) may be made either vertically in the midline or paramedially, extending up the head in a curvilinear fashion if more lateral exposure is required. Self-retaining superficial retractors are inserted and the nuchal muscles separated by cutting diathermy in the midline down to the occipital bone in the arch of the atlas. A larger, deeper, self-retaining retractor is then inserted. A burr hole is made in the occipital bone on each side of the midline and, after separating the dura, the bone is nibbled away with rongeur forceps downwards to include the posterior margin of the foramen magnum, upwards as far as the transverse sinus and laterally to the mastoid process. The arch of the atlas may also be removed. If the dura is tense the ventricles should be punctured and aspirated before it is opened. The occipital sinus runs in the midline and should be divided between ligatures. The sitting-up position, whilst reducing intracranial tension and facilitating exposure, has a very considerable danger of air embolus and with good anaesthesia is no longer necessary.

BRAIN TUMOURS

Brain tumours are either extrinsic, such as meningiomas, acoustic neuromas and pituitary tumours, or intrinsic, such as metastatic tumours and gliomas.

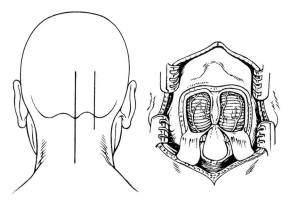

Fig. 9.20 Posterior fossa midline and lateral incision

Meningiomas

Three arise usually in the neighbourhood of dural sinuses, compressing the cerebral cortex and often invading the overlying bone. Meningiomas commonly arise from the falx (parasagittal meningiomas), the sphenoidal ridge and over the convexities. *Parasagittal* meningiomas are exposed by craniotomy extending to or over the midline. For the occasional operator the safest method of removal is to gut the tumour with diathermy loop and then dissect out the shell. If the tumour lies on the convexity the dura can be incised around the margin and removed with the tumour. *Parasagittal* meningiomas are treated similarly but they often invade the sagittal sinus, and again the occasional operator should confine himself to diathermying the involved dura only. *Sphenoidal wing* meningiomas are closely related to the middle cerebral artery and complete removal is difficult.

Acoustic neuromas

These are situated in the cerebellopontine angle on the posterior aspect of the petrous temporal bone. A paramedian posterior fossa craniectomy is performed and the cerebellum on the affected side retracted medially or partially excised to expose the tumour. If possible the tumour is completely removed otherwise it is incised and its contents evacuated.

Pituitary tumours

These compress the optic nerves and distort the carotid. Their successful removal requires meticulous technique and experience. Frontal craniotomy is performed and the frontal lobe elevated to reveal the optic nerve and tumour. An incision is made into the capsule and the contents aspirated or curetted away.

Small or entirely intrasella pituitary tumours are best removed through a transethmoidal or transphenoidal approach. In the transphenoidal route (Fig. 9.21) the upper lip is everted and an incision made in the gingivolabial sulcus. The mucoperiosteum is displaced upwards until the floor of the nose and nasal septum are exposed and the submucous resection of the septum is performed. The resection is carried backwards along the vomer to the roof of the nasopharynx and the anterior wall of the sphenoidal air sinus is removed with punch forceps to expose the sella which is penetrated and the gland removed piecemeal.

Metastatic tumours of the brain

These are often well encapsulated and, if sufficiently large, can be well localized and removed by an incision over them and careful separation around the tumour.

Gliomas

These are infiltrating tumours of the brain without encapsulation. The patient's condition can sometimes be

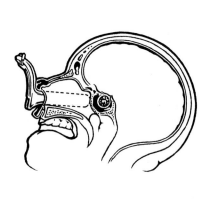

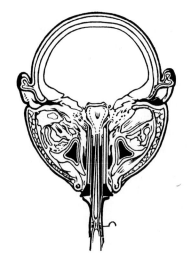

Fig. 9.21 Transphenoidal hypophysectomy

dramatically improved by puncture of a neoplastic cyst or by the partial removal of the tumour by incising the cortex (in an area which is functionally unimportant) and then removing the tumour piecemeal by suction and forceps (the so-called internal decompression).

BRAIN ABSCESS

Brain abscesses occur in association with infections of the frontal or mastoid sinuses. They also occur in the frontal and temporal lobes and in the cerebellum, the latter two in association with middle ear disease. In the early stages of cellulitis antibiotics may prevent progression into a definite abscess cavity. If an abscess forms, however, it constitutes a surgical emergency and drainage should be provided as a matter of urgency. The site of the abscess can be diagnosed from the source of the infection and from the physical signs. Frontal abscesses often present with lethargy, confusion and finally coma, and temporal lobe abscesses present very acutely with a deepening coma and a contralateral hemiplegia. Cerebellar abscesses may show nystagmus and inco-ordination and in all three there may be papilloedema.

Frontal and temporal lobe abscesses (Fig. 9.22) are best drained by making a frontal or temporal burr hole, opening the dura in a cruciate fashion to reveal the bulging brain and inserting a ventricular cannula directly through the brain into the abscess. The wall of the abscess, which is often encapsulated, is felt as a characteristic resistance and when this is penetrated pus oozes out under pressure through the needle. The needle should be carefully retained in position and antibiotics instilled. If a C A T scan is not available for subsequent examination of the progress of the abscess, a small quantity of sterile micropaque is introduced together with the

antibiotic. This will be taken up by the abscess wall and subsequently can be revealed by plain skull X-rays. Failing this a small quantity of air may be injected. After the removal of the pus, small abscesses rapidly shrink, a process that can be observed radiologically. Large chronic abscesses which have developed a firm capsule will require more than one aspiration of pus. Needling may be replaced by the insertion of a small rubber tube-

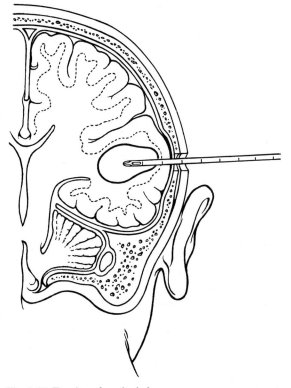

Fig. 9.22 Tapping of cerebral abscess

drain. Such large abscesses, however, frequently require formal craniotomy and excision as they are unlikely to heal satisfactorily by simple aspiration.

Sub-dural empyema

The formation of pus in the subdural space is now much commoner than cerebral abscess formation but is associated with the same primary infections. Patients are often toxic and present focal signs such as hemiplegia or epilepsy due to inflammation in the underlying cortex and veins. The pus should be evacuated and antibiotics instilled as soon as possible. Burr holes are made bifrontally and biparietally to allow the removal of the usually small amount of pus and the placement of two to three small catheters in each burr hole for the administration of antibiotic. Some surgeons, however, favour a wide craniotomy with removal of the pus and placement of a few catheters in the space. Epilepsy is common in this condition and all patients should be treated with prophylactic anticonvulsants.

OPERATIONS FOR TRIGEMINAL NEURALGIA

If drug treatment becomes ineffective in the relief of trigeminal neuralgia, an operation on the nerve is indicated. The older procedure of partial division of the sensory root of the fifth nerve is now rarely performed, having been replaced by either alcoholic or radiofrequency destruction of the trigeminal ganglion. This is performed under local anaesthesia with sedation or general anaesthesia, the needle being inserted about 2.5 cm from the corner of the mouth and directed towards the pupil and the middle of the zygoma. The needle enters the cave of Meckel and cerebrospinal fluid can often be aspirated, confirming the position of the needle, which is further confirmed by A-P and lateral radiographs. 0.5 to 0.8 ml of absolute alcohol is then injected or a current passed through an insulated needle.

INTRACRANIAL ANEURYSMS AND SUBARACHNOID HAEMORRHAGE

Intracranial aneurysms are largely confined to the circle of Willis (Fig. 9.23) and the middle cerebral artery at its first primary branching in the stem of the lateral fissure. The patient complains of sudden onset of severe headache and neck stiffness and a lumbar puncture shows evenly blood stained fluid. If the patient survives this initial haemorrhage he is at grave risk of further haemorrhage which is often more serious. Angiography confirms the existence of an aneurysm and its site. If the patient's condition is satisfactory operation is performed at the earliest opportunity. The operative treatment depends

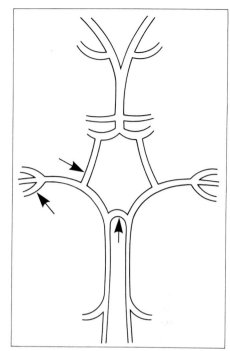

Fig. 9.23 Diagram of the circle of Willis. Arrows indicate the commonest sites for an intracranial aneurysm

upon the site of the aneurysm. The ideal treatment is occlusion of the neck of the aneurysm with a clip, so that it is excluded from the cerebral circulation; if this is not possible the aneurysm sac may be strengthened by fibrous reaction induced by gauze wrapping. Aneurysms of the intracranial part of the internal carotid artery can be dealt with by common carotid ligation but before this is performed a good cross circulation must be demonstrated by angiography.

Carotid cavernous fistula

This is treated by ligature of the internal carotid artery in the neck. If this is unsuccessful due to retrograde filling, the intracranial part of the artery is occluded distal to the fistula just above the cavernous sinus by means of a silver clip. With the exception of the ophthalmic branch this completely isolates the affected segment of the artery. Unfortunately, the collateral circulation to the eye maintained by the anastomosis between the maxillary artery and the orbital plexus of the ophthalmic artery may result in a recurrence of symptoms. Recent approaches to this problem have been by intracarotid balloon obliteration via a catheter inserted through the common carotid artery in the neck.

CHRONIC SUBDURAL HAEMATOMA

This condition may occur after an apparently trivial

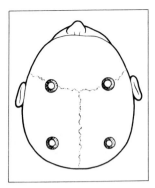

Fig. 9.24 The 'four burr hole' method of diagnosis and treatment of subdural haematoma

injury and manifest itself a considerable time later. Characteristically the patient has a fluctuating course of lethargy or coma and there may be a contralateral or ipsilateral hemiparesis. Diagnosis and treatment can be made by burr holes (Fig. 9.24). These are made under local anaesthesia in the midpupillary line at the coronal suture and parietal eminences. If at one or more of the openings the dura is found to be dark in colour it is incised and the underlying haematoma, which is usually fluid, is evacuated by irrigation and suction. Unless there is radiological evidence to the contrary the procedure should be repeated on the opposite side since bilateral collections are common.

CRANIAL DEFECTS

These may be due to the removal of bone fragments in comminuted or depressed fractures, and less frequently the result of exploratory or decompression operations. Repair of the defect may be desirable for cosmetic or psychological reasons or to protect the brain from possible injury at work or play. It is advisable to wait for at least 6 months after the wound has been soundly healed to ensure the absence of infection. The defect may be filled with autogenous bone graft taken from the ribs or ileum, by the implantation of a tantalum plate or more conveniently by acrylic plastic.

STEREOTACTIC SURGERY

Many procedures which were formerly only possible through craniotomy can now be done by stereotactic instrumentation. There are many stereotactic instruments available but in general all follow the same principles of secure instrument fixation to the head, the taking of X-rays to reveal the ventricular contours outlined by radio-opaque dye and the establishment of their relationship to the stereotactic instrument, which usually has radio-opaque rulers incorporated. After identification of the target the probe is introduced and this destroys tissue either by freezing or heat coagulation using a radiofrequency current. Stereotaxy is now used in the treatment of such diseases as movement disorder, mental disorder, and pain.

FURTHER READING

Gardjian   Operative neurosurgery. Williams and Wilkins, Baltimore

Hitchcock E, Teixeira M, Pinto J 1983 Percutaneous trigeminal radio-frequency rhizotomy. Journal of the Royal College of Surgeons of Edinburgh 28: 74

Schmidek H H, Sweet W H (eds) 1976 Current topics in operative neurosurgery. Grune and Stratton, New York

Smith R R 1980 Essentials of neurosurgery. Lippincott, Philadelphia

Symon L 1982 Neurosurgery. In: Dudley H, Pories W J (eds) Rob and Smith's Operative Surgery. 4th edn, Butterworth, London

10
Operations on the spine and spinal cord

E. R. HITCHCOCK

SPECIAL DIAGNOSTIC PROCEDURES

Lumbar puncture

Lumbar puncture is undertaken for a wide variety of diagnostic and therapeutic purposes and for the induction of spinal anaesthesia. It provides an opportunity to detect purulent or blood stained c.s.f. and to obtain cerebrospinal fluid for laboratory measurements, including cell count, gram stain, culture and antibiotic sensitivity. In addition, protein, glucose and immune globulins and serology may be measured.

In difficult cases or sometimes in very obese patients, the procedure is facilitated by having the patient seated and the spine bent but it is more usual to perform the procedure with the patient lying on his side. In either case, the spine must be flexed as much as possible in order to open out the interlaminar spaces through one of which the puncture is made. Spinal flexion is achieved by having the patient with knees flexed and drawn up to the chest and the neck flexed. This position can be steadied by an assistant. A fine calibre spinal needle is preferable because it produces only a small tear in the dura and minimizes the risk of post puncture headache. It should be very sharp with a short bevel into which the stylet fits accurately. A line joining the highest points of the two iliac crests crosses the interval between the fourth and fifth lumbar spines (Fig. 10.1) and the puncture may be made in this space or one above or below.

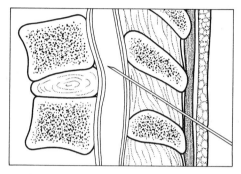

Fig. 10.2 Lumbar puncture needle introduced between the spinous processes

After cleansing the skin a local anaesthetic is injected into the skin and subcutaneous tissues and the lumbar puncture needle then inserted midway between the spinous processes (Fig. 10.2). It should be advanced strictly in a sagittal plane with the point directed slightly towards the head. Immediately after the skin is pierced the resistance of the tough supraspinous ligament is encountered and overcome. At a further depth of about 4 cm the lesser resistance of the ligamentum flavum and of the dura mater is felt. Thereafter entry of the needle point into the spinal canal is denoted by a sudden sensation of decreased resistance. As soon as this is felt the stylet is withdrawn and cerebrospinal fluid should escape in drops. When the needle appears to have been introduced to the required depth but no fluid appears it has probably deviated laterally and the needle should be withdrawn and reinserted. Normal cerebrospinal fluid is colourless and crystal clear.

Cisternal puncture

This is rarely necessary and is a dangerous procedure, best left in the hands of the expert. On the rare occasions when cisternal myelography is necessary because of failure to introduce contrast from below, or patients with multiple blocks, cisternal puncture may be necessary. The procedure is best done with the patient in the sitting posture with the neck strongly flexed. The puncture site is exactly in the midline in the plane of the two mastoid

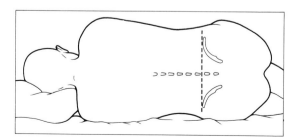

Fig. 10.1 Left lateral position for lumbar puncture. Line joining iliac crests indicates 4th/5th interspace—the usual site for insertion of needle

processes and the needle is directed upwards and forwards in the sagittal plane to strike the under surface of the occipital bone. The point of the needle is then depressed until the needle is felt to penetrate the posterior occipito-atlantal ligament immediately below the posterior margin of foramen magnum. This is encountered at approximately 5 cm depth and cerebrospinal fluid should escape when the stylet is withdrawn.

Spinal manometry

Lumbar fluid pressure is a reasonably accurate measurement of intracranial pressure provided that the head and vertebral column are in the same strictly horizontal plane Apart from some cases with benign intracranial hypertension, where an intracranial space occupying lesion has been excluded, there is no indication for spinal manometry in patients with increased intracranial pressure and its value in indicating a spinal block is debatable whilst it may very well precipitate complete block.

Myelography

The spinal cord and canal can be demonstrated by the introduction of contrast medium into the spinal subarachnoid space. The medium is usually introduced by lumbar puncture after the removal of 5 ml of cerebrospinal fluid for laboratory studies. After a small amount of contrast medium has been injected, an X–ray is taken to ensure that it is in the subarachnoid space. If this is satisfactory the remaining contrast medium, usually about 3 ml of *Myodil*, is injected and, with the patient in the prone position, the X–ray is taken with the patient's head lowered to visualize the flow of contrast medium. If it is arrested by any obstruction within the spinal canal the level is accurately determined and, after examination, as much as possible of the *Myodil* is removed by aspiration.

Water soluble media such as *Conray* or *Metrizamide* have largely replaced the use of *Myodil*.

Isotope scan

The spine may be scanned in a similar fashion to cerebral isotope scan (Fig. 9.14) following the intravenous injection of a suitable intravenous isotope.

SPINA BIFIDA

Spina bifida is a congenital defect in the bony wall of the spinal canal through which the canal contents may protrude. It is almost invariably posterior, usually in the lumbosacral region, less often in the cervical and most rarely in the thoracic region.

Meningocoele

This is saccular protrusion of dura mater often covered completely or incompletely with skin and containing cerebrospinal fluid. The cord is normal and not displaced but the spinal nerve roots are often caught up in the wall of the sac and frequently these patients will have flaccid paralysis of leg muscles and sphincters. The result of surgical repair is poor but, if the sac is ulcerated or rupture is threatened, repair can be done. A transverse elliptical incision is made along the sides of the sac and the surrounding skin undermined. The sac is then opened about 3 cm from the base and inspected to see if there are any nerve roots within it. If possible these are freed and replaced in the canal. The redundant part of the sac is either cut away and the remaining portion repaired with fine sutures or, after tapping, the sac is inverted into the defect and the fascia and skin closed in layers over it. The muscles are approximated in the midline, so as to give a strong repair, but rotation flaps may be needed to ensure adequate skin cover.

Myelomeningocoele

In myelomeningocoele the cord is within the sac and there are invariably serious neurological disabilities. Excision of the sac is usually not possible but it can be emptied by tapping and then replaced in the bony defect and the muscle and fascia closed over it as for simple meningocoele.

A common postoperative complication is *hydrocephalus* which may require separate treatment by ventricular shunting. This is done by inserting a cannula into the dilated lateral ventricles of the brain and passing the catheter, usually via some flushing device, through another silicon catheter with some form of valve. The drainage end is passed down the jugular vein into the heart (*ventriculo-atrial shunt*) or passed down over the chest wall into the peritoneum (*ventriculoperitoneal shunt*).

SPINAL INJURIES

Operation may be indicated in dislocations and fracture/dislocations of the vertebral column, especially when these are associated with neural damage or where there is gross instability with the risk of increasing the neurological deficit. Such interventions are designed to (i) stabilize unstable fractures or (ii) remove compressions, such as prolapsed disc fragments or vertebral fragments. The neurological signs may be due to injury to cord or nerve roots or a combination and these may be partial or complete. Careful neurological examination is mandatory and X–rays should be taken in both anteroposterior and lateral planes to reveal fractures or displacements.

In general lesions above the tenth thoracic vertebra can be considered as causing predominantly cord lesions. If the transection is complete, as is   unfortunately commonly the case in thoracic lesions, then no recovery can be expected since central nervous system fibre injury does not regenerate. On the other hand injuries below that level, even complete motor and sensory paralysis, may be due mainly or entirely to root lesions which are potentially recoverable. After cord injury there is an immediate loss of function below the level of the transection. This may last for several weeks before the return of reflex activity but without the return of voluntary power or sensation.

It is reasonable to take the view that complete loss of power and sensation below the level of the transection does indeed imply a complete and irrecoverable cord damage but, if the injury is partial or predominantly a root injury, immediate measures should be taken to ensure that no further injury occurs. This is particularly important in cervical spine injuries where often unstable fracture/dislocations are unrecognised before serious damage occurs. In all suspected cases of cervical spine injury the neck should be immobilized with a simple collar and if an unstable fracture is demonstrated cervical traction should be instituted.

Skull traction for cervical spine injury

There are various types of skull traction apparatus available but the simplest is the Gardner tongs which can be applied in the dressing room very simply under local anaesthesia. The penetrating points are applied about 6 cm above the ear, just in front of the parietal eminence.

In fracture/dislocations of the cervical spine steady traction may reduce a partial dislocation. It should in any case be used to immobilize and stabilize cervical fractures. Cervical traction is best used on the Stryker frame so that the patient can be turned without interfering with the traction. Unstable cervical fractures should be stabilized by posterior fixation or by anterior fusion. In both cases grafts are taken from the superior iliac crests. In the posterior approach the spines and vertebrae of the cervical spine are exposed. Split portions of iliac crest are laid on either side of the cervical spines across the unstable segment and wired in place. The patient must be maintained in traction. Anterior fusion produces more immediate fixation (see p. 216) and traction can often be dispensed with, providing a secure collar is used. Locked fracture/ dislocations at the cervical level are difficult and dangerous to reduce. Usually, a part or whole of the locked articular facet must be removed and such patients are best dealt with in a neurosurgical centre.

Thoracic and lumbar spine

In thoracic and lumbar injuries with complete transection, reduction of the dislocation prevents gross angulation (a cause of bed sores) and stabilizes the spine to facilitate rehabilitation.

In the lumbar spine, where the damage is entirely root

damage, exploration may be indicated if myelography reveals any evidence of compression.

In *missile* wounds of the spinal column the cord may be compressed by in-driven fragments of bone or by retained missile and, if X-ray examination suggest this, a laminectomy should be performed without delay. After removal of the lamina and exposure of the dura, a search should be made for the displaced fragments and foreign bodies.

Stability depends on whether the ligaments are divided or not. Wedge fractures and compression fractures are usually associated with intact ligaments and are stable but dislocations and fracture/dislocations invariably have ligamentous rupture and are unstable.

Recovery

Attention should be predominantly directed, however, to the prevention of complications which endanger life or render it intolerable (urinary infections, bed sores and contractures). This can be achieved by correct nursing and careful attention to bladder drainage until reflex control of micturition is established. Immobilization of the patient on a Stryker frame reduces the risk of these complications and facilitates nursing. Later, physiotherapy, education in the use of supportive apparatus and general rehabilitation may restore the paraplegic patient to a useful rôle in society.

LAMINECTOMY

Laminectomy or excision of the spinal lamina can be performed at cervical, thoracic or lumbar levels and provides a wide exposure of the spinal dura and underlying cord or nerves.

The procedure is essentially the same at each level.

The patient is usually positioned prone with the spine flexed by placing pillows or sand bags under the upper part of the chest and hips or placing the head in a head holder so that the neck may be flexed. It is important to ensure that the abdomen is unobstructed and that respiration is not impeded. The skin and muscles are infiltrated over the full extent of the midline incision which should extend at least one vertebral level above and below the desired lamina exposure. The skin is incised and held apart by self-retaining retractors and the fibromuscular attachments to the spinous processes are separated by sharp dissection down to the bone. The incision is continued down to the base of the spinous process on each side and an osteotome is used to scrape away the periosteum and retract the muscles laterally. Further self retaining retractors are inserted and, after haemostasis has been achieved, the spinous processes are first removed using rongeurs and then the lamina until the dura is exposed. Particular care should be taken in inserting the under blade of the rongeurs beneath the lamina especially if there is a mass displacing the dura. Extradural masses such as metastases or discs are cautiously removed piecemeal using the rongeurs; intradural masses are removed by carefully incising the dura and retracting the edges by sutures attached to the sides of the wound. The dura is then sutured with a continuous fine suture and the muscles apposed by strong sutures, closing the gap left by the bony excision. Drainage is rarely required.

INTERVERTEBRAL DISC PROTRUSION

This can occur at any level but is most common in the lower lumbar discs. In the cervical region acute disc prolapse is rare.

Most cases of severe and persistent sciatica and many cases of severe low back pain are caused by a protrusion of an intervertebral lumbar disc. The protrusion occurs backwards and usually to one side into the vertebral canal where it presses on the nerve roots, or in the case of the rare thoracic protrusion, into the cord itself. The most common sites are between L5 and S1, and L4 and L5. The primary treatment is immobilization by strict bed rest but if there is evidence of bladder involvement then there is an urgent need for removal of the disc. It is usual to confirm the diagnosis by myelography although the surgeon should be aware that a negative myelogram does not exclude a disc lesion. A limited laminectomy, with the removal of the whole of the fifth and the lower half of the fourth lumbar laminae, gives good access to the lower two intervertebral discs although a neurosurgeon would generally prefer the *fenestration* (Fig. 10.3) procedure in which access is gained through an interlamina space. The ligamentum flavum bridging the space is excised and the margins of the contiguous laminae are nibbled away to reveal the nerve root. The theca and nerve root are gently retracted which brings the protruded disc into view. The annulus fibrosis covering the protrusion is excised and the interior of the disc thoroughly curetted and all degenerated and readily detachable tissue removed. Specially angled scoops and pituitary rongeur forceps are useful. This lateral approach is sufficient for the common unilateral disc protrusion but if there is a large central disc it is safer to form a partial laminectomy. Spinal fusion is unnecessary after this procedure.

Thoracic disc protrusions are difficult and dangerous and the operation has a high morbidity rate. On this account the procedure should not be performed by the inexperienced.

Cervical disc compression
Although acute disc prolapse is uncommon, chronic

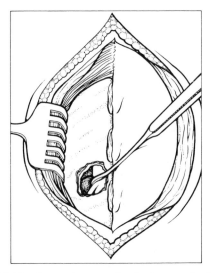

Fig. 10.3 The fenestration operation for intervertebral disc protrusion. The ligamentum flavum and the contiguous margins of the two laminae have been removed on the affected side. The nerve root and the main theca have been retracted to expose the protrusion

degenerative changes in the disc are frequently seen. A combination of ligamentous hypertrophy and osteophytic formation produces cord or root compression. Acute prolapse occurs in the younger age groups, and may produce a sudden quadriparesis or quadriplegia. An emergency laminectomy will decompress the cord and cautious retraction of the root will allow the removal of the prolapsed fragment. A safer procedure is the anterior cervical decompression and fusion procedure of Cloward. The disc is approached from the front by an incision in the neck. The carotid sheath is retracted laterally and the larynx, trachea and oesophagus medially to reveal the anterior aspect of the cervical column. The affected disc is identified by lateral X-ray using a marker thrust into the anterior part of one of the discs. Thereafter the affected disc and a portion of the upper and lower vertebrae around it are reamed out, with a special instrument, down to the dura. The disc fragments are removed en route and a careful search made for any loose fragment. The defect in the bone is filled with a plug of bone taken from the iliac crest.

SPINAL COLUMN INFECTION

Pus may arise in the extradural space following local skin infection, such as boils. The patient is acutely ill with fever and complains of severe back pain, usually with limitation of straight leg raising. Myelography demonstrates an extradural compression. A decompressive laminectomy should be performed as soon as possible and the pus aspirated and antibiotic solution instilled. It is unnecessary and unwise to open the dura to see if the infection has spread but tubes may be inserted into the extradural space for the subsequent administration of antibiotics.

TUBERCULOSIS OF THE SPINE

Tuberculous infection of the spine (Pott's disease) is only a local manifestation of a generalised disease and it is essential to deal with the primary focus of infection. Before the advent of specific chemotherapy active surgical intervention was limited to stabilizing operations which were only undertaken when the acute infection had been overcome at a comparatively late stage in the disease. The risk of introducing secondary infection discouraged attempts to excise an active tuberculous focus—or even evacuate an abscess by open exposure. The risks of such intervention are now very much less due to specific chemotherapy, and it is generally accepted that better results can be obtained by judicious surgical intervention in association with intensive chemotherapy.

Operative treatment in spinal tuberculosis attempts: (1) to provide drainage of abscesses; (2) to remove all necrotic material including sequestra, and also tuberculous granulation tissue; (3) to remove any source of spinal cord compression either by necrotic debris or bony deformity and (4) to stabilize the spine to encourage healing or prevent further deformity.

Abscesses occur in approximately 50% of patients with spinal tuberculosis. Although aspiration is the ideal treatment, often the pus is too thick to be evacuated in this way. Drainage is then by open operation under antibiotic control to prevent secondary infection. At the time of drainage an attempt should be made to eradicate the primary focus and local chemotherapy applied and the wound closed without drainage. Cervical abscesses are approached through an incision behind the sternomastoid, avoiding the accessory nerve. Thoracic abscesses are drained by costotransversectomy or anterolateral decompression and lumbar abscesses through a nephrectomy incision. About 10% of patients with spinal tuberculosis become paralysed, usually because of cord compression by abscess or debris although in a small number pressure from a sequestrum or a bony deformity is responsible. If the paresis does not improve under conservative treatment or becomes worse then operation is indicated.

Anterolateral decompression (Fig. 10.4)
This is a radical method of removing the local focus of disease and is particularly indicated in patients with developing paralysis. An oblique incision is made for thoracic lesions through a left thoracotomy incision and

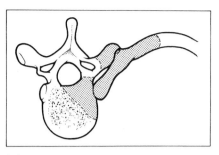

Fig. 10.4 Anterolateral decompression. Drawing to show extent of bone removal

the posterior ends of the affected ribs are removed together with the related transverse process as in the operation of costotransversectomy but in addition the pedicles in the adjacent part of the bodies of the affected vertebra are excised. Thoracolumbar lesions are best excised through the bed of the tenth rib and a similar, but lower, oblique incision is made for lumbar lesions. The articular process in the lamina should be left intact since otherwise lateral spinal subluxation may occur. All necrotic débris including sequestra and degenerate disc material is removed and the walls of the cavity lightly curetted. The cavity is then liberally sprinkled with streptomycin·powder and if there has been considerable bone loss, as is often the case, the cavity is filled with cancellous chips taken from the iliac crest. The wound is then closed by primary suture and antibiotics continued for several months after the procedure. This operation is a major procedure often with considerable blood loss so that it should not be attempted by the inexperienced, except in the most dire emergency.

Costotransversectomy
This can be used for evacuation of abscesses in the thoracic region. If the abscess appears to be bilateral the side of the larger abscess is chosen for operation. An incision about 8 cm in length is made along the posterior part of the appropriate rib which is cleared of periosteum and divided about 5 cm from its medial end. The medial fragment is then avulsed and the related transverse process is chiselled off during which the abscess is usually opened, or if not it is located by blunt dissection close to the vertebral body. After the pus has been evacuated streptomycin is introduced into the cavity and the wound is sutured without drainage. This procedure may relieve cord pressure and reduce toxicity without weakening the spinal column, whilst further collections of pus tend to come to the surface at the operation site. Unfortunately, the exposure, though adequate for the simple evacuation of an abscess, is insufficient to permit the removal of more solid necrotic material which may well be responsible for cord compression and constitute a serious obstacle to healing. The method, therefore, is less

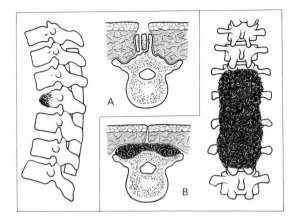

Fig. 10.5 Two methods of spinal fusion. In Albee's operation (A) a compact graft is placed between the split spinous processes. In Brittain's operation (B) cancellous bone chips are packed against the posterior surfaces of the vertebrae, which have been denuded of cortical bone

frequently employed than the anterolateral decompression but in an emergency it may be the safer procedure for the inexperienced operator.

Spinal fusion (Fig. 10.5)
After the active stage of the tuberculosis is passed and healing is in progress vertebral fusion may be helpful to speed healing and prevent further deformity. When deformity is increasing under conservative treatment or appears to be the cause of paralysis, arthrodesis may also be indicated before the disease is under control and many surgeons would advocate spinal fusion routinely after drainage of paravertebral abscesses or relief of cord pressure. At least five vertebrae should be fused, two above and two below the one or more which are involved by the disease. The procedure of choice at the present time depends upon the use of cancellous bone chips to secure osseus union between the vertebrae. The entire posterior surface of the vertebrae to be fused are exposed and cleared of all soft tissue including the capsules of the facet joints. Spinous processes are removed at their bases and the posterior surfaces of the laminae and transverse processes are denuded of cortical bone. A large quantity of cancellous bone chips taken from the iliac crest is evenly distributed over the denuded area and the overlying muscle and aponeurosis sutured to enclose the grafts firmly in their bed. Postoperatively the spine must be kept immobilized until consolidation occurs.

SPINAL NEOPLASMS

Spinal tumours are either extradural, such as secondary deposits in vertebral tumours, or intradural. Intramedullary tumours, that is tumours of the cord itself, are rare and the majority of spinal tumours arise either from the arachnoid (*meningiomata*) or nerve roots (*neurinomata*). These tumours are extramedullary but frequently embed themselves in the cord. Diagnosis is made by clinical examination and confirmed by myelography and operation should be carried out as soon as possible because of the risk of developing paraplegia. Having identified the site of the tumour the spines and laminae of the affected area are removed. The presence of the tumour is often revealed by swelling of the dura, evident as soon as the lamina has been removed, and if the tumour has obstructed the cerebrospinal fluid dural pulsation is frequently absent below that level. Small tumours may only be located after the dura has been opened. Meningiomata are removed along the involved area of dura and nerve root neurinomata require sacrifice of the involved root. Intramedullary tumours are rarely amenable to radical surgery and no attempt should be made to remove the whole of extradural metastatic tumours, the operator being satisfied with a decompression and removal of the posterior and lateral portion of the tumour only. Attempts to remove the anterior portion and rotation of the cord or dura may result in serious cord damage. In such cases radiotherapy can be given subsequently.

ANALGESIC SPINAL SURGERY

Certain severe intractable pains, such as those due to cancer, can be relieved by sectioning the posterior nerve roots or spinothalamic tract.

Posterior rhizotomy
Because of the considerable overlap it is insufficient to sever a single root for one dermatomal or sclerotomal involvement and it is usual to plan for the section of two roots above and below, as well as the affected root, to achieve satisfactory anaesthesia. Roots are exposed by complete laminectomy and identified as they emerge through the intervertebral foramen. They are severed halfway between the exit foramina and the cord, after being carefully separated from the anterior root.

Spinothalamic tractotomy or cordotomy
This is a very effective analgesic operation and can be performed in the thoracic or cervical region. Most neurosurgeons prefer the cervical level because of the more uniform distribution of fibres, less limited space and less need to rotate the cord. The operation is performed in the prone or lateral position and a midline incision made over the occipital bone and upper three cervical vertebrae. The incision is deepened in the midline to the arch of the atlas which is removed and the dura opened. The dentate ligament is identified and severed at its attachment to the lateral wall and heavy

artery forceps clamped on it up to its insertion into the cord. A pointed scalpel blade is inserted 3 mm into the cord and brought round circumferentially to the anterior root. The technique of this operation is not standardized and some operators will prefer to use the older thoracic exposure. Sphincter disorder, transient paresis and skin injury due to unnoticed trauma are well recognized but small risks of the procedure. Many cordotomies are performed percutaneously, inserting a needle laterally into the spinal theca and then passing a fine electrode through the needle into the spinothalamic tract. It has the advantage that the procedure can be done under local anaesthesia which is a useful approach for patients where general anaesthesia is dangerous.

FURTHER READING

Gardjian Operative neurosurgery. Williams and Wilkins, Baltimore

Lipton S 1981 Intractable pain—the present position. Annals of the Royal College of Surgeons of England 63: 157

Schmidek H H, Sweet W H (eds) 1976 Current topics in operative neurosurgery. Grune and Stratton, New York

Smith R R 1980 Essentials of neurosurgery. Lippincott, Philadelphia

Symon L 1982 Neurosurgery. In: Dudley H, Pories W J (eds) Rob and Smith's Operative Surgery, 4th edn. Butterworth, London

11

Operations on the face, mouth and jaws

A. G. D. MARAN & M. N. TEMPEST

WOUNDS OF THE FACE

The chief aim in the treatment of all facial wounds is to reduce disfigurement to the minimum. Most cases of extensive injury will eventually require the attention of a skilled plastic surgeon and it is the responsibility of the surgeon carrying out the initial repair to do nothing which will interfere with such specialized later treatment. His main concern should be to avoid unnecessary scar formation by careful cleansing of the wound, débridement and accurate repair of the tissues in layers with fine sutures.

Because of the great vascularity of the face, primary suture is usually a safe procedure, especially when combined with modern chemotherapy and antibiotics. Irregular lacerated wounds should be trimmed with a sharp knife or fine scissors. Formal excision of a wound is usually unnecessary and could result in unjustifiable sacrifice of healthy tissue. It is important however to remove all ingrained dirt and gravel rash by deliberate scrubbing with a hard brush under general anaesthesia. Only in this way can one avoid leaving the pigmented anthracotic scars that are so disfiguring and difficult to remove adequately later. Bleeding is usually controlled by pressure, forceps and ligation of vessels with the finest available material or diathermy, preferably with the bipolar coagulator.

Wounds with skin loss

Since the facial skin is so elastic, 'skin loss' is often more apparent than real, the wound gaping in a frightening manner due to muscle retraction and oedema. Often it will be found at operation that there is little or no tissue missing once the 'jigsaw' puzzle has been completed. If, however, skin, muscle or vermilion border is missing, it may be possible to rearrange the local tissues and achieve a reasonable closure of the wound, but in most instances the help of the plastic surgeon should be sought. The wound can be covered with a moist pack, bandaged and then repaired any time within the next 36–48 hours with specialist help. Flap repairs should *not* be attempted in the casualty department or even as a

primary procedure in a recent facial injury. Even free grafts (split-skin or full-thickness grafts) need careful choice, planning and design and are best left to the expert. Where the whole thickness of the lip or cheek is missing, skin should be united to mucous membrane around the margins of the defect (the so-called 'skin to mucosa' suture). This procedure, by obviating a raw area, usually promotes rapid healing with minimal scar formation or deformity and facilitates the formal definitive repair that can be carried out later.

Methods of skin suture (Figs. 11.1 & 11.2)
To minimize scarring, needles and suture materials to close the skin should be of the finest available (6/0 nylon, prolene or dexon), and any subcutaneous sutures of 4/0 chromic catgut or 5/0 dexon should be carefully inserted without tension. Each suture should be tied without strangulation of the tissues and the knots placed

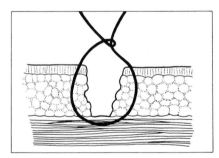

Fig. 11.1

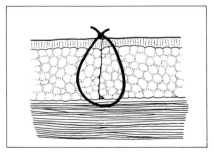

Fig. 11.2

Figs. 11.1 & 11.2 Method of suturing the skin of the face; designed to cause the minimum amount of scarring

in such a position that their removal is simple. Where possible, a single subcuticular running suture of 4/0 to 5/0 nylon can be inserted and removed 14–21 days later. A small 'twist nylon' drain can be inserted at one end of the wound and removed within 24–36 hours. No dressings are usually required, but the suture line must be kept free of crusts as these will encourage local sepsis and ugly stitch marks. The wound edges may be supported by strips of micropore adhesive tape (steristrips (see Fig. 1.16) once the skin has been cleaned and then dried with a swab soaked in ether.

Skin sutures are usually removed on the 3rd–5th day, subcuticular sutures after 14–21 days. All sutures must be removed with the patient lying flat, occasionally sedated or even anaesthetized and in a good light, with the right instruments and by a competent person.

In the case of wounds involving the whole thickness of the lip or cheek, the mucous membrane, muscles and skin should be sutured separately. In wounds of the eyelid, the tarsal plate must be identified and sutured to reduce the risk of distorting the margin of the eyelids. Careful attention should be paid to the possibility of damage to the canthal ligaments and the nasolacrimal ducts in wounds near the inner canthus. Damage to the parotid duct and facial nerve branches may be found in wounds of the cheek and these structures should be identified at the initial operation and repaired by someone who is practiced in the use of the operating microscope.

FRACTURES OF THE JAW AND CHEEK BONE

Fractures of the mandible

Most fractures of the mandible are compound into the mouth even if they are not compound externally. Because of this, a low grade infection in the wound is not unusual particularly if dental hygiene is poor. A considerable degree of displacement is frequently encountered especially with bilateral fractures. The muscles that close the jaw, being attached posterior to the fracture line, cannot control the anterior fragment of the mandible which is pulled downwards and backwards by the muscles of the floor of the mouth and the effects of gravity. This distorts the dental occlusion, is painful and makes eating difficult. The fracture must be reduced accurately to allow bony union in good position, restore the dental occlusion and enable the patient to eat normally. The danger with bilateral fractures is obstruction of the airway caused by the tongue falling backwards, and by increasing oedema of the floor of the mouth. This is particularly liable to happen if the patient is unconscious and is allowed to lie supine. Conscious patients can be nursed sitting up or prone or lying on their

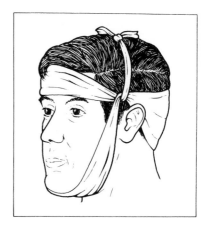

Fig. 11.3 Method of bandaging to support a fractured mandible

side. If unconscious, they *must* be nursed prone or on their side. Only rarely will an urgent tracheostomy be required: often an endotracheal tube will be a safer and better alternative. A suitable bandage (Fig. 11.3) will be adequate to give support to many jaw fractures as a first-aid measure and if the patient still has difficulty with the tongue falling backwards, a simple tongue stitch can be inserted, taking a good bite of tongue muscle with a suture of 3/0 or 4/0 nylon leaving the ends long, tied and held with an artery forceps.

The reduction and fixation of mandibular fractures may need help from a specialist dental surgeon trained in maxillofacial work. If the upper jaw is intact, it acts as a point of fixation to which the lower jaw can be supported and splinted. Indeed in some cases of fracture of the lower jaw all that may be needed for definitive treatment is a simple barrel-bandage support.

Other methods of fixing mandibular fractures include:

1. Interdental 'eyelet' wiring

This can be used if there are healthy teeth in the adjacent upper jaw. Stainless steel wire (gauge 26–32) is used to make eyelet wires that are twisted around teeth and then linked by another set of wires inserted through the eyelets (Fig. 11.4). By tightening this last set of wires the jaws are fixed together by 'intermaxillary fixation' (IMF). The 'linking' wires can be cut in an emergency and a pair of wire cutters should be kept fixed to the patient's bed for use in an emergency.

2. Arch bars

These are slender bars of malleable metal, which can be bent to fit against the outer surfaces of the teeth, to which they are secured by wiring. In this way only the actual fracture is immobilized and a certain amount of jaw movement is possible.

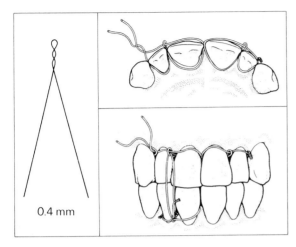

Fig. 11.4 The 'eyelet' method of interdental wiring for fractured mandible

3. Cap splints
These take the form of metallic bridges which are attached to the crowns of the teeth on either side of the fracture. Made by the dentist to a plaster cast, they fit accurately and can be cemented firmly in position. They also allow some jaw movement.

4. Gunning splints
These are used for edentulous patients. They are made of vulcanite or acrylic and resemble dentures without teeth. They can be wired in position for better stability.

5. Open-reduction and direct wiring
Of the fractured bone (Fig. 11.5).

6. Open reduction and plating of the fracture
By using small plates and screws. Some surgeons even encourage the use of compression (AO) plates (see p. 119).

Fractures of the ramus or condylar part of the mandible are seldom associated with much displacement.

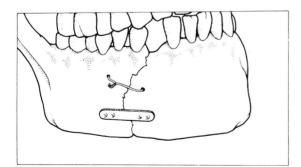

Fig. 11.5 Illustrating two methods of mandibular fracture fixation—wiring and plating

Mastication is encouraged, since this preserves mobility and helps to restore normal occlusion. If serious malalignment of the teeth is present, the mandible should be splinted by one of the methods described. Some condylar fractures are followed by joint stiffness and it may then be necessary to excise the condyle, in order to obtain a false but more mobile joint.

Fractures of the mandible with soft-tissue damage
Such injuries result from gunshot wounds and from the more serious road accidents. There may be widespread destruction both of soft tissue and of bone.

The main danger in such fractures is asphyxia. This may be due to aspiration of blood into the respiratory passages, or to mechanical blockage from falling back of the tongue which is deprived of its normal anterior support. The essentials of first-aid surgery are to arrest haemorrhage and to ensure that the tongue is held forward.

Whenever possible such cases should be sent to a *faciomaxillary* centre, where treatment is carried out jointly by the plastic surgeon and by the specialist dental surgeon. The general surgeon must, however, be familiar with the principles of plastic repair, for in most cases he will be responsible for the initial treatment, and on this much depends. His main aims should be to arrest haemorrhage and to guard against the complication of asphyxia during transit by ensuring a good airway and by aspirating secretions as required. In general, he should be careful to do nothing which may jeopardize the chances of a good final result in more expert hands.

Exploration and excision of the wound is carried out as soon as possible. Intratracheal anaesthesia should always be employed and the pharynx packed-off around the tube to prevent aspiration of blood into the respiratory passages. In certain cases tracheostomy may be required. The wound is carefully explored, foreign bodies, loose teeth and completely detached fragments of bone being removed. Soft-tissue loss is dealt with by stitching mucous membrane to skin around the margin of the defect. Fixation of the mandibular fragments may be effected by interdental wiring, direct wiring, plating or external pin fixation. Defects in the bone can be made good by bone grafting at a later date.

Fractures of the maxilla
Those occurring as part of a complicated middle third facial fracture in particular, are important because of the risk to adjacent structures such as the orbit, the nasolacrimal apparatus, the nose and the ethmoidal region. An associated fracture of the anterior cranial fossa may be complicated by CSF rhinorrhoea. Injuries involving the alveolar segments of the maxilla are relatively simple to treat and mal-alignment of the alveolus and teeth can

be corrected by interdental wiring, or a variety of dental splints.

Damage to the orbital floor and roof, the eye itself, the nasolacrimal apparatus, nasal bones and anterior cranial fossa is a far more complicated injury and needs the full co-operation of the plastic surgeon, ophthalmologist, neurosurgeon and specialist oral surgeon. These are not operations to be embarked upon by ill-trained surgeons with poor facilities under local anaesthesia in the accident unit. The repair of these injuries must observe two cardinal principles:

1. Adequate exposure in ideal surroundings.
2. Recognition that the bony fragments must be reduced and stabilized by wiring, pinning or packing before any soft tissue reconstruction begins.

Fractures of the zygomatic bone

These may be easily missed if the soft tissues are badly bruised or oedematous. The zygomatic bone is usually separated from its normal attachments and displaced forwards, downwards and inwards. A palpable 'step' deformity in the infra-orbital margin, facial flattening, diplopia, anaesthesia in the distribution of the infra-orbital nerve, epistaxis and difficulty in opening the jaw fully (MacLennan, 1977) are symptoms that should suggest a displaced fracture of the zygoma. Special X-ray views will confirm the extent of the fracture and its degree of comminution.

The Gillies approach is normally used to correct the displacement. Under general anaesthesia, a small incision is made in the temporal region inside the hairline and carried down through the temporalis fascia to display the temporalis muscle fibres. A lever (Bristow elevator or even a screwdriver) is then inserted through the incision and directed downwards beneath the zygomatic arch. Using a rolled up swab as a fulcrum, the zygoma is then levered into its normal position usually with an audible click. If the fracture cannot be reduced or is unstable, an open reduction with exploration of the orbital floor and direct wiring at several sites may be needed. The maxillary antrum is packed if there is gross comminution of the orbital floor.

Fractures of the nasal bones

Displaced fractures of the nasal bones are usually clinically obvious (Mayell, 1973) and no X-rays are required unless there is suspicion of other fractures in the naso-maxillary complex. Displacement of the nasal septum must be ascertained and corrected; hence there is no place for blind manipulation with or without local anaesthesia in the casualty department. The fracture must be reduced under general anaesthetic with an endotracheal tube in place, a throat pack inserted and in a good light with full theatre facilities to deal with bleeding. The nasal bones and septum are reduced under direct vision, the nostrils packed with ribbon gauze soaked in Whitehead's varnish (Pigmentum Iodoform Co. BPC) and a small external plaster of Paris splint applied.

INFECTIONS

Infections of dental origin

Alveolar abscess is due to periodontal infection. It is treated normally by a dentist, and usually subsides rapidly after extraction of the offending tooth.

Sub-periosteal abscess may follow an alveolar abscess which is untreated; it may appear either on the internal or external surface of the bone. The abscess should be drained into the mouth by an incision in the mucoperiosteum parallel to the alveolar margin. Drainage from the skin surface should always be avoided.

Ludwig's angina represents usually a further spread of the infection, resulting in a cellulitis within the submental and submandibular triangles. Its treatment is considered on page 238.

Osteomyelitis of the jaws

This may be due to spread of some local condition such as dental sepsis or infection of the maxillary sinus. Most cases subside under antibiotic therapy. Operation is indicated if a fluctuating abscess forms, and is then limited to incision and drainage. This may be carried out either from the mouth or from the skin surface, according to the conditions present. If necrosis of bone occurs sequestrectomy may be required.

Parapharyngeal abscess

Parapharyngeal abscess may complicate tonsillitis and is considered on page 238.

BENIGN CONDITIONS

Protruding ears—Otoplasty

This operation is performed for protruding ears. There are many variations in technique but the one described here does not involve cutting cartilage.

Operation (Figs. 11.6 & 11.7)

The protruding ear is bent so that the missing antehelical curve becomes visible. It is marked with methylene blue and then divided into four equal sections. Four points are marked in each section 7 mm from the line of the antihelix and 4 mm apart. A needle is passed through each of the points (8 in each side of the antihelix) so that it appears through the posterior surface of the ear. It is touched with methylene blue and pulled back on each occasion so that the cartilage is tatooed.

An elliptical incision is made on the posterior surface of the ear and the skin discarded. The cartilage is exposed and the tatooed dots identified. Using 2/0 white silk (so that it is not seen under the skin of the lateral surface of the ear) horizontal mattress sutures are inserted in

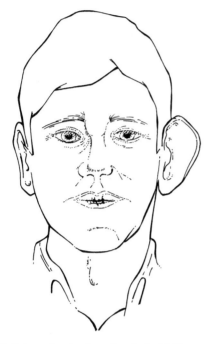

Fig. 11.6 Bat-ear showing loss of antihelical fold

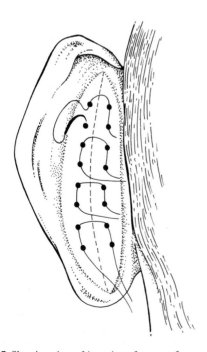

Fig. 11.7 Showing sites of insertion of sutures for otoplasty

each of the groups of four dots. When these are tied the curve of the antihelix is found. The skin edges of the ellipse are brought closer together and can be stitched without tension with 3/0 silk.

A pressure dressing is put on and left for a week, at which time the stitches are removed. Care has to be taken not to pull the ear forwards for at least three months after the operation lest the stitches are torn through the cartilage.

Haematoma of the auricle

If a haematoma is not aspirated almost immediately, it will deform the auricle and lead to the so-called wrestler's or cauliflower ear. The skin which is normally very adherent to the cartilage is pulled away and in a remarkably short time cartilage is resorbed by the pressure of a haematoma.

If the haematoma does not evacuate with a large bore needle, multiple incisions must be made. Once all the clot has been removed a pressure dressing is applied using wet cotton wool to fill all the contours of the ear. The ear must be examined daily because further accumulations of fluid will occur for many days.

Rhinophyma

This is a hypertrophic condition of the nasal skin due to a diffuse adenomatosis of the sebaceous glands. Operative treatment consists in shaving off the redundant masses with a sharp knife until the normal shape of the nose is restored. Great care is taken not to open into the nasal cavity; to ensure against this a finger is kept within the nostril during the shaving process. Haemorrhage is controlled by hot packs. Healing occurs with surprising rapidity, epithelium spreading from the retained parts of the glands.

Dermoid cysts

Facial dermoids occur commonly in the lateral part of the superciliary region, where the classical term *external angular dermoid* applies or at the root of the nose. Not infrequently they are attached to the bone, and may even have fibrous connections through bone diploë with dura mater, so that their removal may present some difficulty.

Sublingual dermoids protrude both below the chin and upwards in the floor of the mouth. They should be excised through a horizontal incision in the submental region. The mylohyoid is divided in the line of the incision to expose the cyst, which can usually be enucleated with surprising ease. If not, a finger placed within the cyst cavity acts as a useful guide to its extent and connections. It is distinguished from a thyroglossal cyst by its suprahyoid position. No sign of a duct is seen and there is no need to remove the hyoid bone.

Removal of leukoplakia

Leukoplakia is a Greek word meaning a white patch, and it is impossible to identify its biological potential other than by histopathology. Even although only 5% turn malignant, leukoplakia must be biopsied.

From the lip (Figs. 11.8–11.10)

The condition, when it affects the lip (usually the lower), is called actinic cheilitis. To remove this requires replacement of the vermilion of the lip or else an ugly deformity results. The incision is made along the muco-cutaneous junction and the vermilion dissected free of the underlying orbicularis oris. The dissection is continued down into the gingivo labial sulcus. The mucosa can then be pulled forwards and the leukoplakic edge excised. The clean mucosa is then stitched to the skin at the excision site with multiple sutures of 5/0 prolene.

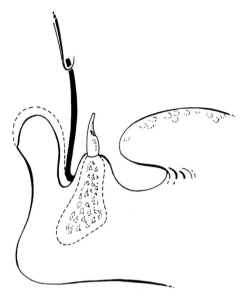

Fig. 11.10 Cross section showing extent of dissection

The lip swells greatly after this procedure but with the help of ice-packs it should look reasonably normal within two weeks.

From the buccal mucosa

Leukoplakia, or any small lesion here, should be removed in the transverse axis as closure is easier and contraction less.

From the tongue

Under general anaesthesia, the tongue is pulled forwards with a tongue clip and the leukoplakia excised. It is nearly always possible to close the area primarily with chromic catgut sutures.

Excision of ranula

Any cyst on the floor of the mouth appears blue domed and tense resembling a frog's belly and so can be called a ranula. A mucous retention cyst is excised locally after incising over the dome and dissecting it out taking care not to damage the submandibular duct. Each oral cyst should be sent to the pathology department however because tumours of minor salivary glands, half of which have a malignant potential, present in this way.

Ranulas which are lymphangiomas present a greater problem. It is impossible to excise them completely and so residual lymphangiomas can recur shortly after excision. It is for this reason that marsupialisation is occasionally performed. Excision of a lymphangioma can be fairly complete from the oral route, however, provided its form (a central body with peripheral pseudopodia) is kept in mind during the dissection. Obviously not all of the pseudopodia can be removed because some

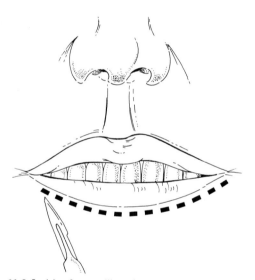

Fig. 11.8 Incision for vermilion advancement

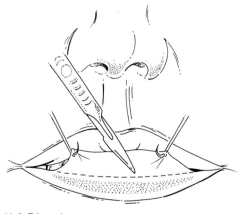

Fig. 11.9 Dissection

will travel deep into the neck and possibly as far as the axilla. A fairly complete dissection is performed and the mucosa of the floor of the mouth closed with chromic catgut after taking care not to include the submandibular duct in any stitch.

Thyroglossal cysts

Lingual varieties of these, situated in the posterior part of the tongue, may bulge upwards into the mouth. They can be enucleated through a median longitudinal incision, the tongue being drawn forward as far as possible. Haemorrhage is likely to be profuse and the operation is not an easy one. The treatment of thyroglossal cysts presenting in the neck is considered on page 241.

Papillomata

Papillomata of the lips, palate, tongue or mucous surface of the cheek should be excised, since they usually increase in size, and it is impossible to exclude the possibility of malignant change.

Submandibular calculus

A stone impacted in the submandibular duct should be removed through an incision in the floor of the mouth. If the calculus lies within the submandibular gland removal of the entire gland should be carried out (p. 267).

Affections of the mandibular joint

'Clicking' jaw

This occurs usually in young women. The cause is obscure, but it probably lies in some irregularity or laxity of the disc. Indications for operation are pain and persistent locking which are greatly relieved by *meniscectomy*. The superficial temporal vessels may be encountered and require ligature. The posterior part of the masseter is detached from the zygomatic arch, and the joint is opened by division of the lateral ligament in the line of its fibres. The articular disc is drawn laterally with a fine hook or forceps, and is removed in its entirety. Care is taken to avoid injury to the upper branches of the facial nerve. The auriculotemporal nerve, which runs laterally behind the joint, between it and the parotid gland, is usually not endangered.

Painful joint disorders

Degenerative changes occur as a result of unnatural occlusion following loss of permanent teeth when abnormal forces occur. Pain can be relieved by high condylectomy if simple measures fail.

Recurrent dislocation

This may be assoociated with a torn disc, and can be treated effectively by meniscectomy, since this allows the mandibular head to sink more deeply into the articular fossa.

Ankylosis of the joint

This may be a sequel to intra- or peri- articular infections or to osteo- or rheumatoid arthritis. Intra-articular ankylosis is treated by excision of the head and neck of the mandible (Rowe, 1982) although some success has been reported using bovine cartilage grafts. Ankylosis due to peri-articular cicatrisation can be treated by the excision of a wedge-shaped segment of mandible just in front of the angle, so that a false joint is formed in this situation.

MALIGNANT DISEASE

General considerations in treatment

The advent of high energy irradiation has greatly improved the prospects of curing the primary condition although major advances in methods of repair following radical excision have made surgery preferable in many cases. Since any major removal of tissue from the head and neck results in mutilation, the emotional response to treatment is to use radiotherapy in the first instance. There are, indeed, sites where radiotherapy gives a much better response than surgery provided this is the sole treatment. A policy of primary radiotherapy followed by salvage surgery is not advocated since the surgery then differs from planned primary excision. *If surgery fails* to eradicate a tumour, it fails at the periphery and recurrence is reasonably easily detected. *If radiotherapy fails*, it fails at the centre of the tumour where the oxygen tension is least. Thus, viable tumour is left within a capsule of fibrous tissue. As this viable tumour expands, so does the capsule, and biopsy revealing recurrent tumour is difficult to obtain. This delays the possibility of salvage surgery and is, therefore, to the patient's detriment. Furthermore, radiotherapy causes periarteritis and the viability of surrounding tissues is affected. Methods of primary wound closure (such as pedicle grafting) are prone to ischaemic necrosis and breakdown. Thus, instead of the patient being in hospital for 2–3 weeks with primary surgery, he may have to stay for 2–3 months undergoing a series of flap repairs because of fistulae. Radiotherapy is particularly noxious with regard to bone. Bone grafting after radiotherapy is usually not possible and so, in the oral cavity, primary surgery is usually the method of choice.

Various combinations of surgery and radiotherapy have been attempted in the past. Controlled trials, however, have shown that preoperative radiotherapy followed by elective surgery six weeks later has no greater effect on the survival rate than either modality used alone. At the moment trials are in progress to determine the effect of postoperative radiotherapy but the impression is that the results will not show any advantage.

There is evidence to show that surgery in combination with chemotherapy gives better results than surgery alone, but irradiation in combination with chemotherapy is worse than irradiation alone. In epithelial tumours chemotherapy has no place as a primary treatment.

Indications for excision

No general agreement has been reached on the indications for operative removal of malignant disease of the face, mouth and jaws. Much may depend upon the facilities for irradiation therapy, and upon the experience of the surgeon concerned. Early tumours of the facial skin and of the lip can usually be cured without serious disfigurement by excision, and this treatment should always be considered when irradiation is not readily available. Radical surgery should always be advised when a growth has invaded the bone, or when it has recurred after irradiation therapy.

Biopsy

Biopsy is essential when the diagnosis is in any doubt. It may be performed as routine in all cases, since it affords valuable information as regards prognosis, and may sometimes indicate the most appropriate treatment. The more anaplastic tumours are usually radio-sensitive, and show a good *immediate* response to irradiation therapy; at the same time they are more malignant, since dissemination occurs early and the prognosis is correspondingly more grave. The biopsy should always be taken from the growing margin of the lesion.

Lip tumours

Wedge excision

Up to one third of the lower lip can be excised with this

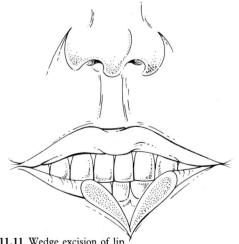

Fig. 11.11 Wedge excision of lip

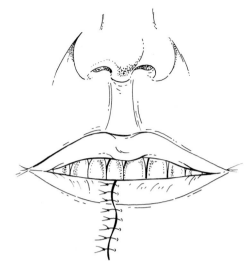

Fig. 11.12 Lip closure

procedure and primary closure is accompanied by no deformity and minimal scarring (Fig. 11.11). The margins of excision are marked at least 0.5 cm from each edge of the tumour. The vermilion edge is marked with a needle and methylene blue. From these marks a V is drawn on the inner and outer surfaces. The sides of the V are curved in order to avoid a decrease in the depth of the lip after suture (Fig. 11.12). The excision is performed along these lines in a through and through manner and the inferior labial artery is clamped and tied. Closure is begun by opposing the orbicularis oris and when this is completed the oral mucosa is stitched with interrupted sutures of 3/0 chromic catgut. The skin and vermilion is closed with 4/0 prolene taking care to appose accurately the vermilion edges.

Buccal mucosa

Small tumours (Fig. 11.13) can be removed with a good margin preserving the facial skin. A split thickness skin graft from the thigh is sewn into place using the quilting technique. This is to ensure a good take because intraoral skin grafts are prone to displacement and haematoma formation due to normal movements. The quilting technique involves placing multiple sutures 1 cm apart stitching the graft to the underlying muscle. The end result resembles a quilt and thus the name.

An alternative method is to stitch the edges of the graft leaving long ends and tying them over a bolster of flavine wool. A similar bolster is placed on the lateral surface of the cheek and the two are attached by through and through sutures so that the skin graft is sandwiched.

If the tumour is placed more posteriorly, then it is difficult to gain access unless a cheek flap is used. For

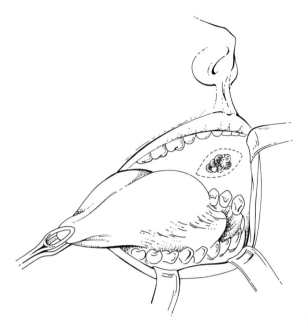

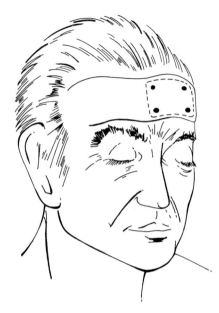

Fig. 11.13 Horizontal elliptical incision is better than vertical for removal of small tumours of the buccal mucosa

Fig. 11.14 Preparation of lined forehead flap. The split thickness skin graft is sewn onto the under surface of the forehead skin and held for seven days by buttons

this purpose a Weber Fergusson incision is used from under the eyelid, down the side of the nose and under the appropriate ala and then down through the centre of the lip. When the incision is extended intraorally in the gingivo buccal sulcus it allows the cheek to be reflected back off the maxilla. Access to posteriorly placed tumours is then easy and a quilted skin graft is applied as before.

Large tumours
These require a through and through excision of buccal skin. It is difficult to achieve closure of this defect with a pectoralis myocutaneous flap and so either a lined forehead flap (Fig. 11.14) is used or, if the patient has not had a radical neck dissection a sternomastoid myocutaneous flap.

If a lined forehead flap (Fig. 11.15) is required it should be prepared two weeks prior to the cheek excision. The end of the forehead flap is lifted and a split thickness skin graft is stitched to its undersurface. The flap is then resutured into place in order to give the split skin time to attach. The flap is lifted when required after the through and through excision and the split skin is sewn to the remaining buccal mucosa and the forehead skin to the facial skin.

After three weeks the pedicle is divided, the upper part of the defect is sewn into place and the remaining forehead skin is returned to its original site, removing the split thickness skin which was used as a temporary cover for the aponeurosis. Only a small defect remains

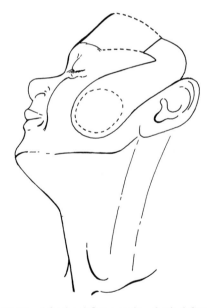

Fig. 11.15 Lined forehead flap covering cheek defect

at one side of the forehead lined with split thickness skin.

Tongue
In operating on the tongue for tumour, several principles must be borne in mind.
1. Due to the spaces created by the intrinsic tongue muscles and also the milking action of the tongue move-

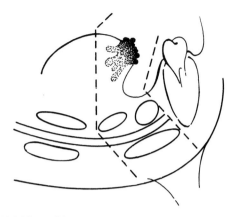

Fig. 11.16 In excising a tongue tumour the lines of excision should not be wedge shaped or else deep tumour will be left. Dotted lines show incisions for removal of tongue tumour in continuity with neck glands

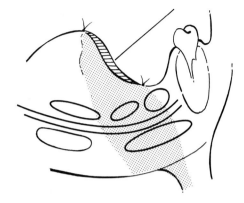

Fig. 11.18 Cross section showing pectoralis major flap in position following the excision indicated in Figure 11.16

ment, cancer can spread widely and in general terms at least a 2 cm excision margin is required.

2. As long as 1 cm of floor of mouth mucosa can be preserved, the tongue will retain a lot of mobility and dentures can be worn or teeth preserved which will help articulation.

3. Free skin grafts do badly in the oral cavity because they are difficult to place and they tend to contract.

4. Up to half a tongue can be removed with no loss of function but half a tongue or more should be replaced with soft tissue or else the oral cavity will be crippled.

Partial glossectomy

A radical or a partial neck dissection is performed and the pedicle is left attached to the submandibular region. The tongue can be approached either from the oral cav-

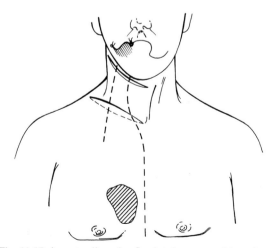

Fig. 11.17 A pectoralis major flap has been passed into the mouth to cover the defect following excision of tongue tumour and neck glands

ity or by splitting the ramus of the mandible. For the occasional mouth surgeon the former route is preferable.

In order not to disseminate tumour into fresh tissue the exophytic or ulcerative surface is coagulated with diathermy (Fig. 11.16). The margin of excision is tatooed with methylene blue and the tatoo marks are embedded deeply into the tongue so that they will be visible during excision. An accurate assessment of spread of the tumour is therefore essential. The actual excision along these marks is done with cutting diathermy. The lingual artery will be divided and requires ligation. When the excision line is cut it is deepened towards the neck dissection space and the whole mass is removed in continuity. A pectoralis major flap is used if any appreciable amount of tongue tissue is removed (Fig. 11.17). It is passed under the neck flaps and sutured to the tongue muscle and also to the tongue mucosa taking care to create as good a sulcus as possible because, if the patient can wear teeth after surgery, morbidity is minimal (Fig. 11.18).

A nasogastric tube is passed and is held in place for 10 days at which time it should be obvious whether or not the pedicle flap has taken. If it has then normal feeding can be resumed. If the flap begins to necrose then it will continue to do so for up to 10 days. The necrotic tissue should be removed but it is unnecessary to remove and replace the flap (as it would be if a forehead or delto pectoral flap was used) because the muscle should scar and provide bulk and also a surface which can later epithelialize. If it is kept free of necrotic debris with frequent débridement then maximal saving of muscle tissue is possible.

Total glossectomy

This operation may on rare occasions be necessary for tumours of the central tongue base that have not responded to radiation. It is on its own a difficult operation with which to obtain cancer clearance since tumours at the base of the tongue spread around the hyoid and via the vallecula into the pre-epiglottic space of the larynx. Thus the more logical procedure is a total glossolaryngectomy but, since this leaves the patient with absolutely no possibility of communication, even the hardiest quail at the prospect.

The actual excision of a whole tongue is simply performed with cutting diathermy going around the floor of the mouth and through the vallecula. The body of the hyoid must be removed to get some access to the pre-epiglottic space even if the larynx is left. The operation should be accompanied by at least an upper neck dissection so access is combined from the mouth and neck.

The large hole remaining in the mouth is closed with a pectoralis myocutaneous flap. This is not mobile but its bulk makes it superior to other flaps and swallowing is not too difficult. Speaking on the other hand is difficult since it takes a great deal of skill to learn new tricks of articulation.

The flap is stitched to the remaining mucosa of the floor of the mouth and to the vallecular remnant. The nasogastric tube can be removed usually at the 10th day and normal swallowing commenced.

Tumours of the floor of the mouth
Tumours of the floor of the mouth (or of tongue which involve the floor) present quite different problems of repair than those confined to the tongue alone.
1. The mandible survives irradiation poorly. If any surgery is performed on an irradiated mandible it can only be excisional. Reconstruction is unlikely to be successful. Osteoradionecrosis presents a real threat both early and late.
2. If a mandible is involved by tumour it needs to be excised and if not involved it does not need to be excised. The problem is that very often the tumour extends to mucosa on or near to the mandible and so there is often considerable doubt as to whether the mandible is involved or not. In these cases it is now common practice to do partial mandibulectomy and this avoids the necessity of a graft.
3. Bone grafting in tumour cases is different from bone grafting in benign disease. Patients with tumours requiring mandibular excision have dirty infected mouths and the degree of mandibular involvement is often in doubt. It is unreasonable to expect a bone graft to take as well here as in excision for benign disease. If a bone graft is used after mandibular excision then the best graft is a composite sternomastoid clavicle myocutaneous flap. It is however not the author's preference to use this flap if a neck dissection is performed since it severely compromises removal of the upper deep jugular lymph nodes. Thus if a tumour is big enough to warrant mandibular excision and not a neck dissection, then it is a rarity.

4. Secondary bone grafting is preferable to a primary graft since conditions are better and one can be sure about adequacy of two margins. It is still rarely done for the following reasons:
   a. The patient realizes that the defect left from a limited mandibular excision is minimal
   b. It is not certain that with a successful bone graft he will eat, speak and look better
   c. Patients often turn down 6–8 weeks of fixation for dubious benefits
5. There is a difference between taking bone from the lateral mandible or from the anterior arch. Defects of the lateral mandible are minimal but defects of the anterior arch are crippling and must be primarily grafted.

The following points apply to soft tissue replacement:
1. The aims are to produce a mobile tongue remnant and a sulcus so that dentures can be fitted.
2. A myocutaneous or axial flap produces mobility and fills out bulk but is very difficult to fashion into a sulcus into which dentures can be fitted.
3. Although split thickness grafts contract, they can be kept stretched in a sulcus provided a denture is worn. This technique of epithelial inlay is useful, and is described below.

Removal of floor of mouth tumour
A neck dissection will have been performed and the specimen left attached to the submandibular region. The tumour is fulgurated and a safe margin marked and tatooed. If the tumour is up to the mandible then a partial mandibulectomy with remnant of the lingual plate is planned.

The excision is performed intraorally and it is joined on to the neck dissection. This leaves everything pedicled on the mandible. Using a fissure burr the mandible is divided vertically a safe distance in front of and behind the tumour. Finally it is split vertically between the inner and outer plates so that the two vertical incisions are joined and the specimen can be removed. The edge of tongue is sewn to the mucosa remaining over the alveolus and cheek. This fixes the tongue laterally and speech is affected quite badly.

In six weeks when everything has healed, the patient is anaesthetized again and a skin graft is taken from the thigh (Fig. 11.19). A denture is prepared with a larger than usual lingual flange which is also bulky so that the graft can be pressed and fixed into place. The tongue/cheek anastomosis is then divided and when haemostasis has been secured the skin is put into the defect and held with the denture. This frees the tongue and since the patient now has a denture, both speaking and eating are improved.

The denture is wired into place for 10 days. Thereafter the dentist goes through various models until an acceptable final denture is created. From the start, how-

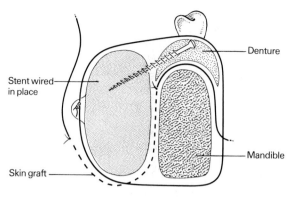

Fig. 11.19 Showing method of fixation of an epithelial inlay in the mouth

ever, the patient must wear the denture both day and night.

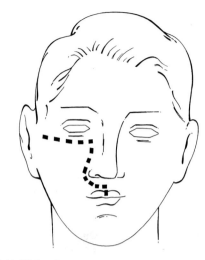

Fig. 11.20 Weber Fergusson incision

Palate

The palate is, according to the UICC, part of the oral cavity. Benign tumours are related to minor salivary glands and are usually pleomorphic adenomas. Malignant tumours are rarely primary on the hard palate and more usually represent spread from the nose and sinuses.

Removal of benign tumours

These present as smooth palatal swellings. They should be excised as pleomorphic adenomas and this includes the overlying mucosa. A bare area is left on the palate which is covered in the first instance with gauze impregnated with Whitehead's varnish. This is removed at 10 days, and the area left to epithelialise on its own.

Removal of malignant tumours

In malignant tumours of the palate the antrum must be removed but the orbit can be preserved.

Incisions. A Weber Fergusson incision is made (Fig. 11.20), starting at one of the creases lateral to the orbit and continuing for 4 cm below the lower eyelashes to the medial canthus. It then goes down in the nasojugal crease to the nasal ala. From here it goes under the nostril to the philtrum of the lip down which it turns to split the lip just to one side of the midline. It is completed by incising the gingivo buccal sulcus back to the tuberosity of the maxilla. The flap is dissected from the face of the maxilla with cutting diathermy because the facial muscles are very vascular. Dissection is continued backwards until the pterygo maxillary groove is identified.

Excision. The first step is to pass a Gigli saw through the nose into the nasopharynx. It is grasped here with Mixter forceps and drawn into the mouth. Keeping to one side of the tumour with a good margin the hard palate and alveolus are split. Using a chisel the nasal

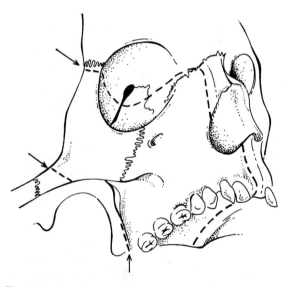

Fig. 11.21 Showing sites of bone cuts in maxillectomy

process of the frontal bone is split up to the frontonasal suture line which is the surface marking of the anterior fossa (Fig. 11.21). The chisel is turned at right angles here, and cuts through the ethmoids are made. The zygomatic arch is cut with a Gigli saw and the maxillary process of the zygoma is divided in a similar manner through the inferior orbital fissure. Finally, using a 5 cm osteotome in the pterygo maxillary fissure the maxilla is freed and removed. The bleeding from the maxillary artery is easily controlled and bleeding from the pterygoid plexus of veins is stopped by packing. The eye position is preserved if the lateral canthus, the periosteum of the orbital floor and the medial canthus are preserved.

Closure. It is better to have a prosthedontist present

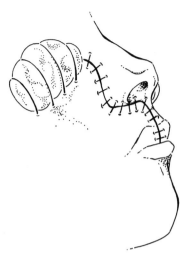

Fig. 11.22 Final closure following excision of maxillary tumour with pack in orbital cavity

to fit a denture and obturator immediately, but failing this the whole cavity can be packed with gauze soaked in Whitehead's varnish. The cheek flap is grafted with a split thickness graft to stop contraction and is returned to its original position. If an obturator is not fitted immediately it must be applied when the pack is removed at about the 10th day (Fig. 11.22).

Tumours of the external ear
Radiotherapy is the primary treatment of tumours of the auricle but surgery is preferable if cartilage is involved. If the tumour is on its commonest site, i.e. the helix, the incision is V-shaped. It is then easy to close the edges provided a little more cartilage than skin is ex-

cised. Closure can only be in the skin layer and 3/0 prolene is used (Figs. 11.23 & 11.24).

If the tumour is in the concha of the ear then primary closure is impossible without severely deforming the ear. A full thickness skin graft is necessary to fill the defect. This is best taken from the post auricular skin crease and primary closure in this site is very easy even after a large amount of skin is excised. The skin graft is stitched into the conchal defect with multiple 5/0 silk sutures and tied over a bolster of acriflavine wool which is left for one week.

CONGENITAL ABNORMALITIES

Cleft lip
This deformity is usually unilateral, occasional bilateral and very rarely median. It is due to failure of fusion between the maxillary process of one side (the lateral element) and the medial nasal process, which forms the central area or philtrum. (A median cleft is rare and is usually in reality a bilateral cleft with failure of development of the median part of the lip from the medial nasal process. Clefts of the lower lip are excessively rare and usually associated with gross facial maldevelopment.)

Clefts may involve the lip only: the lip, alveolus and palate as far as the incisive foramen (the so-called primary palate): or even the full length of the palate as far back as the uvula, i.e. the secondary palate. Clefts of the lip may be incomplete, that is affecting only the lower part of the lip and adjacent vermilion, or extend the full height of the lip involving the floor of the nostril in which case there are associated deformities of the ala of

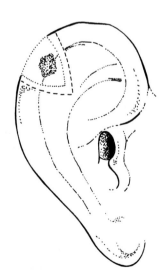

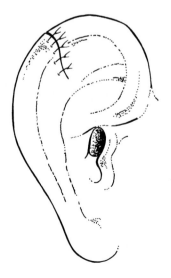

Figs. 11.23, 11.24 Wedge excision of ear tumour. Broken line indicates limit of cartilage excision

the nostril, displacement of the nasal septum and mal-alignment of the alveolar margin.

Closure of the cleft lip, especially the more complicated variety, should be attempted only by those who have had special experience and training. The general aims are to restore the normal symmetry of the upper lip, as gauged by the anatomical landmarks, to provide a mobile lip, close the nasal floor and anterior palate and correct any distortion of the alveolar arch. A well-repaired lip will go a long way towards improving any asymmetry of the nose.

Timing of the operation

Most surgeons prefer to delay repair of the cleft lip until the age of 3 months or so when the child is obviously thriving, gaining weight and has a haemoglobin level of at least 10 gm %. The intervening period allows one to exclude or treat other serious congenital malformations that could be a threat to life, i.e. oesophageal or intestinal atresia, heart defects, imperforate anus etc. The time interval also allows our orthodontic colleagues to carry out any presurgical orthodontic treatment that may be required and which can make the surgical closure simpler and more rewarding. There is no place whatever for immediate repair of the cleft lip and palate in the newly born infant. Surgery should be postponed if there is any doubt about the child's condition and if oral or nasal swabs show the presence of pathogens such as group A β-haemolytic streptococci. Surgery is best done under general anaesthesia with a flexometallic oral endotracheal tube in place and the pharynx carefully packed. It is a wise precuation to know the child's blood group and have some serum ready for cross matching and also to exclude the existence of any abnormal haemoglobin, particularly in patients in tropical countries or likely to have one of the various mediterranean forms of thalassaemia.

Various operations have been devised but they all entail paring the edges of the cleft and identification and dissection of the abnormally placed fibres of the orbicularis oris muscle. These fibres on the lateral side of the cleft will be found sweeping upwards and gaining an attachment to the bone at the piriform opening and on the medial side the same similar bundles of fibres will be found sweeping upwards and gaining an attachment to the base of the columella. These bundles must be detached, brought down to a more horizontal position and sutured across the lip to form a new orbicularis oris sphincter. The skin closure can take the form of a simple straight line repair (possibly incorporating a small Z-plasty) or alternatively both the muscle and the skin can be rotated or transposed as composite units to form a triangular flap repair (Tennison technique 1952) a quadrilateral flap repair (Le Mesurier technique 1949) or a rotation advancement type of repair (Millard technique 1958). For the bilateral clefts of the lip, combinations of the above repairs can be carried out on the opposite side at a second operation or preferably the repair can be carried out in one stage using the Manchester technique, which in practice proves to be the most simple and effective of all the methods hitherto described.

The mucosal layers of the lip and palate are closed with 4/0 black silk, the muscle in the lip is closed with 4/0 chromic catgut or dexon and the skin closed with interrupted 6/0 nylon sutures. At the end of the operation it is prudent to apply short splints to the arms to prevent the child from placing his or her fingers in the mouth and normal bottle or breast feeding is resumed as soon as possible. The sutures from the skin are removed under basal sedation or intravenous ketamine anaesthesia in 5–7 days time.

Cleft palate

Cleft palate is due to failure of the palatal processes of the maxilla to fuse with each other and with the premaxilla which is developed from the medial nasal process and which carries the 4 upper incisor teeth. The anterior (primary) palate, is usually closed at the same time as the lip repair. This is the part of the palate which extends forwards from the incisive foramen and passes through the alveolus on each side just lateral to the lateral incisor tooth. The secondary palate which may be cleft from the uvula as far forwards as the incisive foramen is usually closed in one stage most often between the age of 12–18 months. The aim of this operation is to provide an intact roof to the mouth and a mobile soft palate capable of providing competent velopharyngeal closure that will allow the child to speak well. If this function is not achieved, the characteristic cleft palate speech will remain. Numerous operations have been employed over the years to close palatal defects. The principles of surgical closure were laid down as the result of observations meticulously recorded by Veau (1931). He showed that not only must the palatal repair involve accurate suture of the nasal and oral mucosal lining to reduce scarring and prevent fistula formation but the palatal muscles must be sutured accurately across the midline after detaching their abnormal insertion into the posterior margin of the hard palate. Only in this way can the levator muscle sling act properly and move the soft palate backwards and upwards to provide adequate velopharyngeal closure. Most operations begin with paring of the edges of the cleft and this is followed then by mobilization of mucoperiosteal flaps raised from the oral surface of the palate on each side of the cleft with the help of relaxation incisions so that they can be slid immediately to meet in the midline without tension.

A more useful technique is to raise two flaps on each side and peel these back off the bony surface of the hard

Figs. 11.25–11.28 *Method of cleft palate repair*

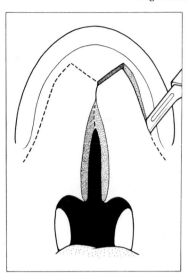

11.25 Skin flaps are raised from the hard palate

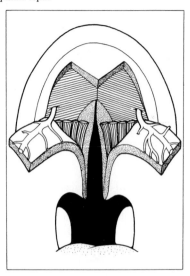

11.26 The posterior palatine arteries have been preserved and the levator palati muscles detached

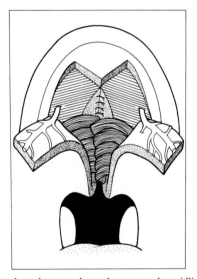

11.27 Muscle ends sutured together across the midline

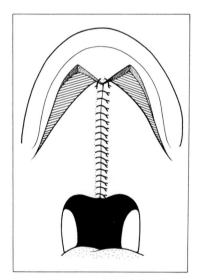

11.28 Oral mucosal layer sutured in the midline

palate (Figs. 11.25 & 11.26). This allows the surgeon to identify the posterior palatine arteries and carry out a careful dissection in each lateral recess, freeing the muscle attachment from the pterygoid plates and if need be fracturing the hamular process to release tension and allow the tensor palati muscle to act as an additional levator muscle. The posterior palatine arteries can be divided (some surgeons do this as a routine) but it is probably wise to preserve them and make a note to this effect in the operation record in case a palatal island flap is required later. With this kind of approach it is simple to detach the levator palati muscle from its abnormal attachment to the posterior border of the hard palate and bring the muscle ends across the midline where they can be sutured together with 4/0 chromic catgut (Figs. 11.27 & 11.28). The nasal lining over the full length of the palate is then closed with interrupted sutures of 4/0 chromic catgut and the oral mucosal layer is enclosed with interrupted 4/0 black silk sutures. At the end of the operation a simple pack of haemostatic gauze (Oxycel) can be placed in each lateral recess to act as a splint and control bleeding. After this operation the child's arms should be splinted to prevent the infant from inserting objects into the mouth and disturbing the palate. Oral feeding should be restarted as soon as possible, taking care after each feed to give the child plenty of water to wash out the palate and prevent food lodging in each lateral recess. There is no need to remove the black silk sutures from the palate as these will disintegrate and separate on their own spontaneously.

The aim of cleft lip and palate surgery is, as Professor Kilner used to stress, to make the child 'look well, eat well and speak well'. Many of these children may require secondary operations in later childhood and adult life to improve the appearance of the lip and nose, to deal with any fistulae which cause trouble and to carry out secondary operations if velopharyngeal closure is incomplete. Speech therapy will be required for most children with cleft palate. Hearing problems may need the attention of the ear, nose and throat specialist and dental problems of occlusion and normal dental care require the attention of our dental colleagues. A team approach is essential and it must be organized with care and compassion.

REFERENCES

Le Mesurier A B 1949 A method of cutting and suturing the lip in the treatment of complete unilateral clefts, Plastic and Reconstructive Surgery 4: 1

MacLennan W D 1977 Fractures of the malar (zygomatic) bone. Journal of the Royal College of Surgeons of Edinburgh 22: 187

Mayell M J 1973 Nasal fractures. Their occurrences, management and some late results. Journal of the Royal College of Surgeons of Edinburgh 18: 31

Millard D R 1958 A radical rotation in a single harelip. American Journal of Surgery 95: 318

Rowe N L 1982 Ankylosis of the temporo-mandibular joint. Journal of the Royal College of Surgeons of Edinburgh 27: 67

Tennison C W 1952 Repair of unilateral cleft lip by stencil method. Plastic and Reconstructive Surgery 9: 115

Veau V 1931 Division Palatine, Paris, Masson Cie

FURTHER READING

Burston W R 1958 The early orthodontic treatment of cleft palate conditions. Dental Practitioner 9: 41

Edwards M, Watson A C H 1980 Advances in the management of cleft palate. Churchill Livingstone, Edinburgh

Maisels D O 1974 The influence of presurgical orthodontic treatment upon the surgery of cleft lip and palate. British Journal of Orthodontics 1: 15

Papers of the Society of Head and Neck Surgeons 1982 American Journal of Surgery 144: No. 4

Rowe N L, Williams J L 1985 Maxillo-Facial injuries. Churchill Livingstone, Edinburgh

12

Operations on the neck and salivary glands

J. M. S. JOHNSTONE, A. G. D. MARAN & R. F. RINTOUL

GENERAL TECHNIQUE

Anaesthesia

This is maintained by tracheal intubation and has special advantages in cervical operations. It obviates the necessity for a face mask, the harness of which may encroach upon the operation field. It allows the anaesthetist full control from a distance, and ensures an adequate airway whatever the position of the head.

Preparation and draping of the part

All hair below the level of the ear on the affected side should be shaved off. Female patients should have their hair completely enclosed with a close fitting cap. Sterile towels must be applied according to a planned technique, by which it is virtually impossible for them to slip, and by which the patient's face and the anaesthetic apparatus are completely excluded from the field of operation. A satisfactory method of draping is shown in Figures 12.1 and 12.2.

Avoidance of disfigurement

Unless they are planned correctly and are sutured with care, incisions in the neck are liable to heal with widely stretched unsightly scars. Such scars, especially in female patients, may constitute a serious disfigurement. The measures necessary to minimize scarring do not normally detract from the efficacy of the operation; they involve the expenditure of a little more time and trouble on the part of the surgeon, but will be most gratefully appreciated by the patient.

Incisions

Unless wide access is of paramount importance (as in the case of operations on the air passages or for the removal of malignant glands), all incisions should be made transversely so that they lie in the natural creases or cleavage lines (Langer's lines) of the skin (Figs. 12.3 & 12.4). These represent the direction in which the skin splits, if punctured with a round instrument. The disposition of skin tension is such that, when an incision is made in the cleavage lines, there is little tendency for the wound

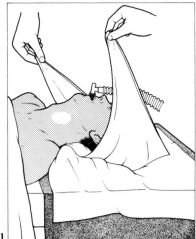

Fig. 12.1

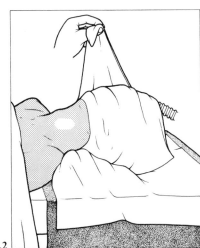

Fig. 12.2

Figs. 12.1, 12.2 Method of draping for operations on the neck. A sterile waterproof sheet and two sterile towels are laid beneath the head and neck. The uppermost towel is then folded across over the point of the chin, to cover the face and the anaesthetic tube

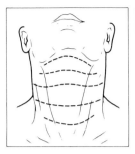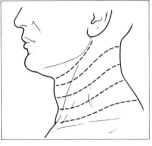

Figs. 12.3 & 12.4 Lines of the natural creases (*Langer's lines*) in the skin of the neck. All skin incisions should, if possible, be made parallel to these lines

edges to separate, so that the scar may become almost invisible. If a single transverse incision gives insufficient access, two such incisions at different levels may be employed (p. 253). Skin and superficial fascia are reflected to expose the underlying platysma, which is then divided in the same line, preferably at a slightly different level. Identification of the platysma as a separate layer is facilitated if the fibres overlying the sternomastoid are divided first.

Closure of the wound
The platysma is sutured as a separate layer. Fine needles and suture material are selected, and interrupted sutures are employed throughout. Each skin stitch is made to traverse the surface close to the wound, and is tied with only sufficient tightness to bring the edges into apposition. Michel clips are especially suitable for neck operations. Both stitches and clips should be removed on the 3rd or 4th day.

Avoidance of haematoma formation
This is most essential, since a haematoma, besides predisposing to infection, may result in a disfiguring scar due to subcutaneous fibrosis. All haemorrhage should therefore be arrested by ligature or diathermy coagulation, and as an additional safeguard the wound should usually be drained for 24–48 hours. *Redivac* drainage (p. 2) is especially useful in neck operations.

WOUNDS OF THE NECK

Cut-throat
This is due most commonly to attempted suicide. Since the head is thrown back at the time of wounding, the great vessels usually escape injury. In most wounds of any depth, however, the air passages are opened, either the thyrohyoid membrane or the thyroid cartilage itself being divided.

Operative repair should be carried out as soon as the

initial shock has been overcome. Where there has been extensive damage to the larynx, a tracheostomy should be performed in order to ensure that post-traumatic oedema will not obstruct the airway. If possible the tracheostomy is performed through an incision separate from the main wound. It may be done as the first step in the operation, and anaesthesia can then be maintained by way of the tracheostomy tube. When tracheostomy is not considered to be necessary, intratracheal anaesthesia is employed in the normal manner throughout the operation. The skin wound is enlarged sufficiently for adequate access to be obtained. Bleeding vessels (usually branches of the superior thyroid and lingual arteries) are secured. If the internal jugular vein has been damaged it should be ligatured above and below the site of injury. General débridement is carried out, and the severed structures, which may include the thyroid cartilage, are repaired as accurately as possible with interrupted sutures. The skin wound is closed by suture, a small drain or gauze pack being left in position to allow the escape of serum.

In wounds of greater depth, especially those above the thyroid cartilage, the cavity of the pharynx is sometimes opened. The pharyngeal wall should then be closed as accurately as possible with interrupted sutures. If the epiglottis is severed it is repaired in a similar manner. Because of the risk of infection, the superficial part of the wound (skin and platysma) may be left open and packed with gauze; it can then be closed by delayed primary suture after 2 or 3 days. In cases of gross damage, a nasogastric tube is passed into the stomach for feeding.

Homicidal cut-throat
The wound is usually in the lower part of the neck, and, if it is of any depth, it is likely to be fatal, because of injury to the great vessels. Treatment is on the lines already described.

Other wounds of the neck
Stabs, gunshot wounds, etc., occur only very occasionally in civilian practice. When vital structures escape immediate damage, the main danger is that of infection in the tissue spaces of the neck. The treatment is according to general surgical principles. Careful débridement is carried out, adequate access being obtained by enlargement of the wound, and by division of sternomastoid if necessary.

INFECTIONS OF THE NECK

Abscesses can occur in any of the fascial spaces of the neck. Up to 27 fascial spaces have been described but, since 'fascia' is merely a subjective assessment of the thickness of connective tissue, much of this is academic. There are only three important spaces in the neck where infections can occur and these are the retropharyngeal space, the paraphyngeal space and the submandibular space.

Retropharyngeal abscess

The retropharyngeal space lies between the pharynx and the posterior layer of the deep fascia which bounds the prevertebral space. It separates the pharynx from the vertebral column and extends from the base of the skull to the posterior mediastinum as far as the bifurcation of the trachea. Anteriorly it connects with the pretracheal space so that infections can spread via this latter space to the anterior mediastinum. In infants, the abscess is due to lymphadenitis secondary to an upper respiratory tract infection and in the adult usually signifies a tuberculous infection of the cervical spine.

Operation

In the child the abscess is best incised per orum. The child is placed in the supine position with the head extended and, using a tonsil gag with a tongue plate, the bulging posterior pharyngeal wall is easily seen. A vertical incision is made in the midline and the pus is evacuated. Using finger dissection, the space is opened up so that any loculated areas are drained. *In the adult* the space is best approached from the lateral direction. A horizontal incision is made, one finger breadth below the angle of the jaw. The tail of the parotid gland is dissected from the sternomastoid and this latter structure is retracted. The carotid sheath is identified and retracted posteriorly. The superior constrictor is then identified and, by passing a finger lateral and posterior to the pharynx, the retropharyngeal space can be entered. The loculated area is broken down with blunt finger dissection and the pus evacuated. A drain is inserted into the space and brought out through the lateral side of the neck. The drain is gradually shortened over a period of three or four days and, when confirmation has been received of the tuberculous origin, the appropriate chemotherapy should be commenced.

Parapharyngeal abscess

The parapharyngeal space lies lateral to the pharynx connecting with the retropharyngeal space posteriorly. Laterally, it is bounded by the lateral pterygoid muscle and the parotid gland. It extends from the base of the skull to the level of the hyoid bone where it is limited by the fascia over the submandibular gland. Posteriorly is the carotid sheath. Infection gains access to this space from either a dental or a tonsillar infection. The origin of the infection should be identified and dealt with prior to drainage of the space. Some 60% of patients have an associated tonsillitis and so the tonsil should be re-

moved. The remainder of the patients have an infected lower third molar tooth which should be extracted.

Operation

A horizontal incision is made on the anterior border of the sternomastoid muscle (Figs. 12.5–12.7) and the muscle is retracted posteriorly. The deep cervical fascia is usually found to be thickened due to the infection and this must be broken down in order to gain access to the space. Once the pus is evacuated blunt finger dissection should open the space widely from the base of the skull to the hyoid. A drain is inserted and the appropriate chemotherapy commenced. The drain is shortened over a period of three or four days and, once the tonsil or tooth has been dealt with, recurrence is unlikely.

Submandibular space infections (Ludwigs angina)

The submandibular space is bounded above by the mucous membrane of the floor of the mouth and tongue and below by the deep fascia, and extends from the hyoid to the mandible. It is divided into two by the mylohyoid

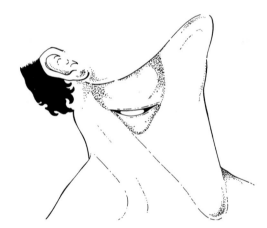

Fig. 12.5 Incision for parapharyngeal abscess

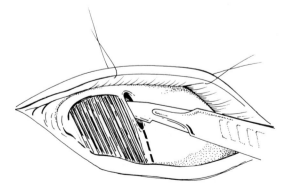

Fig. 12.6 Incising the fascia at the anterior border of sternomastoid

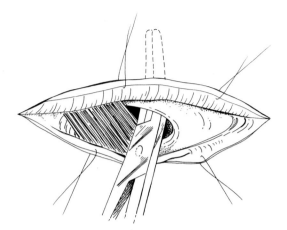

Fig. 12.7 Opening into parapharyneal space

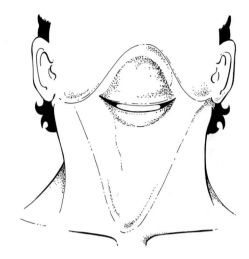

Fig. 12.8 Incision for submandibular space abscess

muscle and so the submandibular gland, which is wrapped around the mylohyoid muscle, extends into both parts of the space. The space superior to the mylohyoid muscle is called the sublingual space and contains the sublingual gland; the space inferior to the muscle is the submandibular space and contains the body of the submandibular gland. Anteriorly lies the submental space between the two anterior bellies of digastric.

Operation
The vast majority of infections of this space are of dental origin. The offending tooth should be identified and removed. Incision of the space is not usually rewarded by evacuation of much pus. There is generally cellulitis of the floor of the mouth and submandibular space but, by merely opening the space after removal of the tooth and the administration of the appropriate antibiotic, resolution is usually rapid.

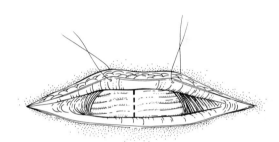

Fig. 12.9 Midline vertical incision in mylohyoid

urged that the swollen and degenerated segment of muscle should be excised although it often resolves spontaneously. If the diagnosis is not made until the age of 5 or 6 when muscle-shortening has occurred, operation may then be advised before facial asymmetry and secondary changes in the cervical spine develop.

Operation
A horizontal incision 5 cm in length is made with its centre over the lower part of sternomastoid 2.5 cm above the clavicle. Under direct vision both heads of the muscle are then divided, together with the deep cervical fascia, and are allowed to retract. If scalenus anterior is shortened and is found to be preventing correction of the deformity, it also is divided, together with the carotid sheath if necessary. The internal jugular vein and phrenic nerve should be identified and safeguarded. The platysma and skin are sutured, a small drain being left in the wound.

After treatment is most essential in order to prevent recurrence of the deformity. Physiotherapy is started two or three days after operation with suitable analgesia. This involves manipulating the head and neck through a full range of movements four times each day.

CONGENITAL ABNORMALITIES

Congenital torticollis
This is generally regarded as being due to a birth injury causing either rupture of the fibres of sternomastoid or of the vessels supplying it. Degeneration of the affected fibres occurs, and is followed by fibrous tissue replacement, which results in contracture (or failure of normal growth) of the muscle. If the condition is untreated the other muscles of the affected side and the deep fascia become shortened as well. An alternative view is that the condition is due to a developmental aplasia of the muscles and other soft-tissue structures on the affected side of the neck.

When the condition is diagnosed shortly after birth, at the stage of the 'sternomastoid tumour', it has been

Branchial cyst

A branchial cyst is derived from the second branchial pouch; it is lined with ciliated epithelium and gradually accumulates a cholesterol rich medium. The cyst commonly presents in early adult life as a painless, globular swelling beneath the angle of the jaw at the anterior border of sternomastoid, roughly one third of the distance between the mastoid process and sternum. Cysts can, however, occur anywhere in the neck without any communication with the pharynx, which gives rise to speculation that a branchial cyst is, in fact, an epithelial cyst within a lymph node.

Treatment is by excision unless the lesion is secondarily infected in which case incision and drainage may be necessary.

Operation

The patient is placed supine, with the head and the neck slightly extended and the chin rotated to the opposite side (Fig. 12.10). A skin crease incision is made over the swelling at least 2 cm below the angle of the jaw (so as to avoid the cervical branch of the facial nerve) and carried deep through platysma. The deep cervical fascia is incised along the anterior border of the sternomastoid and the muscle is retracted posteriorly. The cyst can then be enucleated with ease but care should be taken on the deep surface which may lie between the internal and external carotid arteries (Fig. 12.11). Occasionally, a track passes between these two vessels and can be traced up to the base of the tonsil, although there is no necessity to open into the pharynx.

Branchial fistula

A branchial fistula is probably derived from incomplete obliteration of the precervical sinus, an epithelial lined space formed by down growth of the second branchial arch over the second, third and fourth branchial clefts to fuse with the fifth arch. The small opening of the fis-

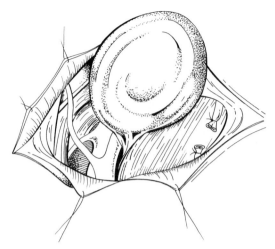

Fig. 12.11 Branchial cyst extending deeply between the internal and external carotid arteries

tula lies over the lower third of the anterior border of the sternomastoid and the tract, if complete, runs upwards to the pharangeal wall at the level of the palatine tonsil. The fistula lies between structures derived from the second and third branchial cleft and therefore passes between the internal and external carotid arteries. More often however the tract extends for a variable distance upwards and ends blind and should therefore be termed a sinus. Occasionally the fistula is derived from the first branchial cleft; the opening then lies over the anterior border of the upper third of sternomastoid and runs towards the external auditory meatus in close relation to the facial nerve.

The small opening of the branchial fistula intermittently discharges a glairy, mucinous substance and may be recurrently inflamed. The extent of the lesion may be demonstrated by a sinogram using lipiodol. Treatment is by excision of the fistula and this must be complete so as to avoid recurrence.

Operation

The patient is positioned as for excision of a branchial cyst. Methylene blue is injected into the fistula as this will be seen if the tract is inadvertently divided during dissection. Two skin crease incisions may be used (Fig. 12.12); the first is an eliptical incision around the opening of the fistula and the second is made above the upper border of the thyroid cartilage. Through the first incision the tract is traced deep through the cervical fascia at the anterior border of sternomastoid and it is then traced upwards towards the carotid bifurcation. The fistula is then passed up from the first to the second incision for the remaining part of the dissection. If complete, the tract leads deep between the internal and external carotid arteries (Fig. 12.13) and between the

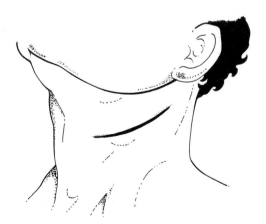

Fig. 12.10 Incision for branchial cyst

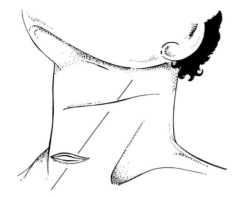

Fig. 12.12 Two incisions for branchial fistula (see text)

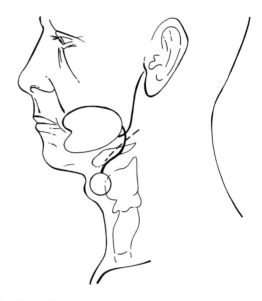

Fig. 12.14 Showing position of thyroglossal duct or the track of a fistula

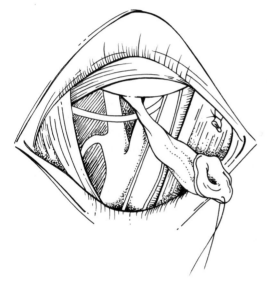

Fig. 12.13 Branchial fistulous track passing between internal and external carotid arteries

hypoglossal and glossopharyngeal nerves, and is divided flush with the pharyngeal wall. A finger introduced into the mouth and pushed against the inside of the pharyngeal wall aids the last stage of dissection. Finally a drain should be laid along the length of the wound and the tissues closed in layers.

Thyroglossal cyst and fistula

The thyroid gland develops from the caudal end of a diverticulum known as the thyroglossal duct. The duct grows downwards in the midline from the foramen caecum and is closely related to the posterior aspect of the hyoid cartilage (Fig. 12.14). Incomplete regression of the duct may result in a thyroglossal cyst or fistula.

A cyst may lie above or, more commonly, below the hyoid bone and is found in the midline unless pushed to one side by the thyroid cartilage. The lesion is spher-

ical, tense, sometimes inflamed and moves with swallowing or protrusion of the tongue. It may resemble ectopic thyroid and, if necessary, must be differentiated by a thyroid scan. A fistula probably forms after spontaneous discharge or drainage of an infected thyroglossal cyst. The opening lies in the midline and intermittently discharges a glairy mucinous substance.

Treatment of both cyst and fistula is by excision. To prevent recurrence the remnant of the thyroglossal duct must be traced back to the foramen caecum at the junction of the middle and posterior third of the tongue.

Operation

An endotracheal tube should be passed and the patient is placed supine with a sandbag under the shoulders and the head on a ring. A skin crease incision 4 cm long is made over the prominence of the cyst and carried deep through platysma. The deep cervical fascia is divided longitudinally in the midline to expose the cyst which can then be mobilized by blunt dissection. It must be assumed that a connection persists between the cyst and the foramen caecum. A core of tissue from the deeper aspect of the cyst is therefore traced to the inferior border of the hyoid bone (Figs. 12.15 & 12.16), the middle 1 cm of the bone is carefully mobilized from the underlying thyrohyoid membrane and excised with bone nibblers. The core with the adherent excised segment of bone can then be traced towards the foramen caecum. A finger introduced into the mouth to push the posterior part of the tongue downwards and forwards aids the last part of the dissection. The wound should be closed with a drain in place.

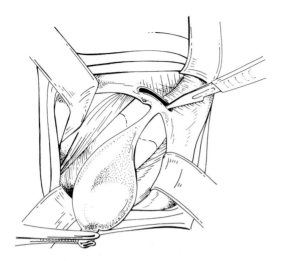

Fig. 12.15 Thyroglossal tract passing deep to the hyoid, the central part of which is being excised

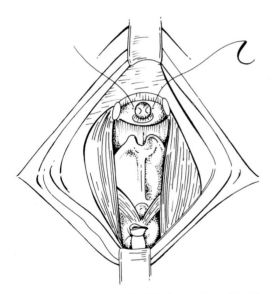

Fig. 12.16 Closure of vallecula following excision of hyoid

Dissection of the thyroglossal fistula may be carried out through two small skin crease incisions both for convenience of access and improved cosmetic appearance. First, the fistulous opening is excised with a transverse elliptical incision and the tract followed proximally through the deep fascia towards the inferior border of the hyoid bone. A second incision is then made at the level of the hyoid and the dissected tract passed up from below. From that point the dissection is described above.

Lymphangioma

Lymphangiomas or tumours of lymph vessels, are of

three clinical types: simple lymph cysts, cavernous lymphangiomas and cystic lymphangiomas. The latter (known as cystic hygromas) are extremely rare but quite dramatic on presentation in the newborn child. The aim of treatment is to remove as much as possible without damaging the child but, before treatment is commenced, a chest X-ray should be taken to make sure that there is no mediastinal extension which could complicate an anaesthetic. The parents should be warned that much of the cyst will remain at the end of the first operation and that several operations will be needed over the ensuing few years, before final eradication of the cyst is accomplished. The main structures at risk during the operation are the facial nerve, the internal jugular vein and, to a lesser extent, the carotid artery.

Operation

In a large cystic hygroma, an incision is made in the skin crease lines over the maximum convexity of the cyst (Fig. 12.17). The skin is dissected very carefully off the thin walled cyst and, at the end of the operation, redundant skin is excised. Blunt finger dissection is used to mobilize as much of the cyst as possible. The position of the facial nerve has to be identified for complete excision but not during this initial operation. A child's mastoid is not well developed and the facial nerve is not protected by the mastoid in the newborn. Dissection should therefore stop 2.5 cm inferior to the mastoid in order to preserve the nerve. Extensions of the cyst can go into the floor of the mouth, the axilla, the pectoral region, the retropharyngeal space and the parapharyn-

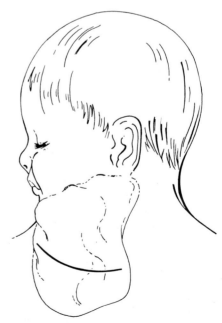

Fig. 12.17 Incision for cystic hygroma

geal space. Not all of these can be excised at the initial operation. There is little point in injecting sclerosing fluid into the remnant because the cyst is multilocular and the sclerosant will have little effect.

Laryngocoele

Lower animals often have air sacs to enable them to submerge for long periods. The remnant of these air sacs in the human is the ventricle and saccule of the larynx. This area can be small or it can be very large. In the latter instance if the patient takes up a hobby such as blowing an instrument, air will distend the saccule pushing it out through the thyrohyoid membrane and creating an airsac in the neck. This diagnosis must be kept in mind for any neck cyst which shows air on plain X-ray. A diagnosis of gas gangrene is often made in error on seeing this radiographic finding.

Operation

An incision is made over the air sac at the level of the thyrohyoid membrane. Skin flaps are elevated and the sac is always seen anterior to the sternomastoid muscles. The sac is mobilized to the thyrohyoid membrane where it will have a very broad base. If it is merely excised at this point in the operation, recurrence will be inevitable because a large portion of the sac will remain within the larynx. The upper half of the thyroid ala is therefore removed (Fig. 12.18) and when this is done the narrow neck of the sac, as it enters the ventricle of the larynx, is seen. It can be transected and ligated at this point and the sac removed. The ligated point can be reinforced by stitching the strap muscles to the remnants of the thyro-

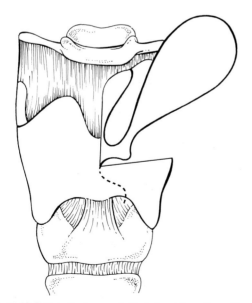

Fig. 12.18 Removal of upper half of thyroid cartilage allows laryngocoele to be removed at its neck

hyoid membrane. A drain is inserted and the wound is closed in two layers.

Cervical rib and the 'scalenous syndrome'

The mechanism by which a cervical rib can give rise to vascular or neuritic manifestations in the upper limb is in considerable dispute. The usual explanation is that stretching and friction occurs as the lower trunk of the brachial plexus arches over the cervical rib, or over the fibrous band extending forwards from an incomplete rib. This explanation, however, will not fit all cases since identical symptoms can occur in the absence of any demonstrable bony abnormality. In such cases it is thought that the nerve trunk or artery may be chafed or otherwise irritated by hypertrophy, spasm or abnormal insertion of one of the scalene muscles (scalenus anterior or scalenus medius). *Postfixation* of the brachial plexus has also been held responsible.

Operative treatment is indicated in patients whose symptoms are sufficient to incapacitate them, and who are unrelieved by exercises and physiotherapy (Roos, 1982).

Excision of a cervical rib

This is usually carried out where this anomaly is present. A sandbag is placed between the patient's shoulders, and the arm is drawn strongly downwards. The customary approach is through an incision extending laterally from the clavicular attachment of sternomastoid to the anterior border of trapezius at the junction of its middle and lower thirds. The lateral border of sternomastoid is then retracted medially and the phrenic nerve is sought. When this nerve has been exposed, it is elevated from the surface of scalenus anterior, which is then divided at its insertion into the first rib (or into the cervical rib if this is complete). The knife edge is kept against the bone, so that the subclavian artery and the thyrocervical trunk are not endangered. The suprascapular nerve is then sought and is used as a guide to identification of the trunks of the brachial plexus (p. 71). The plexus is retracted gently downwards and forwards; the posterior (or lateral) border of scalenus medius is defined, and the fibres of this muscle inserted into the cervical rib (and possibly burying it from sight), are erased from it. The rib is next disarticulated at its attachment to the seventh cervical vertebra, or is divided as far posteriorly as possible, and is then removed.

Scalenotomy

This may be considered as an alternative to excision of a cervical rib, and it is the procedure of choice in cases where no cervical rib is present. Division of scalenus anterior alone may be successful in relieving symptoms; this acts by allowing the subclavian artery and brachial plexus to slide forwards to a lower level on the first rib, so that stretching, compression, or friction may thereby be abolished. The operation should comprise more, however, than simple division of the scalenus anterior. The subclavian artery and the lower trunk of the brachial plexus should be examined carefully and freed from any chafing or other irritation. If the nerve trunks appear to be stretched over the medial tendinous fibres of scalenus medius, these fibres also should be divided.

OPERATIONS ON THE PHARYNX

Nasopharynx

The nasopharynx lies behind the nose and extends from the base of the skull to the level of the soft palate.

Adenoidectomy

Excision of the nasopharyngeal tonsils (adenoids) is indicated when chronic infection leads to obstruction and persistant mouth breathing.

Operation. The child's trachea is intubated with an oral tube and the head is extended. A gag is inserted in the mouth and the adenoid pad is pushed into the midline as far as possible. A Laforce adenotome is inserted behind the palate and the adenoids are pushed into the cup. On closing the blade the adenoids are removed and the bleeding is easily controlled with packing.

Removal of angiofibroma of the naso-pharynx

The diagnosis is made by angiography and from this investigation, the main feeding vessels can be identified. If facilities exist, a radiologist may be able to embolize the vessel making the subsequent excision less vascular. If this facility does not exist then the maxillary artery should be clipped. The approach to this vessel is through the anterior wall of the maxillary sinus via an incision in the gingivolabial sulcus. The posterior wall of the sinus is removed and the fat of the pterygo maxillary fossa is dissected until the tortuous artery is seen. A clip ligature can be applied to it at this point.

A transpalatal approach is then commenced. An incision is made medial to the course of the palatine arteries anteriorly and behind the greater palatine foramen posteriorly (Figs. 12.19 & 12.20). The flap is dissected from the hard palate and, at the posterior end of the hard palate, the nasopharynx is entered. The tumour then usually bulges down into the wound and it is removed by finger dissection. When dissection is commenced there usually is copious bleeding. No attempts should be made to stop this bleeding because it will fail; the only way to stop the bleeding is to remove the tumour as quickly as possible and to pack the nasopharynx.

When bleeding has stopped a postnasal pack is inserted and the palate replaced and sewn in place with

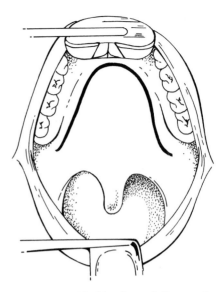

Fig. 12.19 Transpalatal incision for angiofibroma of nasopharynx

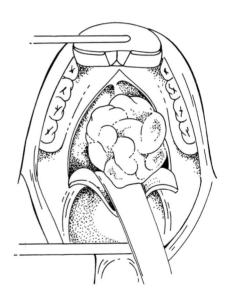

Fig. 12.20 Angiofibroma seen through transpalatal incision

chromic catgut. The postnasal pack is removed after 72 hours.

Oropharynx

The oropharynx extends from the level of the soft palate to the hyoid bone, communicating freely with the mouth.

Tonsillectomy

Apart from tonsillitis uncontrolled by antibiotics, this operation is performed in order to biopsy a tonsil suspected of being affected by lymphoma. It is also performed to obtain histology of a tonsil when there is a malignant neck node with no other discernible primary site; it is becoming increasingly clear that small tumours of the tonsil can present with metastatic neck nodes.

Operation. The patient is anaesthetized with a nasal endotracheal tube and placed supine with the head extended. The tonsil is grasped with volsellum forceps and pulled towards the midline. The mucosa is incised with a number 12 blade. Using blunt dissection with Metzenbaum scissors, a plane is opened up in the peritonsillar space between the tonsil capsule and the superior constricter. Bleeding is controlled by diathermy and dissection is continued down until a tonsil pedicle is established at the base of the tongue. It is then removed.

Removal of the lateral wall of the oropharynx for carcinoma (Commando Operation)

This operation is performed for carcinoma invading the tonsil, palate or base of tongue. It is always combined with a radical neck dissection and the name Commando Operation reflects this; it involves combined excision of mandible and oropharynx.

Incision. The access to the oropharynx and mandible is obtained via the upper neck incision (p. 253). The neck dissection specimen is pedicled on to the angle of the mandible and the upper flap is dissected over the angle and up to the interdental line. The masseter is divided from its insertion onto the mandible and, using a periostial elevator, all the soft tissue (masseter and parotid) is elevated subperiostially up to the coronoid process, the notch and the mandibular neck. Anteriorly a similar elevation is performed up to the mental foramen.

Excision. The temporalis muscle is divided from the coronoid process with Mayo scissors. The neck of the mandible is divided with a Gigli saw (Fig. 12.21). No attempt should be made to remove the head of the mandible as this often causes bleeding from the pterygoid plexus of veins which is troublesome. With a Gigli saw the horizontal ramus of the mandible is divided posterior to the mental foramen.

The oral cavity is entered at this point and the mandible is swung laterally. The tumour is seen and, using cutting diathermy, the tongue is incised 2 cm from the tumour margin. Once the lateral edge and base of the tongue have been incised, the diathermy incision continues up the posterolateral wall and finally the soft palate, always staying 2 cm away from the tumour edge. This leaves the specimen pedicled on to the parapharyngeal space (Fig. 12.22). With a finger protecting the carotid artery in this space the specimen is finally removed, in continuity with the neck dissection.

Closure. While the wound can be closed primarily this is not advised since it cripples the oral cavity and causes difficulty in swallowing. Fresh tissue should be brought in and primary reconstruction using the pectoralis major musculocutaneous flap is favoured.

In order to cut this flap a line is drawn from the acromion to the xiphisternum. A perpendicular is dropped from this line to the midpoint of the clavicle (Fig. 12.23). This new surface marks the course of the thoraco-acromial artery which supplies the flap. At the lower end of this line, approximating the lower edge of pectoralis major, an area of skin the required size is incised. A plane is made deep to pectoralis major and the pectoralis major is incised. A thin muscle pedicle following the line of the artery is created and dissected subcutaneously up to the clavicle. The muscle pedicle with the attached myocutaneous island is passed under the neck skin and placed in the defect where it is sewn in place using 2/0 dexon in two layers.

Two suction drains are inserted and the neck wound is closed as for a radical neck dissection (p. 255).

The gap in the chest wall from which the flap was taken can be closed primarily by undercutting and approximating the edges.

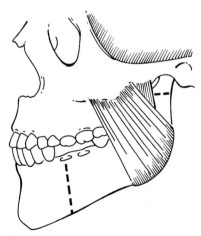

Fig. 12.21 Showing sites on bone cuts for excision of mandible

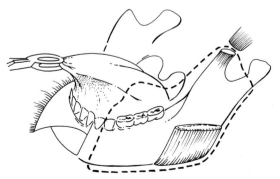

Fig. 12.22 Showing the extent of tissue removal in Commando Operation

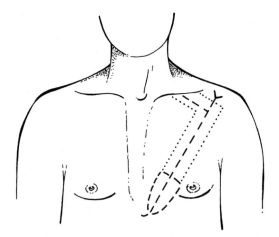

Fig. 12.23 Markings for pectoralis major myocutaneous flap

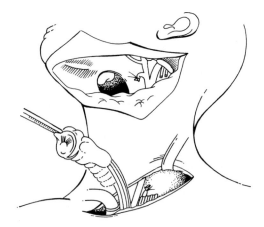

Fig. 12.24 The larynx has been freed leaving an orostome. Oesophagus is transected in the upper third

After care and complications. A nasogastric tube is passed and feeding commenced when bowel sounds are heard. It is removed a week after it has been established that fluid can be drunk with no fistula being apparent. If a fistula is noted the nasogastric tube is left in place until the fistula closes. Fistulae are very rare with a myocutaneous flap because of the muscle bulk that is brought in and also because of the excellent blood supply. If a large fistula develops it must be allowed to stabilize itself and it can then be closed after about a month using local skin to supply inner lining and a pectoral flap for outer lining.

Hypopharynx

The hypopharynx extends from the hyoid level to the cricopharyngeus muscle. It consists of a posterior wall, the piriform sinus and the post cricoid region. Tumours in these sites are treated with radiation unless a neck gland is palpable when primary surgery is the treatment of choice. Tumours of the piriform sinus and post cricoid regions form 90% of tumours of the hypopharynx, and although some of the piriform sinus tumours can be dealt with by laryngectomy and partial pharyngectomy, the majority require a total laryngopharyngectomy or laryngo-pharyngo-oesophagectomy.

Laryngopharyngectomy

Incision. If the patient has had an initial radical neck dissection the head is turned back into the midline and extended. A tracheostomy is performed between the second and third rings after dividing the thyroid isthmus. A number 12 tracheostomy tube is inserted and general anaesthesia continued via this route.

Excision. The sternomastoid on the unoperated side is retracted laterally and a plane is developed medial to the carotid sheath down to the prevertebral fascia. From this plane it is easy to free the laryngopharynx from base

of tongue to the oesophagus. The strap muscles are divided at the lower end and the lobe of the thyroid on the affected side is left attached to the specimen. The other lobe is freed from the specimen and retracted laterally with the blood supply intact.

The upper end of the specimen is divided above the hyoid bone and the base of the tongue is transected through the vallecula. The transection is completed through the posterior pharyngeal wall. The specimen is swung downwards and the oesophagus is transected at least 3 cm distal to the tumour (Fig. 12.24). Resection is completed by cutting the posterior wall of the trachea at the level of the tracheostome.

Closure. The tracheostome is brought out through the lower skin flap and stitched in place as described on page 250. The gap between the tongue and the oesophagus is best filled with a deltopectoral flap (p. 14).

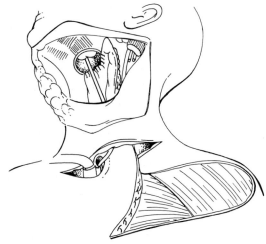

Fig. 12.25 Upper end of deltopectoral flap being sewn to posterior pharyngeal wall

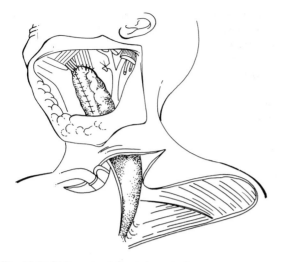

Fig. 12.26 Deltopectoral flap being tubed

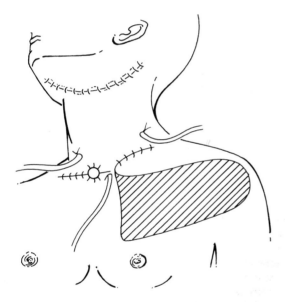

Fig. 12.27 Completion of laryngopharyngectomy. Split skin graft is applied to the chest wound

The upper end is sutured to the tongue and posterior pharyngeal wall in two layers with 2/0 dexon (Figs. 12.25–12.27). The flap is tubed, skin surface in, with the same material making sure the edges of the skin are inverted into the tube. The lower end is stitched end to side to the oesophageal remnant. A nasogastric tube is passed and the skin is closed in two layers. The chest wound is skin grafted and, after three weeks, the tube is divided and the remnant returned to the chest wall.

After care and complications. If the blood supply remains intact then the nasogastric tube can be withdrawn about the 10th day. Nearly always there is a small leak from the lower anastomosis but this will self heal in about a week.

After two weeks the tracheostomy tube can be removed and either a silastic stoma button can be used or else the stoma left open. It is rare to establish oesophageal speech after this operation.

Total laryngo-pharyngo-oesophagectomy

If the tumour goes from the post cricoid area further than 3 cm down the oesophagus then a limited laryngopharyngectomy is not sufficient and a total oesophagectomy is required. This allows of replacement by a viscus such as colon, stomach or revascularised jejunum. Since transposing the stomach only involves one anastomosis, i.e. in the neck, this is preferred (p. 303).

After the pharynx has been transected or the base of the tongue and the larynx divided from the trachea, the specimen is pedicled on the oesophagus. This can be dissected with a finger down as far as the aortic arch; via a midline abdominal incision the stomach is pedicled on the right gastric artery and the first part of the duodenum is freed. The vagi are transected and the oesophagus is dissected up to the arch. The stomach can then be pulled up into the neck through the posterior mediastinum. The oesophagus is divided from the stomach and the cardia is closed in two layers. The fundus is opened to the appropriate size and this is sewn in layers to the posterior pharyngeal wall and tongue base.

Feeding by mouth can usually be started by the 10th day.

Removal of a pharyngeal pouch

A pharyngeal pouch is an outpouching of the mucosa of the posterior wall of the hypopharynx through the weakest part of the wall. Food passes into it more readily than into the oesophagus and some degree of obstruction inevitably develops.

As a preliminary to the operation a wide oesophagoscope is passed so that the pouch, the oesophagus and the intervening bar can be seen at the one time. The pouch is then packed with gauze soaked in acriflavine in order to facilitate dissection. The gauze pack is brought out through the mouth so that it can be pulled out when the pouch is excised. It is also advisable to pass a nasogastric tube into the stomach.

Excision. A horizontal incision is made on the left side of the neck at the level of the cricoid cartilage (Fig. 12.28). The sternomastoid is retracted and the carotid sheath is identified. The middle thyroid vein should be ligated and divided to open the access. The pouch is often firmly attached to the oesophagus but a plane can usually be found quite easily and the pouch dissected up to its pedicle. It is unwise to remove the pack prior to this being achieved. The pedicle is

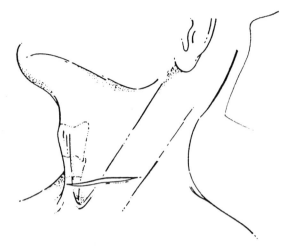

Fig. 12.28 Incision for removal of pharyngeal pouch.

OPERATIONS ON THE LARYNX

Laryngotomy

Since tracheostomy is a difficult operation for the inexperienced, acute airway obstruction is best dealt with by a laryngotomy. The cricothyroid membrane is just below the skin surface and may be palpated easily. The thyroid is distant and only the strap muscles separate it from the skin.

The head is extended and an incision is made with a number 10 scalpel blade above the upper border of the cricoid cartilage (Fig. 12.29). This is deepened into the cricothyroid membrane and an airway is established. The blade is then turned through 45°. No tube should be inserted into this slit but it does give time for proper arrangements to be made for a tracheostomy or intubation.

transected and sutures placed at each end of the opening into the pharynx as holding sutures.

A cricopharyngeal myotomy is an essential part of this operation. A finger is inserted into the oesophagus in between the sutures and passed through the cricopharyngeus. As far posteriorly as possible in order to avoid damaging the recurrent laryngeal nerve, the criopharyngeus is incised with a number 11 blade down to the mucosa. In order to accomplish a good myotomy it must be at least 4 cm long. The opening in the pharynx is then closed with inverting sutures to the mucosa using 3/0 chromic catgut. The muscle layer is sutured with 3/0 dexon. A suction drain is inserted and the wound closed in layers. The nasogastric tube can be removed in five days provided the wound is airtight, and feeding commenced.

Alternative operations for pharyngeal pouch
1. Dohlman's method
   This requires special instruments including a Dohlman's endoscope with two beaks one of which fits into the pouch and the other of which enters the mouth of the oesophagus. The bar between the two is then seen and can be incised using the special diathermy forceps.
2. Inversion of the pouch
   This is a satisfactory method provided a myotomy is also performed. The pouch is identified and inverted into the oesophagus and the inversion site oversewn with dexon.
3. Diverticulopexy
   This involves dissecting the pouch and stitching the fundus as high as possible so that the neck is directed downwards.

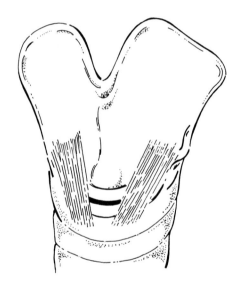

Fig. 12.29 Incision for laryngotomy

Laryngectomy

In this section only the operation of total laryngectomy will be described. Depending on where the tumour is in the larynx, a number of operations have been devised to preserve or reconstruct enough of the larynx to provide voice and to avoid the need for a tracheostomy. There are also a number of variants of the total laryngectomy which create a fistula between the trachea and oesophagus so that voice may be produced. All these operations are, however, very specialized and the general surgeon would not expect to do them. Total laryngectomy is the operation of the choice in cases which are not suitable for one of the partial operations and in whom radiotherapy has failed to eradicate the tumour.

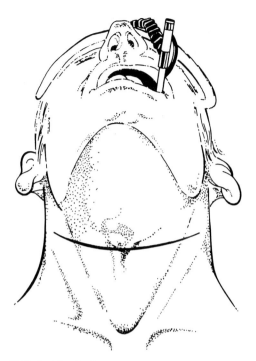

Fig. 12.30 Incision for laryngectomy

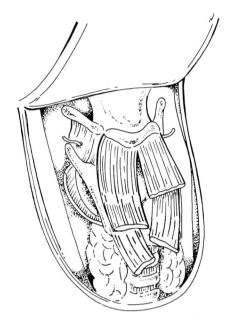

Fig. 12.31 Dissection completed showing horns of hyoid and thyroid

It is also the first line of treatment in T3 and T4 laryngeal tumours with palpable neck nodes. In these latter instances it will be performed along with a radical neck dissection.

Incision (Fig. 12.30)
If the operation is to be performed with a radical neck dissection, then a horizontal incision is made at the level of the thyroid prominence. If a neck dissection is performed then a Schechter incision (p. 253) is used giving basically the same approach to the larynx. In the suprasternal notch, the midline site of the permanent tracheostomy is marked.

Excision
The strap muscles are divided at their lower end and the thyroid isthmus identified and ligated. One lobe of the thyroid gland must be excised in T3 and T4 tumours. The sternomastoid muscle on each side is retracted and a plane created between the carotid sheath and the larynx. The suprahyoid muscles are dissected from the body of the hyoid. The latter is grasped with Allis forceps and drawn forwards so that the lesser horns can be dissected out. The stylohyoid ligament is cut on each side and the hyoglossus is divided from the greater horn on each side. The thyrohyoid ligament is then divided to display the tip of the greater horn (Figs. 12.31 & 12.32). The muscles are carefully dissected in the midline until the outline of the epiglottus is seen. This is grasped

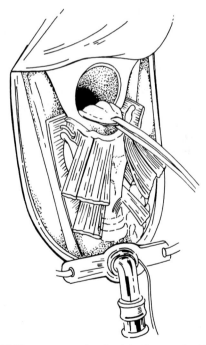

Fig. 12.32 Pharynx opened and epiglottis grasped with Allis forceps

with Allis forceps and pulled forwards. Entry into the pharynx is made through the vallecula and the tip of the epilottis is then seen.

The first cut is made from the tip of the epiglottis to the tip of the greater horn on each side. The second cut is from this point to the tip of the superior cornu of the thyroid cartilage, identifying and ligating the superior laryngeal artery as it crosses the cornu. At this point, the tumour can be seen and assessed by pulling the larynx forwards. The constrictor muscles are next divided from the posterior lamina of the thyroid cartilage and this also divides the mucosa of the pyriform fossa.

The level for the permanent tracheostomy can now be established and the trachea is transected. A tracheostomy tube is inserted, the endotracheal tube withdrawn and general anaesthesia continued via this route. This allows the larynx to be drawn further forwards and the post cricoid mucosa is divided in an easily found plane posterior to the posterior crico-arytenoid muscle. From here the trachea is dissected from the oesophagus to the site of the tracheostomy. The lobe of the thyroid to be saved is dissected from the specimen, and, on the side to be removed, the inferior and superior thyroid vessels and the middle thyroid veins are ligated and divided. The specimen can now be removed by transecting the posterior tracheal wall slightly higher than the anterior level since it is to be turned forwards.

Closure and tracheostomy
The pharynx is reconstructed around a previously passed nasogastric tube with an inverting Connell suture (p. 320) of 3/0 dexon. The closure is reinforced by two more layers of submucosa and constrictor muscle, sutured with the same material. An ellipse of skin of a size to admit an index finger is excised from the previously marked midline site. The trachea is brought out through this hole and the first layer of sutures (3/0 chromic catgut) joins the fascia around the trachea to the subcutaneous tissue. The second layer of 3/0 prolene joins the mucosa to the skin. Two suction drains are inserted and the wound closed in two layers, with catgut and prolene.

After care and complications. Feeding is commenced via the nasogastric tube when bowel sounds return. Fluid diet is given at 10 days and the nasogastric tube is removed, provided there is no leakage. A fistula of less than 2 cm in diameter which persists for a month can be closed with local skin flaps, while one over 2 cm will probably require to be closed with a pectoralis myocutaneous flap (Weingrad, 1983).

Speech therapy is started when the nasogastric tube is removed. About half the patients learn usable speech.

OPERATIONS ON THE TRACHEA

Tracheostomy

Indications
Tracheostomy assists respiration in the following ways. (1) It relieves any upper airway obstruction; (2) it re-

duces the dead space; (3) it affords direct access to the tracheobronchial tree and enables this to be readily cleared by aspiration of secretions; (4) with the aid of a cuffed tube, it allows positive pressure respiration to be maintained for a prolonged period. These objectives can be achieved, to some extent, by the use of an endotracheal tube in the first instance (p. 283). Tracheostomy is thus reserved for those occasions where access to the bronchial tree is required for more than a few days or in circumstances where an endotracheal tube is not available.

Anatomy
The trachea begins as a continuation of the larynx at the lower border of the cricoid cartilage. As it descends it becomes more deeply placed so that at the base of the neck it lies 2–4 cm from the skin. Superficial relations are: skin; superficial fascia; the investing layer of deep fascia splitting above the sternum to enclose the suprasternal space; sternohyoid and sternothyroid muscles; pretracheal fascia; the isthmus of the thyroid gland, which overlies its 2nd, 3rd and 4th rings. Veins which lie superficial to the trachea are (a) anastomosing veins connecting the two anterior jugulars; (b) an anastomosing vein connecting the two superior thyroids, above the thyroid isthmus; (c) the inferior thyroid veins descending vertically from the isthmus. In children the trachea is more superficial than in adults, but it is also smaller and more mobile, so that it may be more difficult to locate. The innominate artery and left innominate vein may be anterior relations of the trachea in the neck, as also may the thymus gland.

Operation
Tracheostomy is not an easy operation and, performed wrongly, leads to chronic stenosis of the upper airway. The only complete ring in the upper respiratory tract is the cricoid and, since it is cartilage, it has an inherent elasticity. Damage to part of this ring does not result in a hole but rather in the cricoid striving to maintain its ring like state and closing over the defect. The loss of integrity of the ring can be due to actual excision of the cricoid or to dissolution of the cartilage by perichondritis as a result of an adjacent tracheostomy through the first ring. The other difficult feature is that the trachea goes in the opposite direction from the sternum (i.e. inferiorly and posteriorly). This means that as one gets closer to the sternum so the trachea gets further from the surface and the inexperienced operator is forced upwards and may do an incorrect high operation. Cricoid stenosis may not always be apparent as an actual difficulty in breathing or stridor. Due to the reduction in air flow, patients can develop recurrent lower respiratory tract infections and no reason for this recurrence may be obvious to the chest physician treating the case.

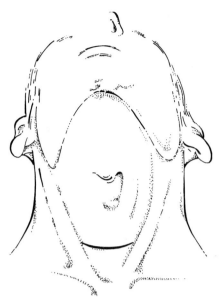

Fig. 12.33 Incision for tracheostomy

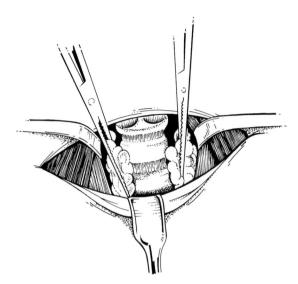

Fig. 12.34 Strap muscles retracted and thyroid isthmus divided

Incision (Fig. 12.33)

It matters little whether the skin incision is horizontal at the level of the 3rd tracheal ring or vertical. Neither makes the procedure appreciably easier but the horizontal wound often heals better. It certainly makes revision of the scar easier if the patient wants this after a few years. Small skin flaps are elevated and the strap muscles separated in the midline.

Approach

The strap muscles are retracted and the trachea is palpated under the pretracheal fascia along with the isthmus of the thyroid gland. The isthmus should always be tied (Fig. 12.34); if it is not, then the operator may go too high and if it is pushed upwards then it can slip down obliterating the stoma causing difficulty in changing the tube.

Occasionally thyroid veins are seen coming down from the isthmus and these must be tied meticulously or else blood welling up from behind the sternum can be troublesome. The isthmus is freed from the trachea by blunt dissection and divided between clamps. The ends are oversewn with 3/0 chromic catgut. The cricoid and first ring are identified. A vertical midline incision is made from the space below the second ring to the space below the fourth ring. At this point the anaesthetist is advised to withdraw his endotracheal tube (if the procedure is being performed under general anaesthesia) to the level above this cut. If the tracheal cartilages are not calcified then semicircles can be excised on either side of the vertical split with a scalpel (Fig. 12.35) but if they are calcified then a chonchatome should be used to punch out semicircles. The tracheostomy tube (size

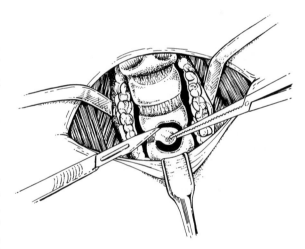

Fig. 12.35 Excision of tracheal rings

11 or 12) is inserted (Fig. 12.36) and retractors withdrawn.

Closure (Fig. 12.37)

It is unwise to suture the wound tightly or else the first cough will cause surgical emphysema. It is also wise to suture the tracheostomy tube in place until the first change after 3 or 4 days or else displacement can occur and replacement of the tube will be difficult if no tract is established.

After care

Humidification. The trachea is lined by columnar epithelium and is used to receiving warm humified air from the upper respiratory tract. A tracheostomy by-

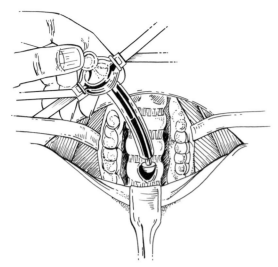

Fig. 12.36 Insertion of tracheostomy tube

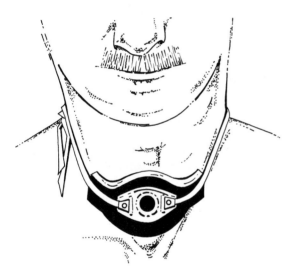

Fig. 12.37 Tracheostomy tube in position with tapes round the patient's neck

passes this and, until the epithelium metaplases or becomes adjusted to the new airflow, crusting is a danger, both within the trachea and the tube. Humidification is therefore essential. It is best done via a tank humidifier from which warm wet oxygenated air is blown over the stoma via a cup fitting over the tube.

If this is not available, an excellent and well tried method is to put 5 ml of normal saline down the tube via a syringe, then to suck out the secretions and then to instil another 5 ml of saline which is left. This should be repeated every two hours for the first 48 hours; then four hourly for the next five days.

Clearance of secretions. This is an essential step and should be done as often as outlined above. The nurse

should wear a mask and gloves when the tracheostomy is new. A Y-connection is used, a sterile tube is attached to the lower end of the Y and suction to one of the upper limbs of the Y. The tube is inserted as far down the trachea as possible and then she puts her finger over the open end of the Y and this creates the suction. The tube is then withdrawn over a period of three seconds. On no account should the tube be inserted with suction on because it will be sucked on to the tracheal wall causing abrasions and coughing.

Replacement of tube. This should not be done before 3 or 4 days until a tract is established and a doctor should be present. The danger especially in a fat person, whose trachea if far from the surface, is that the tube is placed anterior to the trachea. If this risk exists, then a tube with a larger neck should be obtained. If the tube is placed anterior to the trachea it may erode the brachio cephalic artery and this would be fatal. Therefore, great care should be taken to see that the tube is correctly placed. Some air will come out of the stoma, and even the tube, if it is anterior since the stoma is open to the surrounding tissue. A good airflow therefore must be apparent if the tube is in the correct place.

Thereafter the tube should be replaced daily.

Care of cuff. With the widespread availability of low pressure cuffs there should be much less trouble from this source than formerly. Low pressure cuffs do not need to be deflated and there is apparently no danger of tracheal stenosis. If these are not available, the cuff should be let down five minutes every hour. This is not so much to protect the mucosa as the cartilages since ischaemic mucosa will re-epithelialize normally after the tube is withdrawn. What is dangerous, however, is for the cartilage to necrose; the trachea will then collapse on inspiration due to lack of support or it will form a more permanent stenosis.

OPERATIONS ON MALIGNANT GLANDS OF THE NECK

One in 5 patients with a head and neck cancer will present with a lymph node on one side of the neck. One in 20 will have lymph nodes on both sides and one in 20 will have a lymph node which is fixed. The radical neck dissection operation is designed to remove *en bloc* all of the 80 lymph nodes which are normally present on one side of the neck, and it can be unilateral or bilateral. The prognostic significance of bilateral neck glands in the presence of a head and neck primary is so grave that the results of bilateral neck dissection make the operation hardly worth performing. Similarly, the removal of a fixed gland depends on what it is fixed to. If it is fixed to the mandible, the skin or the external carotid artery then removal along with this structure presents little problem. If, however, it is fixed to the pre-vertebral fascia, the brachial plexus, the common carotid artery or the base of the skull, then removal by surgery is often impossible and the operation should not be attempted.

Partial neck dissection is not recommended except in the instance of thyroid carcinoma (p. 261). If the aim of the operation is to remove the entire lymph draining field on one side of the neck then to cut through it compromises the clearance and is not advocated. Similarly, the so-called functional neck dissection which preserves the sternomastoid muscle, the internal jugular vein and the accessory nerve, is not recommended unless the surgeon has trained with an expert in this particular technique. If it is attempted incorrectly then the clearance of the metastatic lymph nodes will be incomplete.

The operation described here is the classical, radical neck dissection first described by Crile in 1921.

Biopsy
When several glands are enlarged, a single discrete gland may be removed for histological examination. In this way the diagnosis can be confirmed before block dissection is considered. Biopsy is not recommended in the case of a fixed swelling which is incapable of removal, since the findings are likely to be of academic interest only and the operation may lead to fungation of the tumour on the skin surface.

Radical neck dissection

Preparation
Following endotracheal intubation, the patient is laid supine with the head extended and turned to the opposite side. A flat pillow is placed under the ipsilateral shoulder to make dissection of the posterior triangle easier. It is advisable to stitch the skin towels in place because it is difficult to isolate the area posterior to the trapezius muscle by using towel clips alone.

Incisions
An incision for neck operations must conform to the following criteria:
a. It must provide adequate access to the structures to be operated on
b. It must be capable of extension during the operation or later so that any present or future eventuality can be dealt with
c. It must not damage vital structures in or beneath the skin
d. It must always heal well producing a scar that is cosmetically acceptable.

The blood supply to the skin of the neck comes down from the face, up from the chest, around from the trapezius and also from the external carotid on the other

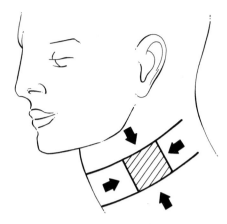

Fig. 12.38 Showing the area of the neck most prone to ischaemic necrosis

side. The most poorly vascularised area in the neck (Fig. 12.38) is in the middle over the common carotid artery. A poorly designed incision placed vertically in this area is liable to break down especially if the patient has been irradiated. This means that the carotid artery becomes exposed after surgery and this puts the patient at risk of a carotid artery rupture. It is best, therefore, to avoid 3 point junctions and vertical incisions in the centre of the neck.

The incisions recommended for radical neck dissection are firstly the *MacFee incision* (Fig. 12.39) which consists of 2 horizontal limbs. The first begins over the mastoid process, curving down to the hyoid bone and up again to the point of the chin. The second lies about 2 cm above the clavicle, starts laterally at the anterior border of the trapezius and ends medially at the midline. The second type is the *Schechter incision* (Fig. 12.40). The vertical limb of this comes from the mastoid process to the point where the trapezius meets the clavicle. It,

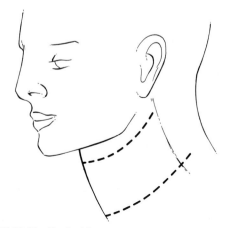

Fig. 12.39 MacFee incision

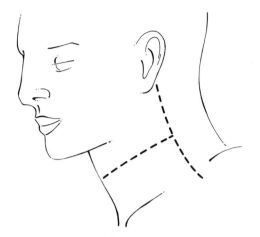

Fig. 12.40 Schechter incision

therefore, runs down the anterior border of the trapezius. Exactly half way down this line a horizontal incision is marked to reach the prominence of the thyroid cartilage. The choice between these incisions depends on the operator's experience and also the shape of the patient's neck.

When the incisions are made the skin flaps are elevated, the platysma being included. This preserves the blood supply and also increases the strength of the skin flaps by up to 10%. In the submandibular area, in order to preserve the cervical branch of the facial nerve, the plane of elevation is deepened onto the body of the submandibular gland and the investing fascia of the neck is lifted off the submandibular gland along with the platysma.

Dissection of the inferior margin
The sternomastoid muscle is divided with a knife. Both the sternal and the clavicular heads are divided and no vessels need to be ligated at this point. The carotid sheath is now visible and the dissection is continued down to the wall of the internal jugular vein. In order to isolate the internal jugular vein to ligate it, it is important to go as close to the wall as possible. Nontoothed dissecting forceps and Metzenbaum scissors are used. Before passing any instruments around the vein the vagus nerve should be identified to make sure that it will not be damaged with this manoeuvre. Mixter forceps are eased around the vein and 3 strands of 2/0 silk are passed. These are tied and a further suture ligature is added at the lower end. The vein is then divided. If the vein is torn during these manoeuvres there is a risk of air embolus. In the event of a tear, the hole should be occluded and the vein dissected above and below the hole so that it may be ligated safely.

The omohyoid muscle is then identified and divided. The fat pad lying between the internal jugular veins and

the omohyoid is dissected and pushed upwards. Underneath the prevertebral fascia one can then identify the phrenic nerve running laterally to medially. When this is identified the correct plane is entered and dissection can proceed laterally superficial to the brachial plexus thus preserving it from injury. A tunnel is created laterally in front of the prevertebral fascia on the brachial plexus to the anterior border of the trapezius. The external jugular vein must be divided in the dissection of this fat pad. Lying between the prevertebral fascia and the fat pad is the transverse cervical artery and vein and these should be preserved if possible.

Dissection of the posterior margin
The transverse cervical artery gives a vertical branch which runs up anterior to the anterior border of the trapezius. This can cause troublesome bleeding and so it should be divided and ligated before this part of the dissection is begun. Again, using blunt dissection, a tunnel can be made up the anterior border of the trapezius and the fat dissected from the structure (Fig. 12.41). In the upper third of the trapezius it is crossed by the sternomastoid muscle and these fibres are divided with sharp dissection. This continues up to the lateral surface of the mastoid bone. During this dissection the accessory nerve is divided as it enters trapezius at the junction of its middle and lower thirds.

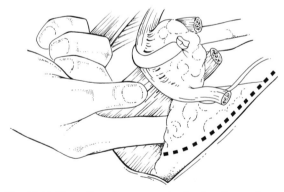

Fig. 12.41 Blunt dissection up anterior border of trapezius to create a tissue plane

Dissection of the anterior margin
The omohyoid is followed up to its insertion into the hyoid bone. This forms the anterior part of the dissection and again by making a tunnel along the omohyoid, this dissection can be done very quickly. It is divided from the hyoid bone, and the submental fat pad is divided in the midline until the anterior belly of the diagastric muscle is identified.

Deep dissection
The posterior margin of the dissection is grasped in Allis

forceps and turned forwards. The fat pad is dissected from the prevertebral fascia and the underlying muscles, the levator scapulae and the scalenes. It is tethered down by the three cutaneous branches of the cervical plexus, namely the anterior cutaneous nerve of neck, the great auricular nerve and the lesser occipital nerve. These neurovascular bundles are identified and divided and ligated well away from the phrenic nerve. This allows the specimen to be swung forward and the internal jugular vein is once again identified. Following this superiorly using Metzenbaum scissors, the carotid sheath is divided up to the jugular foramen. It is important to identify the transverse process of the atlas and, just above this, the posterior belly of diagastric will be found. This is retracted upwards and the upper end of the jugular vein is then seen. It is freed of its fascial connections and Mixter forceps are passed round it. Three 2/0 silk sutures are passed around the vein and tied and an additional suture ligature is applied at the upper end. The vein is then divided and the rest of the sternomastoid can be cut. It is important to cut this muscle in a line extending from the tip of the mastoid process to the angle of the jaw. If one goes above this line then the facial nerve is at risk. As the jugular vein is dissected out of the carotid sheath the vagus nerve will be seen closely applied to the common carotid artery. It must be preserved throughout the dissection. Once the upper end of the jugular vein has been divided the hypoglossal nerve can be seen coming inferiorly from the hypoglossal foramen, crossing just above the bulb of the carotid artery. It is crossed by three pharyngeal veins which join the pharyngeal plexus to the internal jugular vein. These must be ligated and divided (Fig. 12.42) because if they are torn they tend to slip underneath the hypoglossal nerve, putting this at risk during the subsequent attempt at haemostasis.

Dissection of the superior margin
The anterior edge of the submandibular gland is intermingled with the submental fat and the submental artery can cause troublesome bleeding if it is not identified and ligated. The edge of the gland is dissected posteriorly from the lateral surface of the mylohyoid muscle. When the posterior edge of the mylohyoid muscle is seen it is retracted forwards and, if the submandibular gland is pulled inferiorly at this point, the lingual nerve will be seen. It is freed from the gland and the submandibular duct can be ligated safely. The facial vessels entering the gland superiorly, one finger's breadth anterior to the angle of the mandible, are divided and the cervical branch of the facial nerve is safe because it should have been included in the initial dissection of the fascia of the submandibular gland. The lower end of the facial artery can be seen entering the inferior border of the submandibular gland just above the posterior belly of the diagastric. When this is divided the specimen can be removed. Two suction drains are inserted and the incision is sutured in two layers.

Complications
Immediate complications. Bleeding may require re-exploration for identification of the bleeding point. *Pneumothorax* is diagnosed radiologically and under water seal drainage may be necessary. *Raised intracranial pressure* is prevented by avoiding dressings around the neck and not allowing the patient to hyperextend the neck, and by sitting the patient up as soon as possible after the operation. If it occurs then the patient should be given 200 ml of 25% mannitol intravenously as quickly as possible.

Intermediate complications. Chylous fistula occurs following unrecognized operative injury to the thoracic duct. It may not manifest itself until the patient is being given tube feeds. At this time the suction drainage increases dramatically in amount and may reach 500 ml a day, the drainage consisting of thick white fluid resembling milk. The patient must be returned to theatre and the injured duct should be oversewn with 4/0 silk. *Seroma*, or a collection of serum under the neck flaps, can be prevented by using suction drainage for at least five days. The seroma should be aspirated and a pressure dressing applied to avoid failure of skin healing. *Carotid artery rupture* is usually the combination of several complications, namely wound breakdown, infection, fistulae, stripping of the adventitia of the artery and drying of the artery. If the skin breaks down, complete débridement should be carried out and the carotid artery covered with a skin flap at the earliest opportunity. Until

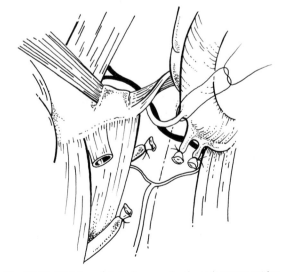

Fig. 12.42 Division of 3rd pharyngeal vein as it passes under the hypoglossal nerve

this is possible the artery should be kept moist with soaks. Ligation of the common carotid artery for rupture is followed by a 20% mortality and a 50% morbidity rate.

Late complications. Frozen shoulder is a common complication after a radical neck dissection since the accessory nerve is always cut. The reason for the shoulder stiffness is that the shoulder girdle falls forward and it becomes impossible for the patient to abduct the arm in the usual fashion. This causes adhesions in the capsule of the shoulder joint and a subsequent frozen shoulder. It should be prevented by starting shoulder exercises as soon as possible after the operation. *Hypertrophic scar and keloid* are similar and the difference is really only one of time and degree. Fortunately they are uncommon in head and neck surgery but they may occur if a vertical incision is used in the middle of the neck. The scar should be excised and the tension removed by a z-plasty repair.

Reticuloses and primary lymphatic tumours

Certain of these may be included among 'malignant' conditions of the cervical glands. They are not as a rule amenable to surgery, but in the case of a strictly localized swelling, operative removal may be the best procedure, even if only to establish the diagnosis. When the glandular swellings are more widespread, a single discrete gland may be removed for biopsy. Radiotherapy and chemotherapy now play a major role in the treatment of lymphatic tumours and gland biopsy is vital in staging the disease.

TUBERCULOUS CERVICAL ADENITIS

This condition is not common in Europe but is still common in Asia and Africa. The bacillus which is usually the bovine variety, reaches the lymph nodes by direct drainage, usually from the tonsil. It is very rare for patients with tuberculous cervical adenitis to have an associated pulmonary tuberculosis. Some 20% of cases have discharging sinuses, 10% a cold abscess and 10% are adherent to skin. Some 90% are unilateral and 90% involve only one gland group, the commonest being the deep jugular chain, followed by the nodes in the submandibular region, and then those in the posterior triangle.

Operation

Diagnosis usually necessitates removal of the glands especially when chemotherapy has been ineffective or is unavailable. If the glands are very large and matted, local removal is dangerous since they are often attached to the wall of the internal jugular vein and indeed can sometimes form the wall of the vein. If this is borne in

mind, then removal of the gland is straightforward through a horizontal neck incision. If bleeding from the internal jugular vein is encountered, it can be stopped with finger pressure while the vein is dissected above and below the matted glands so that it can be ligated and the segment of vein excised with the glands.

In cases where the whole neck is full of glands and the vein is extensively involved, a functional neck dissection is performed. This involves removal of the fat with the associated lymph nodes in the posterior triangle and the anterior triangle of the neck preserving the sternomastoid muscle, and the accessory nerve and, as far as possible, the internal jugular vein.

If removal is not followed immediately by appropriate chemotherapy, sinuses can form with persistent drainage and unsightly scars. Since it is almost certain that infection has spread from the ipsilateral tonsil, this should be removed either at the same operation or later.

OPERATIONS ON THE THYROID GLAND

Anatomy

The thyroid gland

This lies in the lower part of the front of the neck, clasping the trachea and overlapping the sides of the larynx. It consists of a right and a left lobe united across the front of the trachea by the isthmus. Each lobe is piriform in shape with its apex upwards; it extends above to the level of the middle of the thyroid cartilage, and below almost to the clavicle. The isthmus, which is about 2 cm deep, overlies the 2nd, 3rd and 4th rings of the trachea. The gland is enclosed in a sheath of pretracheal fascia, so that it moves up and down with swallowing. Between the gland and its sheath are networks of anastomosing blood vessels.

Relations. The gland is covered superficially by sternohyoid, sternothyroid, and the upper part of omohyoid, and is overlapped in its lower part by sternomastoid. Medially, it is related to cricoid cartilage and inferior constrictor above and to trachea and oesophagus below. Posteriorly it lies on the carotid sheath and the prevertebral muscles.

Blood supply. The superior thyroid artery arises as the first branch of the external carotid; it passes under cover of the infrahyoid muscles and enters the upper pole of the thyroid lobe. *The inferior thyroid artery* arises from the thyrocervical trunk, a branch of the subclavian. It ascends along the medial border of scalenus anterior as far as the level of the 6th cervical vertebra. It then turns medially behind the carotid sheath to reach the middle of the back of the thyroid, and runs down alongside the gland for a short distance before entering its substance. *The superior thyroid vein* emerges from the upper pole of the lobe and runs backwards across the carotid arteries to enter the internal jugular vein. *The middle thyroid vein* emerges from the lower part of the lateral border of the lobe and crosses the common carotid artery, to join the jugular. *The inferior thyroid veins* emerge from the isthmus or lower medial part of the lobe, and descend in front of the trachea to end in the left innominate vein.

Associated nerves. The external laryngeal nerve, which is a terminal division of the superior laryngeal branch of the vagus, runs downwards on the inferior constrictor, to end by supplying the cricothyroid muscle. Near its termination it is in fairly close proximity to the superior thyroid artery, and is liable to injury when this vessel is secured.

The recurrent laryngeal nerve supplies all the intrinsic muscles of the larynx. It arises from the vagus—on the right side as it crosses the subclavian artery, and on the left side as it crosses the aorta. It hooks round the artery, and ascends into the neck in the groove between trachea and oesophagus. Just before it enters the larynx it lies against the posterior surface of the thyroid gland, within its sheath and closely related to the termination of the inferior thyroid artery; it is therefore liable to be injured during the ligation of this vessel.

The parathyroid glands

These are two pairs of reddish brown glands each about the size of a small pea and ellipsoid in shape. They are situated usually in relation to the posterior aspect of the thyroid lobes.

The superior gland is fairly constant in position, lying behind the upper third of the lobe and related to the lateral surface of the trachea. It is stated to lie invariably between the true capsule of the gland and its fascial sheath. It may, however, be placed relatively far forwards, in which case it is liable to be accidentally removed in the operation of subtotal thyroidectomy.

The inferior gland is situated usually behind the lower part of the lobe, either above or below the inferior thyroid artery as it enters the thyroid substance. Considerable variations, however, exist. The gland may be found behind the oesophagus, either in the neck or in the posterior mediastinum, or it may lie in the anterior mediastinum in relation to the thymus. Occasionally it may be situated within the thyroid substance.

Indications for operation

Simple diffuse goitre

Patients with this condition seek operation for cosmetic reasons or to relieve pressure symptoms related to adjacent structures. Such pressure affects usually the trachea, the oesophagus or the large veins at the root of the neck. These mechanical effects are always more evident when there is a retrosternal prolongation of the goitre,

since there is then less room for expansion. It should be noted that simple diffuse enlargement of the thyroid in young adolescents (*pubertal goitre*) usually resolves spontaneously without treatment.

Simple nodular goitre

In this type of goitre there are additional and much stronger reasons for advising operation, for in the course of time such goitres not infrequently become toxic, and are always liable to undergo malignant change. The estimated risk of malignancy in nodular goitre ranges from 5–30% of cases, this discrepancy being due to the difficulties of interpreting the very varied histological patterns which may present in different parts of the gland. Further confusion has arisen from the fact that most statistics showing the incidence of carcinoma are based on the examination of glands that have been removed, and take no account of the large number of nodular thyroids that are not operated upon. Although, however, the dangers of carcinoma have doubtless been exaggerated, they are inescapably present. When carcinoma is diagnosed only by histological examination after thyroidectomy, the prognosis is incomparably better than when it is diagnosed by the clinician before operation. There can therefore be few logical reasons for withholding surgery. An exception may be made in women in the older age groups, especially in the goitrous districts, where nodularity of the thyroid is relatively common. Operation may then be reserved for cases where hardness of the nodules, fixation, or recent increase in size is suggestive of malignant change.

Solitary thyroid nodules

Until a clinically solitary thyroid nodule has been exposed at operation, it is not possible to be certain that it *is* solitary (Taylor, 1979a) or that the other lobe is normal. Unexpected malignancy can only be detected by excision and it is, therefore, a sound policy to advise exploration of any isolated thyroid swelling, even when it is not causing symptoms. *The uptake of radioactive iodine* by a nodule has been suggested as a method of excluding malignancy since increased uptake (known as a 'hot nodule') is seldom malignant (Husband & McCready, 1979) whereas a 'cold nodule' may or may not be malignant. However, this is of no practical benefit in the euthyroid patient since it does not influence the decision in favour of operation. Conversely, *ultra sound scanning*, in skilled hands, can determine which nodule represents a simple cyst and this allows the surgeon to defer operation or to evacuate the contents with a hollow needle (Sykes, 1981). Some clinics now advise needle aspiration or drill biopsy of all solitary nodules for preoperative cytological or histological diagnosis but this procedure requires the help of an experienced pathologist (Wade, 1983).

Toxic diffuse goitre (primary toxic goitre)

Thyrotoxicosis, diagnosed clinically and confirmed bio-chemically, may be associated with *no* enlargement of the thyroid gland or with a diffuse goitre. Treatment may be carried out by antithyroid drugs, by surgery or by radioactive iodine, and these may be employed separately or in combination. The antithyroid drugs act either by inhibiting the synthesis of thyroxine, or by blocking iodine uptake by the gland. The drugs most commonly used in the United Kingdom at present are *carbimazole (neomercazole)* and *potassium perchlorate. Propranolol* may be added to these drugs or used on its own (Lee, 1973) although this drug merely acts on the target organs to control symptoms resulting from excess circulating thyroid hormones. In certain cases the use of drugs has replaced surgery, in that complete remission of thyrotoxic symptoms can be obtained. The younger the patient, the more likely the response to antithyroid drugs, but if this fails, and symptoms recur after completion of a year's treatment, operation should be advised. The realization that some patients with thyrotoxicosis also have auto immune thyroiditis (as indicated by raised antibody titres) will influence the surgeon in withholding operation. In these cases, destruction of functioning tissue by the immune process will lead eventually to control of the toxic state but operation should not be withheld on these grounds alone. In properly selected cases, and when preceded by correct medical treatment, the operation of subtotal thyroidectomy can usually be relied upon to effect a cure, more rapidly, more certainly and more safely, than is possible by medical treatment alone despite a siginificant incidence of recurrent hyperthyroidism (Noguchi, 1981). Young adults (between 18 and 40) with diffuse hyperplasia of the gland often respond well to antithyroid medication, but are likely to be impatient for cure, and may find the prolonged treatment tedious and unacceptable. Sometimes they develop further gland enlargement while under such treatment due to the increased TSH output by the pituitary which follows reduction in circulating thyroid hormones. Older people respond less readily, but they are likely to be more tolerant of prolonged treatment. All cases of thyrotoxicosis should be regarded as a combined medicosurgical problem, and should be assessed by a physician before operation is considered. All should receive medical treatment in the first instance, whether this be employed in the expectation that by itself it will be curative, or merely as a preoperative measure to make the patient safe for surgery. It is obvious that the decision will depend upon a number of factors, including the initial response obtained. Indications for operation are (1) lack of response to antithyroid therapy; (2) toxic effects of the drug; (3) relapse after apparent cure; (4) a gland which is large and cosmetically disfiguring, or which is causing pressure symptoms, especially if these are due to a retrosternal prolongation. Contra-indications to thyroidectomy exist when there has been a failure of response to preoperative treatment, and when the cardiac condition is unsatisfactory. In such cases it is advised that the patient should be given a complete rest from specific antithyroid medication for 6 to 8 weeks, after which an alternative course of preoperative treatment is prescribed.

Treatment by radioactive iodine has great possibilities, and there are some who believe that it is the best and safest treatment for most forms of the disease. Its limitations are not yet fully understood, however, and there are grounds for believing that it may have carcinogenic properties although its use in children has been reported by Hayek (1970). In the majority of centres this form of therapy is used only in cases selected from the following groups (Wayne, 1965): (1) patients over 45 years of age, or those whose life expectancy, because of associated disease, does not exceed 20 to 25 years; (2) patients of any age who have not reacted to antithyroid drugs, and who are either bad surgical risks or have refused operation; (3) all patients who have relapsed after thyroidectomy.

Toxic nodular goitre (secondary toxic goitre)

This shows little response to the antithyroid drugs, although good results have been claimed in some centres by the use of radio-iodine. Most surgeons will have little hesitation in advising operation, especially in the coarsely nodular types of goitre, or if a single localized nodule appears to be present, for such goitres are likely to be resistant to any form of conservative treatment, and to develop a high degree of toxicity. Medical treatment is advised, therefore, only as a preliminary to operation, and in patients who are bad surgical risks. In preparation for operation, a radioactive isotope scan is occasionally of value in detecting excessive activity in one part of the gland thus allowing the surgeon to concentrate his efforts on removing the affected lobe.

Pre-operative treatment

Adequate preparation by medical treatment is essential before surgery on any toxic thyroid and Riddell (1970) recommends that this include routine laryngoscopy.

When the thyrotoxicosis is moderate, adequate preparation can usually be achieved by the administration of iodine, which stimulates colloid storage, so that activity and vascularity of the glands are diminished. Potassium iodide 30 mg three times daily is generally used. Propranolol alone, 40 mg three times daily, is now being used extensively for rapid preoperative preparation (Michie, 1975; Yawhan, 1983) although this is not recommended in the severely thyrotoxic patient (Feely, 1981).

In the case of patients with severe thyrotoxicosis, the

benefits of the antithyroid drugs should not be withheld. Carbimazole may be administered in a total daily dosage of 20 to 45 mg depending upon the severity of the thyrotoxicosis. Potassium perchlorate is more slow acting; its use is restricted to those patients who have adverse reactions to the other drugs. Treatment is kept as short as possible, but should be continued until the patient is symptom-free, or until the maximal lowering of the pulse rate has been obtained. Mason (1969) advises carbimazole for four to six weeks followed by 10 days of iodine, since the latter is credited with reducing the vascularity of the gland. Riddell (1970) states that antithyroid drugs increase thyroid congestion and add to the risks of haemorrhage during surgery. The majority of his patients can be made euthyroid preoperatively with rest, sedation and iodine alone. Iodine is definitely contra-indicated when potassium chlorate has been used in the patient's pre-operative treatment.

Subtotal thyroidectomy (Fig. 12.43)

This implies the removal of the greater part of the enlarged gland, the operation being a bilateral one, leaving an equal and symmetrical amount of gland tissue on each side. The proportion of gland to be removed depends upon the condition present. *In simple goitre* it is advisable (because of the risk of myxoedema) to leave an amount of gland on each side equal at least to a normal lobe. *In toxic goitre* there is a general tendency to leave very little thyroid tissue since the risk of recurrent thyrotoxicosis is greater than that of myxoedema. The amount suggested is 3–4 g on each side (assessed as cm³) depending partly on preoperative antibody levels. When the gland is greatly enlarged, as much as $\frac{7}{8}$ of it may therefore be removed. It is safer to err on the side of leaving too little rather than too much, since recurrent thyrotoxicosis is a less desirable and less easily managed

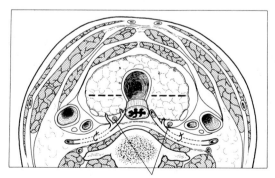

Recurrent laryngeal nerves

Fig. 12.43 Transverse section of neck to illustrate the amount of gland left in situ at the operation of subtotal thyroidectomy. The inferior thyroid arteries, the recurrent laryngeal nerves and the parathryoid glands are shown in their relationship to the remaining gland segment

complication than myxoedema. The latter may recover without medication (Noguchi, 1981) while recurrent hyperthyroidism can be troublesome unless there is an element of thyroiditis. The part of the gland left in situ is a strip of the posterior surface of each lobe. This surface is closely related to the recurrent laryngeal nerve and (usually) to the parathyroid glands, and if it is left undisturbed these structures are unlikely to be injured (Ross, 1966).

Premedication and anaesthesia

In all toxic cases effective premedication is most important, in view of the effect of emotional stress on thyroid activity. The patient should have had a good night's sleep prior to operation and reach the operating theatre in a calm state of mind. General anaesthesia is normally favoured in this country. Endotracheal intubation, advisable in all cases, is essential when deviation or constriction of the trachea has been produced since the ensured airway reduces venous congestion. The neck veins can be further emptied by tilting the operation table and patient some 15 degrees head up.

Technique

A small pillow or sandbag is placed between the shoulders so that the neck is extended and rotation of the head is avoided if the patient's head is supported on a ring. The skin incision can be marked by pressing a length of thread onto the skin just before using the scalpel, keeping in the line of the skin creases, 2–3 cm above the sternum. The 'collar' incision is then made, extending to the lateral borders of the two sternomastoid muscles. (With larger goitres the incision is made a little higher). In order to give a neater scar, the platysma is divided at a slightly higher lever than the skin. The flaps of skin, superficial fascia and platysma are then reflected upwards to the level of the thyroid cartilage, and downwards to the sternum. The anterior jugular veins are divided between ligatures. The investing layer of deep fascia is incised vertically in the mid line, any anastomosing veins being secured, and the interval between the infrahyoid muscles is opened up to expose the sheath of pretracheal fascia covering the gland (Fig. 12.44). The sheath is now incised, and a finger is passed over the front of each lobe to ascertain its size and extent. As a rule the larger lobe is dealt with first, and by retraction of the infrahyoid muscles and fascial sheath the greater part of its anterior surface is exposed. This is facilitated if the surgeon stands on the opposite side to the lobe being mobilized. Improved access can be obtained by division of the infrahyoid muscles (high up, so as to cause the minimum damage to their nerve supply) but this step is not always necessary. The lateral surface of the lobe is cleared by the finger (Fig. 12.45), during which procedure the middle thyroid vein, if pres-

Fig. 12.44–12.49 *Subtotal thyroidectomy*

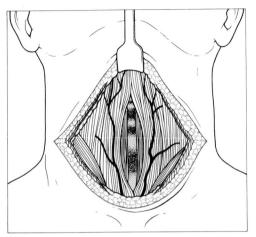

Fig. 12.44 Incision of deep fascia in the midline

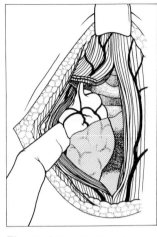

Fig. 12.45 Mobilization of the right lobe

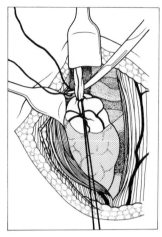

Fig. 12.46 Ligating of superior thyroid vessels

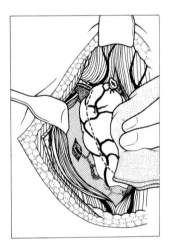

Fig. 12.47 Exposure of the inferior thyroid artery

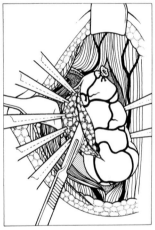

Fig. 12.48 Division of the gland

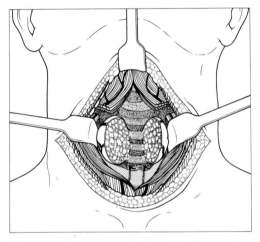

Fig. 12.49 Appearances after the subtotal removal

ent, is divided between ligatures. The muscles are retracted strongly in an upward and lateral direction, and the upper pole of the gland is delivered at the wound, when the vascular pedicle comprising the superior thyroid vessels becomes apparent. These vessels are divided between ligatures, the lower being tied first (Fig. 12.46) so as to provide countertraction for accurate placing of the upper ligature. If possible, a double ligature should be applied to the upper stump. A finger is then swept round the lower pole of the lobe which is delivered forwards, after the inferior thyroid and other veins have been secured. The lobe, which should now be completely mobilized, is drawn forwards and medially, and search is made behind it for the inferior thyroid artery. This vessel should be ligatured *well away from the gland*

in order to prevent injury to the recurrent laryngeal nerve. Its identification at a safe distance from the gland may be somewhat difficult from this approach within the fascial sheath, but careful incision of the fascia at the level of the cricoid cartilage will reveal the artery as it emerges from behind the common carotid (Fig. 12.47). At this point a ligature is applied in continuity. Unfortunately, this does not guarantee the avoidance of damage to an anomalous recurrent laryngeal nerve on the right side and it is preferable to identify and safeguard the nerve in all cases. This manoeuvre is essential if the whole lobe is to be removed (p. 261). A flat dissector is now insinuated between the isthmus of the gland and the trachea, and these structures are gently separated. The decision having been made as to the amount of gland tissue to be left behind (p. 269) several pairs of forceps are applied to the capsule of the lobe on its posterolateral aspect along the line of proposed section. These serve to steady the gland and to arrest haemorrhage.

The lobe is then sectioned from lateral to medial side (Fig. 12.48), in a plane towards the front of the trachea. An ordinary scalpel should be used in preference to the diathermy knife, in view of possible injury to the trachea or to the recurrent laryngeal nerve. When both thyroid arteries have been ligatured there is surprisingly little bleeding from the flat cut surface of the gland, and what little there is can usually be controlled by ligatures.

The opposite lobe of the gland is then treated in a similar manner, an equal amount of gland tissue being left behind. All haemorrhage is arrested, either by fine ligatures or by diathermy coagulation. If the infrahyoid muscles have been divided they are repaired by suture (Fig. 12.49). The wound is then closed, drainage being provided by Redivac suction (p. 2) for 24–48 hours.

Removal of retrosternal goitre

The diagnosis will usually have been made or at least suspected before operation—either from the severity of dyspnoea or from radiological examination. Fortunately the retrosternal prolongation of the gland has seldom any vascular connections within the thorax so that its blood supply is readily controlled from above. The cervical part of the gland is mobilized as far as possible, the superior thyroid vessels and middle thyroid vein being secured. A finger is then insinuated downwards behind the intrathoracic extension, and is used to free it from surrounding structures. By pressure from the finger below, aided by slight traction from above, the retrosternal part of the gland can usually be delivered upwards into the wound. The cavity is packed with gauze while the inferior thyroid artery is secured and the customary resection carried out. The gauze packing is now withdrawn and is replaced by a drain, after which the wound is closed.

Postoperative treatment

With adequate preoperative preparation, thyroid crisis after thyroidectomy for toxic thyroid should not occur. It does no harm, however, to keep the patient in a quiet room, well sedated with morphine or allied drugs, and to continue the preoperative drugs for a few days.

Hemithyroidectomy (Lobectomy)

The lobe of thyroid to be resected is mobilized as in the first stage of the subtotal operation (p. 259). It is particularly important to trace the recurrent laryngeal nerve throughout its visible course and to divide branches of the inferior thyroid artery without damaging the nerve. Ligature of the artery in continuity is not essential but

it may help in the avoidance of damage to the nerve by reducing haemorrhage as branches of the artery are divided close to the nerve. The parathyroids are preserved, preferably with their blood supply. The entire thyroid lobe is then removed together with the isthmus and a thin slice from the front of the opposite lobe to give a better cosmetic result (Taylor, 1969a).

Total thyroidectomy

The technique of this procedure is essentially a bilateral version of the hemithyroidectomy already described. If it is not possible to preserve the parathyroid glands intact, it is preferable to reimplant them within the sternomastoid muscle rather than to remove them completely. Total thyroidectomy may be successful in effecting cure of a carcinoma, and should be advocated in those cases where the growth is sufficiently mobile or if tumour is found in one of the lymph nodes outside the thyroid (Hargreaves, 1981). If the tumour is of papillary type and is confined to one lobe, lobectomy with removal of the isthmus is usually sufficient (Taylor, 1969a). Dissection of lymph nodes need only be carried out when they are involved by tumour. The discovery of isolated lymph node metastases from a carcinoma of the thyroid which is undetectable clinically (lateral 'aberrant' thyroid) requires total or hemithyroidectomy combined with removal of all laterally placed nodes (Taylor, 1969b).

Excision of isthmus

Excision of thyroid isthmus and medial part of each lobe may be required for the relief of pressure on the trachea caused by carcinoma or chronic thyroiditis. Operation is also of value in obtaining tissue for histological diagnosis in the hope that radiotherapy (in the form of radioactive iodine) may help to control a growth if it is not amenable to surgical excision. Autoimmune thyroiditis (lymphadenoid goitre or Hashimoto's disease) should not be confused with carcinoma clinically since antibodies are detectable in the serum, whereas chronic thyroiditis (Riedel's Struma) is indistinguishable from carcinoma without biopsy and is not associated with serum antibodies.

Complications of thyroid surgery

With adequate preoperative treatment and a careful operative technique, immediate complications are rare but later problems arise.

Haemorrhage. Excess bleeding, which does not pass along the drainage tube, may result in accumulation beneath the infrahyoid muscles and may lead to serious dyspnoea from pressure on the trachea or on the recurrent laryngeal nerves. It should be noted that the neck may show no obvious swelling on clinical examination. Instruments should be available at the patient's bedside so that the wound can be opened up. The patient is returned to theatre for evacuation of clot and securing of the bleeding vessel. If carbimazole has been given preoperatively, it may be responsible for a tendency to bleeding; this can be counteracted by the administration of vitamin K (Holl-Allen, 1967).

Respiratory obstruction. Laryngeal oedema may follow tension haematoma and result in obstruction of the airway. The obstruction may be further aggravated if one or both vocal cords has been paralysed by damage to the recurrent laryngeal nerve. Passage of an endotracheal tube should be placed in the hands of one skilled in this procedure.

Recurrent laryngeal nerve paralysis. This may result from pressure on the nerve by blood clot or by oedema in which case recovery can be anticipated. Provided that the nerve has been seen and avoided at operation, any paralysis can be considered as temporary. The prognosis as regards recovery of function after organic injury is poor.

Hypothyroidism. This is encountered after operations for simple goitre or for thyrotoxicosis but rarely after hemithyroidectomy where there may be hypertrophy of the residual lobe. Treatment consists in the administration of the synthetic *L-thyroxine*, using thyroid function tests to control the dosage.

Recurrent thyrotoxicosis. This is due either to inadequate removal of thyroid tissue or to subsequent hyperplasia of the tissue that has been left. It is not uncommon in primary toxic goitre, but very rare in the secondary form of the disease. In cases where there is autoimmune thyroiditis, recovery can be expected after a course of antithyroid drugs. Further operation should be avoided if possible and the administration of radioiodine may be considered as an alternative to antithyroid drugs.

Postoperative hypoparathyroidism. This may be caused by removal of or injury to the parathyroid glands, with resultant lowering of the serum calcium. Frank *tetany* is uncommon and usually transient. It is treated by the intravenous administration of 20 ml of 20% calcium gluconate. Some degree of parathyroid deficiency may persist permanently (Wade, 1972), and may lead to a variety of indefinite symptoms. Treatment consists in the administration of pharmacological doses of vitamin D (Tomlinson, 1978).

Parathyroidectomy

Overactivity of one or more of the parathyroid glands, a solitary adenoma or multiglandular hyperplasia, gives rise to the condition of hyperparathyroidism. This, by increasing the metabolism of calcium, may be the responsible factor in the development of skeletal decalcification (osteitis fibrosa), or in the formation of calculi in the urinary tract (Barnes, 1984). Removal of the affected gland or glands will normally bring about a complete cure of the condition. Exploration is indicated when the provisional diagnosis of parathyroid tumour is confirmed by a high calcium content in the serum, and by other biochemical findings indicating deranged calcium metabolism. It is only rarely that any swelling can be detected on clinical examination.

Clinics which specialize in parathyroid surgery use selective venous catheterization of the neck veins for preoperative localization purposes. Parathyroid hormone levels at various sites in the veins draining the thyroid gland are assessed in determining the site of a parathyroid tumour (Hsu, 1983). If this is not available to indicate the site of the tumour, the entire thyroid gland should be exposed in the manner described for subtotal thyroidectomy. To ensure unrestricted access the infrahyoid muscles should as a rule be divided. Both lobes of the gland are then mobilised sufficiently to allow exploration of their posterior surfaces, and a thorough search is made in all the normal situations of the parathyroid glands. A tumour of the superior parathyroid is as a rule easily located, since this gland is fairly constant in its position, behind the upper third of the thyroid lobe, and within the fascial sheath (Taylor, 1979b). The best way to locate the inferior parathyroid (if this is in its normal position) is to identify the inferior thyroid artery as it approaches the back of the lobe, and then to follow it downwards, when the gland should be found, crossed by its branches. The recurrent laryngeal nerve should be identified and safeguarded. As an aid to location of the parathyroids, methylene blue may be used to stain the glands: a dilute solution containing 5 to 7.5 mg/kg lean body weight is injected intravenously one hour preoperatively.

If no tumour is found in the normal situations for the parathyroid glands, the surgeon should be prepared to extend his search into the upper part of the thorax, splitting the sternum if necessary. Both the retrosternal space and the retro-oesophageal space should be explored. Approach to the latter is obtained by incising the deep fascia above the inferior thyroid artery, and by inserting a finger downwards and medially, behind the oesophagus. If it is possible to identify a branch of the inferior thyroid artery running downwards into the thorax this may point the way to a parathyroid tumour. Parathyroid glands may even be found in or adjacent to thymic tissue according to Wang (1976) who has made a detailed study of their anatomy.

When the enlarged gland has been found it can be removed without difficulty, after small vessels supplying it have been secured. Peroperative frozen section examination is useful in confirming parathyroid identity (Cooke, 1977) although the density test of Wang and Rieder (1978) is necessary to distinguish between an adenoma and multigland disease.

OPERATIONS ON THE SALIVARY GLANDS

Anatomy

The parotid gland

This fits into the space behind the mandible, below the external ear and in front of the mastoid process. It overlies the posterior belly of digastric below, and deeply it is applied to the styloid process and its muscles. It is enclosed by a sheath which is derived from the deep cervical fascia, and which sends processes into the gland substance dividing it into lobules. Its *upper pole* lies just below the zygomatic arch, and is wedged between the meatus and the mandibular joint. The superficial temporal vessels, temporal branches of the facial nerve, and the auriculotemporal nerve are found entering or leaving the gland near the upper pole. The cervical branch of the facial nerve, and the two divisions of the posterior facial vein emerge from its *lower pole*. Its *anterior border* overlies the masseter; from it emerge the parotid duct and the zygomatic, buccal and mandibular branches of the facial nerve.

The external carotid artery grooves the deep surface of the gland, and may pass through its substance; it terminates behind the neck of the mandible by dividing into maxillary and superficial temporal arteries.

The facial nerve, after emerging from the stylomastoid foramen, is intimately related to the parotid gland but its course and branches within the gland conform to a standard pattern. The main trunk, after emerging from the stylomastoid foramen, almost immediately enters the posteromedial surface of the gland at a deep level. It soon splits up into its two main sub-divisions: the *temporo-facial* and the *cervico-facial*, from which the terminal branches arise. The most important feature of the anatomical pattern is that the branches of the nerve lie with remarkable constancy in one plane, and that they all pass superficial to the *posterior facial vein*. This vein is formed within the substance of the gland, mainly by the continuation of the superficial temporal vein, and emerges, usually in two branches, at the lower pole. The plane in which the vein and the branches of the facial nerve lie has been designated by Patey (1957) the *facio-venous plane*. In this plane the gland can be split sagittally into two parts, one superficial to the plane and the other deep, so that the intervening nerve branches can be preserved intact.

The parotid duct emerges from the anterior border of the gland, runs horizontally across the masseter, and pierces the buccinator to open on the mucous membrane of the mouth opposite the second upper molar tooth.

The submandibular gland

This is situated partly below the mandible and partly deep to it. The main part of the gland lies on mylohyoid and hyoglossus, and overlaps both bellies of digastric inferiorly. It is enclosed in a loose sheath of deep cervical fascia. The *superficial surface* is covered only by platysma and deep fascia. The *medial surface* lies on mylohyoid, hyoglossus and pharyngeal wall from before backwards. Between the gland and hyoglossus are the lingual nerve, the submandibular ganglion and the hypoglossal nerve. The *deep part* of the gland is a prolongation extending from its medial surface under cover of mylohyoid.

The submandibular duct emerges from the medial surface of the main part of the gland, accompanies the deep part under cover of mylohyoid, and opens into the mouth on the sublingual papilla at the side of the frenum of the tongue.

The facial artery ascends in a deep groove on the posterior end of the gland, and then turns downwards and laterally between the gland and the mandible to enter the face at the anterior border of masseter.

Indications for operation

Acute suppurative parotitis (parotid abscess)

Incision and drainage should be carried out if the infection does not subside rapidly with antibiotic therapy. Fluctuation should not be awaited, since it is masked by the tense parotid fascia. Delay in providing drainage may lead to spread of the infection to the deep tissue planes of the neck.

A small incision is made over the most prominent part of the swelling. Pus is located by sinus forceps, and a small drain is inserted.

Simple tumours of the parotid

The most common is the so-called 'mixed' tumour, which, although essentially benign and enclosed within a well formed capsule of compressed parotid tissue, tends to recur after local removal. This appears to be due to the fact that the growth not infrequently permeates the capsule, giving rise to 'island' tumours in the surrounding gland. Local removal of the tumour by *enucleation* carries a considerable risk of recurrence, but it is claimed that this risk can be reduced if the excision is combined with irradiation. Many workers, however, believe that radiotherapy has little effect on these tumours, and opinion has now swung over in favour of the operation of *conservative parotidectomy*, which is defined as partial or total removal of the parotid gland with preservation of the facial nerve. This can only be achieved by identifying and exposing the nerve and its branches throughout the gland (Hobsley, 1981; Stevens, 1982). The operation is made possible by the realization that the gland can be split sagittally, in the plane of the facial nerve, into superficial and deep parts which can be removed separately, while the intervening nerve and its branches are preserved intact. The great majority of 'mixed' tumours are situated in the superficial part of the gland, and can be removed very adequately by superficial parotidectomy.

Chronic parotitis (parotid sialectasis)

This is due most commonly to infection or duct obstruction, or to a combination of the two. In the event of failure of conservative treatment, which may include duct irrigation and radiotherapy, removal of the affected gland by conservative parotidectomy is advocated.

Carcinoma of parotid

Total conservative parotidectomy may be practicable in carcinoma of the gland, if some at least of the branches of the facial nerve are free of the growth and can be preserved. When removal of the tumour necessitates sacrifice of the entire facial nerve, this need not occasion undue regret if there is a reasonable prospect of cure, for it is otherwise certain that nerve function will eventually be destroyed by the tumour. Where the growth as a whole is irremovable, partial excision combined with radiotherapy gives the best prospect of palliation.

Uncommon parotid conditions

Parotid calculi are uncommon. Since the symptoms which they cause are more suggestive of infection, and because of their small size, they are frequently missed. They may become impacted either at the hilum of the gland or at the bend of the duct at the anterior border of the masseter (Patey, 1965). If a calculus is palpable from the mouth, it may be removed by an incision made directly upon it through the mucous membrane. An approach from the skin surface may be necessary, but carries the risk of causing an external fistula.

Parotid fistula. A *gland fistula* is an uncommon sequel to operation on the gland or to rupture of an abscess. It usually closes spontaneously.

A *duct fistula* results most commonly from injury to the duct. If the injury is recognized at the time, immediate end-to-end suture of the duct should be carried out over a nylon thread, which is left projecting into the mouth. More often the condition is not recognized until a chronic fistula has formed. It is then unlikely to be cured by anything less than a conservative parotidectomy, and this operation is therefore the procedure of choice.

Enucleation

Removal of a parotid lump by enucleation is not recommended since the proximity of the growth to the facial nerve cannot be determined and its malignant potential is unknown. Hence, there is risk of injury to the nerve and of incomplete tumour removal. After local

excision of a 'mixed' tumour, postoperative radiotherapy is probably advisable in all cases, and is regarded as essential if the capsule has ruptured during the dissection.

Superficial parotidectomy

It is an advantage if the anaesthetist can provide hypotensive anaesthesia and also elevate the head of the table to reduce venous congestion. If a nerve stimulator is to be used (and it is advised for the less experienced surgeon) then the whole side of the face up to the profile line must be seen. A transparent adhesive drape is therefore preferable and is easy to use.

Incision

Many incisions are available, the only real point of difference being what they do under the ear lobe. The skin overlying and just anterior to the mastoid process is very thin and is devoid of underlying muscle which brings its main blood supply. Three point junctions and loops are to be avoided here to prevent ischaemic necrosis. The incision advised is shown in Figure 12.50. It starts at the top of the helix and dips into the tragal notch. It then proceeds inferiorly immediately in front of the ear and turns back gently under the ear lobe to 1 cm inferior to the tip of the mastoid bone. From there it goes down to the tip of the greater horn of the hyoid bone, following the line of the skin creases.

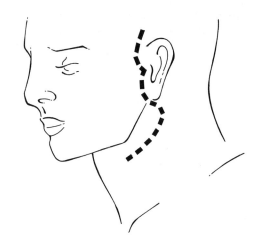

Fig. 12.50 Incision for parotidectomy

Excision

The skin flap is dissected off the parotid gland as far forwards as the anterior border of masseter muscle, taking care not to damage the peripheral branches of the facial nerve. The tail of the parotid is lifted off the surface of the sternomastoid muscle. The great auricular nerve is found entering the gland at the anterior border of sternomastoid. It is divided as close to the gland as possible so as to hasten recovery of sensation in the area. The sternomastoid is then retracted and a search is made for the posterior belly of digastric muscle. This is followed upwards to the mastoid bone into which it is attached. The facial nerve bisects the angle made by the digastric muscle and the tympanic plate. Thus once the digastric muscle is traced to the mastoid bone, one landmark has been established.

The next landmark which must be sought is the point of the tragal cartilage. The dissection is carried deeply along the perichondrium of the tragal cartilage and parotid tissue is separated from it. The cartilage ends in a pointer which points to the facial nerve, 1 cm medially and inferiorly (Fig. 12.51). Once the pointer is found and the digastric dissection completed, a bridge of parotid tissue will be seen overlying the facial nerve. This bridge can confidently be elevated down to the level of the digastric muscle. Thereafter more care must be taken but the position of the nerve is remarkably constant. Once the nerve is found, it is followed forwards but it runs rapidly to the surface and account has to be taken of this in the dissection. After about 2 cm it divides into an upper and lower division. The upper division is dissected out first and, using small artery forceps passed along the line of the nerve (Fig. 12.52), the parotid tissue is cut away from the nerve. The most superior branch is followed first and will be found to cross the mid point of the zygoma. It then divides into its terminal branches to the forehead and eyebrow. The parotid is swung down and the next division (to the corner of the eye) is dissected, swinging the parotid down off this. The next branch is to the lower lid and then a major branch is found running parallel to the duct, the buccal branch which supplies the nose, upper lip and lower eyelid. It usually arises from the upper division but can arise from the lower one. At this stage half of the gland should have been dissected from the nerve and

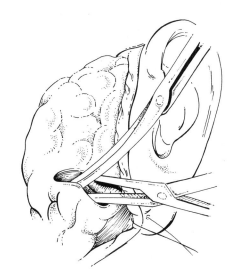

Fig. 12.52 Parotid tissue is lifted from the nerve by the opened blades of mosquito forceps and cut with fine scissors

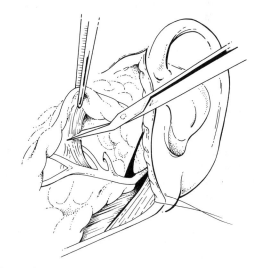

Fig. 12.53 Between each branch of the nerve a bridge of parotid tissue passing between the superficial layer and the deep layer is being divided

turned downwards (Fig. 12.53). The lower branch of the nerve is dissected in the same way and branches to the upper lip, corner of mouth and lower lip must be identified and dissected. The superficial lobe can then be removed leaving the facial nerve exposed on the masseter and retromandibular portion of the gland (Fig. 12.54). If a stimulator is available, it should be used at this point to make sure that all the branches are intact. In the event of postoperative paralysis the patient can be reassured that, in the light of a positive stimulation test, function will eventually return.

Diathermy should not be used for haemostasis unless it is the bipolar type. Unipolar diathermy spreads and

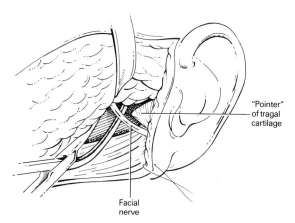

Fig. 12.51 Showing position of the facial nerve in relation to the tip ('pointer') of the tragal cartilage

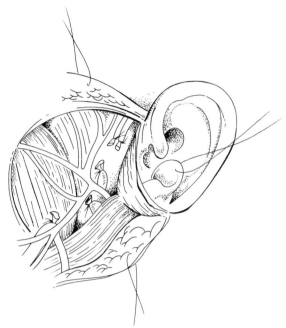

Fig. 12.54 Facial nerve displayed after removal of parotid gland

so heat injury to the nerve is possible. Adrenalin soaks are useful and in this way multiple ties can be avoided. Finally, the skin wound is sutured in two layers with one or possibly two suction drains. Having the drains over the exposed nerve does not seem to increase the risk of facial paralysis.

Complications
The main complication is *facial nerve paralysis*. Partial weakness of the facial muscles is quite common and is recoverable if the facial nerve has been identified and preserved at operation. If paralysis is total then it is useful to know that, if the nerve stimulation test at the end of operation was satisfactory, the lesion is neurapraxia and no treatment is indicated. If no stimulation was checked at the end of operation, the wound must be reopened and the nerve examined. If a division is found it should be repaired by primary suture using 10/0 silk under the microscope. There is no immediate treatment for a partial facial paralysis; function ought to return if some movement is present after the operation. *Bleeding* is rare and is usually venous from the posterior facial vein. It can be easily recognized and religated. A not infrequent late complication (after a month) is *Frey's Syndrome*. When the parotid is removed, the secreto-motor fibres are divided and they subsequently grow back into the skin, given that the parotid is now missing. They supply the blood vessels and sebaceous glands and so when smell and taste are stimulated vasodilatation and sweating occur. Most cases resolve spon-

taneously over a period of six months and only 10% require treatment. The latter is designed to interrupt the reflex arc and is best done through the middle ear, turning back the ear drum and dividing Jacobsen's nerve which runs over the promontory.

Total parotidectomy with preservation of the facial nerve
This is necessary for tumours of the retromandibular portion of the parotid gland which lies in the parapharyngeal space. The operation proceeds as above (p. 264) until the attachment between superficial and deep lobes becomes apparent. This can be in one of two places, namely between the upper and lower divisions of the facial nerve or below the lower division. If the attachment is between the two main divisions, then the dissection of the superficial lobe from the facial nerve should be performed from below upwards so that the superficial lobe is pedicled on the tumour. At this point using blunt pointed scissors the main trunk, upper and lower divisions and distal branches of the nerve are dissected from the underlying tissue. This allows access to be obtained between the two main divisions which can be retracted. The parapharyngeal space contains much loose areolar tissue which allows of easy finger dissection. The posterior facial vein always requires to be ligated and divided but the external carotid artery has usually been pushed deeply into the space by the tumour and rarely presents any problems. If the tumour presents inferior to the lower division of the nerve, the superficial lobe dissection can be continued down to this point and only the lower division with its distal branches needs to be dissected to allow access to the parapharyngeal space. Once this branch of the nerve is free, it can be retracted upwards and finger dissection of the space is simple. Again the posterior facial vein needs to be ligated but seldom the external carotid artery.

Total parotidectomy with sacrifice of the nerve and nerve graft
This is usually the procedure required for the excision of malignant disease of the parotid. The commonest malignant tumour is the adenoid cystic carcinoma and, since its main route of spread is along perineural sheaths, wide removal of the nerve is required. Depending on the position of the tumour and its extent, consideration may have to be given to removal of the temporomandibular joint, the external auditory meatus, the zygoma or mastoid bone and skin overlying the growth.

Details of nerve grafting lie beyond the scope of this book but the following principles should be observed:
1. The best suited graft is the great auricular nerve: it is easily accessible; up to 8 cm can be removed; it has two branches, and the diameters are correct

2. There should be no tension
3. No scar tissue should intrude at the anastomosis and so the sheath should be cut back and only a minimal number of sutures used. Fixation of each junction within a collagen tube is recommended
4. The use of the operating microscope is advisable

Removal of calculi from the submandibular duct

If calculi can be felt in the duct, intraoral removal is possible, using local anaesthetic infiltration or a dental block. In order to prevent the calculi from sliding back into the gland as a result of the manipulations, a silk suture is passed round the duct behind the stone and retracted upwards (Fig. 12.55). With a number 11 blade, the duct is incised directly over the stone (Fig. 12.56). The tissue is thicker than normal due to the irritation caused by the stone and often up to 1 cm of soft tissue must be incised before the stone is found and removed. If the duct is then left to heal by primary

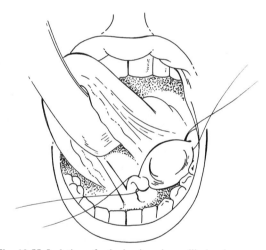

Fig. 12.55 Isolation of calculus in submandibular duct

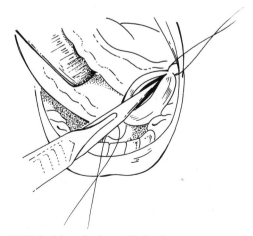

Fig. 12.56 Incision of submandibular duct

intention duct stenosis may result. It is best therefore to marsupialize the lining of the duct with two sutures of catgut on each side.

Removal of the submandibular gland for calculi

This is advised when the gland is chronically inflamed or is the site of stone formation. Tumours of the gland itself are comparatively rare, but secondary carcinoma of the related lymph glands is commonly encountered. Many of these lymph glands are inseparable by dissection from the salivary gland, and in any operation for their removal the salivary gland must be included in the excision.

Incision

The area is prepared and draped so that the corner of the mouth and angle of jaw are visible as well as the upper half of the neck. A horizontal skin crease incision is made two finger breadths below the ramus of the mandible. The incision should be deepened to the body of the submandibular gland before raising skin flaps. The aim is to avoid damaging the cervical branch of the facial nerve which lies in the plane between the platysma and the investing fascia of the neck. As the tissues superficial to the investing fascia are lifted off the body of the gland in the formation of a flap, so is the nerve protected. This flap is developed up to the ramus of the mandible and is then stitched to the upper skin edge to keep it out of the way.

Excision

2.5 cm anterior to the angle of the mandible, the bone is grooved by the facial vessels. These are also crossed by the cervical branch of the facial nerve and so to tie the vessels prior to the development of the fascial flap is to put the nerve at risk. Although the facial artery grooves the gland rather than passes through it and can be dissected out, this course is tortuous and ligation and division of each end is the simpler procedure. Once the artery and vein have been divided at the upper end, the gland is dissected bluntly off the ramus into the sub-mental area. The submental vessels are tied and the sub-mental fat pad and the anterior part of the gland are then dissected backwards off the surfaces of the anterior belly of digastric and the mylohyoid muscle. At the pos-terior border of mylohyoid a Langenbeck retractor is inserted to pull the muscle forwards. This reveals the duct, the hypoglossal nerve running along just above the greater horn of the hyoid and, when the gland is pulled postero inferiorly, the lingual nerve (Fig. 12.57). With this manoeuvre the lingual nerve is pulled down in a U-shape and is attached to the gland by the submandibular ganglion. A small vessel accompanying the ganglionic attachment must be clamped carefully to free the gland from the nerve. The duct is then tied with catgut and

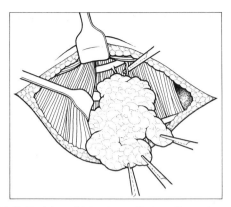

Fig. 12.57 Excision of left submandibular salivary gland

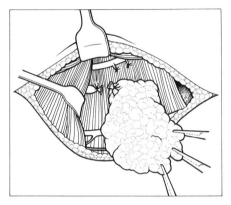

Fig. 12.58 The lingual nerve and hypoglossal nerves are displayed deep to the gland. The submandibular duct has been divided

divided (Fig. 12.58). If the operation is being performed for calculi within the gland, make sure that the duct is removed as far forwards as possible or else stones dislodged into the duct from the operative manipulation may pass into the patient's mouth several days after the operation. (Explanations for this are apt to be confusing and embarrassing.) The only attachment of the gland now is the proximal end of the facial artery entering its postero inferior margin just at the superior border of the posterior belly of digastric. The artery should be identified and suture ligatured with silk, after which it is divided and the gland removed. One suction drain is usually sufficient and it is tucked up underneath the mandible. Since a stab wound leaves an ugly mark in a very visible part of the neck if brought out underneath the incision, it is best brought out as far posteriorly as possible.

Complications
The drain is removed after 72 hours but it is best then to apply a pressure dressing for 24 hours because the operative site is essentially a dependent area and seroma

collection is not infrequent. If this occurs it should be aspirated daily and pressure dressings applied until its ceases. If the cervical branch of the facial nerve has been contused or cut the mouth will be pulled to the opposite side by the normal muscle tone. This is an ugly deformity and is made worse by voluntary movement such as smiling and talking. If the nerve has been contused, the mouth will probably be straight in the resting position. If it has been divided, the mouth will be squint even at rest. Whatever the deformity, six to nine months should elapse prior to offering further treatment. This quite simply aims to equalize tone on the lower lip by cutting the equivalent branch on the other side. No functional defect results.

If the lingual or hypoglossal nerves are damaged little disability results and there is no specific treatment, but every effort should be made to avoid such injury.

The most likely site of dangerous postoperative bleeding is the proximal end of the facial artery and this is why it should be suture ligatured.

Removal of the submandibular gland for tumour

Most benign tumours of the submandibular gland are pleomorphic adenomas and provided one keeps as far from the surface of the tumour as possible, the operation described above is quite suitable. There is no place for enucleation. If the tumour is malignant, then possibly a full radical neck dissection will be required. The least that is acceptable however is an upper neck dissection or a suprahyoid dissection. This is described on p. 253, but involves the additional removal of the digastric muscle and the associated fat and lymph nodes up to the mastoid process and including the tail of the parotid gland. Malignant tumours of the submandibular gland involving the mandible are usually secondary metastatic nodes and should be recognized as such. A search for the primary tumour is necessary so that the tumour can be treated as a whole. Metastatic nodes attached to the mandible in this site will necessitate a partial mandibulectomy in order to obtain adequate removal.

Other conditions and operations

Ectopic salivary tumours
These tumours are rare and between 80 and 90% occur within the buccal cavity, the commonest site being the hard palate. Some 60% are *cylindromata*, this being a designation referring to the unique histological pattern. These tumours are locally invasive and may also metastasise; they therefore carry a grave prognosis, although not so grave as that for carcinoma in similar sites (Harrison, 1956). About 40% of ectopic salivary tumours are of the 'mixed' type similar in behaviour to those arising in the parotid gland.

Preliminary biopsy is advised in order to establish the

diagnosis. The treatment of choice in cylindromata is radical diathermy excision, including a wide margin of healthy tissue, if this is practicable. In the case of palatal tumours an obturator will usually be required to occlude the defect produced by the excision. For surgically inaccessible tumours irradiation probably offers the best palliation. In the case of 'mixed' tumours, simple enucleation is usually adequate.

REFERENCES

Barnes A D 1984 The changing face of parathyroid surgery. Annals of the Royal College of Surgeons of England. 66: 77

Cooke T J C, Boey J H, Sweeney E C, Gilbert J M, Taylor S 1977 Parathyroidectomy: Extent of resection and late results. British Journal of Surgery 64: 153

Feely J, Crooks J, Forrest A L, Hamilton W F, Gunn A 1981 Propranolol in the surgical treatment of hyperthyroidism including severely thyrotoxic patients. British Journal of Surgery 68: 865

Hargreaves A W 1981 Surgical aspects of carcinoma of the thyroid gland. Annals of the Royal College of Surgeons of England 63: 322

Harrison K 1956 A study of ectopic mixed salivary tumours. Annals of the Royal College of Surgeons of England 18: 99

Hayek A, Chapman E M, Crawford J D 1970 Long-term results of treatment of thyrotoxicosis in children and adolescents with radioactive iodine. The New England Journal of Medicine 283: 949

Hobsley M 1981 Surgery of the parotid salivary gland. Annals of the Royal College of Surgeons of England 63: 264

Holl-Allen R T J 1967 Haemorrhage following thyroidectomy for thyrotoxicosis. British Journal of Surgery 54: 703

Hsu F S F, Clark O H, Serata T Y, Nissenson R A 1983 Rapid localisation of parathyroid tumours by selective venous catheterisation and parathyroid hormone bioassay. Surgery 94: 873

Husband J E, McCready V R 1979 Scanning: which technique? British Journal of Hospital Medicine 21: 618

Lee T C, Coffey R J, Mackin J, Cobb M, Routon J, Canary J J 1973 The use of propranolol in the surgical treatment of thyrotoxic patients. Annals of Surgery 177: 643

Mason A S 1969 Treatment of thyrotoxicosis. Journal of the Royal College of Surgeons of Edinburgh 14: 264

Michie W 1975 Whither thyrotoxicosis? British Journal of Surgery 62: 673

Noguchi S, Murakami N, Noguchi A 1981 Surgical treatment for Graves' disease: A long-term follow up of 325 patients. British Journal of Surgery 68: 105

Patey D H, Ranger I 1957 Some points in the surgical anatomy of the parotid gland. British Journal of Surgery 45: 250

Patey D H 1965 Inflammation of the salivary glands with particular reference to chronic and recurrent parotitis. Annals of the Royal College of Surgeons of England 36:26

Riddell V H 1970 Thyroidectomy: Prevention of bilateral recurrent nerve palsy. British Journal of Surgery 57: 1

Roos D B 1982 The place of scalenectomy and first rib resection in thoracic outlet syndrome. Surgery 92: 1077

Ross D E, Castro E C, Wharton C F 1966 Complete thyroidectomy. American Journal of Surgery 112: 34

Stevens K L, Hobsley M 1982 The treatment of pleomorphic adenomas by formal parotidectomy. British Journal of Surgery 69: 1

Sykes D 1981 Solitary thyroid nodule. British Journal of Surgery 68: 510

Taylor G W 1979b The surgery of hyperparathyroidism. In: Lumley J S P, Craven J L (eds) Surgical review 1, Pitman Medical, London, p 137

Taylor S 1969a The solitary thyroid nodule. Journal of the Royal College of Surgeons of Edinburgh 14: 267

Taylor S 1969b Carcinoma of the thyroid gland. Journal of the Royal College of Surgeons of Edinburgh 14:183

Taylor S 1979a Surgical treatment of thyroid disease in modern perspective. Annals of the Royal College of Surgeons of England 61: 132

Tomlinson S, O'Riordan J L H 1978 The parathyroids. British Journal of Hospital Medicine 19: 40

Wade J S H 1972 Clinical Research in thyroid surgery. Annals of the Royal College of Surgeons of England 50: 112

Wade J S H 1983 The management of malignant thyroid tumours. British Journal of Surgery. 70: 253

Wang C A 1976 The anatomic basis of parathyroid surgery. Annals of Surgery 183: 271

Wang C A, Rieder S V 1978 A density test for the intra-operative differentiation of parathyroid hyperplasia from neoplasia. Annals of Surgery 187: 63

Wayne E 1965 The assessment of thyroid function. British Journal of Surgery 52: 717

Weingrad D N, Spiro R H 1983 Complications after laryngectomy. American Journal of Surgery 146: 517

Yawhan L, Gyi K M, Paw K, Brang L, Oo M, Myint H 1983 Propranolol in the surgical treatment of thyrotoxicosis. Journal of the Royal College of Surgeons of Edinburgh 28: 365

FURTHER READING

Freund H R 1979 Principles of head and neck surgery, 2nd ed Appleton-Century-Crofts, New York

Stell P M, Maran A G D 1978 Head and neck surgery, 2nd ed Heinmann, London

13

Operations on the breast

R. F. RINTOUL

Anatomy

Extent

The breast lies embedded in the superficial fascia of the chest wall. It extends vertically between the 2nd and the 6th costal cartilages, and horizontally from the edge of the sternum nearly to the mid-axillary line. A process of the breast, known as the *axillary tail*, extends upwards and laterally along the lower border of pectoralis major into the axilla, where it reaches as high as the 3rd rib; this process, unlike the rest of the breast, lies below the deep fascia. The breast lies upon three muscles—pectoralis major, serratus anterior and external oblique, but is separated from these by deep fascia.

Structure

The secretory acini of the gland are embedded in a fairly dense fibrous stroma, and are grouped in *lobules*. Aggregations of lobules form the *lobes* of the breast (15–20 in number), which are arranged in a radiating manner. Each lobe is drained by a single duct, which is formed by coalescence of the ducts of the component lobules; these ducts converge to open on the summit of the nipple. There is no fascial capsule to the gland as a whole. The lobes are partly separated from each other by irregular and incomplete fibrous septa which are continuous with the gland stroma. Bands of fibrous tissue pass from the stroma both to the skin (ligaments of Cooper) and to the deep fascia. These fascial bands are accompanied by lymphatics which are of importance in the spread of carcinoma.

Blood supply

Arteries supplying the breast are the lateral thoracic (from the 2nd part of the axillary artery), perforating branches of the internal mammary artery, and lateral branches of the 2nd, 3rd and 4th intercostal arteries. The *veins*, which form a plexus beneath the areola, drain mainly to the axillary and internal mammary veins.

Lymphatic vessels

The glandular acini are surrounded by plexuses of small lymphatic vessels. These communicate by vessels accompanying the ducts with the *subareolar plexus*, and also by vessels passing deeply with the plexus on the deep fascia underlying the breast. Cutaneous lymphatics draining the skin surface communicate directly with the subareolar plexus, and, by means of vessels accompanying the ligaments of Cooper, with the lymphatics of the gland stroma. From both superficial and deep plexuses channels pass to the regional lymph glands.

Axillary lymph glands

Lymph glands abound in the axilla, and they all directly or indirectly receive lymph from the breast. Their arrangement is irregular, but they may be divided arbitrarily into five chains or groups.

The *anterior chain* lies under cover of the pectoral muscles, forming the anterior wall of the axilla. The *posterior chain* lies on the posterior wall of the axilla alongside the subscapular vessels. The *lateral chain* lies along the upper part of the humerus on the medial side of the axillary vessels. Glands of the anterior chain (*pectoral nodes*) are usually the first to become involved in breast cancer; they are in actual contact with the axillary tail of the gland and may become involved by direct infiltration. The posterior and lateral chains drain respectively the scapular region and the upper limb, but they have numerous connections with the anterior chain, and are potential sites of spread in carcinoma.

The *central group* of glands lies embedded in the fat in the central part of the axilla, and receives afferents from all three chains. The *apical group* is found at the extreme apex of the axilla, in the space between pectoralis minor and the clavicle, and is covered by the clavipectoral fascia. Afferents reach these glands from all three chains and from the central group. Some vessels come directly from the breast, so these glands may be the first to become involved in carcinoma. Afferents from the apical glands drain mainly to the blood stream at the origin of the innominate veins, but some pass to the supraclavicular glands.

Other associated lymph glands

The *supraclavicular glands* lie in the lower part of the posterior triangle, and belong to the lower group of deep cervical glands. They receive afferents from the apical glands, and also from the internal mammary glands.

The *internal mammary glands (anterior mediastinal or parasternal glands)* lie alongside the artery of the same name, one or two small glands being found deeply placed in each of the upper three or four intercostal spaces close to the sternum. They receive afferent vessels which originate in the lymphatic plexus of the deep fascia, and which pass deeply along the course of the perforating branches of the internal mammary artery. Their efferents pass mainly to the innominate vein, but communicate also with the cervical glands.

CARCINOMA OF THE BREAST

General considerations

Mode of spread of carcinoma

The long and widely held concept that breast carcinoma spreads in an orderly fashion from a recognisible primary tumour to lymphatics and hence to the blood stream is no longer acceptable. Many clinical trials and the observations of surgeons and radiotherapists over the past 20 years have led to the conclusion that, at the time of diagnosis, breast carcinoma is often a systemic disease with small non-detectable secondary growths (*micrometastases*) already present elsewhere in the body. Involved axillary lymph nodes need not necessarily be detected clinically and there may be no evidence of local lymphatic spread within the breast. Alternatively, there may be widespread changes in the vicinity of the primary growth without any distant metastases.

Spread of the tumour within the breast itself may be by direct infiltration or by permeation along the periacinar and periductal lymphatics. The involvement of surrounding structures—the skin or pectoral muscles—occurs either by direct extension of the growth, or by permeation along lymphatic channels. Such permeation occurs along the vessels which accompany the ligaments of Cooper towards the skin surface; contraction of these growth processes leads to fixation or actual dimpling of the overlying skin, and later to the development of cutaneous nodules. Permeation towards the pectoral fascia results in fixation of the tumour on its deep aspect. At any stage, extension to the regional lymph glands by embolism or by permeation may occur in an unpredictable fashion. This is mainly to the axilla but lymphatic spread occurs also to the internal mammary glands or to the peritoneal cavity, and both thoracic and abdominal organs may become involved.

Clinical staging

It is usually considered essential to have some clinical method of classifying the stage to which the disease has progressed in order to make comparisons between various methods of treatment and to judge the patient's progress. Such methods of classification are based upon clinical findings alone, although these may be assisted by radiological and other preoperative investigations. Findings obtained at operation or by histological examination are not included.

Unfortunately, experience has shown that individual patients do not pass from one stage to the next as their disease progresses although any method of staging suggests that this should be the case. In addition to the unpredictable nature of the disease, there are considerable limitations in the methods of clinical assessment. Lymph nodes may be enlarged because of hyperplasia rather than tumour involvement and the presence of lymph nodes may be disputed even between experienced clinicians. Clinical examination also ignores possible spread to the internal mammary glands. Evidence for lymph node hyperplasia comes from histological examination of palpable nodes and from the regression of axillary lymph nodes in patients who, as part of a multicentre trial arranged by King's College Hospital, London (Edwards, 1972), had simple mastectomy without radiotherapy. It was suggested that regional lymph nodes played an important part in the patient's resistance to the tumour (Baum, 1973) and it is now accepted that host reaction, in the form of hyperplasia of regional lymph nodes, indicates a relatively favourable prognosis (Forrest, 1981).

In all methods of clinical staging the accuracy of the axillary examination is important. In particular, differentiation between Stages I and II depends upon the examiner's impressions regarding the presence of palpable axillary lymph nodes and McNair & Dudley (1960) have cast very grave doubts about the validity of any such assessment. Five senior clinicians (surgeons and radiotherapists) were asked to examine the axillae of 10 patients whose breasts were concealed. In 6 of these the breasts were normal, and there was no reason for expecting the axillary glands to be enlarged; 3 of the remaining 4 suffered from breast carcinoma, and 1 from a breast abscess. Thus 100 axillary examinations (10 patients, 20 axillae, 5 examiners) were available for study. There was an altogether astonishing lack of agreement between the examiners. In the patients without breast pathology, positive findings were recorded in 48% of the examinations (20% by one examiner, 73% by another). In the patients with breast pathology, the findings were almost identical—again 48% of positive findings, and a range of 20–80% between the different examiners. These figures seem to indicate that staging by clinical impressions of palpable axillary glands is both valueless and misleading.

Recent methods of investigation have not solved the difficulty in staging. While *mammography* is helpful in the early detection of a previously unsuspected cancer (Millis,

Table 13.1 International Union against Cancer Classification

Stage I
Tumours less than 5 cm in greatest diameter. Skin fixation absent or incomplete. No fixation to underlying muscles. Axillary nodes not palpable.

Stage II
As for Stage I, but with palpable mobile nodes in the homolateral axilla.

Stage III
Tumours more than 5 cm in greatest diameter
or skin fixation complete
or skin involvement wide of the tumour
or peau d'orange
or fixation to underlying muscles
or palpable and immobile nodes in axilla
or palpable supraclavicular nodes
or oedema of arm.

Stage IV
Distant metastases present, regardless of condition of primary tumour and regional lymph nodes.

Table 13.2 Manchester Classification

Stage I
Growth confined to the breast

Stage II
Palpable mobile axillary nodes in addition to Stage I

Stage III
Growth extends *locally* beyond breast tissue

Stage IV
Growth extends *beyond* the breast area and beyond Stage II

1976), *bone scanning*, using a radio-isotope, has resulted in early detection of skeletal metastases. Thus, patients initially considered to have an early tumour may, in fact, be more accurately placed in Stage IV. However, these methods for the detection of spread lack sensitivity and a reliable biochemical 'marker', in the form of an abnormal serum protein which would detect micrometastases and their response to treatment, is not yet available.

The most commonly used classification is that proposed by the International Union against Cancer in 1960 (Table 13.1). The Manchester Classification has four similar stages (Table 13.2). The TNM system is based on clinical observations related to tumour (T), regional lymph node (N) and distant metastases (M).

Prognostic factors
One of the major advances in breast cancer during the last decade has been the realisation that some tumours, when grown in tissue culture, will take up the hormone oestradiol. The test, available in specialised centres, estimates the oestrogen receptor (ER) status of the patient and hence the likelihood of any residual tumour to respond to hormone manipulation (Hawkins, 1980). In general, ER positive tumours have a better prognosis than those which are ER negative (Forrest, 1981). The histological state of the axillary lymph nodes is, at present, the best indicator of likely metastatic spread (Forrest, 1979; Baum, 1980) and hence an indicator of prognosis. Hyperplasia of the regional nodes is favourable whereas the involvement of lymph glands by growth indicates an increasing risk of tumour recurrence as the number of affected glands increases. Assessment by isotope scans of liver and bone, CT brain scans and biochemical tests did not contribute further to the definition of those with

a bad prognosis in almost 200 patients attending the Edinburgh clinic of Forrest (1979) over a 4 year period.

Choice of treatment
The apparently unending controversy as to the best treatment of breast cancer—and the widely varying procedures adopted in different clinics—takes on a new perspective when it is appreciated that the value of surgery to the breast area is limited to local control of the disease. In the 1930s the standard treatment was the classical radical operation of Halsted which included careful clearance of the axilla. This operation was subsequently extended by Dahl-Iversen (1963) to include removal of the parasternal and supraclavicular lymph nodes but the results did not show any advantage over more conservative procedures. During the past 20 years, there has been a trend away from the radical forms of mastectomy although some centres in America currently advise removal of internal mammary nodes in selected cases (Robbins, 1978). No longer does radical surgery entail removal of all pectoralis muscle (Hayward, 1980) and studies have shown that radical surgery is not required if radical radiotherapy follows simple surgery (Forrest, 1980). In fact, some surgeons are content to remove only the actual tumour together with a reasonable margin of breast tissue and to follow this with radiotherapy (Taylor, 1971). To a large extent, radiotherapy offers the same prospect of disease control as excisional surgery with the additional benefit that irradiation can reach the parasternal and supraclavicular nodes with less morbidity than surgery. The move away from radical surgery towards conservative surgery has been accompanied by trials of systemic adjuvant therapy (p. 274). The results are most encouraging but no patient with breast cancer has yet been cured by chemotherapy (Hughes, 1978).

It is difficult, therefore, to lay down any firm principles for guidance in the treatment of breast carcinoma, but the following method of correlating the treatment with the clinical stage of the disease has found fairly general acceptance, and may be taken as representing the majority view at the present time. To a large extent, the treatment of breast cancer is a highly individual matter

(Burn, 1980) and it is important that treatment should be *for the patient* rather than *of the disease*.

In Stage I and II cases, complete removal of breast tissue—total mastectomy—is advisable in the great majority of patients, together with exploration of the axilla. The extent of axillary dissection depends on the surgeon's preference and may involve simple excision of a pectoral node for histological examination *or* complete clearance of the axillary contents in the form of a modified radical mastectomy. In the more conservative surgical approach, the state of the axillary glands is assessed during the operation and a decision to refer the patient for radiotherapy is reinforced in the light of histological evidence of involved axillary nodes. In addition, some surgeons chose to obtain lymph glands from the internal mammary chain for histological examination so as to help in determining the prognosis of the disease.

In Stage III cases, total mastectomy is advised provided that this will result in complete removal of the breast tumour (and involved underlying muscles) and allow for adequate skin closure. The extent of axillary dissection will depend more on the disease than the surgeon's preference and the operation will most likely be followed by radiotherapy if the excision has been inadequate. In the *more extensive Stage III case*, irradiation may precede surgery, the aim being to prevent fungation of the tumour and provide local control of the disease.

In Stage IV cases, treatment can be no more than palliative. Mastectomy may be advised, in order to deal with or to prevent fungation. Pleural effusions or isolated metastases in bone are best dealt with by radiotherapy, which is often effective in relieving pain in such cases. When there is fungation of the growth, radiotherapy may reduce the offensive discharge and allow the ulcer to heal. Progress of the disease may be controlled by hormone therapy, by endocrine surgery, by the administration of antimitotic drugs, or by a combination of these methods.

Hormone manipulation for progressive disease. The hormone control of breast cancer (like that of normal breast development) is exceedingly complex. About 40% of breast cancers are hormone-dependent (Barlow, 1968) in that arrest of growth or regression may be obtained by altering the patient's hormone balance. Unfortunately, in spite of intensive research, there is as yet no reliable method of determining which patients are most likely to respond to endocrine therapy, although interesting comparisons have been made between the levels of various urinary steroids in successful and unsuccessful cases (Atkins, 1966). Measurement of the ER (oestrogen receptor) content of breast tumour tissue, however, provides a predictive test for the selection of patients for therapy. The collected results of studies throughout the world provide clear evidence that receptor analysis is of value

in the management of advanced disease (Griffiths, 1981). More than 94% of all patients with ER negative tumours failed to respond to endocrine therapy whereas more than half of those with ER positive tumours responded (McGuire, 1975). The most striking effects are relief of pain, improvement in nutrition, and regression of local lesions. Thus, osteolytic lesions may calcify and pathological fractures heal. The effects, however, are only temporary, since, after a varying interval, the tumour cells lose their hormone dependence, and thereafter the disease progresses rapidly. No claims for permanent cure have been recorded, nor are they at present anticipated although remission may last for several years in some cases.

In pre-menopausal patients, whose tumours are ER positive, removal of the ovaries will frequently delay progress of the disease, and such patients may be advised to submit to oöphorectomy at the first sign of recurrence. Ovarian irradiation is an alternative to this operation. Remission of the disease following removal or irradiation of the ovaries implies that the tumour is sensitive to hormone deprivation but failure of response suggests that further endocrine therapy is unlikely to be rewarding.

In post-menopausal patients, the anti-oestrogen drug *Tamoxifen* is of proven value. It binds to the oestrogen receptor in tumour cells but has very little oestrogenic activity and very low toxicity. Use of the drug gives rise to good objective remission in about 30–40% of patients with metastatic breast cancer. When used in pre-menopausal patients—where it is equally effective—amenorrhoea may result and appropriate advice should be offered regarding the avoidance of pregnancy. *Aminoglutethimide*, an agent which inhibits steroid (especially oestrogen) synthesis by the adrenal and other tissues, will give rise to similar objective remissions in post-menopausal women with acceptable toxicity (Powles, 1981).

Adrenalectomy and hypophysectomy were introduced about 1953 as a method of obtaining hormone deprivation but their value has been largely undermined by the use of anti-oestrogen drugs since oestrogens can still be detected in the serum after adrenalectomy but not after Tamoxifen. Both operations are major procedures, associated with a considerable mortality and morbidity. Although they offer a 50% chance of relief of pain, there is no more than a 30% prospect of worthwhile remission of the disease (Wallace, 1975). One naturally hesitates to advise an operation which may have so little to offer, since, unless the patient, who has probably only a few months to live, is having severe pain unrelieved by analgesics, she may well be happier left in peace at home with her family.

Combination cytotoxic chemotherapy. The use of three or more potent drugs, aimed at reducing the bulk of tumour tissue, should be reserved for the patient with recurrent breast cancer who is unresponsive to endocrine manipulation or whose tumour is ER negative. A number of drug regimes has been devised, mainly in the form of intermittent or 'pulsed' doses involving one intravenous injection each 2–4 weeks. Although many useful remissions have been obtained, the result is, at best, temporary and side effects may be unpleasant.

Adjuvant therapy. In the management of 'early' breast cancer, it is anticipated that the survival rates will be improved by the use of cytotoxic and anti-oestrogen drugs *at the time of the initial surgery.* The basis for this treatment lies in the fact that micrometastases may be undetected and are likely to be destroyed by chemotherapy. Such a response in post-menopausal patients has been reported by Nissen-Meyer (1978) and further studies are now in progress (Cooke, 1982). It is now accepted that Tamoxifen should be prescribed routinely.

Diagnosis of malignancy

It is often impossible to differentiate with certainty on clinical evidence between a simple swelling and an early malignant one. A period of observation is then unjustifiable, since the delay in treatment may allow the disease to spread. Investigation by mammography is justified only in the doubtful lump since the surgeon would find it difficult to refuse biopsy of an 'obvious' carcinoma even if mammography did not confirm the diagnosis.

Needle puncture is of value in solitary swellings thought to be cystic when aspiration of fluid confirms the diagnosis (Murley, 1976). Cytological examination of the aspirate for malignant cells will detect the occasional carcinoma but refilling of a cyst which has been evacuated, or persistence of a lump, is suspicious.

Aspiration biopsy. This term implies the microscopic examination of cellular material removed from a solid lump through an aspirating needle (Salter, 1981). Its value depends on the availability of a skilled cytologist to interpret films made and stained at the time of aspiration.

Needle biopsy. A core of tissue can be removed with a *Tru-cut* needle under local anaesthetic but the accuracy is less than 75% (Owen, 1980). Unfortunately, needle biopsy is of least value in the small doubtful tumour where it may be impossible to obtain a representative sample for the histologist.

Excision biopsy for histological examination (paraffin sections) may be advised as a preliminary operation so that, if malignancy is confirmed, the patient can be prepared for definitive treatment. Some patients prefer this approach whereas others would rather avoid the delay between the initial biopsy and the more major procedure. There is no evidence that any delay affects the eventual outcome. It is important that the skin incision should lie *within* the ellipse required for mastectomy should this become necessary.

Diagnostic incision. To make an incision directly into the substance of the swelling, and to reach a diagnosis from the character of its cut surface is an entirely rational procedure. In the hands of an experienced surgeon, it is probably as reliable as frozen section histology, in which a definite possibility of error must be accepted although many hospitals now have pathologists skilled in this type of diagnosis. On section with the knife a carcinoma feels hard and gritty 'like an unripe pear'. Its cut surface is seen to merge imperceptibly into the surrounding fat; it has a striated appearance, and becomes concave owing to retraction of fibrous tissue. An area of fibrocystic dysplasia, or a fibroadenoma, has a more rubbery consistence and becomes convex on section; the former may show areas of cystic formation, while the latter is clearly encapsulated. Small swellings should be completely excised with a good margin of healthy breast tissue, before being cut into. In the case of large swellings, it is better to make an incision through the overlying skin, and to deepen it so as to cut directly into the centre of the tumour in situ. (If excision is carried out, a large cavity is left and may well contain cancer cells; this cavity may be opened and the cells dispersed over the wound, if the local excision is followed by mastectomy.) Should the naked-eye appearance and frozen section indicate malignancy, the exploratory wound is closed and, after gloves and towels have been changed, the appropriate elective treatment is at once carried out. This approach assumes that the patient has been suitably prepared and has given her consent.

Operative staging

During mastectomy for breast carcinoma, the axillary content can be more accurately examined than was possible before the operation and nodes are removed for histological examination. Unless the surgeon is confident that he has cleared all nodes from the axilla, the finding of involved glands will necessitate radiotherapy. Thus, the patient may be put in operative *stage A* if local surgery is all that is required, *stage B* if local surgery must be supplemented by radiotherapy because of massive local tumour or positive nodes (indicating high risk malignancy), or *stage C* where treatment is of a general and palliative nature for widespread disease.

Local excision

The ideal treatment for breast cancer is to have breast conservation and cure of the disease. Local excision of a tumour, with a clear margin of breast tissue, is not yet standard treatment unless as part of a controlled trial. It may, however, be suitable for the elderly patient in order to minimise her stay in hospital and avoid any risk of poor wound healing. A large series has been reported by Calle (1978) with good results.

Simple (total) mastectomy and axillary sampling

Treatment of the primary disease is important for adequate local control and for staging of carcinoma. Removal of the breast as a whole may also be advised when the gland is the seat of a simple tumour of large size, such as an intracanalicular fibroadenoma, or of widespread fibrocystic disease. It is the operation of choice in duct papilloma in patients over 40 years of age where the site of the tumour cannot be determined and where the risk of undetected malignancy exists. When it is performed in the treatment of carcinoma, and is to be followed by radiotherapy, the following points in the technique are important.

1. Iodine should not be used for preparation of the skin, nor should adhesive strapping be applied post-operatively, since any irritation produced lowers the skin tolerance to irradiation.

2. While the skin of the nipple and areola and that overlying the tumour must be excised, the total amount of skin removed should be as limited as possible. Tightly-stretched skin, and areas which have healed by granulation or grafting do not tolerate irradiation well. If such conditions are present, the dosage may require to be reduced.

3. In order that the irradiation may be concentrated on as small an area as possible, undermining of skin flaps and opening-up of tissue planes around the breast are reduced to a minimum.

4. The pectoral fascia, unless the growth is adherent to it should not be removed. Retention of the fascia lessens the risk of post-irradiation fibrosis in the muscles, and allows the maximum dose of therapy to be employed.

5. Drainage, if not of the 'vacuum' type (p. 2), should be carried out through the lower end of the main wound, rather than through a stab-wound placed lateral to it. In this way the operative field and the area consequently requiring irradiation, are more confined.

6. In Stage III cases, where the tumour is fixed to the pectoral muscle, part of the muscle should be removed along with the breast.

Technique of operation

During the operation the arm is placed on a rest or is supported by an assistant in the abducted position. It is an advantage to have the head of the table elevated 15–30 degrees to reduce venous congestion.

Incision. In the incision generally employed the central part is made in the form of an ellipse, which includes both the nipple and the skin overlying the tumour. The axis of the ellipse depends, therefore, on the relationship of the tumour to the nipple. Whenever possible, the axis of the ellipse should be transverse so that no part of the scar is visible above normal clothing (Fig. 13.1). The extent of the ellipse will vary with the size of the breast.

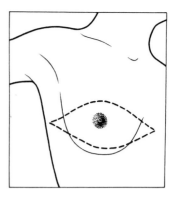

Fig. 13.1 Transverse incision for simple (total) mastectomy.

The skin flaps should be just adequate for covering the chest wall after the gland has been removed. Any upper extension of the incision should not lie too close to the margin of the axillary fold, or a 'bridle' scar may result.

Excision. The skin is raised from the breast substance and is reflected back on each side. There is no clear plane between skin and breast, but prior infiltration of a 1 in 300 000 adrenalin solution serves as a guide during dissection and also diminishes blood loss. The thickness of the skin flaps is increased as the dissection progresses. It is usually desirable that the entire breast (and not only the visible protuberant part) should be removed. For this the flaps must be reflected sufficiently to expose the full anatomical extent of the gland and the axillary tail (Fig. 13.2). When these limits have been defined, the breast is freed by sharp dissection from the underlying pectoral fascia starting just below the clavicle. Bleeding occurs from perforating branches of the internal mammary and intercostal arteries. Most of these vessels

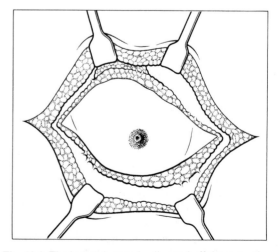

Fig. 13.2 The breast about to be dissected off the pectoral fascia and the axillary tail defined.

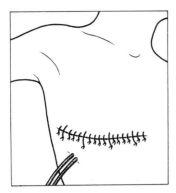

Fig. 13.3 Closure of the wound

require ligature or diathermy coagulation, since haemostasis must be as complete as possible. When the breast
has been freed from the anterior surface of the pectoralis
major muscle, the axillary tail can be clearly defined and
traced upwards to allow gland sampling and full examination of the axilla. Branches of the lateral thoracic vessels require to be secured as axillary contents are freed
and removed along with the breast. Removal of a piece
of tumour for oestrogen receptor assay can now be done
before the excised breast is sent to the pathologist. The
skin wound is sutured, drainage being provided by a
small strip of plastic or by two *Redivac* tubes
(Fig. 13.3).

Modified radical mastectomy

Objectives

This operation, pioneered by Patey (Handley, 1975) is
used by many surgeons for primary treatment of breast
cancer as an alternative to postoperative radiotherapy for
involved axillary glands. It is also justified if adequate
radiotherapy is not available. The pectoralis major is
widely retracted and the pectoralis minor removed. This
gives adequate exposure to allow the axillary contents to
be cleared as completely as in the Halsted operation. Its
main advantage over radical mastectomy is cosmetic, in
that the axillary fold is maintained and there is no hol-
lowing below the clavicle. It also gives a stronger and
more useful arm.

Technique

The incision employed is an elliptical one as for simple
(total) mastectomy (Fig. 13.4). The breast, together with
the deep fascia, is dissected laterally off the pectoralis
major (Figs 13.5 and 13.6). This muscle is now made to
relax by an assistant raising the arm so that the elbow
points towards the ceiling; its lower margin is cleared,
and a retractor is placed against its deep surface. When
this is drawn forwards, it enables the dissection to be
carried upwards in the plane between the two pectoral

Figs 13.4–13.7 *Modified radical mastectomy*

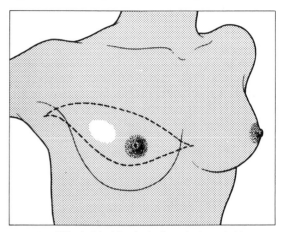

Fig. 13.4 Elliptical incision including nipple and skin
overlying the tumour

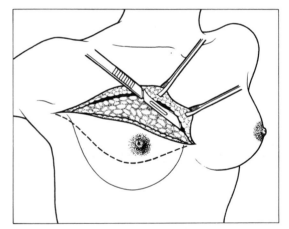

Fig. 13.5 Dissection of the upper skin flap

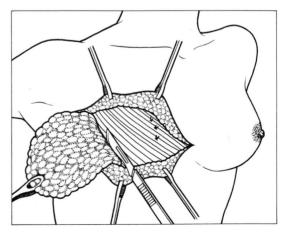

Fig. 13.6 The breast is dissected laterally off the pectoralis
major

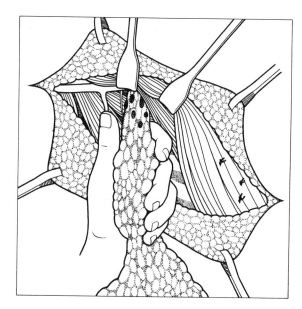

Fig. 13.7 Mobilisation of apical glands and axillary tail using the breast for traction. It is not always necessary to sacrifice the pectoralis minor muscle as in this case

muscles. Pectoralis minor and the clavipectoral fascia are now exposed. This muscle is divided at its insertion and is reflected medially; a branch of the thoraco-acromial artery and the lateral thoracic artery, which run respectively along its upper and lower borders, require to be secured. The pectoralis minor can then be drawn downwards and erased from its costal origin. The axilla is now uncovered, and the dissection of its contents can be commenced. The fascial sheath of the axillary vessels is incised from the clavicle to the lower border of latissimus dorsi. The lower leaf of this fascia, and all fatty and glandular structures which lie below and medial to the vein, are stripped downwards by gauze dissection, i.e. by using the finger covered with several thicknesses of gauze. The apical glands, which lie in the fat at the medial side of the axillary vein just below the clavicle, are removed in this way, as also are the lateral chain of glands which are medial to the vein at a lower level (Fig. 13.7). The stripping process is continued downwards until the muscles of the posterior axillary wall (subscapularis, teres major and latissimus dorsi), and the serratus anterior (forming the medial wall) are completely cleared of all fascial, fatty and glandular tissue. In this part of the dissection, the nerve to latissimus dorsi on the posterior wall, and the nerve to serratus anterior on the medial wall, are identified and carefully preserved. The upper branches of the axillary artery and their companion veins are usually sacrificed; the subscapular vessels are preserved only if the surrounding fatty tissue which harbours the posterior chain of glands can be cleared

without difficulty. The intercostobrachial nerve is divided as it emerges from the second rib space.

Radical mastectomy

The classical operation of radical mastectomy (Halsted) was designed to remove the breast containing a tumour and the entire system of lymphatic glands en bloc which involved sacrifice of at least part of pectoralis major and the whole of pectoralis minor muscles in addition to other structures. The assumption that such a radical procedure would remove all possible tumour cells is no longer accepted and it has no advantages over the other procedures already described.

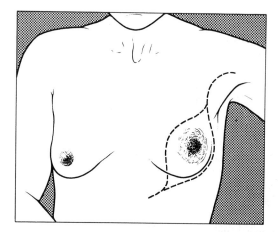

Fig. 13.8 The extent of incision required for radical mastectomy

BENIGN BREAST DISEASE

Certain simple lesions of the breast are dealt with adequately by local excision. This is carried out usually through an incision placed directly over the swelling, and in a line radiating from the nipple, because of the supposed risk of dividing the lactiferous ducts. Some surgeons, however, prefer to place their incisions *transversely* to the radial line, pointing out that no harm results from possible division of the ducts, and that the cosmetic result is much better.

Breast cysts
Many isolated breast swellings, which do not at first appear to be cystic, prove to contain fluid when aspiration is attempted. Repeated aspiration of breast cysts is a safe procedure (Hinton, 1981) provided that the lump disappears completely and no malignant cells are found on cytological examination.

Fibrocystic disease

Operation is indicated when discomfort or mental unrest persist after reassurance, or when malignancy cannot absolutely be excluded. A cyst or a localised area of fibro-adenosis is too adherent to be shelled out like a fibro-adenoma; as a rule it should be removed along with an elliptical segment of breast tissue (partial mastectomy). The long axis of the ellipse is placed radially in order that unnecessary destruction of the lobar systems may be avoided. Haematoma formation is common, and, unless the cavity is a small one and can be completely obliterated by sutures, drainage for 24–48 hours is advisable.

Fibroadenoma

This tumour, which is usually small and encapsulated, can be enucleated without injury to the surrounding breast tissue. To enable this to be done, the incision must be carried through the capsule of the tumour exposing its substance, and the enucleation is carried out in the plane between the tumour and its capsule. It is impossible to enucleate cleanly round the capsule, since this is firmly attached to the fibrous stroma of the gland. With a giant fibroadenoma occupying the greater part of the breast, simple mastectomy may be the best procedure.

Duct papilloma

This condition, which is situated usually in one of the larger ducts deep to the areola, should be suspected when there is serous or sanguineous discharge from the nipple. The formerly held view that it is a pre-cancerous lesion is not now substantiated. The tumour may be felt beneath the areola, or its presence may be determined at a point where local pressure produces the discharge; in 80% of cases this can be localised to one duct (Atkins, 1964). When its site can be identified, local excision is the treatment of choice in all cases. At operation the dilated duct is located by introducing the blunt end of a fine straight needle, which should then pass into the cavity containing the papilloma (Fig. 13.9). The affected duct system is now excised through an incision extending around the margin of the areola, while the needle is held in position. If no tumour or site of bleeding can be detected, it is advisable, in women over 40 years of age, that simple mastectomy should be performed; in younger women, an expectant policy is justified (Forrest, 1966). If examination of any tissue removed shows malignant change, mastectomy is at once performed.

Gaillard Thomas's method

This method is advised in young women who desire an inconspicuous scar. It is also used in young men who request excision of gynaecomastia involving the whole breast tissue. (Gynaecomastia underlying the nipple is removed through a circumareolar incision). An incision is made round the circumference of the inferolateral

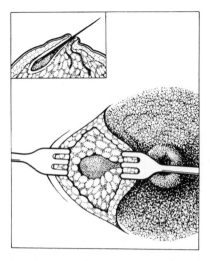

Fig. 13.9 Local excision of a duct papilloma. Inset shows needle in duct used as a guide to the location of the tumour

quadrant of the breast following the submammary sulcus. The deep surface of the gland is freed by dissection from the pectoral fascia, and the breast as a whole is turned upwards (Fig. 13.10). The tumour is then identified, and dealt with from the deep aspect, after which the breast is allowed to fall back and the incision is sutured. Drainage for 24 hours should always be employed.

The approach described is applicable to tumours in any part of the breast, and not, as is frequently stated, only to those in the lower half. Indeed, the method is perhaps most useful in the case of tumours in the superomedial quadrant, where the scar of a direct approach might be visible during the wearing of evening dress. There is no difficulty in throwing up the mamma sufficiently for the necessary access to be obtained.

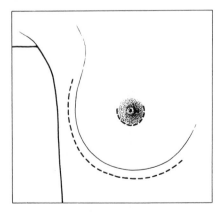

Fig. 13.10 The Gaillard Thomas approach for the removal of simple lesions of the breast. Para-areolar incision for a localised excision is also shown

BREAST ABSCESS

Acute inflammation of the breast (acute mastitis) occurs during lactation, the infection entering through a crack in the nipple. A broad spectrum antibiotic is advisable at the stage of cellulitis since the causative staphylococcus is liable to be resistant to penicillin, but the formation of pus must be anticipated. By retarding tissue necrosis or pus formation, an antibiotic can alleviate both local pain and systemic disturbance, but it denies to the patient the more prompt and lasting benefit that might be obtained from surgical drainage. Furthermore, by promoting excessive fibrosis around the inflammatory lesion, it prevents the abscess cavity from collapsing after incision, and delays final resolution (Ellis, 1969).

Operation should not be delayed until there is fluctuation, for this sign will be elicited only when the abscess has become superficial, and by that time the breast may have suffered irreparable damage. If, after two or three days of antibiotic therapy, tenderness, induration or other signs of inflammation show no signs of subsiding, it is almost certain that deep-seated pus is present, and an operation for drainage should no longer be delayed.

Technique

The incision, which should lie over the area of maximum tenderness, may be placed radially or transversely according to preference (p. 277). When pus is encountered the gloved finger is introduced and the abcess cavity is explored. This is usually partially loculated from the presence of permeated and softened fibrous septa. Such septa, which are nonresistant to the finger, are gently broken down so that the loculi communicate freely. Any loculus which cannot be laid open in this way must be drained by a separate incision. If the abscess appears to be *pre-mammary*, i.e. situated in the subcutaneous tissue, a communicating loculus within the breast substance should be sought.

If the abscess cavity extends deeply into the gland, counterdrainage or dependent drainage is advisable. A pair of forceps is introduced into the cavity, and is gently pushed towards the nearest point on the periphery of the breast. The second incision is made by cutting down on the point of the forceps. A strip of corrugated plastic is then passed between the two openings (Fig. 13.12). Alternatively, if drainage through the second incision is considered to be adequate, the primary incision may be sutured.

Retromammary abscess occurs in the cellular tissue between the breast and the deep fascia. The gland itself is usually not involved but is pushed forward by the swelling. An incision is made along the submammary sulcus, and sinus forceps are introduced. After pus has been evacuated, a search is made for any intramammary prolongation of the abscess, or for a focus of infection in the sternum or ribs. Such abscesses may be tuberculous, in which case the skin incision should be closed, and appropriate chemotherapy instituted.

Chronic subareolar suppuration

Such suppuration occurs most commonly in one or more of the major ducts (Fig. 13.13) and is likely to result from blockage of the duct orifice by inspissated secretion, or from involutionary changes leading to chronic dilatation (*ectasia*). It may be the cause of persistent or intermittent discharge from the nipple; alternatively, by pointing on the skin of the para-areolar region, it may give rise to a *mammillary fistula*.

Operations for drainage, or local excision of the affected duct, are apt to be unsatisfactory, and Thomas

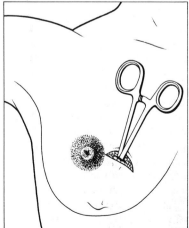

Fig. 13.11

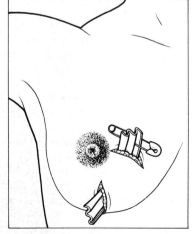

Fig. 13.12

Figs 13.11 & 13.12 Method of draining a breast abscess

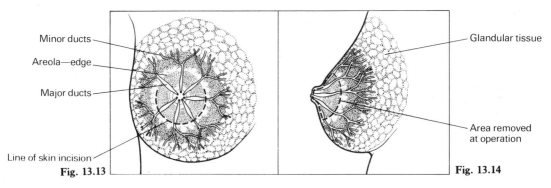

Figs. 13.13 & 13.14 Schematic drawings to show the anatomy of the major lactiferous ducts of the breast, and the extent of an operation for their removal (After Hadfield)

(1982) advises excision of the nipple and major ducts as an alternative.

Hadfield (1969) has described an ingenious operation to excise the entire major duct system, with preservation of the nipple and with little or no reduction in the size of the breast. It is designed to bridge the gap between local operations on a single duct, and the alternative (which is probably unnecessarily radical) of local mastectomy.

Technique of excision of major duct system

An incision is made along the lower half of the areolar margin, and any sinus present is excised. The areolar flap is reflected upwards from the underlying breast tissue, the lactiferous ducts being divided as they enter the nipple. The block of tissue containing the major ducts can then be excised as a roughly conical mass, with long axis of 2.5–4 cm and with a base (lying deeply) of approximately the same diameter as that of the areola (Fig. 13.14). Any obvious ducts entering the mass are closed by ligature or by diathermic coagulation as they are divided, and the cavity in the breast substance is obliterated by deep sutures. The nipple, if previously indrawn, is everted by a purse-string suture applied round the deep surface of its base. The areolar flap is sutured back in position, a small drain being left beneath it for 24 hours. The breast is kept well supported by strapping or by a firm brassière, during healing of the wound.

According to Hadfield, future pregnancies cause no undue disturbance in a breast which has been subjected to this operation—except possibly for a little local tenderness if the pregnancy occurs within 12 months of surgery.

PLASTIC OPERATIONS ON THE BREAST

Correction of indrawn nipples may be indicated in order to permit breast feeding; occasionally, it may be

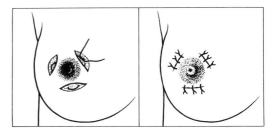

Figs. 13.15 & 13.16 Ashford's operation for retraction of the nipple

requested on aesthetic grounds. It can usually be effected by a simple plastic procedure.

In the operation of Ashford the nipple is drawn outwards with a transfixing stitch. Three elliptical segments are excised from the areolar or periareolar skin, the long axis of each ellipse being placed tangentially (Fig. 13.15). A purse-string suture of silk is passed subcutaneously between the three wounds, and is tied with sufficient tightness to prevent retraction of the nipple, but must not strangulate it. Suture of the incisions tightens the areolar skin, and assists in preventing recurrence (Fig. 13.16).

Reconstruction of pendulous and hypertrophic breasts

Operation may afford great relief to patients who suffer physically from excessively heavy breasts, or who are socially or economically embarrassed by their condition.

Meticulous planning of the operation is essential. Detailed measurements must be taken in order that smoothly contoured and symmetrical breasts may be obtained, and special precautions are necessary to ensure that the blood supply to the nipple and skin flaps is preserved. The operation, therefore, is one of some magnitude, and should not normally be undertaken by those without special training or experience in plastic work.

A number of different operations have been described. Of these, the following two have proved satisfactory:

1. The nipple and areola may be transplanted as a free graft. No attempt is made to conserve the function of the breast, and the operation is indicated therefore in women who are approaching the menopause, or who have very pendulous (and probably functionless) breasts. Firstly, the nipple and areola are excised in the manner employed for raising a free whole-thickness skin graft (p. 13). The incision is extended transversely to each side, and the lower part of the breast is amputated. The upper part is left in situ, and is trimmed suitably to form the new prominence. Redundant skin is excised, and adjustments are made so that the sutured wound lies in the submammary sulcus. Finally, the nipple and areola are grafted on to a circular bed prepared in the appropriate position. A carefully applied pressure dressing is essential to survival of the graft.

2. The nipple may be transplanted at the apex of a pedicle of breast tissue; this is cut in such a way that the nipple remains attached to its lactiferous ducts, and its blood supply is not endangered. In the operation devised by Biesenberger, a circular incision is made around the areola, which is then anchored by four stitches to the underlying breast tissue. A second incision is made down to the submammary sulcus, skin flaps are reflected, and the greater part of the breast *lateral* to the areola is removed. (Adequate blood supply to the medial part of the breast should be assured from branches of the internal mammary artery.) The lower part of the remaining breast segment is mobilised, rotated medially, and sutured to the upper part. In this way the breast is considerably reduced in size and elevated, while the nipple remains situated at its most prominent part. Redundant skin is removed so that the wound can be sutured accurately round the areola and in the submammary sulcus.

Reconstruction following mastectomy

Immediate reconstruction is carried out in some clinics where the surgeon has the combined skills of a cancer specialist and plastic surgeon. Most surgeons will select, for referral to the plastic surgeon, patients who particularly request the operation and who have survived at least two years since the mastectomy. The objectives of reconstruction are volume replacement, maintenance of a cleavage between the breasts, absence of visible scars with normal clothing and unrestricted arm mobility. A *silicone prosthesis* may be placed subcutaneously (Burnand, 1980) but is liable to ulceration or capsule formation. A *latissimus dorsi flap* uses skin overlying this muscle to replace the deficiency following mastectomy and the muscle itself to occupy the space resulting from breast excision. The combined flap of muscle and skin is based on the subscapular artery which must be carefully preserved. A *rectus abdominis flap* may be employed in a similar manner and a thoraco-abdominal flap may be used to restore deficient skin cover.

REFERENCES

Atkins H 1966 Carcinoma of breast. Annals of the Royal College of Surgeons of England 38: 133
Atkins H, Wolff B 1964 Discharges from the nipple. British Journal of Surgery 51: 602
Barlow D, Meggitt B F 1968 Clinical indices to the response rate of advanced breast cancer to bilateral adrenalectomy and oophorectomy. British Journal of Surgery 55: 809
Baum M 1973 Immunological considerations. Journal of the Royal College of Surgeons of Edinburgh 18: 351
Baum M 1980 Carcinoma of breast. Annals of the Royal College of Surgeons of England 62: 35
Burn I 1980 Selective policy in the treatment of early breast cancer. Annals of the Royal College of Surgeons of England 62: 49
Burnand K G, Bulman A S, Nash A G 1980 The place of subcutaneous mastectomy with immediate silicone prosthetic implantation in diseases of the breast. Annals of the Royal College of Surgeons of England 62: 449
Calle R, Pilleron J P, Schlienger P, Vilcoq J R 1978 Conservative management of operable breast cancer. Cancer 42: 2045
Cooke T 1982 The clinical application of oestrogen receptor analysis in early cancer of the breast. Annals of the Royal College of Surgeons of England 64: 165
Dahl-Iversen E 1963 An extended radical operation for carcinoma of the breast. Journal of the Royal College of Surgeons of Edinburgh 8: 81

Edwards M H, Baum M, Magerey C J 1972 Regression of axillary lymph nodes in cancer of the breast. British Journal of Surgery 59: 776
Ellis H 1969 The place of antibiotics in surgical practice today. Annals of the Royal College of Surgeons of England 45: 162
Forrest A P M et al 1979 Is the investigation of patients with breast cancer for occult metastatic disease worthwhile? British Journal of Surgery 66: 749
Forrest A P M 1980 Conservative management of breast cancer. Annals of the Royal College of Surgeons of England 62: 41
Forrest A P M 1981 Primary management of breast cancer In: Breast cancer. Update, London, p 14
Forrest H 1966 Intraduct papilloma of the breast. British Journal of Surgery 53: 1028
Griffiths K, Nicholson R I 1981 Steroid receptors In: Breast cancer. Update, London, p 33
Hadfield G J 1969 The pathological lesions underlying discharges from the nipple in women. Annals of the Royal College of Surgeons of England 44: 323
Handley R S 1975 Carcinoma of the breast. Annals of the Royal College of Surgeons of England 57: 59
Hawkins R A, Roberts M M, Forrest A P M 1980 Oestrogen receptors and breast cancer: Current status. British Journal of Surgery 67: 153
Hayward J L 1980 Radical breast surgery. Annals of the

Royal College of Surgeons of England 62: 43

Hinton C P, Hughes R G 1981 Repeated aspiration of breast cysts—a safe procedure. British Journal of Surgery 68: 45

Hughes L E, Forbes J F 1978 Early breast cancer: Part I: Surgical pathology and pre-operative assessment. British Journal of Surgery 65: 753

McGuire W L, Carbone P P, Vollmer E P (eds) 1975 In: Estrogen receptors in human breast cancer. Raven Press, New York

McNair T J, Dudley H A F 1960 Axillary lymph nodes in patients without breast carcinoma. Lancet 1: 713

Millis R R, McKinna J A, Hamlin I M E, Greening W P 1976 Biopsy of the impalpable breast lesion detected by mammography. British Journal of Surgery 63: 346

Murley R S 1976 Treatment of benign breast disease. Annals of the Royal College of Surgeons of England 58: 385

Nissen-Meyer R, Kjellgren K, Malmio K, Mansson B, Norin T 1978 Surgical adjuvant chemotherapy. Cancer 41: 2088

Owen A W M C, Anderson T J, Forrest A P M 1980 Closed

biopsy for breast cancer. Journal of the Royal College of Surgeons of Edinburgh 25: 237

Powles T J 1981 Adjuvant therapy of breast cancer In: Breast cancer. Update, London, p 20

Robbins G F 1978 Indication for radical and extended radical mastectomy. In: Surgical Clinics of North America 58: No. 4. Saunders, Philadelphia, p 755

Salter D R, Bassett A A 1981 Role of needle aspiration in reducing the number of unnecessary breast biopsies. Canadian Journal of Surgery 24: 311

Taylor H, Baker R, Fortt R W, Hermon-Taylor J 1971 Sector mastectomy in selected cases of breast cancer. British Journal of Surgery 58: 161

Thomas W G, Williamson R C N, Davies J D, Webb A J 1982 The clinical syndrome of mammary duct ectasia. British Journal of Surgery 69: 423

Wallace I W J 1975 Bilateral adrenalectomy for advanced breast cancer. Journal of the Royal College of Surgeons of Edinburgh 20: 374

FURTHER READING

British Journal of Hospital Medicine 1980 23: 1
  Forrest A P M, Roberts M M Screening for breast cancer, p 8
  Hughes L E, Webster D J T The treatment of early breast cancer, p 22
  Baum M The management of advanced breast cancer, p 32
  Bonadonna G Adjuvant chemotherapy in breast cancer, p 40
Cooperman A M, Esselstyn C B (eds) 1978 Symposium on

breast cancer. Surgical Clinics of North America 58: No. 4. Saunders, Philadelphia

Hadfield G J 1981 Cancer of the breast: retrospect, circumspect and prospect. In: Hadfield J, Hobsley M (eds) Current surgical practice, vol. 3. Arnold, London, ch 19

Ward C M 1981 Breast reconstruction after cancer—aesthetic triumph or surgical disaster. British Journal of Plastic Surgery 34: 124

14

Operations on the thorax

J. M. S. JOHNSTONE & P. R. WALBAUM

INJURIES AND WOUNDS

Most civilian thoracic injuries are due to crushing or bruising accidents following deceleration of motor vehicles or falling masonry. As a result, there may be disruption of the chest wall (ribs, sternum or diaphragm), and damage or delayed ill-effects may be suffered by the viscera within. Penetrating wounds result from stabbing assaults or bullet injuries (Ferguson 1978).

Clinical impressions in chest injuries can be dangerously deceptive, and they frequently engender an unwarranted degree of optimism. Even a comparatively mild degree of thoracic trauma may give rise to the condition of 'wet lung', in which fluid accumulates in the alveoli, in the interstitial spaces and in the bronchial tree. Because of pain, these secretions cannot easily be coughed up, and their accumulation leads to CO_2 retention and to a vicious cycle of respiratory depression. Owing to the rapidity with which this may progress to a fatal issue, priority in the case of multiple injuries should always be given to those which affect the chest.

The immediate and most important aims in treatment are the maintenance or restoration of adequate pulmonary ventilation. For this, the first essential is a clear airway, and bronchoscopy is invaluable for the removal of obstructing blood or mucus. If bronchoscopy fails to give immediate and lasting relief, there should be no hesitation in passing an endotracheal tube. This allows for further removal of secretions and permits the use of positive pressure respiration if necessary, particularly in the treatment of paradoxical respiration. Measurement of the arterial blood gases is the safest guide to the necessity for this form of management. With modern plastic endotracheal tubes, a decision regarding tracheostomy need not be made for at least a week. If there is compression of the lungs by air or blood in the pleural cavity, urgent measures may be required to promote their re-expansion.

Wounds of the thoracic wall are treated by excision or débridement, according to the general principles laid down in Chapter 7. Bleeding from an intercostal vessel may necessitate thoracotomy to enable the vessel to be secured. Penetrating wounds—whatever the possibilities of damage to the intrathoracic viscera—do not necessarily demand surgical intervention, except in the presence of certain fairly well-defined indications as detailed below.

The dangerous thoracic *emergencies*, which demand immediate surgical attention are:

1. Pneumothorax. (As a rule this requires urgent treatment only if there is any loss of function in the opposite lung). *Tension pneumothorax* and *open pneumothorax* constitute definite emergencies requiring immediate attention.
2. Haemothorax with massive or continuing bleeding.
3. Large chest wall defects.
4. Suspected thoraco-abdominal injuries.
5. Wounds of the heart.
6. Rupture of the aorta or great vessels.

Pneumothorax may occur in chest injuries in which contusion of the lung, or its laceration by a rib fragment, allows air to escape from the bronchopulmonary tree into the pleural cavity. It may also, however, occur spontaneously (p. 285). There is dyspnoea, due to compression of aerating lung tissue, and a tympanitic note is present over the affected side of the chest; confirmation is readily obtained by X-ray examination. Associated surgical emphysema may be present.

Treatment is not usually a matter of urgency unless it is a single functioning lung that is being compressed or unless positive pressure respiration is being contemplated. In mild and uncomplicated cases the pneumothorax is steadily absorbed until the lung is fully re-expanded, the time required being directly proportional to the size of the pneumothorax. If there is respiratory embarrassment or if the extent of the pneumothorax is increasing, air should be evacuated from the pleural cavity in the manner described for tension pneumothorax.

Tension (valvular) pneumothorax

This results when the opening into the pleural cavity permits the entrance of air during inspiration, but prevents its exit during expiration. As the volume of air in the pleural cavity increases, the lung collapses and the mediastinum moves towards the opposite side with displacement of the apex beat. Dyspnoea is followed by cyanosis, tachycardia and restlessness. If the condition remains untreated, a fatal outcome will ensue.

Treatment

As an emergency measure, a short wide-bore needle is inserted into the pleural cavity through the second intercostal space 4 cm from the sternum, and is connected to a water-seal through which air is allowed to bubble away (Fig. 14.l). It should normally be replaced by a self-retaining catheter as soon as possible. The catheter is introduced through a 1 cm incision, and with the aid of a trocar and cannula (Fig. 14.3), after infiltration of the intercostal space with local anaesthetic and after checking by aspiration that the underlying pleural space is free. It may be advisable to introduce a second catheter through a lower intercostal space posteriorly; this accelerates re-expansion of the lung and allows any effusion to escape. The catheter or catheters should be retained for 24–48 hours after there is radiological evidence of full lung re-expansion. If leakage of air continues after 4 or 5 days of pleural drainage, thoracotomy may be necessary. The damaged segment of lung is then dealt with by repair or resection.

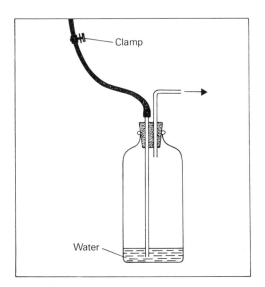

Fig. 14.1 Closed drainage by water-seal

Open pneumothorax occurs when there is a penetrating wound of the chest wall admitting air into the pleural cavity. It constitutes a serious emergency, especially if the diameter of the opening is greater than that of the trachea, for the lung then collapses, owing to the fact that air is drawn through the wound into the pleural cavity,

rather than through the glottis into the lung. A serious degree of respiratory insufficiency develops and may rapidly prove fatal. Diagnosis of the condition presents no difficulty, since it is obvious, on inspection of the wound, that air is being sucked into the pleural cavity at each inspiration (and possibly escaping at expiration). Discharge of frothy blood from the wound indicates lung damage.

Treatment

All perforating wounds of the thoracic wall should be closed as soon as possible, the urgency depending upon the size of the opening. As a temporary measure, any method which produces an airtight closure is effective. One or two skin stitches may suffice; if these are not available, a pad of gauze covered with *Elastoplast* is often adequate. It is advisable to insert an intercostal drain in all cases. At a later stage, and under optimum conditions, exploration and surgical toilet may be carried out, either through the existing wound or through a separate thoracotomy incision.

Haemothorax— bleeding into the pleural cavity—may be caused by any chest injury, and often occurs in association with pneumothorax when the term *haemopneumothorax* is applied. The bleeding may have arisen either from a laceration on the lung surface, from rupture of an intrapleural adhesion, or from damage to an intrathoracic vessel or intercostal artery. The patient shows the classical signs of internal haemorrhage and X-ray confirms the diagnosis. Except when a pneumothorax is also present, there is dullness over the affected side of the chest. As the condition progresses, the patient becomes cyanosed and the neck veins distend.

Treatment

Emergency treatment consists in sedation to relieve pain, transfusion to restore blood volume, and tube-drainage through the 6th or 7th intercostal space in the posterior axillary line. If the patient does not respond to such measures, thoracotomy should be advised; this is particularly necessary if the bleeding is massive and continuing. The chest is opened through the bed of the 5th, 6th or 7th rib; the pleural cavity is cleared of blood, the lung is gently freed and is re-inflated by the anaesthetist. A search is made for a bleeding point on the lung surface, for a torn intrapleural adhesion, or for a torn major or intercostal vessel, and the bleeding is arrested. The lung is then re-expanded, and the pleural cavity is drained to a water-seal. The high mortality in haemothorax has been attributed to a reluctance to operate, but after the initial resuscitation, the patient is in a better condition for operation than he will be for a long time if the bleeding is allowed to continue. *The real risk lies, not in operating, but in not operating* (Borrie).

Chest wall defects

When several ribs are broken both anteriorly and posteriorly, as frequently occurs in severe crushing injuries, a segment of chest wall moves independently from the rest, and is said to be flail. It is thus liable to be sucked-in during inspiration, and so compresses the homolateral lung, driving air from it into the opposite lung. The converse then occurs during expiration. This *paradoxical respiration* leads to inefficient and inadequate ventilation, and results in a dangerous degree of hypoxia and CO_2 retention.

Treatment must be energetic in order to be effective. Mild cases without serious respiratory embarrassment may be treated simply by firm strapping of the chest wall and by oxygen therapy. An open sucking wound of the chest must be closed immediately by suture or firm packing with a wet dressing (Owen-Smith, 1978). More serious cases should be treated by endotracheal intubation and positive pressure respiration. Any major chest wall defect must be repaired as circumstances allow in order that the pleural space can be closed.

Thoraco-abdominal wounds

Owing to the fact that the dome of the diaphragm extends far upwards into the thorax, combined thoracic and abdominal wounds are not uncommon. In nearly all injuries of the upper abdomen the possibility of intra-thoracic damage should be envisaged, and the chest should be X-rayed in the erect position.

As a rule signs of the abdominal injury will predominate, and such signs usually demand surgical exploration (p. 329). It is normally better that the thorax should be explored first—either by enlarging the existing wound or by a separate thoracotomy incision in the 7th, 8th or 9th interspace. By this approach wide exposure of the upper surface of the diaphragm is obtained, and by enlarging any wound found therein the upper abdomen can be explored. 'It is easier to explore the upper abdomen from the chest, than it is to explore the lower part of the chest from the upper abdomen.' (Tudor Edwards). Wounds of the liver, stomach and spleen can usually be dealt with effectively through the diaphragmatic opening. If necessary, the thoracic incision can be extended downwards through the costal margin to provide a combined thoraco-abdominal exposure. If there is found to be damage to the intestine or kidney, it is best to repair the diaphragm and thoracic wall, and then to perform laparotomy.

Ruptured diaphragm may occur from crushing injuries, without any penetrating wound. It is diagnosed on the X-ray finding of air-containing viscera within the chest or the presence of a high and fixed dome of diaphragm. Immediate operative repair is indicated as soon as the initial shock has been overcome. A transthoracic approach is preferred unless there are clear indications for laparotomy.

Wounds of the heart are considered on page 294.

Traumatic rupture of the aorta follows either rapid deceleration or direct chest injury. The most frequently damaged site lies lateral to the left subclavian artery where the descending thoracic aorta lies close to the vertebral column (Keen, 1972). X-ray shows widening of the mediastinum (Keen, 1974) due to bleeding in that area. Aortography should, if possible, be carried out prior to thoracotomy so that any repair of the aorta may be planned. Local bypass of the area is usually required to protect the spinal cord and kidneys from ischaemia.

SPONTANEOUS PNEUMOTHORAX

In 30–40% of cases, pneumothorax occurs spontaneously, without any history of injury or of previous lung disease, but the onset may coincide with heavy lifting or with some other form of muscular strain. It is due usually to the rupture of a bullous cyst (which may be either congenital or emphysematous) on the surface of the lung, especially in the upper lobe. Occasionally, the rupture of a tuberculous cavity on to the lung surface has been responsible. There may be an associated haemothorax, the bleeding having occurred usually from an intra-pleural adhesion which has been torn by the collapsing lung. The onset is sudden and is associated with pain in the chest, together with a sensation of compression or constriction.

Treatment

All but the mildest cases, in which symptoms abate as air is gradually absorbed, should be treated by intercostal drainage. If tension develops, as it not infrequently does, or if there is an associated haemothorax, urgent treatment may be required (see p. 283).

Chronic or recurrent pneumothorax

Persistence or recurrence of the pneumothorax indicates usually the presence of a bronchopleural fistula. The treatment then advised (Ferguson, 1981) is by thoracotomy and excision of bullae or over-sewing of the leak. An alternative form of treatment to pleurectomy is *chemical pleurodesis*. In the latter, iodised talc or kaolin is insufflated (into the pleural space) through a cannula from which the trocar has been removed after insertion through an intercostal space. *Pleurectomy* requires thoracotomy for removal of the parietal pleura in order to provide an extensive raw surface to which the visceral pleura will adhere, thus obliterating the pleural space.

PLEURAL EMPYEMA

The term *empyema* is used to denote a frankly purulent effusion within the pleural cavity. Some difficulty in its application to the acute case arises from the fact that most purulent effusions are preceded by serous or haemorrhagic effusions, in which varying numbers of pus cells can be detected. The time which elapses before frank pus is apparent varies from case to case, depending upon the organisms responsible and upon the efficacy of treatment employed. In most cases the empyema is secondary to some inflammatory condition of the lung—lobar pneumonia, bronchopneumonia or lung abscess. It may sometimes be secondary to suppuration below the diaphragm. In a small proportion of cases, some disease of the lung, such as bronchiectasis or carcinoma, is the primary factor. A pneumococcal or staphylococcal effusion is likely to be purulent from the outset, whereas an effusion due to streptococci or *E. coli* may remain watery in consistence for several days.

Choice of treatment
The availability of antibiotics has led to a considerable reduction in the incidence of empyema. Needle aspiration of fluid for culture and sensitivity will allow the appropriate drug to be prescribed with maximum benefit.

When the pus is thin—and remains thin—many cases can be treated successfully by aspiration combined with the instillation of antibiotics, but any infected effusion generally needs a tube. When *thick pus* is recognised, most surgeons will insert a drain. In the chronic case, decortication may be required or, rarely, thoracoplasty.

Pleural aspiration
The puncture should normally be made in the first instance in the 8th or 9th intercostal space, in the posterior axillary line. Introduction of some contrast medium (*lipiodol*) at this site will locate the lower limit of the cavity on X-ray and allows the aspirating needle to be placed with some accuracy. The patient's arm is abducted so as to displace the scapula (Fig. 14.2). A large needle is required, but its insertion can be rendered quite painless if all tissues from the skin to the pleura at the site of puncture are infiltrated with 1% local anaesthetic solution, injected through a fine needle. In the search for a pleural effusion exploration may be made further afield, but spaces lower than those given should be avoided, or entered with the greatest care. Pus rarely collects in the lowest part of the pleural cavity (*the costodiaphragmatic recess*), since the layers of pleura forming this recess are normally in contact, and become fused together in inflammatory conditions. A needle inserted into the 10th or 11th space is therefore liable to penetrate

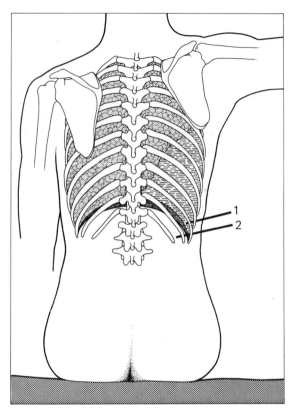

Fig. 14.2 Schematic drawing to show the customary site for drainage of an acute pleural empyema. A needle introduced into the 10th or 11th intercostal space is liable to penetrate the diaphragm and to enter the abdominal cavity. Correct (1) and incorrect (2) positions of the needle are shown

the diaphragm and to enter the abdominal cavity (Fig. 14.2). If it is necessary to explore the pleural cavity through these spaces, the needle should be entered only for a short distance, and should be inclined in an upward direction.

After as much fluid as possible has been removed, a solution of antibiotic may be instilled, or it may be preferred to rely on systemic administration.

Closed drainage by intercostal tube
This method is indicated when, for any reason, aspiration is unsuccessful in preventing the accumulation of fluid within the pleural cavity. The tube advocated is a Malecot's self-retaining catheter, which is available in various sizes. It is introduced by means of a trocar and cannula of suitable calibre. An Argyle catheter does not block so readily and is supplied with its own trocar but it is more difficult to insert with any precision.

The operation may be performed under local anaesthesia, and with the patient seated. The classical site for insertion of the tube is the 8th or 9th intercostal space between the posterior axillary and scapular lines depend-

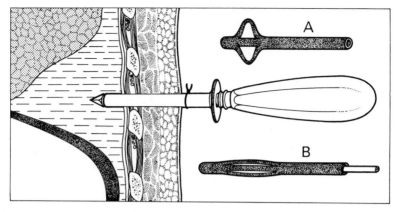

Fig. 14.3 Method of closed drainage of the pleural cavity by means of a Malecot self-retaining catheter, introduced by trocar and cannula through an intercostal space. Note the suture placed around the cannula to mark the proposed depth of penetration

ing on the X-ray taken after injection of contrast medium.

Local anaesthetic is infiltrated at the chosen site, using the needle to confirm the presence of fluid and its depth. An incision 1 cm in length is made in the overlying skin, and the trocar and cannula are introduced by a steady thrusting movement accompanied by rotation. The instrument is kept as close as possible to the rib below in order to avoid the intercostal vessels (Fig. 14.3).

The trocar is withdrawn, and the stretched catheter (or Argyle catheter without its trocar) is immediately introduced. The cannula is then removed, followed by the introducer; the catheter which has now expanded should fit tightly in the wound. As soon as its placing has been confirmed by the escape of pus, the tube is clamped until such time as it can be placed under a 'water-seal' (Fig. 14.1) or connected to suction. It is now withdrawn until its flange comes to lie against the chest wall (Fig. 14.4).

After-treatment
The patient is encouraged to cough, breathing exercises are prescribed, and are carefully supervised. Air-tight

fitting of the tube can normally be maintained for 7 to 10 days, by which time sufficient adhesions will have formed to nullify the effects of atmospheric pressure. The tube should not be discarded until there is clear evidence that the empyema cavity has been obliterated, except along the actual line of the tube track, by contact between visceral and parietal pleura.

Drainage by rib resection
This operation is indicated in cases where the pus is too thick or contains too much organised fibrin to be evacuated by intercostal tube, or where such a tube cannot be placed to drain the lowest part of the cavity. It is safe only if the pus has loculated since, otherwise, pneumothorax could result. Until thick pus has loculated, it is better to do a limited thoracotomy with intercostal drainage. This allows for adequate opening of the space to remove fibrinous clots and an open drain is inserted through the wound one week later, by which time the lung has become adherent. This two stage procedure limits the need for decortication later.

It is possible to carry out the operation under local anaesthesia but general anaesthesia, using a cuffed endotracheal tube and positive pressure, is preferable and is more comfortable for the patient. It is customary to resect 5–7 cm of a rib overlying the lower part of the empyema cavity. The most suitable rib, and the part to be resected, is chosen after diagnostic aspiration has been carried out and contrast medium introduced. The latter indicates which rib should be removed to allow accurate placing of the drain *above* the lower limit of the cavity.

If local anaesthesia is to be employed, the overlying skin and muscles, and the intercostal space above and below the rib selected, are infiltrated with 1% solution. A 10 cm incision is made in the line of the rib (or vertically if two rib spaces are required) and is carried down to the periosteum. A further injection of local anaesthetic

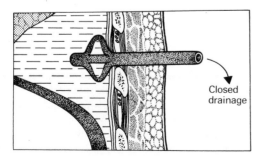

Closed drainage

Fig. 14.4 Malecot catheter lying with its flange against the chest wall

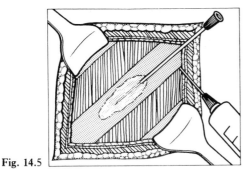
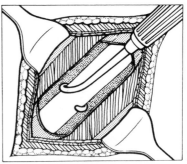

Fig. 14.5

Fig. 14.6

Figs. 14.5 & 14.6 Rib resection under local anaesthesia. Injection of solution below the periosteum, which, after being stripped upwards and downwards, is cleared from the deep surface of the rib by means of a curved elevator

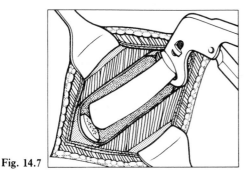
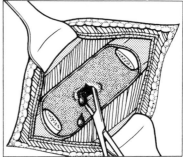

Fig. 14.7

Fig. 14.8

Figs. 14.7 & 14.8 Drainage of empyema after rib resection. Division of rib with special guillotine. Exploration of pleural cavity by sinus forceps introduced through incision in deep periosteum of rib and parietal pleura

is then made subperiosteally on the superficial aspect of the rib, and also just deep to its lower border in the posterior end of the wound, in order to block the intercostal nerve. The periosteum is incised longitudinally, and the section of rib is cleared subperiosteally—first on its superficial surface with a periosteal elevator and then on its deep surface with the special rib-stripper. It is now divided at each end of the wound with rib shears and is removed. The intercostal vessels and nerves are protected by the periosteum and should not normally be damaged in the resection. A final injection of anaesthetic solution is made into the floor of the wound, composed of the deep periosteum of the rib and the adherent parietal pleura. Aspiration with a fine needle will confirm the presence of fluid and its depth. The empyema cavity is now opened by removing a disc of rib bed and thickened parietal cortex. The cavity is vigorously cleaned with gauze to break down any loculi and remove clot which is liable to block the drain.

A tube of at least 2 cm external diameter is employed for drainage. 8 cm of its length should be placed within the empyema cavity, lying along its base, and should have two or more lateral openings cut in it. A short oblique cut is made at the internal end of the tube for subsequent recognition that the whole tube has been

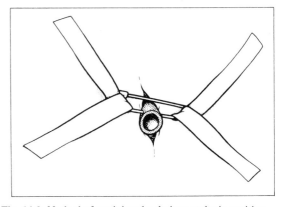

Fig. 14.9 Method of retaining the drainage tube in position

removed. A transfixing safety pin is inserted into the tube outside the skin. The wound is closed by through-and-through stitches on each side of the tube; this is secured by some method to the dressings, which are strapped to the chest wall (see Fig. 14.9).

After treatment is on the lines already described on page 287. Water-seal drainage is not necessary where the empyema cavity is localised and the patient can remain ambulant after the operation. Suction has no effect in expanding the lung, but it helps to remove discharge from the pleural cavity, and obviates the necessity for frequent dressings. Irrigation of the cavity may be carried out if desired. A *pleurogram*, at intervals of 2–3 weeks, is used to assess the reduction in size of the cavity. The tube is not shortened but is retained until X-ray shows obliteration of the whole cavity other than the tube itself.

Decortication

This operation is indicated when simpler drainage has failed and a fibrous lined cavity has formed. It aims at promoting re-expansion of the lung by removal of the densely fibrosed visceral pleura which covers and constricts it. In addition, it should include removal of the thickened membrane covering the diaphragm and chest wall in order to restore mobility to these surfaces. At the same time the lung should be mobilized from the diaphragm and from the mediastinum, so that there may be no hindrance to its complete expansion.

Technique of decortication

The customary approach is by a *posterolateral thoracotomy*—either through the bed of the 7th or 8th rib, which is resected from transverse process to costochondral junction, or through a corresponding intercostal space. Where wide access is required, the rib either above or below may be divided posteriorly. The empyema cavity is mobilized extrapleurally with the aim of removing it intact, starting with the chest wall or diaphragm. The plane of cleavage separating it from the lung is opened up by a combination of blunt and sharp dissection as required. In this way the 'peel' is removed from the collapsed segment of the lung, or from the entire lung if this is necessary to allow complete expansion. This process is helped by inflation of the lungs by the anaesthetist, who should also ensure complete re-expansion of the lung by the end of the operation. When all bleeding has been arrested, a drainage tube is brought out through a convenient intercostal space at the lower limit of the cavity and the thoracic wound is closed. The drainage tube is connected to a water-seal, or preferably to suction; it is removed in 2–3 days if X-rays are satisfactory.

Thoracoplasty

This term denotes an operation to mobilise the chest wall so that it can fall inwards against the collapsed lung or segment of lung, thus obliterating the intervening pleural space. The operation is now rarely required. Indications for a total thoracoplasty may arise in cases of empyema following pneumonectomy. Small persistent cavities may be treated by complete *deroofing*, i.e. by excision of overlying ribs to leave a saucerised cavity which is packed with gauze and allowed to heal from within outwards by granulation.

OPERATIONS FOR PULMONARY TUBERCULOSIS

The introduction of specific chemotherapy has revolutionised the surgery of pulmonary tuberculosis and has led to a steady reduction in the number of patients requiring surgical treatment. Operation is rarely required in U.K. at present but may be indicated when social reasons prevent adequate medical treatment or when chemotherapy has failed due to drug resistance. In addition, there will continue to be patients with undiagnosed pulmonary tuberculosis who have the diagnosis made during exploratory thoracotomy for a pulmonary opacity. Operation represents no more than one part of a carefully controlled regime which includes general measures, rest and intensive chemotherapy.

Surgical treatment takes the form either of resection or, in an exceptional case, of collapse therapy. Resection, with complete removal of the focus of disease, aims to excise the minimum of tissue consistent with maintaining lung function. The object of collapse therapy is to cause relaxation of a diseased segment of lung, so that, by rest and by the obliteration of cavities, healing may occur.

Excisional surgery for pulmonary tuberculosis may take the form of *segmental resection, lobectomy* or *pneumonectomy.* The operation of segmental resection has found increasing acceptance over the past 25 years and has had frequent applications. This method of excision, which conserves as much healthy lung tissue as possible, is the treatment of choice for all relatively small and localised lesions, especially if they are bilateral. Ideally, of course, the resection should ablate the disease without transecting tuberculous tissue. More extensive but still localised lesions will be treated by lobectomy. Pneumonectomy is reserved for cases where there is gross involvement of one lung alone. The technique of these operations is described on pages 290–292.

Thoracoplasty

This term implies an operation for subperiosteal resection of two or more ribs on the affected side of the thorax, so that the chest wall falls inwards on the lung. Thoracoplasty has now largely fallen out of use although it is the only method of collapse therapy still used on occasion. The modern operation is a limited or selective one, designed to preserve as much functioning lung as possible. It is employed, if resection is contraindicated, in the treatment of upper lobe cavities. The chest wall collapse is effected by dividing the 2nd to 4th ribs at their necks and anteriorly. The 5th rib is removed and wound repair fixes the chest wall in its new position.

Operations for tuberculous empyema

The principles are very similar to those which apply to pyogenic empyema, but intensive treatment by antituberculous drugs is an essential prelude to surgery. Open drainage should be avoided, in view of the risk of secondary infection. Decortication, combined if possible with complete excision of the empyema cavity, is the treatment of choice, and is carried out under full antibiotic cover. If active disease is present in the lung, the whole lung or the affected part may be removed together with the thickened pleura.

OPERATIONS FOR LUNG RESECTION

Indications for lung resection

The commonest indication is carcinoma then inflammatory disease—bronchiectasis, tuberculosis and lung abscess, being occasionally treated surgically.

Lung cancer is now the commonest malignant tumour affecting males in U.K. although its incidence appears to be decreasing. The results of excisional surgery, which offers the only known prospect of cure, are not unsatisfactory, when compared with those obtained for many malignant growths elsewhere in the body—but they are none the less disappointing. In patients in whom it is practicable to carry out resection—and these are the early and favourable cases—the 5-year survival rate is less than 30%. X-ray is vital in the diagnosis but bronchoscopy should be carried out in all cases, in an attempt to obtain histological confirmation; only about 50% of tumours, however, can be seen at bronchoscopy (Belcher, 1981) even using the fibreoptic instrument. Percutaneous needle biopsy may also be done under X-ray control for tissue diagnosis when the advisability of operation is in doubt. Signs of an irremovable growth are recurrent laryngeal paralysis, extension to cervical or mediastinal glands, involvement of the trachea, phrenic nerve palsy and distant metastases. In order to establish operability, the minor operations of scalene node biopsy or mediastinoscopy are often employed. In the presence of palpable nodes in the posterior triangle of the neck lying on the scalene muscles, the scalene pad of fat with enclosed enlarged lymph nodes is removed through a small 5 cm transverse skin incision. The platysma is divided and the sternomastoid retracted medially to expose the enlarged nodes. Glands on the anterior scalene muscle are removed as they lie just lateral to the jugular vein which must be avoided. *Mediastinoscopy* is done through a transverse incision above the sternum with vertical division of the cervical fascia to expose the rings of the trachea below the cricoid cartilage. The finger is inserted along the trachea. Laterally lies the pleura and anteriorly the right innominate vein while lower down the innominate artery and aortic arch can be felt. Through the special endoscope, the right and left tracheobronchial nodes and the subcarinal nodes can be seen and dissected bluntly so that a biopsy can be made. The azygos vein is often seen and must not be damaged. Complications are rare but pneumothorax, recurrent nerve palsy and bleeding are reported.

The investigation of mediastinal spread by mediastinoscopy allows a more rational approach to be made in the treatment of lung cancer. Nohl-Oser (1972) has used his extensive experience of the method to describe the anatomy of the glands likely to be involved by tumour. In an analysis of 320 cases, Gunstensen (1972) and his colleagues found that the presence of mediastinal node metastases indicates a poor prognosis in the patients with bronchial carcinoma, and they were able to reduce their unnecessary thoracotomies from 28% to 15%. Despite this investigation, however, an exploratory thoracotomy will still be necessary in certain cases of suspected malignancy in order to establish the diagnosis, or, when a tumour is found, to determine its resectability. Segmental resection or lobectomy should be carried out if possible (Bates, 1981), particularly for patients suffering from peripheral tumours without mediastinal node involvement. Pneumonectomy is used for tumours which involve all lobes or the hilar structures, but has a higher mortality than conservative surgery. Elderly patients (over 70 years of age) have an increased risk in pulmonary resection, and poor respiratory function (as judged by a *Forced Expiratory Volume* of less than 1 litre in 1 second) is a contraindication to pulmonary surgery in younger patients.

Bronchiectasis

Although the mortality of this condition has been greatly reduced by modern chemotherapy, serious complications such as empyema or amyloid disease are always liable to supervene, and, provided that the disease can be eradicated, excisional surgery offers the best prospect of cure. Segmental resection, which is designed to excise only those segments that are actually diseased, and to preserve healthy lung tissue, may be required if there is failure of antibiotic control and if the disease is limited to one lung. This operation may be carried out on both sides although this is rarely done. If the disease is confined to one lobe, and occupies the greater part of that lobe, lobectomy is then the ideal treatment. When extensive unilateral lung destruction is present, pneumonectomy may, rarely, be advocated.

Lung abscess may follow respiratory infection or result from a septic pulmonary embolism. Conservative treatment consists in postural drainage, chemotherapy and bronchoscopic aspiration of the abscess. Segmental resection or lobectomy is occasionally required if the condition does not clear up under conservative treatment.

General principles of lung resection

Access is usually obtained by a posterolateral thoracotomy at the level of the 5th, 6th or 7th ribs, depending upon the site of the proposed resection.

The main dangers of resection operations are (1) spill-over infection into the opposite lung; (2) infection of the pleural cavity, due to the escape of infected sputum from the cut bronchus; (3) the development of a bronchopleural fistula from failed closure or leakage from the bronchial stump. One lung anaesthesia, using one of the bronchus-blocking endotracheal tubes, reduces the risk of spill-over and aids hilar dissection. All manipulations should be carried out very gently. The *individual ligation or suture technique* of the hilar structures is always done, the supplying bronchus and all accompanying vessels being exposed at an early stage of the dissection. If excessive secretions are present, the bronchus should receive prior attention, in order to prevent any spill-over into the opposite lung. Thereafter, the vessels are isolated one by one and are divided between ligatures. The bronchus is now divided close to its parent stem, so as not to leave a blind end, and the separated lung tissue is removed. Particular attention is paid to closure of the bronchial stump, in order to reduce the risk of bronchopleural fistula. All bronchi, including those divided in segmental resections, require careful suture with interrupted nonabsorbable sutures. Crushing clamps should not be used for the proximal bronchial stump since this may cause devitalisation and predispose to leakage.

Segmental resection

This operation is rendered practicable by the anatomical pattern by which there is a relatively avascular plane of cleavage between the various bronchopulmonary segments, each having its own individual artery and bronchus, although the venous drainage may be shared with other segments. The first step in dissection is towards isolation of the segmental bronchus and its accompanying artery. The bronchus is then clamped, whereupon inflation of the lung delineates the segment to be removed, since this remains collapsed. The pleura is divided along the line of the intersegmental plane, and the resection is then effected by a combination of blunt and sharp dissection, the vessels being secured individually. The bronchus is divided *proximal* to the clamp, and is then closed by suture. Raw areas are covered by healthy lung tissue, drawn against them by a few sutures.

Lobectomy

In a healthy lung each fissure may extend nearly to the hilum, but fissure depth is variable and, unfortunately, often incomplete. In diseased conditions the lung is very often adherent to the parietal pleura, especially on the diaphragmatic surface, and adhesions between the lobes may make their separation difficult. The affected lobe is held under a moist pack and is drawn towards the thoracotomy wound. Surrounding adhesions are divided with scissors and the lobe is isolated by opening up the interlobar fissure down to the hilum, further adhesions being dealt with as they are encountered. If it is the lower lobe that is being removed, the pulmonary ligament requires to be divided. The visceral pleura is incised around the hilum of the lobe; the lobar bronchus is isolated and is controlled by a clamp, and the vessels are divided individually between ligatures. The bronchus is then divided *proximal* to the clamp and close to its origin from the main-stem bronchus in order to avoid the formation of a blind end, which owing to its poor blood supply might give way. Closure is effected by the 'open-bronchus' technique, the use of a clamp on the bronchial stump being avoided, so that no crushed or devitalised tissue is included in the suture line. Interrupted sutures of unabsorbable material are employed, and as much of the stump as possible is closed before the division is finally completed (Fig. 14.10). The stump is then securely buried by over-sewn flaps of mediastinal pleura.

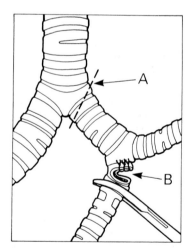

Fig. 14.10 Site for division of bronchus—(A) in pneumonectomy, and (B) lobectomy. The method of suturing the bronchial stump is shown

Pneumonectomy

After parietal adhesions have been divided, the entire lung is drawn gently outwards towards the wound. The pleura is divided around the pulmonary root, and the structures comprising the root are isolated individually. There are certain advantages in isolating and controlling the main-stem bronchus first, but, because of malignant invasion of the root or for other reasons, it may facilitate the dissection if the vessels are dealt with as the first stage

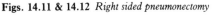

Figs. 14.11 & 14.12 *Right sided pneumonectomy*

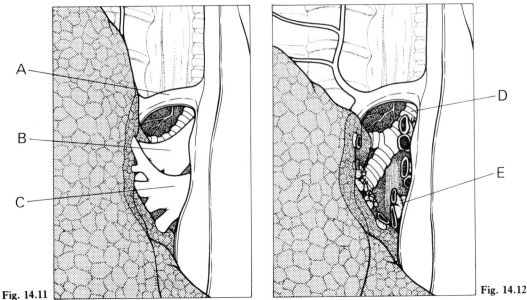

Fig. 14.11

Fig. 14.12

Fig. 14.11 Dissection of the hilum from the front. The right pulmonary artery is seen overlying the main bronchus, with the upper pulmonary vein below it. **Fig. 14.12** The major vessels have been divided between ligatures and the main bronchus is about to be divided: A—azygos vein. B—R. pulm. artery. C—Upper pulm. vein. D—main bronchus. E—Lower pulm. vein. (After Rob and Smith.)

of the dissection. Owing to the risk of tumour emboli being displaced into the pulmonary veins, these may be divided first between transfixing ligatures. The pulmonary artery is closed with a continuous suture. Division of the bronchus is effected close to the bifurcation of the trachea, so that no blind end remains, and closure is carried out in the manner described for lobectomy.

Intrapericardial dissection
In cases of carcinoma where the growth may have extended towards the mediastinum, a more radical dissection can be carried out if the pericardium in front of the hilum is opened to expose the vessels. In this way, the vessels can be dealt with as centrally as possible, and affected lymph nodes in the hilum and in the adjacent mediastinum can be removed at the same time.

OPERATIONS ON THE HEART AND GREAT VESSELS

Surgical approach to the heart
The heart, like other hollow muscular organs, can now be subjected to a wide variety of surgical procedures aimed at maintaining or improving its function. When it has stopped beating, it can be stimulated or massaged in order to restore its function and the life of the patient. Penetrating wounds of its walls can be sutured and foreign bodies removed. Obstruction at the valvular open-

ings can be relieved, and fistulous communications between the two sides of the heart, or between chambers and vessels, can be closed. Furthermore, diseased heart valves can be repaired or replaced with prosthetic valves under vision, with the support of cardiopulmonary bypass, and surgical operation on the coronary arteries is similarly performed.

Methods of exposure
Left thoracotomy is used for closed operations on the heart, for closure of the patent ductus arteriosus, for resection of aortic coarctation and for urgent exposure of the heart. With the patient partly on his side, the incision is made in the 4th or 5th intercostal space extending from the left margin of the sternum to the posterior axillary line. In urgent cases, e.g. cardiac arrest or wounds, the incision is deepened directly through the intercostal space, and the pleural cavity is opened in the same line. In elective cases a better approach, associated with less bleeding, is through the deep periosteum of the rib above the incision (but without rib resection) after detaching the periosteum from its upper border and deep surface. Improved access is readily obtained by dividing the costal cartilage above or below close to the sternum. For wider access, the incision can be extended transversely (*trans-sternal thoracotomy*), dividing the sternum with a Gigli saw and necessitating division and suture ligation of the two internal mammary arteries. *Median sternotomy* (Fig. 14.13) gives the best approach to all

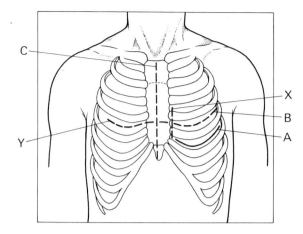

Fig. 14.13 Incisions for exposure of the heart. A & B—the most generally useful incisions in the 5th and 4th intercostal spaces on the left side. Either incision can be enlarged by carrying its medial end upwards along the sternal border (X), or by extending it across the sternum into the corresponding intercostal space on the opposite side (Y). C—incision for exposure of heart by median sternotomy

other operations on the heart, particularly those with cardiopulmonary bypass. The vertical incision extends from the sternal notch to below the xiphoid. The sternum is split with a sternal chisel or pneumatic or electrical saw. A very careful closure using heavy wire sutures to fix the sternum is needed.

Cardiac arrest is a catastrophe which may occur during any operative procedure, major or minor. The patient's survival depends upon prompt action by means of external or internal cardiac massage in order to restore the flow of oxygenated blood in the coronary and cerebral circulations.

Even the most inexperienced house-surgeon should be familiar with the techniques of cardiac resuscitation, for he may be required to undertake it at any time. He must not be deterred by the apparent risks, for the brain at normal temperatures can tolerate no more than 3–4 minutes deprivation of its blood supply, and, if the patient is to survive, the circulation must be restored within this period. He should, preferably, know the location of the special equipment with its supply of drugs and he should know where skilled assistance can be obtained.

After instituting external cardiac massage, the next essential in the emergency situation is to provide adequate pulmonary ventilation, for without this any form of cardiac resuscitation must inevitably fail. An airway is at once introduced, and mouth-to-mouth resuscitation is instituted. Initially, this is entirely adequate, but, as soon as skilled help is available, endotracheal intubation and inflation of the lungs with pure oxygen provide much more efficient oxygenation.

External cardiac massage should always be employed in the first instance. The principle of the method is that pressure on the lower part of the sternum compresses the heart between it and the spine, and forces blood into the arterial system. Relaxation of the pressure then allows the heart to refill. It is carried out by rhythmic pressure with both hands, about 60 times per minute, against the lower sternum, (Fig. 14.14), the patient lying on a firm surface (i.e. either with fracture boards beneath the mattress, or on the floor). Such treatment can at once produce a good systolic blood pressure, with an adequate flow of oxygenated blood to the coronary and cerebral vessels—an effect which can be gauged by palpation of the femoral pulse. While the external cardiac massage is being carried out, adequate pulmonary ventilation must, of course, be maintained, either by mouth-to-mouth respiration or by tracheal intubation. The external massage, if energetically carried out, carries some risk of damage to the ribs or costal cartilages or of bruising of the liver, but in the special circumstances, such risks are entirely acceptable.

When applied by an experienced operator, external cardiac massage will normally produce an adequate circulation. Should it fail to do so, as indicated by the absence of peripheral pulses and by dilating pupils, the surgeon should proceed to internal cardiac massage without delay. Internal massage is also required in arrest after a wound of the heart.

Internal cardiac massage
So great is the urgency that sterility may be disregarded. An incision is made in the 4th or 5th intercostal space

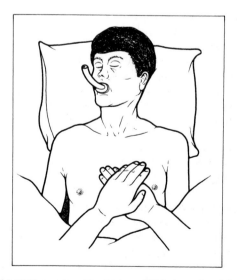

Fig. 14.14 External cardiac massage. With the patient lying on a firm surface, the sternum is pressed rhythmically towards the vertebral column 60 times per minute

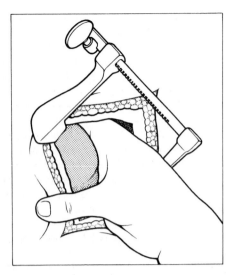

Fig. 14.15 Internal cardiac massage. Through an incision in the 5th intercostal space, the hand is introduced behind the heart and is used to compress it against the sternum

on the left side. This is then opened up by rib-spreaders, if available, or simply by manual retraction, sufficiently for a hand to be introduced into the thoracic cavity. The heart is then compressed through the intact pericardium against the sternum. If rhythmic contractions are not rapidly restored, the pericardium is opened widely, and the fingers are passed into the pericardial sac behind the heart. Rhythmic compression is now exerted upon it, between the fingers and the posterior surface of the sternum. The thumb should not be used to exert direct pressure on the myocardium, since it may cause rupture; it should rather be kept outside the wound, and used to provide counter-pressure against the skin overlying the sternum (Fig. 14.15). Fatigue is best avoided (and prolonged massage may be required) if the surgeon stands on the *right* side of the patient when using his *right* hand.

If arrest of the heart's action occurs during laparotomy, internal cardiac massage may be carried out through an incision in the diaphragm, but this is necessary only if external cardiac massage fails.

Drugs
Probably the most valuable drug for use in cases of cardiac arrest is sodium bicarbonate. It is given to counteract the acidosis which results from the tissue anoxia, and which is an important factor in perpetuating the arrest. 25 ml of molar (8.4%) solution may be given intravenously every five to ten minutes of arrest. 5 ml of 10% calcium chloride, or 1 to 2 ml of 1 : 1000 adrenaline, injected directly into the heart chambers may promote contractions. Under such treatment the heart may either resume normal rhythm, or may go into ventricular fibrillation.

Electrical defibrillation may be effective in restoring normal rhythm, in conditions of ventricular fibrillation. If the heart has been exposed, this is recognised by irregular twitching or writhing of the entire musculature; alternatively, it may be shown by an electrocardiographic tracing. Restoration of normal rhythm can often be effected by a series of electric shocks, which render the heart muscle refractory, so that the fibrillary contractions cease. Two types of apparatus are available—an *external* defibrillator, the electrodes of which are applied to the chest wall, and an *internal* defibrillator, which has electrodes designed for direct application to the heart itself, and may be used in conjunction with internal cardiac massage. The techniques of defibrillation vary according to the type of apparatus available.

It is difficult to state for how long the attempt at resuscitation should be pursued. It can only be recorded that an effective heart-beat has been achieved after two and a half hours. Neurological damage rarely occurs if an adequate circulation can be maintained by the cardiac massage, provided that treatment was initiated promptly after the arrest.

The thoracotomy wound should not be closed as soon as normal contractions have been resumed, for the patient is by no means out of danger, and further massage, injections or shock therapy may be required. After 10–15 minutes of normal rhythm the pericardial wound may be loosely sutured or left open; the internal mammary artery, which owing to the state of shock would not bleed at the time of incision, is secured and the pleural cavity is closed with water-seal drainage.

Wounds of the heart
Most wounds which penetrate the chambers of the heart are associated with massive bleeding which may take place both to the exterior and into the pleural cavity. Many of such wounds are rapidly fatal, and no treatment is of any avail. If, however, the pericardial wound is small, blood may accumulate under tension in the pericardial sac giving rise to the condition of *cardiac tamponade* (compression of the heart). While this causes serious embarrassment of the heart's action and cannot long be tolerated, it has at least some beneficial effect in arresting or reducing haemorrhage, so that the patient, even although in extremis, may sometimes be resuscitated and subjected to urgent thoracotomy.

Cardiac tamponade is diagnosed if, in association with a possible wound of the heart, there is a marked degree of collapse out of proportion to the amount of bleeding; tachycardia and falling arterial pressure coexist, together with cyanosis and venous engorgement, this latter being the most important single sign. X-ray is seldom helpful in diagnosis but echocardiography, if immediately available, may be advised provided that the circulation is not yet seriously compromised. Treatment by aspiration may be a useful emergency measure.

The best operative approach is probably through a generous incision in the 4th or 5th intercostal space, on the side of the external wound. If necessary, the incision can be extended to give wider access by one of the methods described on page 292. The pleural cavity is opened and the ribs retracted widely by a rib-spreader. The pericardium, which is seen to be purple in colour and pulsating feebly, is incised freely and all contained blood is evacuated. The wound in the heart is sought, and a finger is placed upon it to control bleeding while stitches are inserted. It is recommended that the pericardial wound should not be sutured, since it is better that any further bleeding should take place into the pleural cavity, from which it can easily be withdrawn, rather than into the closed pericardial sac. The chest wall is repaired, the internal mammary artery being secured, and the pleural cavity is drained to suction or to a water-seal.

Open heart surgery

Major advances in cardiac surgery have taken place since the development of *extracorporeal circulation* about 30 years ago. The first successful ligation of a patent ductus arteriosus had taken place in 1938 and, in 1947, mitral stenosis had been treated by closed valvotomy. In the latter type of procedure, access to the heart is obtained by the introduction of the finger or specialised instruments through a small opening in the heart wall. Such closed methods are still employed for mitral stenosis in certain circumstances. In other conditions, however, they are necessarily somewhat haphazard, and there has been a steadily increasing trend in the development of open techniques, which allow safer and more accurate work, since 'bypass' was introduced in the early 1950s. As the result of measures which provide for temporary arrest of the heart's action, operations can now be carried out under direct visual control, with the lesion fully exposed in a heart which is both empty and flaccid.

At normal temperatures circulation through the heart cannot be arrested for more than 3 or 4 minutes without residual damage to the brain from anoxia—and few operations can be effectively performed within this time. The foundations of open heart surgery are built upon certain techniques which allow the operative time to be extended. Firstly it was found that, if the body temperature was lowered to 30°C (*hypothermia*), the period of occlusion could be prolonged to 7 or 8 minutes without fear of brain damage. An alternative method consists in the installation of an *extracorporeal circulation*. This provides for the heart and lungs to be completely bypassed during the operation by a 'heart–lung' machine, in which a mechanical pump substitutes for the heart, and some type of oxygenator for the lungs. Such equipment maintains adequate perfusion of oxygenated blood within the

vital organs during intracardiac procedures. Problems of the technique such as air embolism and coagulation defects have now, in the main, been overcome.

Hypothermia

The technique is now used less frequently on its own. The first method was to immerse the anaesthetized patient in iced water, until the requisite degree of cooling had been obtained but this can now be achieved by the administration of drugs to prevent shivering and to promote heat loss. At about 30°C, which reduces the body metabolism by about 50%, both superior and inferior venae cavae can be clamped, thus producing inflow arrest of the heart for 6–8 minutes. This usually allows sufficient time for minor intracardiac procedures to be carried out. The method is suitable for the repair of *ostium secundum* defects in the atrial septum, although its use in this condition is becoming less frequent, owing to the increasing safety of cardiopulmonary bypass. In most cardiac units, hypothermia has been replaced by methods of extracorporeal circulation, which allow the heart's action to be arrested for much longer periods, and enable more unhurried and precise techniques to be employed.

Extracorporeal circulation

The general principle of this method is that all systemic blood entering the heart is diverted by catheters or cannulae placed in the superior and inferior venae cavae. From these vessels the blood is led through an oxygenator, in which it is spread out as a film exposed to gaseous oxygen; it is then led to a pump which returns it to the body via an artery—usually the ascending aorta—although the femoral may be used. Thereafter it perfuses the patient's systemic circulation, but is prevented from entering the heart by closure of the aortic valves. The metabolic requirement of the heart can be decreased by the technique of *cold cardioplegia* in which 1 litre of potassium containing solution at 4°C is injected into the ascending aorta. This may be repeated each 45–60 minutes as required or the coronary arteries may be perfused intermittently with the solution if the aortic valve is being replaced. The increasing safety of 'bypass' techniques during the past three decades has extended the scope of cardiac surgery and operations are now being done which were not previously possible.

Hypothermia combined with extracorporeal circulation has been employed with two objects in view. Firstly, by the incorporation of a heat exchanger in the circuit, accurate control can rapidly be effected, thus achieving with safety lower temperatures than would be permissible under hypothermia alone. Secondly, adequate circulation can be maintained if the return of cardiac function is delayed as a result of hypothermia. Using surface induced deep hypothermia (Subramanian, 1974), the patient can be cooled to 20°C and circulatory arrest is employed for up to 60 minutes, while precise intra-cardiac operations are carried out.

Cardiac operations under cardiopulmonary bypass

Congenital cardiac defects

The most important congenital conditions now considered suitable for surgical treatment under bypass are atrial and ventricular septal defects, and pulmonary stenosis. This last condition is commonly one of a group of four defects, collectively designated the tetralogy of Fallot. Transposition of the great vessels is also correctable by open heart surgery (Mok, 1982) and some cases of total anomalous pulmonary venous return may be suitable for operation (Subramanian, 1974).

Atrial septal defects are probably the most common of all congenital abnormalities, and are due to maldevelopment of the interatrial septum. The larger the defect, the greater is the blood flow from the left atrium (in which the pressure is higher) into the right atrium, and thence round the pulmonary circulation. The strain imposed by the abnormal shunting leads to heart failure or the lung vessels may become sclerosed, cause obstruction and add to the right-sided heart failure. Pulmonary vascular disease results in reversal of the shunt and inoperability thus occurs in a small proportion of cases. The simplest type of defect (*ostium secundum* or *fossa ovalis defect*) is placed centrally in the septum (Fig. 14.16) and its closure can be effected by an open operation conducted under hypothermia although many clinics now prefer to use bypass. The right atrium is opened by a longitudinal incision, and the defect is repaired by silk sutures, which usually secure accurate coaptation of the margins without difficulty (Fig. 14.17). The *ostium primum defect* is situated low down on the atrial septum in close proximity to the tricuspid valve and is often associated with a ventricular septal defect as well.

It requires insertion of a patch of synthetic material.

Ventricular septal defects. These defects, which are relatively common, permit the shunting of blood from the left ventricle to the right ventricle, with consequent overloading of the pulmonary circulation. As in the case of atrial septal defects, increasing resistance may develop in the lung vessels, and most large defects, if untreated, progress to right heart failure. Repair is effected usually by suturing a patch of pericardium or synthetic material against the defect, access being obtained by an incision in the right ventricle (Fig. 14.18).

Pulmonary stenosis may be *valvular*, or it may be situated in the upper part of the right ventricle (*infundibular*). Relief was previously obtained by division of the constriction through a small opening in the wall of the right ventricle, but the method was unreliable, and surgeons now prefer to carry out a more precise operation in which the pulmonary trunk is opened to expose the valvular area. If infundibular stenosis coexists or is present independently, it will require ventriculotomy with excision of the strictured area.

Tetralogy of Fallot. This designation is applied to a group of four congenital defects which may coexist. They are (1) pulmonary stenosis or atresia; (2) a ventricular septal defect; (3) dextro-position of the aorta, which straddles the defect and therefore receives blood from both ventricles; (4) hypertrophy of the right ventricle. Cyanosis is a marked feature of the condition—hence the popular term 'blue babies': it is due to the fact that the aorta receives deoxygenated blood from the right ventricle, in addition to its normal complement of blood from the left ventricle. Palliative treatment is usually advised without delay in infants if the disability is severe unless the patient is suitable for primary correction. Blalock's operation consists in an anastomosis between the proximal end of the right subclavian artery and the side of the right pulmonary artery (Fig. 14.19). Waterston's

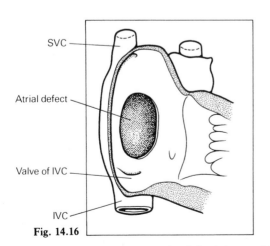

Fig. 14.16

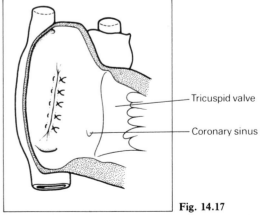

Fig. 14.17

Figs. 14.16 & 14.17 *Ostium secundum* defect in inter-atrial septum: method of closure by direct suture

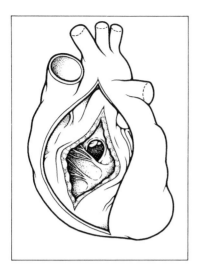

Fig. 14.18 Interventricular septal defect as seen through incision in wall of right ventricle

operation (1972) in which the ascending aorta is anastomosed to the right pulmonary artery (Fig. 14.20), may be used as an alternative during the first year of life when operation is urgently required. The immediate effect of these operations is often most dramatic as regards relief of cyanosis and increased tolerance to exercise, but the final results in most cases have proved disappointing. Following these 'shunt' operations, repair of the tetralogy may be undertaken at a later date but Subramanian (1974) makes a plea for early complete correction of operable defects as a one stage procedure. Unfortunately, not all cases are suitable, for the combined mortality of shunt with later repair is greater than for the single procedure alone. The latter consists in open relief of the pulmonary stenosis and patch closure of the septal defect

which results in a normal outflow of blood from the ventricles.

Acquired heart disease

Ischaemic heart disease. Coronary bypass surgery now forms a major part of the work of a cardiac surgeon. Atherosclerosis of the coronary arteries with thrombosis formation is the cause of angina pectoris, myocardial infarction and ventricular aneurysm. With the development of selective coronary angiography and ventriculography, the sites and extent of coronary artery obstruction can be accurately identified. Reversed saphenous vein bypass grafts from aorta to the peripheral coronary arteries can be made using cardiopulmonary bypass so that the anastomoses of the graft can be made under optimal conditions (Wheatley, 1981). An oblique anastomosis is made between the graft and the coronary arteries distal to the obstruction. Relief of intractable anginal pain is usually obtained. Aneurysmectomy, with excision of extensive aneurysms of the left ventricle and closure of the ventricular wound with supported mattress sutures is advised in cases where cardiac failure cannot be relieved by medical measures.

Mitral stenosis. Mitral valve replacement is indicated when stenosis is associated with (1) calcification (2) dense sclerosis of the cusps and (3) more than trivial regurgitation. Previous systemic embolism from the valve is a possible additional reason to advise replacement which is a good procedure now preferred by most cardiac surgeons. It is usual to excise the diseased valve and insert a prosthetic mechanical valve such as the Björk-Shiley tilting disc (Fig. 14.21) or the Starr-Edwards caged ball valve. The operative mortality is around 10%.

Mitral incompetence. When this is the dominant lesion, it can only be dealt with under cardiopulmonary bypass. Modern techniques of *annuloplasty* have achieved accur-

Figs. 14.19 & 14.20 *Operations for the tetralogy of Fallot.*

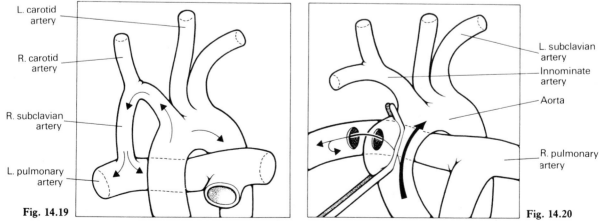

Fig. 14.19 Blalock anastomosis between right subclavian and pulmonary arteries. **Fig. 14.20** Waterston anastomosis between ascending aorta and right pulmonary artery

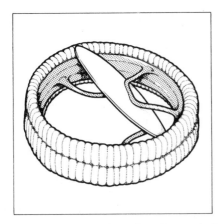

Fig. 14.21 The Björk–Shiley tilting disc valve prosthesis

ate suturing and preservation of the mitral valve in suitable cases. With the help of Carpentier rings, the separated valve cusps are approximated unless there is calcification or associated stenosis which requires valve replacement.

Aortic valve disease. Aortic stenosis, congenital or acquired, may be associated with extensive calcification of valve tissue and aortic ring. It is a dangerous and usually progressive condition which demands urgent relief. Aortic incompetence is less likely to be associated with calcification, but it also is a crippling and dangerous condition, leading to progressive enlargement of the left ventricle.

Both stenosis and incompetence may now be treated successfully by open operation under cardiopulmonary bypass with a mortality of less than 5% (Oakley, 1982). The aorta is clamped just below the origin of the innominate artery, and is opened between this and the valve. Perfusion of the coronary circulation is instituted by the introduction of catheters into both coronary arteries for cold cardioplegia (p. 295). Satisfactory results follow replacement of the valve by a mechanical prosthesis (Björk, 1971) or by a porcine heterograft valve mounted on a flexible stent. Most mechanical valves have a good record of reliability but tissue valves have a lower risk of embolism.

Cardiac operations without bypass

Congenital heart disease

Patent ductus arteriosus. This abnormality consists in the persistence of the fetal channel of communication between the arch of the aorta and the pulmonary artery. Since the abnormal shunt of blood takes place from the systemic to the pulmonary circulation, cyanosis is absent—unless at a very late stage of the disease, when, if the ductus is large, cardiac failure may supervene. The condition may be associated with retarded growth and signs of cardiac insufficiency but many patients are asymptomatic. Bacterial endocarditis, however, is a major risk in these cases. Surgical closure of the ductus is now a standard procedure, and should be considered in all cases where the diagnosis is established. It is indicated especially when bacterial endocarditis is present, for it has been shown to be capable of curing this otherwise serious complication. A left transpleural approach through the 4th or 5th interspace is normally employed. The mediastinal pleura is incised vertically between the phrenic and vagus nerves, and, by dissection between the arch of the aorta and the pulmonary artery, the ductus is exposed. The recurrent laryngeal nerve is identified; it is followed down behind the ductus, and is carefully preserved. The ductus is then isolated in its whole length by gentle dissection, the pericardium being opened if necessary. Closure of the ductus can sometimes be obtained by ligature in continuity, but complete division with suture of the cut ends is more effective in preventing recanalisation, and is now the method of choice. The division should be carried out between special clamps (*Pott's multi-point clamps*) which provide a very firm grip, since slipping of a clamp might well be disastrous.

Coarctation (stenosis) of the aorta. The constriction (which may cause almost complete obliteration of the lumen) is located usually in the arch of the aorta, just beyond the origin of the left subclavian branch at the ligamentum arteriosum. The circulation to the head and upper limbs is normal although in a state of hypertension. The circulation to the abdomen and lower limbs is surprisingly normal although at a lower pressure despite its dependence upon a collateral circulation from anastomoses between the internal mammary, subscapular and intercostal vessels. Resection of the stenosed segment of aorta, with end-to-end anastomosis, is the operation of choice (Fig. 14.23).

Acquired heart disease

Mitral stenosis. 'Closed' mitral valvulotomy is restricted to selected cases of stenosis uncomplicated by calcification, cusp sclerosis or incompetence. The incidence of rheumatic heart disease, the main causative factor, is decreasing in U.K. but the operation may still be required in countries with rheumatic conditions. It is designed to effect separation of the fused cusps of the valve along the line of the commissures, i.e. where the fusion has occurred. When the valve is mobile and there is no gross deformity of the cusps or shortening of the chordae tendinae, almost complete normality may be restored. In favourable and carefully selected cases, the mortality is less than 1%, and the results are excellent.

The method of transventricular dilatation, introduced by Logan in 1959, is now generally used and constituted an important technical advance. An incision is made in

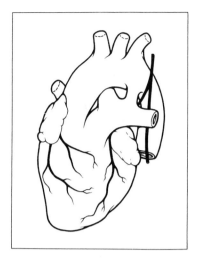

Fig. 14.22 Patent ductus arteriosus. Treated by division of the ductus, and closure of the cut ends by suture

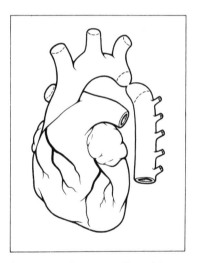

Fig. 14.23 Coarctation of the aorta. Treated by resection of the stenosed segment and end-to-end anastomosis

the left atrium, and the right forefinger is entered, the opening around it being controlled with a purse-string suture. The valve is palpated, and gentle pressure is applied with the finger to enlarge the opening by splitting, which normally takes place in the line of the commissures. If this fails, as it may do if there is a sclerotic ring around the orifice, a small incision is made in the wall of the left ventricle near the apex; a dilator held in the left hand is introduced, and its head is accurately placed in the valve orifice, under the guidance of the atrial finger. The plane in which the dilator is made to expand is immaterial, since the opening will always tend to split along the line of the commissures. The dilator is opened just far enough to overcome the resistance offered

by the valve (the ideal spread is 3.5–5 cm), and is withdrawn so that its effect can be assessed digitally. When the dilator is withdrawn, bleeding from the ventricular wound is controlled by pressure with the thumb until the wound is sutured.

Acute suppurative pericarditis is frequently associated with a septicaemic or pyaemic condition, in which surgical treatment may be of little avail.

Aspiration is carried out for diagnostic purposes, the needle being introduced either at the costoxiphoid angle, or through the 5th intercostal space.

Antibiotic instillation, following aspiration of the effusion, may be employed in the first instance, but, if the patient's condition does not rapidly improve, surgical drainage should be carried out. Operation for drainage is transpleural or upper midline abdominal splitting the xiphoid and detaching the combined origins of the transversus and diaphragm from the deep surface of the costal margin. The pericardium is exposed and can be opened on its inferior surface, so that dependent drainage is provided.

Constrictive pericarditis. In this condition, which is usually of tuberculous origin, the pericardium (mainly the fibrous layer) becomes thickened and rigid, with obliteration of the pericardial space. Venous obstruction with liver enlargement and ascites may progress steadily towards a fatal issue; operation, therefore, should not be withheld.

The aim of operation is to free the ventricles from constriction by excision of the pericardium covering the anterior surface and left border of the heart, within an area bounded by the coronary sinus, the inferior border of the heart, and the phrenic nerves. The pericardium covering the atria is left intact.

The approach is by median sternotomy or bilateral transverse thoracotomy through the 4th or 5th spaces. A plane of cleavage is sought between the visceral pericardium and the heart muscle; both layers of pericardium (usually fused together) are elevated within the limits described, by a combination of blunt and sharp dissection, and are removed. The pericardium covering the coronary sulcus and the interventricular groove is left undisturbed lest the coronary vessels should be damaged.

THE THYMUS GLAND

The association between the thymus gland and myasthenia gravis is now well established, although not many myasthenics have a thymoma. Such tumours show a wide range of histological pattern, and vary very considerably in their behaviour. Only the oval-celled *thymomata* appear to be simple in nature; they form slowly-growing circumscribed masses, which can be successfully removed without recurrence (Olanow, 1982). In the others, all degrees of malignancy are represented, and the prognosis is uniformly bad.

Thymectomy in myasthenia gravis is an empirical form of treatment, justified in cases where the tumour has the appearance of being simple, i.e. where it is circumscribed and has shown no signs of rapid growth. The thymus gland, which varies considerably in size and shape, is exposed by splitting the sternum in the mid line, the two halves being separated by a rib-spreader. The gland is often adherent to the pleura, and to the pericardium and great vessels, so that its removal entails very careful dissection to avoid damage to these structures.

There is no doubt that the best results are obtained in young patients with a short history, and in whom there is no thymic tumour. The presence of tumour indicates a much worse prognosis.

CARCINOMA OF THE OESOPHAGUS

Carcinoma of the oesophagus is one of the less aggressive malignant tumours, and for a long time is no more than locally invasive. Thus, many growths, if diagnosed at a sufficiently early stage, are technically removable and surgery offers the greatest chance of cure (Roberts, 1980). The tumour is exposed through a transthoracic or abdominothoracic incision. The diaphragm can be widely incised, so that simultaneous exposure of both abdominal and thoracic cavities is obtained. Continuity after resection may be restored by bringing the stomach (converted into a long straight tube), or a mobilized loop of jejunum or colon, upwards into the thorax (or even into the neck), so that it can be anastomosed at any level with the upper segment of the oesophagus. In order to obtain the best results, an experienced team is essential but, even then, operative mortality is high and long-term survival disappointing (McKeown, 1985).

Radical excision
Radical surgery remains the best treatment for squamous or adenocarcinoma but is inappropriate if there is clinical evidence of dissemination or if the oesophageal tumour is more than 10 cm in length. The upward submucous spread of squamous carcinoma necessitates a wide resection and McKeown (1979) suggests a line of section 7 cm above the apparent upper margin of growth. A review of 83 783 patients from the world literature gives an overall operative mortality of 13%, resection rate of 39% and 5 year survival of 4% (Earlam, 1980a). Adenocarcinoma occurs usually at the gastro-oesophageal junction, and has probably originated in the gastric mucosa. Operative mortality is lower although prognosis worse than for squamous carcinoma.

Irradiation therapy
Following the introduction of the linear accelerator in 1956, Pearson (1971) reported that megavoltage irradiation was no less effective than surgery for squamous carcinoma in the lower oesophagus. However, his 21% 5 year survival following radiotherapy has not been confirmed by other series in U.K. although collected data on 8489 patients from the world literature gives an overall 5 year survival of 6% (Earlam, 1980b). Attempts are now being made to improve the results of surgery by combining it with radiotherapy and/or chemotherapy.

Palliative procedures
It must be admitted that the proportion of patients who can be helped either by surgery or by radiotherapy remains comparatively small. Many of the patients are old, and they are often enfeebled by semi-starvation. If complete dysphagia is present, measures must be taken to provide adequate nourishment, either in preparation for surgery, or until the possible benefits of radiotherapy can be obtained. An adequate calorie intake can be achieved by using one of the proprietary liquid food preparations, infused, if necessary, through a 1 mm bore tube (see p. 312) passed through the stricture endoscopically.

Resection with anastomosis, or a short-circuiting operation alone, carried out by the methods about to be described, may be advocated in cardio-oesophageal growths, which are usually adenocarcinomata, and therefore resistant to irradiation therapy. It may provide an acceptable degree of palliation except in advanced cases with widespread metastases.

Intubation
By this method a tube is passed through the malignant stricture, and is left in situ. It keeps the passage open, and allows the patient to swallow fluid or soft foods in relative comfort, for as long as he may live. Endoscopic placement of a tube avoids the need for open operation (Jones, 1981) but the tube is more liable to be dislodged (Bache, 1982).

Celestin's tube (1959), made of flexible polythene, is oval on cross-section, with a lumen diameter of about 9 mm by 14 mm. It is 25 cm in length, with the upper 5 cm forming a barrel-shaped funnel. For attachment to the tube, there is a slender pilot bougie, made of solid polythene and 60 cm in length. With the aid of an oesophagoscope, this is piloted through the stricture, and is passed well down into the stomach, after which the oesophagoscope is withdrawn over it. The tube is then plugged on to the bougie, and is anchored securely by a stitch passed through the holes provided. The abdomen is opened, and a small incision is made in the anterior wall of the stomach just below the cardia. The pilot bougie is located, and is gently withdrawn until the upper funnel-shaped end of the tube impacts against the stricture. Finally the excess of tube within the stomach is cut off and the gastrotomy wound is closed. The *Mousseau-Barbin tube* (1956) is an alternative one-piece tube which includes the bougie.

Souttar's tube (1924) is of value in terminal cases with severe dysphagia. The tube is made of spirally wound silver wire, and is introduced through a rigid oesophagoscope, after dilatation of the stricture. It is as effective as a *Celestin's tube*, except with very large tumours, and its introduction does not require a laparotomy.

Oesophageal resection—the approach

The abdominothoracic approach is used for carcinoma below the arch of the aorta in the lower two-thirds of the oesophagus. It is also the approach of choice for high gastric tumours which often extend into the lower oesophagus. It allows a radical dissection of the lymphatic field below the diaphragm to be carried out, and permits the spleen or part of the pancreas to be removed if necessary. The patient is placed in the right lateral position with a slight dorsal tilt. The incision passes obliquely upwards from a point just above the umbilicus to the left costal margin, and is then carried backwards along the 8th intercostal space—if necessary as far as the vertebral border of the scapula (Fig. 14.24).

The abdominal part of the exposure can be used as an exploratory procedure if it is suspected that an inoperable gastric extension of the tumour is present. It is usual, however, for the thoraco-abdominal incision to be completed in the first instance. The cartilaginous costal margin is divided and the pleural cavity is entered, the 8th

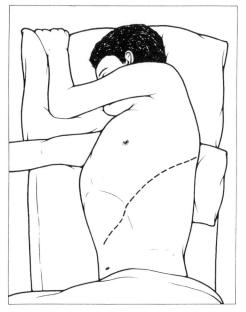

Fig. 14.24 Position of the patient for a combined abdominothoracic approach to the stomach or lower oesophagus. The line of incision is shown

intercostal space being opened widely by a rib spreader. If wider access is desired the 8th or 9th rib may be resected. The diaphragm is separated from its costal attachments over a short distance on each side of the transcostal incision. This is preferable, particularly in elderly patients, to a radial incision since it retains integrity of movement of the diaphragm.

First the lung is mobilised by division of the pulmonary ligament, and is retracted forwards. The oesophageal neoplasm is carefully palpated to assess the degree of involvement of adjacent structures such as aorta, pericardium and main bronchus. If it is decided that the growth is removable, the diaphragm is incised around the oesophageal hiatus or radially from chest wall to hiatus depending on circumstance. If the liver is free from secondary deposits, the stomach is mobilized by division of its peritoneal attachments along the greater parts of both curvatures. The left gastric artery is exposed and ligatured near its origin from the coeliac axis and the short gastric arteries are divided. The right gastric and right gastro-epiploic vessels are carefully preserved. This should allow the stomach to be stretched into a long tube, extending without tension well up into the thorax, and capable of being anastomosed at any level to the upper segment of the oesophagus after resection (Fig. 14.25B).

Right-sided thoracotomy

This approach, described by Lewis (1946), is favoured by the majority of surgeons for the treatment of growths in the upper one-third of the oesophagus. It obviates the difficult and nearly blind dissection required to free the oesophagus from the arch of the aorta, which obscures it from a left-sided approach. On the right side, the oesophagus is crossed only by the azygos vein—and this structure can easily be divided between ligatures. A disadvantage of the right-sided approach is that it must be preceded by an abdominal laparotomy in order to mobilise the stomach, since it is not possible to do this working from the right side of the chest. The abdominal part of the operation should be completed first and the wound closed, before the thorax is opened. Should it now be found that the tumour is irremovable, the mobilised stomach can be used to bypass the obstruction.

Left-sided thoracotomy provides a limited exposure for lesions in the lower two-thirds of the oesophagus and has now largely been replaced by the abdomino-thoracic approach.

Extent of resection and methods of anastomosis

The concept of radical operation is that in all cases the tumour-bearing area, *together with the entire oesophagus below this level*, should be removed *in continuity*. The upper limit of resection and the type of anastomosis to be performed must depend upon the situation and extent of the growth.

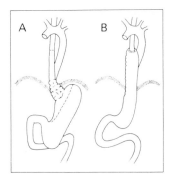

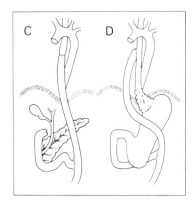

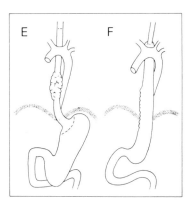

Fig. 14.25 Operations for carcinoma of the oesophagus. A—carcinoma of the cardia showing extent of resection. B—tube constructed from gastric remnant, and joined to upper oesophagus by sub-aortic anastomosis. C—total gastrectomy. Continuity restored by oesophagojejunal anastomosis, with formation of *Roux* loop. D—irremovable carcinoma of the cardia, treated by a short-circuiting oesophago-jejunostomy with *Roux* loop. E—carcinoma near middle of oesophagus showing extent of resection. F—whole stomach preserved to form gastric tube. Anastomosis performed through *right* thoracotomy

Carcinoma of the gastro-oesophageal junction

If the growth appears to have originated in the oesophagus, the lower part of the oesophagus and the cardia of the stomach are removed (Fig. 14.25A), together with as much of the lymphatic bed as appears necessary. In more extensive growth, the whole of the upper part of the stomach may require to be removed, in continuity with the spleen, the body of the pancreas, and retroperitoneal lymphatic tissues. The remaining part of the stomach is closed to form a tube and the pylorus is stretched or a pyloromyotomy is carried out since a vagotomy will, of course, have resulted from the resection. The tube of stomach is brought up to be joined to the upper segment of the oesophagus just below the arch of the aorta as a *sub-aortic anastomosis* (Fig. 14.25B). To effect such an anastomosis, the mobilised stomach is turned upwards, and, at the level selected for section, its posterior wall is united to the gastric tube below its upper pole, by a row of interrupted sutures. An opening (a *circular* one being recommended by some surgeons) is then made into the gastric tube to match the size of the oesophageal lumen, and, after division of the oesophagus, the anastomosis is completed by two layers of interrupted nonabsorbable suture. Special care is taken with the stitching of the mucosa; this is the toughest coat of the oesophageal wall, and the only one in which sutures can obtain a firm hold. In experienced hands, the circular stapling device can be used with benefit as an alternative to sutures. On completion of the anastomosis, the gastric fundus is anchored posteriorly by stitching it to the mediastinal pleura, and anteriorly it is folded over in order to reinforce the suture line. For still more extensive tumours involving a considerable part of the stomach, total gastrectomy should be performed, and continuity established by an oesophagojejunal anastomosis. For this, the uppermost loop of jejunum is transected; its distal part is anastomosed end-to-end with the upper oesophagus, and its free proximal end is implanted end-to-side into the distal segment below the anastomosis (*Roux loop*) (Fig. 14.25C). If the growth is irremovable, it may be left in situ, and short-circuited by an oesophagojejunostomy (Fig. 14.25D).

Carcinoma of the lower third of oesophagus not involving the cardia

In such cases the whole stomach can be preserved and its fundus used for the anastomosis. The oesophagus is divided at the cardiac orifice, which is closed and invaginated by suture (Fig. 14.25E). A sub-aortic anastomosis is then carried out on the lines described above.

Carcinoma of the middle third of the oesophagus

The advantages of a right thoracotomy for the approach to such tumours have already been referred to. By the simple expedient of dividing the azygos vein, the whole length of the thoracic oesophagus is displayed and can be mobilised from the aorta for anastomosis to a tube of stomach as a *supra-aortic anastomosis* (Fig. 14.25F). This is a technically difficult procedure, since adequate mobilisation of the upper thoracic aorta is impeded by the presence of its intercostal branches.

Carcinoma of the upper thoracic oesophagus is fortunately rare, since this region is relatively inaccessible both from the thorax and from the neck. McKeown (1972) has described the technique of three stage total oesophagectomy for growths in the upper middle third of the oesophagus and for those above the aortic arch. In addition to the abdominal and right thoracotomy wounds, the oesophagus is exposed on the right side of the neck. The growth is excised through the neck wound so as to avoid contamination of the abdominal or thoracic cavities and the anastomosis is made without difficulty in the neck (Fig. 14.25F). Ong (1975) advises that the tube used for such reconstruction, or for palliative bypass, should be laid in a subcutaneous tunnel in front of the sternum in order to avoid compression at the thoracic inlet by recurrence of the tumour. Also, any leakage that does occur at the anastomosis is unlikely to cause mediastinitis, which is usually a fatal complication.

Sometimes the vascular pattern of the jejunum may make it difficult to mobilise an adequate length of bowel for the preparation of a *Roux* loop. In such cases, the transverse colon, from hepatic flexure to upper descending, may be isolated and transplanted to form a channel of communication between the upper oesophagus and the jejunum. It usually retains a good blood supply from the upper branch of the left colic artery, the middle colic artery having been divided. The transverse colon, based on middle colic artery, is used for short segment interposition.

Repair of the diaphragm is effected with interrupted sutures, enough room being left posteriorly for the stomach to pass through. In order to minimize tension on the anastomosis from contraction of the diaphragm, the stomach is drawn firmly upwards, and the margins of the new hiatus are stitched around it as low as possible.

Bypass procedures may be considered as a palliative measure, when the growth is found at operation to be irremovable. The most satisfactory operation is probably an oesophagojejunostomy, by means of a *Roux* loop, the tumour together with the stomach being left in situ (Fig. 14.25D).

OTHER OESOPHAGEAL CONDITIONS

Oesophageal atresia

Oesophageal atresia is one of the more common congenital abnormalities, the incidence being one for 3250 live births. Although the problem continues to challenge the surgeon, few conditions can be more rewarding to treat.

Embryogenesis

The respiratory system develops from a diverticulum which first appears in the embryo at four weeks as a longitudinal groove on the ventral surface of the foregut. Lateral ridges in the wall of the foregut on either side of the groove fuse in the midline so as to separate the two structures. The process of separation starts at the caudal end of the groove and extends incompletely to the cranial end. Oesophageal atresia and tracheo-oesophageal fistula are probably established at this early date and this would explain the high incidence of associated anomalies.

The structural form of the anomaly is variable (Figs 14.26–14.29). In 70% of babies, oesophageal atresia is associated with a fistula between the trachea and

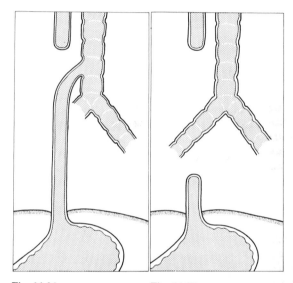

Fig. 14.26   Fig. 14.27

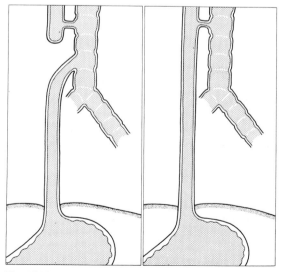

Fig. 14.28   Fig. 14.29

Figs 14.26–14.29 Anatomical variations of oesophageal atresia and tracheo-oesophageal fistula

the distal limb of the oesophagus. In 10% oesophageal atresia is present without fistula; these babies have a characteristically scaphoid abdomen as the bowel is empty of gas. In a few there may be fistulae between the trachea and both proximal and distal segments of the oesophagus and, in others, a tracheo-oesophageal fistula may be present in the absence of an atresia.

Clinical presentation

The condition is apparent soon after birth. Maternal hydramnios and low birth weight are common. The baby collects excessive frothy saliva in the mouth and inadvertent feeding causes choking and respiratory distress. An unsuccessful attempt to pass a firm 12 French gauge nasogastric catheter will confirm the diagnosis. The major risk to the baby is that of atelectasis and pneumonia from overspill of saliva and, in the presence of a fistula, reflux of gastric secretion. The risks can be reduced by continuous suction of the nasopharynx, by physiotherapy and by nursing the baby horizontal in either a prone or lateral position. A plain X-ray should be taken of both chest and abdomen. A radio-opaque catheter in the oesophagus will indicate the length of the upper pouch and gas in the bowel will confirm the presence of a fistula and may demonstrate an associated intestinal abnormality.

Operation

In a fit baby an attempt should be made to close the fistula and repair the oesophagus during the first thirty-six hours of life. It may, however, be necessary to delay the procedure either to treat respiratory problems or to investigate further an associated anomaly. At operation the mediastinum is reached by an extrapleural approach using a right thoracotomy incision through the bed of the 4th rib. The proximal and distal segments of the oesophagus are mobilized with care so as to preserve both the blood supply and the right vagus which runs along the lateral wall of the distal segment. The fistula, which normally lies between the distal segment and the lateral wall of the trachea just above the carina, is transfixed and divided. Continuity of the oesophagus is achieved by an end-to-end anastomosis of the two segments with fine interrupted sutures (Fig. 14.30). A fine silastic catheter placed down the lumen of the oesophagus allows easy feeding. Finally the wound is closed with a drain in place.

In some babies the gap between the two segments of the oesophagus may be too great to allow a primary anastomosis and a feeding gastrostomy should then be fashioned. This situation is common in babies with atresia but no fistula, as the distal segment of the oesophagus tends to be short. If the discrepancy preventing a primary anastomosis is marginal, a further attempt may be made at a later date as growth of the oesophagus during the interval and daily stretching of the proximal segment with a bougie may enable the gap to be closed. Alternatively, if a second attempt is unlikely to be successful, a left sided cervical oesophagostomy is fashioned to allow swallowing. After an interval of 12 months the gap between proximal oesophagus and stomach is either interposed with a segment of colon (Fig. 14.31) (Waterston, 1964) or bridged with a gastric tube fashioned from the greater curvature (Cohen, 1974).

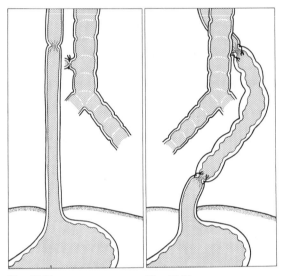

Fig. 14.30   **Fig. 14.31**

Fig. 14.30 Primary anastomosis of oesophagus and ligation and division of fistula.
Fig. 14.31 Colonic interposition between proximal and distal oesophagus.

Benign stricture of oesophagus

The majority of strictures are in the distal third of the oesophagus and are peptic in origin, being the result of reflux oesophagitis. When the diagnosis has been established by careful endoscopic biopsy (repeated as necessary) the initial aim is to manage the stricture by dilatation. An antireflux operation may be required for an associated hiatus hernia, where reflux dominates the clinical picture (Williamson, 1975) and a small number of patients will require resection if dilatation is difficult or is required frequently. Endoscopic dilatation can be effected by a variety of instruments which are reviewed by Earlam (1981). The advantage of the recently developed Eder-Puestow dilators is that a flexible guide wire may be passed through the stricture under local anaesthesia using a flexible fibreoptic endoscope and its position confirmed radiologically. Graduated dilators are then passed over the guide wire (the endoscope having been removed) under X-ray image intensification for greater safety.

Cardiospasm (oesophageal achalasia)

In this condition benefit is often obtained by forcible dilatation with a *hydrostatic bag* which aims to disrupt muscle fibres and weaken the lower sphincter. Relief may be only temporary and most surgeons prefer to proceed to operation without delay.

Heller's operation resembles that of Ramstedt for congenital pyloric stenosis. A high midline or left paramedian incision is made, and the left lobe of the liver is mobilised by division of the left coronary ligament. The peritoneum covering the oesophageal hiatus is incised, and the hiatus is gently stretched with the finger. A longitudinal incision 5 cm in length is made over the oesophagogastric junction, and is carried down through the muscular wall until the submucous layer is reached. The muscle fibres are carefully dissected apart, so that the intact mucosa bulges through. Mucosal perforation, which is a not infrequent immediate complication, is easily repaired with fine catgut sutures and is managed by post-operative parenteral feeding for 5 days. A transthoracic approach is used by some surgeons (Menzies-Gow, 1978), and repair of an associated hiatus hernia, possibly by *fundoplication*, is also adivsed.

This operation effectively relieves regurgitation of food and dysphagia but retrosternal pain may persist. The less severe the obstruction the better are the results likely to be. The operation seems to cause no more than temporary incontinence of the sphincter in some patients although reflux may occur.

DIAPHRAGMATIC HERNIA

Congenital malformations

The diaphragm is formed in the fetus between 8 and 10 weeks from the middle part of the septum transversum, the pleuroperitoneal folds and the dorsal mesentery of the foregut. A hernia is most commonly associated with failure of fusion of these components and the persistence of the pleuroperitoneal canal though, on occasions, the hernia may lie within the foramen of Morgagni or the posterolateral foramen of Bochdalek (Sutton, 1982). The left dome of the diaphragm is more commonly affected than the right, presumably because the latter is protected by the liver. The underlying lung is hypoplastic and bowel fixation is abnormal. In eventration of the diaphragm, abdominal viscera lying within the thorax are covered with a hypoplastic structure and this condition mimics a true diaphragmatic hernia.

Clinical presentation

The incidence of diaphragmatic hernia is approximately one per 5000 live births. The condition presents with respiratory distress in the newborn. There is limited movement of the affected side of the thorax, the medias-tinum is displaced to the opposite side and the abdomen appears scaphoid. A chest X-ray shows bowel within the thorax and an abdominal film may show reduced bowel content. The condition is perhaps the foremost emergency in neonatal surgery. The accumulation of gas in bowel lying in the thorax reduces the ventilatory capacity and aggravates the mediastinal displacement. For the immediate management a nasogastric tube is passed to empty the stomach and the baby nursed on the affected side in an incubator. Positive pressure ventilation through an endotracheal tube may be necessary. A face mask should not be used since it results in more gas being introduced into the stomach.

Operation

The diaphragmatic hernia is repaired through a transverse upper abdominal incision. The bowel is gently withdrawn from the thorax through the deficit in the diaphragm. Incomplete rotation is inevitable and the duodenum may be partly obstructed by Ladd's bands (see p. 426). The hernial sac, if present, should be either excised or plicated, the underlying hypoplastic lung inspected and a thoracotomy drain placed in position. The anterior and posterior rims of the diaphragm can then usually be defined and brought together without difficulty using interrupted nonabsorbable sutures. However, occasionally the posterior rim is absent and it is then necessary to suture the anterior rim to the lower ribs. Only rarely is it necessary to mobilise a flap from the anterior abdominal wall or use prosthetic material to fashion a diaphragm.

Postoperative care

After operation, the nasogastric tube is left in position to ensure that the stomach remains empty and an intravenous infusion continued. Respiratory function is monitored by serial blood gas and bicarbonate analysis and assisted ventilation may be necessary. Sudden collapse in the postoperative period may be due to a pneumothorax on the normal side of the chest and is an indication for an immediate chest X-ray. The mortality rate amongst babies who require surgery in the first 12 hours of life remains high although those treated after that period normally survive. In the former group, the babies often survive the operation only to die during the next 24 hours from cardiorespiratory problems related to pulmonary hypoplasia and shunting of blood as a result of increased pulmonary vascular resistance.

Oesophageal hiatus hernia

The different types of oesphageal hiatus hernia can be classified, not only according to anatomical variations, but also according to the effects produced on sphincteric control at the oesophagogastric junction. It is now believed that such control, which serves mainly to pre-

vent regurgitation of gastric contents into the oesophagus, is due to angulation of the oesophagus at the point
where it passes through the diaphragmatic hiatus; this
lies between the fibres of the right crus, which hitches
the oesophagus down to the lumbar spine. It is doubtful
if there is any true sphincter, since intrinsic muscle fibres
which might fulfil this role can seldom be demonstrated.

In *sliding herniae* (85% of cases) the oesophagogastric
junction passes upwards through the diaphragmatic hiatus into the posterior mediastinum, and comes to lie at
or near the highest point of the stomach. The resultant
loss of the normal angulation of the oesophagus allows
postural regurgitation to take place, giving rise to an
intractable form of oesophagitis, with or without
ulceration.

In *para-oesophageal herniae* (10% of cases) the fundus
of the stomach protrudes upwards through the diaphragmatic hiatus in front of the oesophagus (possibly into a
preformed sac of peritoneum), by a process of rolling-
up of its anterior wall. The cardiac orifice may lie in its
normal sub-diaphragmatic position, but even if it also is
displaced upwards along with the gastric fundus, the
oesophagus still enters the stomach at an oblique angle,
and pressure upon it by the fundus is maintained, so
that regurgitation does not occur. Oesophagitis is therefore absent, but a variety of other symptoms may be
produced.

Congenitally short oesophagus, as a cause of hiatus hernia, is uncommon (less than 5% of cases). Like an
acquired hernia of sliding type, it is subjected to gastric
regurgitation, and may, therefore, develop oesophagitis
with ulceration. A short oesophagus which persistently
maintains the cardia within the thoracic cavity is not
necessarily congenital, but may be the result of post-
inflammatory fibrosis following an acquired hernia
of sliding type.

Operation should not be advised when the diagnosis
is reached as an incidental finding. It should be reserved
for patients who do not respond to medical treatment,
and in whom no other cause for the symptoms can be
found. The method of approach is best determined by
the experience of the operator.

The transabdominal approach makes it possible to evaluate or to deal with any conditions such as peptic ulcer
or cholelithiasis, which may coexist. The most essential
part of the operation, after reduction of the hernia, consists in narrowing the hiatus in the right crus by two or
three stitches which approximate the muscle fibres—
behind the oesophagus, in order to restore its normal
angulation at this level. The hiatal repair may be combined with the operation of *fundoplication* described by
Nissen (Rossetti, 1978). A large stomach tube having
been passed, in addition to the customary duodenal tube,
the gastric fundus is mobilized by incision of the peritoneum around it, and by division of the upper part of
the lesser omentum. It is then pushed round the back of
the oesophagus, to emerge in the space which has been
created on its medial side (Fig. 14.32). The two folds of
fundus are then united across the front of the oesophagus
by three or four stitches, after which the larger tube,
which has now served its purpose in preventing the
oesophagus from being too tightly constricted, is removed (Fig. 14.33). This operation is designed, firstly
to prevent reflux by creating a valve-like effect from
burying of the terminal oesophagus in the stomach wall;
secondly, the buttress formed by the plicated fundus
renders recurrent herniation unlikely.

The transthoracic approach provides better access, but
imposes a greater strain on elderly patients. It is the
method of choice when the hernia has recurred after a
previous abdominal repair. The approach is generally
made through the bed of the 8th rib on the left side. The

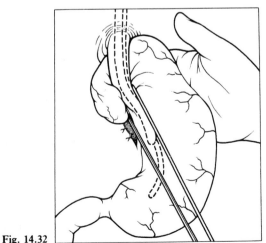

Fig. 14.32

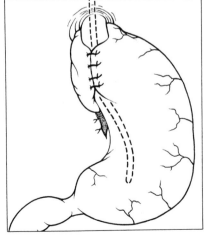

Fig. 14.33

Figs. 14.32 & 14.33 The operation of *fundoplication* in the treatment of oesophageal hiatus hernia

lower part of the oesophagus immediately above the cardia is exposed by incision of the overlying pleura, and it elevated by a sling. A radial incision is made in the left dome of the diaphragm; two fingers are introduced through this and are passed upwards through the hiatus alongside the herniated portion of the stomach. The coverings of the protrusion—the stretched phrenico-oesophageal ligament (fascia reflected from the under surface of the diaphragm to blend with the fascia propria of the oesophagus), and the peritoneal reflection—are then divided from the thoracic aspect around the front and sides of the stomach 1–2 cm below the cardia. The excess, together with any retroperitoneal fatty tissue lying within the hiatus, may be excised. The cardia is drawn downwards into the abdomen, and, through the diaphragmatic incision, the cut edge of the attached peritoneum and fascia is stitched to the under surface of the hiatus on the front and sides. The oesophageal hiatus is then repaired as in the trans-abdominal approach with the addition of an antireflux procedure.

Traumatic herniae result usually from a crushing injury which has caused rupture of the diaphragm. They are commoner on the left side, where the diaphragm is unsupported by the liver. Immediate repair should be undertaken, a combined abdominothoracic approach being employed.

REFERENCES

Bache J R, Bentick B, Mercer J L 1982 Oesophageal intubation. A review of 100 cases. Journal of the Royal College of Surgeons of Edinburgh 27: 26

Bates M 1981 Surgical treatment of bronchial carcinoma. Annals of the Royal College of Surgeons of England 63: 164

Belcher J R 1981 Carcinoma of the bronchus. In: Hadfield J, Hobsley M, (eds) Current surgical practice, vol. 3. Arnold, London, p 280

Björk V O 1971 Aortic valve replacement with the Björk-Shiley tilting disc valve prosthesis. British Heart Journal 33 supplement: 42

Celestin L R 1959 Permanent intubation in inoperable cancer of the oesophagus and cardia: a new tube. Annals of the Royal College of Surgeons of England 25: 165

Cohen D A, Middleton A W, Fletcher J 1974 Gastric tube oesophagoplasty. Journal of Paediatric Surgery 9: 451

Earlam R, Cunha-Melo J R 1980a Oesophageal squamous cell carcinoma: 1 A critical review of surgery. British Journal of Surgery 67: 381

Earlam R, Cunha-Melo J R 1980b Oesophageal squamous cell carcinoma: 2. A critical review of radiotherapy. British Journal of Surgery 67: 457

Earlam R, Cunha-Melo J R 1981 Benign oesophageal strictures: historical and technical aspects of dilatation. British Journal of Surgery 68: 829

Ferguson D G, Stevenson H M 1978 A review of 158 gunshot wounds to the chest. British Journal of Surgery 65: 845

Ferguson L J, Imrie C W, Hutchison J 1981 Excision of bullae without pleurectomy in patients with spontaneous pneumothorax. British Journal of Surgery 68: 214

Gunstensen J, Wade J D 1971 Mediastinoscopy. An analysis of 320 consecutive cases. British Journal of Surgery 59: 209

Jones D B, Davies P S, Smith P M 1981 Endoscopic insertion of palliative oesophageal tube in oesophagogastric neoplasm. British Journal of Surgery 68: 197

Keen G 1972 Closed injuries of the thoracic aorta. Annals of the Royal College of Surgeons of England 5l: 137

Keen G 1974 Chest injuries. Annals of the Royal College of Surgeons of England 54: 124

Lewis I 1946 The surgical treatment of carcinoma of the oesophagus, with special reference to the new operation for growths of the middle third. British Journal of Surgery 34: 18

Logan A, Turner R 1959 Surgical treatment of mitral stenosis. Lancet 2: 874

McKeown K C 1972 Trends in oesophageal resection for carcinoma. Annals of the Royal College of Surgeons of England 51: 213

McKeown K C 1985 The surgical treatment of carcinoma of the oesophagus. A review of the results of 478 cases. Journal of the Royal College of Surgeons of Edinburgh 30: 11

Menzies-Gow N, Gummer J W P, Edwards D A W 1978 Results of Heller's operation for achalasia of the cardia. British Journal of Surgery 65: 483

Mok C K, Lee J W T, Nandi P L, Cheung K L, Ong G B 1982 Early correction of cardiac anomalies using extracorporeal circulation. Journal of the Royal College of Surgeons of Edinburgh 27: 33

Mousseau M M, LeForestier J, Barbin J, Hardy M 1956 Place de l'intubation a demeure dans le traitment palliatif du cancer de l'oesophage. Archives Francaises des Maladies de l'Appareil Digestif et des Maladies de la Nutrition 45: 208

Nohl-Oser H C 1972 An investigation of the anatomy of the lymphatic drainage of the lungs. Annals of the Royal College of Surgeons of England 51: 157

Oakley C M 1982 Long-term complications of valve replacement. Leading article. British Medical Journal

Olanow C W, Wechsler A S, Roses A D 1982 A prospective study of thymectomy and serum acetycholine receptor antibodies in myasthenia gravis. Annals of Surgery 196: 113

Ong G B 1975 Unresectable carcinoma of the oesophagus. Annals of the Royal College of Surgeons of England 56: 3

Owen-Smith M S 1978 High velocity missile injuries. In: Hadfield J, Hobsley M (eds) Current surgical practice, vol.2. Arnold, London, p 218

Pearson J G 1971 The value of radiotherapy in the management of squamous oesophageal carcinoma. British Journal of Surgery 58: 794

Roberts J G 1980 Cancer of the oesophagus—how should tumour biology affect treatment? British Journal of Surgery 67: 791

Rosetti M E, Hell K 1978 Sliding hiatus hernia: Fundoplication or Nissen repair. In: Nyhus L M, Condon R E (eds) Hernia, 2nd edn. Lippincott: Philadelphia, ch 40

Souttar H S 1924 A method of intubating the oesophagus for malignant stricture. British Medical Journal 1: 782

Subramanian S 1974 Early correction of congenital cardiac defects using profound hypothermia and circulatory arrest. Annals of the Royal College of Surgeons of England 54: 176

Sutton P P, Longrigg N 1982 Strangulated Bochdalek hernia in an adult. Journal of the Royal College of Surgeons of Edinburgh 27: 58

Waterston D J 1964 Colonic replacement of the oesophagus (intrathoracic). Surgical Clinics of North America 44: 6

Waterston D J, Stark J, Ashcroft K W 1972 Ascending aorta-to-right pulmonary artery shunts: Experience with 100 patients. Surgery 72: 897

Wheatley D J, Penhall J R H 1981 The place of surgery in coronary artery disease. Journal of the Royal College of Surgeons of Edinburgh 26: 54

Williamson R C N 1975 The management of peptic oesophageal stricture. British Journal of Surgery 62: 448

FURTHER READING

Moghissi K 1979 Reflux stricture of the oesophagus and its surgical treatment. In: Lumley J, Craven J (eds) Surgical review 1. Pitman Medical, London, p 167

Sellors T H 1976 A review of cardiac surgery for the general surgeon. In: Hadfield J, Hobsley M (eds) Current surgical practice, vol 1. Arnold, London, ch 2

15

Abdominal operations

J. M. S. JOHNSTONE & R. F. RINTOUL

GENERAL CONSIDERATIONS AND TECHNIQUE

Preparation

During the outpatient investigation of a patient who is to be admitted to hospital for an abdominal operation, the surgeon will have already offered advice regarding preparation of a general nature. In many cases, the patient need be admitted only one day prior to his operation, but this assumes that his fitness for anaesthesia has been considered and that little further preparation is required. Patients who require complex assessment or preparation for surgery will be admitted to hospital several days before operation and will then have the opportunity to become accustomed to their surroundings. In emergency conditions any scheme of preoperative treatment must necessarily be curtailed, but conditions such as shock and water or salt depletion should receive adequate correction.

Teeth and oral hygiene. Oral or pharyngeal sepsis predisposes to postoperative respiratory infection or to the less common complication of parotitis. Abdominal operations, unless urgent, are best postponed until infected teeth or tonsils have been removed.

Respiratory complications are among the most common after abdominal surgery. It is a wise precaution to postpone a non-urgent operation in a patient with respiratory infection, and to X-ray the chest in such cases and in all patients being prepared for major procedures.

Diet. A patient admitted to hospital on the day prior to operation follows an unrestricted diet except for a light supper. Fluids are withheld after he retires for the night if operation is arranged for the following morning. Those patients who require longer preparation may take the opportunity to improve their nutrition with a well balanced normal diet or with one of the many fluid substitutes now available (p. 312). In cases where hepatic dysfunction may be present, e.g. in biliary disease (p. 385), a high carbohydrate diet should be prescribed in order to ensure adequate stores of liver glycogen. Glucose may be given orally—100 to 200 g daily for 2—3 days before operation.

Gastric aspiration and lavage. Whenever there has been much vomiting, and in all cases for operation on the stomach or duodenum, a nasogastric tube should be passed in order that all stomach contents can be withdrawn before the patient is taken to the theatre. The tube is left in situ during the operation, so that further aspiration can be carried out as required. This is a valuable precaution in preventing vomitus being inhaled during induction of anaesthesia. When there has been gastric stasis, thorough lavage of the stomach is indicated, and, if possible, should be repeated two or three times before operation; for this it may be necessary to use a large-bore tube passed by the mouth.

Bowel action. Provided that the bowel action has been regular, it is unnecessary to give an aperient. Where indicated, however, some mild laxative such as Mist. Cascara Co. or Dorbanex may be prescribed not later than the morning of the day prior to operation. It is common practice to give suppositories on the evening before operation; this may be given as routine, or only when it is thought that a normal evacuation has not been obtained. For all operations on the colon or rectum where resection is likely to be carried out, special preparation (p. 436) is required.

Urinary system. Estimation of the specific gravity of the urine, and examination for albumin and sugar, will be carried out as part of the routine clinical examination, and such investigations normally suffice in the preparation for most abdominal operations. In conditions where the fluid or electrolyte balance may be disturbed (see below) a fluid balance chart should be kept. If it is suspected that any urinary disease may complicate the abdominal condition, a full urological investigation must, of course, be carried out.

Blood. Any suspected anaemia should be investigated by red and white cell counts and by haemoglobin estimation. In many cases the underlying disease or nutritional disturbance leads to a degree of anaemia, which it may be necessary to correct by transfusion, so that the patient is submitted to operation in the optimum condition to withstand blood loss. In all major abdominal cases a full blood examination should be carried out as routine; in addition the blood group should be determined prior to operation, and an individual compatibility test done against the blood of a prospective donor. Blood transfusion plays an integral part in saving life, and the blood may not be available when it is most urgently required unless the need is anticipated. In such cases it is an advantage to set up an intravenous infusion of glucose or saline on the morning of operation, using a standard 'giving set', so that blood transfusion may be substituted quickly and easily during operation should this prove necessary. Investigation of the blood chemistry is indicated in conditions of fluid and electrolyte imbalance, and in hypoproteinaemia. Preoperative measurement of blood urea should be routine since a high level requires investigation and correction if postoperative renal failure is to be avoided.

Fluid and electrolyte therapy is now accepted as a valuable and indeed essential part of modern surgical treatment, both pre- and postoperative. Since it attains its greatest importance in abdominal surgery, it is conveniently considered here.

The essentials of such therapy are (1) to make good any fluid deficit already incurred, (2) to ensure an adequate balance between the daily intake and output of fluid, replacing any continuing losses as they arise, and (3) to administer fluids which contain in solution the appropriate mineral constituents according to the patient's needs.

Dehydration. By far the commonest cause of dehydration is abnormal loss of fluid from the gastrointestinal tract. Such losses may occur before operation, and are then likely to be due to the primary condition which brings the patient to treatment, e.g. the profuse vomiting of pyloric obstruction, or the severe and prolonged diarrhoea of ulcerative colitis. Alternatively the fluid loss may occur as a complication of operation, e.g. prolonged aspiration of gastric contents or discharge from fistulae. In either case the deficit should be assessed, if possible, from the clinical state, from the haematocrit, or from the estimated amount of fluid lost. Serum analysis is not always helpful initially but is a guide to progress. (When fluid losses are large, laboratory analysis of each *fluid* is of value). Early replacement of deficiencies should be the aim, firstly to ensure that the patient is in the best possible condition to withstand surgery, and secondly because the difficulties of replacement are greatly increased thereafter. As soon as the deficiency has been assessed, replacement should begin, the method and the quantity administered depending upon the circumstances of the case. If adequate fluid can be administered orally (but this is rare in surgical patients), few difficulties will arise. As a rule administration must be by the intravenous route, and the fluids to be infused must then be selected with care.

Solutions. The simplest solutions for intravenous infusion are isotonic (0.9%) saline and 5% dextrose solution. Some of each solution is necessary each day depending on losses likely to be sustained. In general, the *normal* requirement of the body for salt is in the region of 5 g per day, and this will be met very adequately by 600 ml of isotonic saline solution. When the patient's main need is for water alone, any additional fluid should be given in the form of glucose solution. Proportionately much larger quantities of saline will, however, be required when there is actual loss of gastrointestinal secretions, for in general such losses should be replaced with saline. Certain alternative solutions are mentioned in the following sections.

Quantity to be administered and rate of flow. When the fluid loss has been severe, it is obviously desirable to replace this as expeditiously as possible, and large quantities of intravenous fluid may then be required. Using central venous pressure measurements, over- and under-infusion can be avoided in such cases. (For central venous pressure measurement, a long *Portex* nylon cannula is inserted into an arm vein—see p. 55—and advanced towards the heart. A 'drip' is set up including a side tube for use as a manometer.) Adequate replacement can also be judged by the patient's clinical state, a useful guide being a urine output of 1—2 ml per minute. Serum electrolytes should be measured frequently. Any marked degree of water and salt depletion leads to nitrogen retention, so that the blood urea level is a most useful and most sensitive index of the degree of depletion and the efficacy of replacement (le Quesne, 1967). The optimal basal intake of fluid in *average* conditions is in the region of 2–3 litres in the 24 hours, 0.75 to 1 litre for 'insensible' loss (via the expired air and by evaporation from the skin), and 1–2 litres to allow for an adequate urinary output, of which the acceptable minimum is 500 ml. If fluid cannot be taken orally, the whole amount should usually be given intravenously. Since the *normal* daily requirement of the body for salt is about 5 g, this will be adequately met by 600 ml of isotonic saline solution; thus two or three ½-litres of glucose solution should be given for every one ½-litre of saline. Any abnormal losses by vomiting, etc., should be compensated for by a corresponding increase in the amount of saline infused, so that a daily balance is achieved (see below). For the first 24–48 hours after a major operation when urinary output is reduced, the amount of fluid infused should not normally exceed 2 litres per day unless it is necessary to compensate for abnormal losses. The rate of administration—in drops per minute—can be determined by multiplying the required number of litres per day by 11. Intravenous therapy should be discontinued when 2½ litres (i.e. 100 ml per hour) can be taken orally.

Daily fluid balance. The keeping of a daily fluid balance chart is an essential safeguard whenever a patient is being treated by continuous intravenous infusion—

whether this be pre- or postoperatively. An exact record must by kept throughout the 24 hours of all fluid intake—by stomach (orally or by gastric 'drip'), and by intravenous infusion. The output—by urine, by vomiting or by gastric aspiration, by fistulous discharges or by diarrhoea—must be similarly recorded. (The fluid content of solid faeces can be disregarded.) To the total amount of the recorded output must be added 0.75 to 1 litre for 'insensible' loss. The intake and output should be compared after each 12 hours, and any fluid debt or *negative balance* should be replaced during the ensuing 12-hour period. A more frequent balance should be kept where losses are high, and in all cases a cumulative balance should be made daily, taking into account gains or losses during the preceding days of the infusion.

Alkalosis. Continued vomiting or aspiration of gastric secretions over a prolonged period leads to a state of alkalosis, since gastric juice normally contains excess of chlorides over sodium and potassium, and there is therefore a greater loss of acid radicles. When vomiting has continued for more than a few days, there is a considerable loss of sodium and potassium, but this appears to be due to loss in the urine, rather than in the vomit. The alkalosis leads to an increased bicarbonate concentration in the plasma, and therefore in the glomerular filtrate. In consequence there is an increased secretion of bicarbonate in the urine, and kation (sodium and potassium) is excreted in proportionate amounts, in order to maintain the electrochemical neutrality of the urine. The loss of water, chlorides and sodium is replaced very adequately by the infusion of isotonic saline solution. For the correction of potasium deficiency (see below), it is recommended that potassium chloride should be added to the solution in divided doses.

Acidosis (diminished alkali reserve) is commonly caused by loss of the more alkaline secretions of the alimentary tract below the stomach—as may result from the vomiting of high intestinal obstruction, duodenal fistula, ileostomy or prolonged diarrhoea. The main deficiencies, besides that of fluid are of sodium and potassium. When, as is usually the case, the sodium loss predominates, there will be an associated fall in the plasma bicarbonate level, a fall in the CO_2 combining power, and a resulting acidosis. The administration of isotonic saline replaces losses in water and sodium, but not in potassium; it provides an excess of chlorides, which, although partly removed by renal excretion, may increase the tendency to acidosis. In severe acidosis, 500 ml of 5% sodium bicarbonate may be given by intravenous infusion over a period of four hours. Alternatively, Hartmann's solution or Ringer-lactate solution, each of which contains sodium chloride, sodium lactate and potassium chloride, may be used.

Potassium deficiency. The importance of potassium deficiency in postoperative states is now generally appreciated. A certain proportion of the deficit may be due to direct loss of potassium from prolonged vomiting or loss of intestinal secretions, but indirect losses are probably more important. Following all operations, and in direct proportion to their severity, there is an increased loss of potassium in the urine, indicative of mobilisation of intracellular potassium. It would seem that the most important loss follows the prolonged intravenous infusion of solutions containing no potassium, since this is secreted in larger quantities in the urine because of the resulting diuresis. There is probably little risk of potassium deficiency during the first 48 hours of infusion. When, however, this is continued for a longer period, it is wise to give potassium, either orally or added to the infusion. Potassium deficiency, which presents clinically by intense drowsiness deepening to coma, muscular weakness and incoordination, should be suspected whenever there has been prolonged or severe loss of gastrointestinal secretions or if an intravenous infusion has been in use for over 48 hours. Replacement should not await laboratory confirmation of the deficiency, which being mainly intracellular will not be accurately represented by the serum level. Potassium should be given orally if possible because of the risk of arrhythmias occurring from too rapid a rise in the plasma concentration. If oral administration is practicable the recommended dosage is 1 g of potassium chloride 4-hourly for the first 24 hours, followed by 2 g 4-hourly until the serum potassium reaches normal levels. If intravenous administration is necessary, 1 to 2 g of potassium chloride should be added to 500 ml of glucose solution, and infused over a period of four hours. Provided the urinary output is over 600 ml per day, further potassium infusion is safe although the total dosage should not normally exceed 5 g per day. Magnesium deficiency may accompany potassium loss. It is recognized by serum measurement and is easily amenable to replacement therapy.

Protein deficiency

Many patients who require surgery, particularly as an emergency, are depleted of plasma proteins. Rapid depletion can result from severe haemorrhage or from serious burns or other injuries. Gradual depletion may be due to inadequate ingestion of protein, resulting either from starvation or from defective absorption, as may occur in malignant disease, and in conditions such as Crohn's disease and ulcerative colitis. The deficient protein content of the plasma gives rise to a decrease in the colloid osmotic pressure, so that, provided that severe dehydration is not present, extruded tissue fluid fails to return to the circulation, and some degree of oedema results. Such conditions give rise to increased susceptibility to infections and to diminished healing power. They, therefore, add considerably to the risk of operation and retard convalescence.

The normal level of plasma proteins is 65–85 g per litre, including 35 g per litre of albumin. Estimations made during protein deficiency may give a misleadingly high figure on account of the dehydration which may coexist, and this factor must be considered.

Acute protein deficiency cannot be corrected by blood transfusion although plasma, or plasma substitutes, are used in the treatment of burns to correct the colloid osmotic pressure and maintain the circulation. Chronic deficiency of protein can be treated by the administration of a high protein diet, comprising 200–250 g of protein daily. This should be combined with vitamin C in doses up to 1 g daily. If the patient cannot take food normally by mouth, protein hydrolysates may be given by 'drip' through a nasogastric tube. Proprietary solutions can now be administered through a fine bore (1 mm) tube which has been passed into the stomach and which is well tolerated once it is in position (Fig. 15.1).

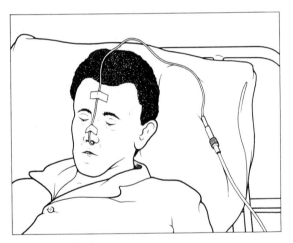

Fig. 15.1 Fine bore (1 mm) tube for nasogastric feeding

It should be noted that all major operations lead to a considerable amount of protein catabolism, and, if hypoproteinaemia exists preoperatively, a serious deficiency may develop. It is obvious, therefore, that any protein replacement required should be effected if possible before operation.

Parenteral nutrition may be considered to combat postoperative or post-traumatic negative nitrogen balance where normal feeding will be delayed for more than a few days (Johnston, 1977), or preoperatively in an emaciated patient. *Fat emulsions* and ethanol provide essential calories and are necessary for correct utilization of *amino-acid solutions* (Hadfield, 1973). Side-effects are few, the main being thrombosis of the drip vein. This can be minimised by use of a 'two-drip' technique, mixing separate infusions of fat emulsion and amino-acid solution in the cannula or by adding a small dose of heparin to the lipid infusion. Use of a central venous cannula must be attended by strict asepsis.

Position for operation

For most abdominal operations the patient is placed in the supine position. The arms may be laid alongside the body and anchored by the simple apparatus shown in Figure 15.2. The hands should not be placed beneath the buttocks since damage to the circulation or nerve supply of the fingers may result. For lower abdominal operations the arms may be folded across the chest and secured by the safety-pinned bed-jacket.

Recognition that the deep veins of the calf are a common site for postoperative thrombosis has led to the routine practice of raising the heels on a sponge rubber pad (Fig. 20.7) or using intermittent calf compression during operation; subcutaneous heparin is also being used.

Operations on retroperitoneal structures such as the kidney and sympathetic trunk are performed usually with the patient in the lateral position.

Trendelenburg position. Downward tilting of the head-end of the table is employed frequently in operations on the pelvic organs. Its effect is to cause the more mobile organs to gravitate towards the diaphragm so that a less obstructed view of the pelvis can be obtained. The rubber mattress supplied with the modern operating table is ridged so as to prevent the patient from sliding headwards (Fig. 15.3)

ABDOMINAL INCISIONS

Anatomy of abdominal wall

Muscles

The muscles of the anterior abdominal wall are external oblique, internal oblique, transversus abdominis and rectus abdominis. (The pyramidales muscles are frequently absent and are of no surgical importance.) In general the first three of these arise at the side of the trunk—from the lower ribs, lumbar fascia or iliac crest. As they traverse the front of the abdomen they become aponeurotic, and are inserted mainly into the *linea alba*, a band of fibrous tissue extending in the mid line from the xiphoid process to the pubis. Before they reach the linea alba they combine to form a sheath for the rectus muscle. Above the umbilicus the linea alba is 1–2 cm wide, but in its lower part it is much narrower.

External oblique runs mainly downwards, forwards, and medially, but its upper fibres are nearly horizontal, its lower ones (inserting into the iliac crest) nearly vertical. Its lower free border forms the *inguinal ligament* which stretches from the anterior superior spine to the pubic tubercle.

Internal oblique runs mainly in a slightly upward direc-

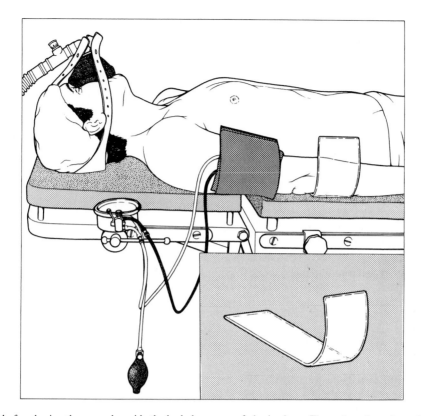

Fig. 15.2 Method of anchoring the arms alongside the body by means of plastic plates. These plates (one shown in inset) are introduced transversely between the patient and the mattress, where they are firmly secured by the patient's weight. Sphygmomanometer is shown in position for the purpose of blood pressure recording during the operation

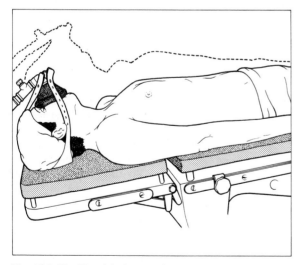

Fig. 15.3 The Trendelenburg position

tion but its lower fibres, which descend to the pubis, are nearly vertical.

Transversus abdominis runs mainly horizontally, but its lowest fibres run downwards along with those of internal oblique. Its deep surface is lined by transversalis fascia; between this and the peritoneum there is a thin layer of extraperitoneal fat.

Rectus abdominis lies alongside the linea alba, stretching from the front of the pubis to the xiphoid process and to the 5th, 6th and 7th costal cartilages. Its substance is traversed by three horizontal *tendinous intersections*— one opposite the umbilicus, another near the xiphoid, and a third midway between these.

Rectus sheath

This is formed by the aponeuroses of external oblique, internal oblique and transversus, the last two of which are arranged in a somewhat complicated manner.

The *anterior sheath* is complete from rib margin to pubis. In its upper three-fourths it is formed by external oblique and by the anterior lamina of internal oblique. In the lower one-fourth it is formed by all three aponeuroses. It is adherent to the tendinous intersections of the rectus muscle.

The *posterior sheath* is complete only as far down as a point midway between umbilicus and pubis, where it ends as a free border, the *linea semicircularis*. Below this level the sheath is deficient, the rectus being separated

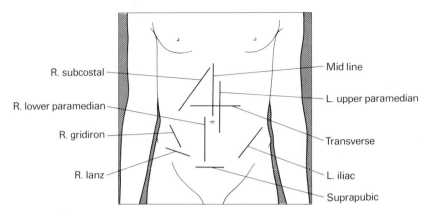

Fig. 15.4 Abdominal incisions

from the peritoneum by transversalis fascia alone. It is formed by the posterior lamina of internal oblique fused with transversus. Some fleshy fibres of transversus appear in the upper part of the posterior sheath.

Vessels

The *inferior epigastric vessels* are the only ones of surgical importance. The artery, arising from the external iliac, runs upwards and medially from just above the midinguinal point; it then passes under cover of the lateral margin of the rectus and enters its sheath. The companion vein joins the external iliac vein.

Nerves

The nerves of the abdominal wall are the *lower five intercostal*, the *subcostal*, the *iliohypogastric* and the *ilioinguinal*. These run an oblique course in the abdominal wall, lying mainly between transversus and internal oblique. All except the last two enter the rectus sheath and pierce rectus to end as cutaneous branches.

All incisions should be planned to give adequate access to the operative field, but at the same time to inflict the minimum of damage to the abdominal wall, so that a strong and durable scar will result. Provided that the necessary access can be obtained, splitting of a muscle in the line of its fibres (fleshy or aponeurotic) is preferable to division. Healing then occurs much more readily, there is no tendency to disruption of the scar, and subsequent function is unimpaired. In children, the skin incision should conform to Langer's lines (p. 236), otherwise the scar becomes increasingly unsightly with age. With few exceptions, a transverse skin incision can be used for all abdominal surgery in children.

The midline incision

In the upper abdomen the midline incision is suitable for most operations on the stomach and duodenum. It traverses the linea alba, which is practically avascular, so that

the abdomen can be both quickly opened and quickly closed. It is, therefore, a popular incision for emergency operations.

After the skin has been incised the linea alba is divided to expose the peritoneum, which is covered by the thin transversalis fascia. These are usually divided as one layer. This division should be made a little to one side of the midline, or the knife may pass between the layers of the falciform ligament.

In the lower abdomen the midline incision is less satisfactory, unless particular care is taken with suture of the wound. It is not recommended for routine use unless nylon, or similar strong suture, is available. The linea alba is both thin and narrow below the umbilicus, and incorrect suturing results in an incisional hernia.

The midline incision can be readily enlarged if required. If the umbilicus is encountered the incision should be carried round one side of it. Major exposure for aorto-iliac reconstruction may be obtained by a midline incision from the xiphisternum to pubis.

Closure of the incision is effected by three layers of sutures—approximating respectively the peritoneum (together with transversalis fascia), the linea alba and the skin. The 'mass closure' technique is now equally acceptable for routine wound repair, provided sutures are inserted at least 1 cm from the edge of the incision and monofilament nylon is used (Bucknall, 1983).

The paramedian incision

This is the most widely used incision for all general purposes, and is applicable to both the upper and the lower abdomen. Its chief advantage lies in the exceptionally strong scar which results.

The incision is made parallel to the midline, and at a distance of 2–3 cm from it. The anterior rectus sheath is divided in the line of the skin incision. Forceps are placed on the medial cut margin, which is retracted to expose the medial edge of the rectus muscle. In the upper abdomen the anterior sheath must be freed by sharp dis-

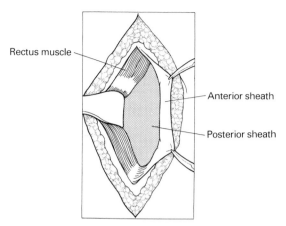

Fig. 15.5 Paramedian incision. The rectus muscle has been retracted laterally to expose the posterior sheath, which is then incised together with the peritoneum

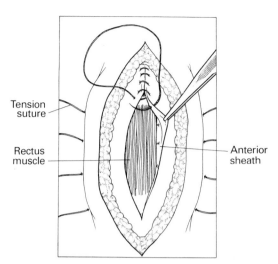

Fig. 15.6 Closure of paramedian incision. The rectus muscle covers the suture line in the posterior sheath. Tension sutures have been inserted. The anterior sheath is being repaired by a continuous suture

section, since it is adherent to the tendinous intersections which traverse the muscle. The rectus is then displaced laterally (Fig. 15.5) to expose the posterior sheath, which in the upper part shows fleshy fibres of the transversus. The posterior sheath is incised in the line of the skin incision, together with transversalis fascia and peritoneum.

Closure. The incision is sutured in three layers—firstly peritoneum and posterior sheath as one layer, secondly anterior sheath, and thirdly skin. Tension sutures may be passed down to but not penetrating the posterior sheath: these are inserted before the anterior sheath is

sutured, but are not tied until the end of the operation (Fig. 15.6). The strength of the repair lies in the fact that the intact rectus muscle covers and gives support to the incisions into the anterior and posterior sheaths.

Instead of the rectus being displaced laterally it may be split in the same line as the skin incision. This method provides more rapid access to the abdominal cavity although troublesome bleeding from the muscle may occur. The scar is not so strong as in the classical para-

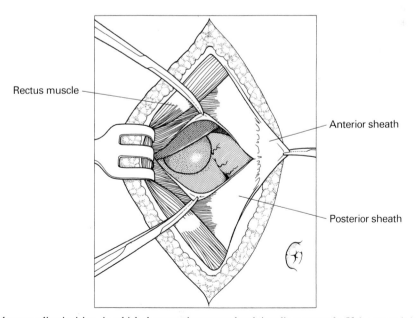

Fig. 15.7 Modified paramedian incision, in which the posterior rectus sheath is split *transversely*. If the access is inadequate, this is easily rectified by converting the incision into an ordinary paramedian

median incision, not only because the rectus is split, but also because the narrow medial strip of the muscle is deprived of its nerve supply. *A modified paramedian incision*, in which the posterior rectus sheath is split transversely in the line of its fibres (Fig. 15.7), instead of being incised vertically, is preferred by the writer for many cases of uncomplicated cholecystectomy. It is especially applicable to adipose patients with flabby musculature, in whom incisional hernia is a comparatively frequent sequel to operation. This incision is very simply closed, since the split posterior sheath tends to fall together without tension, and the repair is an extremely strong one. If the access is found to be inadequate, the incision is very easily converted into an ordinary paramedian one by vertical incision of the posterior sheath.

The gridiron incision

This is the incision most commonly used for removal of the appendix. It gives only limited access, but can readily be enlarged by the method described below.

The incision, 7–10 cm in length, lies at right angles to the line joining the anterior superior spine and the umbilicus. Classically its centre should be placed at McBurney's point, i.e. at the junction of the lateral and middle thirds of that line. It is the normal practice, however, to vary the position of the incision according to the supposed situation of the appendix, as judged from the site of maximum tenderness or muscle guarding.

External oblique aponeurosis is split in the line of its fibres (which is the same as that of the skin incision). If the incision is high or laterally placed, fleshy fibres of the muscle are encountered and are split along with the aponeurosis. Both margins of the split are held aside with haemostats or with small retractors, leaving exposed the fleshy fibres of internal oblique running transversely and slightly upwards. This muscle, together with transver-

sus, the fibres of which run in approximately the same line, is then split by blunt dissection. The closed end of a Mayo's scissors or the handle of a scalpel is used for the initial separation, and the split is widened by stretching it between the two forefingers. The fingers are then replaced by small retractors (Fig. 15.8), after which transversalis fascia and peritoneum are picked up as one layer and are incised.

Closure. The peritoneal incision being small can be closed effectively with a running suture, the ends of which are tied together. The split fibres of transversus and internal oblique are very loosely approximated by one or two stitches which pick up both muscles (Fig. 15.9). Alternatively, each muscle split may be closed by suture of the overlying fascia. The external oblique aponeurosis is then sutured, and finally the skin.

Enlarging the gridiron incision. If more access is required in a medial direction the split in internal oblique and transversus is extended into the rectus sheath. If extension is required in an upward or downward direction, these muscles may be divided at right angles to their fibres. The muscles cut in this manner are repaired without difficulty with interrupted stitches. No special liability to postoperative hernia has been recorded.

The Lanz incision is a minor modification of the gridiron. The skin incision is made more or less transversely and curves so that it lies in the interspinous crease. Thereafter the muscles are divided as in the classical gridiron approach. The method has a definite cosmetic value in producing an almost invisible scar, but difficulties are encountered if the incision requires to be enlarged.

Muscle-cutting iliac incision (Rutherford Morison)

This incision is employed in such operations as exposure of the ureter or external iliac vessels; it is favoured by

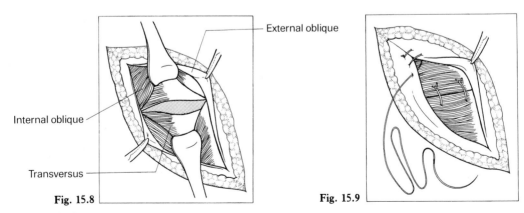

External oblique

Internal oblique

Transversus

Fig. 15.8

Fig. 15.9

Figs. 15.8 & 15.9 Gridiron incision, in which the muscles are not divided, but are split in the line of their fibres—external oblique in the line of the skin incision, internal oblique and transversus in a more or less transverse direction. The muscles are held apart by retractors, to expose transversalis fascia and peritoneum, which are then incised as one layer. The method of closing the incision is shown

some surgeons for removal of the ascending colon or for access to the pelvic colon or rectum on the left side. In general the skin incision is similar to that of the gridiron, but all muscles are cut in the same line.

Closure. The cut muscles are sutured in layers. If this is carefully done there is no tendency to hernia.

Subcostal incisions are most useful in operations on the gall bladder or spleen, or on the flexures of the colon, especially in adipose patients with a wide costal angle.

Kochers' incision begins in the midline below the xiphoid process, and runs downwards and laterally 2.5 cm below and parallel to the costal margin (Fig. 15.4). All muscles, including the rectus, are divided in the same line. The 8th, 9th and 10th intercostal nerves are found running downwards and medially between internal oblique and transversus. Not more than one of these nerves should be divided: the others are carefully retracted and preserved.

Closure is effected in three layers. The first layer comprises peritoneum, posterior rectus sheath and (more laterally) internal oblique and transversus. The anterior rectus sheath and the external oblique are now repaired, and, finally, the skin. No attempt is made to suture the rectus muscle itself—see below.

Transverse incisions may be employed in both upper and lower abdomen. Two distinct types of such incision can be described.

Transverse division of all layers. Both anterior and posterior rectus sheaths are divided transversely—in the line of their fibres. The recti also are divided transversely, so that excellent access is obtained (Fig. 15.10). Division of the recti in this manner causes no interference with their nerve supply, which has a segmental distribution. The method is most suitable for use in the upper abdomen where the rectus is adherent at its tendinous intersections to the anterior sheath. For this reason the cut rectus muscle does not retract, and accurate suture of its

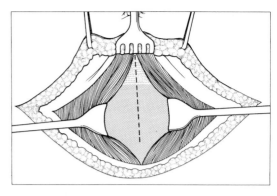

Fig. 15.11 Lower abdominal transverse incision with vertical separation of the recti. The incision is curved so as to lie in the skin creases. After the anterior sheaths have been incised, and the superior flap elevated upwards, the recti are separated and held apart by retractors. Transversalis fascia and peritoneum are then incised in a vertical direction

sheath is all that is required in the way of repair. The incision may be used for cholecystectomy (p. 387) or pancreatic operations (p. 400).

With vertical separation of the recti (Pfannenstiel). This method is more suited to the subumbilical region, where the recti have no tendinous intersections and are more mobile within their sheaths. The skin and anterior rectus sheaths are incised transversely. The anterior sheaths are elevated from the underlying recti both upwards and downwards by sharp dissection. The recti are widely separated and held apart by retractors (Fig. 15.11), and transversalis fascia and peritoneum are then incised in a vertical direction. For bladder exposure, these layers are swept upwards and the prevesical fascia is divided.

The lower abdominal transverse incision, placed close to the pubis, is popular for gynaecological operations where limited access is required and a good cosmetic result is considered important. An incision 2 cm above the pubis is favoured by many urologists and provides adequate exposure of the bladder.

The low pararectal incision is described in the section on femoral hernia where access to the peritoneal cavity *and* to the femoral canal may be required.

Transverse incisions in children

In the newborn, the transverse upper abdominal incision provides good access to the entire peritoneal cavity and is suitable for all operations other than those on the distal large bowel and bladder. Blood loss is critical and can be reduced by cutting with diathermy. In the older infant and child, an upper transverse abdominal incision provides good access to structures lying up to the level of the diaphragm (Fig. 15.12A).

Upper abdominal. A transverse skin incision is made across the width of the recti-abdominis at a level one-

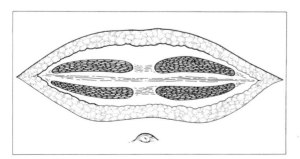

Fig. 15.10 Upper abdominal transverse incision, with division of rectus muscles. Note that the cut muscles do not retract, and that accurate suture of their sheaths is all that is required in the way of repair

Figs. 15.12–15.14 *Abdominal incisions in children.*

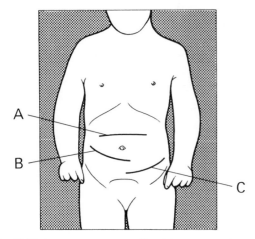

Fig. 15.12 A—transverse upper. B—right transverse lower placed high in the iliac fossa. C—left transverse lower placed low in the iliac fossa

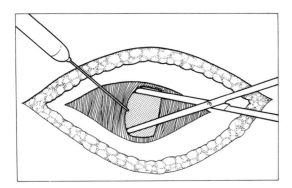

Fig. 15.13 Muscle fibres lifted by artery forceps and cut with diathermy

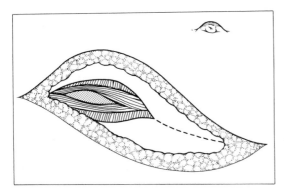

Fig. 15.14 Right transverse lower incision extended by dividing the rectus

third of the distance from the umbilicus to the xiphisternum. Subcutaneous fat and anterior rectus sheath are divided in the line of the incision. Muscle fibres are lifted from the posterior rectus sheath with artery forceps and the fibres can then be safely cut with diathermy between the open blades (Fig. 15.13). Posterior rectus sheath and peritoneum are gripped with two artery forceps and a fold is lifted clear of underlying structures. A small incision is made in the fold with a scalpel and extended under direct vision with scissors along the full length of the wound. In the newborn, the umbilical vein lying in the free margin of the falciform ligament must be identified and divided between ligatures.

Lower abdominal. A transverse lower abdominal incision started in the right iliac fossa and extended towards the left (Fig. 15.12B) gives access to the distal half of the ileum, the caecum and ascending colon and a similar incision in the left iliac fossa extended to the right (Fig. 15.12C) gives access to the sigmoid colon and rectum. However, when extensive mobilisation of the colon is anticipated a transverse incision may be inadequate, particularly in the older child and a left paramedian approach is preferred. A *right-sided transverse lower abdominal incision* is made high in the right iliac fossa. The skin incision is started on the right side of the abdomen and extended towards the mid-line, crossing a point one-third of the distance from the umbilicus to the superior iliac spine. The external oblique aponeurosis is divided obliquely in the line of the incision and the muscle fibres of internal oblique and transversus split by blunt dissection towards the lateral margin of the rectus sheath. The fascia transversalis and peritoneum are then divided transversely to give access to the peritoneal cavity. The incision can be extended with ease across the midline by dividing the rectus muscle with cutting diathermy (Fig. 15.14). A *left-sided transverse lower abdominal incision* is placed low in the iliac fossa so as to cross a point two-thirds of the distance from the umbilicus to the superior iliac spine. In other respects the incision is identical to the approach from the right side. In the newborn it must be remembered that the bladder extends up towards the umbilicus, the apex being tethered by the urachus flanked on either side by an umbilical artery.

Closure. According to preference the muscle layers of an abdominal wound may be closed with Dexon or interrupted monofilament nylon. If the latter method is used the knot should be tied deep and buried to prevent discomfort under the scar. Skin closure with a fine subcuticular suture will avoid ugly cross hatching. With the introduction of mass closure of an abdominal wound with interrupted monofilament nylon, tension sutures should rarely, if ever, be necessary.

For operations on the urinary tract the approach is similar to that used in the adult. A loin incision is used for a retroperitoneal approach to the kidney, a muscle splitting incision in the iliac fossa for the lower part of the ureter and a Pfannenstiel incision for the bladder.

GENERAL TECHNIQUE

Screening of the skin

The skin around the incision should be covered with side towels. This is not only a part of the customary aseptic ritual; in addition it prevents irritation of the delicate serous surface of the bowel from contact with the iodine or other antiseptic which has been used for skin preparation.

Opening of the peritoneum

The utmost care must be taken to ensure that no underlying viscus is wounded during incision of the peritoneum. When the peritoneum has been exposed a small bite is taken with dissecting or artery forceps, and is lifted forwards. It is an advantage to do this during a period of expiration, when the viscera tend to fall away from the abdominal wall. The fold which is lifted up may be given a gentle shake to dislodge any adherent structure, or it may be pinched between finger and thumb so that its thickness can be estimated. A second pair of artery forceps is then applied alongside the first, and the fold is carefully incised (Fig. 15.15). If an opening into the peritoneal cavity is not immediately apparent the forceps should be taken off and reapplied.

When the initial opening has been made, it is enlarged upwards—usually by cutting with scissors under direct vision. It is enlarged downwards by cutting with a knife against two fingers of the left hand which protect the bowel (Fig. 15.16).

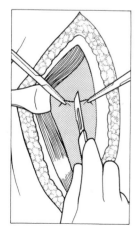 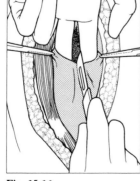

Fig. 15.15   **Fig. 15.16**

Figs. 15.15 & 15.16 Method of opening the peritoneum. Injury to the underlying viscera is avoided by the technique depicted

Gentle handling and care of the bowel

Gentle handling is an essential part of all abdominal operations. Forcible traction on the gut or on its mesentery is never permissible. If the incision gives insufficient access it must be enlarged or a fresh incision employed. Bowel is slippery to hold, and a firm grasp is most easily obtained with the aid of a large swab; this should be wrung out in hot saline, for dry gauze may abrade the delicate serous surface.

Bowel is very readily damaged by *chilling* or *drying*, and no more than is necessary should be brought out of the wound. If a coil of bowel has to be retained on the surface for even a short time, it should be covered with a hot moist towel which is renewed frequently.

Separation of adhesions

All adhesions should be separated as far as possible under direct vision. For the most filmy adhesions, the finger covered with a moist swab may be used as a blunt dissector. Stronger adhesions should be cleanly divided with fine curved dissecting scissors, the curve being directed *away* from the structure which is more likely to suffer from damage. If there are widespread adhesions, as may occur after a previous operation, they should not be disturbed more than is necessary, for they are likely to reform—possibly over a wider area. Separation is carried out only in those adhesions which may give rise to trouble (e.g. by kinking of the gut), or which prevent the necessary access from being obtained.

Re-peritonisation of raw surfaces

The separation of an adhesion involving bowel often leaves a raw area on the serous surface. In order to prevent the adhesion reforming, and to repair what is potentially a weak area in the bowel wall, the affected part may be invaginated by means of continuous or interrupted Lembert sutures (Fig. 15.18). An alternative method is to stitch a piece of omentum over the raw surface.

Prevention of soiling of peritoneal cavity.

In operations for any condition of localised intraperitoneal sepsis, one of the first cares of the surgeon is to prevent the infection spreading to other parts of the peritoneal cavity. Whenever a mass is encountered, and there is even a suspicion that it is inflammatory in origin, the rest of the peritoneal cavity should be carefully *packed-off* before the mass is disturbed. This necessitates the insertion of large abdominal swabs or packs placed in such a manner as to surround the mass, so that any septic exudate will be diverted to the surface or will be absorbed by the gauze, before it can permeate to other parts of the peritoneal cavity.

Any operation which entails opening the lumen of the gut carries a risk of contaminating the peritoneal cavity.

Figs. 15.17 & 15.18 *Method of suturing bowel in two layers.*

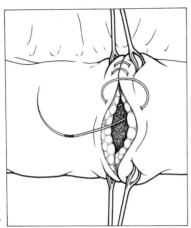 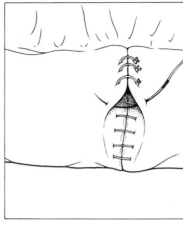

Fig. 15.17   **Fig. 15.18**

Fig. 15.17 *Through-and-through* stitches transfixing all coats and inverting the mucosa.
Fig. 15.18 *Lembert* or seromuscular sutures which do not penetrate the mucosa. They are used to invaginate the previous suture line, and to bring serous surfaces into firm and even contact

This risk is minimised: (1) by bringing the gut outside the abdomen while it is being opened; (2) by completely surrounding it with gauze packs, so that no septic material can enter the wound; (3) by the use of a clamp which will prevent the escape of intestinal contents; (4) by careful suturing of the gut afterwards, and (5) by discarding all instruments, packs, etc., which have become potentially contaminated, and by using clean gloves and towels for subsequent stages of the operation.

Danger of retained swabs
Abdominal packs should have tapes sewn on to them. Forceps are attached to these tapes, and also to any swabs which are introduced into the wound or placed in its vicinity. All swabs put out for an abdominal operation should be of large size. Any swab used for mopping is not left lying near the wound, but is immediately discarded. In most operating theatres the sister is responsible for knowing the exact number of swabs that have been issued, and for checking these at the end of the operation. *Raytex* swabs, which are radio-opaque, may be used as routine; they can be demonstrated on X-ray examination if there is a discrepancy in the swab-count. These, however, should be no more than *additional* safeguards; the surgeon should aim at a technique which will make it almost impossible for a swab to be retained within the abdomen.

Methods of suturing gut
It is customary for any incision which opens the lumen of the gut to be repaired by two layers of sutures. The deeper sutures are *through-and-through* ones transfixing all coats. (As they are effective in arresting haemorrhage

from the gut wall they are also called *haemostatic* sutures.) They may be either continuous or interrupted. A special variety of through-and-through suture is known as the 'loop on the mucosa' (*Connell*) suture; in this the needle is passed twice in succession through each cut edge (first from without-inwards and then from within-outwards). It is effective in preventing eversion of the mucous membrane. A simpler and equally effective inverting suture is shown in Figure 15.17. This continuous suture is started within the lumen and finishes at the same point (after apposition of the two bowel ends) so that the knot disappears into the lumen. The anterior layer of the anastomosis is treated as an extension of the posterior layer, the needle being passed from one lumen to the other before tightening the thread. By any method the sutures, since they penetrate the lumen of the gut, are potentially infected, and should be covered over. This is done by the insertion of a second row of sutures which invaginate the first suture line by bringing together over it the bowel wall on each side. These sutures, which are known as *Lembert* sutures, take up the serous and muscular coats on each side of the deep suture line and about 5 mm distant from it, but do not penetrate the mucous membrane (Fig. 15.18). The serous surfaces thus brought into contact are gummed together by lymph exudate, and the junction rapidly becomes organised and water-tight. For incisions of any length a continuous Lembert suture may be employed.

Needles
Fine round-bodied needles are used throughout—straight or curved according to individual preference. *Atraumatic* needles have a tubular end instead of an eye, and into this the suture material is suaged by the man-

ufacturers. They inflict the minimum of trauma on the bowel wall, and make for smooth suturing.

Suture materials
Fine catgut is probably best for through-and-through sutures, since the persistence of an unabsorbable suture on the mucous surface may predispose to ulceration. For Lembert sutures either catgut, linen or silk may be used. Dexon, or alternative absorbable material, provides a useful alternative which can be used for both layers.

Reposition of viscera and repair of incision
The edges of the peritoneal incision are grasped with forceps and are lifted away from the patient. Provided that there is no distension and the abdominal wall is relaxed the viscera should fall back into the abdomen almost of their own accord. Should a distended coil of bowel fail to go back easily it should be gently compressed to empty it of gas. If the intestines or omentum interfere with suture of the peritoneum they may be covered with a moist abdominal pack which is held down with a spatula or with a special depressor. When the suture line is nearly complete the pack and depressor are withdrawn. If the suturing is being carried out under tension, and the stitches tend to cut out, the needle may be made to pick up muscular fibres along with the peritoneum, or each bite may be taken from the *inner* surface of the peritoneum, parallel to the cut edge. Alternatively, a continuous mattress suture may be used, placing several sutures before tightening up and approximating the edges of the wound. When the tension is due to incomplete anaesthesia the surgeon should cover the wound with a towel, and wait until the necessary relaxation is obtained. Whatever method of suturing is preferred, it is essential to insert the needle at least 1 cm from the wound edge and place the loops of suture about 1 cm apart.

Suture materials
Catgut, as it is absorbed by the body, is the material most commonly employed for sutures which approximate peritoneum and the adjacent layer of abdominal wall. Catgut is also satisfactory for the muscular or aponeurotic layers in small wounds particularly in a thin, young, well nourished patient where difficulty in wound healing is not anticipated. Nonabsorbable material such as linen, silk or monofilament nylon is essential for repair of the linea alba in midline incisions and may also be used in the superficial layers of the abdominal wall in elderly patients, the obese or those liable to put strain on the wound postoperatively as a result of coughing.

Drainage of the peritoneal cavity is essential in cases of severe peritoneal sepsis, since, by allowing the escape of

inflammatory exudate or of frank pus, it reduces toxaemia and the likelihood of paralytic ileus.

Prior to insertion of a drainage tube, antibiotic lavage may be carried out to cleanse the most contaminated area and then the entire peritoneal cavity (Stewart, 1980).

In choosing the type of drain and siting it in the abdominal wall, consideration must be given to the nature and quantity of drainage which is likely to occur within the next 72 hours. Pus which forms *after* the operation must be able to drain freely, as should any bowel content, in the event of intestinal leakage.

When a localised abscess is present it is drained by the shortest possible route—usually through the incision used for exposure. *The wound should be closed very loosely around the drain*, so that any exudate from the layers of the wound, as well as from the peritoneal cavity, can readily escape to the surface. It should be possible, therefore, to insert a finger alongside the drain (Wilkie). Either a tube or a strip of plain or corrugated material may be used. The drain is usually left in situ until discharge is minimal, but is shortened at intervals.

Suction drainage
The *Redivac* drainage system is now generally available and can be used to advantage in any part of the abdominal cavity. Unless pus is viscid, it will pass through the larger size of *Redivac* tube. Suction is applied from 'vacuum' bottle to numerous holes in that part of the tube which lies within the patient. Suction cannot be applied to a single tube drain, since its action would be to draw surrounding bowel and omentum against the tube; not only might these structures be damaged, but all drainage would cease immediately. Should suction be required, 'sump' drainage is instituted by inserting one tube within the other (Fig. 15.19). The outer tube projects for 2–3 cm outside the wound; the inner tube is longer and

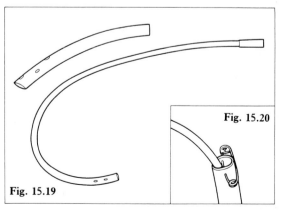

Figs. 15.19 & 15.20 Two plastic tubes, the narrower placed within the wider, for 'sump' drainage by suction to the inner tube. Figure 15.20 shows method of securing the inner tube. The safety-pin compresses slightly but does not transfix the inner tube

Figs. 15.21 & 15.22 *Double-tube suction drainage (sump drainage) applied to the peritoneal cavity*

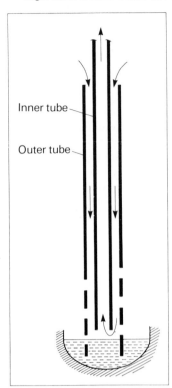

Inner tube

Outer tube

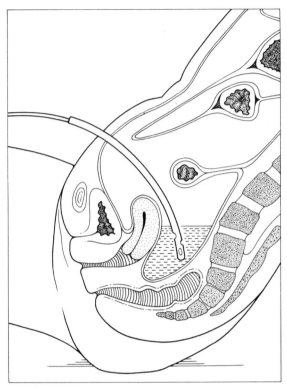

Fig. 15.21 Diagram to illustrate the mechanics of the method. A continual current of air, activated by the suction, passes down through the outer tube and up through the inner tube. Any fluid collecting in the outer tube is immediately sucked away, but no suction occurs at the openings in this tube. For the sake of clarity the internal end of the inner tube is shown at a slightly higher level than that of the outer tube, but it may be difficult to maintain the tubes in this position. A similar effect is obtained by introducing both tubes to the same depth and by cutting a single hole in the inner tube 1–2 cm from its end

Fig. 15.22 Diagram to show the method in use for drainage of fluid from the recto-uterine pouch, the patient being nursed in the propped-up position

is connected to suction. A number of holes are cut in the lower part of the outer tube, and the inner tube has a single hole cut in it close to its end, as shown in Figure 15.21. A continual current of air, activated by the suction, passes down through the outer tube and up through the inner tube. Any fluid collecting in the outer tube is immediately sucked away. No suction occurs at the openings in the outer tube, so that the surrounding tissues are not drawn against it. This method of suction drainage may be applied to any part of the peritoneal cavity where it is thought that fluid may collect—below the diaphragm, in Morison's pouch or in the pelvis. For drainage from the pelvis the patient should be nursed in the propped-up position (Fig. 15.22).

Drainage of the wound

The wound in the abdominal parietes is less resistant to

infection than is the peritoneal cavity, and wound sepsis is a common cause, not only of prolonged convalescence, but also of postoperative hernia. The risks of wound infection are present in all cases of peritoneal sepsis or potential sepsis (e.g. in the presence of an inflammatory exudate). Such risks may be reduced by the employment of local antibiotic spray or solution or by systemic chemotherapy, but the additional precaution of a small drain can do no possible harm and may be an essential factor in the balance between a clean and a badly infected wound. A narrow strip of corrugated plastic is adequate; this is placed down to the peritoneum, and the wound is closed *loosely* around it. (If it is closed tightly around it, the whole purpose of the drainage is defeated.) In cases where the advisability of drainage is in doubt, it is as well to observe the maxim—*close the peritoneum, but drain the wound.*

ANASTOMOSIS OF GUT

Anastomosis between segments of gut may be required in order to short-circuit some obstructive or other lesion, or to re-establish continuity after resection has been carried out.

The junction may be effected in one of two ways—*lateral anastomosis, or end-to-end anastomosis*. The latter method is applicable mainly to the intestines, and is dealt with in a later chapter (pp. 429–431). The first method has a wider application, and will be described here.

Lateral (side-to-side) anastomosis

Most surgeons use clamps for this operation, in order to steady the gut, to control haemorrhage and to prevent escape of contents, but others prefer to rely on a skilled assistant. The clamps must be of the light *occlusion* type, which will cause the minimum of trauma to the gut. The blades may be protected by rubber tubing, but if they are sufficiently light this is unnecessary.

For a *gastrojejunostomy* a segment of each viscus 8–9 cm in length is included in the clamp; for an *enteroanastomosis* about half this length will suffice. A long swab is laid between in order to absorb any escaping contents, and the clamps are approximated. They are secured either by a locking device (Fig. 15.23) or by tying together. Adjacent loops of bowel are returned to the peritoneal cavity, and gauze packs are placed around the clamps, so that no escaping intestinal contents can enter the wound.

The anastomosis is carried out usually by a relatively standardised technique which employs either four or six layers of sutures. A classical description of the 4-layer method is as follows:

1. Posterior serous suture

This is a continuous Lembert suture of thread or fine catgut, which unites the adjacent surfaces of the two loops of gut. A short end is retained in forceps at the start of the suture (Fig. 15.23), and the thread is tied when the first layer has been completed.

The lumen of each segment is now opened, within the limits of the posterior serous suture, by an incision parallel to the suture line and approximately 5 mm from it. In the first instance the incision should be made through serous and muscular coats only; the mucosa is then picked up with forceps and incised separately. This limits soiling of the cut edges. As soon as the lumen has been opened intestinal contents are carefully mopped away with small gauze pledgets held in forceps. For a gastrojejunostomy the length of each opening should be 5–6 cm.

2. Posterior all-layers suture

Catgut or Dexon may be used. The suture begins at one extremity of the incision and unites the posterior cut edges, traversing all coats of the gut. The short end is held in forceps. An ordinary overhand continuous suture

is employed, but, after every five or six stitches, a lock stitch is inserted to prevent a possible purse-string effect being produced. When the other extremity of the incision is reached, the suture is carried round the corner and is continued in the reverse direction as the anterior all-layers suture (Fig. 15.23).

3. Anterior all-layers suture

This begins as a continuation of the posterior layer, the needle passing from one lumen to the other as before excepting that the wall of each gut edge must be traversed separately. As the suture is tightened towards the start of the suture (held in forceps), the mucosa is inverted by the loop of thread which has just been inserted. The suture is continued in this manner, to complete the junction between the cut edges of gut, and is tied to its own end.

The anastomosis should now be water-tight, and the clamps are removed so that any bleeding points can be identified. These are dealt with by the insertion of additional interrupted sutures.

4. Anterior serous suture

This is required to cover the previous suture line which is potentially infected, and to bury any tags of mucous membrane which may be pouting between the stitches. A continuous Lembert suture is employed; during its application the bowel is held taut between the ends of the posterior serous suture, which have been retained in forceps (Fig. 15.25).

It should be noted that there are numerous minor variations from the technique described above. Some surgeons prefer a simple over-and-over suture for the third layer but, although taking a shorter time to complete, this method is much more likely to result in eversion of mucosa with a consequently greater risk of leakage. In cases where difficulty in suturing the corners is anticipated, it has been recommended that the all-layers suture should be threaded with a needle at each end, and that a start should be made in the middle of the posterior cut edges; the needles are then made to sew in opposite directions until they meet again anteriorly.

A six-layer anastomosis has certain advantages in that it effects a neater junction, with more effective control of bleeding. The first and sixth layers are Lembert sutures, the second and fifth unite the seromuscular cut edges, and the third and fourth are reserved for mucosa alone. Since this last is joined as a separate layer, there are no mucosal projections which require to be invaginated by the final Lembert suture. Because of the ease with which the separate muscular and mucosal layers fall together, longer stitches can be employed, so that the anastomosis takes very little more time to perform than by the four-layer method.

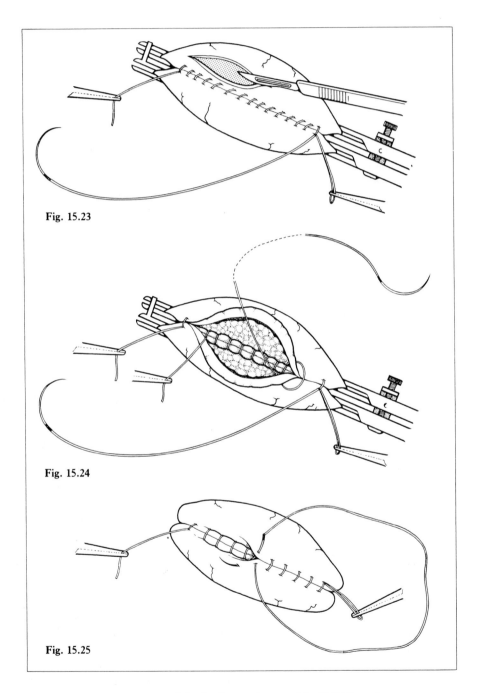

Fig. 15.23

Fig. 15.24

Fig. 15.25

Figs. 15.23–15.25 Technique of lateral anastomosis by four layers of sutures. **Fig. 15.23** Posterior serous suture completed. Bowel wall being incised—serous and muscular coats only in the first instance. **Fig. 15.24** Posterior through-and-through suture completed. Anterior through-and-through suture in progress. **Fig. 15.25** Anterior serous suture (the final layer) nearing completion

AFTER TREATMENT IN ABDOMINAL OPERATIONS—SEQUELAE AND COMPLICATIONS

General measures

Careful case selection and preoperative preparation will forestall later problems but good postoperative care is an essential adjunct to abdominal surgery if unpleasant sequelae and complications are to be minimised.

Position in bed

When returned to bed after operation the patient should be placed in the semi-prone position, in order to obviate the risk of vomitus being inhaled into the respiratory passages. As soon as consciousness returns he may be turned on to his back, and this position is maintained until hypotension, if present, is corrected; if necessary the foot of the bed is raised on blocks. When the condition permits, and usually on the evening of the day of operation, the patient may be allowed to adopt any position which he finds most comfortable. Old people, and those who have undergone major operative procedures, should as a rule be propped up in order to allow of maximum pulmonary ventilation.

Sedation

With modern anaesthetics, skilfully administered, patients may pass imperceptibly from the state of anaesthesia to that of sleep, and may awake several hours after operation, feeling little the worse for their experience. In many cases, however, this happy ideal is not attained; the patient becomes conscious or semi-conscious soon after his return to bed, and pain and restlessness develop. Such cases may be treated effectively by intravenous injection of morphine 10 mg or heroin 5 mg or alternative synthetic analgesic. The dose can be titrated to meet the patient's needs by diluting the drug to 10 ml and injecting slowly until the desired effect is achieved. A similar dose, or a slightly larger one (morphine 15 mg or heroin 10 mg), is usually given intramuscularly on the first and second nights after operation and may be repeated if necessary. Thereafter restful nights can usually be obtained by use of a hypnotic combined with a milder analgesic. Continued administration of morphine or heroin should be avoided if possible, unless actual pain is present, since, by diminishing the cough reflex, it favours the development of pulmonary complications.

Diet and fluid intake

Even after operations on the stomach and duodenum the necessity for withholding fluids by mouth is no longer accepted. 'Unless the surgeon can make his anastomosis milk-proof and water-proof, a patient will not live to take a diet at all' (Dunlop, 1949). It is now customary to allow sips of water as soon as bowel sounds return, provided that the patient does not vomit. In most major cases intravenous infusion is given as routine, in order to replace fluid lost during the operation and to supply the daily fluid requirement. When intravenous infusion has been instituted preoperatively for the correction of fluid and electrolyte deficiency, it will usually be continued during and after operation. Balanced saline solution, plasma expanders or blood transfusion may be given according to the needs of the patient. It is essential to note all fluids on a balance chart so that the patient receives the correct type and volume of fluid for his requirements (p. 310). Intravenous infusion is continued until an adequate oral intake of fluid has been achieved. Diet is then gradually increased through the stages of fluid and semisolids until a normal diet is attained. Any protein or vitamin deficiency (p. 311) should be corrected at the same time. It is the modern practice to regulate dietary progress by the needs and reactions of the patient, rather than by the arbitrary rules of former years.

Bowel action

One of the benefits of early ambulation (see below) is that the normal bowel function may be attained within 2 or 3 days of operation without the necessity for aperients. A mild aperient may, however, be prescribed as routine; it is given usually on the second or third night after operation, but in the case of major operations or those involving the lower bowel, it may be delayed for several days longer. Colicky pains, due to flatulent distension of the bowel, are a frequent source of discomfort during the first 2 or 3 postoperative days. Relief from these can usually be obtained with the help of suppositories.

Exercises and period of bed rest

During recent years the principles of early ambulation have become more and more widely accepted. After many 'minor' abdominal operations (appendicectomy, herniotomy, etc.) the patient may be encouraged to get up for a little while on the evening of operation, and, if possible, to walk to the toilet. In most major cases he can be helped into a chair by the first or second postoperative day. The benefits of such early activity are considerable. Cardiac, respiratory and excretory functions are stimulated, and there is less time for muscular weakness to develop. Complications such as respiratory lesions and retention of urine have been rendered much less frequent. The psychological benefits are incalculable—especially to male patients to whom the necessity of having to ask a nurse for a bed pan may be a greater ordeal than the operation itself. Young patients recovering from some simple operation such as an uncomplicated appendicectomy will often appreciate being allowed to return home on the third or fourth postoperative day with their stitches in situ. Indeed, if their bowels have moved, and if there has been no rise of temperature or pulse rate, there would seem to be no reason why they should not do so. In major cases or where ambulation is likely to be delayed, deep breathing exercises should be commenced as soon as possible after operation. The patient should be encouraged and helped to change his position in bed at frequent intervals, and active exercises for the abdominal and limb muscles should be carried out. Such treatment should, if possible, be under the instructions and supervision of a trained physiotherapist.

Complications

Vomiting

After modern anaesthesia vomiting does not normally occur or is no more than transient. Persistent vomiting may indicate the threat of some serious complication such as paralytic ileus or acute dilatation of the stomach, a condition which requires prompt gastric decompression. In nervous patients, however, vomiting may persist for no detectable reason. Anti-emetic or sedative drugs may be tried, but the only really effective treatment is to keep the stomach empty as far as possible by intermittent or continuous aspiration through a nasogastric tube. If large quantities of gastric secretion are removed by aspiration, replacement of fluid and electrolytes must be carried out by intravenous administration (pp. 310–311).

Retention of urine

Difficulty in initiating the act of micturition occurs chiefly in older men, especially after operations on the pelvic organs. It frequently responds to simple remedies which include reassurance and allowing the patient to sit or stand at the side of the bed, while attempting to urinate. If these measures fail, a hot drink, suppositories or the injection of some parasympathetic stimulant such as *Carbachol* may be effective. Catheterization should be employed only if all other methods fail and if obvious distension of the bladder is present, for there is a considerable likelihood that the catheter will need to be retained until the patient is fully ambulant. Even then, he may be unable to pass urine when the catheter is removed. If the patient can be induced to pass water naturally he seldom has any further trouble unless some organic cause for the obstruction exists. When the operation is of such a nature that difficulty with micturition may be anticipated—e.g. excision of the rectum—a urethral catheter may be left in situ for 2 or 3 days.

Hiccough is now fairly uncommon after abdominal operations and does not usually occur when the stomach is kept empty by aspiration through a nasogastric tube. If it fails to respond to simple remedies or sedation, the inhalation of 5% carbon dioxide may be of benefit.

Abdominal distension

In its mild form this may be regarded as a sequel to abdominal operation, rather than as a complication, since some temporary inhibition of peristalsis is inevitable. It is rarely of any serious significance, but should not be ignored lest it prove to be a warning of some serious complication such as acute dilatation of the stomach or paralytic ileus. Treatment is by gastric aspiration, either intermittent or continuous. This is effective in relieving distension, not only of the stomach, but also of the greater part of the small bowel, since intestinal peristalsis is inhibited by gastric distension, and is restored when this is relieved. The tube should normally be retained until there is evidence of peristaltic activity as shown by bowel sounds on auscultation or by the passage of flatus per rectum. Distension after lower abdominal operations is due often to colonic stasis, and can usually be relieved by suppositories or enemata. The treatment of true ileus is described on page 422.

Pulmonary complications

These include conditions such as bronchitis, pneumonia and pulmonary atelectasis. They are most liable to occur after upper abdominal operations in older patients, but are infrequent with modern methods of anaesthesia and with insistence on deep breathing exercises early in the postoperative period. In general, treatment is on medical lines including physiotherapy, but bronchoscopy may be employed to remove liquid secretions or plugs of mucus from the bronchi: endotracheal intubation, possibly with artificial ventilation, is indicated in cases where severe respiratory embarrassment exists, and may be a life-saving measure (p. 283). Pulmonary embolism is very commonly secondary in phlebothrombosis in the veins of the lower limb or of the pelvis.

Phlebothrombosis is a relatively common complication after abdominal operations. Its apparently increased incidence is due probably to the fact that it is now more frequently recognized. It occurs usually in the deep veins of the calf (posterior tibial veins), and less commonly in the femoral and iliac veins. Its significance lies in the danger that pulmonary embolism may result from detached fragments of clot entering the circulation. It becomes manifest usually between the third and tenth day after hospital admission. Routine examination daily, or the occurrence of minor elevations of temperature or pulse rate, will lead to early diagnosis. Various measures used in the prevention of phlebothrombosis include compression stockings, subcutaneous heparin 5000 I.U. subcutaneously two or three times daily (starting before operation and continuing until the patients is ambulatory), intermittent compression of the legs during operation, protection of the leg veins from pressure during and after surgery, intravenous dextran and by exercises in the postoperative period. When phlebothrombosis or pulmonary embolism has actually occurred, the best treatment is by a combination of rest, elevation of the limb and anticoagulant therapy (p. 38). Ligation of the femoral or iliac veins, or even of the inferior vena cava, has been practised in some clinics, but the value of such procedures has not been established. When the condition is quiescent and the patient is about to become ambulant, the limb should be provided with support, by an elastic stocking or by bandaging, in order to prevent recurrent swelling.

Postoperative peritonitis
This term is usually restricted to peritonitis which develops unexpectedly after operation. It may be due to accidental contamination during the operation; more frequently, it results at a later stage from leakage of bowel content at a suture line. The onset is insidious and the diagnosis difficult, for the classical signs of peritonitis (pain and muscular rigidity) are lacking, and little abnormal may be found on examination, except for some elevation of temperature and pulse rate. Later, the clinical picture may become that of paralytic ileus (p. 419),

when there is progressive distension of the abdomen with profuse vomiting. The prognosis must then be guarded for the patient's condition may steadily deteriorate. Treatment is that of the paralytic ileus (p. 422), combined with intensive chemotherapy. Operative intervention is seldom indicated unless to drain collections of pus which may have become localised, e.g. subphrenic or pelvic abscesses.

Postoperative renal failure
This very serious complication has a mortality of about 50% (Marshall, 1971). It may follow severe sepsis or prolonged hypotension such as may be associated with extensive injury or operations on the cardiovascular system. 50 ml of 25% mannitol given intravenously over 3–5 minutes may rapidly increase the urinary output but if renal failure persists, the fluid intake should be restricted so as to maintain the daily fluid balance (pp. 310 & 545). Haemodialysis or peritoneal dialysis may then need to be considered.

Burst abdomen
Disruption of the abdominal wound is in danger of occurring in elderly or debilitated subjects, especially if they are suffering from advanced malignant disease, pro-

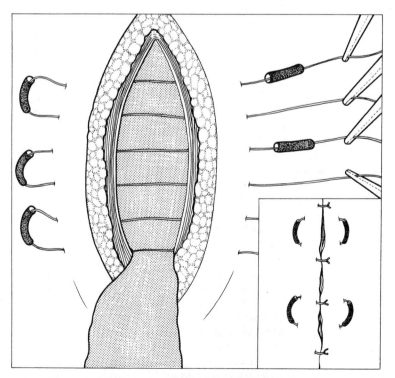

Fig. 15.26 Method repairing a disrupted abdominal wound by means of through-and-through mattress stitches of strong silk, stainless steel wire or nylon. The stitches are made to pass through all layers of the abdominal wall about 2.5 cm from the wound edge, and are passed through pieces of rubber tubing to prevent them from cutting into the skin. A few additional sutures are inserted to coapt aponeurosis and skin.

tein or vitamin C deficiency or uraemia, and also in those who have been treated by corticosteroids. Persistent cough, vomiting or abdominal distension may be contributing causes. The disruption is most likely to occur about a week or 10 days after operation. As a rule it develops suddenly, in which case the patient complains that 'something has given way,' and the surgeon is summoned hastily because one or more coils of intestine are seen to have prolapsed on to the abdominal wall. In many cases there is no warning of the catastrophe, but sometimes the patient may have complained of some discomfort in the wound, and a serosanguineous discharge may have been noted. Immediate operative repair is advisable. First-aid treatment, while the theatre is being prepared, consists in covering the parts with sterile towels wrung out of warm saline; these in turn are covered with abundant cotton wool and a firm binder is applied. The patient is warned to avoid coughing if at all possible. At operation the protruding abdominal contents are wrapped in fresh packs wrung out of warm saline, and are carefully protected while the wound surfaces and surrounding skin are cleansed and disinfected; after the skin

has been towelled-off, they are washed gently with saline, and are returned to the abdomen, where they are retained by the introduction of a moist pack into the wound. Repair of the wound is carried out by the use of through-and-through stitches of thick silk, monofilament nylon or stainless steel wire, which are made to traverse all layers of the abdominal wall from skin to peritoneum about 2–3 cm from the wound edge. Mattress sutures are used as giving the most secure closure; they may be tied over small swabs or rubber tubing (Fig. 15.26), so that they cannot cut through the skin. Care must be taken that bowel is not trapped in the wound as these sutures are tightened. To avoid such an accident the retaining pack is left in position until the last stitch is about to be tied. Additional sutures may be inserted to draw together the aponeurosis and skin, but accurate coaptation of these layers should not be attempted lest drainage from the wound be impeded.

Parotitis is now an uncommon complication after abdominal operation. As a rule it is readily controlled by antibiotic therapy, but occasionally an abscess may form and require drainage (p. 263).

REFERENCES

Bucknall T E 1983 Factors influencing wound complications: a clinical and experimental study. Annals of the Royal College of Surgeons of England 65: 71

Dunlop D M 1949 Changing concepts in therapeutics. Edinburgh Medical Journal 56: 146

Hadfield J 1973 Parenteral feeding of surgical patients. Annals of the Royal College of Surgeons of England 53: 40

Johnston I D A 1977 Parenteral nutrition In: Taylor S (ed) Recent advances in surgery, no. 9. Churchill Livingstone, Edinburgh, ch 6

leQuesne L P 1967 Fluid and electrolyte balance. British Journal of Surgery 54: 449

Marshall V C 1971 Acute renal failure in surgical patients. British Journal of Surgery 58: 17

Stewart D J 1980 Generalised peritonitis. Journal of the Royal College of Surgeons of Edinburgh 25: 80

FURTHER READING

Maingot R 1980 Abdominal operations, 7th edn. Appleton-Century-Crofts, New York, Ch 1

16
Exploratory laparotomy

R. F. RINTOUL

An exploratory laparotomy is carried out in conditions where the need for operation is recognized, but where a definite diagnosis cannot be made until the abdomen has been opened. Such conditions arise most characteristically in cases of suspected intraperitoneal injury, whether this is due to crushing or bruising of the abdomen or to a penetrating wound. An accurate preoperative diagnosis is usually impossible; if the evidence suggests that any intraperitoneal viscus has been injured the abdomen must as a rule be explored.

Exploratory laparotomy may be required also in the various emergencies which constitute the 'acute abdomen.' Whenever possible, an attempt should be made to arrive at an accurate diagnosis before the operation is commenced, since this allows preoperative treatment and the method of approach to be planned, and increases the likelihood of a successful operation. In many cases, however, it may be impossible to reach any diagnosis other than that of 'acute abdomen' and the surgeon must proceed to exploratory laparotomy. Where such doubt about the diagnosis exists, an attempt should be made to decide at least whether it is the upper or the lower abdomen which requires to be opened. Frequently the final preoperative diagnosis is made only after the patient is under the anaesthetic, when palpation of the relaxed abdomen may bring fresh evidence to light.

If the abdomen has been opened by an unsuitable incision, it is usually best, especially in septic cases, to close that incision and to reopen the abdomen in the optimum situation. Prolongation of the original incision is permissible only if adequate access can thereby be obtained without excessive retraction on the wound margins and without pulling on the gut. In general two small incisions are preferable to one large one. A large incision is more difficult to sew up, especially in the presence of intestinal distension; it is more liable to infection, and the results of infection are more serious.

LAPAROTOMY FOR INTRAPERITONEAL INJURIES

It is safer to look and see than to wait and see.
                                    Sir Cuthbert Wallace

In bruising and crushing injuries of the abdomen any intraperitoneal organ may be ruptured without the association of superficial trauma. All penetrating wounds of the peritoneal cavity are likely to cause internal damage (Donaldson, 1981). The external wound is not necessarily situated in the anterior abdominal wall—it may be in the thorax, the loin, the buttock or the perineum.

The clinical picture in cases of intraperitoneal injury varies considerably, and may even be misleading when multiple injuries are present. It is advisable to explore the abdomen in doubtful cases unless injury can be excluded with reasonable certainty. Paracentesis, carried out in the four quadrants of the abdomen, may help in this decision (Powell, 1982; Shepherd, 1971) and is of particular value in multiple injuries where the interplay of many factors produces a confusing clinical picture. The mortality, without operation, in injuries of the hollow viscera approaches 100%, and injuries of the solid viscera are only slightly less serious. Shock is usually present and is likely to be severe; it is not in itself a sign of diagnostic value, but if it persists after resuscitative treatment it is strong evidence of internal injury (Trunkey, 1980). Another sign of even greater importance is a rising pulse rate. The detection of free gas or fluid (usually blood) in the peritoneal cavity is diagnostic. Pain, tenderness and rigidity are present in varying degree. The abdomen may not become boarded until general peritonitis has developed, and the diagnosis must not be delayed until this sign has appeared. Injuries to the urinary tract, which are most likely to be extraperitoneal, can usually be excluded by the passage of a catheter.

The prognosis in cases of intraperitoneal injury depends very largely on the length of time that is allowed to elapse before operation is carried out. The patient must first, however, receive adequate intravenous therapy, which will often include blood transfusion. The aim of resuscitation is to make the patient fit for anaesthesia and full blood replacement should not be attempted until the start of operation.

Late cases. When the patient comes to treatment 24 hours or longer after the injury, laparotomy is usually contraindicated. If the patient has survived in reasonable condition for that time, it is likely that haemorrhage has been arrested spontaneously, and that ruptured viscera have become sealed off by adhesions, in which case operative interference might result in spreading of the infection. Treatment is carried out on the Ochsner-Sherren lines (p. 414). Laparotomy should, however, be performed if there are signs of general peritonitis, or of continued or recurrent intraperitoneal haemorrhage.

Technique of exploration

In the absence of any localising signs it is usual to open the abdomen through a midline or right paramedian incision in the region of the umbilicus; through this most of the abdominal organs can be investigated. The incision may be enlarged either upwards or downwards, or by cutting across one rectus muscle. Alternatively, a second incision may be made. When a wound is present in the anterior abdominal wall, it is a good practice to excise the wound and to use that approach to the peritoneal cavity—at least for the preliminary exploration. A stab wound, the depth of which is unknown, is best explored through a separate incision so that inspection of the damaged area is unimpeded by blood escaping from the laparotomy wound.

If any viscus has been injured there will usually be a certain amount of haemorrhage in the peritoneal cavity. A large collection of blood suggests damage to a solid viscus—spleen, liver, mesentery and omentum being the structures which are most commonly injured. These are, therefore, investigated first in order that the source of bleeding may be located and dealt with.

If the gut has been ruptured, turbid or bile-stained fluid, or (in the case of the colon) faecal matter may be present in the peritoneal cavity. In small perforations, however, owing to the sealing effect of pouting mucous membrane, little or no escape of contents may occur. *A 'clean' peritoneal cavity in no way excludes such injuries.*

The small intestine is injured more commonly than all the other hollow viscera, and it must be systematically examined throughout its entire length. The examination may be commenced either at the duodeno-jejunal flexure or at the caecum. No more than one loop should be withdrawn from the wound at one time; it is examined carefully from both sides, and as soon as it has been passed as being intact it is returned by the assistant to the abdomen. If a perforation of the gut is discovered it is closed with a clamp or with light tissue forceps. The affected loop is retained on the surface, covered with a moist towel, while the rest of the gut is examined. It is most important, especially in penetrating wounds where there may be multiple intestinal injuries, to ascertain the full extent of the damage before undertaking the repair of any single lesion, for the discovery of further injuries will often determine the treatment which is to be

adopted, e.g. it may be necessary to resect a segment of bowel.

The stomach and duodenum are brought into view by gentle traction on the omentum and are examined both visually and by palpation.

The transverse colon is examined at the same time as the stomach. By suitable retraction and by packing off of coils of small bowel, the other parts of the colon are then investigated in turn. The presence of a retroperitoneal haematoma in relation to the fixed vertical parts of the colon suggests a rupture in its posterior wall. The suspected area should not be explored from the peritoneal cavity, since a generalized peritonitis might thereby be produced; it is better that the original incision should be closed, (perhaps after a colostomy has been made—p. 433) and the colon approached retroperitoneally through an incision in the flank.

Injuries of the spleen

The spleen is very commonly ruptured as the result of crushing injuries or of blows on the flank. Suture of the rent is rarely possible and *splenectomy* (p. 368) is the standard procedure. If blood for transfusion is not available, unclotted blood from within the peritoneal cavity, after being filtered through gauze and citrated, may be returned to a vein.

Injuries of the liver

Penetrating wounds of the liver may be treated on conservative lines, provided that the surgeon feels secure in his belief that no other organ has been damaged. Liver wounds as a whole, however, are usually associated with severe intraperitoneal haemorrhage, and it is on this account that laparotomy is likely to be required. Both upper and lower surfaces of the liver should be carefully examined. If the operation field is obscured by profuse haemorrhage, this may be arrested by temporary compression of the hepatic artery as it lies in the free border of the lesser omentum—either digitally or with a light bowel clamp. Wounds involving the upper or posterior aspects of the liver may be inaccessible from an abdominal approach. They are then best exposed transdiaphragmatically through a right thoracotomy, the chest being opened in the 8th or 9th intercostal space. Wounds which are recognized preoperatively to be thoracoabdominal should as a general rule be explored, in the first instance, through the chest (p. 285). When the tear has been identified it should be gently but firmly packed with gauze, which is left in situ for 2 or 3 minutes. After removal of the gauze, spouting vessels in the liver substance may be picked up and coagulated, or occluded by suture. Tears are best repaired with deeply placed stitches of thick catgut or other absorbable material carried on a round-bodied needle. If the stitches tend to cut out, they may be supported by a flap of falciform ligament or by a free transplant from the rectus sheath, which is laid on the liver surface. In extensive injuries, devitalised liver tissue should be removed and in some cases, there may be no alternative to hepatic lobectomy for the control of bleeding (Blumgart, 1980). Drainage to the exterior should always be provided using corrugated plastic or suction, as there is likely to be leakage of bile. In some cases, packing of the liver for up to 48 hours may be a life saving measure (Calne, 1982).

Injuries of the mesentery

If spleen and liver are intact, laceration of the mesentery is the next most likely cause of haemorrhage. This is a serious injury since the blood supply of the related segment of bowel may be endangered, especially if the tear lies parallel and in close proximity to the gut (Fig. 16.1). Smaller tears and those placed radially to the gut are not so serious, and can as a rule be treated effectively by simple suture; the production of further haemorrhage is avoided if the needle, threaded in the usual way, is passed *eye-first* through the mesenteric tissue. The operator must be satisfied that the blood supply of the gut has not been interfered with; either pallor, cyanosis or oedema is a dangerous sign, and may demand resection.

Haematoma of the mesentery results when a vessel is ruptured without laceration of the peritoneal layers. The blood should be evacuated through a small incision, and if necessary the bleeding vessel is ligatured. The related segment of bowel should be examined carefully to ensure that its blood supply is adequate.

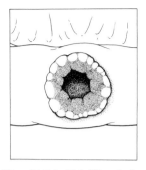
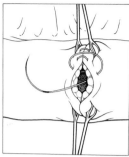

Figs. 16.2 & 16.3 Wound of small bowel, such as may be caused either by a penetrating missile or by a crushing injury. The method of repair in the transverse axis is shown

Injuries of the small intestine

The systematic examination of the small intestine has already been described.

Simple suture of wounds should be carried out whenever possible. Very small perforations can be closed by a single purse-string suture of Lembert type. Larger wounds are repaired by two layers of sutures. If the edges of the tear are ragged or bruised they may be excised. It is an advantage to stitch up the tear *transversely* (Fig. 16.3), in order that narrowing of the lumen will be prevented. It is probable, however, that the dangers of narrowing have been exaggerated; since the contents of the small intestine are fluid, it is unlikely that obstruction will occur unless the narrowing amounts almost to complete occlusion. If the patency of the gut is in doubt the affected segment may be short-circuited by a lateral anastomosis, or, alternatively, resection may be performed. Areas of bruising on the gut wall (without perforation) should be infolded by Lembert suture, or covered with an omental patch.

Resection with anastomosis (p. 429) is associated with a considerable mortality, and should be avoided wherever possible. It may be advisable, however, when there are multiple injuries confined to one segment of the gut, or when laceration or bruising is extensive; it is essential if the blood supply of the gut has been destroyed or seriously endangered by associated mesenteric injury.

In most cases of intestinal rupture drainage of the peritoneal cavity should be provided.

Injuries of the colon

Rupture of the colon as the result of crushing or bruising injuries is not uncommon. When caused by a penetrating wound it is usually associated with injuries of other viscera. Sometimes there is no more than bruising of the gut wall, but secondary perforation is a likely sequel. Bruised areas should, therefore, be infolded carefully or covered with omentum. Severely injured colon should always be excised (Parks, 1981).

Intraperitoneal ruptures should as a rule be treated by

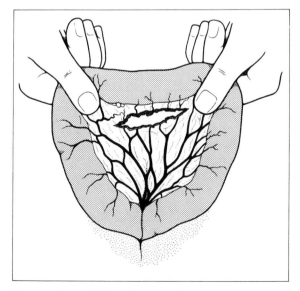

Fig. 16.1 A tear of the mesentery lying parallel and in close proximity to the bowel makes resection imperative, since the blood supply of the gut is seriously endangered

exteriorisation. The affected loop is mobilized if necessary (p. 438); it is brought to the surface and a Paul's tube is tied into its lumen. When, however, the perforation is clean-cut and the bowel wall little damaged, as may occur with stab wounds or traversing bullet wounds, careful suture of the tear or resection with anastomosis may be performed (Owen-Smith, 1978). In all such cases a drain should be left in position against the sutured bowel, so that any escape of contents will take place towards the surface.

Retroperitoneal rupture is more likely to occur in the fixed vertical parts of the colon. It is probably even more serious than intraperitoneal rupture, owing to the great vulnerability of the retroperitoneal tissues to infection—especially anaerobic infection. If this type of injury is suspected at laparotomy the anterior incision must be closed, and the affected part approached retroperitoneally through an incision in the flank. An attempt may be made to repair the rupture, but, owing to bruising and to the absence of a peritoneal covering, the suturing is often inadequate. It is of much greater importance to provide free drainage by the retroperitoneal route. If a wound is present in the flank, it should be utilised as the route for exploration.

Except in cases where the damaged segment of colon has been exteriorized, the advisability of a caecostomy or of a proximal colostomy should be considered. When adequate repair of an intraperitoneal rupture is thought to have been achieved, a caecostomy may suffice, but in other cases a proximal colostomy of *defunctioning* type (p. 433) is a better safeguard against leakage and subsequent infection.

Injuries of the stomach and duodenum are uncommon except in penetrating wounds, when they are usually associated with damage to other viscera.

Both surfaces of the stomach should be examined—the posterior, through an opening made into the lesser sac, either through the anterior layers of the greater omentum or through the transverse mesocolon. Repair is effected by two layers of suture. Wounds of the curvatures of the stomach are accompanied by profuse haemorrhage, and the divided vessels require to be ligatured.

Wounds of the duodenum are likely to implicate surrounding structures such as the pancreas, the common bile duct, the portal vein or the hilum of the kidney, or they may give rise to extensive retroperitoneal extravasation. They are, therefore, usually fatal.

Injuries of the pancreas
Tears in the pancreas should be repaired accurately by suture. Sometimes, in association with a ruptured spleen, the tail of the pancreas is torn completely across. The severed portion should then be removed. Drainage of the lesser sac is advisable in all cases (Robbs, 1980).

Injuries of the gall bladder and bile ducts
These will be suspected if there is a large collection of bile in the peritoneal cavity. A ruptured gall bladder or cystic duct is best treated by cholecystectomy. A torn common bile duct may be repaired by suture over a T-tube (p. 396).

Injuries of the kidney
Renal damage is confirmed by intravenous pyelography which demonstrates delay in function or leakage of dye on one side. The associated retroperitoneal haemorrhage may, by sympathetic stimulation, result in an ileus which, unfortunately, adds to the difficulty of interpretating the abdominal signs. Operations for renal injuries are discussed on page 552.

Intraperitoneal rupture of the bladder
The tear, which is necessarily situated on the peritoneal surface of the bladder, is repaired by two layers of suture. The peritoneum, after careful mopping up, may be closed. The bladder is kept empty by an indwelling urethral catheter (see also pp. 512 & 576).

LAPAROTOMY FOR PERITONITIS

The necessarily incomplete diagnosis of 'acute abdomen' will be made when the clinical evidence suggests no more than the existence of peritonitis. If there is any reason to believe that the peritonitis has resulted from perforation of the gut, e.g. from a gangrenous appendix or from a perforated peptic or typhoid ulcer, immediate laparotomy is imperative. When this possibility can be excluded with reasonable confidence, operation may be deferred and treatment on the Ochsner-Sherren lines instituted (p. 414), in the hope that the infection may become localized. When advanced generalized peritonitis is present, and when the pulse is rapid and thready, it is always advisable to delay operation for 2 or 3 hours, while the patient's general condition is improved by intravenous infusion, antibiotics and gastric aspiration.

Principles of operative treatment
Unless the appendix has previously been removed it usually will be suspect. In all cases it is a good plan to open the abdomen through a right gridiron incision. Should the appendix be healthy it will often be possible through this incision to determine the cause or nature of the peritonitis. If no operative treatment other than peritoneal drainage is indicated, the incision is utilised to guide a drainage tube, introduced through a suprapubic stab wound, down to the rectovesical pouch. If further access is required the gridiron incision can be enlarged. Alternatively, if a second incision is indicated the gridiron is easily and rapidly closed (p. 355). When the

appendix can be excluded as the source of infection, a long midline or right paramedian incision centred over the area of suspected pathology will as a rule be employed.

The priority in all cases of peritonitis is rapid evacuation of toxic exudate—preferably by suction. The surgeon may then concentrate his attention on the source of the infection and carry out appropriate definitive treatment such as removal of a gangrenous appendix. Antibiotic peritoneal lavage, using 1–3 litres of tetracycline solution (1 g per litre), is useful in dealing with residual infection (Stewart, 1980). The fluid is directed into the recesses of the abdomen by the exploring hand and trapped debris is aspirated.

Nature of the peritoneal exudate. Brownish-coloured fluid with the putrid smell of bowel organisms is almost diagnostic of a perforated appendix, or a perforated diverticulitis. Milky fluid with flakes of lymph—often bile-stained—suggests a gastric or intestinal perforation. In pneumococcal peritonitis the exudate is characteristic; it is greenish-yellow in colour, creamy and odourless. In streptococcal peritonitis the fluid is turbid and sometimes blood-stained. A tuberculous effusion is clear and straw-coloured.

Pneumococcal peritonitis is usually a primary infection. It occurs most commonly in female children under the age of 10, when it may be associated with a pneumococcal vaginitis.

Conservative treatment may be employed, provided that other causes of peritonitis can be excluded with reasonable certainly. It is usually safer, however, to open the abdomen—even if only to verify the diagnosis, since the risks of missing a gangrenous appendix with general peritonitis greatly outweigh those of operation.

The approach should be through a small gridiron or rectus-splitting incision. The diagnosis will be made usually from the character of the exudate, and from the failure to find any primary focus of infection within the abdomen. As much as possible of the exudate is removed by suction and the abdomen is closed—preferably with drainage.

Streptococcal peritonitis is treated on similar lines to those described for pneumococcal peritonitis, but, since the exudate is more toxic, drainage is advisable in all cases.

Peritonitis due to salpingitis

As a rule the peritonitis is localised to the pelvis. Laparotomy is contraindicated, but sometimes the diagnosis is not made until the abdomen has been opened. It is usually advised that the inflamed tube should be left in situ (p. 639). Peritoneal drainage may be instituted, but unless the exudate is present in considerable amount, it is often better to close the wound.

Ruptured ectopic pregnancy is discussed on page 637.

Tuberculous peritonitis

The acute type is uncommon; it occurs usually as a flare-up of a previously unsuspected chronic condition, and is unlikely to be diagnosed before the abdomen has been opened. The condition is then apparent from the presence of clear straw-coloured exudate and of tubercles. As much fluid as possible is removed; a sample is sent for bacteriological examination, and one or more peritoneal nodules are removed for histology (Lambrianides, 1980). The abdomen is then closed *without drainage*. If the condition is suspected prior to laparotomy, the diagnosis may be confirmed by peritoneoscopy, biopsy or culture of peritoneal fluid (Addison, 1983).

Chronic tuberculous peritonitis. In the *fibrous* or *adhesive* type of tuberculous peritonitis, laparotomy may be carried out in order to establish the diagnosis, or to deal with intestinal obstruction.

REFERENCES

Addison N V 1983 Abdominal tuberculosis – a disease revived. Annals of the Royal College of Surgeons of England 65: 105

Blumgart L H 1980 Hepatic resection. In: Taylor S (ed) Recent advances in surgery no. 10. Churchill Livingstone, Edinburgh, ch 1

Calne R Y, Wells F C, Forty J 1982 26 cases of liver trauma. British Journal of Surgery 69: 365

Donaldson L A, Findlay I G, Smith A 1981 A retrospective view of 89 stab wounds to the abdomen and chest. British Journal of Surgery 68: 793

Lambrianides A L, Ackroyd N, Shorey B A 1980 Abdominal tuberculosis. British Journal of Surgery 67: 887

Owen-Smith M S 1978 High velocity missile injuries. In: Hadfield J, Hobsley M (eds) Current surgical practice, vol. 2. Arnold, London, ch 12

Parks T G 1981 Surgical management of injuries of the large intestine. British Journal of Surgery 68: 725

Powell D C, Bivins B A, Bell R M 1982 Diagnostic peritoneal lavage. Surgery Gynaecology and Obstetrics 155: 257

Robbs J V, Macintyre I M C 1980 Pancreatic and duodenal injuries. Journal of the Royal College of Surgeons of Edinburgh 25: 110

Shepherd J A 1971 Trauma to the abdomen: Diagnosis. Annals of the Royal College of Surgeons of England 48: 11

Stewart D J 1980 Generalised peritonitis. Journal of the Royal College of Surgeons of Edinburgh 25: 80

Trunkey D D 1980 Massive abdominal injury. In: Hardy J D (ed) Critical surgical illness, 2nd ed. Saunders, Philadelphia, ch 8

FURTHER READING

Maingot R 1980 Abdominal operations, 7th edn. Appleton-Century-Crofts, New York, Ch 1

17

Operations on the stomach and duodenum

D. C. CARTER & J. M. S. JOHNSTONE

Anatomy

The stomach begins at the gastro-oesophageal junction 2–3 cm below the diaphragm, deep to the sternal end of the 7th costal cartilage. It varies greatly in its shape and disposition within the abdomen. For example, the lowest part of the greater curvature may be as high as T12 or as low as S1, while the pylorus may lie at any level between T12 and L5.

The *cardia* is the indefinite region around the gastro-oesophageal junction while the *fundus* is that part of the stomach above the cardiac incisura. The *corpus* or *body* of stomach lies more or less longitudinally and extends from the level of the cardiac incisura to the level of the angular notch. The remainder of the stomach is formed by the *antrum* and ends at the *pylorus* where the circular muscle condenses to form the *pyloric sphincter*. The pylorus is recognized at laparotomy by a small pre-pyloric vein or veins on its anterior aspect. Although its vertical disposition varies greatly, the pylorus is usually located in or near the mid-line.

The stomach

The stomach is lined throughout by mucus-secreting columnar epithelium. The cardiac gland area is a ring of about 1–4 cm wide around the gastro-oesophageal junction. Its glands secrete mucosubstances only and do not contain peptic or oxyntic (parietal) cells. The glands of the body are lined by oxyntic cells which secrete hydrochloric acid and intrinsic factor, and by peptic cells which contain granules of pepsinogen, the precursor of the proteolytic enzyme pepsin. The mucus cells of the glands in the antrum are interspersed with G cells which secrete gastrin. It is important to appreciate that the antral mucosa may extend for a variable distance up the lesser curvature above the angular notch.

The duodenum

The duodenum is intimately associated with the head of the pancreas, although its first part is not bound to the gland. The first part of duodenum is 5 cm long and passes backwards and to the right. A variable length of the first part is mobile by virtue of its omental attach-ments, but the final portion is fixed to the posterior abdominal wall. The hepatic artery passes along the upper border of the first part of the duodenum; the gastroduodenal artery, portal vein and common bile duct pass behind it. The second part of the duodenum descends almost vertically for 10 cm on the right side of the vertebral column to the level of L3 or L4. It is crossed by the root of the transverse mesocolon, and its concave medial wall receives the common bile duct and main pancreatic duct. Posteriorly it is related to the right kidney and inferior vena cava. The third part of the duodenum extends horizontally for 7.5 cm, passing from the right to left side of L3. It is crossed anteriorly by the superior mesenteric vessels and root of the mesentery, and is related posteriorly to the inferior vena cava and aorta. The fourth part of the duodenum is 2.5–5 cm long and ascends on the left of the aorta to the level of L2 where it becomes the duodeno-jejunal flexure. A number of peritoneal recesses may be found around this flexure and on rare occasions they are the site of internal herniation.

Peritoneal attachments of the stomach. Apart from a small area on its posterior wall just below the gastro-oesphageal junction, the stomach is completely invested by peritoneum. At the lesser curvature the peritoneum covering the anterior and posterior walls forms the *lesser omentum* which passes upwards to the liver in the region of the porta hepatis. At the greater curvature, the peritoneal layers meet to form the *greater omentum*, the *gastrosplenic (lieno-gastric) ligament*, and the *gastrophrenic ligament*. The greater omentum arises from the greater curvature of the antrum and lower portion of the body of stomach, and extends downwards in front of the transverse colon (Fig. 17.1). As the greater omentum returns over the transverse colon its posterior surface fuses with the anterior surface of the transverse meso-colon.

The lesser sac lies behind the caudate lobe of the liver, lesser omentum and stomach. It extends for a variable distance into the greater omentum in front of the transverse colon but in most adults this part of the lesser sac is obliterated (Fig. 17.1). Surgical access to the lesser sac may be obtained by creating a window in the lesser

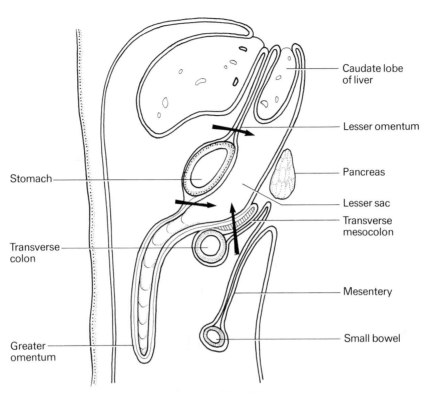

Fig. 17.1 Sagittal section through the abdomen to show the disposition of the omentum and lesser sac. Arrows indicate the means of access to the lesser sac

omentum, transverse mesocolon or gastrocolic portion of the greater omentum. Although the lesser omentum is avascular close to the liver, generous access to the lesser sac is prevented by the structures in the free edge of the lesser omentum (hepatic artery, portal vein and bile duct). Exposure through the mesocolon is limited by the middle colic artery. When it is necessary to create a window as for example in posterior gastrojejunostomy, it is usually best to divide the mesocolon to the left of the middle colic vessels. The incision runs parallel to the vessels and can extend from the marginal artery to the root of the mesocolon. When wide exposure of the lesser sac is needed, as for example in operations involving the pancreas, the gastro-colic portion of the greater omentum is incised widely in a line parallel to the greater curvature of the stomach. The incision lies outwith the gastro-epiploic vessels and individual omental vessels are divided between ligatures. Avascular adhesions between the posterior wall of the stomach and front of pancreas have to be divided to allow unrestricted access to the lesser sac.

Blood supply. The *arteries of the stomach* are all derived from the coeliac axis, and form arches which run along the greater or lesser curvature between the layers of the omenta. The greater curve arch is formed from the right gastro-epiploic branch of the gastroduodenal artery, and

from the left gastro-epiploic branch of the splenic artery. The lesser curve arch is formed from the descending branch of the left gastric artery and the right gastric branch of the common hepatic artery. The blood supply of the greater curve is supplemented by four or five short gastric branches of the splenic artery which travel in the gastrosplenic ligament to the fundus and upper part of the body of stomach (Fig. 17.2).

The *arteries of the duodenum* are derived from the coeliac and superior mesenteric vessels. The first part of the duodenum receives branches from the right gastric, gastroduodenal and right gastro-epiploic arteries. The superior pancreaticoduodenal artery is one of the two terminal branches of the gastroduodenal (Fig. 17.2) and runs downwards in the concavity of the duodenum to anastomose with the inferior pancreaticoduodenal branch of the superior mesenteric artery. The vessels form an arcade on the front of the head of pancreas, and there is also a posterior pancreaticoduodenal arcade behind the head of the gland. In about 10% of subjects, the superior mesenteric artery gives off a right hepatic branch which ascends behind the pancreas and is usually the sole supply to the right lobe of liver. In 2–3% of individuals, the entire hepatic artery arises from the superior mesenteric.

The *veins from the stomach and duodenum* accompany

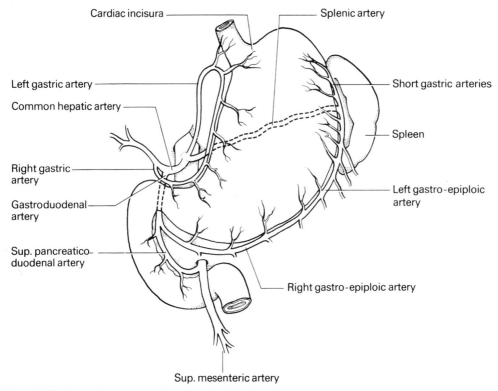

Fig. 17.2 Arterial blood supply to the stomach and proximal duodenum

the arteries and drain into the portal system via the splenic or superior mesenteric veins.

Lymphatic drainage. The lymphatics of the stomach anastomose freely in the submucosa, communicate with intermuscular lymphatics, and then drain into a subserosal network. This network drains in turn into large lymphatic vessels which accompany the four main arteries to the lesser and greater curvatures. The submucosal lymphatics of stomach and lower oesophagus communicate freely, facilitating spread of carcinoma from one organ to the other. There is debate as to the degree of communication between antral and duodenal lymphatics across the pylorus. Material injected into the wall of the stomach spreads evenly in the gastric submucosa but stops abruptly at the pylorus. However, the proximal duodenum may become involved by carcinoma arising in the distal stomach, and as direct spread is unusual retrograde spread from subpyloric nodes may be responsible.

Classical descriptions of the lymphatic drainage of the stomach stressed that there were four drainage zones demarcated by watersheds. This concept of zonal drainage has been over-emphasized, and free submucosal communication allows carcinoma to spread widely from 'zone' to 'zone'. The largest area of stomach drains predominantly into nodes along the lesser curve, and then to the left gastric nodes (Fig. 17.3). Lymph from the upper part of the pyloric region drains predominantly into right gastric nodes, and from there to hepatic nodes lying in the course of the common hepatic artery and hepatic artery proper. The fundus drains to paracardial nodes which also receive lymph from the oesophagus. The remainder of the fundus and upper portion of the greater curve drain predominantly to pancreaticosplenic nodes alongside the short gastric and left gastro-epiploic vessels, and from there to the coeliac nodes by lymphatics running with the splenic vessels along the upper border of the pancreas. The distal greater curve drains to right gastro-epiploic nodes which lie in the greater omentum, often as much as 3–4 cm from the greater curve. There is an important group of subpyloric nodes which lie on the pancreas close to the bifurcation of the gastroduodenal artery, and which receive lymph from the distal stomach and proximal duodenum. All of the gastric lymphatics drain ultimately to coeliac nodes around the coeliac axis. It must be stressed that the pattern of lymph node involvement cannot be predicted accurately from the location of the primary tumour, and that lack of lymph node enlargement at laparotomy does not mean that the nodes are tumour-free.

The lymphatics of the duodenum anastomose freely within the submucosa. Those of the anterior collecting vessels pass to nodes along the anterior branch of the

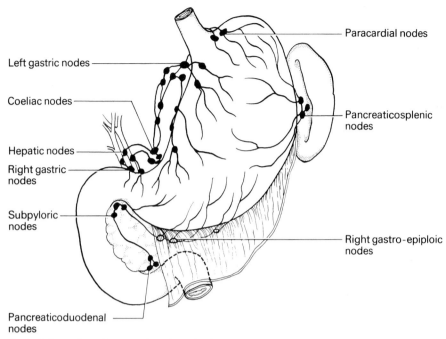

Fig. 17.3 Lymphatic drainage from the stomach and proximal duodenum

superior pancreaticoduodenal artery and drain upwards to the subpyloric and coeliac nodes. The posterior collecting vessels pass to nodes behind the head of pancreas and drain to pancreaticoduodenal nodes associated with the superior mesenteric vessels.

Nerve supply. (1) *Parasympathetic nerve supply.* The vagi descend through the thorax in the posterior mediastinum forming the oesophageal plexus just below the root of the lung. This plexus gives rise to anterior and posterior vagal trunks which pass through the oeso-

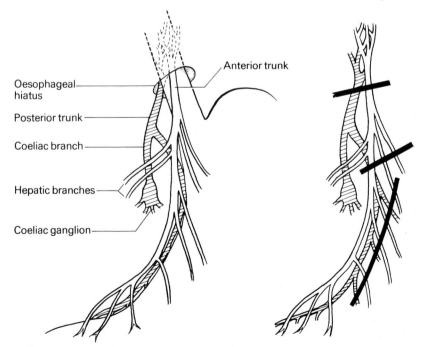

Fig. 17.4 Diagrammatic representation of the disposition of the vagus nerves. The three bars indicate the levels of section in truncal vagotomy (1); selective vagotomy (2); and highly selective vagotomy (3)

phageal hiatus to enter the abdomen (Fig. 17.4). The anterior trunk lies on the anterior aspect of the oesophagus whereas the posterior trunk lies in loose connective tissue some distance behind the back of the oesophagus, even as far as some centimetres away on the front of the right crus. The anterior and posterior nerve trunks may exchange fibres as they descend into the abdomen and frequently divide into two or more branches which descend to the stomach to the right of the cardia, in front of or behind the oesophagus, or even to the left of the oesophagus.

The anterior trunk gives off a hepatic branch (or branches) near the oesophagogastric junction. This hepatic branch passes within the lesser omentum to supply the liver and gall bladder, and gives off some twigs which descend to supply the pylorus. The continuation of the anterior trunk along the lesser curvature is known as the anterior gastric nerve (anterior nerve of Latarjet) and supplies branches to the front of the gastric corpus and antrum.

The posterior vagal trunk gives off the posterior gastric nerve (posterior nerve of Latarjet) which descends along the lesser curvature supplying the posterior aspect of the stomach. The remainder of the posterior trunk constitutes the coeliac branch and passes to the coeliac plexus around the coeliac axis. Vagal fibres from this plexus accompany branches of the coeliac and superior mesenteric arteries to the duodenum, pancreas, small intestine and large intestine as far as the distal transverse colon.

(2) *Sympathetic nerve supply*. The sympathetic nerve supply reaches the stomach by travelling from the coeliac ganglion with branches of the coeliac axis.

Applied gastric physiology

Regulation of acid and pepsin secretion
Separation of the roles of acid and pepsin in ulcerogenesis is impossible. Pepsin is only active in an acid milieu and in general, secretion of acid and pepsin is linked so that their outputs rise and fall in parallel. Pepsins are stored and secreted as inactive pepsinogens and on exposure to acid solution (pH < 5) fragments cleave from the molecule to leave active proteolytic pepsins. All pepsins are inactivated irreversibly at neutral or slightly alkaline pH.

The role of the vagus and gastrin in stimulating gastric secretion is established but that of histamine is controversial.

1. Vagal stimulation. The vagus stimulates secretion by direct and indirect means. Direct stimulation is achieved by liberation of acetylcholine from postganglionic vagal terminals in the immediate vicinity of the secretory cells, while indirect stimulation is effected by vagal release of gastrin from G cells in the pyloric antrum.

2. Stimulation by gastrin. Vagal release of gastrin is usually overshadowed by gastrin release triggered by protein and protein digestion products in the antrum and by antral distension. A negative feedback mechanism normally prevents excessive acid-pepsin secretion in that gastrin release diminishes as pH falls in the gastric lumen. A luminal pH of around 1.0 suppresses gastrin release completely, but even at pH 2.5 the acid secretory response to a protein meal is halved.

3. Stimulation by histamine. Histamine may serve as a 'paracrine' regulator of acid secretion, the term 'paracrine' implying a chemical messenger released by cells in the immediate vicinity of the parietal cell. Recent studies with isolated parietal cells suggest that gastrin, acetylcholine and histamine each have distinct receptors at the parietal cell, but that interaction between receptors allows each agent to increase the secretory response to any of the others. Conversely, blockade of any receptor diminishes the secretory response to the agent concerned, and reduces the response to other stimulants by removing a background 'tonic' effect. For example, H_2 receptor antagonists such as cimetidine reduce not only the acid secretory response to histamine, but also that induced by gastrin or vagal stimulation. Similarly by removing the tonic influence of acetylcholine, surgical vagotomy may render the parietal cell less amenable to stimulation by gastrin or histamine.

Gastric and duodenal defences against acid-pepsin digestion
These defence mechanisms may be summarized as follows: (1) excessive and inappropriate acid-pepsin secretion is normally prevented by negative feedback involving reduced secretion of the hormone gastrin (see above). Other hormonal and neural factors may reduce acid-pepsin secretion but have not been well characterized; (2) the gastric mucosa prevents back-diffusion of acid and pepsin from the lumen. The covering layer of mucus serves as an unstirred layer which retards back-diffusion of acid and traps the alkaline secretion of the surface epithelium. Other factors on which the gastric mucosal barrier depends include integrity of the apical cell membrane, normal mucosal acid-base balance, and an appropriate mucosal blood flow. Destruction of the barrier allows acid and pepsin to enter the underlying tissues leading to gastritis, erosion formation and ulceration. Agents capable of damaging the barrier include bile salts, alcohol, and non-steroidal anti-inflammatory drugs such as aspirin and indomethacin; (3) gastric emptying is normally regulated so that excessive amounts of acid-pepsin do not enter the duodenum (see below); (4) acid in the duodenum is rapidly neutralized

by the combined alkaline secretions of the pancreas, biliary tract and duodenal mucosa. Release of the hormone secretin by acid in the duodenal lumen is instrumental in stimulating alkaline secretion by the pancreas.

Gastric motility

The stomach receives and accommodates ingested food, mixes it thoroughly with gastric secretion, grinds it to semi-fluid consistency, and delivers it at a controlled rate into the duodenum. Meals are accommodated by receptive relaxation of the body (corpus) and fundus, while mixing, grinding and emptying are achieved by gastric peristalsis. The 'gastric slow wave' (or pacesetter potential) occurs at intervals of about 20 seconds and is an inherent property of gastric muscle. The slow wave does not cause muscle contraction unless associated with 'electrical response activity', in which case a contraction wave appears in the body of the stomach and moves distally. The contraction band widens and accelerates as it moves distally and the terminal 3–5 cm of antrum contracts powerfully as a single unit. This 'antral mill' activity is particularly important in grinding and mixing, and in propelling food into the duodenum when the pyloric sphincter opens.

The rate of emptying of gastric contents into the duodenum is regulated by the following factors:

1. Nature of contents. Gastric emptying is slowed if luminal pH falls in the proximal duodenum. Fat delays gastric emptying by a mechanism which may involve release of a hormone ('enterogastrone') from the duodenum, while osmoreceptors in the duodenum and proximal jejunum slow emptying if the expelled gastric contents have a high osmolarity. In general, fluids empty from the stomach more rapidly than solids.

2. Neural control. The stomach wall contains intrinsic myenteric and submucous plexuses which control gastric contractility. The extrinsic parasympathetic and sympathetic nerve supply is not essential for motility, but influences the intrinsic system.

The vagal parasympathetic fibres are preganglionic and approximately 80% are afferent. Cholinergic fibres excite motor activity, while receptive relaxation is controlled by inhibitory non-cholinergic, non-adrenergic fibres which are probably purinergic.

The sympathetic postganglionic fibres are adrenergic. The sympathetic supplies vasomotor fibres to the gastric blood vessels, inhibits gastric motility but is motor to the pylorus, and serves as the main pathway for gastric pain fibres.

3. Hormonal control. Many gastro-intestinal hormones can influence gastric motility and emptying. For example, motility is inhibited by gastrin, secretin, CCK, VIP and pancreatic glucagon but increased by motilin. It is uncertain whether these are physiological actions.

Effect of surgery on gastric motility and emptying

1. Truncal vagotomy and drainage. Vagal denervation of the corpus and fundus abolishes receptive relaxation and the postprandial rise in intragastric pressure may restrict meal size. Vagal denervation of the antrum leads to loss of antral mill activity and may cause gastric stasis unless combined with a drainage procedure.

Loss of receptive relaxation increases the rate of emptying of liquids, and a gastric drainage procedure further accelerates emptying by reducing gastric outflow resistance. On the other hand, solid meals empty slowly after truncal vagotomy and pyloroplasty, although emptying rates usually return to normal within 6 months.

2. Highly selective vagotomy. Receptive relaxation is abolished with some increase in the rate of emptying of liquids. Emptying of solid food is not affected significantly, and sequelae such as dumping and diarrhoea are less common after this form of vagotomy.

3. Partial gastrectomy. Receptive relaxation still occurs if the body and fundus are vagally innervated but meal size may be restricted if the gastric remnant is small. Gastric incontinence and rapid emptying may be associated with dumping, late hypoglycaemia, diarrhoea and malabsorption.

Investigation of gastroduodenal disease

A detailed history and full physical examination are essential. The following specialized investigations may be helpful when gastroduodenal disease is suspected.

1. Barium swallow and meal examination

Barium swallow is used primarily in the investigation of oesophageal disorders whereas barium meal is intended to display the lower oesophagus, oesophagogastric junction, stomach, pylorus and proximal duodenum.

In patients with peptic ulceration, abnormal motility is often apparent during screening. The ulcer crater may be visible 'en face' or in profile, and surrounding oedema and radiating mucosal folds may be seen. In some patients an ulcer crater is not detected but ulceration (past or present) is inferred from scarring and deformity.

In patients with gastric neoplasia the radiological appearances depend upon the type of lesion. Proliferative carcinoma produces a filling defect which encroaches on the gastric lumen, infiltrative lesions produce mucosal irregularity and rigidity of the stomach wall, and ulcerating lesions produce a crater. Radiological discrimination between benign (peptic) and malignant ulceration is often difficult. Malignant ulcers tend to be large, have raised or rolled edges, frequently involve areas outwith the lesser curvature, do not have mucosal folds radiating from the craters edge, and when see in profile, the ulcer base usually lies within the line of the wall of the stomach. Benign gastric ulcers are often smaller; do not have raised or rolled edges; are particularly common on the lesser curvature; may have radiating mucosal folds; and when seen in profile, the base of the ulcer crater usually projects outwith the line of the wall of the stomach. These guidelines are sufficiently inaccurate to make fibreoptic endoscopy and biopsy necessary in all patients found to have a gastric ulcer on barium meal examination.

2. Fibreoptic endoscopy

As with barium meal examination, accuracy depends on the skill and experience of the individual carrying out the examination. Endoscopy has the advantages that the lesion is seen directly, biopsy or brush cytology is possible, and any source of upper gastrointestinal bleeding can be determined. Either investigation can be used in the diagnosis of duodenal ulcer. Given a firm diagnosis of duodenal ulcer with one technique, there is no need routinely to employ the other. While either investigation can be used to diagnose gastric ulceration, endoscopy allows multiple biopsy of the ulcer and its surroundings and is essential to exclude malignancy. In the event that a gastric ulcer appears benign and medical treatment is employed, vigilance must still be maintained with repeat endoscopy after 4 to 6 weeks to confirm ulcer healing.

3. Acid secretory testing

Definition of maximal acid output by testing with pentagastrin (or histamine) has little value in the diagnosis of peptic ulceration or gastric cancer. While it is true that duodenal ulcer patients often have a high acid output; that patients with gastric ulcer often have a low output; and that gastric cancer is associated with hypochlorhydria or achlorhydria, there is considerable overlap between the groups. Diagnosis is achieved with much greater accuracy by radiology and/or endoscopy. Acid secretory tests were once used to select the type of operation to be performed for duodenal ulcer but are now seldom employed in this context.

The insulin test was used widely to check the completeness of surgical vagotomy and assess patients thought to have recurrent ulceration. The associated hypoglycaemia is often unpleasant and is potentially dangerous. The ready availability of radiology and endoscopy has made the insulin test obsolete in most centres although both insulin and pentagastrin tests are still used as research tools to assess new antisecretory drugs or new ulcer operations.

4. Basal and stimulated serum gastrin

Measurement of fasting serum gastrin levels is used to screen patients in whom the Zollinger-Ellison syndrome (ZES) is suspected. Other conditions associated with hypergastrinaemia include pernicious anaemia, retained antrum after Polya gastrectomy, hyperparathyroidism, and antral G cell hyperplasia. When the ZES is suspected in patients with borderline hypergastrinaemia, a further rise in serum gastrin can be provoked by intravenous secretin injection, intravenous calcium infusion or ingestion of a protein meal. Injection of secretin (2 units/kg by bolus i.v. injection) is recommended (McGuigan & Wolfe, 1980) and in the ZES provokes a 50% rise in serum gastrin within 10–15 minutes of injection. When the ZES has been confirmed, the tumour may be localized and its resectability assessed by venous sampling from a catheter inserted into the portal venous system by the percutaneous transhepatic technique.

SURGERY FOR PEPTIC ULCER

Indications for operation

Duodenal ulcer

Duodenal ulcer is becoming less common in North America and Europe. Its aetiology remains obscure. In general, patients with duodenal ulceration have more parietal cells than normal individuals; secrete more acid; are more responsive to stimulation by gastrin; and have less effective inhibition of gastrin release when antral contents become acid. Excessive acid-pepsin secretion cannot be demonstrated in a substantial proportion of patients and other factors such as defective duodenal mucosal resistance to acid-pepsin digestion must be invoked.

The clinical diagnosis of duodenal ulceration must be confirmed by fibreoptic endoscopy or barium meal examination. The results of 'ulcer surgery' are particularly poor when operation is carried out in the absence of an ulcer or significant scarring. Given a firm diagnosis, the following indications for operations are suggested as guidelines but are by no means universally accepted. Each decision to recommend operation is based on the clinical judgment of the surgeon as applied to the problem of an individual patient.

1. Chronicity and failure of medical therapy. The classical course of duodenal ulceration is one of periods of relapse interspersed with longer periods of remission. Few surgeons advocate operation unless the patient has experienced symptoms for more than one year and has undergone an adequate course of medical treatment. Measures now available include H_2 receptor antagonists such as Cimetidine and Ranitidine, carbenoxolone and colloidal bismuth, and ulcer healing can be expected after a 6 to 8 week course of treatment in about 80% of patients. The histamine H_2 receptor antagonist cimetidine (*Tagamet*) has been used most widely in this context in doses of 1000–1200 mg/day, and healing can be maintained by prolonged maintenance therapy (e.g. 400 mg nocte). Although cimetidine has reduced the number of patients undergoing ulcer surgery, it remains an open question whether the drug will affect the proportion of patients coming to ulcer surgery in the long-term. For the moment, failure of medical therapy may be defined as failure to respond to a course of full-dose cimetidine, relapse after ceasing medical therapy or completing a course of maintenance therapy, or (rarely) development of a complication which precludes continued cimetidine treatment. It should be stressed that recrudescence of symptoms does not necessarily indicate ulcer recurrence, and endoscopy is used to establish the diagnosis if doubt persists. The decision to advocate surgery is strengthened if the patient has a past history of perforation or haemorrhage. Conversely, the decision to persist with effective medical treatment may be strengthened if the risks of operation are increased by intercurrent disease. Factors influencing the decision include amount of time lost from work, amount of sleep lost, dietary incapacity and the less definable factor of impairment of the quality of life.

2. Development of complications of duodenal ulcer. Emergency or urgent surgery may have to be undertaken for patients who develop haemorrhage, perforation or pyloric stenosis (see below).

Gastric ulcer

Gastric ulcers which occur in the pylorus or immediate prepyloric area are frequently associated with acid-pepsin hypersecretion and are regarded as a variant of duodenal ulcer from the point of management. Gastric ulcers which occur in association with duodenal ulcers are thought to be secondary to duodenal ulceration; are often associated with hypersecretion; and may be expected to heal with effective surgical treatment of the duodenal ulcer. The remainder of this discussion is devoted to the chronic gastric ulcers of the body, fundus or antrum of the stomach.

The incidence of gastric ulceration is declining but less sharply than the fall in incidence of duodenal ulcer. A few patients exhibit gastric hypersecretion but the majority have acid-pepsin outputs within or beneath the normal range. A number of factors contribute to this apparent hyposecretion; the functioning parietal cell mass may be reduced by associated gastritis and some secreted acid may leak from the lumen by back-diffusion across a damaged mucosa. Current concepts of pathogenesis stress the importance of damage to the gastric mucosa by bile reflux. Other agents which can damage the mucosa include non-steroidal anti-inflammatory drugs such as aspirin and indomethacin. Acid and pepsin secretion is still essential to exploit the weakened mucosal barrier and cause ulceration. Despite isolated reports of benign gastric ulceration in patients with achlorhydria, the dictum 'no acid no ulcer' is still valid.

The indications for operation are:

1. Failure of medical therapy. Failure of adequate medical therapy (e.g. cimetidine, carbenoxolone) including bed rest if necessary, to induce healing within 6 weeks increases the suspicion of malignancy as a cause of ulceration. It is now accepted that malignant transformation of a benign gastric ulcer is extremly rare, but that problems frequently arise in distinguishing between benign and neoplastic ulcers in their early stages. The problem is complicated by reports that early neoplastic ulcers can sometimes heal during medical therapy, and a good symptomatic response does not necessarily exclude malignancy. Given that surgery is contra-indicated by other factors in the patient's general condition, one may persist with medical treatment provided that the ulcer shows some reduction in size and repeated endoscopy fails to furnish histological evidence of malignancy. Otherwise, failure of medical therapy is a strong indication for operation.

2. Development of complications of gastric ulcer. Emergency or urgent surgery may have to be undertaken for patients who develop bleeding, perforation or stenosis (see below).

Recurrent or anastomotic ulcer

Failure of surgery to reduce acid and pepsin secretion sufficiently is the prime cause of recurrent or anastomotic (stomal) ulceration. In a few cases the operation has been conducted satisfactorily but proves inadequate, whereas in the majority, the operation has not been performed correctly. For example, the operation of gastroenterostomy alone for duodenal ulceration carried an unacceptably high recurrence rate as it did not reduce acid-pepsin secretion sufficiently. On the other hand, the recurrence rate of about 10% following truncal vagotomy and drainage is due almost entirely to the surgeon failing to divide all vagal fibres. In general, the incidence of recurrent ulceration is lowest following combination of vagotomy with partial gastric resection in that both the vagal and gastrin drive to secretion are abolished.

Indications for operation. The clinical diagnosis of recurrent or anastomotic ulceration may be confirmed by barium meal examination but fibreoptic endoscopy is much more reliable. Acid secretory studies with pentagastrin or insulin may support the suspicion that previous vagotomy has been incomplete but add little to diagnosis or to the ultimate decision regarding operative management. It is good practice to screen all patients with recurrent ulceration for the ZES by determination of fasting serum gastrin levels.

Medical treatment with cimetidine allows ulcer healing in the majority of cases and can be maintained if there is a specific contra-indication to re-operation. In the absence of any contra-indication, surgery is usually recommended.

Choice of operation

Duodenal ulcer surgery

Acid and pepsin secretion can be reduced by partial gastric resection, vagal denervation or a combination of the two. Partial gastrectomy for ulceration implies resection of two-thirds to three-quarters of the distal stomach and reduces secretion by removing the antrum (the major source of gastrin production) and a variable amount of acid-pepsin secreting mucosa. Less extensive resection is needed if truncal vagotomy is carried out as in vagotomy and antrectomy. More radical (i.e. subtotal) gastrectomy is usually reserved for the treatment of gastric carcinoma although total gastrectomy may be used in the rare Zollinger-Ellison syndrome.

Truncal vagotomy is usually combined with a drainage procedure to avoid gastric stasis and on clinical grounds there is little to choose between pyloroplasty and gastro-enterostomy (Kennedy et al, 1973). Selective vagotomy was introduced in the hope of reducing the incidence of incomplete vagotomy and symptoms due to vagal denervation of other abdominal viscera. A drainage procedure was also required and the operation is now seldom performed. Highly selective vagotomy (syn. parietal cell vagotomy, proximal gastric vagotomy) denervates the acid-pepsin secreting mucosa but spares the innervation of antrum and pylorus so that a drainage procedure is not needed (De Vries, 1983). The operation of lesser curve seromyotomy developed by Taylor (1982, 1985) is currently under review as an alternative to highly selective vagotomy.

The ideal ulcer operation is safe, cures the ulcer and is without side effects; none of the operations available fulfils these aims. Although experienced surgeons may achieve lower mortality rates, it is estimated that some 2–5% of patients would succumb if partial gastrectomy were employed routinely. The risk of mortality is lower when resection is avoided; it should be less than 1% after truncal vagotomy and drainage and is only 0.3% after highly selective vagotomy (Johnston, 1975).

The estimated overall risk of recurrent ulceration is less than 1% after truncal vagotomy and antrectomy, between 2–5% after partial gastrectomy and between 4 and 15% after truncal vagotomy and drainage. It seems likely that the overall risk of recurrence after highly selective vagotomy will be similar to that of truncal vagotomy and drainage.

With regard to side effects, highly selective vagotomy is attended by fewer sequelae of disturbed gastro-intestinal function. Although gastric resection was thought to lead to more side effects than truncal vagotomy and drainage, the Leeds-York trial showed that good results (Visick grades I + II) were achieved in 77% of male patients after Polya partial gastrectomy, in 78% after truncal vagotomy and antrectomy, and in 70% after truncal vagotomy and gastroenterostomy (Goligher et al, 1968, 1972).

In general, surgeons in the United Kingdom have opted for safety, accepting that truncal vagotomy with drainage and highly selective vagotomy carry a greater risk of ulcer recurrence. As highly selective vagotomy appears to carry a lower incidence of side effects such as dumping, diarrhoea and bilious vomiting, this is now the procedure of choice. It can be argued that recurrent ulceration after vagotomy is easier to deal with than severe dumping and diarrhoea. Truncal vagotomy and drainage is reserved for obese patients and those with overt pyloric or duodenal stenosis. It should be stressed that many surgeons do not adopt this approach and truncal vagotomy and antrectomy retain popularity in many centres particularly in North America.

Gastric ulcer surgery

Reduction of acid-pepsin secretion is also the objective of surgery for gastric ulcer. The same considerations of safety, risk of recurrence and incidence of side effects apply but there is the added problem of excluding malignancy if the ulcer is not resected. The choice of operation for most surgeons lies between partial gastrectomy (usually with gastroduodenal anastomosis) or truncal vagotomy with drainage. Patient variables are important and the problems of surgery in a frail elderly patient with ulceration high on the lesser curve are obviously different from those of a younger otherwise healthy patient with ulceration at the incisura. Collective reviews reveal that mean operative mortality is 1.4% after vagotomy and drainage as opposed to 1.8% after partial gastrectomy, while ulcer recurrence rates are 5.2% and 1.8% (Duthie, 1970). Functional results after vagotomy and drainage have not proved superior.

In the author's practice, Billroth I partial gastrectomy remains the elective procedure of choice for benign gastric ulcer unless the patient is elderly, ill from intercurrent disease or has an ulcer high on the lesser curve which poses significant technical problems. Under these circumstances he opts for truncal vagotomy and pyloroplasty provided that preoperative endoscopy and biopsy confirm that the ulcer is benign. Even with these precautions he prefers to excise the ulcer at operation or at least excise its edge for frozen section examination.

Vagotomy

Access

Successful vagotomy demands adequate access to the abdominal oesophagus and upper stomach. A long upper mid-line or paramedian incision is used with upward extension through or alongside the xiphisternum. Access to the cardia is improved if the lower end of the sternum is retracted upwards using a device of the type described by Goligher (1974). A hook or retractor is placed in the upper end of the wound and the surgeon lifts the retractor and lower sternum as strongly as possible. Upward retraction is maintained by connecting the retractor to the rigid crossbar of the anaesthetist's frame. A self-retaining retractor is then used to retract the sides of the incision, and the table is tilted head-up by some 20–25 degrees.

The spleen and intestine are packed off if necessary. The retractor system described avoids forcible retraction of the costal margin by the assistant and reduces the risk of splenic injury. The left lobe of liver must still be retracted to allow access to the lower oesophagus. It can be retracted to the right after division of the left triangular ligament, but adequate access is frequently obtained by simple upward retraction of the left lobe using a deep bladed Lloyd Davies pelvic retractor or Kelly liver retractor. If the left triangular ligament is divided, care must be taken not to extend the incision too far to the right and cause troublesome bleeding from phrenic veins.

Transabdominal truncal vagotomy

Gentle downward traction is applied to the cardia and lesser curve of the stomach; forcible downward traction on the greater curve predisposes to splenic injury. A small transverse incision is made with a long handled knife in the peritoneum in front of the oesophagus some 2 cm below the inferior edge of the diaphragm. The operator's right index finger is passed from left to right behind the oesphagus so that it emerges into view on the right side. Gentle blunt dissection is required and the nasogastric tube serves as a guide to the correct dissection plane. Perforation of the oesophagus is a potentially lethal complication of vagotomy and is more likely to occur in patients undergoing re-operation. Failure to appreciate that perforation has occurred is the real tragedy, and direct palpation of the tube no longer separated from the finger by the thickness of the oeso-phageal wall means that the situation can still be retrieved by direct primary repair.

Once the index finger has encircled the oesophagus, a soft umbilical catheter or tape is placed between the right thumb and index finger and passed from right to left behind the oesophagus, serving as a useful retractor in subsequent dissection. The anterior vagus nerve or

nerves are sought as they pass downwards on the anterior wall of the oesophagus. A 3–5 cm length of each major trunk is caught in three long forceps and the section of nerve held in the middle forceps is excised. Ligation or clipping of the cut proximal and distal nerve ends may not be necessary in every patient but it is good practice to ligate them routinely. A right angled nerve hook is useful in mobilizing smaller vagal fibres which can be dealt with by diathermy before division. The posterior vagus nerve or nerves lie in loose areolar tissue separated by a small interval from the posterior wall of the oesophagus. The posterior nerve trunks are identi-fied by palpation and divided as described above.

The vagal system enters the abdomen as two distinct trunks in only 75% of individuals and a meticulous search for undivided fibres is essential to avoid incom-plete vagotomy. Aids to complete vagotomy have been described. The so-called selective nerve stain, leucometh-ylene blue, has proved disappointing and non-selective, while intraoperative pH testing and intraoperative electrical stimulation testing have not gained wide acceptance. The surgeon's unaided ability to achieve complete vagotomy undoubtedly improves with experi-ence but some surgeons become better vagotomists than others. The importance of a thorough unhurried search for individual fibres cannot be overemphasised. It is salutory to recall that some 40% of patients have positive insulin tests six months following 'vagotomy' and at re-operation for recurrent ulceration, no less than 85% of patients have substantial and apparently untouched vagal trunks which are more often found posteriorly (Fawcett et al, 1969).

Transthoracic truncal vagotomy

This approach is only employed when the transabdomi-nal approach would be rendered difficult by adhesions from previous gastric surgery. Left thoracotomy is used so that if necessary, access can be had to the stomach by incising the diaphragm. The patient is placed on his right side, a long incision is made in the 7th, 8th or 9th interspace, and the ribs are spread widely. The lung is allowed to collapse and is displaced forwards. The parietal pleura overlying the oesphagus is incised from the aortic arch down to the diaphragm and a soft cath-eter is passed around the oesophagus for use as a retractor. The two vagus nerves and their plexuses are dissected clear of the oesophageal wall from just below the tracheal bifurcation to the hiatus, and are then resected. The chest is closed with underwater seal drainage (see Fig. 14.1).

Selective vagotomy

This operation was introduced in an attempt to reduce the incidence of incomplete gastric vagotomy and avoid some of the sequelae attributed to vagal denervation of other abdominal viscera. The technique entailed sparing the hepatic branch of the anterior vagus and the coeliac branch of the posterior vagus, but as with truncal vagotomy, a gastric drainage procedure was also performed. The operation is more time-consuming than truncal vagotomy and showed little or no advantage with regard to the incidence of recurrent ulceration or other sequelae of surgery. It has been abandoned in most centres and will not be considered further.

Highly selective vagotomy

The operation divides individual vagal branches passing to the upper two-thirds of the stomach while sparing the vagal supply to the antrum and pylorus, so obviating the need for a drainage procedure. This objective is attained by preserving the continuation of the anterior and posterior nerves of Latarjet which innervate the distal stomach.

Some surgeons prefer to begin the operation by displaying the main anterior and posterior vagal trunks on the lower oesophagus in the manner described above for truncal vagotomy. This preliminary step is not essential but may be helpful while one is acquiring experience of the operation.

Unless the patient is obese, the anterior nerve of Latarjet can usually be seen clearly some 1–2 cm from the lesser curve of the stomach. On reaching the antrum it fans out in a manner likened to a crow's foot (Fig. 17.5). The lesser omentum is incised in its avascular portion so that a hand can be passed into the lesser sac behind that portion of the lesser omentum which contains the nerves of Latarjet (Fig. 17.5). The anterior leaf of lesser omentum is drawn to the right so that nerves and vessels passing from the nerves of Latarjet to the lesser curve are put on the stretch. This manoeuvre is facilitated if the assistant grasps the distal stomach in a gauze swab and pulls it gently downwards and to the left. The anterior leaf of lesser omentum is then divided close to the lesser curve commencing at a point just above and to the left of the crow's foot some 7 cm from the pylorus. Rather than leave innervated parietal cells, the point of commencement can be extended into the heel of the crow's foot. This means that only 5–6 cm of antrum remain innervated but this does not appear to compromise gastric emptying. Each vessel passing to the lesser curve is divided between ligatures. Alternatively the vessel may be doubly clipped with artery forceps prior to division and ligation. Some surgeons use Cushing clips or Ligaclips but care must be taken to avoid dislodging the clips by swabbing later in the procedure. The line of dissection proceeds upwards alongside the lesser curve before inclining across the front of the cardia to the cardiac incisura (Figs. 17.5 & 17.6).

Before commencing division of the posterior leaf of the lesser omentum, a plane of intermediate loose connective tissue must be divided. This layer contains fine vessels and nerves which must be ligated carefully and one must resist any temptation to hurry this stage of the operation. Attention is then turned to the posterior layer of the lesser omentum and division is commenced by passing a pair of Mayo scissors or Lahey forceps backwards through the posterior leaf and having them re-emerge 1–2 cm higher up so that the leash of vessels is displayed and can be divided. It may be

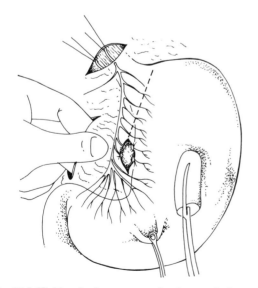

Fig. 17.5 Highly selective vagotomy showing crow's foot and commencement of division of anterior leaf of lesser omentum. The dotted line indicates the line of separation to be used at a higher level (after Figs. 6, 8 and 9 in Goligher J C. British Journal of Surgery, 61:337)

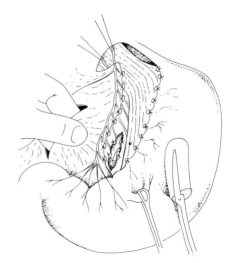

Fig. 17.6 Highly selective vagotomy showing separation of posterior leaf of lesser omentum and window created into lesser sac (after Goligher, 1974)

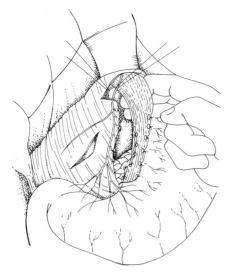

Fig. 17.7 Highly selective vagotomy: finished dissection showing extent of oesophageal clearance (after Goligher, 1974)

helpful to begin this dissection by creating a window in the gastrocolic omentum, turning the stomach upwards, and dividing the first leash of vessels from behind. It is important to keep close to the lesser curve to avoid damage to the posterior nerve of Latarjet. Division of the posterior leaf continues upwards and as the oesophagogastric junction approaches, the bulk of tissue to be divided increases. Access is improved by drawing the lower oesophagus forwards and to the left, taking care not to damage either nerve of Latarjet (Fig. 17.7). Clearance must extend for 7–8 cm up the lower oesophagus to ensure that there are no residual vagal fibres passing downwards on the wall of the oesophagus to reach the stomach. Failure to complete this part of the dissection is a major cause of incomplete parietal cell vagotomy.

The operation is completed by checking the amount of distal stomach which remains innervated. As mentioned above, the uppermost branch from the crow's foot is divided if the innervated portion seems too large. Many surgeons cover the bare strip of the lesser curve by suturing the cut edges of peritoneum in the hope of reducing the risk of the rare complication of lesser curve necrosis.

Gastric drainage procedures

Pyloroplasty

Pyloroplasty was one of the first procedures used for the surgical treatment of duodenal ulcer. Ineffective alone, it is now used as a gastric drainage procedure in conjunction with truncal vagotomy. The operation has the theoretical advantage over gastrojejunostomy that

the normal continuity of the gastro-intestinal tract is retained. The procedure is particularly useful when ulceration is complicated by bleeding as the gastroduodenal mucosa can be inspected and the ulcer base transfixed. It is also used in the surgery of perforated duodenal ulcer, the perforation site being incorporated in the incision through the pylorus.

Technique of pyloroplasty. (1). Heineke-Mikulicz. The original Heineke-Mikulicz pyloroplasty consisted of a 5 cm longitudinal incision through all coats of the anterior wall of the pyloro-duodenal region. The incision was closed transversely with multiple rows of interrupted silk sutures but excessive infolding of tissue frequently narrowed the lumen. Weinberg's modification of the Heineke-Mikulicz technique avoids narrowing by employing only one layer of interrupted sutures.

Two stay sutures are inserted deeply 1 cm apart on the anterior aspect of the pyloric ring. The pyloroduodenal wall is incised longitudinally to open the lumen for approximately 3.5 cm on the gastric side and

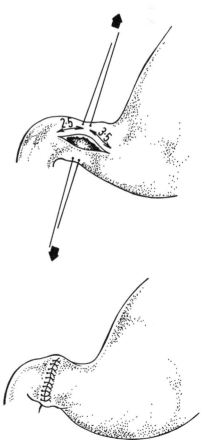

Fig. 17.8 The operation of Heineke-Mikulicz pyloroplasty using one layer of interrupted sutures to close the incision. The stitch for inversion of the mucosa is not essential and may be replaced by a simple through-and-through all coats stitch

2.5 cm on the duodenal side of the pylorus. If an anterior ulcer is present, the incision is made right through it. Ulcer excision should not be attempted. Traction on the stay sutures converts the longitudinal incision to a diamond-shaped opening which is closed transversely, commencing at its upper end (Fig. 17.8). Non-absorbable sutures of 3/0 silk were at one time preferred to absorbable material such as catgut, but a single layer of 3/0 polyglycolic acid (Dexon) sutures is now my material of choice. The sutures are placed some 3 mm apart and include all layers of the gastric and duodenal wall. No attempt is made to infold the 'dog-ear' projection at the upper and lower ends of the suture line so as to avoid narrowing of the lumen. It is unnecessary to cover the suture line with omentum as leakage is extremely unlikely.

(2). *Finney.* Finney's technique is strictly speaking a gastroduodenostomy rather than a pyloroplasty. It demands thorough mobilization of the pylorus and first three portions of the duodenum by Kocher's method. The peritoneum and fascia propria on the outer aspect of the duodenum are divided, any adhesions are freed, and the duodenum and pylorus are lifted forwards and to the left by gauze or finger dissection. The greater curve of the distal stomach is then applied to the first two parts of the duodenum by three stay sutures of 3/0 silk (Fig. 17.9) which are knotted and clipped. A posterior continuous Lembert suture of 3/0 Dexon is commenced at the pylorus and extends to just beyond the furthest stay suture. An inverted U-shaped incision is made through all coats of the stomach, pylorus and duodenum and passing around the suture line (Fig. 17.9). A posterior all coats suture of 3/0 Dexon is then applied, commencing at the divided pylorus. From the lower angle of the incision the suture is carried upwards as a Connell or loop-on-the-mucosa stitch to approximate the anterior walls of the stomach, duodenum and pylorus. The gastroduodenal anastomosis is completed by taking up the posterior seromuscular stitch and continuing it anteriorly to invaginate the all coats layer (Fig. 17.9).

Finney's operation is seldom performed today. The Heineke-Mikulicz pyloroplasty is simpler and less time consuming, and if difficulty is anticipated with this form of pyloroplasty most surgeons elect to carry out posterior gastrojejunostomy for drainage purposes.

Gastrojejunostomy

Anastomosis of the stomach to a loop of jejunum may be used as a gastric drainage procedure in conjunction with truncal vagotomy, and is occasionally used for palliation in patients with unresectable carcinoma obstructing the distal stomach. Gastrojejunostomy alone was once used to treat duodenal ulcer but carried a high incidence of recurrent ulceration and is no longer recommended. In general, posterior gastrojejunostomy

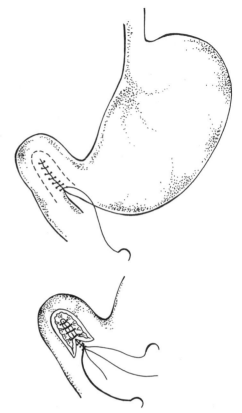

Fig. 17.9 The operation of Finney gastroduodenostomy showing insertion of the posterior seromuscular layer and the commencement of the posterior all coats layer

drains the stomach more effectively and is preferred in ulcer surgery.

Posterior gastrojejunostomy. The greater omentum, transverse colon and lower part of the stomach are brought out of the wound and turned upwards. A hand is passed along the root of the transverse mesocolon to the left of the spine to identify the proximal jejunum as it leaves the duodeno-jejunal flexure. This loop is withdrawn and two pairs of light tissue forceps (e.g. Babcock's forceps) are applied to its antimesenteric border at distances of approximately 10 and 20 cm from the duodeno-jejunal flexure.

While the assistant holds up the transverse colon, the surgeon pushes the dependent portion of the distal stomach against the transverse mesocolon which is incised vertically in an avascular area, usually to the left of the middle colic artery. The incision is enlarged with dissecting scissors to a length of about 10 cm and the posterior wall of the dependent portion of gastric antrum is grasped with light tissue forceps and pulled gently through the window. Once sufficient stomach has been made available for anastomosis, the margins of the defect in the mesocolon are sutured to the stomach by

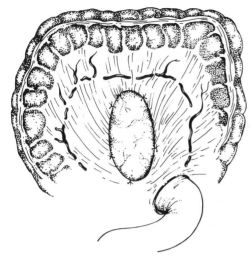

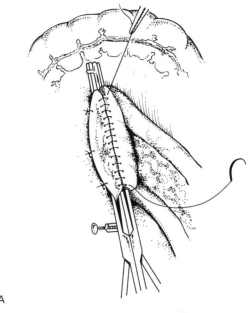

Fig. 17.10 Posterior gastrojejunostomy. The stomach has been drawn down through a window in the transverse mesocolon, and the window should now be closed around it. A segment of jejunum some 15–20 cm from the duodenojejunal flexure has been selected for the anastomosis

A

interrupted sutures (Fig. 17.10). These sutures prevent herniation of the small intestine through the window and it is simpler to insert them before constructing the anastomosis.

The selected portions of stomach and jejunum are then held up by the tissue forceps, brought into apposition by locking anastomosis clamps such as Lane's, Dott's or Swanson's clamps, and the tissue forceps are removed. The eventual opening in the stomach may lie vertically, obliquely or horizontally and the anastomosis may be isoperistaltic or antiperistaltic. There is little to choose between these methods although most surgeons favour an oblique isoperistaltic anastomosis (Fig. 17.11). Regardless of the method employed, the anastomosis is placed in the most dependent region of the stomach to ensure efficient drainage. The transverse colon, greater omentum and any protruding loops of small bowel are replaced in the peritoneal cavity, and the segments of gut to be anastomosed are surrounded by moist packs. Lateral anastomosis is carried out (p. 323), many surgeons opting to use two layers of continuous absorbable suture such as polyglycolic acid (Dexon).

In obese patients with a short thick mesocolon and relatively fixed stomach, it may prove difficult to perform a posterior gastrojejunostomy in the conventional manner. In this event, the gastrocolic omentum is divided between ligatures to gain access to the lesser sac and the selected loop of jejunum is drawn upwards through a window in the transverse mesocolon. Anastomotic clamps can then be applied and the anastomosis performed with relative ease above the transverse colon. On completion, the anastomosis is drawn down through

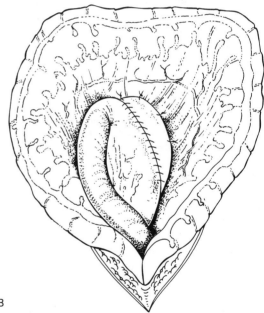

B

Fig. 17.11 Posterior gastrojejunostomy completed showing the closed window in the transverse mesocolon and an oblique isoperistaltic anastomosis

the mesocolon window, the margins of which are sutured to the stomach with a series of interrupted sutures. It should be stressed that this method still creates a posterior gastrojejunostomy using the posterior wall of the most dependent portion of stomach.

Partial gastrectomy

When partial gastrectomy is performed for peptic ulceration the line of proximal transection lies across the body of the stomach, its level and angle depending on the size of the organ, the site of any gastric lesion, and the type of anastomosis envisaged. The distal transection line passes through the first part of the duodenum. When operating for duodenal ulcer it is sometimes safer to divide the duodenum proximal to the ulcer, rather than attempt to remove the ulcer-bearing area with difficulty in closing the duodenal stump and increased risk of damage to the common bile duct, hepatic artery or pancreas.

Types of gastrectomy

In Billroth's first operation described in 1881, only the pyloric part of the stomach was excised with end-to-end anastomosis between the remaining stomach and duodenum. It is now customary to resect more of the stomach but the term Billroth I operation is retained when gastroduodenal anastomosis is performed.

In the Polya operation (Fig. 17.12) described in 1911, the duodenal stump is closed and the remaining stomach is anastomosed end-to-side with the jejunum. Most modern forms of gastrectomy with gastrojejunal anastomosis are modelled on this operation. The proximal loop of jejunum may be brought through an opening in the transverse mesocolon (retro-colic anastomosis) or in front of the transverse colon (ante-colic anastomosis). A longer loop of jejunum (20–25 cm) is required for an antecolic anastomosis. The other major variation relates to whether the afferent loop of jejunum is brought to the lesser or greater curvature, giving 'isoperistaltic' or 'antiperistaltic' anastomosis respectively. No one method is superior and the choice of technique is dictated by the operative findings and personal preference. It has been suggested that obstructive complications are more frequent after antecolic anastomosis but many surgeons simply place the jejunum in the position in which it lies most conveniently. Although the jejunum is brought through the mesocolon for a retrocolic anastomosis, the stomach should be drawn down through the window on completion and the defect closed

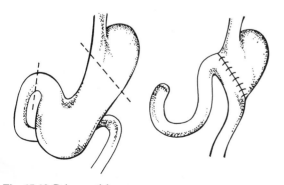

Fig. 17.12 Polya partial gastrectomy

around *the stomach* with interrupted sutures. Failure to close the window may allow jejunum to herniate into the supracolic compartment of the abdomen, or kink and obstruct as it passes through the mesocolon. An antecolic anastomosis is preferred when there is a small gastric stump or the mesocolon is unusually short or loaded with fat.

The valvular (small-stoma) anastomosis introduced by Finsterer in 1913 can be used in both retrocolic and antecolic forms of the Polya operation. The upper part of the cut end of stomach is closed before anastomosis of the lower part to the jejunum. This reduces the size of the stoma and it is claimed that the valve (see Fig. 17.16) directs both gastric and duodenal contents into the efferent loop of jejunum with minimal reflux. Many surgeons do not employ the small stoma technique.

Technique of the Polya operation

The technique to be described for duodenal ulceration may differ from that used for gastric ulcer or gastric carcinoma (see p. 359). After opening the abdomen by a long mid-line or paramedian incision, the duodenum is carefully examined and the mobility of its first part is determined. The stomach is drawn out of the wound and the extent of resection is planned. The mesocolon and first loop of jejunum are examined and a decision is made as to whether a retrocolic or antecolic anastomosis is to be performed.

Mobilization of the stomach. The greater omentum is detached from the stomach, dividing its contained vessels between successive pairs of ligatures. It is not necessary to preserve the main gastro-epiploic arch and it is less tedious to divide the gastrocolic omentum beneath the arch, ligating the main right and left gastroepiploic vessels at the lower and upper resection lines respectively. Division of the greater omentum continues to the right, to the middle of the first part of the duodenum, and to the left to the level selected for transection; this usually entails dividing the lower of the short gastric vessels. The stomach is lifted forwards and avascular adhesions between its posterior wall and pancreas are divided with dissecting scissors. The lesser omentum is next incised in its avascular portion. The right gastric artery is identified just above the point where it reaches the upper border of the first part of the duodenum. The artery is doubly ligated and divided. Division of the lesser omentum continues parallel with the lesser curvature but stops before reaching the left gastric artery as the vessel is dealt with more conveniently at a later stage. The stomach is lifted forwards and the inferior border of the first part of duodenum is separated from the pancreas, ligating all vascular adhesions before their division. If possible the duodenum is freed for 1 cm beyond the area of ulcer

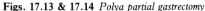

Figs. 17.13 & 17.14 *Polya partial gastrectomy*

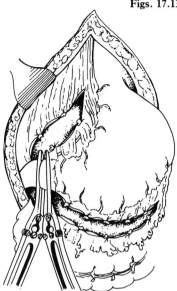

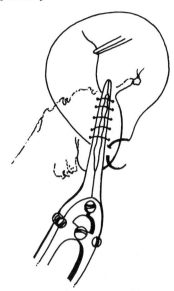

Fig. 17.13 Division of the first part of duodenum between crushing clamps after mobilization

Fig. 17.14 Closure of the duodenal stump commencing with a continuous invaginating seromuscular stitch passed from side to side over the clamp

scarring to facilitate subsequent closure of the duodenal stump. Ligation of the gastroduodenal artery is seldom required and must never be attempted before the common bile duct and hepatic artery have been displayed and safeguarded. If a posterior wall ulcer has penetrated deeply into the pancreas and partial gastrectomy is still considered the operation of choice, the duodenum is dissected free leaving the ulcer crater attached to the pancreas. Attempts to excise an adherent ulcer carries substantial risks of subsequent pancreatitis and fistula formation.

Division of the duodenum and closure of the stump. There are many acceptable methods for carrying out this part of the operation. One traditional method entails placing two straight crushing clamps across the selected transection line (Fig. 17.13), packing off the operative field, and dividing the bowel with a scalpel or diathermy. The proximal cut-end is covered with a gauze swab and the stomach is turned back over the left side of the wound. The duodenal stump is usually closed in two layers. A continuous seromuscular stitch can be used to pick up the duodenal wall first on one side of the clamp and then on the other, passing over the clamp but not under it (Fig. 17.14). This invaginating stitch is tightened as the clamp is removed and is reinforced by a second continuous or interrupted seromuscular stitch. An alternative method of suture closure uses a 'sewing machine' stitch for the first layer (Fig. 17.15). The choice of suture material is a matter of personal preference but many surgeons employ polyglycolic acid

for both layers or use nonabsorbable material for the outer layer.

Many surgeons now employ the Auto Suture GIA

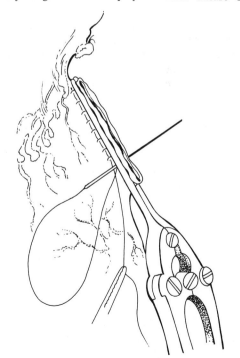

Fig. 17.15 The 'sewing machine' stitch used to close the duodenal stump; a secure method when the stump is short and may be difficult to invaginate

stapling device to divide the duodenum. The row of staples on the duodenal stump are buried by a layer of interrupted seromuscular stitches of 2/0 polyglycolic acid. Regardless of the method of closure employed, the suture line is covered with a convenient tag of omentum or buried by stitching it against the pancreas. Leakage from the duodenal stump is one of the major complications of the Polya operation and a tube drain is placed down to the stump routinely. Over-zealous closure and insertion of sutures under tension increases the risk of leakage by impairing duodenal vascularity. Indeed, in the rare event that tissue friability precludes secure closure it may be safer to suture the duodenum around the tube drain and elect to manage a controlled fistula in the postoperative period. Given that there is no distal obstruction to flow down the small intestine this fistula closes readily and the approach exposes the patient to much less risk than development of stump necrosis and uncontrolled leakage.

Transection of the stomach and retrocolic anastomosis. The stomach is turned back over the left costal margin to identify the left gastric artery as it reaches the lesser curvature just below the oesophagogastric junction. The vessel is divided and doubly ligated. Both curvatures of the stomach should be entirely bared of omentum at the level selected for anastomosis. The proximal loop of jejunum is brought through the transverse mesocolon and placed alongside the stomach in the position in which it seems to lie most conveniently, although most surgeons prefer to bring the afferent loop to the lesser curvature. The length of afferent loop employed should be such that it is neither too tense nor too lax. Two pairs of Babcock's tissue forceps are applied to the jejunum to mark the points for anastomosis to the lesser and greater curvatures. A light occlusion clamp is placed across the stomach proximal to the level of section and a similar clamp is applied to the selected length of jejunum (Fig. 17.16). Locking twin clamps such as Lane's clamps usually facilitate anastomosis. A continuous seromuscular stitch is used to unite the adjacent surfaces of the two viscera and a crushing clamp is then applied to the stomach 1 cm distal to the suture line. The stomach is divided with a scalpel run along the underside of the crushing clamp so that the clamp remains on the excised segment.

If a full length stoma is to be made, the jejunum is incised for a distance which corresponds to the length of the cut-end of the stomach. The anastomosis is then completed in the classical manner (p. 323).

If a valvular anastomosis is preferred, the jejunum is incised for only 3–4 cm opposite the lower part of the cut-end of the stomach. The upper part of the open stomach is closed by through-and-through sutures (the 'sewing machine' stitch is a convenient method) and only the lower 3–4 cm is anastomosed to the open

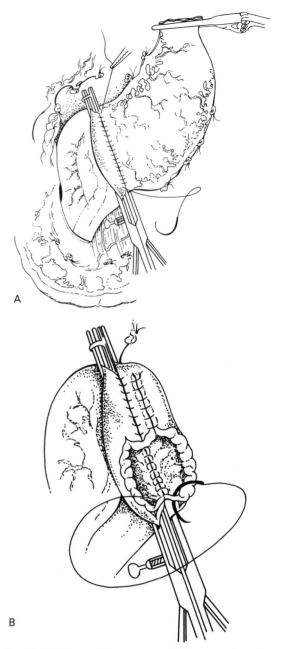

Fig. 17.16 Polya partial gastrectomy with construction of a retrocolic valvular (short stoma) anastomosis. (A) proximal loop of jejunum brought through a window in the transverse mesocolon. Twin locking clamps have been used in anastomosis and the posterior seromuscular stitch has been inserted. (B) the stomach has been transected and the upper part of the stump has been closed. The lower part only of the cut-end of stomach is being used for the anastomosis

jejunum. The anterior seromuscular layer of sutures is used to anchor the intact jejunum to the upper sutured part of the stomach. The extremities of the suture line at the greater and lesser curvature may be reinforced with omentum. The anastomosis is drawn down through the defect in the mesocolon, the margins of which are attached to the stomach wall by interrupted stitches placed about 1 cm above the suture line.

Technique of the Billroth I operation

The stomach and first part of the duodenum are mobilized as described for the Polya operation. It is vital to confirm that the duodenum beyond the proposed resection line is healthy and of sufficient calibre for gastroduodenal anastomosis. The duodenum is divided between clamps as in the Polya operation, gastric mobilization is completed, and the stomach is transected with the aid of the two clamps placed at an angle to each other.

The lower clamp encloses a portion of the gastric

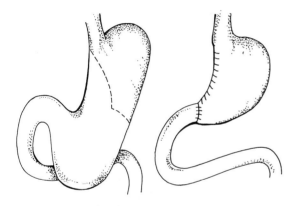

Fig. 17.17 Billroth I partial gastrectomy

lumen suitable in size for anastomosis with the duodenum, while the cut-end of stomach held in the upper clamp is closed in two layers to create a new 'lesser curvature' (Fig. 17.17). Alternatively the gastric stump can be closed with a TA90 Auto Suture stapling device. The jaws of the instrument are placed across the stomach at the level of transection, the locking pin is screwed into place, the jaws of the instrument are tightened, and the staples are fired. Before removing the instrument a crushing clamp is placed on the specimen side and the stomach is divided with a scalpel using the edge of the TA90 as a cutting guide. Any bleeding from the staple line is dealt with by under-running the bleeding point with a suture. A portion of the gastric stump staple line is excised on its greater curve aspect for anastomosis to the duodenum (Fig. 17.18). In a variation of the stapling technique the greater curvature aspect of the stomach is divided between crushing clamps before using the TA90 or TA55 stapling device to staple and transect the remaining portion of stomach. Many surgeons also employ stapling techniques when dividing the stomach in the Polya operation.

Provided that the greater curvature has been mobilized adequately, the gastric remnant can usually be brought across for anastomosis with the duodenum without tension. If necessary the duodenum can be mobilized by incising the peritoneum along the lateral aspect of its first and second part. When clamps have been used the gastroduodenal anastomosis is commenced by uniting the posterior walls of the gut with interrupted seromuscular sutures of 3/0 silk or polyglycolic acid leaving a stay suture at each end of the suture line for

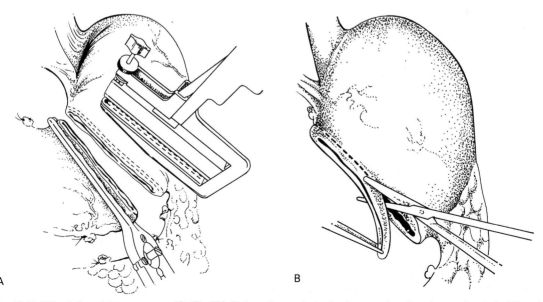

A   B

Fig. 17.18 Billroth I partial gastrectomy. (A) The TA 90 Auto Suture device has been used to close the gastric pouch. (B) excision of a portion of the staple line on the greater curve aspect for anastomosis to the duodenum (courtesy of Auto Suture UK Ltd.)

use as retractors. The small rim of stomach enclosed in the Payr crushing clamp is then excised, the clamp on the duodenum is removed, and the posterior wall of the anastomosis is completed by an all-coats continuous suture of 3/0 polyglycolic acid. This suture is continued forwards as the inner layer of the anterior aspect of the anastomosis. The outer layer of the anterior suture line consists of a series of interrupted seromuscular stitches of 3/0 silk. It is advisable to reinforce closure of the 'angle of sorrow' between the lesser curvature of the stomach and superior border of the duodenum by inserting a purse-string suture across the junction. A portion of greater omentum may be drawn across the anastomosis. Many surgeons do not leave a drain to the anastomosis but I prefer to leave a suction drain in this area. Routine use of a nasogastric tube in the postoperative period is equally controversial but it is my own practice to pass the tube through the anastomosis before leaving the abdomen.

Partial gastrectomy for gastric ulcer. When the ulcer lies in the pyloric antrum or lower part of the body of stomach it can be removed as described above with the excised portion of stomach. The Billroth I operation is the procedure of choice but the Polya operation is preferred when the duodenum has been distorted by existing or previous ulceration. If the gastric ulcer is adherent to the pancreas it can often be pinched off between finger and thumb. If the ulcer has penetrated deeply it is simpler to incise the stomach wall so that the ulcer base is left in situ and covered with a piece of omentum. Frozen section examination of the ulcer margin is advisable to ensure that the ulcer is benign.

When the gastric ulcer is situated so high on the lesser curve or posterior wall that clamps cannot be applied easily across the resection line, the Pauchet manoeuvre may be helpful. Two small Payr crushing clamps are applied to the greater curvature and the stomach between them is divided with a scalpel. The stomach is surrounded by packs and held upward with the Payr clamps so that short segments of both the anterior and posterior wall can be incised with scissors. The walls of the gastric stump are sutured together by a continuous through-and-through suture of 3/0 polyglycolic acid (Dexon) before proceeding to cut the next segment on the transection line. The line of the cut can be altered to remove more or less of either the anterior or posterior wall to excise the ulcer. Provided that each incised segment is sutured immediately, soiling and bleeding are kept to a minimum. When the new 'lesser curvature' has been created, the suture line is inverted by continuous or interrupted seromuscular sutures. A gastro-jejunal anastomosis is usually preferred if the gastric stump is small so as to avoid tension on a gastro-duodenal anastomosis.

Postoperative management

Intravenous infusion is used to maintain fluid and electrolyte balance until adequate oral intake is re-established. As indicated earlier, opinions vary greatly regarding the need for a nasogastric tube and the duration of its use. I remove the tube on completion of highly selective vagotomy but retain it for 24 hours after truncal vagotomy and drainage or partial gastrectomy. Water is allowed on the day of removal and the amount is increased gradually from 15 ml hourly to permit free fluid intake and ingestion of a light diet by the fourth or fifth day. The tube is reinserted in the uncommon event of abdominal distension, ileus or repeated vomiting. Many surgeons do not employ a nasogastric tube routinely and encourage water and food intake from an earlier stage.

Complications

Detailed consideration of the complications of ulcer surgery is outwith the scope of this volume, but the management of major specific early and late complications will be outlined.

Specific complications in the postoperative period

1. Haemorrhage. Intraperitoneal haemorrhage is rarely a problem and any bleeding from suture or staple lines should be under-run with a stitch. Bleeding into the gut lumen is most often due to faulty anastomotic technique and is usually reactionary, becoming manifest in the hours following operation. Aspiration of blood-stained fluid is common after gastric surgery but continued aspiration of frank blood, the onset of haematemesis or melaena, and development of shock reflect significant blood loss into the gut lumen. Morphine is given to relieve anxiety, blood is transfused, a nasogastric tube is inserted if not already in place, and vital signs are monitored. Re-operation is indicated if bleeding continues. When a pyloroplasty has been performed the suture line is opened remembering that in some cases the duodenal ulcer rather than the suture line is responsible for bleeding. When the patient has a gastrojejunal anastomosis the anterior suture line can be re-opened but it may prove simpler to incise the front wall of the stomach so that the suture line can be inspected from above and any bleeding point under-run.

2. Obstruction. Obstruction at the site of a pyloroplasty or Billroth I anastomosis usually reflects poor operative technique with luminal narrowing by excessive inversion of the suture line, or poor choice of operation if the duodeno-pyloric region was scarred. Obstruction after gastrojejunostomy or Polya partial gastrectomy may be due to faulty anastomotic technique, kinking or volvulus of the jejunal loop, herniation of small intestine through a defect in the mesocolon or behind an antecolic anastomosis, or retrograde jejunogastric intussusception (although this is more often a late complication). Stomal oedema is often advanced as the explanation for persisting postoperative gastric outlet obstruction but must be accepted with great caution. Obstruction which persists for more than 3–5 days after gastric surgery should always be taken seriously. A nasogastric tube is inserted, intravenous fluids are continued, and the patient should be investigated by endoscopy and/or radiology in the form of plain abdominal films (erect and supine) and gastrografin instillation. Re-operation should not be deferred if contrast or the endoscope do not pass through the stoma. Obstruction in or around the anastomosis after Polya partial gastrectomy carries added dangers as a blocked afferent jejunal loop becomes grossly distended with resultant necrosis and potentially fatal 'blow-out' of the duodenal stump.

3. Anastomotic or suture line leakage. Leakage from a gastrojejunal anastomosis, gastroduodenal anastomosis or pyloroplasty is unusual following good operative technique. Leakage from the duodenal stump is a recognized complication of the Polya operation and is prone to occur when there is any obstruction in or around the gastrojejunal anastomosis. Development of duodenal necrosis is often signalled by otherwise unexplained pyrexia or tachycardia, but frank leakage may not become manifest until about the fifth postoperative day. The drainage tube down to the duodenal stump should be retained for at least 5 days. The principles of management are: (1) ensure free external drainage from the leaking stump; (2) protect the surrounding skin; (3) maintain fluid and electrolyte balance; (4) provide parenteral nutrition; (5) stop oral intake; and (6) ensure that there is no distal obstruction that will prevent the fistula from closing spontaneously. Suction sump drainage often aids management and Stomahesive or Baltimore paste can be used to protect the skin. The majority of duodenal fistulae close on conservative management in the absence of distal obstruction.

Late sequelae of ulcer surgery

1. Recurrent ulceration (see Stabile & Passaro, 1976). Medical therapy with antisecretory drugs (e.g. cimetidine) usually allows ulcer healing but surgery remains the definitive form of management. The choice of procedure is controversial. When ulceration recurs after highly selective vagotomy or vagotomy and drainage the choice of procedure lies between revagotomy, partial gastrectomy and a combination of the two. I always attempt to divide any residual vagal fibres but also resect part of the distal stomach to decrease the risk of further ulcer problems. If further vagal trunks are discovered and divided the resection is limited to antrectomy; if not, resection is extended to a 70% partial gastrectomy.

If ulceration recurs after partial gastrectomy, I carry out vagotomy at re-operation and may resect more

stomach if there is a substantial gastric remnant. If the recurrent ulcer is in the gastric stump and there is pronounced bile reflux and gastritis at endoscopy, re-anastomosis using a Roux loop of jejunum may be advisable.

2. Entero-gastric reflux (see Alexander-Williams, 1981). The patient frequently complains of post prandial fullness, nausea, pain and vomiting of bitter bile-stained fluid. Enterogastric reflux can be demonstrated on barium meal and quantified by measurement of bile acids in gastric aspirate or scintillation scanning using labelled material (e.g. $^{99}Tc^m$ HIDA) excreted in bile. Endoscopy reveals an angry hyperaemic mucosa, gastritis being most marked near the stoma. Surgery should not be employed prematurely as many patients improve within 1 to 2 years. Severe intractable reflux is treated by Roux-en-Y reconstruction if the patient has previously had a Polya gastrectomy or vagotomy and antrectomy, and the length of the Roux loop should be at least 45–50 cm. Interposition of an isoperistaltic jejunal loop between stomach and small intestine has also been used but may have a higher morbidity and the results are less predictable. In patients with biliary gastritis after vagotomy and gastroenterostomy, simple closure of the gastroenterostomy may be worthwhile if there is no pyloroduodenal narrowing.

3. Dumping (see Hobsley, 1981). Early dumping occurs within 30 minutes of eating a meal and is distinguished from the syndrome of hypoglycaemia which occurs 60–90 minutes after eating. The dumping symptoms are abdominal fullness, nausea, vomiting and diarrhoea, in association with weakness, sweating and palpitation. Symptoms often improve with time and may be minimized if the patient takes small dry meals and avoids drinking with them. Surgery is undertaken if severe dumping persists and consists of conversion of a Polya operation to a Billroth I anastomosis, or interposition of an isoperistaltic or retroperistaltic jejunal loop between the gastric remnant and the intestine to slow emptying. This is a complex area of surgery and patients with dumping problems are best referred to specialist surgeons.

4. Diarrhoea. Diarrhoea is common after operation involving truncal vagotomy but is only severe in 2–5% of cases. It may be continuous or episodic and its aetiology is unknown. The symptoms improve with time and some patients learn to avoid articles of diet associated with diarrhoea. Surgery is rarely recommended and the effect of interposition of a reversed jejunal loop is unpredictable.

5. Metabolic upsets and anaemia. Such upsets include malabsorption, weight loss, osteomalacia, and both iron deficiency and megaloblastic anaemia. Although more common after extensive resection, lesser upsets may follow vagotomy and drainage. Medical management is usually indicated although on rare occasions, conversion of a Polya type of gastrectomy to a Billroth I operation will remove a blind loop causing megaloblastic anaemia.

6. Gastrojejunocolic fistula. This complication is now extremely rare with the decline of gastroenterostomy alone as an ulcer operation, the increased use of operations not involving gastroenterostomy, and the prompt management of recurrent ulceration. The fistula develops when an anastomotic or jejunal ulcer following gastroenterostomy or Billroth II gastrectomy erodes the wall of the overlying transverse colon. Severe and intractable diarrhoea results with malabsorption and rapid weight loss. Diarrhoea is not due to passage of food and acid into the colon, but to gastritis, duodenitis and jejunitis caused by faecal organisms entering the upper gastrointestinal tract. The pain of ulceration usually eases with fistula formation possibly because acid secretion falls following the development of severe gastritis.

The diagnosis can sometimes be confirmed by barium meal or endoscopy, but barium enema is much more reliable. The condition was once managed in three stages: preliminary proximal colostomy to improve the general condition; subsequent repair of the transverse colon, resection of the affected jejunum and antrum, and gastrojejunal anastomosis; and finally, closure of the colostomy. With nutritional support and bowel preparation a one-stage resection of the affected transverse colon, jejunum and antrum is now usually recommended. It may be possible to avoid formal resection of a segment of transverse colon and merely excise a V-shaped margin of colon at the fistula site (Fig. 17.19).

7. Retrograde jejunogastric intussusception. Retrograde intussusception of one or occasionally both loops of jejunum is a late complication of gastro-enterostomy or Polya partial gastrectomy. There is usually acute epigastric pain and vomiting, visible peristalsis, and a palpable epigastric mass, although the condition can present on a more chronic basis. Barium meal reveals a gastric filling defect caused by intussuscepted coils of jejunum, or endoscopy can be used to clinch the diagnosis. Operation is essential. Gangrenous jejunum demands resection with revision of the anastomosis. If gangrene is not present the intussusception is reduced and an entero-anastomosis can be performed between the efferent and afferent loops of jejunum. Revision of the anastomosis may also be undertaken but the only guarantee of avoiding recurrence is to carry out a Billroth I conversion.

8. Gastric cancer. It is now accepted that development of cancer in the gastric stump is a long-standing complication of gastrectomy and may prove to be a complication of vagotomy and drainage. Endoscopy is the mainstay of diagnosis and the cancer is treated by further gastric resection.

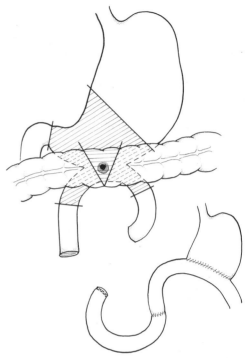

Fig. 17.19 Surgery for gastrojejunocolic fistula. The shaded areas indicate the portions of gut resected and the inset illustrates the restoration of upper gastrointestinal continuity

COMPLICATIONS OF PEPTIC ULCERATION

Perforated gastric or duodenal ulcer

Diagnosis

Perforation of a peptic ulcer usually presents as an acute surgical emergency. On rare occasions the perforation is sealed so rapidly by omentum and adhesions to neighbouring viscera that peritoneal contamination is minimal and localized, with eventual resolution or formation of a chronic abscess. The majority of patients have a preceding history suggestive of chronic ulceration but about one-third have no history of dyspepsia or one which extends for only a week or two. The clinical diagnosis of perforation can be confirmed radiologically in some 80% of cases by demonstrating free gas beneath the diaphragm when the patient is erect or sitting. If free gas is not apparent perforation may be demonstrated by instilling 50–100 ml of 50% gastrografin down a nasogastric tube. It should be stressed that the decision to operate is based on clinical findings and many surgeons do not use gastrografin unless there is a strong desire to avoid operation or treat the perforation conservatively.

Principles of operative management

Perforated peptic ulcer is usually treated by operation

but on rare occasions may be managed conservatively.

Pre-operative preparation. Mortality can be reduced if precipitate surgery is avoided and 2–3 hours are spent in active resuscitation. Pain and anxiety are relieved by intravenous injection of morphine or pethidine. A naso-gastric tube is passed and the stomach is kept empty by regular hand suction. Lavage is contraindicated but a large bore tube should be used if the patient has eaten recently. A free-flowing intravenous line is established to treat dehydration and shock but blood transfusion is not needed unless the patient is grossly anaemic or has the relatively rare combination of ulcer perforation and haemorrhage. Pulse and blood pressure are monitored regularly, a urinary catheter is inserted and hourly urine output is recorded in the presence of shock. Central venous pressure (p. 310) monitoring may be particularly helpful when resuscitating the elderly and patients with cardiovascular disease.

Operative technique. The abdomen is opened by an upper mid-line or upper right paramedian incision if perforation is suspected. If acute appendicitis is thought more likely, it is advisable first to inspect the appendix by a small gridiron or skin crease (Lanz) incision in the right iliac fossa. If the appendix is normal but bile-stained free fluid is apparent, the gridiron incision is closed and a separate incision is made in the upper abdomen. Removal of an acutely inflamed appendix through an upper abdominal incision is often difficult despite extending the incision and frequently requires a second incision in the region of the appendix.

In patients with perforation, gas and turbid bile-stained fluid often escape as the peritoneum is incised. Free fluid is aspirated from the peritoneal cavity and the perforation is sought. The anterior aspect of the first part of the duodenum and distal stomach are inspected first. A retractor is inserted beneath the liver and the stomach is drawn down, first by gentle traction on the transverse colon and gastrocolic omentum, and then by grasping it with a moist pad (Fig. 17.20). Overlying omentum is gently peeled away by blunt dissection with a pledget or gauze swab. Flakes of creamy fibrin often adhere to the gut near the perforation and are a useful guide to its location. If perforation of the proximal duodenum or distal stomach is not apparent, the remainder of the anterior aspect of the stomach and distal oesophagus is inspected. On rare occasions, the stomach has perforated into the lesser sac and fluid and gas may be seen through the gastrohepatic omentum or issuing from the epiploic foramen. In this event, one should gain access to the lesser sac by dividing part of the gastrocolic omentum.

The quickest method of dealing with the perforation is simple closure. Control of the stomach is handed to the assistant, retractors are arranged to give the best possible access and any viscera which intrude are packed

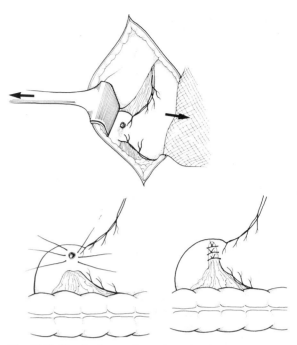

Fig. 17.20 Simple closure of a perforated duodenal ulcer showing insertion of three sutures to close the perforation. The omental tag is secured in place with the same sutures

off. Closure is achieved by inserting 3 or 4 gauge 0 sutures of an absorbable material such as chromic catgut or Dexon which transfix the entire thickness of the gut wall (Fig. 17.20). The central suture which crosses the perforation is inserted (or at least tightened) last so that it is less likely to cut out of the oedematous gut wall. The sutures are inserted in the long axis of the gut to avoid narrowing of the lumen. An additional layer of seromuscular Lembert sutures is unnecessary and increases the risk of narrowing the lumen, but a portion of omentum is used to reinforce closure (Fig. 17.20). If scarring makes pyloric or duodenal obstruction inevitable after closure, pyloroplasty or gastro-enterostomy may be unavoidable (see below).

In cases where the induration is so marked that all stitches tend to cut out, the perforation can be closed with omentum alone, or in extreme circumstances the margins of the perforation may be approximated around a Portex tube or large Foley catheter led through a stab incision to the exterior.

Closure of the perforation is followed by meticulous peritoneal toilet. The subphrenic spaces, kidney pouches, paracolic gutter and pelvis are all cleared of fluid by suction and a specimen is sent for bacteriological culture and sensitivity determinations. Lavage is advisable if there has been significant peritoneal contamination and is carried out with warm saline to which tetracycline (1 g/l) may be added if there is purulent peritonitis. The abdomen is closed without drainage unless there is anxiety about the security of perforation closure or frank pus has been present in a specific area of the peritoneal cavity. Antibiotic therapy is usually reserved for specific indications such as proven bacterial peritonitis or significant chest infection.

Definitive ulcer surgery. The role of emergency definitive ulcer surgery remains controversial. Approximately one-third of patients treated by simple closure remain symptom-free and definitive ulcer surgery is contra-indicated when a history of dyspepsia is absent or of only a few weeks duration, and at operation there is a small punched-out perforation without scarring. In patients with a significant dyspeptic history and scarring at operation, definitive surgery is considered if:
1. anaesthetic and surgical facilities are ideal
2. the surgeon is experienced in carrying out definitive ulcer surgery
3. the patient's general condition is such that the extra time needed for definitive surgery does not impose an unacceptable additional risk
4. purulent peritonitis is not present.

The case for definitive emergency surgery is strengthened:
1. when closure of a stenosed duodenum or pylorus would cause obstruction
2. when the patient has had a previous perforation treated by simple closure
3. when the patient has a perforated gastric ulcer and malignancy is suspected
4. when perforation and bleeding occur together.

The definitive operation usually advocated for a perforated duodenal, pyloric or pre-pyloric ulcer is truncal vagotomy with drainage. The choice between pyloroplasty and gastro-enterostomy is dictated by conditions prevailing in the pyloroduodenal area. Where possible the perforation is incorporated in a pyloroplasty, but significant stenosis may mean that simple closure with gastro-enterostomy is preferred. Partial gastrectomy is no longer recommended in this context.

Perforation of a gastric ulcer should always raise the suspicion of malignant ulceration, particularly in the elderly. Given favourable circumstances the preferred operation is partial gastric resection (including the ulcer) with gastroduodenal anastomosis. Given less favourable circumstances it may be wiser to temporise. For example, an elderly patient with perforation of an apparently benign ulcer high on the lesser curve may be better served by excision biopsy of the ulcer margin with simple closure alone, or closure with truncal vagotomy and drainage if definitive surgery is indicated.

Non-operative management
Conservative management of perforated peptic ulcer is now seldom employed. The principal indications are:

1. when the patient is so elderly or infirm that the risks of general anaesthesia and surgery are unacceptably high
2. when the patient presents 24 hours or more after perforation and continuing clinical evaluation suggests that leakage and infection have been contained
3. when adequate surgical and anaesthetic facilities are lacking

Conservative therapy suffers from the disadvantage that the diagnosis may remain in doubt (despite radiology including gastrografin instillation) or the site of perforation and nature of underlying ulceration (peptic or neoplastic) remain uncertain. Conservative management consists of continued nasogastric aspiration, nil by mouth, intravenous fluids, administration of an antisecretory drug such as cimetidine, and appropriate sedation. Antibiotic cover is generally advised and combination of gentamicin and ampicillin may be used. Conservative therapy is abandoned in favour of operation if clinical deterioration suggests continued leakage and worsening peritonitis.

Prognosis
Recognition of the importance of active adequate resuscitation before operation has reduced reported operative mortality from around 25% to as little as 2–5% over the past 50 years. Nevertheless, perforated peptic ulcer remains a potentially dangerous condition particularly in the elderly and those ill from intercurrent disease, and mortality rates recorded in the surgical literature may not represent the general experience. The mortality of conservative management was about 10% when it was applied widely but may be much higher when only the very ill and elderly are managed in this way.

Bleeding gastric or duodenal ulcer

Diagnosis and management
The three cardinal principles of management of patients with upper gastrointestinal bleeding are: (1) vigorous resuscitation to stabilize the circulation and prevent exsanguination, (2) prompt investigation to define the source of bleeding and (3) institution of appropriate measures to arrest bleeding and prevent further haemorrhage. The great majority of patients bleeding from gastritis, erosions or frank peptic ulcers settle when treated conservatively, and it has been traditional to admit all patients to medical rather than surgical wards. In some hospitals these patients are now managed by a 'haematemesis team' of physicians and surgeons, while in other centres all patients are admitted directly to surgical wards. The policy adopted is dictated largely by local circumstances but it is clear that mortality can only be reduced if these patients are managed by experienced

clinicians, if resuscitation and investigation are carried out with a sense of urgency, and if an experienced surgeon is involved from the time of admission so that operation can be undertaken if and when appropriate.

Vigorous resuscitation. Blood is grouped and cross-matched so that 4–6 units are available. A free-flowing line is established to allow *rapid* transfusion; peripheral veins are inadequate for this purpose and a cannula is placed in the subclavian, jugular or basilic veins. If the patient is shocked, plasma or plasma substitute is used until blood is available; otherwise normal saline is infused in the first instance.

A nasogastric tube (FG 16) is passed to keep the stomach empty, prevent vomiting, and monitor continued or renewed bleeding. Pulse and blood pressure are monitored every 15 minutes, a urinary catheter is inserted to monitor hourly output if the patient is shocked, temperature is monitored 4-hourly, and haematocrit is checked daily. A separate central venous pressure (CVP) line (p. 310) is an invaluable guide to the rate of fluid replacement in the elderly and those with myocardial insufficiency. Oxygen is given to all shocked patients at 4 l/min through a well-fitting Hudson mask, unless there are anxieties regarding carbon dioxide retention. Periodic checks on arterial H^+ concentration, pO_2 and pCO_2 are used to monitor gas exchange and detect derangement in acid-base balance.

Impaired haemostasis is anticipated in patients needing massive transfusion and in those with deranged liver function. Stored blood transfusion quickly results in deficiencies of labile factors V and VIII, but these defects can be restored by fresh frozen plasma (FFP–one pack for every 3 litres of blood transfused). Regular clotting screens to determine thrombin time, prothrombin time, kaolin-cephalin coagulation time and platelet count are of value in patients with massive bleeding. Vitamin K_1 is given routinely to all jaundiced patients when prothrombin time is prolonged (5–50 mg i.v.), but FFP is needed in patients with liver disease who are unresponsive to vitamin K (see p. 61).

Prompt investigation. The patient's history and findings on physical examination provide valuable clues to the source of bleeding but can mislead and should be interpreted with caution. Upper gastro-intestinal endoscopy has now replaced barium meal examination as the investigation of choice and defines the source of haemorrhage in 80–90% of emergency admissions. Barium meal examination suffers from the disadvantages that: it defines lesions without necessarily defining whether they are the source of bleeding; may not define mucosal lesions such as gastritis; may make for difficulty in interpretation of subsequent endoscopy or angiography; and may prove difficult to mount as a 24-hour emergency service. Endoscopy should be performed by an experienced endoscopist within 12 hours of admission as the diagnostic yield falls as the interval between admission and endoscopy increases. Ideally, endoscopy is undertaken as soon as the circulatory state has been stabilized, accepting that it may have to be undertaken more urgently in the relatively rare situation where massive continued bleeding threatens exsanguination. It must be admitted that the impact of endoscopy on mortality has been difficult to define, and much of the reduction in mortality in specialized centres is related to vigorous resuscitation and appropriate timing of surgery by experienced clinicians. Nevertheless, accurate diagnosis of the source of bleeding remains a cornerstone of rational management.

Appropriate measures to arrest bleeding. Conservative measures including intensive antacid therapy (e.g. magnesium trisilicate 15–30 ml and alternating hourly with aluminium hydroxide 15–30 ml) and/or cimetidine therapy (e.g. 300–400 mg i.v. 6-hourly) are indicated for patients found to be bleeding from gastritis, duodenitis or erosions. Operative intervention is rarely necessary. On the other hand, medical management appears to have little influence on the risk of continued or further bleeding from frank gastric or duodenal ulceration, and some 10–20% of these patients still require operation. In general the risk of continued or recurrent bleeding is greater in patients with gastric ulcer, in the elderly, and in those who were shocked on admission to hospital. The risk of further bleeding requiring operation increases markedly if certain endoscopic stigmata are present; these include a vessel protruding from the ulcer base, red or black spots in the ulcer base, and evidence of active bleeding or recent haemorrhage in the form of fresh clot.

The decision to undertake surgery and time it correctly requires considerable clinical judgment. Operation is obviously indicated as a matter of urgency in patients who are clearly continuing to bleed; the major problem is posed by patients who appear to settle and then have evidence of further haemorrhage. In general, conservative management is indicated in those who have settled clinically and have no endoscopic evidence of continued bleeding. Operation is usually advised when such patients have clinical evidence of re-bleeding, and the indications for operation are stronger in patients over the age of 55 years. It may appear paradoxical to strengthen the recommendation for surgery in older patients but these are the individuals who are least able to withstand the repeated episodes of re-bleeding. In future, endoscopic techniques such as laser photocoagulation or electrocoagulation may provide an alternative means of arresting haemorrhage but these modes of therapy require further evaluation.

Nature of surgery

Once the decision to operate has been taken, vigorous

resuscitation is continued to counter circulatory insufficiency prior to inducing anaesthesia. Adequate amounts of blood must be available and an experienced anaesthetist is essential. Every effort is made to evacuate the stomach through a wide-bore nasogastric tube and a cuffed endotracheal tube is passed quickly to prevent inhalation of clot and gastric secretion.

The stomach and duodenum are carefully examined for external evidence of ulceration even if endoscopy appears to have defined the source of bleeding. If necessary the lesser sac is opened to inspect the posterior surface of the stomach.

If a *gastric ulcer* is the cause of bleeding, the alternatives are partial gastrectomy including removal of the ulcer, or gastrotomy with undersewing of the bleeding point, excision biopsy of the ulcer margin (to exclude malignancy) and closure of the gastrotomy followed by truncal vagotomy and a drainage procedure. The risks of failing to appreciate that the ulcer is malignant cannot be overemphasized, particularly in elderly patients. In general, partial gastrectomy with Billroth I gastroduodenal anastomosis is preferred given that the patient is in good general condition, the lesion is not situated high on the lesser curve requiring an extensive gastrectomy, and the surgeon has the necessary experience.

For bleeding *duodenal ulcer* the choice lies between Polya partial gastrectomy, truncal vagotomy and antrectomy, or truncal vagotomy with pyloroplasty and underrunning the ulcer base to arrest haemorrhage. Although operations involving gastric resection may carry a lower incidence of re-bleeding, the lesser procedure of truncal vagotomy and pyloroplasty is now preferred by most surgeons. The ulcer is under-run by two or three sutures of strong silk all of which are inserted deeply through the edges and base of the ulcer before being tied (Fig. 17.21). A 'fish hook' needle is particularly helpful where access to the ulcer is difficult.

If the patient is bleeding from *gastritis, duodenitis or*

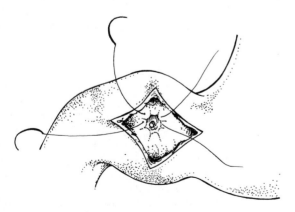

Fig. 17.21 Method of arresting bleeding by under-running the ulcer during the operation of pyloroplasty

erosions operation is necessary only if massive bleeding continues. The interior of the stomach is inspected to confirm that there is no other source of haemorrhage which may have been missed at endoscopy. The choice of operative procedure remains controversial but truncal vagotomy is accepted as an essential component. The risk of re-bleeding is lower if vagotomy is combined with partial gastrectomy and given that the patient's condition is satisfactory, an experienced surgeon may prefer resection to a drainage procedure.

If the cause of bleeding has not been defined endoscopically and no abnormality is apparent on inspecting the surface of the stomach and duodenum, 'blind' partial gastrectomy should not be performed. The interior of the stomach and proximal duodenum are inspected to make certain that an ulcer, neoplasm, area of gastritis, Mallory-Weiss tear or varices have not been missed at endoscopy.

Pyloric stenosis

Patients presenting with pyloric stenosis have frequently lost weight and are dehydrated with metabolic alkalosis. Some days should be spent in preparation and intravenous infusion of normal saline to which potassium chloride is added will counter dehydration, alkalosis and hypokalaemia. A wide-bore nasogastric tube is used to empty the stomach and lavage may be necessary to remove food debris. Operation is undertaken once fluid and electrolyte balance have been restored and truncal vagotomy and pyloroplasty is usually preferred to partial gastrectomy. Where conditions preclude a satisfactory pyloroplasty, gastrojejunostomy is a reasonable alternative.

CARCINOMA OF THE STOMACH

Gastric carcinoma remains a disease of poor prognosis with an overall 5 year survival rate of 5–10%. Five-year survival rates following gastric resection range from 10–25%; when resection is carried out for apparently localized disease they range from 25–50%; and when cancer is confined histologically to the mucosa or submucosa 5-year survival rates are as high as 90%. Few symptomatic patients have such superficial lesions. Indications that the disease is advanced include a growth which is palpable and fixed, palpable metastases in the liver, peritoneum or supraclavicular nodes, ascites, jaundice, and radiological evidence of skeletal or pulmonary metastases. Laparotomy offers little or no prospect of cure in such individuals and although palliative resection or by-pass may prolong life when performed for obstruction, it is doubtful whether palliative surgery otherwise affects survival duration. When radical surgery is contemplated it should be remembered that operative mortality following subtotal gastrectomy is around 3–5% but rises to the order of 10–30% following total gastrectomy.

Choice of operation

The choice of operation is influenced by the findings on clinical examination, the endoscopic findings with regard to extent and histological nature of the lesion, and the findings at laparotomy. When the lesion appears amenable to resection and cure the choice of radical operation lies between subtotal and total gastrectomy. Lesions confined to the distal stomach are treated by radical subtotal gastrectomy with en bloc resection of 80–85% of the stomach and a Polya type of gastro-jejunal anastomosis. The Billroth I procedure is seldom employed as anxieties regarding anastomotic tension may compromise the extent of proximal resection and a 15% incidence of obstruction at the gastroduodenal anastomosis significantly impairs the quality of survival. When the lesion is in the proximal half of the stomach, total gastrectomy is indicated with oesophagojejunal anastomosis to restore intestinal continuity. Malignant lesions at the cardia may be squamous cell carcinoma or adenocarcinoma and deserve special mention. Squamous cell lesions may be regarded as oesophageal lesions which have extended down to the cardia whereas adeno-carcinomas do not differ from lesions of the body of the stomach with regard to their behavioural character-istics. The lymphatics of the oesophagus and stomach are in free continuity across the cardia and upward submucous extension of tumour into the oesophagus frequently exceeds the macroscopic extent of growth. Oesophagogastrectomy is the radical treatment of choice for malignant lesions of the cardia and usually entails total gastrectomy. When the lesion is of the squamous cell type or obviously localized to the cardia, the distal portion of the stomach may be retained for anastomosis to the oesophagus.

Radical operation implies en bloc resection of the greater and lesser omentum with removal of as many regional lymph nodes as possible (p. 336), splenec-tomy, and removal of the first part of the duodenum. The proximal and distal resection lines should be at least 2.5 cm from the tumour margin and when dealing with lesions of the cardia, the line of oesophageal transection must be at least 5 cm above the obvious extent of growth. Even this precaution can prove inadequate and some surgeons request routine frozen section examin-ation of the specimen resection margins before completing the anastomosis. While it is now accepted that survival prospects are dictated more by the presence of distant metastases outwith the reach of radical surgery, local recurrence in or around the anastomosis represents a distressing but often avoidable complication of radical surgery.

When laparotomy reveals that a gastric carcinoma is resectable but incurable, palliative partial gastrectomy is the procedure of choice for distal lesions and offers better prospects for relief of symptoms than anterior gastroenterostomy. Proximal gastric lesions pose greater problems as palliative total gastrectomy is contraindi-cated because of the substantially increased risk of operative mortality and postoperative sequelae if a cuff of stomach is not available for anastomosis to the jejunum. Intubation may be used for obstructing lesions of the cardia (p. 300) or a Roux loop of jejunum may be used for oesophagojejunal anastomosis if the lesion is deemed irremovable (p. 303).

Exploration of the abdomen
Lesions of the distal stomach are dealt with through a long mid-line or paramedian incision. The position and extent of the growth are determined and its degree of fixation to surrounding structures is assessed. The regional nodes in the greater and lesser omentum are examined and both lobes of the liver are inspected and palpated by passing a hand over their surfaces. The parietal peritoneum and mesentery are examined and a hand is passed into the pelvis to detect any tumour deposits.

Lesions in the proximal stomach may be approached in the same way but the optimal approach to lesions of the cardia is through an abdominothoracic incision with the patient placed in the right lateral position. The hips and knees are flexed and the left arm is drawn forwards and upwards (Fig. 17.22). A transverse or obligue incision is made from a point midway between xiphi-sternum and umbilicus to cross the left costal margin,

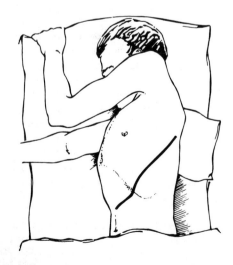

Fig. 17.22 Position of the patient and incision employed for abdominothoracic approach to total gastrectomy

the left rectus sheath and enclosed muscle are divided, and a hand is inserted into the abdomen to determine resectability before opening the chest.

Radical sub-total gastrectomy

The operation is similar to that described for peptic ulceration – except that 80–85% of the stomach is removed, care is taken to remove all involved regional lymph nodes, and the spleen is removed routinely. The greater omentum is first reflected upwards and commencing at the splenic flexure, its avascular attachment to the transverse colon is divided with dissecting scissors. The right gastro-epiploic vessels are divided between ligatures at their origin beneath the pylorus and the subpyloric nodes are dissected so that they remain attached to the portion of gut to be removed. Similarly, the node-bearing tissue in the duodenohepatic pedicle is dissected so that its contained nodes will remain attached to the resection specimen. Following double ligation and division of the right gastric artery the duodenum is transected and its stump oversewn. The lesser omentum is divided as close to the porta hepatis and liver as possible, safeguarding vital structures in its right free border. The coeliac nodes are dissected free and the left gastric artery is divided as close to its origin as possible. The spleen is left attached to the greater curvature by the short gastric vessels but is mobilized

(p. 368) so that the splenic artery and vein can be doubly ligated and divided. On occasions it is advisable to remove the tip of the tail of pancreas to ensure removal of all nodes in the splenic hilus, while extension of posterior wall growths of the stomach may entail distal pancreatectomy. Under these circumstances care is taken to ligate the main pancreatic duct with a silk ligature. The stomach is then divided with construction of an antecolic or retrocolic gastrojejunal anastomosis.

Radical total gastrectomy (Figs. 17.23 & 17.24)

Radical total gastrectomy can be carried out through a long left paramedian incision when the growth does not extend to within 5 cm of cardia and extensive resection of the oesophagus is not required. Mobilization of the lower oesophagus by gentle finger dissection through the diaphragmatic hiatus usually allows some 5–8 cm of oesophagus to be drawn down into the abdomen. Once the stomach has been mobilized, it is turned upwards so that the posterior wall of the oesophagus comes into view. The first loop of jejunum can then be brought up in front or behind the transverse colon to enable oesophagojejunal anastomosis. The author prefers to bring

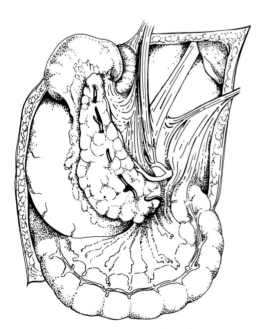

Fig. 17.23 Total gastrectomy by the abdominothoracic approach. The diaphragm has been incised from the rib margin into the oesophageal hiatus. The mobilized spleen and stomach have been turned forwards and to the right exposing the splenic and left gastric arteries at their origin from the coeliac axis

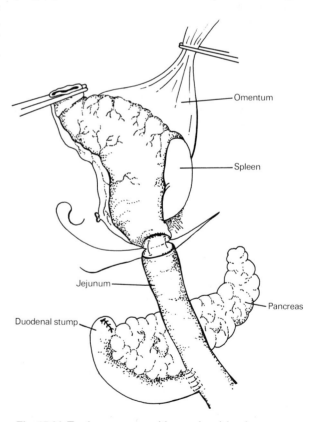

Fig. 17.24 Total gastrectomy with oesophagojejunal anastomosis. The mobilized stomach and spleen have been reflected upwards and a Roux loop of jejunum has been brought up for anastomosis to the oesophagus

a Roux loop of jejunum through a window in the transverse mesocolon and construct an all coats one-layer anastomosis of interrupted 3/0 silk sutures between the end of the oesophagus and side of the jejunum. The GIA Autosuture stapling device is used to facilitate division of the jejunum when constructing the Roux loop and the proximal cut-end of jejunum is implanted into the side of the distal jejunum in the infracolic compartment. There are numerous alternative techniques and many surgeons employ two layers of sutures or use staplers such as the EEA Auto Suture device for the oesophagojejunal anastomosis. Various techniques are described in which a pouch of jejunum is created distal to the anastomosis in the hope of forming a food reservoir (Maingot, 1980) but I do not employ them. It is essential that the anastomosis lies without tension and it is helpful to anchor the jejunum to the undersurface of the diaphragm with some interrupted polyglycolic acid sutures. A nasogastric tube is placed through the anastomosis prior to closure of abdomen and the mesocolic window is closed around the Roux loop.

When the lesion is located at or close to the cardia an abdominothoracic approach is advised. Once resectability has been confirmed, the transverse or oblique abdominal incision is extended over the desired intercostal space or rib as far back as the edge of the erector spinae muscle. Incision through an intercostal space usually allows adequate access and the rib above or below the space can be divided to give greater exposure if required. The choice of intercostal space is dictated largely by convenience and the decision to open the seventh, eighth or ninth space is taken while exploring the abdomen. Some surgeons still prefer to enter the chest through the bed of a rib after periosteal elevation and removal of the rib from behind its angle to the costal margin. Division of the overlying muscles may be attended by considerable blood loss and each bleeding point is ligated or coagulated by diathermy. The cartilage of the costal margin is divided and excision of a few centimetres of the posterior part of the intercostal nerve beneath the resected rib helps to diminish postoperative pain. If rib resection is not employed it is good practice to inject long-acting local anaesthetic (e.g. Marcaine) around the appropriate nerve before closing the incision. The pleural cavity is entered and the wound edges are protected by sterile towels. The intercostal space is opened widely with a large rib spreader as the diaphragm is incised down to the oesophageal hiatus. Diaphragmatic vessels including the inferior phrenic artery require ligation as the diaphragm is divided. Adhesions to the lung base and the lower part of the pulmonary ligament are divided so that the lung can be retracted upwards. The stomach is mobilized as described above and the lower oesophagus is freed through a longitudinal incision in the pleura between aorta and

pericardium. There may be one or two small oesophageal arteries passing forward and downwards from the aorta but one should only divide vessels essential for adequate oesophageal mobilization. The oesophagus is encircled by a tape which can be used for retraction. Division of the diaphragm is now completed but a ring of diaphragm may have to be removed if the growth is adherent.

Total gastrectomy with oesophagojejunal anastomosis is usually performed but some growths of the cardia can be dealt with by anastomosing the oesophagus to the retained distal portion of stomach. Numerous techniques for oesophagogastric anastomosis are available; it is my own practice to transect the stomach with a TA90 Auto Suture stapling device and use one layer of all coats interrupted sutures of silk to implant the oesophagus in the anterior wall of the gastric pouch. If oesophagogastric anastomosis is employed it is important to mobilize the duodenum thoroughly and it is advisable to carry out a simple pyloric myotomy (as in the Ramstedt operation) or pyloroplasty to avoid gastric stasis.

The diaphragm is closed with interrupted stout linen or polyglycolic acid sutures. An intercostal drainage catheter is placed in the dependent part of the pleural cavity for subsequent underwater seal drainage and the lung is reinflated. Closure commences with the posterior rectus sheath and peritoneum, followed by the pleura and intercostal muscles, and then by the anterior rectus sheath, thoracic muscles and skin. Polyglycolic acid sutures (gauge 0) can be used to re-approximate the edges of the costal margin.

SARCOMAS OF THE STOMACH

Sarcomatous lesions account for only 1–3% of malignant gastric lesions. Most gastric sarcomas arise from lymphoid tissue or smooth muscle (leiomyosarcoma) but rare examples arise from other tissues (e.g. fibrosarcoma, haemangeiopericytoma, neurofibrosarcoma). Lymphoid tumours are more often manifestations of systemic lymphoma than primary localized gastric lymphomas.

All patients thought to have gastric lymphoma should undergo laparotomy unless investigation shows diffuse systemic involvement with positive bone marrow biopsy. Unless diffuse metastatic disease is obvious the gastric lesion is excised radically as described for carcinoma. A full staging laparotomy is also indicated with added wedge biopsy of both lobes of liver, biopsy of glands in the para-aortic and iliac chains, and use of Ligaclips to mark the splenic pedicle and gland biopsy sites for subsequent radiographic identification. The patient should be considered for postoperative radiotherapy, particularly in the lymphocyte predominant type of lesion. Chemotherapy is reserved for patients with diffuse systemic involvement or recurrence after irradiation.

Other forms of gastric sarcoma are also treated by radical excision whenever possible. These neoplasms are usually radioresistant but improved survival has been reported following the use of adjuvant combination chemotherapy.

MINOR GASTRIC OPERATIONS

Gastrotomy

Gastrotomy may be used to remove benign gastric neoplasms or sharp foreign bodies or bezoars which are unlikely to pass spontaneously. The stomach is delivered through a small upper mid-line incision, surrounded by packs, and its anterior wall is incised longitudinally between stay sutures or Babcock's forceps. The offending lesion or agent is removed and the gastric wall is closed with two layers of continuous polyglycolic acid sutures.

Gastrostomy

The indications for gastrostomy have decreased in recent years. Gastrostomy was never a satisfactory form of palliation for patients with obstructing gastric or oeso- phageal neoplasms and some form of by-pass operation or intubation with a Celestin tube is preferred so that the patient can swallow. In the context of feeding, parenteral nutrition and the long-term use of non- irritant fine-bore nasogastric or naso-enteric tubes (see Fig. 15.1) has reduced the need for feeding gastros- tomy or jejunostomy. Gastrostomy is still useful as an alternative to nasogastric intubation when protracted gastrointestinal hold up is anticipated, as for example in patients with severe acute pancreatitis and its compli- cations, and is also used as a temporary measure in pa- tients with trauma or acute inflammation of the pharynx or oesophagus.

The operation can be carried out under local or general anaesthesia. A small mid-line or left subcostal incision is used and two pairs of Babcock's tissue forceps are applied to the anterior gastric wall on either side of a point midway between the greater and lesser curve. The stomach is incised to allow insertion of a FG 12–14 Foley catheter, the ballon of which is then inflated. Leakage alongside the catheter is minimized in one of two ways. In *Stamm's method* two purse string sutures of polyglycolic acid are inserted at distances of one and two centimetres from the tube. When drawn tight these sutures create an 'inkwell' effect with invagination of the

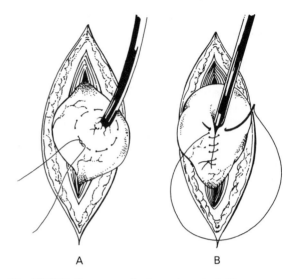

Fig. 17.25(A) Gastrostomy by Stamm's method. The purse string suture closest to the tube has been tied, and the second purse string has been inserted and is about to be tied.
(B) Gastrostomy by Witzel's method showing the tube being buried in a tunnel of stomach wall by continuous suture

catheter. In *Witzel's method* a valve is created by burying the tube in a short tunnel in the stomach wall (Fig. 17.25). The tube is usually brought through a stab incision in the anterior abdominal wall and interrupted sutures are used to anchor the stomach to the posterior rectus sheath and parietal peritoneum.

Gastrostomy in children

In paediatric surgery a gastrostomy is normally a temporary procedure performed in a baby either to provide gastric decompression after surgery for a congenital high intestinal obstruction or to allow feeding during a staged operation for oesophageal atresia.

Unless the abdomen has previously been opened a transverse incision three centimetres long is made in the left hypochondrium. Two concentric purse string su- tures are placed high in the anterior wall of the stomach. The wall is then incised with a pointed scalpel, the mar- gins of the opening are held apart with forceps so that a 10 Malecot catheter can be introduced with ease and the sutures are tied so as to invaginate the stomach wall around the catheter. The stem of the catheter is then brought out through a separate stab wound, the stomach wall sewn to parietal peritoneum around the catheter to prevent leakage and the incision is closed in layers. Finally the catheter should be withdrawn so that the bulbous expansion lies flush against the inner aspect of the stomach wall and the stem of the catheter fixed to abdominal skin with a silk suture. Unless adequately se- cured the catheter may be passed down the stomach to obstruct the pylorus.

CONGENITAL CONDITIONS

Congenital hypertrophic pyloric stenosis
This condition presents in babies within the first 5 weeks of life. Boys are four times more commonly affected than girls and the first born child is relatively at risk. The circular muscle of the pylorus is hypertrophied to produce a fusiform tumour between 1 and 2 centimetres in diameter causing partial or complete occlusion of the pyloric canal.

Diagnosis
The classical features of pyloric stenosis are forceful vomiting after feeds, visible gastric peristalsis and a palpable pyloric tumour. At the start of the illness the baby is otherwise healthy, but with time becomes progressively weaker from lack of nourishment and fluid loss. Both gastric peristalsis and the pyloric tumour become more obvious when the baby is fed. The tumour is most easily felt when the nurse feeding the baby sits with the infant cradled in the left arm, the surgeon sits on the left side of the nurse and palpates the baby's abdomen with the left hand. The middle finger of the left hand is placed over the right rectus muscle, half way between the xiphisternum and umbilicus and pressed both deep and medially. The tumour has a characteristic feel, likened to the tip of the nose.

Pre-operative care. The baby's fitness for surgery is assessed and any dehydration or electrolyte imbalance corrected by intravenous infusion. A nasogastric tube is passed to allow gastric lavage and free drainage of stomach content.

Pyloromyotomy—Ramstedt's operation
The purpose of the operation is to split the hypertrophied muscle in the long axis of the pylorus leaving the underlying mucosa intact. The procedure is normally carried out under general anaesthetic but local anaesthesia is a practical alternative.

According to preference a small transverse (Fig. 17.26) or longitudinal incision is made in the right upper quadrant of the abdomen and the peritoneum opened through a rectus muscle splitting approach. The liver lies well below the costal margin in the new-born and must be retracted upwards. The stomach wall, which lies deep and medial to the incision, is lifted through the wound with blunt dissecting forceps and held with the aid of a wet gauze swab. The proximal part of the stomach is drawn down through the wound to provide extra mobility which allows the pylorus to be delivered with greater ease. The thickened pylorus is pinched between the finger and thumb so as to stretch the anterior wall and a 2 mm incision is made along the full

Figs. 17.26–17.30 *Pyloromyotomy for congenital pyloric stenosis*

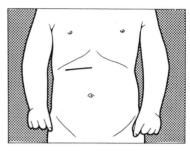

Fig. 17.26 Transverse incision high in right upper quadrant of abdomen

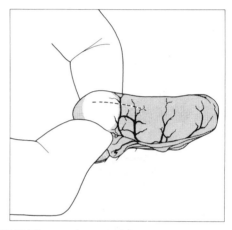

Fig. 17.27 The posterior part of the tumour pinched with finger and thumb to stretch the antimesenteric border. Dotted line indicates incision

length of the tumour in the avascular upper border (Fig. 17.27). The points of blunt curved artery forceps are introduced into the incision and spread from side to side to split the brittle muscle down to mucosa (Fig. 17.28). The remaining fibres can be broken with a blunt dissector. Care is taken not to damage the mucosa, particularly distally where the fornix of the duodenum lies close to the serosal surface (Fig. 17.29). When the dissection is complete the mucosa bulges freely into the base of the incision (Fig. 17.30). Main bleeding points are coagulated with diathermy. The more general ooze from venous congestion will stop when the stomach is returned to the abdominal cavity. Finally the wound is closed in layers.

Postoperative care. A healthy breast fed baby can be suckled 4 hours after operation and a bottle fed baby offered Dextrose Saline. In both it may be possible to establish a normal feeding pattern within 24 hours. However, vomiting after pyloromyotomy is common and a more gradual approach may be needed. A debilitated baby should be maintained by intravenous infusion until oral feeding has been well established.

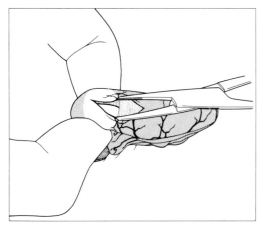

Fig. 17.28 Mosquito artery forceps introduced into incision and spread so as to split the hypertrophied muscle

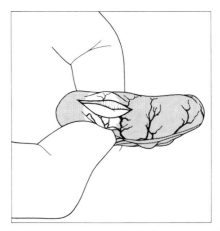

Fig. 17.30 Pyloromyotomy completed. Intact mucosa bulges into base of incision

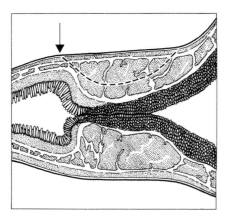

Fig. 17.29 Cross section of hypertrophied pyloric muscle and line of incision. Arrow indicates the point where special care must be taken to avoid penetration of the mucosa

Duodenal atresia and stenosis

The incidence of duodenal atresia and stenosis is 1 per 6000 live births. The lumen of the duodenum develops in the embryo between 6 and 8 weeks after a period of mucosal proliferation and recanalization and the anomaly is probably established at this early stage. The duodenum is usually occluded at the level of the ampulla. The stomach and proximal duodenum are grossly hypertrophied and dilated and the duodenum distal to the obstruction is narrow. Although a wedge of pancreas may partly encircle the narrowed segment of duodenum, annular pancreas probably exists as a separate entity. If the obstructed duodenum has a normal outward appearance a mucosal diaphragm may be present.

Clinical presentation

There is a high incidence of associated abnormalities, 25% of babies having Down's Syndrome. Half of the babies with duodenal atresia are of low birth weight and maternal hydramnios is common. The presenting signs are copious vomiting which may be bile stained depending on the level of the lesion and either constipation or the passage of small, pale meconium plugs. In addition there may be a fullness in the epigastrium due to the dilated stomach and visible peristalsis. An erect abdominal X-ray will demonstrate the classical double bubble appearance of gas lying above one fluid level in the stomach and a second fluid level in the first part of the duodenum. For immediate management a nasogastric tube should be passed to prevent vomiting, an intravenous infusion established and the baby nursed in an incubator.

Treatment

At operation the obstructed segment is usually bypassed with a duodenoduodenostomy between dilated and narrowed duodenum immediately above and below the lesion. However, when the atresic segment is more extensive a duodenojejunostomy may be necessary. Gastrojejunostomy should be avoided because of stasis and ulceration in the proximal duodenum. As there may be a considerable delay in gastric emptying after operation a gastrostomy should be performed. In the absence of an atresic segment a mucosal diaphragm should be considered and this may be demonstrated when an attempt is made to pass a tube through a gastrostomy and down through the duodenum. The duodenum can then be opened longitudinally, the mucosal diaphragm excised circumferentially and the duodenum closed transversely.

As the baby is unlikely to feed normally for 2 or 3 weeks full nutritional needs should be provided early in the postoperative period either by intravenous feeding or, preferably, by giving milk through a fine transanastomotic silastic line introduced alongside the gastrostomy tube.

REFERENCES

Alexander-Williams J 1981 Duodenogastric reflux after gastric operations. British Journal of Surgery 68: 685

De Vries B C et al 1983 Prospective randomised multicentre trial of proximal gastric vagotomy or truncal vagotomy and antrectomy for chronic duodenal ulcer: results after 5–7 years. British Journal of Surgery 70: 701

Duthie H L 1970 Vagotomy for gastric ulcer. Gut 11: 540

Fawcett A N, Johnston D, Duthie H L 1969 Revagotomy for recurrent ulcer after vagotomy and drainage for duodenal ulcer. British Journal of Surgery 56: 111

Goligher J C, Pulvertaft C N, de Dombal F T et al 1968 Five- to eight-year results of Leeds-York controlled trial of elective surgery for duodenal ulcer. British Medical Journal 2: 781

Goligher J C, Pulvertaft C B, Irvin T T et al 1972 Clinical comparison of vagotomy and pyloroplasty with other forms of elective surgery for duodenal ulcer. British Medical Journal 2: 787

Goligher J C 1974 A technique for highly selective (parietal cell or proximal gastric) vagotomy for duodenal ulcer. British Journal of Surgery 61: 337

Hobsley M 1981 Dumping and diarrhoea. British Journal of Surgery 68: 681

Johnston D 1975 Operative mortality and post-operative morbidity of highly selective vagotomy. British Medical Journal 4: 545

Kennedy F, McKay C, Bedi B S, Kay A W 1973 Truncal vagotomy and drainage for chronic duodenal ulcer; a controlled trial. British Medical Journal 2: 71

Maingot R 1980 Subdiaphragmatic total gastrectomy for malignant lesions of the stomach. In: Maingot R (ed) Abdominal operations, 7th edn. Appleton Century Crofts, New York, ch 39, p 597

McGuigan J E, Wolfe M M 1980 Secretin injection test in the diagnosis of gastrinoma. Gastroenterology 79: 1324

Stabile B E, Passaro E Jr 1976 Recurrent peptic ulcer. Gastroenterology 70: 124

Taylor T V, Gunn A A, Macleod D A D, MacLennan I 1982 Anterior lesser curve seromyotomy and posterior truncal vagotomy in the treatment of chronic duodenal ulcer. Lancet 2: 846

Taylor T V, Holt S, Heading R C 1985 Gastric emptying after anterior lesser curve seromyotomy and posterior truncal vagotomy. British Journal of Surgery 72: 620

FURTHER READING

Carter D C 1983 Peptic Ulcer. In: Clinical Surgery International, Vol 7. Churchill Livingstone, Edinburgh

18

The spleen and portal hypertension

C. V. RUCKLEY

Anatomy

The spleen lies between the fundus of the stomach and the diaphragm under cover of the left 9th, 10th and 11th ribs, its long axis being in the line of the 10th. Normally it lies entirely behind the midaxillary line, and does not project below the costal margin.

Its convex medial surface is related to the fundus of the stomach and the tail of the pancreas in front, and to the upper part of the left kidney behind. Its lower part is in contact with the left colic (splenic) flexure.

Peritoneal connections

The spleen is almost completely invested by peritoneum. At its hilum it is connected to the upper part of the greater curvature of the stomach by the *gastrosplenic ligament (omentum)*, and to the posterior abdominal wall in front of the left kidney by the *lienorenal ligament*. These ligaments each consist of two layers, one layer being formed by peritoneum of the lesser sac (Fig. 18.1).

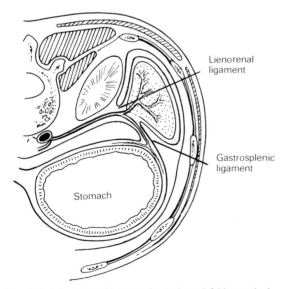

Lienorenal
ligament

Gastrosplenic
ligament

Stomach

Fig. 18.1 Diagram to illustrate the peritoneal folds attached to the spleen, and their contained blood vessels

Vessels

The splenic vessels are large in proportion to the size of the organ, and are very thin-walled. The *splenic artery* arises from the coeliac, and runs a tortuous course to the left along the upper border of the pancreas, crossing the front of the left kidney; it reaches the spleen between the layers of the lienorenal ligament, and divides into five to eight branches which enter the hilum. Other branches, the *short gastric* and *left gastro-epiploic arteries*, pass onwards between the layers of the gastro-splenic ligament to reach the stomach. The *splenic vein* runs to the right behind the pancreas, and joins the superior mesenteric vein to form the portal vein; its tributaries correspond to the branches of the artery.

INDICATIONS FOR SPLENECTOMY

The conditions for which removal of the spleen may be required fall naturally into four main groups:

1. Rupture of the spleen

This is one of the commoner intraperitoneal injuries which may result from blows or crushes to the abdomen. In cases where the spleen is enlarged from disease, rupture may result from comparatively minor injuries. The spleen may be injured also in association with penetrating abdominal wounds. In a typical case signs of increasing intraperitoneal haemorrhage are present, and operation should be undertaken without delay, since it offers the only chance of recovery.

Delayed rupture

This equally dangerous condition may arise when the damage to the spleen is less severe. The laceration may then become temporarily sealed-off by omentum or by blood clot, or the bleeding may at first be confined within the capsule of the organ. In such cases the initial shock may be relieved by treatment and all symptoms subside. After a period of several days (or even of 2 or 3 weeks) symptoms suddenly recur; signs of serious intraperitoneal haemorrhage develop, and the case at once becomes of the gravest urgency. Splenic suture has been recommended in order to conserve the spleen, but is rarely possible for a blunt injury (Chadwick, 1985). Splenectomy is usually required in order to control haemorrhage.

2. Other conditions related to the spleen itself

Cysts, tuberculous infection, abscesses and tumours are rare in the spleen, but when they are confined to that organ, splenectomy should be carried out.

Aneurysm of the splenic artery

This is occasionally encountered, and may be a cause of sudden internal haemorrhage. The diagnosis is made usually at laparotomy in cases where rupture has already occurred. Treatment consists in splenectomy, combined with ligature of the artery on both sides of the aneurysm.

Abnormal mobility of the spleen

This may occur as part of a generalized visceroptosis. When symptoms are referable to the spleen alone splenectomy should be considered. This may be required urgently if torsion of the pedicle occurs.

Total gastrectomy and upper partial gastrectomy

The spleen is usually removed as part of the resection, since this gives better access and allows more radical clearance of the glandular fields. Splenectomy may be included also in the operation of pancreatectomy.

3. Splenomegaly associated with blood dyscrasia

Enlargement of the spleen frequently co-exists in association with various altered conditions of the blood. The enlargement may occur because of congestion of the pulp cords, congestion of the venous sinuses, hyperplasia of the lymphatic tissue or hyperplasia of the red pulp. In some cases, more than one cause may be present. When red blood cells are abnormal, either congenitally as in *congenital spherocytosis*, or from acquired causes (*autoimmune haemolytic anaemia*), the passage of the red cell through the pulp cords is slowed, the cell becomes more fragile and its survival time is reduced. In these haemolytic anaemias the spleen is moderately enlarged because of pulp congestion. In portal hypertension, congestion of the venous sinuses occurs and is accompanied by proliferation of the cellular elements of the spleen. In the bulk of such an enlarged spleen sequestration of erythrocytes, granulocytes and platelets may occur, giving rise to considerable reduction in their numbers in the circulating blood (*hypersplenism*). Lymphatic hyperplasia occurs in the lymphoproliferative diseases and may give rise to a very large spleen with associated hypersplenism. Red pulp hyperplasia is found

in infections, especially with parasites such as leishmaniasis and chronic malaria (*tropical splenomegaly*).

Haemolytic anaemia

In the condition of *congenital spherocytosis* there is an abnormal fragility of the red blood cells, which pass into the circulation in an immature form. In such cases splenectomy is, as a rule, most successful (Devlin, 1970). Although the red cell fragility is usually unaltered by the operation, the excessive blood destruction is arrested, and in most cases lasting cure, both of the anaemia and of the jaundice, is obtained. The optimum time to perform the operation is in late childhood or early adolescence, before liver changes have occurred. Performed in early childhood splenectomy is liable to be followed by acute and very serious infection (Cooper, 1984). The operation is uniformly and permanently successful in relieving the anaemia although the red blood cell abnormality persists (Macpherson, 1973). The gall bladder should be inspected at the time of the splenectomy, and, if calculi are present, they should be removed by cholecystectomy or cholecystostomy; at the same time, the common bile duct should be examined by cholangiography and explored if necessary. In the acquired type of haemolytic anaemia, when the cause cannot be discovered and is, therefore, incapable of control, splenectomy is usually undertaken because of the failure of reasonable doses of corticosteroids to control the haemolysis. Experience shows however that the operation is less effective than in the congenital forms of the disease.

Idiopathic thrombocytopenic purpura

Splenectomy is followed by cessation of abnormal bleeding and restoration of the platelet count to normal in 60 to 80% of cases, the better results being obtained in cases with a short history. The initial treatment should be with corticosteroids up to a maximum of three weeks. Splenectomy is indicated in that time in short history cases and in all those with a long history of repeated relapses. At operation the discovery and removal of accessory spleens is of importance, since these may be responsible for a recurrence of the condition (Holme, 1984).

Other conditions

There are certain other diseases of the blood and reticulo-endothelial system where splenectomy is occasionally (but by no means consistently) successful. When anaemia is present, from whatever cause, splenectomy, by slowing down the rate of blood destruction, may have markedly beneficial effects. Even in conditions such as Hodgkin's disease, Gaucher's disease, and reticulosarcoma, in which splenomegaly with hypersplenism is often a feature, it may be justifiable to recommend splenectomy. Splenectomy is part of 'staging laparotomy' for Hodgkin's disease. The operation includes careful dissection and biopsy of retroperitoneal glands and wedge biopsy taken from both lobes of the liver. Hypersplenism is in fact the main indication for splenectomy even where the primary disease is almost inevitably fatal. Although the operation cannot influence the final outcome of the disease, it may have considerable palliative value by slowing down the rate of blood destruction. Restoration of the blood count to normal often produces a worthwhile effect until such time as the marrow is overwhelmed by invading cells.

4. Congestive splenomegaly (portal hypertension)
Splenectomy in this condition is considered on page 373.

TECHNIQUE OF SPLENECTOMY

Preparation

In nearly all patients requiring splenectomy, blood transfusion, both before and during operation, is valuable if not essential. In cases of ruptured spleen a delay of 1 to 2 hours, especially when used for resuscitation, is not associated with an increased mortality (Sargison, 1968). In the absence of transfusion facilities, the circulation may be temporarily sustained by infusion of dextran or plasma, to be followed by whole blood as soon as this is available.

Incision

The best access to the spleen is obtained by a left rectus-splitting paramedian incision or by an oblique subcostal incision. The first incision may be extended laterally by a transverse cut which divides the outer fibres of the rectus muscle. In cases of ruptured spleen, the abdomen will often have been opened in the midline; this incision, extended laterally if necessary, should give adequate access. If a right paramedian incision has been employed, it may be best to close this and to make a left subcostal incision.

Mobilization of spleen

A hand is passed over the lateral surface of the spleen, between it and the diaphragm; the organ is lifted forwards and medially, and the posterior layer of the lienorenal ligament, which passes from it to the posterior abdominal wall and holds it in position, is divided under vision. The underlying fascia is also divided but the knife must not pass too deeply or the vessels may be wounded. Adequate exposure for this dissection is obtained by strong retraction of the left side of the wound while the spleen is drawn medially (Fig. 18.2). When

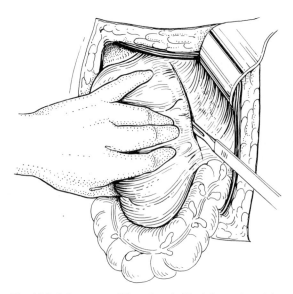

Fig. 18.2 Splenectomy. The spleen is lifted forwards and is mobilized by incision of the peritoneum passing from its lateral surface on to the posterior abdominal wall, i.e. the posterior layer of the lienorenal ligament

the spleen is enlarged numerous vascular adhesions may be encountered. These are divided, if possible, under the guidance of the eye, and all haemorrhage arrested. Next, the gastrosplenic ligament (omentum), stretching between the spleen and the upper part of the greater

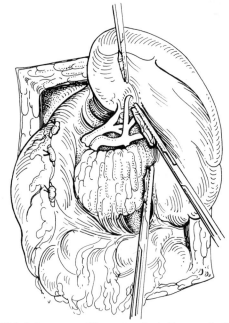

Fig. 18.3 Splenectomy. The gastrosplenic ligament is divided between clamps and ligatured. The thin anterior layer of the lienorenal ligament is then incised to expose the splenic vessels and the tail of the pancreas

curvature, is divided between clamps (Fig. 18.3). This fold contains the short gastric vessels which require to be ligatured. The spleen can then be delivered easily into the wound and the tail of the pancreas is carefully separated from the splenic hilum. Both the fundus of the stomach and the left colic flexure lie in contact with the spleen and must be safeguarded, all avascular fascial connections being divided. The splenic vessels are now exposed and may be approached from in front or behind, the latter usually being safer and easier. The artery and vein are ligatured individually.

Division of splenic vessels
The tail of the pancreas, which may partially obscure the vessels, is gently thrust aside by gauze stripping. A finger is passed behind the vascular pedicle, and the artery and vein are divided separately between clamps or ligatures. Gentle handling is most essential, since the vessels are exceptionally delicate and are easily torn. In Hodgkin's disease, the pedicle is marked by a wire suture for subsequent radiographic identification.

Technique in cases of rupture
When splenectomy is being performed for rupture, a less deliberate exposure of the vascular pedicle is permissible. The spleen is delivered at the wound as rapidly as possible, and a hot moist pack is placed behind it. The combined pedicle—peritoneal and vascular—is then clamped and divided *in small sections at a time*, from below upwards. To obviate the risk of injury to neighbouring organs (particularly the tail of the pancreas), the clamps are applied as close as possible to the hilum.

Search for accessory spleniculi
This is essential when splenectomy is being performed for conditions of hypersplenism; otherwise the spleniculi may enlarge and give rise to recurrence. A single spleniculus may be more or less continuous with the main spleen at either pole or at the hilum, being separated from it only by a constriction. Alternatively, one or more entirely separate spleniculi may be found within the layers of the gastrosplenic ligament.

Peritoneal toilet and closure
When the spleen has been removed, both the pedicle and the splenic bed are examined carefully, and bleeding points are dealt with, either by ligature or by underrunning suture. Drainage is necessary if there has been damage to the tail of the pancreas, or if haemorrhage has not been completely arrested.

Difficulties and complications
Operative difficulties arise in cases where the spleen is enlarged and concern mainly the management of adhesions, since these are easily torn and may bleed alarmingly. For this reason the exposure must be adequate, so that all steps of the operations can be carried out under the guidance of the eye. If haemorrhage cannot be arrested, a gauze pack should be left in position against the bleeding surface.

When severe anaemia is present blood transfusion may be required postoperatively. If the pancreas has been injured, sloughing of the wound may result from the escape of proteolytic enzymes.

Thrombosis may occur after splenectomy, owing to the temporary increase in the platelet content. Treatment is by anticoagulant therapy.

Combined abdominothoracic approach
Technical difficulties in the removal of a grossly enlarged spleen result mainly from inadequate access. Vascular adhesions on its diaphragmatic and posterior surfaces are a source of danger unless dealt with under direct vision, and this may be impossible from a purely abdominal approach.

A combined abdominothoracic approach obviates these difficulties. The abdomen is explored first, and the incision is then prolonged upwards and backwards through the 8th intercostal space as far as the posterior axillary line, the costal margin being divided at the junction of 8th and 9th cartilages. The pleura is opened, and the diaphragm is incised in the same line. Wide retraction is then obtained by a rib-spreader, so that the entire diaphragmatic surface of the spleen is exposed. All adhesions can now be divided under direct vision, and the vessels secured with ease.

This combined approach is well tolerated. The ease of access, and the safer performance of a difficult splenectomy, compensate for the additional time required to make and close the incision. Indeed some surgeons now advise this method as routine in all cases where the spleen is more than moderately enlarged.

PORTAL HYPERTENSION

Increased pressure in the portal circulation, usually associated with enlargement of the spleen is due to an obstruction between the venous drainage of the gastrointestinal tract and the heart. In practice the obstruction is usually situated in the portal system of veins. *Intrahepatic obstruction* is by far the most common and is due usually to cirrhosis of the liver in which the fibrotic changes have led to obliteration of the branches of the portal vein within that organ. *Prehepatic obstruction* occurs in the portal or splenic veins and is found most frequently in children although it may first manifest itself in adult life. It may be due to a congenital abnormality of the affected vein or, more commonly, to thrombosis occurring some years before the onset of symptoms.

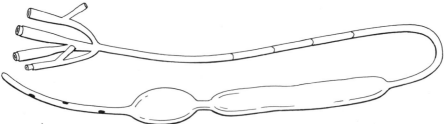

Fig. 18.4 Minnesota tube

Umbilical vein sepsis in the new-born is the commonest cause of such thrombosis. Splenic enlargement and bleeding into the alimentary tract are the only features in the early stages; later atrophic changes develop in the liver. *Posthepatic obstruction* is rare except in tropical countries.

The main effect of portal hypertension is to cause gross engorgement of the anastomosing veins which connect the portal and systemic circulations. This is evidenced particularly by the development of oesophageal varices from which traumatic and devastating haemorrhage can occur. Some 40–50% of cirrhotic patients die from their first haemorrhage. Other effects are splenomegaly; anaemia, leucopenia and thrombocytopenia, due mainly to pooling of blood in the spleen (hypersplenism); and ascites.

Conservative treatment of oesophageal haemorrhage
Bleeding can usually be controlled in the first instance by rest, transfusion, pitressin etc. or by passing a Minnesota tube (Fig. 18.4) which is designed to occlude the varices by direct pressure from a spherical balloon in the stomach and a cylindrical balloon in the lower oesophagus. There are separate channels for aspiration of the stomach beyond the gastric balloon and the oesophagus above the oesophageal balloon. The latter is especially important because of the ever present danger of aspiration. The balloons should not be left inflated for more than 24 hours; the tube is removed 24 hours later if bleeding has not occurred. Should these measures fail to control the bleeding, or should it recur soon after removal of the tube alternative nonoperative measures are available. The first of these is endoscopic sclerotherapy which has gained increased recent popularity following the development of fibroptic endoscopic instruments (Clark, 1980).

An alternative nonoperative method is transhepatic embolization of the left gastric and short gastric veins. This is a highly specialized radiological technique in which a selective catheter is inserted percutaneously through the liver into an intrahepatic branch of the portal vein. The catheter having been guided into the appropriate vein small portions of gelatin sponge soaked in sclerosing material are injected. This has proved to be an excellent method of arresting haemorrhage al-

though it cannot be regarded as a long-term solution (Henderson, 1979).

The development of these techniques means that emergency operative intervention for oesophageal haemorrhage in portal hypertension is less often required than hitherto. Such operations take the form of oesophageal transection rather than portal decompression which nowadays is seldom performed on an emergency basis.

Oesophageal transection
Earlier transthoracic operations, such as the Boerema-Crile and the Milnes Walker procedures have given way to oesophageal stapling (Spence, 1985) as the standard surgical method for the emergency control of oesophageal bleeding (Fig. 18.5). The great advantage of this technique is its avoidance of the need for a thoracic approach in a group of very ill patients. The abdomen is opened through an upper midline incision. The use of

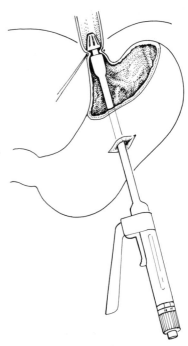

Fig. 18.5 Oesophageal stapling. The staple gun is inserted through a gastrotomy

a manubriosternal elevator as employed in highly selective vagotomy greatly assists exposure. The overlying peritoneum is incised transversely at the point at which it is reflected from the anterior surface of the oesophagus onto the under surface of the diaphragm. The lower oesophagus is mobilized by blunt dissection preserving at least one vagus nerve. A longitudinal incision is made on the anterior surface of the body of the stomach to allow insertion of the stapler. A No. 1 silk ligature is applied round the lower oesophagus approximately 2 cm above the oesophagogastric junction. It is tied to invaginate a cuff of the oesophageal wall between the two halves of the stapling capsule. The stapler is then closed to excise the core of the oesophageal wall and at the same time effect anastomosis with two rows of staples. The staple gun is carefully and gently withdrawn through the anastomosis and the gastrotomy. The latter is closed in routine fashion. The core of oesophageal wall is inspected for completeness. This simple procedure is highly successful in the majority of patients. Occasionally oesophageal stricture develops which may require dilatation at a later date.

Decompression operations

Survival in portal hypertension is determined mainly by the quality of liver function. The operative mortality in Child's (1957) groups A and B is in the region of 5%, whereas in group C it is around 40%. These facts together with the improvements in conservative measures (patients may be very successfully maintained with regular sclerotherapy see Clark, 1980) means that surgeons now tend to be selective in offering decompression operations. Such operations cannot reverse pathological changes in the liver but they may effectively prevent further haemorrhages, which in themselves are a serious menace to life.

There are two types of operations available: total and selective portalsystemic shunts.

Mesenteric arteriography is a valuable investigation if portal decompression is contemplated. It displays the arterial anatomy which may influence the choice of operation (an aberrant hepatic artery may contraindicate portocaval shunt) and, in its venous phase, outlines the portal venous system. If more information is required this may be obtained by either *transhepatic or transplenic venography*. Portal pressures can be measured at the same examination.

Total shunts

Those in which the whole of the portal system is decompressed by anastomosis of a systemic vein. This includes portacaval, mesocaval and proximal splenorenal shunts. Portacaval and mesocaval shunts result in diversion of the blood from the liver through a wide channel. It is associated with a low incidence of recurrent bleeding (10–20%) but a relatively high rate of encephalopathy (approximately 30% in Child's groups A and B). Splenorenal shunt is mainly indicated when there is hypersplenism necessitating removal of the spleen. The anastomosis being of smaller bore it is more liable to thrombosis and therefore to recurrence of oesophageal haemorrhage which occurs in 20–30% but the incidence of encephalopathy is slightly lower than after portacaval anastomosis.

Selective shunt

This concept introduced by Warren (1967) involves decompression of the veins draining the oesophagus without deviation of portal flow from the liver. The main objective is to reduce the incidence of postoperative encephalopathy while decompressing the source of haemorrhage. The spleen is not removed. The splenic end of the divided splenic vein is anastomosed to the left renal vein. By division of left gastric, gastro-epiploic and umbilical veins, the splenic part is further separated from the remainder of the portal system. This is a technically more demanding operation than any variety of total shunt and should not be attempted by an inexperienced surgeon.

Portacaval anastomosis

An extended transverse right subcostal or, provided the patient is not obese or the liver greatly enlarged, a right paramedian incision give satisfactory access. The advantage of the latter is that it is also suitable for a mesocaval shunt should technical difficulty arise. The second part of the duodenum is reflected and the inferior vena cava exposed by incision of the overlying peritoneum. Its anterior surface is exposed from the caudate lobe to the level of the renal veins. The portal vein is exposed in the posterior part of the free border of the lesser omentum and is mobilized as far as possible. It is divided close to the liver and the upper stump is ligated. The lower end is implanted end-to-side into the inferior vena cava which has been partially occluded by an atraumatic clamp (Fig. 18.6).

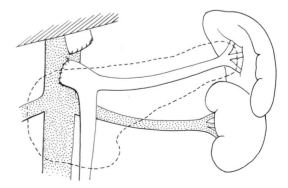

Fig. 18.6 Total shunt: end-to-side portacaval anastomosis

Proximal (standard) splenorenal anastomosis

The operation comprises an anastomosis between the splenic and left renal veins, splenectomy having been performed. It is best carried out through a left thoraco-abdominal incision but a long subcostal incision has proved to be equally satisfactory. After the spleen has been removed the splenic vein is dissected out of its bed in the pancreas, its tributaries being divided between ligatures. The peritoneum over the left kidney is incised so that the renal artery and a segment of the vein may be controlled. An end-to-side anastomosis between the splenic vein and the left renal vein is carried out (Fig. 18.7).

Mesocaval anastomosis

This is probably the easiest procedure for the inexperienced surgeon and the results are not significantly different from those of portacaval shunt. Through a midline incision the superior mesenteric vein is exposed at the lower border of the third part of the duodenum and by direct dissection through the posterior peritoneum the adjacent inferior vena cava exposed. A 20 mm woven or knitted Dacron graft is anastomosed as a bridge between the two vessels (Fig. 18.8).

Selective distal splenorenal shunt

Through a midline incision the small intestine is displaced to the right. The third and fourth parts of the duodenum are mobilized from the aorta to expose the left renal vein. The splenic vein is located by following up the inferior mesenteric vein to its junction. Separation of the distal splenic vein from the posterior surface of the pancreas, by division and ligation of the numerous fine tributary veins, is difficult and time consuming. At its junction with the portal vein the splenic vein is divided. The portal end is ligated and the splenic end anastomosed to the left renal vein (Fig. 18.9).

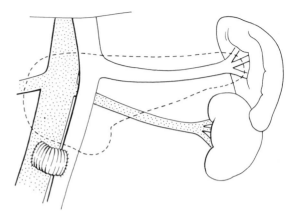

Fig. 18.8 Total shunt: mesocaval dacron 'H' graft

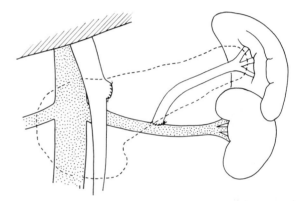

Fig. 18.9 Selective shunt: distal (Warren) lienorenal anastomosis

Complications

The most significant complication in patients who survive one of these shunting operations is *hepatic failure* of which a major manifestation is hepatic encephalopathy. The latter occurs more commonly after a portacaval shunt (where the portal flow is totally diverted) than after a selective splenorenal anastomosis and this knowledge may influence the choice of operation. *Encephalopathy* is due to the toxic effects of breakdown products of protein digestion, which would normally be rendered harmless by deamination processes in the liver, but which, as the result of the shunt, are now poured directly into the systemic circulation. The risks of oesophageal bleeding, however, far outweigh those of encephalopathy. *Thrombosis at the site of anastomosis* occurs in a proportion of cases, particularly in small bore shunts such as the total splenorenal.

Other operations

Transthoracic oesophageal transection (the Milnes Walker operation)

The oesophagus is approached through the left chest.

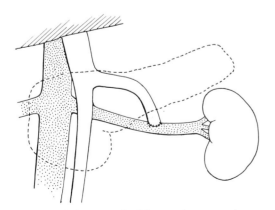

Fig. 18.7 Total shunt: proximal lienorenal anastomosis

It is opened through a longitudinal incision in the muscular layers through which the mucosal layer is separated, divided transversely and rejoined with a continuous catgut suture. This operation has largely been replaced by oesophageal stapling.

Splenectomy alone

This has been employed when the spleen is much enlarged, when the obstruction seems to be confined to the splenic vein, and when the liver is apparently healthy—but this combination is rare. It is now seldom advised, since it precludes the possibility of a splenorenal anastomosis at a later date, and, by encouraging portal vein thrombosis, it may also preclude a subsequent portacaval anastomosis.

Sub-cardiac gastric transection

This operation, as devised by Tanner (1958), is designed to arrest oesophageal haemorrhage by interrupting the venous communications between the portal and azygos (systemic) systems. The stomach is transected 5 cm below the cardia, and, all its vessels having been divided and ligatured, is immediately resutured. This operation carries a high mortality and is seldom performed today.

Oesophagogastrectomy

This may require to be undertaken as an emergency procedure, to arrest bleeding which is derived mainly from gastric varices. It is then a difficult and hazardous operation, but, in the presence of severe bleeding which cannot be controlled by simpler methods, there may be no other alternative. In rare cases, it may be the only elective procedure which is possible.

REFERENCES

Chadwick S J D, Huizinga W K J, Baker L W 1985 Management of splenic trauma: the Durban experience. British Journal of Surgery 72: 634

Child C G, Donavan A J 1957 Current problems in management of patients with portal hypertension. Journal of the American Medical Association 163: 1219

Clark A W et al 1980 Prospective controlled trial of injection sclerotherapy in patients with cirrhosis and recent variceal haemorrhage. Lancet 2: 552

Cooper M J, Williamson R C N 1984 Splenectomy: Indications, hazards and alternatives. British Journal of Surgery 71:173

Devlin H B, Evans D S, Birkhead J S 1970 Elective splenectomy for primary hematologic and splenic disease. Surgery Gynaecology and Obstetrics 131: 273

Graham H K, Johnston G W, McKelvey S T D, Kennedy T L 1981 Five years' experience in stapling the oesophagus and rectum. British Journal of Surgery 68: 697

Henderson J M, Buist T A S, Macpherson A I S 1979 Percutaneous transheptic occlusion for bleeding oesophageal varices. British Journal of Surgery 66: 569

Holme T C, Crosby D L 1984 Elective splenectomy. Indications and complications in 102 patients. Journal of the Royal College of Surgeons of Edinburgh 29: 229

Macpherson A I S 1973 The Spleen. Charles C Thomas, Springfield, Illinois

Sargison K D, Cole T P, Kyle J 1968 Traumatic rupture of the spleen. British Journal of Surgery 55: 506

Spence R A J, Johnston G W 1985 Results in 100 consecutive patients with stapled oesophageal transection for varices. Surgery Gynaecology and Obstetrics 160: 323

Tanner N C 1958 Operative management of haematemesis and melaena; with special reference to bleeding from oesophageal varices. Annals of the Royal College of Surgeons of England 22: 30

Warren W D, Zeppa R, Fomon J T 1967 Selective transsplenic decompression of gastroesophageal varices by distal splenorenal shunt. Annals of Surgery 166: 437

19

The liver and the sub-phrenic space

I. B. MACLEOD

Anatomy

The liver lies immediately below the diaphragm, mainly on the right of the median plane, only its thin left lobe being on the left. It is divided anatomically into two lobes, separated anteriorly and above by the attachment of the falciform ligament. The right lobe is the larger, and is related to the greater part of the right side of the diaphragm. In the recumbent position it is entirely under cover of the ribs; the gall-bladder is attached to its inferior surface. The left lobe stretches across the epigastrium towards the left hypochondrium and within the costal angle it is related to the anterior abdominal wall. The *porta hepatis* is a transverse cleft placed far back on the inferior surface of the right lobe. It transmits the portal vein, the hepatic artery and the hepatic ducts, together with lymph vessels and nerves.

Segmental anatomy

Increasing experience of liver resection for tumour or trauma has emphasized the importance of knowledge of the segmental anatomy of the liver. These segments have a relatively selective hepatic arterial, portal venous and biliary tract supply, and prior ligation and division of these structures allows a relatively bloodless resection of one or more segments (see p. 378).

The segmental anatomy is illustrated in Figures 19.1 & 19.2. It is to be noted that the line of division between the true right and left lobes runs in the plane of the gall-bladder fossa and the inferior vena cava.

The venous drainage of the liver is by hepatic veins draining into the inferior vena cava. The true right lobe of liver is drained by a large right hepatic vein; the lateral segment of the left lobe is drained by a smaller left hepatic vein, while the medial segment is drained by the middle hepatic vein which usually drains into the left hepatic vein to form a common trunk before entering the inferior vena cava.

Peritoneal connections

The liver is clothed with peritoneum except at the 'bare area' on the back of the right lobe where it is in direct contact with the diaphragm. The peritoneum is reflected off the liver in four *double* folds—the coronary, left

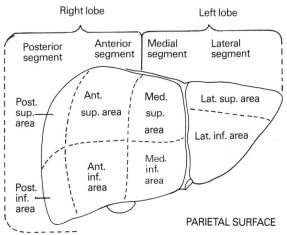

Fig. 19.1 Anatomical lobes and segments of the liver as seen on parietal surface (After Christopher)

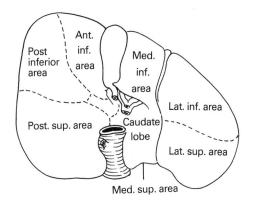

VISCERAL SURFACE

Fig. 19.2 Segments of liver as seen on the visceral surface

triangular and falciform ligaments, and the lesser omentum.

The coronary ligament is formed by the layers of peritoneum reflected on to the diaphragm from the upper and lower margins of the 'bare area'. Its two layers are separated by the vertical width of this area, but meet at its right-hand corner to form a free border to the ligament. The upper layer intercepts the hand which is passed backwards over the dome of the right lobe.

The left triangular ligament connects the upper surface of the left lobe to the diaphragm, and its two layers are in contact. (The right triangular ligament is a redundant name given to the right free border of the coronary ligament).

The falciform ligament lies in the median plane. It is formed by peritoneum reflected from the upper and anterior surfaces of the liver to the diaphragm and linea alba down to the umbilicus.

The lesser omentum stretches from the porta hepatis to the lesser curvature of the stomach and the first 2.5 cm of the duodenum. Its right free border forms the anterior boundary of the epiploic foramen; it contains the hepatic and common bile ducts, the hepatic artery and the portal vein.

The sub-phrenic space

This can be defined as that space which exists between the diaphragm above and the transverse colon and mesocolon below. Previously, considerable emphasis was laid on the division of the space into numerous compartments, but for practical purposes one may simply consider that there is a right and left subphrenic space, that on the right being divided into a supra and a subhepatic compartment.

SUBPHRENIC ABSCESS

A subphrenic abscess may follow perforation of an abdominal viscus or abdominal surgery (especially biliary or gastric surgery) and occasionally may result from direct extension of intrahepatic infection. The right subphrenic space is involved in approximately 70% of patients, with subhepatic collections being more common than suprahepatic collections. Abscesses may be bilateral, a factor which may dictate the operative approach.

The incidence of subphrenic abscess is falling, possibly related to the greater use of prophylactic antibiotics in biliary surgery, improved techniques of bowel preparation, the use of antibiotic peritoneal lavage in combination with powerful systemic antibiotics in patients with a generalized peritonitis, and the recognition of the importance of anaerobic organisms in intraperitoneal infection.

Diagnosis

Clinical presentation of subphrenic abscess is often vague, and in patients on systemic antibiotics the classical features of infection are often suppressed. A persisting temperature, continued leucocytosis and/or elevation of ESR or simply 'failure to thrive' should raise suspicion of the condition. Occasionally patients complain of shoulder tip pain, or hiccoughs. Direct clinical signs are few, though some patients may be tender on percussion of the lower ribs. Associated chest pathology makes interpretation of chest signs difficult.

Screening of the diaphragm may reveal an immobile diaphragm on the affected side, but again a supradiaphragmatic effusion (present in 90% of affected patients) or basal collapse may make recognition of the diaphragm difficult. Fewer than 25% of patients demonstrate the classic radiological features of a raised hemidiaphragm with an effusion and some collapse above, and an air/fluid level below. If present, the appearances are diagnostic.

The preferred method of investigation is by ultrasonic scan, which is highly accurate in detecting fluid collections. Combined isotope lung and liver scan may detect collections in the right suprahepatic space, showing a 'cold' space between uptake in the lung and liver, but will not demonstrate collections elsewhere. Radioisotope scans using Gallium or Indium labelled leucocytes have been recommended to demonstrate intraabdominal pus, but still require evaluation.

If the diagnosis is established, surgical drainage is indicated—delay may permit intraperitoneal rupture with an extremely high mortality. If the diagnosis remains in doubt and the patient is receiving antibiotics, these should be discontinued and the situation allowed to clarify. Persisting uncertainty justifies exploration through an upper mid-line incision. Diagnostic aspiration is not recommended.

Surgical approaches

Previously, great emphasis was placed on the need to avoid encroaching on either the peritoneal or pleural cavity because of the risk of disseminating infection. With the availability of modern antibiotics this risk is minimized and an *upper mid-line incision* is recommended for the majority of patients for the following reasons:

1. Subphrenic abscesses may be bilateral
2. Abscesses may be present elsewhere in the abdominal cavity
3. Anastomoses may be inspected for evidence of persistent leakage.

If the surgeon is certain that only one abscess exists and its position is known a unilateral approach may be performed.

Posterior subpleural approach

Abscesses in the subhepatic space may be drained by this method. The greater part of the 12th rib is removed and the abscess approached from below the pleural cavity. An oblique incision is made along the whole length

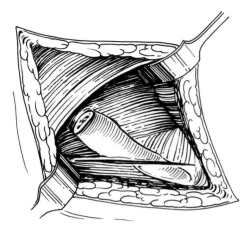

Fig. 19.3 Posterior approach for drainage of a subphrenic abscess through an incision made *transversely* through the centre of the bed of the resected 12th rib. This incision, which divides diaphragmatic fibres arising from the periosteum, should lie safely below the pleura

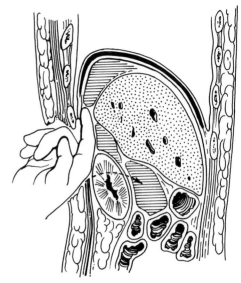

Fig. 19.4 Method of locating a subphrenic abscess by the posterior subpleural approach. The finger passed round the lateral side of the kidney (arrow) can reach an abscess in the hepato-renal pouch

of the 12th rib. The rib is cleared of periosteum as far back as its neck, where it is crossed more or less horizontally by the lower reflection of the pleura; it is divided at this level and is removed. An incision is then made *transversely* at the level of the first lumbar spinous process—across the centre of the bed of the rib (Fig. 19.3). This incision avoids the pleura and divides the diaphragmatic fibres arising from the periosteum of the rib. A finger is introduced deeply into the wound to enter the loose cellular tissue between the upper pole of the kidney and the diaphragm. By working upwards it comes in contact with the bare area of the liver (Fig. 19.4) and by further exploration it can locate an abscess in the related intraperitoneal compartments, since the oedematous and friable peritoneum covering the abscess is readily penetrated. Any abscess located is drained in the usual way.

Lateral approach
This approach may be suitable for a right sided posterior subdiaphragmatic abscess. An incision is made over the 10th rib posterolaterally and a portion of the rib removed. Pleura is sutured to diaphragm around the margins of the wound, and the diaphragm opened within this suture. The abscess is now drained transdiaphragmatically without contaminating the free pleural space.

Anterior extraperitoneal approach
An anterior approach may be considered when the abscess is thought to be situated in front of the liver, or after exploration by the posterior route has been unsuccessful. An incision is made 2 cm below and parallel to the costal margin, and all structures are divided down to, but not including, the peritoneum. A finger is then

passed gently upwards, separating this from the diaphragm until the abscess is felt. The abscess cavity is now entered and the pus evacuated without contaminating the general peritoneal cavity. Large bore tube drains are used for drainage of subphrenic abscesses. Progressive diminution in the size of the abscess cavity may be checked by serial sinogram, and the drain removed when the cavity has closed round it.

SURGICAL CONDITIONS OF THE LIVER

Trauma (see pp. 330 & 378).

Pyogenic liver abscess
In this serious condition there may be a single large abscess or multiple small abscesses. Biliary tract disease is now the commonest source of the infection and elderly patients are most frequently affected. Infection may arrive via the portal system (from appendicitis, diverticulitis, inflammatory bowel disease), the hepatic arterial system (e.g. subacute bacterial endocarditis), or by direct spread from a contiguous organ (e.g. gall-bladder). Abscess formation may follow blunt or penetrating trauma. In about one quarter of patients the source of infection is not determined (cryptogenic). Anaerobic organisms are common in cryptogenic infections and those arising from the portal system; coliforms and streptococci are present in most cases and are particularly common in cases arising from the biliary tract, while bacteraemia is probably responsible for abscesses with

staphylococcus aureus or streptococcus (Lancefield A).

Investigations of suspected liver abscess are similar to those for suspected subphrenic abscess. Technetium sulphur colloid scans and arteriography are useful. C.T. scanning is being increasingly used.

Large abscesses require open surgical drainage with appropriate antibiotic cover for 3 weeks. The site of the abscess may be obvious at laparotomy or may be located by needle aspiration. Loculi are broken down. A large bore (28–32 FG) tube drain is inserted and brought out through the abdominal wall at the nearest convenient point. Micro-abscesses arising from biliary tract disease require antibiotics for 4–8 weeks combined with appropriate biliary tract surgery. Micro-abscesses of haematological or cryptogenic origin may require antibiotic therapy for up to 4 months.

Amoebic abscess

Amoebic abscess is a complication of amoebic dysentery caused by the parasite *Entamoeba Histolytica*. Formerly confined to tropical countries, amoebiasis is occurring with increasing frequency in temperate zones as a result of immigration and intercontinental air travel. Hepatic infection results from migration of trophozoites from the intestine into the portal venous system. Up to 50% of patients with amoebiasis will show some evidence of amoebic 'hepatitis', but the incidence of true abscess formation is approximately 3% (Payne, 1945). It is likely that patients with 'hepatitis' would progress to true abscess formation in the absence of treatment.

The abscess is characteristically single and occupies the right lobe of liver. The histological features suggest that the principal pathology is a coalescence of multiple small areas of necrosis. There is little surrounding tissue reaction, the 'abscess cavity' being lined by only a fine layer of granulation tissue separating it from normal liver. The contents of the abscess are usually bacteriologically sterile, and while the colour is variable the classic description is of 'anchovy sauce'. Trophozoites are identifiable in about 30% of cases.

The onset of symptoms may be sudden or insidious. Right upper quadrant pain and tenderness over the right lower ribs is almost invariable. Fever is present in over three quarters of the patients and may exceed 40°C. Hepatomegaly is detectable in 50%, but surprisingly, clinical jaundice is uncommon. Abnormal physical signs at the right lung base are common.

In patients suspected of the disease, fresh stool samples should be examined for cysts or trophozoites. Radiological investigations are similar to those for pyogenic liver abscess while serological studies are useful in distinguishing amoebic from pyogenic abscess. Diagnostic aspiration may be necessary in some patients but should *always* be preceded by drug therapy (vide infra).

Earlier diagnosis and prompt institution of treatment has reduced the incidence of the highly lethal complication of rupture and metastatic abscess.

Most amoebic abscesses respond to drug treatment, the size of the cavity being monitored by ultrasound or scintiscan. Metronidazole is the drug of choice at present, 800 mg t.d.s. for 10 days. Emetine hydrochloride or dehydroemetine are also very effective though potentially more toxic. Large abscesses may require closed needle aspiration in addition if there is no clear clinical response within 48 to 72 hours, or rupture appears imminent (Dietrick, 1984). A large bore spinal needle is introduced, after local anaesthetic infiltration, either over an obvious mass or through the right 9th intercostal space in the mid-axillary line and directed towards the suspected site of abscess for a distance of not more than 10 cm. Ultrasonic guidance is now often used. Left lobe abscesses, though uncommon, may rupture into the pericardium (a lethal complication) and should be aspirated to prevent this.

Open surgical drainage is rarely required, and is reserved for the few cases who have secondary bacterial infection not responding to therapy, or patients in whom intra-abdominal rupture has occurred. The approach would be dictated by the position of the abscess (see p. 375 pyogenic abscess). If percutaneous aspiration of a left lobe abscess is unsuccessful, needle aspiration at laparotomy should be undertaken as such abscesses frequently develop complications.

The overall mortality of amoebic abscess approximates to 4%.

Hydatid cyst of the liver

Hydatid disease, due to infestation with the *Taenia Echinococcus* is uncommon in Great Britain but is endemic in the great sheep-rearing countries. The cyst commonly develops in the right lobe of the liver, where it may be mistaken for malignant disease or, if it extends upwards, for subphrenic abscess. If it becomes secondarily infected an abscess will result; this may rupture into the pleural space and give rise to empyema.

Chemotherapy with Merbendazole has a limited effect; the most satisfactory treatment is complete excision of the cyst together with its contained parasites. According to the position of the cyst an abdominal or a subpleural approach is employed. By the latter method the 9th or 10th rib is resected, the pleura displaced upwards and the diaphragm incised. After the liver has been exposed and the area packed off, the fluid content of the cyst is aspirated and replaced by 96% alcohol solution; left in situ for 10 minutes, this should be lethal to any free parasites (Hicken, 1966). The liver tissue is then incised along the needle track. The *ectocyst* or adventitious capsule, composed of condensed liver tissue, is opened and the rubbery *endocyst* is brought into view. By blunt dissection the endocyst is separated from the ectocyst, to which it is usually only loosely adherent. Every effort should be made to remove the endocyst intact. If it ruptures during removal the surgeon should satisfy himself, by careful inspection of the cavity, that the entire lining membrane together with any loose daughter cysts has been removed. Finally the cavity is swabbed again with alcohol; it may either be drained by a large tube or may be loosely packed with gauze. A large residual cavity after removal of the cyst wall can be filled with greater omentum (Papadimitriou, 1970).

A new approach to the surgical treatment of hydatid cysts involves local freezing of the cyst's outer layer which allows its contents to be evacuated cleanly into a cone-shaped instrument which has become adherent to the cyst by the freezing process. The residual space is irrigated with 0.5% silver nitrate solution which is non-toxic to tissue and destroys scolices (Saidi, 1977).

RESECTION OF THE LIVER

Provided the liver is basically healthy, extensive resection may be carried out with only temporary biochemical upset as normal liver tissue has considerable powers of regeneration.

Lobar or segmental resection
This may be indicated for:

1. Primary malignant tumours of liver—hepatoma, cholangiocarcinoma or hepatocholangioma. Unfortunately only about 10% of such patients prove technically suitable for resection, either because of the presence of intrahepatic metastases or the co-existence of cirrhosis. The long term survival rate after resection is disappointing, though Foster & Berman (1977) have reported a 36% five year survival rate.

2. Carcinoma of the gall-bladder. Either extended right hepatic lobectomy (Tri-segmentectomy) or middle lobe lobectomy has been recommended.

3. Rarely for solitary hepatic metastases from other organs or for multiple metastases involving one lobe only. Long term survivals have been reported after resection of metastases from colon and from kidney.

4. Some benign tumours of liver, e.g. haemangioma.

5. For blunt trauma causing extensive 'bursting' injury, particularly of the right lobe.

Major resections of the right lobe carry an operative mortality of 10–15%. Resections of the left lobe are less demanding on both patient and operator. Planned resections for tumour should be preceded by extensive investigations to exclude metastatic disease within the liver and elsewhere, and to determine the anatomy of the hepatic vasculature. The operations must be covered by broad spectrum antibiotics, and careful attention must be paid to maintenance of acid base balance and to the

provision of adequate albumin postoperatively. Diversion of the whole of the blood flow through the small liver remnant results in temporary oedema of the remnant and associated impairment of function.

Right hepatic lobectomy
A thoraco-laparotomy incision through the right eighth intercostal space and extending well across the epigastric mid-line is preferred. The abdominal part of the incision is made first, the suitability of the lesion for resection determined, and the incision completed. The right lobe of liver is mobilized by division of the coronary and falciform ligaments and the diaphragm now split radially down to the inferior vena cava. The liver is rotated upwards to display better the porta hepatis. The cystic duct and artery, the right hepatic duct and artery and right branch of the portal vein are divided between ligatures. A clear line of demarcation between the devascularized right lobe and the left lobe is now apparent running in the line of the gall-bladder bed to the inferior vena cava—transection of the liver takes place through this line (Fig. 19.5).

Though not always technically feasible, it is preferable to secure the venous drainage of the right lobe prior to transection. The duodenum is fully Kocherized to expose the inferior vena cava. The liver is further rotated upwards and to the left, and a variable number of small posterior hepatic veins entering the front of the vena cava are ligated and divided and the venous hilum of the liver approached. The right hepatic vein is a large vessel, which is now ligated and divided, preserving the middle and left hepatic veins. Glisson's capsule is incised along the line of demarcation, and the liver substance transected using the 'finger-fracture' technique. Small ves-

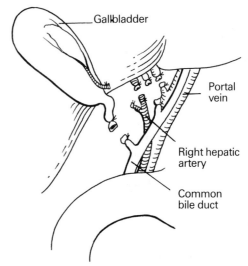

Fig. 19.5 Blood vessels and bile ducts ligated and divided prior to right hepatic lobectomy

sels and ducts crossing the plane of demarcation can be felt, clamped and divided, then ligated or suture ligated with 3/0 Dexon or chromic catgut. Diathermy may also be used, while techniques using laser or cryosurgery are still in the experimental stage. The right lobe of liver is now removed. If prior ligation of the hepatic veins was not performed, they are ligated and divided from the front after transection of the liver, allowing the right lobe to be removed. If right hepatic lobectomy is being carried out for trauma, occlusion of the free border of the lesser omentum by a vascular clamp (or by the fingers—*Pringle's maneouvre*) will reduce blood loss from the liver while the vessels in the porta hepatis are being ligated. Such occlusion may be maintained for up to 20 minutes. The greater omentum may be brought up and sutured to the raw surface of liver to reduce leakage of blood and bile, though this is not an essential step. *Adequate* subdiaphragmatic drainage preferably of the low pressure suction type must be provided, the drains being brought out below the wound. Drainage of the pleural space is via a tube inserted in the 10th intercostal space and connected to an under water seal. The diaphragm is repaired with No. 1 Dexon, and the wound closed.

Extended right hepatic lobectomy (Tri-segmentectomy)

The technique is similar to that of right hepatic lobectomy. Additional steps are—the arterial and portal supply to the middle lobe is ligated and divided in the porta hepatis, and the middle hepatic vein is ligated at the venous hilum. The line of transection is close to the falciform ligament which, after removal of the right and middle lobe, may be used to cover the raw surface of the liver remnant.

Middle lobe lobectomy

This may be indicated for removal of carcinoma of gall-bladder, or a centrally placed benign tumour. Dissection at the porta hepatis is carried a little deeper than with right or left hepatic lobectomy. The primary vessels arising from the right and left hepatic artery and right and left branches of the portal vein, supplying the four median segments, are ligated and divided along with the appropriate draining hepatic duct branches, leaving the main vessels and ducts intact. The liver is transected along the two planes of demarcation, the middle hepatic vein ligated and divided, and the middle lobe (four segments) removed. The residual right and left hepatic lobes are now sutured together using interrupted 2/0 chromic catgut.

Left hepatic lobectomy

This procedure is carried out through an abdominal incision, either a right paramedian or subcostal incision

being suitable. Depending on the nature and size of the lesion in the left lobe, vascular ligation at the porta hepatis may be planned to devascularize the whole of the left lobe (with the demarcation line running from gall-bladder fossa to inferior vena cava) or the lateral segments with the demarcation line in the vicinity of the falciform ligament (left lateral segmentectomy). In the former, the middle and left hepatic veins are ligated and divided in the venous hilum and in the latter only the left hepatic vein.

Wedge resection of liver

This technique may be employed for liver biopsy at laparotomy, for small peripherally located tumours or for tumours of other organs involving the liver by direct spread, e.g. stomach. It is also employed for carcinoma of gall-bladder in patients not considered fit for the more radical procedures of tri-segmentectomy or middle lobe lobectomy. The main difficulties of the operation arise from haemorrhage, which is profuse and difficult to control, and from the fact that stitches tend to cut out. To reduce these difficulties, the liver substance may be divided either with the diathermy knife or simply by pressure with the point of an artery forceps (this latter method facilitating the location of vessels before they are divided). Small segments at a time are divided in order that bleeding can be arrested—by gauze pressure or by the securing of larger vessels as they present. Any sudden bleeding can be controlled by temporary compression of the hepatic artery where it lies in the right free border of the lesser omentum—either digitally or by the use of a light controlling clamp. Another method of arresting haemorrhage is to insert a series of interlocking sutures, carried on a large round-bodied needle, through the liver substance on each side of the segment to be resected. If the excision has been in a V-shaped form (Fig. 19.6), it may be possible to approximate the margins by deeply placed sutures. These may be made to

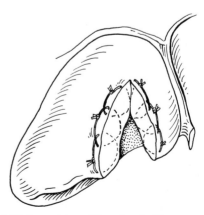

Fig. 19.6 Wedge excision of liver. Interlocking sutures are inserted on each side of the segment to be resected

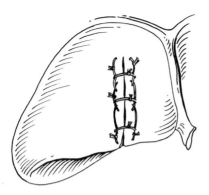

Fig. 19.7 Repair of liver after wedge excision. The resected margins are approximated by further sutures which include those previously inserted

include the interlocking sutures previously inserted (Fig. 19.7); alternatively, they may be supported by transplants of falciform ligament or of rectus sheath laid on the liver surface. If the gap in the liver substance cannot be closed by suture, it may be plugged with omentum. Packing should be avoided if possible, since it may give rise to a biliary fistula (McClelland, 1965).

Needle biopsy of liver

Needle biopsy, in which a small core of liver is removed, is a useful technique in the investigation of liver disease. Three types of needle are commonly used—the Trucut needle, the Menghini needle, and the Vim-Silvermann needle, of which the first two are the most popular. If diffuse liver disease is suggested by isotope scan, the procedure is done by 'blind' percutaneous puncture under local anaesthesia in the right 9th or 10th intercostal space in the mid-axillary line, or, if the liver is palpable, over the most superficial part. The patient must be able to co-operate by holding his breath in expiration while the needle is inserted into liver tissue.

If focal liver disease is anticipated (e.g. metastatic or primary liver tumour), the procedure is best done under vision at laparoscopy (preferably) or at laparotomy so that the needle may be accurately directed to the area under suspicion (*Target Biopsy*). Care should be taken when biopsying a narrow left lobe of liver lest the needle pass through and damage posterior structures.

The procedure is relatively safe, the principal risk being of haemorrhage, and it is essential that any coagulation defects are corrected beforehand. Rarely, haemobilia, or the development of an intrahepatic arteriovenous fistula may follow.

REFERENCES

Davis-Christopher 1982 ed. Sabiston D C Textbook of Surgery, 12th edn. W B Saunders Co., Philadelphia, p 1135
Dietrick R B 1984 Experience with liver abscess. American Journal of Surgery 147: 288
Foster J H, Berman M M 1977 Solid liver tumours In: Major problems in clinical surgery, Volume 22. W B Saunders Co., Philadelphia, p 85
Hicken N F, McAllister A J, Carlquist J H, Madsen F 1966 Echinococcosis of the liver and lungs. American Journal of Surgery 112: 823

McClelland R N, Shires T 1965 Management of liver trauma in 259 consecutive patients. Annals of Surgery 161: 248
Papadimitriou J, Mandrekas A 1970 The Surgical treatment of hydatid disease of the liver. British Journal of Surgery 57: 431
Payne A M M 1945 Amoebic dysentery in eastern India. Lancet 1: 206
Saidi F 1977 A new approach to the surgical treatment of hydatid cyst. Annals of the Royal College of Surgeons of England 59: 115

20

The gall-bladder, the bile ducts and the pancreas

J. M. S. JOHNSTONE & I. B. MACLEOD

Anatomy

The gall-bladder is pear-shaped and about 10 cm long. It is attached to the inferior surface of the right lobe of the liver, and is enclosed within its peritoneal sheath. Its lower end or *fundus* is completely covered with peritoneum, and projects slightly beyond the free margin of the liver opposite the upper end of the linea semi-lunaris. The *body* and *neck* are covered only on three sides with peritoneum. They are attached anteriorly to the liver by loose connective tissue and are easily separated from it. The neck shows a dilatation, the *infundibulum* (Hartmann's pouch), which hangs downwards and is often connected to the duodenum by folds which may be either congenital or inflammatory in origin. The upper end of the neck narrows down to form the *cystic duct* which runs backwards and medially,

and joins the common hepatic duct to form the common bile duct.

The gall-bladder is supplied by the cystic artery, which is usually a branch of the right hepatic (Fig. 20.1).

The bile ducts

The *right* and *left hepatic ducts* emerge from the liver through the porta hepatis, and unite to form the *common hepatic duct*, which is in turn joined by the cystic duct to form the *common bile duct*. This last duct is about 10 cm long; it runs downwards behind the first part of the duodenum, and ends by passing obliquely through the postero-medial wall of the second part. The extreme lower end of the duct is dilated to form the *ampulla of Vater* which lies partly within the duodenal wall.

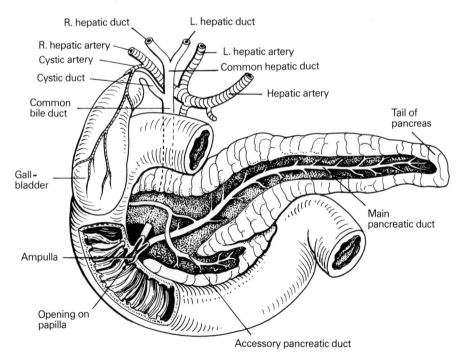

Fig. 20.1 Drawing to show the relations of the gall-bladder and bile ducts to the duodenum and head of pancreas

Relations. The hepatic ducts and the supraduodenal part of the common bile duct lie in the right free border of the lesser omentum. The *hepatic artery* lies on the left side of the common bile duct, and the *portal vein* is behind it, these structures being all contained within the omentum. The *right hepatic artery* crosses behind the common hepatic duct, before it gives off its cystic branch. The lower part of the common bile duct descends behind the first part of the duodenum, and then lies in a groove on the back of the head of the pancreas or may tunnel the gland substance.

Anomalies. The above description of the relationship of the bile ducts and associated blood vessels is that given in the standard textbooks of anatomy. It should be noted, however, that considerable variations may exist; those which occur most commonly are shown in Figure 20.2. A knowledge of such 'anomalies' is of the greatest importance to the surgeon, for failure to recognize them at operation may lead to disaster. Thus, severance of an anomalous or accessory hepatic duct, without ligature of its cut-end, would result in biliary peritonitis, while inadvertent ligature of an abnormally placed right hepatic artery might produce a fatal hepatic infarction. Other anomalies render the right hepatic duct or the common bile duct very liable to injury.

The pancreas

This lies obliquely across the upper part of the posterior wall of the abdomen. Its *head* lies within the concavity of the duodenum, and is closely related to the lower part of the common bile duct. Its *body* lies behind the stomach, separated from it by the lesser sac of the peritoneum; the splenic artery runs along its upper

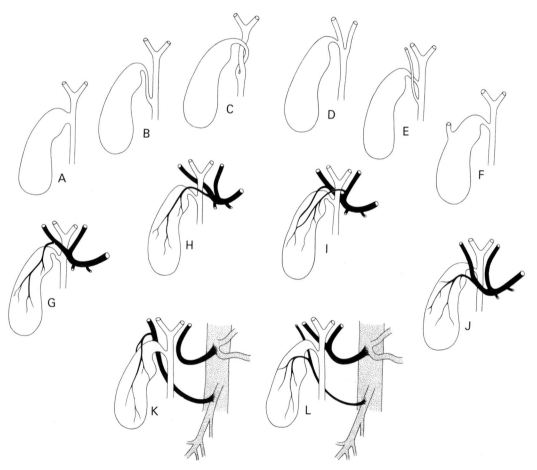

Fig. 20.2 Anomalies of the bile ducts and related arteries (A) short cystic duct; (B) long cystic duct; (C) long cystic duct winding round common hepatic duct; (D) cystic duct joining right hepatic duct; (E) Accessory hepatic duct joining common bile duct; (F) Accessory (*hepato-cholecystic*) duct passing directly into gall-bladder; (G) right hepatic artery crossing in front of common hepatic duct; (H) cystic artery arising low and crossing in front of common hepatic duct; (I) accessory cystic artery from left hepatic; (J) low division of hepatic artery; (K) right hepatic artery arising from superior mesenteric; (L) accessory right hepatic artery from superior mesenteric

border and the splenic vein is behind it. Its *tail* lies in contact with the spleen.

The pancreatic duct traverses the whole length of the gland, and ends by joining the common bile duct, either at the ampulla or at a slightly higher level. An *accessory pancreatic duct* may enter the duodenum about 2.5 cm higher up.

INDICATIONS FOR SURGERY AND CHOICE OF OPERATION

Cholecystitis and gall-stone formation are the most common disorders affecting the biliary tract. The great majority of stones develop within the gall-bladder, and those giving rise to symptoms are usually associated with inflammatory changes in the wall of the viscus.

Removal of the gall-bladder (*cholecystectomy*) is the standard procedure when the gall-bladder is diseased or contains calculi. Simple drainage of the gall-bladder (*cholecystostomy*) combined with removal of any stones present is occasionally indicated if severe inflammatory changes render the anatomy obscure, in very poor risk patients, or for preliminary drainage of the biliary tree obstructed by tumour in patients in whom later resection is contemplated.

Cholecystectomy has definite advantages over cholecystostomy:
1. it removes the site in which most gall-stones form, and thus reduces the risk of recurrence
2. it removes a focus of infection which may persist
3. it obviates the risk of persistent biliary fistula which may follow cholecystostomy
4. it eliminates the risk of carcinoma developing in a gall-bladder which has been the seat of stone formation.

Acute cholecystitis
In the majority of patients acute cholecystitis develops as a complication of gall-stones. *Acalculous* cholecystitis may occur, however, and has been reported in patients with severe multiple trauma, in septicaemia, and rarely as a result of embolization into the cystic artery in patients with atrial fibrillation. The acalculous variety tends to be more rapidly progressive than the calculous type, frequently leading to gangrene of the gall-bladder wall, and early surgery is indicated.

The traditional management of calculous-acute cholecystitis is initially conservative, in the anticipation that in approximately 70% of patients the condition will settle (probably the result of an obstructing calculus disimpacting) allowing later elective cholecystectomy. Pain is relieved, pethidine by i.m. injection being suitable. Oral intake is stopped and adequate fluids given by i.v. infusion. If vomiting is a feature, a nasogastric tube is passed and aspirated hourly. Blood samples are

taken for routine haematology, urea and electrolytes, standard liver function tests and blood culture, and antibiotic therapy started. Gentamicin, Cefuroxime, or Cotrimaxazole are suitable. Pulse and temperature are carefully monitored, and the patient re-examined at 4–6 hour intervals. Early confirmation of the diagnosis by ultrasound scan, or by intravenous cholangiography (provided liver function is satisfactory) should be undertaken in the first 24 hours. Improvement in the patient's condition will normally allow reintroduction of oral intake at 48 hours, discontinuation of antibiotics at 7 days, discharge from hospital at 7–10 days, and an appointment for re-admission for elective cholecystectomy in 8–12 weeks' time. Indications to abandon this conservative regime and proceed to *early surgery* include:
1. failure to improve after 48 hours therapy
2. development of a tender enlarging mass in the right hypochondrium
3. development of rigors
4. features of general peritonitis (uncommon).

In recent years, increasing numbers of surgeons have favoured a policy of early surgery. Treatment is initiated as above, fluid and electrolyte deficiencies corrected, the diagnosis confirmed and, provided there are no specific contraindications to surgery, the patient is prepared for surgery on an elective operating list within 48–72 hours of admission to hospital. Antibiotics are continued for 3 days postoperatively unless it is necessary to explore the common bile duct, when they should be continued for 5 days. Advantages of this policy include:
1. shorter total period of hospitalization
2. prevention of the development of serious complications such as empyema (which carries a mortality of 10%)
3. operation is often technically relatively simple during the first week of the illness, oedema making dissection of tissue planes easier. The operative mortality of *planned* early cholecystectomy is similar to that of elective cholecystectomy
4. approximately 20% of patients leaving hospital after initial conservative therapy require emergency re-admission with a recurrent acute episode prior to their planned elective procedure.

Choice of operation
The writer recommends the policy of early surgery in acute cholecystitis, with the proviso that it is undertaken by a surgeon with considerable experience in surgery of the biliary tract. Cholecystectomy with peroperative cholangiography is the procedure of choice. This is usually possible using the standard technique (see p. 390), but any difficulty in visualizing the anatomy of the cystic duct and Calot's Triangle should dictate that dissection begins at the fundus and works towards the cystic duct. Haemorrhage is a little greater than with

the standard technique, but risk of inadvertent damage to the common bile duct or right hepatic artery is minimized. Espiner has recently described a technique which avoids the necessity of ligation of the cystic artery. Using diathermy, dissection is carried out in the submucosal plane of the gall-bladder working from the fundus towards the cystic duct, which is amputated as soon as tissues in the free border of the lesser omentum are reached. Cholecystostomy is now infrequently practised, but may be indicated in some difficult patients as may be met if an initial conservative policy has failed, and is indicated if the surgeon is inexperienced.

Chronic cholecystitis and gall-stones

The incidence of gall-stones has increased markedly in recent years, this increase being most evident in men and in young women (in whom use of the contraceptive pill may be implicated). Surgical treatment is usually advised once the diagnosis is made, even in those patients in whom the stones are 'symptomless'. Some 50% of such asymptomatic patients will develop symptoms of biliary colic within 5 years, and the possible development of carcinoma of the gall-bladder following squamous metaplasia of the mucosa should always be borne in mind. Patients who have had one or more attacks of biliary colic usually accept readily the advice to undergo surgery, but patients with milder symptoms such as flatulent dyspepsia may not. Such patients, and those who are considered poor operative risks, should be advised about a fat reduced diet and considered for treatment with gall-stone dissolving agents such as chenodeoxycholic acid (*Chendol*) or ursodeoxycholic acid (*Destolit*).

Dissolution therapy is not suitable in the following situations:
1. calcified stones (10–15% of all stones)
2. nonfunctioning gall-bladder, or obstructed cystic duct
3. stones larger than 1 cm diameter
4. liver disease or jaundice
5. inflammatory bowel disease present
6. women of child bearing age.

Diarrhoea is a common side-effect, although reported to be less frequent with *Destolit* than with *Chendol*. Treatment should be continued for 3 months following disappearance of the stones, which may take up to 2 years. Stones may reform after discontinuing therapy, as the underlying lithogenicity of the bile is not permanently altered.

Obstructive jaundice

If an attack of biliary colic is followed by jaundice it is very likely that a stone has entered the common duct. Many such stones pass spontaneously into the duodenum, and initial treatment is medical, anticipating improvement in liver function. Operation is undertaken electively when liver function has returned to normal, or has stopped improving, with a lower morbidity and mortality than operating on the jaundiced patient. Broad spectrum antibiotic cover is advised if it is anticipated that the common bile duct will need to be explored.

Persistent jaundice following biliary colic indicates that a stone has become impacted in the common bile duct. Early operation after careful preparation is indicated to prevent further liver damage from back pressure and from the almost invariable cholangitis. Rigors indicate bacteraemic episodes from *cholangitis*. After obtaining blood cultures, broad spectrum antibiotic therapy is started, the patient is adequately hydrated, and after correction of any coagulation defects (usually an extended prothrombin time ratio) cholecystectomy and exploration of the common bile duct is undertaken. Preoperative confirmation of the diagnosis by percutaneous cholangiography (PTC) is advisable (Gibbons, 1983).

Steadily deepening jaundice, without preceding biliary colic suggests obstruction of the common bile duct by malignant disease or chronic pancreatitis. Malignant disease may be primary in the head of the pancreas, in the bile ducts or in the peri-ampullary region, or may be secondary from a more distant primary. Ultrasound and isotope liver scan will demonstrate the presence of hepatic metastases and show the diameter of the common bile duct.

If these investigations suggest metastatic disease and the common bile duct is of normal calibre it is wise in most patients to obtain a tissue diagnosis by liver biopsy using a Travenol Trucut needle. This is best done under vision provided by a laparoscope to ensure that an appropriate site is sampled.

If extrahepatic obstruction is indicated by a dilated common bile duct the site and nature of the obstruction should be delineated by *percutaneous transhepatic cholangiography* (PTC) (Fig. 20.3) supplemented when necessary by *endoscopic retrograde cholangiopancreatography* (ERCP).

Peri-ampullary carcinomas and carcinomas at the lower end of the common bile duct may be suitable for resection (Whipple's operation q.v.) Many surgeons consider that resection for carcinoma of the head of the pancreas does not yield results sufficiently superior to simple bypass to justify such a major procedure even in those patients in whom it is technically possible. In this condition, in patients with metastatic disease and in patients with benign stricture from chronic pancreatitis, some form of drainage or bypass procedure to relieve the jaundice should be undertaken. Increasingly, the interventional radiologists contribute significantly to the palliation of malignant obstructive jaundice by the percutaneous insertion of a 'pig-tail' drainage catheter (Fig. 20.4) or a biliary endoprosthesis (Fig. 20.5).

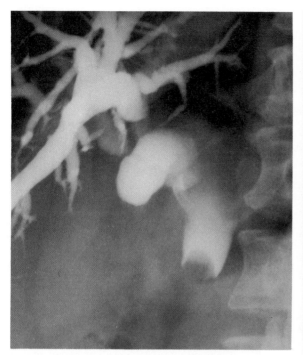

Fig. 20.3 Percutaneous transhepatic cholangiogram showing obstructing calculus at the lower end of bile ducts

Such prostheses may also be inserted in retrograde fashion using an endoscope (Fig. 20.6) and in some patients with small peri-ampullary tumours who are considered unfit for surgery, an endoscopic papillotomy may be undertaken to relieve the jaundice.

GENERAL CONSIDERATIONS IN TECHNIQUE

Preparation for operation

All diseases of the biliary tract are likely to be associated with some disturbance of liver function. As operation is not usually a matter of urgency, some time should be spent in preoperative preparation. A high carbohydrate diet should be prescribed to ensure adequate stores of liver glycogen, and in the iller patient high carbohydrate intravenous infusions employed. Adequate preoperative hydration is important and is particularly so in the jaundiced patient (q.v.) Broad spectrum antibiotic therapy is used in the acute case, and where exploration of the common bile duct is anticipated. Gross obesity, common in patients with gall-stones, is a relative contraindication to elective surgery, and every encouragement should be given to the patient to lose weight before operation. Regrettably, such advice often 'falls on deaf ears', and continuing symptoms necessitate operation in less than ideal circumstances.

Any operation on the biliary tract should be

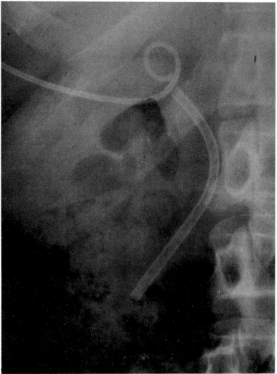

Fig. 20.4 Plain X-ray showing 'pig-tail' drainage catheter and biliary endoprosthesis inserted percutaneously

approached with the maximum possible information and adequate time for investigation should be provided. In elective surgery most of the investigations will have been performed on an outpatient basis. Ultrasound scanning is now the usual 'screening' procedure (Muir, 1983), while oral cholecystography or intravenous cholangiography are less frequently used than formerly. Suspicion that the common bile duct may require to be opened demands accurate delineation of its anatomy by PTC or ERCP or both.

Preparation in jaundiced patients

Both morbidity and mortality are higher following surgery in jaundiced patients than in non-icteric subjects. The increased risks are:

1. *Haemorrhage.* In obstructive jaundice there is impaired absorption of the fat soluble vitamin K due to failure of bile salts to reach the intestine. This leads to failure to synthesize prothrombin, and an extended prothrombin time ratio (PTR). If the PTR is increased, it should be corrected before operation by the parenteral administration of vitamin K; 10 mg per day by i.m. or i.v. injection is normally adequate. In patients with severe intrinsic liver disease there may be a more general failure in synthesis of clotting factors. A full coagulation

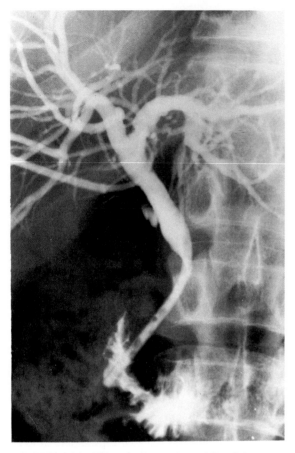

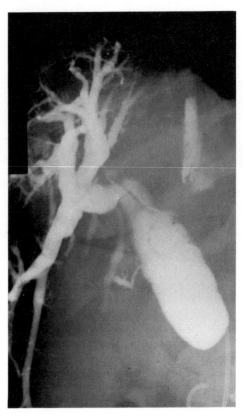

Fig. 20.6 Contrast X-ray showing biliary obstruction, relieved by a 'pig-tail' catheter which has been inserted in retrograde fashion using an endoscope

Fig. 20.5 Contrast X-ray confirming the position of the endoprosthesis within a malignant stricture

screen should be ordered and fresh frozen plasma made available for the perioperative period (p. 61).

2. *Infection.* The majority of patients with obstructive jaundice, and virtually all of those in whom the cause is gall-stones, have infected bile. Antibiotic therapy in the elective case should be administered parenterally, beginning with the premedication and continued for 3–5 days. Gentamicin, Cefuroxime, or Co-trimaxazole are suitable.

3. *Acute renal failure.* Renal tubular function is compromised to a greater or lesser degree in jaundiced patients due to a direct action of bilirubin on the tubules and to a degree of vascular shunting in the kidney leading to relative cortical ischaemia. Episodes of hypotension due to haemorrhage or infection are more likely if the patients, as many of them are, are hypovolaemic prior to surgery. Adequate *preoperative* hydration is essential to minimize the risk of acute renal failure, and frequently obviates the need for peroperative mannitol infusion so favoured by anaesthetists. An intravenous infusion is set up to aim for a minimum urinary output of 2000 ml/day. The patient will frequently require bladder catheterization a day or two preoperatively to ensure accurate recording. All patients should be catheterized once anaesthesia has been induced, in order to monitor urine output during the operation, and hourly in the postoperative period.

4. *Liver failure.* When combined with acute renal failure, the patient has the hepato-renal syndrome. Adequate preoperative carbohydrate intake and hydration, combined with measures to control infection and minimize haemorrhage should reduce considerably the risk of this severe complication.

Position of the patient

The patient should lie supine on an operating table which can accept X-ray casettes for peroperative cholangiography (Fig. 20.7). A careful check should be made that the biliary area lies over the aperture in the casette carrier allowing X-rays to reach the films. The patient should be tilted 15° down to his or her right, either by placing a rubber wedge under the patient's left side or by tilting the table itself. This maneouvre carries the common bile duct away from the line of the vertebrae and allows easier interpretation of cholangiogram films.

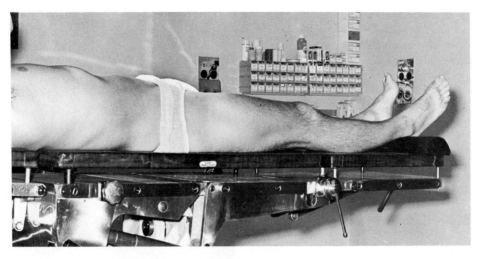

Fig. 20.7 Patient in position for operation on the biliary system. The X-ray translucent operating table top, to allow insertion of X-ray plates for cholangiography, is shown. Note that the ankles are supported by a rubber pad to prevent pressure on the calves (see p. 312)

Incision

Biliary surgery may be undertaken through one of a variety of incisions.

Right paramedian

Either rectus displacing or rectus splitting. This is most suitable for patients with a narrow costal angle, and most easily allows a full laparotomy.

Kocher's subcostal

In stout patients with a wide costal angle this incision allows easier access to deeper structures than the paramedian incision.

Mayo-Robson (Hockey stick)

This is a combination of a paramedian and a medial subcostal incision.

Right upper quadrant transverse

This is the author's preferred incision and provides the most cosmetic scar, a significant consideration when many patients are young women. The incision can be carried across the mid-line if required to improve access.

Upper midline

Some surgeons prefer to operate on the biliary tree through a midline incision while standing to the *left* side of the patient

Preliminary exploration

In the absence of acute inflammation, a careful examination of the entire biliary system should be carried out before any decision is made as to operative procedure. The stomach and duodenum are examined first, and are then packed-off out of the way. The gall-bladder is palpated for calculi, particular attention being paid to the infundibulum in which a calculus may be overlooked, and the condition of its wall is noted. The cystic duct is now brought into view by drawing the gall-bladder upwards and to the right. Any adhesions or peritoneal folds connecting the gall-bladder to the duodenum or colon are divided, and bleeding points are ligatured. The cystic duct is examined by palpation down to the point where it joins the common hepatic duct to form the common bile duct. The condition of these ducts also should be investigated as routine. The supraduodenal part of the common duct lying in the right free border of the lesser omentum is palpated between the index finger in the epiploic foramen and the thumb in front. If the foramen is not patent the duct can be palpated by pressing it backwards against the vertebral column. The retroduodenal part of the common duct may be palpated by placing the finger tips of the left hand along the lateral border of the second part of the duodenum, and by pressing them medially against the thumb, which is placed firmly against the groove between pancreas and duodenum. By this method the consistency of the pancreas can be determined at the same time, and any abnormality noted. If the appendix is accessible it is examined and, if necessary, removed—either immediately or towards the end of the operation.

In the presence of jaundice special precautions must be observed. In view of the risk of haemorrhage, exploration is reduced to a minimum; gentleness is more than usually essential, and even the smallest vessels should be caught and ligatured. Attention is directed mainly to the common duct and to the pancreas, for it is in these situations that the cause of the obstruction is most likely to be found. The appearance of the gall-bladder is a useful guide to diagnosis. If the gall-bladder is contracted and fibrotic the obstruction is most likely to be caused by a stone impacted in the common duct. If the gall-bladder is dilated the obstruction is due usually to some cause other than stone (*Courvoisier's law*). In this latter case particular attention should be paid to the head of the pancreas. If the whole pancreas is enlarged and of rubbery consistency the condition is probably one of chronic pancreatitis. If stony hardness or nodularity is present and affects mainly the head of the pancreas, it is more likely to be due to carcinoma. A palpable nodule at the ampulla suggests a carcinoma of this region.

Choice of procedure as determined by operative findings

Following the preliminary exploration, the next step is to obtain *operative cholangiogram* films, preferably after direct cannulation of the cystic duct. The cystic duct is isolated and its junction with common hepatic duct and common bile duct noted. The cystic duct is clamped or ligated at its junction with Hartmann's pouch. A second ligature of absorbable material is passed around the duct close to its junction with common hepatic duct. The cystic duct is now incised between the ligatures, a metal or plastic catheter introduced, and held in place by tightening the second ligature with one throw. Three films (Fig. 20.8) are usually taken following injection of 2 ml, 3 ml and 5 ml of 25% *Biligram*. Features to note on the films are:

1. evidence of duct dilation (normal diameter < 7 mm)
2. presence of filling defects (stone, tumour, occasionally blood clot)
3. evidence of flow of dye into duodenum
4. particular attention should be paid to the anatomy of the lower end of the common bile duct—more detail may be obtained if necessary by placing a small piece of dental film directly behind the second part of duodenum
5. the configuration of the biliary tree as a whole.

On occasion, because of the tilt of the patient to the right, the left hepatic duct system is underfilled. If doubt exists, further films should be taken after removing the tilt.

Prior isolation of the cystic duct may be difficult or dangerous in a patient with severe acute cholecystitis, or the cystic duct may prove in some patients to be too narrow to cannulate. In such cases, cholangiogram films may be obtained after direct needle puncture of the common bile duct. The puncture wound should then be occluded by a fine suture (e.g. 3/0 Dexon), but even so, postoperative leakage of bile from the puncture site is not uncommon.

Operative cholangiography should be regarded as routine for patients with suspected calculous disease

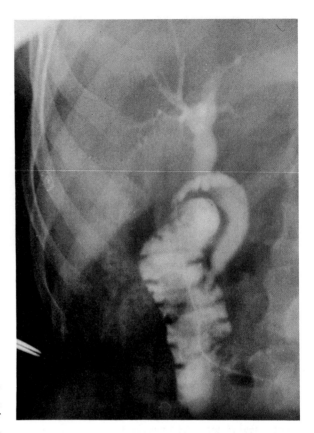

Fig. 20.8 X-ray film of normal operative cholangiogram

(Doyle, 1982). It may be omitted in patients with carcinoma of the head of pancreas with a clear preoperative diagnosis and confirmatory findings at laparotomy in whom the intention is to carry out palliative bypass surgery.

For patients with calculous disease, cholecystectomy should be the aim, with the decision to explore the common bile duct being largely determined by the cholangiogram films, provided these are of reasonable quality. Occasionally, in patients with severe acute cholecystitis, a determined attempt to carry out cholecystectomy will be dangerous, and cholecystostomy with extraction of the intravesical stones is the more prudent course, particularly if the surgeon is inexperienced.

Transduodenal sphincteroplasty, or choledochoduodenostomy may be indicated for an impacted stone at the lower end of the common bile duct, stricture at the ampulla, or multiple stones in the common bile duct. The alternative of a later endoscopic papillotomy should be considered in such patients particularly if the patient is frail.

Obstruction due to chronic pancreatitis will normally be dealt with by a bypass procedure (cholecysto- or choledochojejunostomy). Obstruction due to small ampullary carcinoma without evidence of spread should be treated by pancreaticoduodenectomy if the patient's overall condition permits.

CHOLECYSTOSTOMY

The indications for this operation have already been discussed. In cases of acute cholecystitis, a provisional decision to perform cholecystostomy may be made before the abdomen is opened. The operation may then be planned accordingly; local anaesthesia can be employed if desired, and a small incision (vertical or oblique) made directly over the fundus of the gall-bladder. If the diagnosis of acute cholecystitis is confirmed, adhesions are separated only sufficiently to expose the gall-bladder, and no further exploration is attempted.

The gall-bladder is carefully surrounded with moist packs, and an Oschner aspirator attached to suction inserted into the fundus of the gall-bladder to aspirate the liquid contents. When no more bile can be aspirated, light tissue forceps are applied to the gall-bladder wall on each side of the needle, which is then withdrawn. The opening is enlarged with scissors to a length of 2 to 3 cm, and the remaining contents (usually gall-stones and biliary 'mud') are evacuated with a scoop or with fenestrated forceps, a large spoon or special receiver being held against the opening in order to catch any escaping bile or debris. Two fingers are then passed deeply along the outside of the gall-bladder, and the neck of the viscus and the cystic duct are carefully palpated. Any further calculi detected are milked upwards until they are within reach of the scoop or forceps (Fig. 20.9). Care must be taken not to overlook

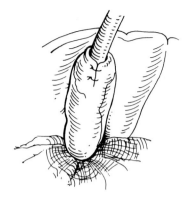

Fig. 20.10 Cholecystostomy. The gall-bladder has been repaired around a drainage tube

a stone impacted in the cystic duct. The interior of the gall-bladder is then explored with the finger, and is dried with a swab held on forceps; this is rotated in order to entangle and remove any small stones which remain.

A 24 FG Latex Rubber Winsbury White or Foley catheter is introduced into the gall-bladder as far as its middle and sutured with 2/0 chromic catgut to the edge of the opening. Closure of the opening around the tube is effected by a purse-string suture of 2/0 chromic catgut or (if the gall-bladder wall is thickened or friable) by one or two interrupted sutures (Fig. 20.10). The tube drain should be brought to the surface through a stab incision separate from the main wound using the shortest route. If the gall-bladder fundus lies close to the parietal peritoneum, it should be attached to it using chromic catgut sutures—alternatively omentum may be brought up and sutured to the fundus. Lavage of the area with an antibiotic solution is advisable prior to closure of the wound, and use of a small suction drain (e.g. *Redivac*) from the subhepatic space is recommended.

After-treatment
The tube is attached to a closed system bile drainage bag and allowed to drain freely for 7–10 days, when a tube cholecystogram should be undertaken to check for the presence of residual stones in the gall-bladder or common bile duct. If the X-rays show no residual calculi and a normal common bile duct, the tube drain may be removed at this stage. In this situation a decision to undertake elective cholecystectomy will be determined by whether or not the patient develops symptoms. More than 50% will be asymptomatic during the next 5 years, so that an expectant policy is justified.

If the cholecystogram demonstrates the clear presence of stones, or blockage of the cystic duct (most likely from a stone) the tube should be left in situ for a further 3 to 4 weeks and consideration given to planned chole-cystectomy (which is likely to be difficult and therefore

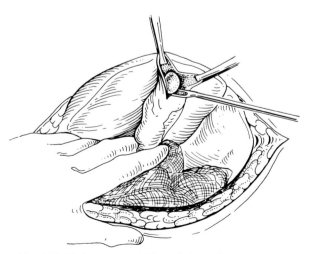

Fig. 20.9 Cholecystostomy. The technique of removing stones from the gall-bladder is depicted

should be undertaken only by an experienced surgeon) or to instrumental removal of the stones through the tube track. Removal of the cholecystostomy tube in the presence of obstruction is likely to lead either to a persisting mucous fistula or to recurrent infection in the gall-bladder.

Should the X-rays reveal a gall-bladder clear of stones or obstruction, but a stone or stones in the common bile duct, the ideal treatment, if the expertise is available, is endoscopic papillotomy and removal of the stones in view of the difficulties of surgery following cholecystostomy.

CHOLECYSTECTOMY

All steps of the operation must be carried out under direct vision. The patients are often obese and access is difficult, so that an adequate exposure is essential. Suitable incisions are described on p. 387.

The first step consists in careful packing-off. At least two large-sized packs are required. The first is placed in the lower part of the wound, displacing downwards duodenum, transverse colon and small intestine; the second is placed medially to cover and retract the stomach. A third pack may be inserted laterally to fill the right kidney pouch. Deep retractors are then placed in position, and are held by the assistant so as to give the best exposure.

There are two principal methods of removing the gall-bladder. In that which is generally advocated (the *retrograde* method), the cystic duct and cystic artery are divided first, and the gall-bladder is then stripped off towards the fundus. In the alternative method the separation of the gall-bladder is commenced at the fundus.

The retrograde method

This has the great advantage that the cystic duct and cystic artery can be clearly identified before division, this part of the operation being carried out at an early stage before the deeper parts of the operation field can become obscured by haemorrhage. The risk of injury to the common duct or to the right hepatic artery are therefore greatly reduced.

When distension of the gall-bladder prevents ready access to the ducts, or if there is thought to be any danger of rupture, the contents should be aspirated, the puncture opening being afterwards closed with a stitch or clamp. A forceps is applied to the infundibulum of the gall-bladder, and is used to draw the viscus gently forwards and to the right (Fig. 20.11). The junction of the cystic and common ducts is now displayed by snipping of the overlying peritoneum and by gauze stripping. This dissection may take some time since the ducts

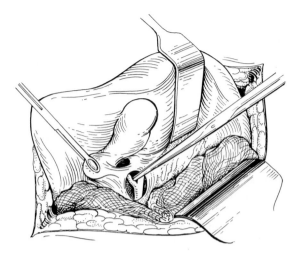

Fig. 20.11 Cholecystectomy by the retrograde method—exposure of the cystic duct at its junction with the common hepatic duct, in the right free border of the lesser omentum

are often obscured by fat or by oedematous connective tissue.

Occasionally the cystic artery runs anterior to the cystic duct, obscuring access. It should then be divided between nonabsorbable sutures, a procedure usually left until later in the operation. An absorbable ligature (Dexon or catgut) is now placed loosely around the cystic duct close to its junction with the common bile duct. Any stones in the cystic duct should be milked towards the gall-bladder and the cystic duct clamped or ligated (Fig. 20.12) close to Hartmann's pouch. The cystic duct is now opened between the ligatures, any stones remaining in the duct removed, a bacteriology swab taken for culture, and the cannula introduced for

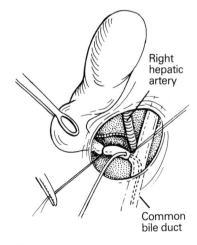

Right hepatic artery

Common bile duct

Fig. 20.12 Cholecystectomy. The cystic duct has been ligated and a cannula has been inserted into the common bile duct for cholangiography. The cystic artery has been identified

operative cholangiography (see p. 388). The cannula is left in place until the films have been viewed, lest further films are required. When satisfactory films are obtained, the cannula is removed, the ligature close to the common bile duct fully tightened and the cystic duct divided.

Gentle traction on the cystic duct and careful sharp and gauze dissection keeping close to the upper part of the gall-bladder neck will now reveal the cystic artery (if not previously divided) in its usual position crossing the triangle of Calot. It should be doubly ligated with silk or linen and divided between the ligatures.

The gall-bladder is now attached by little more than the peritoneal sheath which binds it to the inferior surface of the liver. Its neck is drawn forwards away from the liver and a finger is insinuated between the two. The finger is made to work its way gently upwards separating the gall-bladder from its bed. As the separation progresses the peritoneal reflection on each side is divided with scissors. An attempt is made to retain a fringe of peritoneum on each side, with which the gall-bladder bed can be covered. To enable this to be done, the peritoneum should if possible be stripped for a short distance from the sides of the gall-bladder before being divided. Some haemorrhage occurs from minute vessels which pass directly to the gall-bladder from the substance of the liver, but if the separation is carried out in the correct plane the bleeding is relatively slight and can be arrested by pressure with a hot moist pack or by light coagulation with the diathermy electrode. If an aberrant duct (*hepato-cholecystic duct*) is encountered entering the gall-bladder directly from its bed (see Fig. 20.2) it should be secured and ligatured. It is a good plan to delay the final separation of the gall-bladder until its bed has been dealt with, for the partially separated viscus can be used as a convenient retractor (Fig. 20.13).

If it has been possible to conserve peritoneal fringes at each side of the raw area, these are brought together by continuous or interrupted sutures, if necessary to control haemorrhage, since the raw area seldom if ever produces any harmful effects.

Drainage should be provided as there may be leakage of bile from the cystic duct if the ligature slips, from the gall-bladder bed, or from the common bile duct if it has been punctured for cholangiography. Some postoperative oozing of blood may also occur, particularly if the gall-bladder was badly inflamed, with the potential for development of an infected collection in what is usually a contaminated area. Two *Redivac* suction drains are recommended, one led from the subhepatic and one from the right suprahepatic space, brought out separately from the wound. These drains would normally be removed at 48 hours unless there is continuing drainage of bile (Hoffman, 1985).

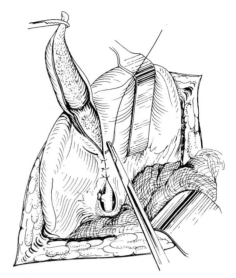

Fig. 20.13 Completion of cholecystectomy by the retrograde method. The partially separated gall-bladder is used as a retractor to allow exposure for haemostasis. Sutures are rarely necessary

Depending on the incision and the surgeon's preference, the wound is closed in layers or by the mass suture technique.

'Fundus first' method

This method is advised only when difficulties (particularly severe inflammatory changes) prevent the ducts being displayed in the first steps of the operation, so exposing them to great danger if dissection near the cystic duct and common bile duct is continued. Paradoxically, however, the fundus first method also carries risks of injury particularly to the common bile duct and right hepatic artery. Excessive traction on the mobilized gall-bladder may pull these structures out of their normal alignment, rendering them liable to be clamped or included in a ligature (Fig. 20.14).

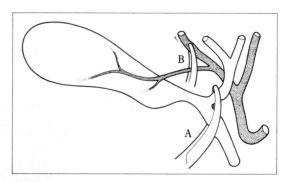

Fig. 20.14 Accidents liable to occur at cholecystectomy—inclusion of the common bile duct (A) or the right hepatic artery (B) in clamp or ligature

Separation of the gall-bladder is commenced at the fundus, the peritoneal sheath being divided with scissors at each side where it is reflected on to the liver. It is most desirable that the cystic duct and cystic artery should be clearly defined before the gall-bladder is removed. If, however, owing to adhesions, isolation of these structures is thought to endanger the right hepatic artery or the common duct, it is far better to leave part of the neck of the gall-bladder in situ. More bleeding is encountered using this technique than using the retrograde method, where the cystic artery is controlled at an earlier stage.

Espiner (1982) has described a modification of the fundus first method which he considers particularly suitable for the very thickened and inflamed gall-bladder, in which the separation of the gall-bladder bed is carried out in the submucosal plane using diathermy. This obviates the requirement to control the cystic artery and minimizes the risk of danger to the common bile duct.

Risks of the operation

The chief danger lies in the possibility of injury to one of the main bile ducts or to the right hepatic artery. Unless the junction between the cystic and common ducts is clearly demonstrated, a segment of the common duct may be inadvertently clamped or included in a ligature (Fig. 20.14), so that biliary obstruction may result. Undetected section of a duct—possibly an abnormally placed or accessory one—may lead to biliary peritonitis or to an external fistula. The right hepatic artery may be ligatured in mistake for the cystic artery, or may be included in the ligature applied to it (Fig. 20.14); this accident may cause a fatal issue owing to massive liver necrosis. To obviate these dangers two simple rules should be observed at any operation for cholecystectomy:

1. The junction of the cystic and common ducts should be displayed beyond the slightest possibility of doubt, before any clamp or ligature is applied.
2. The cystic artery should be ligatured separately, and only after it has been clearly identified by its course to the gall-bladder.

Haemorrhage

Haemorrhage from a torn cystic artery or from a slipped ligature is likely to be profuse, and injudicious attempts to arrest it may damage important structures in the vicinity. A large pack should be placed against the bleeding area, *and left in situ for 2 or 3 minutes*; when it is removed the bleeding vessel can usually be secured without difficulty. If necessary, the hepatic artery may be temporarily occluded by a light bowel clamp placed on the right free border of the lesser omentum.

Accumulation of bile

This may occur in the right subphrenic or subhepatic region, even when provision for drainage appears to have been adequate. Upper abdominal or chest pain associated with tachycardia and a persistently low blood pressure (the Waltman-Walters syndrome), are cardinal signs, and the condition is often mistaken for coronary thrombosis. If there is any suspicion that such an accumulation is present, no time should be lost in re-exploring the abdomen, since immediate and dramatic relief is obtained from evacuation of the bile, and unless this is done the patient's condition rapidly deteriorates.

Cholecystectomy for carcinoma

A very early carcinoma may be detected only after the gall-bladder has been removed and opened up; in such cases the prognosis is reasonably good. More often, however, the gall-bladder is hard and nodular from an infiltrating growth. A segment of the adjacent liver tissue should then be removed along with the gall-bladder (p. 378). When there is naked-eye evidence of extension of the disease to the liver it is probably too late to hope for a cure, but partial hepatectomy may be considered.

CHOLEDOCHOTOMY

Choledochotomy (opening and exploration of the common bile duct) is indicated when the operative cholangiogram reveals filling defects or stricture. If facilities for operative cholangiography have been omitted or are not available, the palpation of a stone is a clear indication for exploration of the duct. Reliance on the classical indications for exploration, for example, a dilated or thickened duct, recent jaundice, multiple small stones in the gall-bladder with a wide cystic duct results in a negative exploration rate of approximately 50%. Negative exploration of the common bile duct increases mortality, morbidity and duration of hospital stay in comparison with simple cholecystectomy.

Supraduodenal choledochotomy

This approach is the method of choice since the supraduodenal portion of the duct, lying in the free border of the lesser omentum, is relatively accessible in most cases. Exploration of the duct is, in the majority of cases, for suspected calculi, and the gall-bladder will have been removed earlier in the operation.

The second part of duodenum should be fully mobilized ('Kocherized') after incision of the peritoneum lying lateral to it. This is usually avascular, though some vessels may require ligation close to the region where the common bile duct passes behind the duodenum. Mobilization of the duodenum and head of the pancreas should be carried as far as the left side of the inferior

length of the common bile duct, and for the second part of duodenum to be brought forward into the wound. A pack is now placed posterior to the duodenum in Morison's pouch.

The peritoneum over the supraduodenal portion of the common duct is incised and the anterior surface cleared of peritoneum and fatty tissue over a distance of 1.5 cm. One or two small vessels in the immediate supraduodenal region may require to be controlled either by fine ligatures or by haemoclips. If, due to gross inflammatory changes, there is some doubt as to the actual location of the common bile duct it may be identified by aspirating bile through a fine bore needle.

Exploration of the duct
Stay sutures of 2/0 chromic catgut are now inserted near the borders of the duct and a 1 cm longitudinal incision made between them into the duct (Fig. 20.15). A bacteriological swab is taken of the bile escaping through the incision, and the bile is aspirated through a fine bore sucker. Some small floating stones may emerge with the first rush of bile, and these should be retrieved. An attempt should now be made *gently* to milk any palpable stones towards the choledochotomy incision, whence they may easily be removed using gall-stone forceps.

Removal of calculi
The duct is now formally explored for residual stones,

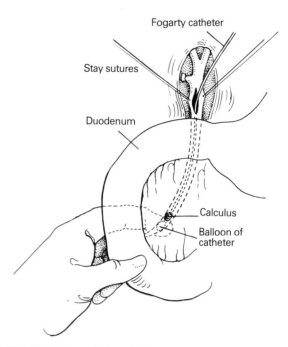

Fig. 20.16 Removal of a calculus in the lower part of the common bile duct using a Fogarty biliary catheter

palpable or otherwise. A wide variety of instruments is available for this purpose. Rigid bougies or forceps (e.g. Maingot's, Desjardins's) are most frequently used, but unless great care is exercised damage to the duct, particularly at its lower end, may result, with subsequent stricture formation. It is therefore recommended that the initial exploration be made with a Fogarty biliary catheter (Fig. 20.16).

Retrograde exploration is undertaken first. The common bile duct is lightly compressed between finger and thumb below the choledochotomy incision. The catheter is passed upwards and guided into the right hepatic duct and advanced as far as it will go. The balloon is now inflated until slight resistance to downward traction is felt, and the catheter is pulled downwards, maintaining inflation to provide slight resistance. Any calculi appearing at the choledochotomy incision are removed by forceps. The procedure is repeated for the left hepatic duct and then for both ducts in turn until the surgeon is satisfied that the upper biliary tree is clear.

Prograde exploration is now undertaken. The duct above the choledochotomy is occluded between finger and thumb, or using light occlusion forceps, and the Fogarty catheter passed into the duodenum (judged by the distance it has passed) and the balloon inflated. Confirmation of its position in the duodenum is made by palpation of the inflated balloon. The balloon is now partially deflated while maintaining upward traction until the balloon is felt to come through the sphincter.

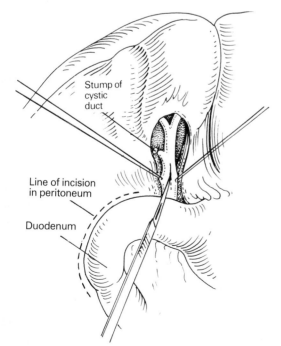

Fig. 20.15 Method of opening the supraduodenal part of the common bile duct by incision between stay sutures

It is then re-inflated to maintain slight resistance to traction and the catheter pulled upwards until calculi, or the balloon, appear at the choledochotomy incision. Calculi are removed. The procedure is repeated until the surgeon is content that no calculi remain.

Should the Fogarty catheter fail to enter the duodenum (usually due to an impacted and palpable stone) further gentle exploration with a metal biliary scoop or Maingot's forceps, using the left hand to guide the instrument into position, will usually result in a successful extraction. Management of the impacted and apparently immoveable stone will be considered later on this page.

Given that at this stage in the operation the surgeon feels that he has cleared the ducts, the common bile duct and hepatic ducts are irrigated with saline to wash out any calculous debris or blood clots and postexploratory cholangiogram films are taken. Dissatisfaction with films obtained by injecting dye through the T-tube, usually due to failure to outline the lower end of the common bile duct because dye does not pass through, because of spasm of the sphincter of Oddi, led Gunn (Fox, 1984) to describe a technique using a fine (8 FG) Foley catheter. The catheter is first inserted upwards through the choledochotomy incision, and the balloon inflated to occlude the common hepatic duct. Dye is now injected to display the upper biliary tree. The balloon is deflated, the catheter inserted downwards, the balloon inflated to occlude the common bile duct and dye injected to display the lower biliary tree. Provided the ampulla is not occluded by a stone, the extra pressure obtained using this technique will allow dye to pass into the duodenum and fully display the lowest part of the common bile duct. Exploration of the duct system under vision using a *choledochoscope* is of added benefit if the necessary equipment and skills are available (Ernst, 1982).

Drainage

Following demonstration of a satisfactory duct system T-tube drainage of the common bile duct should in the author's view be routine. Some surgeons omit this step, especially if the exploration has been negative, but the opportunity subsequently to obtain high quality films of the duct system in the X-ray department is then lost. A relatively fine Latex rubber T-tube (10 or 12 FG) should be used. The long limb of the T-tube is brought out through the *lower* end of the choledochotomy incision (Fig. 20.17), which is closed in one layer of continuous fine absorbable suture (e.g. 3/0 Dexon), and brought to the surface through a stab incision, taking the most direct route.

Antibiotic lavage of the operation area prior to closure of the main wound is recommended, and small bore

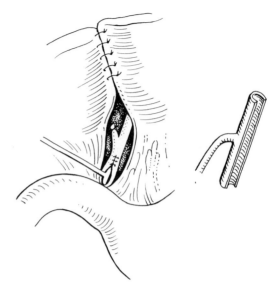

Fig. 20.17 T-tube drainage of the common bile duct. The incision in the duct is sutured *above* the emerging limb of the tube in order to avoid any drag on the suture line when the tube is withdrawn

Redivac drains are led both from the subhepatic and suprahepatic spaces.

Postoperative check films are taken on the 7th–10th day usually following 2 to 3 days of intermittent clamping of the T-tube and, if satisfactory, the tube is removed. There may be a small bile leak following removal which rarely persists for more than 48 hours.

The impacted stone

If, as mentioned earlier, a stone remains impacted at the lower end of the common bile duct despite routine measures to remove it, the surgeon has essentially three choices, determined by the fitness of the patient, or availability of endoscopic skills:

1. To leave the stone where it is, drain the common bile duct by T-tube for 2 to 3 weeks to allow inflammation to settle, and invite an expert endoscopist to carry out endoscopic papillotomy. This has attractions for the very sick patient, but the truly impacted stone does provide the endoscopist with some difficulties, and stones over 15 mm in diameter are not suitable for the technique.

2. Leave the stone where it is and carry out *choledochoduodenostomy* (Figs. 20.18 & 20.19) (Almeida, 1984). A transverse incision is made in the common bile duct as low down as possible, and an incision made in the adjacent duodenum. The anastomosis is performed in one layer of interrupted inverting sutures of 3/0 absorbable material (knotted on the inside). At completion the stoma should have a diameter of 2.5 cm. If the diameter of the common bile duct is insufficient

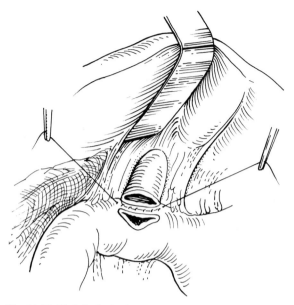

Fig. 20.18 Choledochoduodenostomy by anastomosis between the common duct in continuity and the first part of duodenum

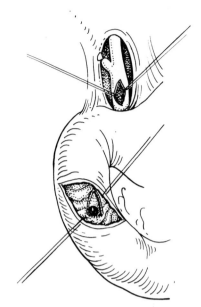

Fig. 20.20 Transduodenal choledochotomy

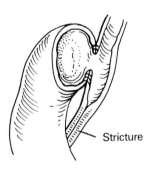

Stricture

Fig. 20.19 Diagramatic cross-section of choledochoduodenostomy

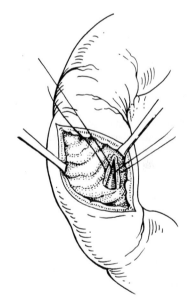

Fig. 20.21 Transduodenal sphincteroplasty

to permit a transverse incision, a vertical incision is made which is then sutured transversely. A T-tube is not usually necessary following this procedure and the choledochotomy incision is closed in one layer of a continuous 3/0 absorbable suture.

3. Remove the stone via a *transduodenal sphinctero-plasty*. An oblique anterolateral incision is made in the second part of duodenum in a position determined by the palpable stone (Fig. 20.20). Stay sutures are now inserted in the medial wall of the duodenum on either side of the ampulla (Fig. 20.21). Using a knife, an incision is made directly over the stone which is then extracted. The incision in the wall of duodenum is now enlarged, using sphincteroplasty scissors, to a minimum length of 1.5 cm and converted to a formal sphinctero-plasty by approximating duodenal and bile duct mucosa using interrupted 3/0 absorbable sutures. Care must be

taken to ensure apposition of mucosae at the apex of the incision. The duodenotomy incision is now closed in its own line in two layers of suture (Fig. 20.22). Supra-duodenal T-tube drainage is not normally necessary following this procedure (Carter, 1983) and the chole-dochotomy incision is closed in one layer using a continu-ous 3/0 absorbable suture.

The retained stone

Despite apparently satisfactory postexploratory films

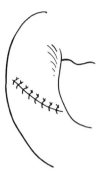

Fig. 20.22 Closure of duodenotomy

obtained at operation, the T-tube cholangiogram obtained 7–10 days after operation may demonstrate one or more stones that had been missed at operation (Fig. 20.23). Again, several management options are available:

1. Leave the T-tube to drain for a further 7–10 days and then repeat the cholangiogram. Up to 40% of filling

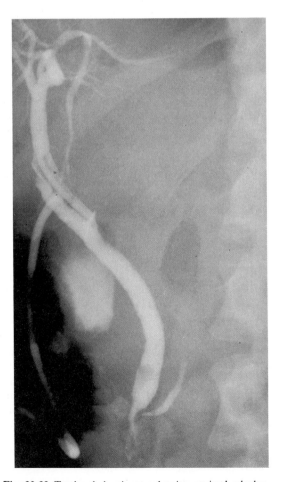

Fig. 20.23 T-tube cholangiogram showing retained calculus

defects will have disappeared, either because they were not stones (e.g. blood clot, air bubble), or, if they were, have passed spontaneously.

2. Institute *irrigation* of the common bile duct through the T-tube. Intramittent irrigation through the T-tube using bile acids has been favoured, and heparin suggested, but there is little hard evidence that they provide better results than irrigation with saline. The method may be continued for up to 3 weeks, but is unlikely to be successful if the retained stone lies in the biliary tree above the level of the T-tube, and is contraindicated if a stone is impacted at the lower end of the bile duct preventing flow of dye into the duodenum. Check cholangiograms are taken through the T-tube every few days to assess progress.

3. *Endoscopic papillotomy* may be undertaken 2 weeks after surgery. The stone may be left to pass spontaneously after papillotomy, or it may be extracted at the time of papillotomy using a Dormia basket, or Fogarty type catheter. This technique is not suitable for stones retained high in the biliary tree, and may be unsuccessful if the stone is very firmly impacted at its lower end.

4. *Instrumental removal via the T-tube tract* (Burhenne, 1976; Irwin, 1985). This technique, which should be delayed for 4 weeks after operation to allow maturation of the T-tube track, may be used for retained stones anywhere in the biliary tree, but is particularly suitable for stones in its upper part. The original injunction to use a large bore T-tube (> 14 FG) so as to permit this technique, no longer prevails, as the T-tube track may be dilated using graduated dilators before introducing the cannula down the track. Under fluoroscopic control, a Dormia basket or Fogarty type catheter is manipulated into position around or beyond the stone, which is then drawn out along the T-tube track.

5. *Re-operation* will be required in the event of failure or non-availability of the preceding techniques. Such reoperations are difficult and supraduodenal re-exploration particularly so, so that preference is given to a transduodenal approach with sphincteroplasty for stones in the lower parts of the duct.

OTHER OPERATIONS ON THE BILE DUCTS

Immediate repair of injuries

Most injuries to the bile ducts follow operative misadventures. They are due usually to failure to isolate and to ligature separately the cystic duct and cystic artery at the operation of cholecystectomy or to lack of care in freeing the duodenum at gastrectomy. The common bile duct is the one most frequently damaged. Such injuries are potentially serious and should be dealt with at once provided that the situation is not aggravated by unskilled attempts at repair.

End-to-end suture

This is the ideal method of repair, but as a rule it is practicable only when the condition is discovered at or very soon after the injury, for at a later date considerable retraction together with periductal fibrosis will have occurred. The cut ends are identified; the upper is usually traced without difficulty from the escape of bile; the lower may have retracted behind the duodenum, which must then be mobilized by division of the peritoneum along its lateral border. This allows the duodenum to be brought up towards the porta hepatis, so that the cut ends of the duct may be approximated without tension. It is advisable that the anastomosis should be effected over a latex rubber tube: this not only forms an effective splint, but also serves to maintain the lumen of the duct. If a T-tube is used, it should be brought out through a separate opening in the lower segment of the duct at least 1 cm below the suture line (Fig. 20.24), and the anastomosis made over its upper limb. The cut ends of the duct are united by interrupted sutures of fine catgut, and the suture line is reinforced by repair of the surrounding fascial layers. Alternatively, a simple tube may be used, and may be brought to the surface by one of the methods described below.

Late repair or reconstruction of ducts

Secondary repair of a severed or stenosed duct is one of the most difficult of operations. The duct is likely to be

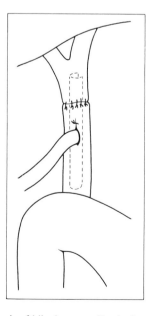

Fig. 20.24 Repair of bile duct over T-tube brought out through opening at lower level

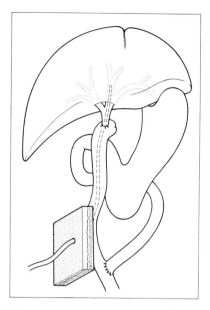

Fig. 20.25 Reconstruction of bile duct by the use of a *Roux* loop of jejunum. A latex tube splints the anastomosis, and is led down through the jejunal loop for about 10 cm before being brought out through the abdominal wall

buried in dense scar tissue, and the ends may be widely retracted.

Experience suggests that the most successful method of reconstruction is to effect an anastomosis between the upper stump of the duct and a defunctioned (*Roux*) loop of jejunum, as shown in Figure 20.25 (Bismith, 1978). This is done by transecting the bowel 25 to 30 cm below the duodenojejunal flexure, and by bringing the lower cut end upwards in front of or behind the transverse colon, to be joined to the upper stump of the biliary duct. Direct suture may be possible to a stump of bile duct or to the left hepatic duct if this can be exposed (Blumgart, 1984). The 'mucosal graft' technique described by Rodney Smith (1980) is applicable where no duct stump remains; by bringing into contact mucosa of bile duct and jejunum, it reduces the risk of re-stenosis. A soft latex tube within the anastomosis and brought out through the abdominal wall (Fig. 20.25) may be extruded by peristalsis and it is preferable to bring the tube to the surface through the liver substance (Fig. 20.26). By this latter method the tube can remain in situ for 6 to 12 months; it can be clamped so that no external leakage of bile occurs; it will stay in place until removed by the surgeon, and until then can be used for irrigation of the reconstructed duct. This method greatly reduces the risk of progressive stenosis, which is always liable to occur after operative repair.

Strictures of the common bile duct

These may result from injury or from fibrosis following

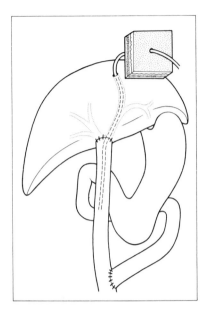

Fig. 20.26 Alternative method of splinting the anastomosis, the tube being led upwards through the liver substance before reaching the exterior

some inflammatory lesion. A common type of stricture occurs at the lower end of the duct, the most likely cause being a stone which has been impacted sufficiently long to set up a fibrotic reaction (see Fig. 20.19).

When stenosis involves only the orifice of the duct, it may be dealt with either by transduodenal surgical sphincteroplasty (see Fig. 20.21) or by endoscopic papillotomy. For sphincteroplasty, a probe is passed into the duct orifice which is then slit upwards for 1 to 2 cm. The mucosal layers of duct and duodenum are then united by two or three stitches on each side.

When the stricture is thought to be too high, too long or too resilient to be treated by simple incision of the duct orifice, short-circuiting operations offer the best prospect of success. The upper part of the duct, which is likely to be much dilated, can usually be anastomosed without undue difficulty to the duodenum by the operation of *choledochoduodenostomy* (see Fig. 20.18). This is attended usually by good results. Alternatively, a *Roux* loop of jejunum may be employed for the anastomosis (Figs. 20.25 & 20.26).

Operations for biliary fistula
The temporary fistula which follows the operations of cholecystostomy and choledochostomy usually closes spontaneously within a week or 10 days after withdrawal of the tube.

A *persistent* fistula may close spontaneously even after a period of several months, so that surgical interference should not be too hastily considered. When, however, serious loss of bile is occurring and especially if there

is evidence that no bile is reaching the intestine, operation should be undertaken without undue delay. The operative procedure will depend upon the conditions present.

A fistula following cholecystostomy is likely to be due to stricture of the cystic duct or to an impacted calculus, in which case the discharge will consist mainly of mucus. Cholecystectomy is usually curative.

Biliary fistula following cholecystectomy may be due to accidental wounding of a duct during the operation. Often the accident becomes evident only after several days, from profuse discharge of bile from the wound, or from signs of a subhepatic collection—the *Waltman-Walters syndrome* (p. 392). When the injury to the duct has been relatively slight, or if it is only a small accessory duct that has been severed, a large proportion of the total bile may pass normally to the intestine, and spontaneous healing may then be expected. If, however, the common duct or one of the main hepatic ducts has been completely severed, spontaneous cure is impossible, and immediate operation is required.

If a fistula persists after choledochostomy, it is likely that the lower part of the common duct is obstructed—possibly by a residual stone, or by fibrosis associated with chronic pancreatitis. If the patency of the duct cannot be restored, an attempt may be made to carry out one of the reconstructive or short-circuiting operations already described.

ANASTOMOSIS OF GALL-BLADDER TO GASTRO-INTESTINAL TRACT

The operations described under this heading are designed to short-circuit irremediable obstruction of the common bile duct, such as may be caused by carcinoma or by chronic pancreatitis. They are seldom applicable to cases of common duct obstruction due to the effects of gall-stones, for the gall-bladder is then likely to be shrivelled and fibrotic, or otherwise unsuitable for anastomosis; in many cases it will have been removed at a previous operation.

Cholecystogastrostomy
This is technically the easiest operation since the distended gall-bladder usually lies in contact with the pyloric part of the stomach. It is now seldom employed, however, since it has certain serious disadvantages: bilious vomiting due to the large quantities of bile which may be passed directly into the stomach, and an irritative cholangitis due to regurgitation of gastric contents into the biliary passages.

Technique
The gall-bladder is emptied by a trocar and cannula

inserted on the inferior aspect of the fundus. Light occlusion clamps are applied to the fundus, and to the nearest portion of stomach. The clamps are laid side by side, and lateral anastomosis is carried out by the standard technique, the first line of sutures being placed so that the opening made by the cannula can be enlarged to form the anastomosis. An opening 2 cm in length is adequate.

Cholecystoduodenostomy

This is technically very difficult, and has no special advantages. It is therefore seldom performed.

Cholecystojejunostomy

By pass using a loop of jejunum is the operation most commonly performed. A loop of jejunum some 45 cm below the duodenojejunal flexure is selected and brought up in front of the colon for the purpose of the anastomosis. The operation is completed by making an entero-anastomosis between the afferent and efferent loops of jejunum (Fig. 20.27). This not only prevents obstruction of the bowel by kinking, but diverts much of the bowel contents from the site of the anastomosis. More complete diversion is obtained by utilizing a defunctioned (*Roux*) jejunal loop of jejunum. Though technically more demanding to surgeon and patient than the standard cholecystojejunostomy it is preferred in the fitter patient and in those whose obstruction is of benign aetiology and consequently have a longer life expectancy.

Tumours of the bile ducts

Carcinomas of the common bile duct are rarely amenable to excision. Occasionally a carcinoma of the lower end of the common bile duct may be resected by *pancreatico-duodenectomy*. Rarely it may be possible to resect a

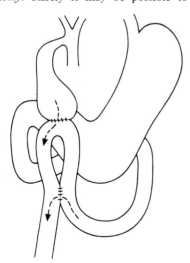

Fig. 20.27 Cholecystojejunostomy with entero-anastomosis

tumour of the common hepatic duct, restoring biliary drainage through a Roux loop of jejunum.

Usually only palliative treatment is possible. In the case of tumours involving the lower common bile duct, cholecyst- or hepatico-jejunostomy may be employed, or drainage provided by percutaneous insertion of a biliary endoprosthesis through the tumour into duodenum. In tumours involving the duct system at the level of the common hepatic duct or above, percutaneous intubation is the palliative procedure of choice (Cameron, 1982), though a Longmire hepaticojejunostomy may be considered.

Some of these tumours may be very slow growing and occasionally prolonged survival follows palliation.

BILIARY ATRESIA

In this text the term biliary atresia is used to include classical extrahepatic biliary atresia, biliary hypoplasia and choledochal cyst. In 10% of babies with biliary atresia a dilated bile duct proximal to an atretic segment is found below the level of the porta hepatis in the free margin of the lesser omentum. In the remainder, hypoplastic or atretic ducts extend proximally within the substance of the liver. The two types of lesion have been described as 'operable' and 'inoperable' respectively. In clinical practice it is important to differentiate between obstructive jaundice of biliary atresia and cholestatic jaundice of neonatal hepatitis. This must be done with some urgency as the treatment of biliary atresia is by operation within 6 to 8 weeks of birth so as to prevent irreversible damage to the liver. The distinction, however, is not always clear as there appears to be an area of overlap between the two conditions. The classical view of biliary atresia and neonatal hepatitis as separate entities is now in doubt and it is more probable that both are part of a spectrum of change in the biliary system from damage either viral or by foetal bile salts.

A diagnosis of obstructive jaundice should be considered in a baby with conjugated hyperbilirubinaemia and acholic stools who becomes icteric within a few days of birth or in whom 'physiological' jaundice fails to clear. Other causes of hepatitis, for example infection, galactosaemia and alpha 1 antitrypsin deficiency must first be excluded. The distinction between biliary atresia and neonatal hepatitis is then made on the basis of I[131] Rose Bengal excretion studies and percutaneous liver biopsy. Excretion of less than 10% of active iodine in the stool is indicative of biliary atresia whereas a greater figure favours a diagnosis of hepatitis. The histological changes of bile ductule proliferation, fibrosis and bile stasis are seen in biliary atresia whereas giant cell transformation is typical of neonatal hepatocytes.

The management of a baby with a diagnosis of biliary

atresia is by operation. An operative cholangiogram is first performed through the fundus of the gall-bladder (Howard, 1983). The free margin of the lesser omentum is then dissected. When an 'operable' lesion is present a dilated duct is found and bile drainage can be achieved by means of a choledochal enterostomy fashioned with a Roux loop. Alternatively the dilated duct can be dissected proximally, divided at the level of the porta hepatis and porto-enterostomy performed. More often however only a hypoplastic or atretic duct is present; the fine stricture is then dissected proximally with great care to an area of fibrous tissue at the porta hepatis. The fibrous tissue at this level may contain fine ductules; the tissue is therefore divided and, once again, a porto-enterostomy performed using a Roux loop (Kasai, 1959). By this means it may be possible to obtain bile drainage even though this type of lesion has, in the past, been termed 'inoperable'. The only other alternative is liver transplantation.

Although there has been some success with Kasai's operation, the earlier results were disappointing. Babies died of liver failure or, in later years, children died of haemorrhage from portal hypertension secondary to cirrhosis. The failure of surgery may have been, in part, related to delay in operation, failure to establish satisfactory bile drainage and ascending cholangitis. Recognition of the importance of early operation and a modification of Kasai's original procedure so as to allow bile drainage through a cutaneous fistula may prove to be an advantage (Lilly, 1975).

OPERATIONS ON THE PANCREAS

In comparison with operations on other upper abdominal organs, operations on the pancreas are relatively infrequently performed, and are often difficult.

Surgery may be indicated for:

1. *Tumours*
   a. Benign
   b. Malignant
   c. Functioning tumours (Apudomas) which may be benign or malignant.
2. *Inflammatory disease*
   a. Acute pancreatitis
   b. Chronic pancreatitis
3. *Trauma*

Surgical approach to the pancreas

In most patients excellent access to the pancreas is provided by a transverse epigastric incision extending from costal margin to costal margin. In patients with a narrow subcostal angle, a bilateral Kocher incision or a midline epigastric incision extended below the umbilicus is preferred.

The head of the pancreas is exposed by displacing the hepatic flexure downwards after incising peritoneal folds lateral and superior to, and by full Kocherisation of the duodenum as described on page 392. This allows visualization and full palpation of the head of the pancreas. The body and tail of the pancreas are exposed by serial ligation and division of the gastrocolic omentum along most of its length, allowing full access to the lesser sac. This permits visualization and palpation of the anterior aspect of the body and tail. Access to the posterior aspect of the body and tail, as may be required for location of a small apudoma, necessitates medial mobilization of the spleen and tail of pancreas after division of the lienorenal ligament. Progressive medial mobilization of the body of pancreas may now be made.

Tumours of the pancreas

Benign tumours of the pancreas

These are relatively uncommon and unless they are functioning tumours (apudomas) rarely require surgical treatment. Cystadenomas may, however, through their cystic component reach a large size and cause pressure effects requiring operation. Local excision (enucleation) is often possible. Alternatively, depending on the location within the pancreas, distal pancreatectomy (for distal tumours) or drainage into a neighbouring organ such as stomach or jejunum may be undertaken.

Malignant tumours

Carcinoma of the pancreas is a common tumour, and its incidence in the United Kingdom appears to be rising.

Carcinomas of the body of pancreas rarely give rise to definable symptoms permitting diagnosis before they are inoperable as a result either of metastatic spread or local invasion. Cystadenocarcinomas may, however, produce symptoms by their size at an earlier stage and be more amenable to resection. The recognition that the maturity onset diabetic has a higher incidence of pancreatic carcinoma may lead to a higher index of suspicion and earlier investigation leading to the diagnosis of a tumour while still operable.

Carcinoma of the head of the pancreas is more common, and for the purpose of surgical discussion, is usually grouped with carcinoma of the ampulla and lower common bile duct. This is because their common presentation (obstructive jaundice), and operative procedures designed to cure and palliate the condition, are similar. Carcinomas of the ampulla and common bile duct however present at an early stage as from their location they rapidly cause obstruction and they are often slow growing; thus they carry an acceptable prognosis following radical resection with a 5-year survival of approximately 40%. The situation is quite different with carcinoma of the head of the pancreas. The presentation is usually late, and the lesion unsuitable for attempts at resection in 80–90% of cases by reason of lymph node or more distant metastases, or because of local invasion (superior mesenteric vein, or the root of the mesocolon). In patients with an apparently resectable lesion, 5 year survival is 7% (Jones, 1985). Many surgeons thus claim that survival prospects following radical resection are little better than after palliative measures and that resection is not justified.

Radical resection

It is usually possible to make a preoperative diagnosis as to whether one is dealing with a carcinoma of head of pancreas or one of the localized tumours. A combination of PTC, ERCP, CT scanning, direct endoscopic biopsy or guided fine needle biopsy under ultrasound scan, coupled with ultrasound or isotope liver scan to exclude (within the limits of the technique) hepatic metastases would normally give sufficient evidence to permit the surgeon to decide that the patient has a lesion potentially amenable to radical resection, and set aside adequate operating time for the procedure. A further investigation is advisable before surgery, namely superior and coeliac angiography with portal venography, for two reasons:

1. To exclude involvement of the superior mesenteric vein or portal vein by tumour (a contraindication to resection)

2. To demonstrate the arterial anatomy—in particular an anomalous origin of the hepatic artery from the superior mesenteric artery, which if unsuspected before operation, may result in damage to the hepatic artery during resection.

Pancreaticoduodenectomy (Whipple's procedure 1946)

This is the radical resection most frequently used (Fig. 20.28).

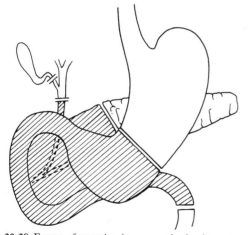

Fig. 20.28 Extent of resection in pancreaticoduodenectomy

Preparation

The procedure is extensive, and adequate preoperative preparation is mandatory. The patient must be adequately hydrated, broad spectrum antibiotic cover provided, and a minimum of 6 units of blood be available for transfusion. A urethral catheter should be in place preoperatively to permit monitoring of urinary output during and after the operation, and a central venous catheter should be inserted by the anaesthetist after induction of anaesthesia. The operation is nowadays usually performed as a single procedure, but in the deeply jaundiced patient, consideration should be given to a period of preoperative external biliary drainage through a percutaneously placed biliary 'pig-tail' catheter (see Fig. 20.4).

Intraoperative assessment of operability

Upon opening the abdomen, the liver is carefully palpated for evidence of metastases. Any suspicious nodules should be biopsied and subjected to frozen section examination. The tumour mass is now palpated and its mobility assessed. The inferior aspect of the transverse mesocolon is inspected for evidence of tumour invasion—a contraindication to proceed with resection. Any enlarged lymph nodes should be removed for frozen section examination and it is good practice routinely to submit the retroduodenal node to this examination. Lymph node involvement, hepatic involvement, or fixity of the tumour are contraindications to resection, and a palliative bypass procedure should be undertaken.

The duodenum and head of pancreas are now fully mobilized as described on page 400 and the tumour palpated bimanually. Particular attention should be directed to see if there is involvement of the superior mesenteric vein—a contraindication to proceed further. If all factors are favourable, the resection may proceed.

The resection (Fig. 20.29)

Some surgeons leave the gall-bladder in situ, but it is good surgical practice to remove it early in the operation. It should certainly be removed if diseased, if the insertion of the cystic duct is low, or if the size of the gall-bladder hampers access. The supraduodenal portion of the common bile duct is now isolated from other structures in the free border of the lesser omentum, and transected below the normal level of insertion of the cystic duct. The gastroduodenal artery is ligated and divided close to its origin from the hepatic artery. The anterior surface of the portal vein is exposed and a blunt dissector passed down its anterior surface and that of the superior mesenteric vein to confirm resectability.

The stomach is transected along the line of junction of body and antrum. The duodenojejunal flexure is mobilized after division of the Ligament of Treitz and, after inspecting the proximal jejunal mesentery for a suitable

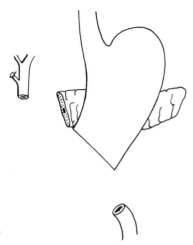

Fig. 20.29 Structures remaining after pancreaticoduodenectomy

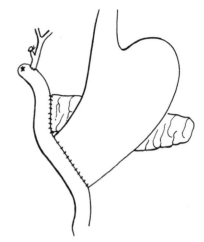

Fig. 20.30 Reconstruction following pancreaticoduodenectomy

vascular arcade, appropriate mesenteric vessels are ligated and divided and the proximal jejunum transected, usually within 10 cm of the duodenojejunal flexure. The proximal jejunum is now drawn to the right behind the superior mesenteric vessels.

A light occlusion clamp is passed gently across the neck of the pancreas, with crushing clamp or forceps to its right, and the neck of pancreas divided between them. An attempt should be made to isolate the main pancreatic duct allowing it to project 1 or 2 mm from the distal cut-end of the gland. Vessels on the distal cut surface should be ligated or suture ligated individually.

Numerous small venous tributaries pass from the head of the pancreas into superior mesenteric and portal veins, and these require careful isolation before dividing them between ligatures or ligaclips. The head of the pancreas is now clear from the veins and all that remains before removal of the specimen is to dissect the unciform process from behind the mesenteric vessels. This may prove tedious, and in some patients it is more expeditious to transect the process and oversew its distal cut-end.

The distal cut-end of jejunum is now closed in two layers and drawn up to the common bile duct through an opening in the transverse mesocolon. The common bile duct, pancreatic stump, and gastric remnant are anastomosed end-to-side to the jejunum, in that order from above downwards (Fig. 20.30). The choledochojejunal anastomosis is best carried out using a single layer of interrupted inverting sutures of Dexon or Vicryl. The pancreaticojejunal anastomosis is the most difficult, and the most likely to leak (producing a fistula) and some surgeons avoid it altogether, either by carrying out a total pancreatectomy (see below) or simply by oversewing the distal cut-end of pancreas, allowing the distal pancreas to atrophy. However the former inevitably pro-

duces diabetes if the patient is not already diabetic, while the latter does carry some risk of producing chronic pancreatitis. Most surgeons will undertake a pancreaticojejunal anastomosis. An incision the length of the cut-end of pancreas is made in the seromuscular layer of jejunum exposing submucosa and mucosa. A small opening is now made in the jejunal mucosa in the centre of the incision, and a direct anastomosis made between jejunum and pancreatic duct using interrupted fine (3/0 or 4/0) sutures of Dexon or silk, the sutures picking up jejunal mucosa and the full thickness of pancreatic duct. This anastomosis may be facilitated by inserting a fine polythene catheter (e.g. umbilical catheter) into the pancreatic duct after completing the posterior row of sutures. The catheter is led out through a stab incision lower down the jejunum and then to the exterior through a stab in the abdominal wall, allowing external drainage of pancreatic juice for the first few postoperative days. The substance of the gland is now sutured to the jejunal seromuscular layer with interrupted 2/0 nonabsorbable sutures. A standard two-layer gastrojejunal anastomosis is then fashioned. Before closure, two fine bore suction drains are led from the vicinity of the pancreaticojejunal anastomosis.

Total pancreatectomy

Total pancreatectomy has been advocated for management of carcinoma of the head of pancreas for two reasons:

1. the tumour might be multicentric so that foci of tumour persist in the body and tail of the pancreas, or in related lymph nodes.
2. the difficult pancreaticojejunal anastomosis is avoided.

The steps of the operation are in general similar to those of Whipple's procedure, apart from the fact that the neck of pancreas is not transected. The body and tail of pancreas, together with spleen, are mobilized medially after division of the lieno-renal ligament. Inferiorly the inferior mesenteric vein requires ligation and division at the lower border of pancreas as it runs to join the splenic vein, and superiorly the short gastric vessels require ligation and division.

Palliative procedures

Increasingly, palliative relief of the obstructive jaundice is being achieved by the percutaneous insertion of a biliary endoprosthesis, inserted following a few days prior drainage using a 'pig-tail' biliary catheter. The technique is very useful in frail patients, and gives a mean survival time of 4 months.

Surgical bypass, however, does provide rather better drainage of the biliary system, and in carcinoma of the head of pancreas where later duodenal obstruction is not uncommon as a result of increasing size of the tumour, affords the opportunity for a prophylactic gastrojejunostomy. It is therefore preferred in the fitter patients.

Cholecystojejunostomy

This is the most frequently performed operation. A loop of proximal jejunum is brought up anterior to the hepatic flexure, and an end-to-side two layer anastomosis made between the fundus of the gall-bladder and the jejunal loop. An enterostomy performed between the afferent and efferent loops is said to reduce the likelihood of contamination of the biliary tree, but this is rather doubtful. In fitter patients, or those with a potentially longer prognosis, a Roux-en-Y cholecystojejunostomy or choledochojejunostomy is to be preferred.

Functioning pancreatic tumours (Apudomas)

A number of functioning pancreatic tumours may produce symptoms. They are uncommon tumours arising in the islet cells but important because of their systemic effects:
1. insulinoma: the commonest
2. gastrinoma: producing the Zollinger Ellison syndrome
3. diarrhoegenic tumour: producing the WDHA (Verner Morison) syndrome
4. glucagonoma: producing a mild form of diabetes and a characteristic skin rash

A detailed discussion of these tumours is beyond the scope of this book. They may be single or multiple, malignant or benign.

Single benign lesions may be dealt with by local excision or enucleation. Single malignant lesions require one of the standard pancreatic resections in the absence of metastatic disease. The lesions are commoner in the body and tail of pancreas than elsewhere and a distal pancreatectomy is indicated in this event, the pancreas

being transected just to the left of the inferior mesenteric vessels.

INFLAMMATORY CONDITIONS OF THE PANCREAS

Acute pancreatitis

Acute pancreatitis is a potentially lethal condition, with a mortality rate of 10–12% in most series. The spectrum of severity is wide, however, and it is worthwhile at an early stage in management attempting to identify the most severe cases using criteria such as those proposed by Ranson (1974) or Imrie (1975).

Although the direct cause of acute pancreatitis is not known, the commonest associated disorder in the United Kingdom is gall-stone disease, followed in second place (with the gap narrowing) by alcohol abuse.

The diagnosis is made by a consideration of the history, the finding (not always present) of an elevated serum amylase and by demonstration of a swollen pancreas by ultrasonography. It is becoming increasingly uncommon to make the diagnosis at laparotomy, and as the initial management is essentially nonoperative, such an 'accidental' diagnosis should be avoided.

The majority of patients' symptoms and signs settle within 48–72 hours, and patients are managed in this expectation. More serious patients require particular consideration. The overall management plan can be simply defined:
1. Establish the diagnosis
2. Control pain and provide adequate fluid replacement
3. Identify and subsequently treat the aetiological factor (e.g. gall-stones, alcoholism, hyperparathyroidism)
4. Monitor for the development of complications, e.g. pseudocyst, abscess, and treat appropriately.

Conservative management

Pethidine is usually recommended for analgesia because of its (debateably) lesser action on the sphincter of Oddi than morphine. A nasogastric tube is passed to provide intermittent aspiration. An i.v. infusion is set up and adequate fluid and electrolyte administered as assessed by the patient's circulation and urinary output. In severe pancreatitis, a CVP line should be set up and a urethral catheter inserted to monitor hourly urine output.

Many patients are hypoxic to some degree, and oxygen should be administered. This is mandatory in the severe case, who may progress to require ventilation. The use of a number of ancillary drugs has been advocated:

Broad spectrum antibiotics

Although there is little evidence that their use prevents

the development of pancreatic abscess, most surgeons use antibiotics—possibly because of the likelihood, at least in gall-stone associated pancreatitis, of infection in the biliary tree.

Anticholinergics

There is no evidence that their use (aimed to 'rest' the pancreas by reducing secretion) favourably alters the course of acute pancreatitis. Side effects such as urinary retention, prolongation of ileus, and eye problems in older patients are not infrequent and their use is not recommended.

Trasylol

An anti-enzyme drug (proteinase inhibitor) greeted initially with much enthusiasm, has now been shown not to influence the course of an attack.

Glucagon

Although infusion of glucagon may afford pain relief through an unknown mechanism, it too appears to have little influence on the outcome of an attack.

More recently, however, Cuschieri (1983), once more exploring the role of proteinase inhibition in management, has suggested the use of naturally occurring proteinase inhibitors in fresh frozen plasma (FFP). The FFP administered over the first 5 days of the illness is claimed to provide a substantial reduction in the morbidity of severe acute pancreatitis.

Investigation and treatment of aetiological factors

Investigations into the aetiology of the pancreatitis begin early in the management phase. The demonstration (usually by ultrasound) of gall-stones raises the question of the timing of cholecystectomy. There is increasing agreement that in the average patient who settles rapidly, cholecystectomy should be undertaken during the second week of the illness.

Investigation and management of complications

The more common complications requiring management are:

Abscess formation

This usually becomes manifest during the second week producing a high temperature and leucocytosis. The diagnosis is confirmed by ultrasound examination and is an indication for drainage. If the abscess is suitably situated, and the appropriate skills are available, drainage may be achieved by percutaneous insertion of a tube drain under radiological control. Alternatively, surgical drainage is required. Secondary haemorrhage from the abscess cavity is not uncommon.

Pseudocyst formation

This should be suspected in the presence of continuing hyperamylasaemia, or persisting pain and again the diagnosis is confirmed by ultrasound. The diagnosis of pseudocyst is not in itself an indication for surgery, and a proportion resolve spontaneously. Persisting pain, or pressure effects caused by the increasing size of the cyst are indications for drainage. The usual pressure effect is on the stomach, producing limited meal capacity and vomiting, but a pseudocyst in the head of the pancreas may compress the common bile duct causing obstructive jaundice, or the duodenum producing vomiting.

External drainage using the percutaneous technique has been used (Colhoun, 1984) but in most patients some form of internal drainage into a neighbouring part of the gastro-intestinal tract is indicated (Boggs, 1982). If possible, surgery should be delayed for 3–4 weeks to allow the cyst wall to thicken and mature so that it will hold sutures better.

Pseudocyst-gastrostomy is the operation most often performed, as the stomach is the organ most likely to be compressed by the cyst, which becomes densely adherent to it. An appropriately placed longitudinal gastrotomy incision is made in the anterior wall of the stomach to expose the mucosa of the posterior wall. A 4 cm longitudinal incision is now made through the full thickness of the posterior wall of stomach and cyst wall into the cyst, the contents of which are rapidly aspirated. Any loculi within the cyst are broken down. Bleeding from the posterior incision is free and should be controlled by full thickness mattress sutures of No. 1 silk placed around the margins of the incision. These sutures also maintain the communication between the cyst cavity and the stomach. The cyst cavity soon closes down, and problems arising from food or other gastric content entering the cyst cavity are surprisingly uncommon.

Occasionally the cyst presents inferiorly, depressing the transverse mesocolon, when the appropriate procedure is a *pseudocystjejunostomy*, preferably of the Roux-en-Y type. If the duodenum is being compressed, a *pseudocystduodenostomy* using a technique similar to that for pseudocystgastrostomy is employed.

Indications for surgery in acute pancreatitis

The indications for surgery in acute pancreatitis may be summarized as follows:

1. *Doubt as to the diagnosis.* In some patients it may prove impossible to exclude other potentially lethal pathology, e.g. intestinal ischaemia, even after full investigation

2. Deteriorating condition of the patient

3. Treatment of complications: abscess formation; pseudocyst formation; persisting obstructive jaundice; haemorrhage

4. Semi-elective surgery for gall-stone disease or hyper-parathyroidism.

Certain situations require further consideration:

The diagnosis has been made at emergency laparotomy
In most cases the surgeon, having established the diagnosis, is advised to close the abdomen without drainage and without undertaking further procedures.

If the gall-bladder is badly inflamed or has multiple stones, it may be removed, or cholecystostomy undertaken, while if the common bile duct is much distended, T-tube drainage may be provided. Formal exploration of the common bile duct should not be undertaken at this stage. In very severe cases the institution of a feeding jejunostomy may be considered as such patients are likely to have a protracted gastric or duodenal ileus, but most surgeons now prefer total parenteral nutrition to cover such an event.

The place of peritoneal lavage
Peritoneal lavage, instituted via a percutaneously placed dialysis catheter, or at laparotomy as above or in the face of the patient's deteriorating condition, has been advocated in the management of the patient with *severe* acute pancreatitis (Kauste, 1983). There is little evidence that this technique, aimed to remove toxic materials from the peritoneal cavity favourably influences the outcome.

The place of emergency pancreatectomy
Formal laparotomy to excise necrotic pancreatic tissue in the severe case has been advocated, particularly by Continental surgeons. The procedure carries a high mortality and has little to commend it.

Chronic pancreatitis
The usual indication for surgery in chronic pancreatitis is relief of pain if more conservative measures, e.g. coeliac or splanchnic nerve block have failed. Less common indications are pseudocyst formation, when the management is similar to that in acute pancreatitis, and haemorrhage from a pseudocyst. Haemorrhage may be into the peritoneal cavity, or along the pancreatic duct to produce apparent intestinal bleeding. The usual cause is a small pseudocyst eroding into an artery. Arteriographic localization of the bleeding area followed by embolization is sometimes successful in controlling the bleeding, but an appropriate pancreatic resection to include the bleeding site may be required.

Pain is usually associated with stricture formation in the pancreatic duct, single or multiple, with dilatation of the duct behind or between strictures. The ductal anatomy is defined at ERCP and surgery appropriate to the findings is undertaken.

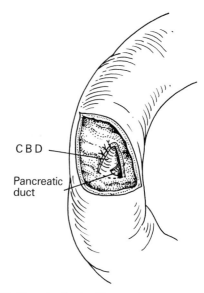

Fig. 20.31 Transduodenal sphincteroplasty of bile duct and pancreatic duct

A single stricture at the ampulla with dilatation
This may satisfactorily be treated by a modified transduodenal sphincteroplasty (Fig. 20.31) (Nardi, 1983).

A formal sphincteroplasty of the lower common bile duct is undertaken as described on page 395. The entrance of the pancreatic duct is now identified and a similar procedure carried out on the pancreatic duct—a sphincteroplasty of 1.0–1.5 cm should be aimed for. The appearances of the anatomy following completion has led to the name 'butterfly sphincteroplasty' being given to the procedure.

In the event of recurrent pain after this operation the option of lateral pancreaticojejunostomy described below remains.

A more distal stricture is present, the proximal duct being normal
In this event, a distal pancreatectomy is undertaken, the line of transection lying to the right of the site of the stricture (Fig. 20.32).

Multiple strictures are present with intervening dilatation (Fig. 20.33).
The gastrocolic omentum is opened to expose the pancreas. The pancreatic duct is entered and opened along its length from the tail of the pancreas and as far into the head as possible (Fig. 20.34). Any calculi are removed. Bleeding is often free, requiring control by multiple suture ligation. A Roux loop of proximal jejunum is constructed, brought up through an opening in transverse mesocolon, and laid alongside the opened duct. A side-to-side pancreaticojejunostomy is now made in two

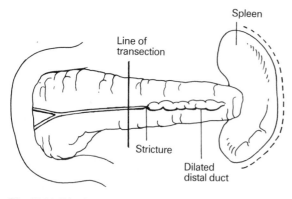

Fig. 20.32 Distal pancreatectomy for stricture

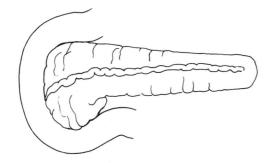

Fig. 20.33 Multiple pancreatic duct strictures

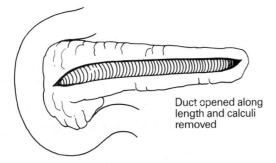

Fig. 20.34 Pancreatic duct opened along its length

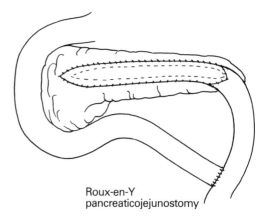

Fig. 20.35 Pancreatic duct drainage

createctomy, preserving the duodenum and pancreaticoduodenal vascular arcade by leaving a small rim of pancreatic tissue attached to duodenum, may be considered.

Overall, the results of surgery for chronic pancreatitis are disappointing. Many patients are alcoholics, with poor compliance with treatment, and it is doubtful whether surgery should be offered without a genuine undertaking from them that they will avoid alcohol permanently.

TRAUMA

Pancreatic trauma may result from penetrating or non-penetrating abdominal injury, and may occasionally occur during abdominal surgery, e.g. splenectomy, difficult gastrectomy.

In the patient with abdominal injury, the presence of hyperamylasaemia should alert the surgeon to the probability of pancreatic damage, and provide an indication for laparotomy if other indications do not already exist. If diagnostic lavage has been employed, a high amylase level in the returned fluid would again provide indication for laparotomy.

At laparotomy, the presence of retroperitoneal haematoma or oedema in the vicinity of the pancreas should lead to a formal exploration of the organ as described on page 400.

The most frequent injury is *contusion* of varying degrees of severity, and the preferred treatment is to provide adequate drainage from the vicinity using one or more drains of the sump-suction type. Severe contusions of the distal body and tail are best dealt with by distal pancreatectomy, with over-sewing of the proximal cut-end of pancreas—this carries less risk of the development of a pancreatic fistula. Severe contusions of the

layers, using interrupted nonabsorbable sutures to unite the seromuscular coat of jejunum with pancreatic substance, and interrupted sutures of Dexon, Vicryl or Merseline to join jejunal mucosa and pancreatic duct. The proximal cut-end of jejunum is now anastomosed end-to-side to the vertical jejunal limb some 40 cm below the mesocolon (Fig. 20.35).

The pancreatic duct is fibrosed along its length
The duct in such cases is not suitable for a drainage procedure. Total pancreatectomy, or a near total pan-

head of pancreas are normally treated by sump drainage (see p. 332), but if severe duodenal damage has also been sustained, a Whipple type of resection is indicated.

Pancreatic *transection* occurs most commonly in the region of the neck of the pancreas as it crosses the spine. Attempts at repair of the transected duct are ill-advised, and the most appropriate management is to resect the pancreas distal to the transection, closing the proximal cut surface of pancreas.

Whatever procedure is undertaken, adequate postoperative drainage should be provided, and broad spectrum antibiotic cover prescribed.

REFERENCES

Almeida A M De, Cruz A G, Aldeia F J 1984 Side-to-side choledochoduodenostomy in the management of choledocholithiasis and associated disease. American Journal of Surgery 147: 253

Bismith H, Franco D, Corlette M B, Hepp J 1978 Long term results of Roux-en-Y hepaticojejunostomy. Surgery Gynaecology and Obstetrics 146: 161

Blumgart L H, Lelley C J 1984 Hepaticojejunostomy in benign and malignant high bile duct stricture: approaches to the left hepatic ducts. British Journal of Surgery 71: 257

Boggs B R, Potts J R, Postier R G 1982 Pancreatic pseudocysts. Five year experience with pancreatic pseudocysts. American Journal of Surgery 144: 685

Burhenne H J 1976 Complications of non-operative extraction of retained common duct stones. American Journal of Surgery 131: 260

Cameron J L, Broe P, Zuidema G D 1982 Proximal bile duct tumours: surgical management with silastic transhepatic biliary stents. Annals of Surgery 196: 412

Carter A E 1983 The transduodenal peri-ampullary approach to common bile duct calculi. Annals of the Royal College of Surgeons of England 65: 183

Colhoun E, Murphy J J, MacErlean D P 1984 Percutaneous drainage of pancreatic pseudocysts. British Journal of Surgery 71: 131

Cushieri A, Wood R A B, Cumming J R G, Meehan S E, Mackie C R 1983 Treatment of acute pancreatitis with fresh frozen plasma. British Journal of Surgery 70: 710

Doyle P J, Ward-McQuaid J N, McEwen-Smith A 1982 The value of routine peri-operative cholangiography—a report of 4,000 cholecystectomies. British Journal of Surgery 69: 617

Ernst D, Windsor C W O 1982 The use of a rigid choledochoscope in exploration of the common bile duct. British Journal of Surgery 69: 463

Espiner 1982 Emergency cholecystectomy: towards guaranteed safety. In: Wilson E H, Marsden A K (eds). Care of the acutely ill and injured. John Wiley, New York, p 385

Fox J N, Gunn A A 1984 Common bile duct exploration by a balloon catheter technique. Journal of the Royal College of Surgeons of Edinburgh 29: 81

Gibbons C P, Griffiths G J, Cormack A 1983 The role of percutaneous transhepatic cholangiography and grey-scale ultrasound in the investigation and treatment of bile duct obstruction. British Journal of Surgery 70: 494

Greenall M J, Gough M H, Kettlewell M G, Nolan D J 1982 Non-operative removal of retained biliary tract stones. Journal of the Royal College of Surgeons of Edinburgh 27: 87

Hoffman J, Lorentzen M 1985 Drainage after cholecystectomy. British Journal of Surgery 72: 423

Howard E R 1983 Extrahepatic biliary atresia: a review of current management. British Journal of Surgery 70: 193

Imrie C W, Whyte A S 1975 A prospective study of pancreatitis. British Journal of Surgery 62: 490

Irwin S T, McIlrath E M, Kennedy T L 1985 Burhenne technique for extraction of retained biliary calculi. Journal of the Royal College of Surgeons of Edinburgh 30: 39

Jones B A, Langer B, Taylor B R, Girotti M 1985 Periampullary tumors: which ones should be resected. American Journal of Surgery 149: 46

Kasai I M, Susuki S 1959 A new operation for 'noncorrectable' biliary atresia; hepatic porto-enterostomy. Shujutsu 13: 733

Kauste A, Hockerstedt K, Ahonen J, Tervaskari H 1983 Peritoneal lavage as a primary treatment in acute fulminant pancreatitis. Surgery Gynaecology and Obstetrics 156: 458

Lilly J R, Altman R P 1975 Hepatico porto-enterostomy (the Kasai operation) for biliary atresia. Surgery 78: 76

Muir B B, Rimmer S, Redhead D N, Buist T A S, Best J J K 1983 The radiological assessment of the obstructed biliary tree. Journal of the Royal College of Surgeons of Edinburgh 28: 233

Nardi G L, Michelassi F, Zannini P 1983 Transduodenal sphincteroplasty. Annals of Surgery 198: 453

Ranson J H C, Rifkind K M, Roses D F, Fink S D, Eng K, Spencer F C 1974 Prognostic signs and the role of operative management in acute pancreatitis. Surgery Gynaecology and Obstetrics 139: 69

Smith R 1980 In: Maingot R (ed) Abdominal operations, 7th edn. Appleton-Century-Crofts, New York, p 1251

Whipple A O 1946 Observations on radical surgery for lesions of the pancreas. Surgery Gynaecology and Obstetrics 32: 623

21

Operations on the appendix

R. F. RINTOUL

Anatomy

The appendix is normally 8–10 cm long and 6–8 mm in diameter, but great variations occur. Its wall has the same coats as the large gut, but contains numerous aggregations of lymphoid tissue. It is attached at its base to the posteromedial aspect of the caecum just below the ileocaecal junction. The three taeniae coli of the caecum converge to end at this point and are used as a guide to the appendix. The surface marking of the base of the appendix is at *McBurney's point*—at the junction of the lateral and middle thirds of the line joining the anterior superior spine and the umbilicus.

In most cases the appendix has a complete peritoneal covering, with a well-formed mesentery, the *mesoappendix*, derived from the posterior layer of the mesentery of the lower end of the ileum. The artery of the appendix, a terminal branch of the ileocolic, runs along the free edge of the mesentery, giving off two or three branches during its course. The mesentery may extend to the tip of the appendix or may terminate about its middle. An additional fold of peritoneum, usually avascular (the inferior ileocaecal or 'bloodless' fold of Treves), may be present, extending from the proximal part of the appendix to the front of the terminal inch of the ileum.

Different positions of the appendix

The base of the appendix is no more than relatively fixed in position, since the caecum enjoys a certain amount of mobility. The rest of the appendix is as a rule freely movable, and may occupy one of several positions: (1) It may curl round the lower pole of the caecum and pass upwards on its lateral side—*paracolic position* (3%). (2) It may pass upwards behind the caecum—*retrocaecal position* (70%). (3) It may extend more or less transversely to the left, passing either in front of or behind the terminal part of the ileum (2%). (4) It may hang downwards into the pelvis—*pelvic position* (25%). The retrocaecal and pelvic positions are the commonest. In the former the greater part of the appendix may be embedded within the serous coat of the posterior caecal wall, or, if this part is not covered with peritoneum, it may lie in the retroperitoneal tissues.

In rare cases the caecum (through developmental arrest of its descent) is absent from the right iliac fossa, and together with the appendix it must then be sought high up below the right lobe of the liver.

INDICATIONS FOR APPENDICECTOMY

Acute appendicitis

In most cases of acute appendicitis which are seen in the

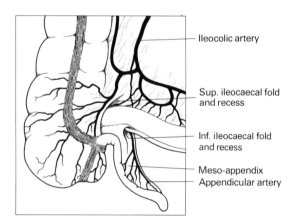

Fig. 21.1 Anatomy of the appendix and ileocaecal region (After Grant)

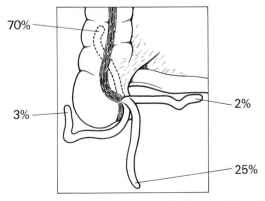

Fig. 21.2 The more common positions for the appendix and the relative frequency with which they are found

early stages of the attack, operation should be carried out without delay. A distinction has been drawn between *catarrhal* appendicitis in which resolution will frequently occur and *obstructive* appendicitis which is likely to progress rapidly to gangrene and perforation. It is usually impossible, however, to determine with any degree of certainty from the clinical examination which type of appendicitis is present, and the risks which are involved do not justify delay. Even when the severity of the attack appears to be declining operation should as a rule be considered, for there is an invariable tendency towards recurrence. A patient who is in pain is usually willing or even eager to undergo operation. If he is advised to have his appendix removed later in the quiescent stage, the advice will often be unheeded, and the next attack may develop when the conditions are less favourable for operation.

An exception may be made in those cases where the attack is obviously passing off, and where, for various reasons, it may be desirable to postpone operation until a more convenient time. Such conditions arise when appendicitis of mild degree develops during an acute illness, or during the first 3 months of pregnancy when appendicectomy is associated with some risk of miscarriage. The risk of appendicectomy during pregnancy must be weighed against the greater risk of peritonitis should the appendicitis fail to settle with conservative treatment.

Late cases

In cases where the patient is not seen until 48–72 hours after the onset of symptoms, *and provided that there are no signs suggestive of general peritonitis*, it is probable either that the attack is passing off or that the infection is being successfully localised. The second alternative requires special consideration, for it constitutes a contra-indication to immediate operation. Definite evidence of localisation is obtained from the palpation of a tender mass in the right iliac fossa—a mass formed by the matting together of omentum and bowel around the inflamed appendix. As long as the infection remains localised there is little danger, whereas any attempt to remove the appendix entails the breaking down of protective adhesions, with the risk of spreading the infection to the general peritoneal cavity. The initial treatment of such a *localizing* appendicitis is conservative, and is described on page 414.

In children and in old people early operation should as a rule be advised since there are special dangers of delay. In children the appendix is thin-walled, and what appears to be a mild catarrhal inflammation may proceed rapidly to gangrene and perforation. Both in childhood and in old age there is less tendency to localisation, and the risks of general peritonitis are very considerable.

Unless, therefore, a definite mass is palpable, operation should not be delayed.

Recurrent or chronic appendicitis

Once the appendix has become inflamed, further attacks at gradually shortening intervals are to be expected. Appendicectomy during the quiescent stage is attended by the minimum of risk and discomfort to the patient, and it should not be delayed until a second attack develops. In a proportion of cases, and frequently in the absence of any acute attack, chronic appendicitis may be diagnosed from the existence of a 'grumbling' pain in the right iliac fossa. In addition there may be general malaise or various digestive symptoms—the so-called *appendix dyspepsia* (Kerr, 1962). Appendicectomy is usually curative in such cases.

Carcinoma of appendix

In a very small proportion of cases a tumour of the appendix is found (Cohen, 1974). Appendicectomy is satisfactory in the treatment of an adenocarcinoma which is confined to the mucosa but its diagnosis depends on routine histology of all appendices.

Carcinoid tumour of the appendix

The appendix is the most common site for gastrointestinal carcinoid tumour. A small tumour of the distal appendix is adequately removed by appendicectomy but, if histological examination shows involvement of the base of the appendix, right hemicolectomy is advisable (Anderson, 1985).

ELECTIVE APPENDICECTOMY

Removal of the appendix between attacks—the so-called 'interval' operation—will be described first, since it is usually a simple procedure and a relatively standardized technique may be employed.

Incision

A right gridiron or *Lanz* incision is commonly employed. A few surgeons, who believe that an operation for the removal of a quiescent appendix should be exploratory, advise a paramedian incision, but the majority prefer to act upon a preoperative diagnosis, and to examine only the organs that lie in the vicinity of the appendix.

Technique

The caecum may present as soon as the peritoneum has been opened, or it may have to be sought for by two fingers introduced into the peritoneal cavity and passed backwards round the lateral wall. It is easily distinguished from small bowel by the presence of taeniae coli.

Occasionally in visceroptotic cases the transverse colon is withdrawn in mistake for the caecum, but it should be recognized at once from the fact that it has omentum attached to it. The caecum is grasped in a moist pack by the left hand and is gently withdrawn towards its lower end, when the appendix should follow it into the wound. Delivery of the appendix is assisted if necessary by the right index finger, which is introduced deeply into the lower part of the wound below the caecum. If the appendix cannot readily be found, the operator should trace one of the taeniae coli of the caecum leading to its base. The appendix is then freed by a finger passed along it towards its tip, any filmy adhesions being gently disrupted. If dense adhesions are present these should be separated or divided under the guidance of the eye, and with the assistance of narrow-bladed retractors. Sometimes, as the result of previous inflammation, the appendix is sharply kinked and is bound down by adventitious bands to the right iliac fossa or to the brim of the pelvis. Such bands can be divided with safety and without risk of causing haemorrhage if the knife is kept to the lateral side of the appendix.

Some difficulty is apt to be encountered when the appendix occupies the retrocaecal position. It may then lie free behind the caecum or it may be bound down to the posterior wall of the gut; often the distal part is extraperitoneal, in which case it may be completely buried behind the caecum. The incision may require to be enlarged upwards and laterally, so that the caecum can be turned over and the appendix dissected free under direct vision.

The part of the caecum to which the appendix is attached is retained outside the wound, while the remainder is returned to the peritoneal cavity. The appendix is raised up and is held taut by a pair of Babcock's forceps applied near its tip. The mesentery is clamped with one or more pairs of artery forceps, and is divided and ligatured. A forceps is momentarily applied to the base of the appendix exactly at the point of its junction with the caecum (Fig. 21.3), and a ligature is tied around the crushed area. It assists in the subsequent control of the stump if the ends of this ligature are kept long and are retained in forceps. A purse-string Lembert suture is inserted in the caecal wall around the base of the appendix (Fig. 21.4). Forceps are then applied to the appendix 5 or 6 mm distal to the ligature, the intervening lumen

Figs. 21.3–21.6 *Technique of appendicectomy*

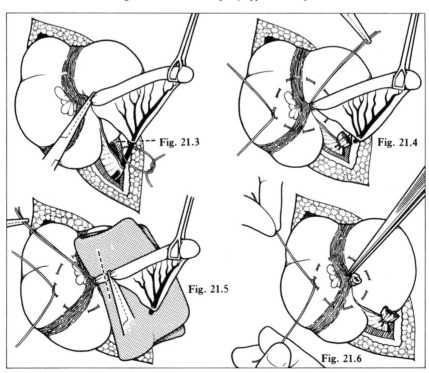

Fig. 21.3 Meso-appendix clamped and divided; base of appendix crushed with forceps.
Fig. 21.5 Appendix clamped distal to ligature and about to be divided against swab.

Fig. 21.4 Meso-appendix tied off; appendix ligatured at base; purse-string suture inserted.
Fig. 21.6 Appendix stump about to be invaginated before tightening of purse-string suture.

having been emptied by pressure of the blades. A swab is placed underneath to absorb any escaping contents, and the appendix is divided close to the forceps (Fig. 21.5). The stump ligature is cut short and the stump is invaginated with slender forceps while the purse-string suture is tightened (Fig. 21.6). The appendix, together with the knife, swab and forceps, which have been contaminated by contact with the mucosa, are placed in a bowl and are removed from the field of operation.

Before the abdomen is closed the ligatured meso-appendix is re-examined for bleeding. The parts within reach are inspected or palpated, particular attention being paid to the lower coils of the ileum and to the ileocaecal lymph glands. In the female the uterus and the right ovary and tube are palpated by two fingers passed downwards into the pelvis. The operation is completed by suture of the wound in layers.

Kinking of the terminal ileum
This condition, described by Lane, occurs within the last 10–12 cm of the ileum. It is due to an adventitious band or adhesion which binds the ileum down to the brim of the pelvis and causes a V-shaped kinking of the bowel. It may occur in association with appendicitis, when it is probably a result of the inflammatory reaction, but sometimes it appears to be congenital. In either case it may cause delayed emptying of the ileum, and can be responsible for any of the symptoms commonly associated with chronic appendicitis. In the 'interval' operation, therefore, this condition should always be excluded by the withdrawal of the terminal coil of ileum. If a kink is found it is rectified by division of the adhesion along the lower border of the bowel with a touch of the knife, and by stripping the bowel gently upwards (Fig. 21.7).

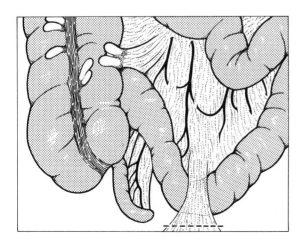

Fig. 21.7 Kinking of the terminal ileum by adventitious band. The site for division of the band is shown

EMERGENCY APPENDICECTOMY

Incision
The gridiron incision is again the one which is most commonly employed. It has been criticized on the grounds that it gives insufficient access, and that the delivery of an acutely inflamed appendix through the limited space available may necessitate harmful manipulation with consequent risk of rupture. It is only in a small proportion of cases, however, that any difficulty is encountered, and *provided that the incision is then enlarged*—which is a very simple matter (p. 316)—these criticisms of its use cannot be sustained.

An alternative approach which is frequently advocated is the muscle-cutting iliac incision (Rutherford Morison). This is, in fact, the incision which results when a gridiron is enlarged, the internal oblique and transversus muscles being divided in line with the fibres of the external oblique (see also p. 416). The advantages of this incision are those of wide access, and the fact that a more direct approach is obtained in cases where the appendix is retrocaecal in position; furthermore, free drainage can be provided with less risk of contaminating the general peritoneal cavity.

The paramedian incision should be condemned for use in acute appendicitis. The appendix is relatively inaccessible by this approach, and the risks of spreading the infection are considerable. *Doubts as to the correctness of the diagnosis do not justify its use.* If the gridiron incision reveals some other condition to which it gives inadequate access, it can be quickly closed, and a second incision made. Two small incisions are preferable to a single one, unduly extended.

Technique
As soon as the peritoneum has been opened there may be an escape of exudate. Unless this is frankly purulent or malodorous it does not indicate that general peritonitis is present. More often the fluid is the result of peritoneal reaction to the local inflammation; it is then odourless, clear or slightly turbid, and is usually sterile. All exudate in the neighbourhood of the wound should be removed by gentle swabbing or by the use of suction, a sample being collected for bacteriological examination.

The caecum is identified and is very gently withdrawn towards its lower end. If the appendix does not come into view it is located by a finger passed along one of the taeniae coli. It may be felt as a tense resistant cord, lying in most cases lateral to or behind the caecum.

The appendix is delivered partly by traction on the caecum, and partly by gentle pressure exerted by a finger below it. If the appendix is adherent, no force must be used to 'hook' it out of the wound. It is necessary in such cases to enlarge the wound, to pack off the rest of the peritoneal cavity, and to free the appendix under direct vision. Omentum which is firmly wrapped round the appendix should not be separated, since it is likely to be involved in the inflammatory process. It should rather be ligatured and divided a short distance away, and the adherent part removed along with the appendix.

Removal of the appendix is then carried out on the lines described for the 'interval' operation. If the meso-appendix is short and oedematous it may be necessary to clamp and divide it within the peritoneal cavity. In such cases care must be taken that the stump of the meso-appendix does not slip out of the forceps while it is being tied-off, and it is an advantage to employ a transfixing ligature. When the inflammatory process has extended into the meso-appendix, this structure should be clamped and divided as far away as possible from the appendix, since the septic thrombosis of its vessels may lead to pylephlebitis. Sometimes the proximal end of the appendix is buried by inflammatory swelling of the caecal wall, and care should then be taken that the entire organ is removed. When the caecal wall is friable or oedematous it is wiser not to attempt to bury the appendix stump, for this procedure may predispose to the development of faecal fistula.

Retrograde removal of the appendix
Frequently the base of the appendix is more accessible than the tip. This is especially likely to occur when the appendix occupies the retrocaecal position—when its inflamed distal end may be adherent to the posterior wall of the caecum, or may even be buried within the serous coat. In such cases the retrograde method of removal may often simplify the operation. Two pairs of artery forceps are insinuated through the meso-appendix and are applied to the base of the appendix 5–6 mm apart. The proximal forceps is removed and the appendix is ligatured in the groove that has been crushed. It is then

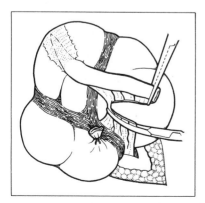

Fig. 21.8 Retrograde appendicectomy—a method to be considered when the base of the appendix is more accessible than the tip

divided close to the distal forceps and the proximal stump is invaginated. The appendix, with its cut end still occluded by the forceps, is now freed by careful dissection, and by successive clamping and clipping of its mesentery from base to tip it is removed (Fig. 21.8).

Drainage in non-perforated cases
If the appendix shows incipient gangrene, if it bursts during removal, or if reactive free fluid is present, the existence of potential contamination must be recognised. The peritoneal cavity is usually able, however, to combat such infection, and drainage is therefore unnecessary, but it is a wise precaution to leave a superficial drain in the wound which is less resistant to infection. This can do no possible harm and may be the means of preventing an infected wound.

ACUTE APPENDICITIS WITH PERFORATION

Localised peritonitis or abscess
When this condition is diagnosed clinically, operation may be contra-indicated (p. 414). Frequently, however, it is discovered only at operation from the presence of a mass of inflammatory adhesions around the appendix. It is probable in such cases that the appendix has perforated, and that pus or septic exudate is enclosed within the mass. The most essential aim of the operation is now to avoid spreading the infection to the general peritoneal cavity. The incision is enlarged if necessary, its medial side is lifted forwards with a retractor, and the mass is carefully surrounded with hot moist packs. Retractors are inserted, and under direct vision the mass is gently explored with the finger in an attempt to identify the appendix. If pus is encountered, it is immediately swabbed away. In the majority of cases the appendix is isolated without great difficulty and is removed in the usual way, but all manipulation should be reduced to a minimum. When the caecum is fixed by inflammatory adhesions the appendicectomy may require to be carried out in the depths of the wound and invagination of the stump should then be omitted. Before the packs are removed the appendix area and wound may be irrigated with 0.1% Tetracycline solution.

Sometimes the appendix is found to have become divided into two parts at the site of perforation; care must then be taken that the entire organ is removed. A faecolith which has escaped through the perforation may be found lying loose in the abscess cavity.

Drainage
The wound is closed around a drain which extends down to the infected area and into the pelvis. Either a tube or a corrugated plastic drain may be employed. When the appendix has been retrocaecal in position, it reduces the risk of peritoneal contamination if the drain is brought

out as far laterally as possible, through the upper angle of the wound. Whatever type of drain is used, the wound should never be closed tightly around it, for it is essential that there should be free egress for infected exudate. This is particularly important when a tube drain is used; there must be room for exudate to escape, not only through its lumen, but also alongside it. Many infected wounds result from neglect of this precaution. Occasionally it may be an advantage to employ a separate stab wound for drainage lateral to the main incision, which also should be drained.

When a large abscess is present or when the appendix is found to be surrounded by friable inflammatory tissues which bleed readily to the touch, appendicectomy entails the risk of inflicting serious trauma or of spreading the infection. *In such cases it is wiser to be content with simple drainage alone.* Appendicectomy can be carried out with comparative safety at a later date (p. 416).

General peritonitis is most likely to occur when the perforation is near the base of the appendix, for this part is not so readily shut-off by adhesions. It may appear also as a later complication, when a collection of pus, which is at first localized, overflows into the general peritoneal cavity.

When appendix peritonitis is diagnosed clinically it is usually advisable that operation should be delayed for an hour or two, in order to allow of treatment which will improve the patient's general condition. Such preoperative treatment consists in the institution of continuous intravenous infusion, gastric suction and antibiotic therapy. Delay in diagnosis without deterioration in the patient's general condition may persuade the surgeon to continue with conservative treatment but it is wiser to explore the abdomen for drainage and antibiotic lavage.

At operation the diagnosis is apparent as soon as the abdomen has been opened, from the presence of frankly purulent or dark-coloured fluid—usually with the putrid smell of bowel organisms.

The existence of general peritonitis—unlike that of localized peritonitis or abscess—demands that every effort should be made to remove the appendix. Simple drainage alone will not suffice, for, since the perforation is not effectively sealed-off, further contamination is usually inevitable. As these patients are gravely ill the appendicectomy should be carried out as expeditiously as possible. Pus is evacuated and the peritoneum washed out with tetracycline solution—see page 333 (Stewart, 1980).

Drainage
If there is much peritoneal exudate, it is best to drain the pelvis by means of a tube brought out through a stab wound above the symphysis pubis—and here *suction drainage* (p. 321) has special advantages. Additional drainage of the appendix area through the main wound is usually advisable; if this is omitted, the wound at least should be drained. A tube from the pelvis should not normally be brought out through a laterally placed incision, since this is a long and an indirect route. The suprapubic drain is usually removed after 48 hours, by which time it will have ceased to function; a local drain is shortened gradually as the discharge diminishes.

Prevention of wound infection
Infection of the wound after appendicectomy in septic cases is a troublesome complication, in that it prolongs convalescence and an incisional hernia may result.

When gross contamination has been unavoidable, the wound is very liable to become infected, and it is particularly important that it should be very loosely sutured around the drain, so that there is ample space for inflammatory products to escape to the surface. The amount of buried suture or ligature material should be reduced to a minimum, for this forms a nidus for bacterial growth. Delayed primary wound closure is contraindicated, even in a grossly infected wound (Pettigrew 1981).

Chemotherapy
The routine use of Metronidazole has reduced the incidence of wound infection. The presence of general peritonitis requires the additional benefits of an antibiotic active against gram negative organisms e.g. Gentamicin or a Cephalosporin.

Postoperative complications
Such complications as may occur after any abdominal operation have already been discussed (pp. 326–328). Those which are associated more specifically with appendicectomy in septic cases may be mentioned briefly here.

Pelvic abscess
This should be suspected if fever or tachycardia persist, and cannot be ascribed to wound infection, or to a pulmonary condition. The diagnosis may be confirmed by rectal examination, when a boggy and tender mass can be detected anteriorly. Most pelvic abscesses resolve under conservative treatment, the pus being absorbed, or alternatively they burst spontaneously into the rectum. Deliberate evacuation per rectum is very seldom required, and should be reserved for cases where the abscess is soft and bulging into the rectal wall (Fig. 21.9). This is done by penetrating the rectal wall with a long haemostat—if possible under direct vision, as can be obtained by the use of a vaginal speculum placed within the anal canal.

Subphrenic abscess and paralytic ileus
The treatment of these conditions is discussed on pages 375 and 422.

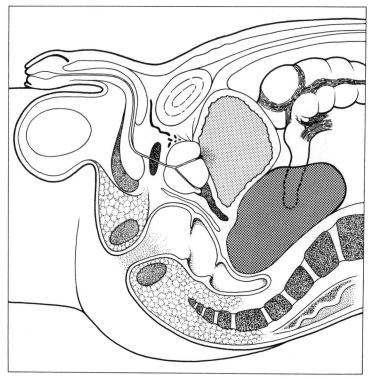

Fig. 21.9 Pelvic abscess bulging into the rectum (After Hamilton Bailey)

Faecal fistula after appendicectomy may result from localised necrosis of the caecal wall. It is not a serious complication; indeed, it may actually be beneficial, in that, by draining distended gut, it may prevent the development of paralytic ileus. The fistula usually heals spontaneously within 2–3 weeks.

APPENDIX ABSCESS OR MASS

The term 'appendix abscess' is applied in a wide sense to include any type of localizing appendicitis where a definite mass has formed in the region of the appendix. This finding is most likely to be present in patients who come to examination 48 hours or longer after the onset of symptoms. The mass is formed by the matting together of omentum and bowel round the inflamed appendix. Unless the mass is situated in the pelvis it can usually be detected on ordinary abdominal palpation.

In most cases the appendix has perforated, and a collection of pus is enclosed within the mass of adhesions. If perforation has not occurred the term 'abscess' is strictly incorrect—the condition is rather one of localized plastic peritonitis. In either case the presence of a mass is an indication that the infection is adequately circumscribed and walled-off from the general peritoneal cavity. The *initial* treatment in such cases should always be conservative, since removal of the appendix entails the risk of damaging the inflamed and friable bowel in the vicinity, and of spreading infection to the general peritoneal cavity. The mortality of cases treated conservatively has been much lower than that of cases subjected to immediate operation, although the latter has been greatly improved by broad spectrum antibiotics.

Conservative treatment

This, as first described by Ochsner and Sherren, is advised for all cases of acute appendicitis where operation, for one reason or another, is withheld. It may be employed, therefore, both in the early case when the attack appears to be subsiding or conditions are unfavourable for operation, and in the late case where it is believed that the infection is being successfully localized.

The details of the method may be summarised as follows:

1. The patient is nursed propped-up, in order to encourage any peritoneal exudate to gravitate towards the pelvis.

2. Intensive antibiotic therapy is instituted if there are signs of toxicity.

3. For the first 24–48 hours nothing is administered by mouth, except sips of water or ice. An adequate fluid intake is maintained by intravenous infusion, and naso-

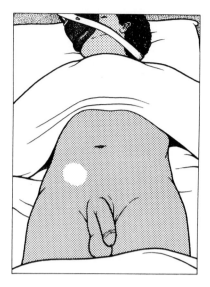

Fig. 21.10 Appendix abscess in contact with the abdominal wall

gastric suction is installed. After 24–48 hours, provided that all symptoms are subsiding and bowel sounds are present, fluid diet is commenced and is gradually supplemented. Solid food is withheld until pulse rate and temperature have returned to normal.

4. A careful record is kept of the pulse rate and temperature. The pulse rate is much the more important; at the commencement of treatment it should be recorded at hourly intervals.

5. Strong analgesics should be avoided if possible, since they may mask symptoms which demand operation.

6. Too frequent examination of the abdomen is avoided, but it is helpful to outline the mass on the patient's abdominal wall so as to compare one examination with the next.

7. Suppositories are administered after the third day. No aperient is given until the pulse rate and temperature have returned to normal.

The majority of cases react favourably to this treatment. The pulse rate and temperature fall and pain is relieved. The lump becomes less tender, shrinks steadily in size and ultimately disappears. Any pus which is present is absorbed. It is most essential, however, that the treatment should be carried out in a hospital or nursing home under the care of the surgeon who has accepted responsibility for the case, for at any moment it may require to be abandoned in favour of operation. When the method is employed in children and in old people, particularly careful supervision is essential.

Indications for operation

Unless *all* symptoms subside, and there is a steady improvement in the patient's general condition, operation should as a rule be considered. *The most dangerous sign is a rising pulse rate*—hence the necessity for frequent recording in the early stages of treatment. If this sign is present, operation should be carried out without delay. A pulse rate which remains high (e.g. above 95 or 100) is also an indication for operation, but is not a matter of such urgency. A raised temperature is of less importance in the early stages, provided that the pulse rate is steady or falling, but a persistently high or swinging temperature indicates that operation will be required. Continued pain, vomiting or diarrhoea usually demands that conservative treatment should be abandoned. If there is spreading tenderness or resistance—signs which suggest an incipient general peritonitis—immediate operation should be undertaken.

In a proportion of cases the abscess, although remaining successfully localized, shows no sign of shrinking. Operation will then be required, but it may with advantage be deferred until the abscess, as shown by a dull note on percussion, has come into contact with the abdominal wall for it can then be approached extraperitoneally. The operation should consist of simple drainage alone, no attempt being made to remove the appendix.

Technique of simple drainage

The best approach is by a small muscle-cutting iliac incision, made just to the lateral side of the summit of the mass. All muscle layers are divided in the line of the skin incision (p. 316). The peritoneum, which is usually thickened and oedematous, is incised with care since it may be adherent to the underlying mass. Its medial leaf is held forwards with a retractor, and a gauze pack is inserted below it. The mass is then gently explored with a finger directed laterally and backwards. The abscess cavity is usually located without difficulty, and a varying

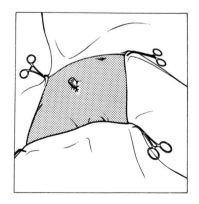

Fig. 21.11 Abscess drained through small incision; drainage tube in situ

quantity of malodorous pus escapes. Adhesions which form loculi within the cavity are very gently broken down with the finger. A soft tube or corrugated drain is inserted into the cavity and the wound is loosely closed around it. *When the abscess is in contact with the abdominal wall*, drainage is a very simple procedure and can be carried out under local anaesthesia. A 3–4 cm incision is made directly over the mass; pus is located with sinus forceps or with the finger, and while it is still flowing, a tube is introduced into the abscess cavity (Fig. 21.11).

Subsequent appendicectomy

The patient must be impressed with the necessity of having his appendix removed at a future date. The operation should be postponed, however, until all inflammatory reaction has subsided unless symptoms recur.

When the abscess has resolved under conservative treatment alone, appendicectomy is performed about 2–3 months later. Where simple drainage has been carried out a period of 3–6 months should be allowed to elapse. There is then usually a remarkable absence of adhesions. The appendix may be reduced to an attenuated cord; sometimes it looks surprisingly normal. In the elderly it may have been destroyed by the inflammatory process so that it is not always essential to persuade such a patient to undergo elective appendicectomy.

REFERENCES

Anderson J R, Wilson B G 1985 Carcinoid tumours of the appendix. British Journal of Surgery 72: 545

Cohen S E, Wolfman E F Jr 1974 Primary adenocarcinoma of the vermiform appendix. American Journal of Surgery 127: 704

Kerr J A 1962 Appendix dyspepsia. British Journal of Surgery 49: 437

Pettigrew R A 1981 Delayed primary wound closure in gangrenous and perforated appendicitis. British Journal of Surgery 68: 635

Stewart D J 1980 Generalised peritonitis. Journal of the Royal College of Surgeons of Edinburgh 25: 80

22

Operations on the intestines

H. A. F. DUDLEY, J. M. S. JOHNSTONE,
I. B. MACLEOD & R. F. RINTOUL

Anatomy

The small intestine

This lies in coils which are found in all parts of the abdominal cavity below the liver and stomach, and which bear no fixed relationship to each other. The coils are covered to a varying extent by the greater omentum which hangs down in front of them. The *jejunum* begins at the duodenojejunal flexure at the left side of the body of the 2nd lumbar vertebra, and is about 2 m in length. The *ileum*, which is 3 m to 4 m long, is continuous with the jejunum and ends in the right iliac fossa by joining the medial side of the caecum. The jejunum, which has a thicker and more vascular wall than the ileum, lies mainly to the left and above, but there is no definite line of demarcation between the two. The small intestine has a complete peritoneal covering, and, being attached by a long mesentery to the posterior abdominal wall, it is freely movable except at its two ends.

The *mesentery* contains between its two layers the blood vessels (*jejunal and ileal branches of the superior mesenteric*), the lymphatics and the nerves of the small intestine. Its root or line of attachment to the posterior wall is no more than 15 cm long; it extends obliquely downwards and to the right from the duodenojejunal flexure. Distally the mesentery fans out to its attachment along the whole length of small gut.

The colon

This can be distinguished from small bowel by its sacculated structure, and by the presence of taeniae coli and appendices epiploicae. The *caecum* normally occupies the right iliac fossa; it is completely clothed with peritoneum, but has no mesentery so that it is relatively fixed in position. The *ascending colon* is bound down to the posterior wall, and is covered with peritoneum only on its front and sides. The *right colic (hepatic) flexure* lies on the right kidney immediately below the liver. The *transverse colon* is freely movable since it has a complete peritoneal investment with a mesentery—the *transverse meso-colon*. It is very variable in position, and may hang down nearly to the pelvis. It is easily recognized from the attachment of the greater omentum to its lower border. The *left colic (splenic) flexure* lies behind the stomach on the lateral border of the kidney and on the diaphragm to which it is attached by the phrenicocolic ligament. The *descending colon*, like the ascending colon, is covered by peritoneum only on its front and sides, and is fixed in positon. Both flexures have a partial peritoneal covering similar to that of the ascending and descending colons; they are the most fixed parts of the large bowel. The *pelvic colon* hangs down as a loop in the pelvis, and forms a reservoir where solid faeces accumulate. Its extremities lie fairly close together— hence its liability to volvulus. It begins at the brim of the pelvis, and ends opposite the middle of the sacrum by becoming the rectum. It is relatively mobile having a complete peritoneal investment and a mesentery—the *pelvic meso-colon*.

Arteries of the colon

The caecum and ascending colon together with the terminal few centimetres of the ileum, are supplied by the *ileocolic* and *right colic* arteries, the transverse colon, by the *middle colic*—all branches of the superior mesenteric. The descending and pelvic colons are supplied by the *upper* and *lower left colic (sigmoid)* arteries, from the inferior mesenteric. Between these arteries there is a free anastomosis by marginal vessels lying close to the bowel.

Lymphatic drainage of the colon (Fig. 22.1)

This is of great importance in regard to the spread of carcinoma (see also p. 435). Glands draining the colon fall into four main groups—*epicolic* glands lying on the surface of the bowel wall; *paracolic* glands between the layers of the meso-colon close alongside the bowel; *intermediate* glands along the branches of the mesenteric arteries; and *central* or *principal* glands around the main trunks of these vessels.

The lymphatic drainage from the different parts of the colon bears a direct relationship to the arterial blood supply. Thus, drainage from the right side of the colon takes place to glands related to the entire course of the ileocolic and right colic arteries, and extending right up to the origin of these arteries from the superior mesenteric. The middle three-fifths of the transverse colon

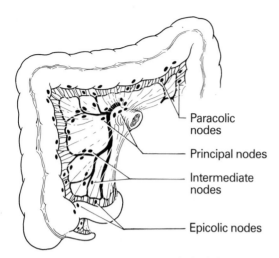

Fig. 22.1 Anatomy of the colonic lymphatic drainage

drains to glands around the middle colic artery. The splenic flexure, the descending colon and the pelvic colon, drain to glands around the branches and main trunk of the inferior mesenteric artery.

INTESTINAL OBSTRUCTION: GENERAL CONSIDERATIONS

Most cases of intestinal obstruction are mechanical in origin, and are due to occlusion of the lumen of the bowel, caused by changes in its wall or by compression or constriction from without. Strangulation of the bowel may complicate this type of obstruction, and adds greatly to the seriousness of the condition. Occasionally, usually in postoperative cases, there is no mechanical obstruction, and the stoppage is due entirely to paralysis of the bowel wall. The effects, however, are very similar.

Before any treatment, conservative or operative, can be planned, it is essential to assess (1) whether the obstruction is mechanical or paralytic; (2) its probable level, and (3) whether any element of strangulation is present. A decision on such points is reached by the taking of a detailed history and by careful examination of the patient, including inspection of the vomitus and material voided after enema. Erect and supine plain abdominal X-rays are mandatory (Figs. 22.2–22.5). In the healthy state the small and scattered collections of gas in the small bowel cast no definite radiological shadow; a variable quantity of gas is seen in the colon, but this is evacuated completely after an enema. When small bowel obstruction is present (unless at an unusually high level) gas-distended loops of bowel above the obstruction are shown lying transversely across the abdomen, and may contain fluid levels. In colonic

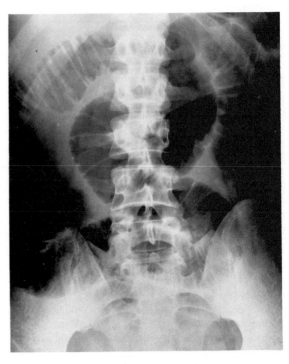

Fig. 22.2 Lower small bowel obstruction; supine X-ray film showing distended loops

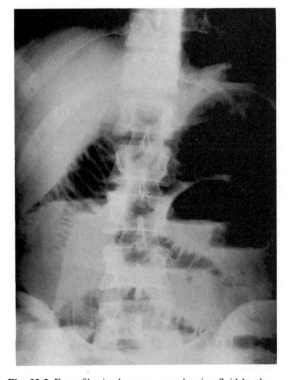

Fig. 22.3 Erect film in the same case showing fluid levels

obstruction large collections of gas may be shown in the colon, both proximal and distal to the obstruction; the larger collection is usually proximal, and is not evacuated after an enema. If gas remains in any part of the colon after an enema colonic obstruction probably exists. In suspected large bowel obstruction, sigmoidoscopy should be undertaken. It may allow confirmation of the presence of carcinoma, and it may prove therapeutic, e.g. in some patients with volvulus of the sigmoid colon.

Mechanical obstruction

This includes simple occlusion and occlusion combined with strangulation. Except when the obstruction is at an unusually high level, it is characterized invariably by colicky pain as the bowel above the obstruction contracts in an attempt to overcome it. In some cases the nature of the obstruction can be determined or conjectured before operation. In others the diagnosis must await laparotomy. The obstructive lesions which give rise to typical diagnostic features are listed on Table 22.1.

Strangulation

This may complicate most of the common types of mechanical obstruction except carcinoma of the colon. Its existence should be suspected in the following conditions:

1. when an irreducible external hernia is tense and tender
2. when the pain is severe and comes in frequent spasms, or becomes constant and localized
3. when there is elevation of temperature and pulse rate
4. when tenderness or rigidity or *rebound tenderness* is present
5. when the white cell count is elevated
6. when a state of shock exists; this suggests that a large segment of bowel is involved, as in mesenteric occlusion. The effects of this last condition are in every way similar to those of strangulation, and it can be considered under the same heading
7. if pain persists for more than 2 hours after effective gastroduodenal suction has been installed.

Level of obstruction

This has considerable bearing on the indications for operation, and on the necessary preparation should operation be considered. The distinguishing features of obstruction at different levels are set out in Table 22.2.

Paralytic ileus

This condition results from paralysis of the intestinal musculature leading to cessation of peristalsis, progressive abdominal distension and profuse vomiting. Colicky abdominal pain is absent, though the patient may be

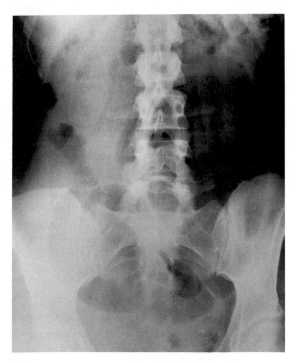

Fig. 22.4 An erect film showing distended caecum due to volvulus

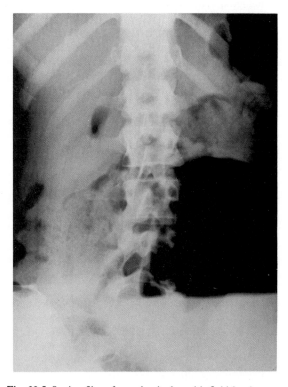

Fig. 22.5 Supine film of caecal volvulus with fluid levels

Table 22.1 Differential diagnosis in intestinal obstruction

Intussusception in infancy	Occurs usually in a healthy child during the first year. Sudden onset of severe colicky pain, followed by passage of blood-stained stool. Elongated mass palpable in umbilical region; RIF 'empty'. Blood on finger after rectal examination
External hernia*	An irreducible swelling at any of the hernial orifices furnishes an obvious cause for obstruction. Examination for such should never be omitted
Adhesive obstruction†	This is at once suspected if there has been any previous abdominal operation—especially if for peritonitis
Gall-stone ileus	Usually in elderly women. Insidious colicky pain. Previous history may suggest gall-stones. X-ray shows distended small bowel and may show gas in the biliary tree. Diagnosis seldom made before laparotomy
Mesenteric vascular occlusion	Should be suspected if the obstruction is accompanied by a shock-like state of collapse—especially if patient suffers from degenerative vascular disease. Blood-stained stool may be passed
Carcinoma of the colon	By far the commonest cause of obstruction in older patients. Insidious in onset. Progressive constipation and distension. Growth may be palpable, or its site determined by radiography
Volvulus of the colon	Usually pelvic colon. Tense tympanitic swelling placed centrally in abdomen. A blood-stained stool may have been passed or an enema may be returned blood-stained. Radiograph shows extreme distension confined to a single loop of bowel, which is often ∩-shaped

* The commonest cause of small bowel obstruction in the Third World
† The commonest cause of small bowel obstruction in the Western World

uncomfortable from the distension, and on auscultation no bowel sounds are heard.

A short period of ileus, usually only a few hours, follows most intra-abdominal procedures. If the ileus persists for more than 48–72 hours it is regarded as 'refractory', and may be due to intra-abdominal sepsis, to hypoxia or to electrolyte imbalance, particularly deficiencies of potassium, calcium or magnesium. Retroperitoneal trauma, either deliberate (as in renal or spinal surgery) or accidental, is frequently followed by ileus, and the mechanism may be reflex through the autonomic nervous system. A similar mechanism may account for the ileus seen in patients immobilized in a spinal plaster cast (The Cast Syndrome). Ileus is a frequent finding in circulatory shock of whatever cause and may be due to a combination of hypoxia and catecholamine overactivity.

Peritonitis, resulting from perforation of an intra-abdominal viscus or abscess produces an ileus due to paralysis of the plexus of Auerbach. A localized ileus is frequently seen in the vicinity of localized intra-abdominal inflammation (e.g. a dilated loop or loops of small bowel in the right iliac fossa in the abdominal X-ray of a patient with appendicitis) and this may occasionally be of sufficient degree to produce the clinical features of mechanical small bowel obstruction.

Intestinal pseudo-obstruction (Ogilvie's syndrome)
The condition of acute colonic pseudo-obstruction was described by Ogilvie in 1948 and the literature recently reviewed by Nanni (1982). It presents with clinical and radiological features of mechanical large bowel obstruction although no obstructing lesion exists. Radiologically, gas may be seen extending down to and including the rectum, but frequently there is a sharp 'cut off' of gas in the transverse or descending colon, making distinction from mechanical obstruction difficult. Inco-ordinated autonomic activity on the colon is thought to be responsible. Gross dilation of the colon is common with risk of caecal perforation, so that a high index of suspicion is required. Some 90% of patients have serious extra-intestinal metabolic or systemic dysfunction. The condition may be chronic or recurrent in some cases and a familial form has been described.

Conservative or preoperative treatment
Certain forms of therapy now used as routine in the preoperative treatment of intestinal obstruction may so relieve the patient's symptoms and may bring about such improvement in his general condition that operation can be deferred indefinitely. In cases of paralytic ileus they have almost entirely replaced operation. Their routine adoption in all cases of intestinal obstruction, combined with the choice of the correct time for operative intervention, has been by far the greatest factor in producing the lowered mortality rates of recent years.

The essentials of conservative or preoperative treatment are suction drainage of the gastro-intestinal tract, and intravenous infusion (Fig. 22.6) to restore fluid and electrolyte balance.

Table 22.2 Diagnosis of the level of obstruction

Level of obstruction	Onset	Pain	Dehydration	Distension	Radiographs
High small bowel	Sudden	Upper abdominal. Variable severity: may be continuous	Extreme	Absent	May show 'gasless' abdomen or may show distension of duodenum or first jejunal loop
Low small bowel	More gradual	Central abdominal, severe, colicky	Less marked	Moderate: central in position	Gasless small loop of small bowel on supine film, usually lying transversely. Fluid levels on erect films
Large bowel	Usually insidious	Central or lower abdominal. May be colicky or generalized; discomfort due to distension	Slight except in late stage	Progressive: extreme in late stage: peripheral except in volvulus	Gas shown in the colon mainly proximal to obstruction: this is not evacuated after an enema

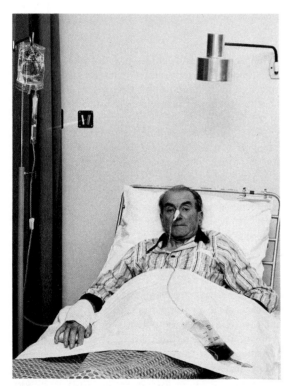

Fig. 22.6 Intravenous 'drip' infusion and nasogastric drainage into a polythene bag to allow for siphonage

Suction drainage

This has, as its object, the removal of fluid and gas from the stomach and upper intestine. By so doing it usually abolishes vomiting and brings about progressive relief of pain and distension. It greatly facilitates operation, should this be required, and obviates the risk of vomitus being inhaled during anaesthesia. Various types of tube, made either of rubber or of plastic, have been devised for this purpose. The Miller-Abbott tube has a double lumen, the larger lumen being used for aspiration purposes, and the smaller for inflation of a rubber balloon which surrounds its distal end, and which enables it to be carried by peristalsis for a considerable distance down the intestinal tract. Cantor's tube, a single lumen tube carrying at its tip a balloon weighted with mercury, is preferred by some surgeons. These tubes pass readily along the small intestine in a healthy individual, but in cases of obstruction they frequently fail to negotiate the pylorus: the more severe the obstruction, and the greater therefore the need for their use, the greater is the difficulty experienced. In this country it is usual to be content with *gastric* or *gastroduodenal* suction by means of a simple plastic tube which can be passed without difficulty through a nostril. This is usually effective in relieving distension not only of the stomach, but also of the greater part of the small bowel—due probably to the reversed peristalsis which commonly exists in the obstructed state, and to the fact that intestinal peristalsis is inhibited by gastric distension, and is restored when this is relieved. Frequent, usually hourly, aspiration may be carried out by syringe, or continuous suction applied using a low-pressure suction pump. If continuous suction is used a double lumen tube, with one lumen to allow air to be drawn into the tube is advised (e.g. the Salem Sump Tube made by Argyle). This will prevent mucosa being sucked into the tube and effectively blocking it.

Intravenous infusion

The patient with acute small bowel obstruction has usually suffered a serious loss of fluid and electrolytes from the out-pouring of intestinal secretions into the distended bowel above the obstruction—whether the fluid stagnates in the bowel, or whether it is lost by vomiting. If he has been sick for several days, the total deficit of water and sodium may run to several litres of water and several hundred millimoles of sodium. Such deficits may have been partly restored by the transfer of intracellular water and by the mobilization of bone sodium. Restoration of the estimated *total* of fluid should not therefore be attempted too rapidly, since overloading of the circulation may result. In the average case of obstruction it will usually suffice to give 1 litre of normal saline and 1 litre of glucose solution before operation is undertaken. Administered at the rate of a fast 'drip', this total of 2 litres can be given in the space of 2 to 3 hours, which is usually both an adequate and justifiable time to spend in preoperative preparation.

High small bowel obstruction
Characterized by profuse vomiting, the patient's greatest need is for fluid and electrolytes. These needs are effectively met by intravenous infusion, while the vomiting is abolished by suction drainage. Alkalosis is likely to be present, since the vomiting of acid gastric juice predominates, but this is satisfactorily corrected by normal saline given intravenously (p. 311). If the obstruction is due to simple kinking of the bowel it may be completely relieved by this treatment. In any case, there is seldom any great urgency for operation since strangulation is rare. If the patient's general condition is improved, and if such improvement is maintained, conservative treatment may be continued for several days if necessary.

Low small bowel obstruction
The need for fluid therapy (except in the late case) is less urgent, but such therapy, together with suction drainage, should always be installed before the patient is submitted to operation. In obstruction due to bands or adhesions, complete (even if only temporary) relief may be obtained by such treatment. Operation can then be undertaken later—and with much greater safety, when the acute symptoms of obstruction have been relieved, and fluid and electrolyte balance has been restored.

Late cases of small bowel obstruction
The fluid loss is too great for the deficit to be made up by the transfer of intracellular fluid. In consequence the blood volume is reduced and the patient exhibits all the signs of shock. The *first priority* in treatment is restoration of the circulatory volume, and, with this object in view, whole blood, plasma or dextran should be administered (Wilkinson, 1973). Electrolyte solutions, given in the stage of shock, will serve only to increase the hypoproteinaemia, and may lead to pulmonary oedema. As soon as the blood volume has been restored, the

patient can, if necessary, be submitted to operation. Electrolyte solutions are then infused during the operation, and are continued into the postoperative period as required. A fluid balance chart must, of course, be kept throughout the period of intravenous therapy (p. 310).

Colonic obstruction
These methods of preoperative treatment have a more limited application here. They should always be employed, however, in cases where vomiting or dehydration have occurred, or where gross distension is present.

In cases of suspected *strangulation* there is no justification for any undue delay, but suction drainage and intravenous infusion should be installed before the patient is taken to the operating theatre. When shock is present, operation should be delayed until the blood volume has been restored by whole blood, plasma or dextran solution.

Paralytic ileus
Suction drainage and intravenous infusion form the basis of modern therapy, and in most cases the condition resolves completely under this treatment. All purgatives and other drugs which stimulate peristalsis are avoided, and the bowel is left completely at rest to recover in its own time. This treatment can be continued for 2 weeks or longer if necessary, until bowel sounds return or flatus is passed. The suction may then be discontinued for a trial period of a few hours; if vomiting occurs it is at once reinstalled. In the reflex type of paralytic ileus the effect of guanethidine and prostigmine may be tried (Neely, 1971): by abolishing sympathetic inhibition this may bring about the return of peristalsis.

Indications for operation
In small bowel obstruction without suspicion of strangulation, the indications for operation depend largely on the response to conservative treatment. The patient's condition is assessed at 2-hourly intervals by clinical examination, which includes measurement of the abdominal girth, and estimation of the fluid loss obtained by aspiration. If the response to treatment is satisfactory, operation may be delayed until conditions are considered to be most favourable. Failure to respond to conservative treatment may well indicate strangulation (p. 419). Shatila (1976) therefore makes a plea for early intervention in these cases since the patient's only hope of survival lies in prompt operative treatment.

In acute colonic obstruction, especially when distension is marked, operation should be carried out without undue delay. Ischaemic rupture of the caecum may occur and is a real risk when the transverse diameter of the caecum on the abdominal film is greater than 12 cm.

Paralytic ileus

Operation is indicated if there is suspicion of intra-abdominal infection or that a mechanical element may exist. In long persisting paralytic ileus (12–14 days) a mechanical element may have resulted from matting together of intestines by fibrinous exudate.

In paralytic ileus, or in intestinal pseudo-obstruction, colonic distension may be so great that rupture of the large bowel becomes a risk. Decompression of the colon by tube caecostomy may be required. Alternatively, in skilled hands, decompression by colonoscopy may be undertaken.

LAPAROTOMY FOR INTESTINAL OBSTRUCTION

Operation for intestinal obstruction—except when this is due to an external hernia—will usually take the form of an exploratory laparotomy. Its primary object is to save life by relieving the state of obstruction which exists. In certain cases this can be accomplished effectively by some simple procedure such as the division of a constricting band or adhesion. Otherwise it may be necessary to deal with the obstruction by short-circuiting or (in the case of the colon) by drainage of the bowel to the exterior. Resection of a segment of small bowel may be rendered necessary by strangulation or by infarction.

In carcinoma of the colon (the commonest cause of obstruction in elderly patients), a second object of laparotomy is to assess the possibility of radical removal of the tumour at a later date, and to plan the most suitable operative procedure. Occasionally, when the obstruction is of moderate degree, it is permissible to remove the growth and perform a primary anastomosis although this should usually be combined with some drainage procedure.

Anaesthesia

A good anaesthetic with complete relaxation is essential in order to reduce the surgeon's difficulties in dealing with distended and unruly coils of bowel. The skilled anaesthetist will probably choose some form of inhalation anaesthetic, with tracheal intubation, and combined with a relaxant drug. Gastroduodenal suction carried out during anaesthesia prevents vomiting or inspiration of stomach contents. When such expert assistance is not available the advantages of spinal anaesthesia should be considered.

Incision

A midline incision centred on the umbilicus is preferred to a paramedian incision and is suitable for most patients with obstruction. A transverse subumbilical incision is satisfactory for patients with small bowel obstruction or obstructing lesions of the colon, and is advised particularly in patients with chronic respiratory problems. Transverse incisions are preferred also in neonates and young infants (see p. 317). Haemostasis should be meticulous and diathermy or staples may be used in division of the rectus.

If the patient already has a suitable previous incision the same site should be used. The new incision should start above or below a previous vertical incision, or lateral to a transverse one, so that the peritoneal cavity may be entered without risk of damaging adherent bowel. Bowel or omentum adherent to the inner aspect of the scar may then be dissected free under direct vision.

A clear peritoneal exudate is usually present when intestinal distension is marked. A bloodstained exudate suggests either some form of strangulation or of mesenteric occlusion, while a seropurulent exudate indicates an inflammatory cause for the obstruction.

Following any operative procedure necessary, it is advised that the incision is closed using a continuous mass suture of No. 1 Prolene or nylon incorporating peritoneum and muscle layers. Continued abdominal distension is common for a few days after operation for intestinal obstruction and chest complications are frequent, so that the strain on the wound is great.

Location of the obstruction

Sometimes the cause of the obstruction is at once apparent—as when the loop of a colonic volvulus presents in the wound. More often, however, nothing can be seen except distended coils of small bowel. In such cases the first step in the operation is to inspect the caecum. This can be done by retracting the right margin of the wound and by packing distended coils of small bowel away to the left.

If the caecum is distended the obstruction must be in the colon. By far the commonest cause of such obstruction is carcinoma. Growths which give rise to obstruction affect usually the left side of the colon; these growths are of the constricting or 'string' type, and may easily be missed if the surgeon is expecting to find a large tumour mass. The colon should, therefore, be methodically examined, and this should always be done *from below upwards*.

If the caecum is collapsed the obstruction is in the small bowel. A search is then made in the right iliac fossa or in the pelvis for a collapsed loop and this is traced proximally until the obstruction is reached. The actual direction in which the bowel must be traced is determined in the following manner. The loop is held in the long axis of the body, and a finger is passed deeply along the left side of its mesentery. If the finger finds itself guided inevitably to the left iliac fossa or to the left

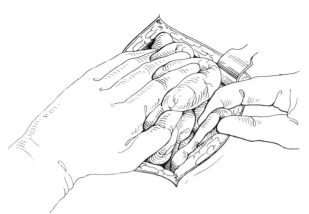

Fig. 22.7 Laparotomy for intestinal obstruction of uncertain origin. Distended coils of small bowel are kept as far as possible within the abdomen, while a search is made for a collapsed loop

side of the vertebrae, the proximal end of the loop lies towards the thorax. If the finger is guided into the right iliac fossa or to the right side of the vertebrae, the loop is inverted, i.e. its proximal end lies towards the feet. During the search for the cause of the obstruction, distended coils of bowel should if possible be kept within the abdomen (Fig. 22.7); any coils which cannot be retained are covered by warm moist packs.

When, as frequently occurs, the operation is impeded by gaseous distension of the small bowel the bowel should be deflated. This is best done by 'milking' back small bowel content from proximal jejunum into the duodenum and thence stomach, from where it may be aspirated through the nasogastric tube by the anaesthetist (Fig. 22.8). It is seldom necessary to carry out needle aspiration of the small bowel.

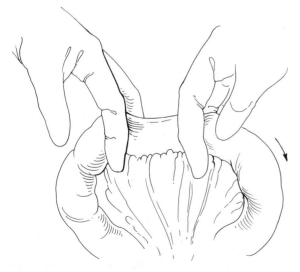

Fig. 22.8 Method of 'milking' back small bowel content

Gross gaseous distension of the colon should be dealt with by inserting a fine bore needle obliquely through a taenia coli in the transverse colon and attaching it to a low pressure suction apparatus—if a transverse colostomy is contemplated the proposed site of the colostomy should be used. Occasionally a further needle may need to be inserted in the sigmoid colon. It is advisable to oversew the puncture sites with a Z suture of 2/0 chromic catgut to minimize the risk of leakage from the site during further manipulations.

Bands and adhesions

These are likely to have resulted from a previous operation—especially if performed for some condition complicated by peritonitis. In other cases they are congenital—as in the case of the band which is sometimes found stretching from the umbilicus to the ileum about 60 cm from its lower end, and which is the remains of the vitello-intestinal duct. The ileal end of the duct may remain open to form a Meckel's diverticulum. A loop of small bowel may become wound round the band or may be ensnared by it.

Bands and small adhesions are divided under direct vision. The remnants of any band or diverticulum should be removed in order to prevent a possible recurrence. The constricted area or the site of adhesion on the gut is examined carefully; if it is damaged it is infolded by *Lembert* suture. If there has been gross distension the bowel may be deflated by aspiration; alternatively a temporary enterostomy may be performed (p. 432).

Where a complicated mass of adhesions is present, separation of the loops of bowel may be difficult and carry an attendant risk of damage to the bowel. When such a situation exists it is better to short-circuit the obstruction by making a lateral anastomosis above and below the involved bowel. Sometimes more than one anastomosis is necessary (p. 431). If the length of bowel to be bypassed is such that there is a risk of producing a short-bowel syndrome, adequate bowel must with great care be dissected free to reduce this risk.

Recurrent adhesive small bowel obstruction

Some unfortunate patients are subject to repeated episodes of adhesive small bowel obstruction. Glove powder has been incriminated in the past, and the modern starch powders are not above considerable suspicion.

In patients with multiple adhesions, where recurrent obstruction is considered to be likely, or in those where it has already occurred, a number of authors consider that some form of plication procedure, allowing the intestine to take regular folds, will reduce the risk of further obstruction. Noble (1937) described his intestinal plication procedure, whereby the small intestinal

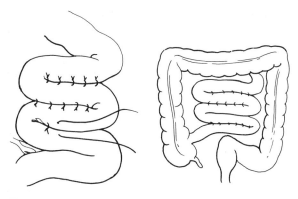

Fig. 22.9 Noble's plication procedure

loops, after lysis of adhesions, are sutured to one another in ordered fashion (Fig. 22.9). The procedure is laborious and carries a risk of intestinal fistula formation. A simpler technique is transmesenteric plication, as described by Childs, 1960 (Fig. 22.10).

Baker (1959), and more recently Munro & Jones (1978), have advocated the use of a jejunal tube brought out through a jejunostomy to act as an internal splint holding the bowel in gentle curves and preventing kinking while adhesions form. The polyvinyl tube,

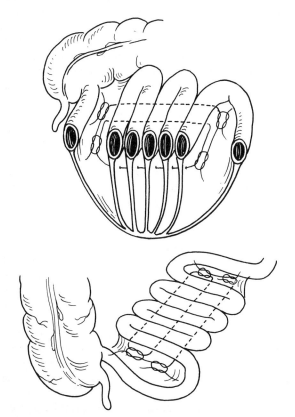

Fig. 22.10 Transmesenteric plication

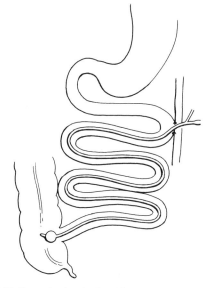

Fig. 22.11 Operative intubation in the treatment of complicated small bowel obstruction

300 cm long, and with a double lumen, one leading to an inflatable balloon and one for drainage, is inserted into the jejunum approximately 20 cm distal to the duodenojejunal flexure. It is then guided along the small bowel into the caecum, when the balloon is inflated (Fig. 22.11). The tube is removed 12 days postoperatively.

Internal strangulation
This term is applicable when the blood supply of a loop of bowel has been endangered by an obstructing constriction. If the bowel is considered to be non-viable (p. 500), resection and anastomosis must be carried out.

Intussusception
Intussusception occurs with invagination of bowel so that the apex is carried distally by peristalsis. Depending on the segment involved, the lesion is described as ileo-ileal, ileocolic or colocolic. The condition is most common in babies between 3 and 9 months who develop an ileocolic intussusception, probably from hyperplasia of Peyer's patches secondary to a virus infection. In older children and adults, a Meckel's diverticulum, Henoch Schönlein's purpura, or a bowel neoplasm may be the underlying cause.

Intussusception presents initially with bouts of colicky abdominal pain which may continue for a variable interval before the signs of bowel strangulation and obstruction develop. During such bouts of pain a baby will scream, go red in the face and draw its knees up to the chest; as the pain subsides the baby lies pale and lethargic. Vomiting may be a feature and constipation follows after bowel content distal to the intussusception has been passed. At a later stage the typical red current jelly stool may be seen. When the abdomen is relaxed between bouts of pain it may be possible to feel a sausage-shaped mass above the umbilicus in the line of the transverse colon. Occasionally the intussusception will progress further along the bowel and the apex can be felt on rectal examination. However, the clinical picture is often inconclusive and the diagnosis can then be confirmed on a barium enema examination which will outline the apex of the intussusception within the lumen of the colon.

Management

Depending on the severity of the presentation it may first be necessary to correct fluid loss and electrolyte imbalance.

In babies, hydrostatic reduction of an intussusception by barium enema can often be successful. The procedure is, however, potentially dangerous and should not be attempted when strangulation of bowel or obstruction are suspected. Furthermore, reduction may be incomplete. In the absence of an experienced radiologist an operation is preferable.

A transverse right sided lower abdominal incision will usually provide adequate access and can, if necessary, be extended towards the left. The thickened mass of the intussusception can be easily felt but, to obtain a better view, it may be helpful to deliver dilated proximal ileum through the wound. The intussusception is reduced by applying firm pressure over the apex, so as to push the intussuscipiens back along the line of the bowel; traction should never be applied to bowel proximal to the lesion. If this manoeuvre proves difficult, the intussusception should be wrapped in warm gauze and squeezed gently along its length so as to reduce oedema. Providing the wall of the caecum is undamaged, an appendicectomy may be performed so as to prevent confusion in the future. When reduction of the intussusception is incomplete or when the ileum is traumatized or ischaemic, the abnormal segment of bowel should be excised and an end-to-end ileocolostomy performed in two layers. Resection of gangrenous bowel may require replacement of blood loss by transfusion.

Small bowel volvulus

This may be primary in infants and young children. In older children and adults the condition is usually secondary to adhesions. Adhesions, if present, are divided, then the loop of bowel derotated. Non-viable intestine must be resected and intestinal continuity restored in end-to-end fashion.

Malrotation of bowel in infancy

Embryology

This condition may present as an isolated anomaly but may also be found in association with a diaphragmatic hernia or exomphalos. Between the fourth and twelfth weeks of pregnancy, the mid-gut is first displaced into the umbilical sac and then withdrawn back into the abdominal cavity. During this period the proximal and distal limbs of the mid-gut rotate in an anti-clockwise direction through 270 degrees about the long axis of the superior mesenteric artery. As a result, the distal part of the duodenum passes behind the artery from right to left and the caecum passes in front of the artery from left to right so that it comes to lie in the right hypochondrium. Thereafter the caecum slowly descends to the right iliac fossa and the ascending colon and duodenum are fixed to the parietal peritoneum of the posterior abdominal wall.

The term malrotation embraces both incomplete and abnormal rotation. The most common situation is that the gut rotates only 180 degrees so that the duodenum lies partly behind or to the right of the superior mesenteric artery and the caecum lies in front of the artery. Adhesions (Ladd's bands) pass from the caecum across the duodenum to the under surface of the liver (Fig. 22.12). Less commonly there may be non-rotation or, after initial rotation, the gut twists in a clockwise direction. Ladd's bands may partly or completely obstruct the duodenum and the narrow root of mesentery of the mid-gut predisposes to volvulus.

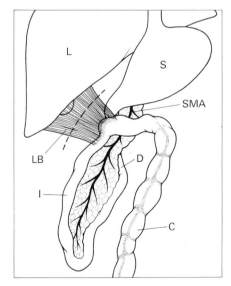

Fig. 22.12 Illustration of the most common type of malrotation. C—colon; D—duodenum; I—ileum; L—liver; LB—Ladd's bands; S—stomach; SMA—superior mesenteric artery

Clinical presentation

Symptoms may develop at any age but are more common in the neonate (Welch, 1983). Partial obstruction of the duodenum and intermittent volvulus may present with bile stained vomiting only, there may be little or no abdominal distension and meconium and changed stools are passed normally. Volvulus may however cause complete obstruction and strangulation. The baby then becomes rapidly ill and in addition to vomiting there is abdominal distension and constipation. A plain abdominal X-ray may show either the 'double bubble' appearance of duodenal obstruction or the more generalized changes of small bowel obstruction. In incomplete obstruction barium studies may demonstrate the abnormal position of the duodenum and caecum; however, the examination should be carried out with dilute medium and only used with caution.

Treatment

In a baby with malrotation the immediate treatment is that of obstruction by nasogastric aspiration, intravenous infusion and correction of fluid and electrolyte imbalance. The underlying anomaly should then be corrected by operation.

The abdomen of the baby is opened through a transverse upper abdominal incision and the bowel delivered through the wound. A volvulus, if present, is usually twisted in a clockwise direction and can easily be corrected. It is important that Ladd's bands are completely divided so that the terminal ileum and

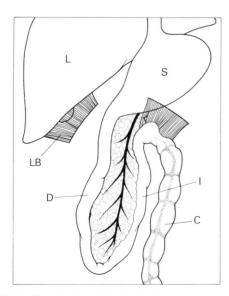

Fig. 22.13 After division of Ladd's bands, the caecum is placed in the left hypochondrium and the duodenum is freed to lie to the right of the vertebral column. C—colon; D—duodenum; I—ileum; L—liver; LB—Ladd's bands; S—stomach

caecum can be placed in the left hypochondrium (Fig. 22.13). This will expose the full length of the duodenum which can then be mobilized so that it lies freely to the right of the vertebral column. Finally, remaining adhesions between loops of bowel are separated. To ensure patency of the duodenum, air can be introduced into the stomach through a nasogastric tube and manipulated into the jejunum. According to preference an appendicectomy may be performed if the caecum is undamaged but caecopexy which was practised at one stage to prevent recurrent volvulus is unnecessary. The abdominal wound is then closed in layers.

The postoperative management of malrotation is usually uncomplicated and oral feeding can be started after a few days.

Small bowel atresia

This condition is probably the result of ischaemic damage rather than a primary developmental anomaly (Louw & Barnard, 1955). It is one of the more common major congenital gastro-intestinal abnormalities, the incidence being approximately one in 2500 live births. Bland Sutton (1889) describes three types. In type I continuity of the lumen of the bowel is obstructed by a membrane; in type II the proximal and distal segments of the bowel are connected by a fibrous cord; and in type III the two segments are separated and there may be a 'V' shaped deficiency in the mesentery. Less commonly, multiple atresias are found or the distal bowel may be vascularized by a branch of the middle colic artery and arranged in a spiral form around a central vessel giving the appearance of 'apple peel'. The proximal bowel in atresia is normally grossly dilated and hypertrophied and the distal part may be partly ischaemic.

The baby born with jejunal or ileal atresia may be of low birth weight and there may be a maternal history of hydramnios. Associated congenital abnormalities may be present but they are less common than in duodenal atresia. The presenting sign is that of bile stained vomiting. Abdominal distension may be a feature particularly when the obstruction is distal. Although normal meconium or pale inspissated plugs may be passed initially, the baby thereafter becomes constipated. A plain erect and supine abdominal X-ray will show features of small bowel obstruction. When the atretic segment is distal the condition must be distinguished from meconium ileus, malrotation and Hirschsprung's disease and a barium enema may be of value.

The immediate management is that of obstruction; a nasogastric tube is passed, an intravenous infusion established and any fluid and electrolyte imbalance corrected. As part of the supportive care the baby should be nursed in an incubator. When the baby's condition is satisfactory a laparotomy is performed using a transverse upper abdominal incision. It is important to exclude further areas of atresia in the distal bowel and this is done by introducing a catheter and injecting saline into the lumen. The dilated part of the proximal bowel is then generously excised as it may fail to develop effective peristalsis (Nixon, 1955). Because of the discrepancy between the dilated proximal and narrowed distal bowel an end-to-end anastomosis is impractical and an end-to-back anastomosis should be performed with a single inverting layer of fine sutures. In a small baby with a proximal jejunal atresia a gastrostomy may be fashioned to ensure gastric emptying and thus prevent vomiting. At the same time a fine silastic trans-anastomotic feeding tube can be introduced alongside the gastrostomy tube and threaded down into the distal segment. In most babies a delay in normal feeding should be anticipated and intravenous nutrition started early in the postoperative period.

Impacted gall-stone or faecalith
On occasion, a gallstone may pass into the lumen of the gut through a cholecystoduodenal fistula which has resulted from unsuspected cholecystitis. The calculus becomes impacted at any narrowing of the gut and causes intestinal obstruction. The diagnosis is suspected when air is noted in the biliary tree in addition to the X-ray features of small bowel obstruction.

Operation
The segment of bowel (usually the lower ileum) in which the concretion has become impacted is withdrawn from the wound; contents are milked away in both directions and clamps are applied. After careful packing-off the bowel is opened, if possible by a transverse incision, and the concretion is removed, either by expression or by the use of stone-holding forceps. The opening is repaired by two layers of suture. If the concretion is not too firmly impacted it may with advantage be moved proximally to a healthier part of the bowel which can be incised with greater safety.

Internal hernia
A coil of small bowel is occasionally imprisoned in a hole in the mesentery or omentum, or in a retroperitoneal fossa. The constricting ring should be gently stretched and the bowel withdrawn, after which the opening is closed by suture. If difficulty is encountered, the distended bowel should be emptied by aspiration (p. 424). Great care must be taken if the constricting ring requires to be divided, for severe haemorrhage may be induced. Strangulation is common in internal hernias, and if present, resection of the involved loop is mandatory.

Mesenteric vascular occlusion
This is a relatively uncommon and frequently fatal cause of intestinal obstruction. The occlusion may be the result of embolism to or thrombosis in the superior mesenteric arteries, or thrombosis in the superior mesenteric or portal vein. In many patients the large vessels are not involved, the occlusion occurring widely in small arteries or veins.

Presenting symptoms and signs are vague in the early stages of the occlusion, so that the diagnosis remains unsuspected until a greater or lesser length of intestine has infarcted, providing the clinical features of peritonitis. Inferior mesenteric artery occlusion presents with severe lower abdominal pain and there may be little to find at laparotomy until bowel necrosis occurs.

On suspicion of the diagnosis, providing time and facilities permit, mesenteric angiography may be very helpful preoperatively, since any major arterial occlusion may be relieved surgically although small vessel or venous thrombosis is not amenable to this.

At laparotomy, if extensive established gangrene is present, attempts to restore arterial flow are not indicated. Resection of the involved intestine is required. In patients with potential for restoration of arterial flow, and intestine which is still viable (or of questionable viability) attention should be directed first to restoration of flow. An embolus is extracted using a Fogarty catheter via an arteriotomy in the main trunk of the superior mesenteric artery. Main stem superior mesenteric artery thrombosis is best dealt with by inserting a graft of saphenous vein or dacron between more distal superior mesenteric artery and the aorta (H-graft). Following successful restoration of flow, areas of dubious viability may become clearly viable and intestinal resection can be lessened in extent, or even avoided. A 'second look' laparotomy after 24 hours has been recommended by some authors.

Operations on patients with mesenteric vascular occlusion should be covered by broad spectrum antibiotics (including an anti-anaerobe agent) and followed by anticoagulation. Adequate fluid replacement is essential, and requirements are particularly high in the patient who has had successful restoration of flow.

Volvulus of colon
Rotation of a loop of bowel on its vascular pedicle occurs most commonly in the *pelvic colon* in the adult. It represents a good example of closed loop obstruction, allowing entry of some intestinal content from more proximal bowel, so that rapidly increasing distension of the loop occurs, while more proximal bowel may not be impressively distended. Compression of the blood vessels in the rotated pedicle compromises the blood supply to the loop, and this, added to the effect of distension, leads to a high risk of strangulation.

In volvulus of the sigmoid colon where there is no suspicion of strangulation, the condition may be treated conservatively by the careful insertion of a flatus tube via a sigmoidoscope into the distal limb of the volvulus. If done successfully, decompression of the loop occurs, allowing time for assessment of the patient and consideration of definitive elective treatment, for the condition, once it occurs, tends to be recurrent.

If the method is unsuccessful, or strangulation is suspected, laparatomy is undertaken through a lower midline or left paramedian incision. As soon as the abdomen is opened, the distended and congested pelvic colon presents. When the loop is only moderately distended it should be gently withdrawn from the abdomen and unwound by rotation between the two hands. When the pedicle can be inspected the direction for rotation is obvious—otherwise it must be discovered by trial and error; usually the twist has been in an anti-clockwise direction. When the loop is too distended to be delivered through the wound there should be no hesitation in decompressing it by aspiration.

If the loop is non-viable, it *must* be resected. If the loop is viable it is still best resected, as recurrent volvulus is common, and various means of colopexy are relatively unsuccessful. If the patient's condition does not permit emergency resection, the sigmoid loop may be drained via a flatus tube inserted per rectum, or by performing a sigmoid colostomy (q.v.) Later elective resection of the sigmoid loop is undertaken when the patient is fit.

Following emergency resection, the surgeon has three choices, determined by local conditions and by the general condition of the patient:

1. To perform an end-to-end reconstitution of colonic continuity. This is the preferred choice. The anastomosis should be in one layer, using interrupted inverting sutures of 2/0 or 3/0 gauge.

2. To bring both cut ends of bowel to the surface—the proximal end as an end colostomy, and the distal end separately as a mucous fistula (Mikulicz operation). Intestinal continuity is restored at a later date.

3. The length of distal bowel available may not permit its cut end being brought to the surface. In this event the distal cut end is oversewn in two layers and returned to the pelvis, while the proximal cut end is brought out as an end colostomy (Hartmann's procedure). Intestinal continuity is again restored at a later date, but the procedure is usually technically more difficult than if a mucous fistula had been formed.

Volvulus of the caecum

This is less common. Right hemicolectomy is the preferred procedure and is mandatory if the bowel has been devitalized. If resection is not undertaken the caecum may be fixed in the right iliac fossa (caecopexy)

by direct suture to parietal peritoneum, by using poly-vinyl alcohol sponge (El-Katib, 1973), or by performing a tube caecostomy.

Postoperative obstruction

This is most liable to occur in cases of peritonitis. It may be either paralytic or mechanical in origin.

Paralytic ileus

The clinical features of this condition, the conservative treatment and the rare indications for operation have been discussed (p. 419). An obvious source of infection should be sought, abscesses should be drained, and a leaking anastomosis repaired or resected. Simple repair of a leaking anastomosis may be unsatisfactory, and if resection is inadvisable for technical reasons a large bore tube drain should be led from the vicinity of the anastomosis to the exterior; this, in the event of further breakdown of the anastomosis, will lead to a controlled fistula rather than recurrent peritonitis. Prior to closure of the abdomen peritoneal lavage using 3 l of a wide-spectrum antibiotic solution is advised. The wound should be closed using a mass suture technique.

Mechanical obstruction

This may be due to oedema of the bowel at the site of an anastomosis, or to kinking or compression by adhesions. Unlike paralytic ileus it occurs fairly late in the postoperative period—usually 5 to 10 days after operation, by which time the bowels may have moved normally. Colicky pains are present, and bowel sounds are heard on auscultation. The guiding principles in treatment are the same as in other types of mechanical obstruction—i.e. early laparotomy if there is no response to conservative treatment.

RESECTION AND ANASTOMOSIS OF SMALL BOWEL

Resection is always attended by some risk and should be avoided wherever possible. The most absolute indication arises when the blood supply of a segment of bowel has been so seriously interfered with that gangrene, if not already present, is considered to be inevitable. Resection may be required also in extensive injuries of a segment of gut, as may occur in penetrating abdominal wounds. The risks of resection are greatly increased in the presence of obstruction, which usually co-exists with strangulation, but when the bowel is considered to be non-viable (p. 500) such risks must generally be accepted.

Resection with end-to-end anastomosis

This is the standard procedure for re-establishing

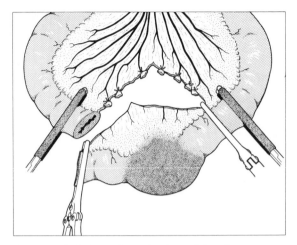

Fig. 22.14 Technique of resection in small bowel

continuity of small bowel. Disparity in the sizes of ends to be joined is corrected by division of the narrower bowel obliquely, the greater length of bowel being, of course, retained on the mesenteric border.

Technique of resection (Fig. 22.14)

In order to ensure a satisfactory anastomosis the level of resection must be well to each side of the devitalized area. The affected loop is withdrawn from the wound until a sufficiency of healthy bowel has been delivered, and the wound and peritoneal cavity are protected with moist packs. At the levels selected for the section a hole is made in an avascular area in the mesentery close to the gut. The mesentery is now divided between these two points, in the line of a shallow V, the apex of which points towards the mesenteric root, the division being carried out by clamping with a succession of artery forceps, and by cutting with scissors. This is most satisfactorily achieved by displaying the vascular pattern of the mesentery by means of a bright light behind it. The forceps are then tied off; they should each contain a relatively small bite of mesentery owing to the danger of a ligature slipping. The segment of bowel to be resected is emptied by milking away its contents, and a crushing clamp is applied at each end. *The tip of this clamp should lie exactly opposite the line of division of the mesentery.* In order to ensure a good blood supply to the anti-mesenteric border it may be placed slightly obliquely, so that more of this border is removed. Light occlusion clamps are now applied to the healthy bowel 2.5 cm away from the crushing clamps. A swab having been placed underneath to absorb leakage, the bowel is divided close to the crushing clamps. The loop is now removed along with the crushing clamps still attached. The open ends of the healthy bowel protruding beyond the occlusion clamps are mopped out with small gauze pledgets held on forceps.

Technique of anastomosis

The occlusion clamps are approximated so that the open ends of bowel lie in apposition. The junction is effected by two complete layers of suture—a layer of through-and-through sutures, and a layer of Lembert sutures which do not penetrate the lumen. It is usually easier to insert the through-and-through suture first. This is commenced at the anti-mesenteric border, and is continued round the circumference of the bowel until the starting point is reached, when it is tied to its own short end. A lock-stitch should be inserted at intervals to prevent a purse-string effect being produced. When the superficial cut edges are being approximated, the Connell type of suture (Fig. 22.15), which prevents eversion of the mucous membrane, may be employed as an alternative to the method shown on page 320. When this suture has been completed the clamps may be removed. The suture line is carefully inspected for oozing or haemorrhage, and additional stitches are inserted if necessary. The line of junction is now invaginated by Lembert suture. Special attention should be paid to the point where the leaves of the mesentery separate to enclose the bowel (the 'mesenteric angle'), for here there is a small area of gut wall which is uncovered by serosa, and from which leakage may occur. It is an advantage to commence the suture at this point, and to pass the needle through both leaves of the mesentery close to the bowel, so that they are included in the first stitch. The suture is then continued round the circumference of the bowel until the starting point is reached, when it is passed through the mesentery and tied to its own short end (Fig. 22.16). Finally, the gap in the mesentery is closed by interrupted sutures; haemorrhage is avoided if the needle, threaded in the usual way, is passed *eye first* through the tissue. Small bites only should be taken, or vessels supplying the gut may be

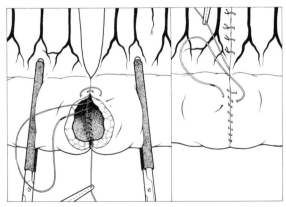

Fig. 22.15   **Fig. 22.16**

Figs. 22.15 & 22.16 End-to-end anastomosis of small bowel by two layers of continuous suture. The *Connell* suture shown in the first drawing prevents eversion of the mucosa

damaged or occluded. The bowel is washed with saline or antibiotic solution before being returned to the peritoneal cavity. Drainage is not required unless there was perforation of the gut before operation.

SHORT-CIRCUITING OPERATIONS ON THE INTESTINES

These operations are carried out, as a rule, by lateral anastomosis, the technique of which has already been described (p. 323). In the case of such an operation on the colon the incision into the lumen should be made along one of the taenia, since the greater thickness of the muscular coat in this line ensures a more satisfactory anastomosis.

Short-circuiting of small bowel
This is the operation of choice when obstruction has been caused by a complicated mass of adhesions as may result from caseating mesenteric glands. Unless the length of bowel to be short-circuited is considered likely to result in 'short-bowel' problems no attempt should be made to free the adherent loops as damage to the bowel, or haemorrhage from mesenteric vessels may result. The anastomosis should be performed as close to the obstruction as possible. Most surgeons prefer a two-layer anastomosis in small bowel, using continuous sutures of 2/0 or 3/0 chromic catgut or Dexon. In some cases more than one anastomosis may be necessary.

Ileotransverse anastomosis (Fig. 22.17)
This is employed most commonly in the treatment of

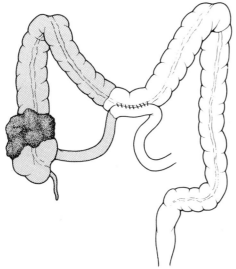

Fig. 22.17 Ileotransverse anastomosis (antiperistaltic) with the ileum in continuity. Stippling shows segment of bowel which is 'defunctioned'

tumours of the caecum and ascending colon. If the growth is removable the anastomosis forms part of the operation of right-sided *hemicolectomy*; alternatively, it may be carried out as a preliminary measure when the hemicolectomy is planned as a two-stage operation. If the growth is irremovable, ileotransverse anastomosis is valuable as a palliative procedure. It may also be used as an effective diverting procedure in ileocaecal tuberculosis with obstructive features, allowing chemotherapy to be used and obviating the necessity of resection.

When the operation is being carried out by itself (not as part of a one-stage hemicolectomy), it is usually best that the anastomosis should be effected with the ileum in continuity (i.e. not divided), in view of the possibility that the colonic lesion might give rise to obstruction—in which case, if the ileum were divided, a 'closed loop' would result. A segment of ileum, as near to the caecum as is found convenient, is brought up to lie without tension alongside the transverse colon at the junction of its proximal and middle thirds, so that a lateral anastomosis may be made. If a hemicolectomy is to be performed later, the direction of the ileum should be such that the anastomosis will be *antiperistaltic*; this will facilitate the second-stage operation by leaving a clearer field for the resection. Otherwise the direction of the ileum is immaterial. The stoma of the anastomosis should be about 4 cm in length.

When no obstruction is anticipated, or when it is planned to carry out a second-stage operation before obstruction can supervene, it may be preferable to divide the ileum, in order to obtain a defunctioning effect on the right side of the colon. By this method the ileum is divided in its terminal part, the distal cut-end is closed, and the proximal cut-end is joined to the transverse colon by end-to-side anastomosis.

In Crohn's disease affecting the terminal ileum and caecum and causing obstruction, right hemicolectomy is the preferred surgical treatment. This may not in some patients be technically feasible at the time of laparotomy. In this circumstance ileotransverse anastomosis with exclusion is preferred to in continuity anastomosis as it is associated with a lower incidence of continued or recurrent activity in the affected area of bowel.

Transverse-pelvic anastomosis (Fig. 22.18).
This is the procedure of choice in irremovable tumours of the splenic flexure, and has obvious advantages over a permanent transverse colostomy. Except in cases where the transverse colon is pendulous, the lower part of the descending colon may require to be mobilized by incision of the peritoneum along its lateral border, in order that the anastomosis can be effected without tension.

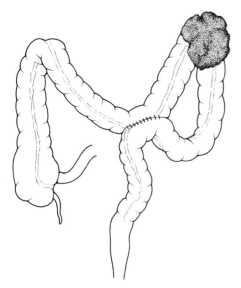

Fig. 22.18 Transverse-pelvic anastomosis, short-circuiting an irremovable tumour of the splenic flexure

OPERATIONS FOR EXTERNAL DRAINAGE OF THE INTESTINES (STOMA)

Drainage of the colon (*colostomy*) may be either temporary or permanent. Temporary drainage is performed for the immediate relief of obstruction or for the protection of a colonic anastomosis following resection of a distally placed tumour: it may be employed also in inflammatory conditions such as Crohn's disease, diverticulitis and intractable fistula-in-ano in order to 'defunction' the distal colon. Permanent drainage (i.e. the making of an 'artificial anus') is inevitable in the case of tumours which are irremovable and cannot be short-circuited, or in which continuity of the bowel cannot be restored after excision. A colostomy may be formed in any mobile part of the colon but is usually either transverse or pelvic.

Ileostomy

Ileostomy following colectomy for inflammatory disease such as ulcerative colitis, is usually permanent (see p. 449).

Ileostomy in children

A temporary ileostomy may be necessary in a baby to relieve obstruction or to defunction ischaemic bowel in necrotising enterocolitis. Normally the decision to perform an ileostomy will be taken during an exploratory laparotomy. A separate stab wound is then made in the right iliac fossa of sufficient size so that a loop of ileum can be drawn through with ease. Within the abdomen the bowel should be fixed by a stitch placed between serosa and parietal peritoneum. On the outside, the loop of ileum is opened longitudinally and sewn to the skin margin with an everting suture so as to raise the stoma 3–4 mm.

The procedure for a permanent spout ileostomy in an older child with ulcerative colitis is the same as that used in the adult.

Management of an ileostomy

The ileostomy does not usually act for 12 to 24 hours after operation. It may then act profusely, however, and the sudden and unaccustomed loss of small bowel contents may lead to dehydration and salt depletion. For this reason, intravenous infusion should be maintained for at least the first 2 postoperative days and longer if oral intake does not replace fluids lost by the ileostomy. It is most important, if at all possible, to prevent excoriation of the skin by the ileostomy efflux, and for this purpose a collecting appliance (*ileostomy bag*) should be fitted immediately after the operation. The ileostomy bags at present in use are designed to fit closely and firmly to the skin around the stoma. In some types there is a flange which can be made to adhere for as long as 3 or 4 days by means of special cement containing either a latex mixture, karaya gum or stomahesive, and to the rim of this flange a detachable or disposable bag is fitted. There are also one-piece disposable bags incorporating a small adhesive area. Other types of bag are not adherent, but depend upon a belt to hold the flange in position around the stoma.

After a week or two, the discharge becomes more solid, but it never develops the solidity of normal stools passed per rectum; it is, however, relatively odourless. In the early days there will be frequent difficulties because of looseness of the efflux, but the patient will soon learn to prevent such troubles by discovering which foodstuffs to avoid. When stability has been reached, the bowel acts shortly after meals, and usually remains quiescent at other times, except at night when it may move freely.

Stoma care in children. In a *baby* it is preferable to cover a stoma with an appliance rather than a dressing or nappy so as to prevent excoriation of surrounding skin and loss of blood from bowel mucosa which may be sufficient to cause anaemia. Suitable appliances, consisting of a flange and clip-on bag, are available in all age groups. The flange is made up of a stomahesive square carrying a 38 mm ring. The flange can be left in position for 2 or 3 days providing the seal is watertight and the bag is changed as necessary. The baby can be bathed in the normal manner and the stoma is cleaned with cotton wool soaked in warm water. The parents must be fully conversant with stoma care before the baby leaves hospital and the support which they received in hospital must be continued at home by a health visitor or district nurse. The important role of the stoma therapist in co-ordinating this care cannot be over-emphasized.

In an *older child*, in addition to the physical problems of the stoma, there may be profound psychological disturbance which may become accentuated with puberty. The disturbance may be such as to cause behavioural problems and this should be recognized. The management of both child and family requires particular skills and understanding. Under favourable circumstances, a child will learn to manage the stoma independently at about the age of 8; he or she should be able to attend a normal school and take part in a full range of outdoor activities including swimming.

Caecostomy

Drainage by caecostomy is now rarely required and is indicated for devitalization of the caecum resulting either from pseudo obstruction (p. 420) or caecal gangrene (p. 445).

Transverse colostomy

The technique for making a loop colostomy is described in the section on colonic carcinoma (p. 446).

Opening the colostomy

In the presence of obstruction, it is usual to open the colostomy at the initial operation. Wound infection can be avoided if the opening is delayed for 2 or 3 days after the operation. To achieve simple and speedy opening, a single blade of a Cope's clamp is applied to the bowel at operation (Fig. 22.19). On removal of the clamp, crushed tissue is trimmed without pain or bleeding.

Defunctioning transverse colostomy

Any colostomy may be regarded as 'defunctioning' if it is so constructed that faeces are prevented from entering the bowel distal to it. This is a most desirable aim if a resection is to be carried out later, for the distal part of the colon bearing the tumour or the inflammatory mass is placed completely at rest; it regains its normal size and tone, and, if faeces from the proximal colon is prevented from entering it, its bacterial content becomes greatly reduced. The operation for resection and primary anastomosis can then be carried out under the best possible conditions—in a defunctioned segment of colon (which is empty, inactive and relatively sterile) although *total* defunctioning may only be obtained by dividing the colon and bringing each end out through a separate opening in the abdominal wall.

Pelvic colostomy

This is most commonly performed as part of the operation of abdominoperineal excision of the rectum for

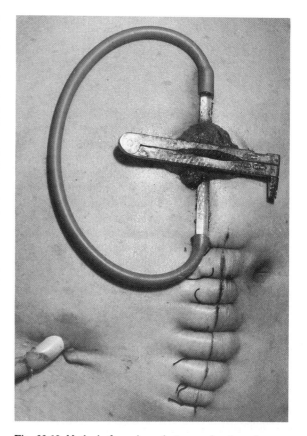

Fig. 22.19 Method of opening colostomy—the clamp is simply removed after 2 or 3 days. (A glass rod was used in this case because of short mesocolon and a tube caecostomy provided immediate drainage)

carcinoma. In such cases it is usually an *end-colostomy* (single stoma), and will, of course, be permanent. The technique is described on page 466.

A pelvic colostomy of *loop* type (with eventually a double stoma) may be indicated as a palliative measure in the case of obstructing and irremovable growths of the rectum. It may be employed also in nonmalignant strictures and gunshot wounds of the rectum, and in intractable cases of fistula-in-ano, when it may be only temporary.

For the simple loop colostomy a small left gridiron incision is used. It should not lie too near the anterior superior spine, lest this interfere with the accurate fitting of a colostomy appliance. The pelvic colon is identified and withdrawn. If it is fixed by a short mesentery it is mobilized by dividing the peritoneum on the lateral side as it is reflected on to the left iliac fossa. The site for the stoma should be in the upper part of the mobile loop of pelvic colon, in order that prolapse of the bowel may be avoided. The loop is retained on the skin surface by sutures to peritoneum and layers of abdominal wall in order to avoid the need for a supporting rod. The colostomy is normally opened after 2 or 3 days (p. 433).

Pelvic colostomy has no place in the treatment of acute obstruction, since, owing to the solid nature of the faeces in this part of the colon, immediate drainage is unsatisfactory.

Care of colostomy

This, like the management of an ileostomy (p. 432), has been made very much easier by the development of disposable plastic bags which can be made to fit very accurately around the stoma, either by an adhesive flange or by the use of a belt. Since, however, the efflux from a colostomy, unlike that from an ileostomy, is solid or semisolid, a watertight junction between skin and collecting appliance is by no means so necessary. Most patients will prefer a close fitting appliance, since it will make the stoma almost odourless and interfere very little with daily activities. It is possible, should appliances not be available, to manage the colostomy with a pad of wool held in position by a belt or by an elastic girdle of the 'roll on' type.

Colostomy in children

A colostomy is most often used in a baby or infant in the management of anorectal agenesis and Hirschsprung's disease both to relieve obstruction and as a preliminary to a definitive operation. It is important to prevent spillover of bowel content; this can be ensured by separating the proximal and distal limbs of bowel so as to form a split colostomy. The construction must be such that the flange of an appliance fits comfortably round the proximal stoma and forms a watertight seal with the surrounding abdominal wall and this includes both distal stoma and wound. Normally the colostomy is placed either in the right hypochondrium using right transverse colon or in the left iliac fossa using descending or sigmoid colon.

A transverse incision 3 or 4 cm long is made through the abdominal wall. The underlying colon is mobilized and a loop drawn through the incision. The bowel is divided transversely at the apex of the loop and the mesentery divided sufficiently so that proximal and distal limb lie without tension at either end of the incision. It is important that both limbs are fixed on the inside of the abdominal wall with stitches placed between serosa and parietal peritoneum to prevent prolapse. The incision between the two limbs is then closed in layers. The proximal limb is sewn to the skin margin with an everting suture to raise the stoma 3 or 4 mm and the distal limb is sutured flush with the skin (see Fig. 22.52).

Stoma care in children
(see p. 432).

Closure of colostomy

This procedure is only applicable where a temporary colostomy has been formed for the relief of obstruction, the protection of an anastomosis or in order to rest or 'defunction' the colon. The safety of the distal bowel to resume its normal function must be ascertained by appropriate examination, possibly including contrast X-ray and endoscopy. The operation may involve intra-peritoneal dissection if the colostomy is other than of the loop type and full bowel preparation is then required. The restoration of bowel continuity in such cases is identical to the methods applicable to primary anastomosis following resection of colonic carcinoma. Limited preparation is appropriate to closure of a loop colostomy.

Operation

An elliptical incision is made around the colostomy opening about 0.5 cm from the mucocutaneous junction (Fig. 22.20). Bowel is separated, by sharp dissection, from the layers of the abdominal wall as far as the peritoneum which is gently separated from the deep layers of the muscles. The edges of the opening in the colon, which still have a narrow margin of skin attached, are excised. The defect in the anterior wall of the colon

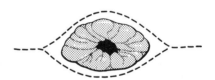

Fig. 22.20 Closure of colostomy—skin incision

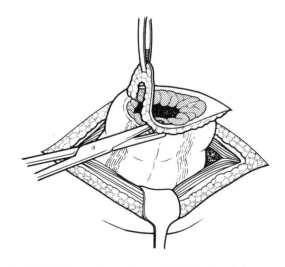

Fig. 22.21 Closure of colostomy—bowel freed and mucocutaneous junctioned trimmed

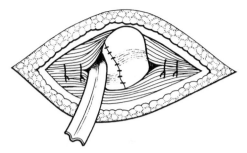

Fig. 22.22 Closure of colostomy—suture in transverse axis and drain inserted

is repaired by sutures placed in the transverse axis of the bowel, inverting the mucosa. The bowel is now allowed to fall back (Fig. 22.21) or is gently pushed into the depths of the wound. If it has been possible to separate the peritoneum in the manner described, the bowel should lie well below the level of the muscles. The wound is repaired in layers, a small drain being left extending down to the suture line in the bowel (Fig. 22.22). Sometimes leakage of faecal matter occurs, but it usually ceases spontaneously within a few days.

CARCINOMA OF THE COLON

Surgery for colon cancer is based upon three premises: an understanding of principles and strategy—of what is right and proper for each situation; an appreciation of the appropriate techniques for colonic mobilization and resection; and the needs of effective reconstruction.

Strategy

It is reasonable to divide the large bowel into right half of colon, left half of colon, sigmoid and colorectum. These areas correspond approximately to vascular-lymphatic supply and drainage. A cancer operation is one which, in addition to the primary and adjacent bowel, removes the lymph node field which is illustrated in Figure 22.1. This involves a wide mesenteric resection and dissection carried up to the feeding artery, irrespective of whether this compromises bowel to a greater extent than would appear necessary. Cancer operations can then be rationally based upon these vascular patterns. For a right sided lesion in caecum or ascending colon a formal right hemicolectomy (Fig. 22.23) will remove the ileocolic vascular territory but permit preservation of the distal ileum and thus of the entero-hepatic bile salt circulation. Even in the presence of an obstructing lesion such a resection can usually be followed by a primary reconstruction (see *Obstruction* below). Right hemicolectomy can be extended to

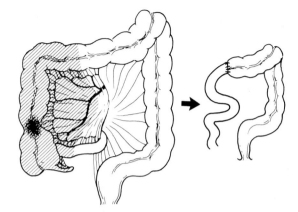

Fig. 22.23 The operative resection for a right sided tumour

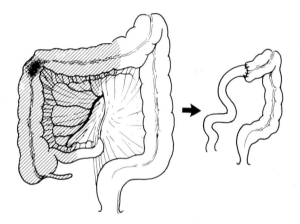

Fig. 22.24 Extended colectomy for a hepatic lesion

embrace the hepatic flexure (Fig. 22.24) and transverse colon (Fig. 22.25) lesion, and the same principles apply. The further this concept is extended, the more water absorbing surface is inevitably removed and thus the greater the likelihood of troublesome diarrhoea for the patient. In consequence, though occasionally a hemicolectomy which embraces splenic flexure, descending colon or even sigmoid carcinoma is expedient (obstruction; synchronous multiple tumours; an unprepared bowel; palliative resection in the presence of metastases), it is more usual to carry out an adequate local procedure (Fig. 22.26–22.28) with reconstruction by colocolostomy. In all instances the resection is based upon the main feeding and draining vessels which are accompanied by lymphatics and lymph nodes.

The more distal the lesion the more difficult it becomes to effect reconstruction, while at the same time undertaking an adequate cancer operation. Until recently it has been accepted that a cancer of the large bowel spreads almost equally distally as proximally and

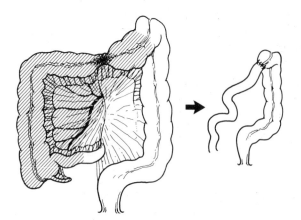

Fig. 22.25 The extent of resection for a transverse colon tumour

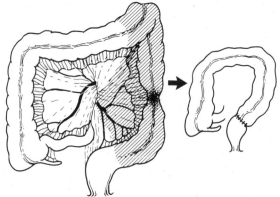

Fig. 22.28 Left hemicolectomy

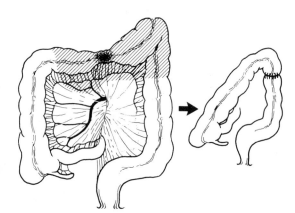

Fig. 22.26 Alternative resection for a transverse colon tumour

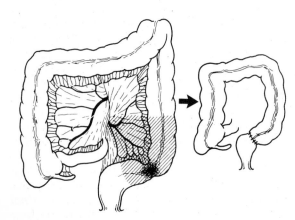

Fig. 22.27 Sigmoid colectomy

that in the rectum a large distal margin is required so necessitating in low tumours an abdominoperineal excision and a permanent colostomy (see Fig. 23.7). The pathological support for this view is not well defined and increasingly a distal rectal stump, perhaps no more than 2–3 cm beyond visible tumour, is being preserved for reconstruction (Williams, 1983). This attitude is additionally supported by the observation that continence is not wholly dependent upon a rectal reservoir but is more a function of extra-rectal receptors. Though the long term outcome is not yet known, resection and reconstruction of tumours as low as 5–6 cm from the dentate line is now being undertaken, assisted by the use of stapling devices (see below).

Tactics

Bowel preparation
Surgery on the colon is, while faeces are present, like stepping into a cesspool. Every effort should be made to have a completely empty colon before surgery. Indeed it is a criterion of excellence that this should be so. An empty bowel can be achieved by:
1. A combination of oral cathartics and repeated high colonic lavages (the composition of which is irrelevant).
2. Antegrade lavage by the use of either:
   a. constant infusion by a nasogastric tube of up to 12 l of saline over 3 hours, or
   b. the oral administration of 2–3 l of 20% mannitol which attracts water into the gut and thus constitutes an endogenous whole gut irrigation.

These methods cannot work in obstructed patients which include not only those admitted as emergencies, but also patients with slowly progressive but high grade stenosis. In such circumstances it is traditional to say that resection is contraindicated, or resection may be undertaken but primary reconstruction is not to be done. Such a view may no longer prevail in that the bowel can be prepared on the operating table (see *The management of obstruction* below).

Perioperative antibiosis

Though oral antibiotics as a method of 'sterilizing' the bowel have been shown to be effective in reducing septic wound complications, they carry the risk of intestinal superinfection and are now not recommended. There is by contrast ample evidence to support the safety and efficacy of perioperative antibiosis, either systemically or by local application. Some form of such prophylaxis should be routine. My present preference is:

Gentamicin 2 mg/kg and

Metronidazole 500 mg

both given i.v. 1.5 h before operation followed by two further doses at 8-hourly intervals. In addition, at the conclusion of the operation the operative site and general peritoneal cavity is washed out with at least a litre of saline containing 1 g/l of tetracycline. Some 200 ml of the same solution are used to irrigate the superficial layers of the wound. There are many alternative techniques for chemoprophylaxis including local use only of high concentrations of, for example, cephalosporins.

Other tactical measures

In large bowel surgery these include: correction of preoperative anaemia; reversal of starvation (though not prolonged preoperative nutritional support) and avoidance of low blood pressure states which adversely affect colonic blood flow.

Operative techniques

Rather than describe each operation, the general surgical techniques appropriate to all colonic surgery will be given. From these the operations can easily be assembled to deal with any individual lesion.

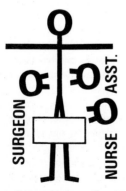

Fig. 22.29 Position of operating team for right hemicolectomy (Reproduced with permission from Dudley, 1977)

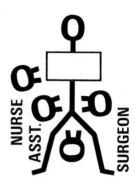

Fig. 22.30 Position of operating team for left colon procedures (Reproduced with permission from Dudley, 1977)

Position on the operating table

For surgery of the right colon the patient lies supine and the surgeon stands to the patient's right (Fig. 22.29). In all other circumstances it is strongly recommended that the lithotomy-Trendelenberg (Lloyd Davies) position is used and that the surgeon is on the patient's left (Fig. 22.30). This not only facilitates assistance—a second assistant if available can be between the legs—but allows the surgeon freedom to change his position or move from, say, a handsewn to a peranal stapled procedure, or even to resort to an abdominoperineal excision (p. 463) as necessary. The disposition of the operating team is shown in Figure 22.30 and though unfamiliar to many at first, has proven most satisfactory in use over the last 20 years.

Incision

Planned right sided surgery can be carried out through a transverse incision at the level of the umbilicus and which must cross both rectus sheaths. Such an approach may even facilitate the dissection of a bulky lesion in the proximal transverse colon from the lower border of the third part of the duodenum. However, all other surgery is best carried out through generous vertical midline incisions both because they provide access to all parts of the abdomen and allow the siting of a stoma laterally, well clear of the incision. Both types of incision are closed with a single layer of heavy (3 metric) nylon with 1 cm deep bites; the author uses interrupted sutures as a routine but a loosely inserted continuous suture is equally acceptable.

Exploration

A full laparotomy is undertaken in a systematic manner, ascertaining in particular the nodal status and the presence or absence of hepatic metastases. Synchronous or other neoplasms in the large bowel have been largely eliminated by preoperative barium enema and/or endoscopy but the colon should be carefully palpated. In circumstances where neither of the preoperative investigations has been done we now routinely insert the flexible fibreoptic sigmoidoscope into the empty residual bowel to ascertain its normality.

Principles of mobilization

The colon is, at the final stage of gastro-intestinal rotation, firmly tucked back against the posterior abdominal wall in the lumbar groove and anchored by the parietal peritoneum of the lateral paracolic gutters. It follows that the only intrinsically free parts are the transverse and sigmoid colons and these are held at the hepatic and splenic flexures and at the junction of distal sigmoid and rectum. Mobilization of the colon requires division of these parietal peritoneal attachments: in the right paracolic gutter in order to free the caecum, ascending and proximal transverse colon (Fig. 22.31); in the left paracolic gutter to mobilize the left half of the transverse and descending colon (Fig. 22.32) where, in addition, a very constant band connecting the left edge of the omentum and the lower pole of the spleen should be divided early in order to avoid tearing the splenic capsule. In the transverse colon the omentum may be detached from the colon along its bloodless union by turning it up and slitting with the scissors along Pauchet's bloodless line; or the omentum may be taken down from the epiploic vessels and incorporated in the resection as shown in Figure 22.32. In either event, it is important to lift the omentum forwards and medially from the splenic flexure so as to divide the highest part

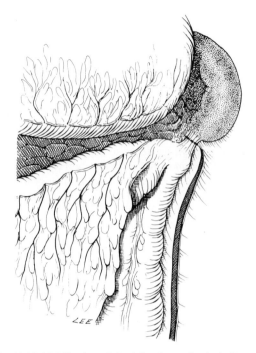

Fig. 22.32 Mobilization of the left colon and splenic flexure Note the 'adhesion' to the lower pole of the spleen

of the peritoneum lateral to and above the colon—the so-called left phrenocolic 'ligament'. Turning the dissection medially at this point allows the operator access to the left end of the transverse mesocolon below the splenic hilum and pancreatic tail. The sigmoid colon and hence the upper rectum are mobilized by incision of the two leaves of the sigmoid mesentery (Fig. 22.33A & B). On the left (A) the common iliac vessels and ureter are found with the gonadal vessels laterally; on the right the dissection begins over the front of the bifurcation (B) and may have been preceded by flush ligation of the inferior mesenteric artery (see below). The distal sigmoid and upper rectum are freed by extending the two sigmoid mesenteric cuts downward and anteriorly across the floor of pelvis behind the bladder in the male and uterus in the female (Fig. 22.34). The late Mr T McW Miller, a colleague of Eric Farquharson's, pointed out that this U shaped incision is best made early in the procedure before the anatomy is distorted.

Once any or all of these incisions in the parietal peritoneum are made—and this should be done by insinuating the blades of the scissors under the peritoneum and raising the layer so that the cut is made under direct vision—the dissection takes place in the *fascia propria*. This is a dense meshwork of connective tissue in which the retroperitoneal structures are embedded; it must be formally entered and opened up. In particular, sweeping the fascia propria away from the

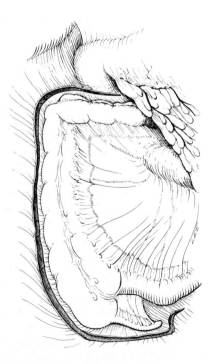

Fig. 22.31 Mobilization of the right colon

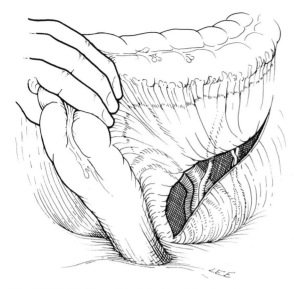

Fig. 22.33A Division of the left side of the sigmoid mesentery

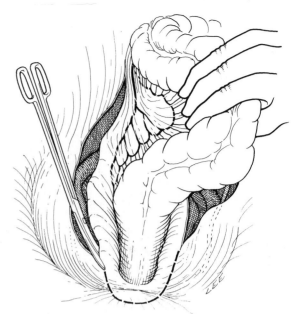

Fig. 22.34 The peritoneal mobilization required to free the rectosigmoid

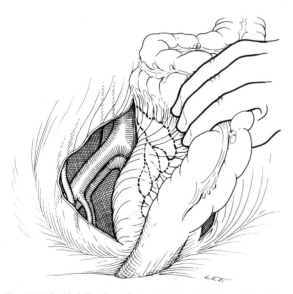

Fig. 22.33B Mobilization of the sigmoid colon from the right

posterior aspect of the mesentery of ascending and descending colons makes sure the gonadal vessels and, more medially, the ureter are displaced on to the posterior abdominal wall. In the case of the ureter such dissection should proceed as required downwards over the iliac vessels and brim of the pelvis so that the ureter is displaced laterally and the mesocolon medially.

Vascular mobilization

The cancer operations of right hemicolectomy, transverse colectomy, left hemicolectomy and sigmoid resection are based upon the above peritoneal mobilizations

and the division of the vascular supply of the segment at its root so that a fan shaped area of mesentery and its contained lymph nodes can be removed in one piece. Wide mesenteric resection is regarded by most as essential. In the classical approach to resection the peritoneal mobilization is done first, traction is applied to the colon so freed, in order that the vascular pedicle can be drawn into view and divided. Some years ago Turnbull, at the Cleveland Clinic, suggested that such a way of proceeding by handling the tumour, invited the detachment and embolization of tumour cells to the liver. He recommended a 'no touch' technique in which vascular and mesenteric division was undertaken first, so isolating the tumour. Though the figures he adduced to support this approach do not stand up to rigorous analysis, the technique is rational, elegant and the present writer's preference. It has the additional advantage that it permits clear delineation of a line of good vascularity in the rare circumstances where the marginal artery and vein are incomplete. In addition, in tumours where it is possible to get beyond the growth before mobilization is begun, the possibility of intraluminal spread by detachment can be guarded against by tying a tape tightly around the bowel 4 cm proximal and distal to the lesion.

Whether the mobilization is done lateromedially or mediolaterally the vessels should be divided as close to their root as is possible. Though the anatomy is moderately constant, no assumption can be made and each vessel is dissected and formally displayed.

For *right hemicolectomy* the middle colic/ileocolic trunk

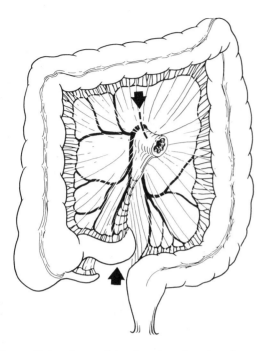

Fig. 22.35 Arteries supplying the colon—branches of superior and inferior mesenteric. Arrows show initiation of right mediolateral colonic mobilization

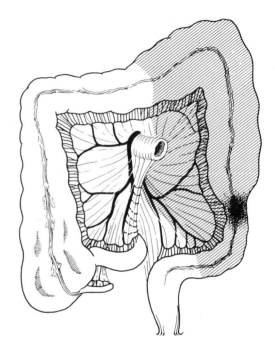

Fig. 22.36 Early ligation of the inferior mesenteric trunk delineates the bowel which must be resected in left colectomy

is identified to the right of the fourth part of the duodenum (Fig. 22.35), a procedure that can be made easier by dividing the peritoneum below the terminal ileum (lower arrow Fig. 22.35) and insinuating the finger upwards behind the ileocolic mesentery. For transverse colectomy the middle colic trunk alone is ligated in the same position. For any tumour at or beyond the splenic flexure it is best, if an adequate node dissection is to be achieved, to make a flush ligation of the inferior mesenteric trunk and to remove bowel as indicated in the shaded area of Figure 22.36. As long as the marginal supply is satisfactory the splenic flexure is mobilized (see above) for more distal tumours rather than resected. To dissect the inferior mesenteric vessels the fourth part of the duodenum is mobilized by dividing the peritoneum which flows from its lower border on to the anterior face of the infrarenal aorta (Fig. 22.37). This exposes the artery on the left antero-lateral face of the aorta with the vein more in the mesenteric substance laterally. When both have been ligated and divided the distal ligatures may be left uncut to provide traction against which the division of the mesenteric leaves laterally is undertaken and the peritoneal mobilization on the right side of the sigmoid mesentery (see Fig. 22.33B) carried down the front of the aorta and over the pelvic brim and sacral promontory in front of the *left* common iliac vein.

We have now completely described colonic mobiliz-

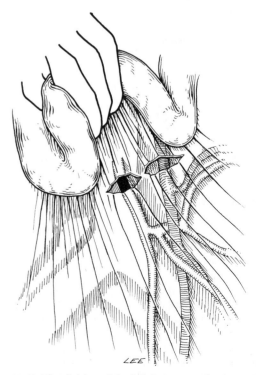

Fig. 22.37 The division of the inferior mesenteric artery and vein

ation with the exception of the two ends. Proximally, the medially-turning branch of the ileocolic artery runs along the upper border of the terminal ileum as a marginal vessel and is simply divided, usually preserving as much terminal ileum as possible so as to maintain the enterohepatic bile salt circulation and so prevent diarrhoea. At the distal end the situation is more complex. When restorative resection of a distal sigmoid tumour is undertaken the bowel will have been mobilized as already described. The rectosigmoid junction is next lifted out of the pelvis by: first mobilizing the whole mass of the bowel and bulky perirectal fat from behind by blunt dissection in the hollow of the sacrum; and second, by entering the plane anterior to the rectum. By these two moves the proximal rectum is brought up but remains enveloped in a fatty/vascular sheath, laterally (lateral rectal 'ligaments') and behind (the superior rectal artery and vein). The former can usually be divided freely but the latter is dissected piecemeal and sectioned between ligatures until only a relatively narrow muscular-mucosal tube of rectum remains. For sigmoid and upper to mid-rectal tumours where a restorative resection is to be done, it is strongly recommended that the splenic flexure is fully mobilized and swung down on to the pelvic brim so, when most if not all the rectum has been removed, to lie in a floppy and redundant manner in the hollow of the sacrum. Failure to do this may result in a stretched and potentially ischaemic bowel.

Restoration of continuity

Sutures. In the last decade or so it has become apparent, particularly thanks to the work of John Goligher (1984), that imperfections in colonic anastomoses are relatively common. Both clinical leaks with either general peritonitis or a faecal fistula occur in upwards of 8–10% of most series and subclinical leaks—detected by radiological contrast examination—in anything from an extra 10 to 50% depending on the site of anastomosis and the skills of the operator. Though many factors—blood supply, the quality of bowel preparation, prolonged operating time and age, for example—have been implicated, it remains fundamental that a technically satisfactory anastomosis without tension is the key to success. Individual series with low radiological leak rates (3–5%) have been published which bear out the importance of technique.

The conventional two layer anastomosis with an inner 'all coats' continuous suture of absorbable material to make the junction haemostatic and watertight with an outer layer of interrupted nonabsorbable material to ensure serosal apposition (when contiguous serosal surfaces are present) has become established as the norm (p. 332). Yet from the days of Halsted there have existed several theoretical, experimental and practical

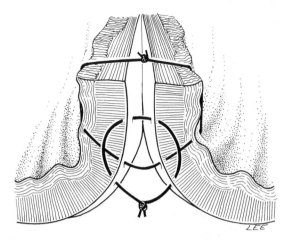

Fig. 22.38 Snagging of the two layers—a danger of conventional anastomosis

arguments against it. The theoretical and experimental is that healing takes place chiefly on the serosal aspect and that all-coats apposition does not contribute to this. Both experimental and practical observations show that continuous full thickness sutures produce linear necrosis by strangulation and that the best clinical results with handsewn anastomoses have been those which did not use a two layer technique but relied simply on an outer interrupted coaptation. An additional factor is that two layer anastomosis may be associated with snagging between the two sutures—inner and outer—(Fig. 22.38) which makes necrosis between the sutures wellnigh inevitable.

These problems suggest that a one layer reconstruction is the ideal. Non absorbable, relatively non irritant material—braided nylon or monofilament polypropylene (marginally more difficult to handle) are the sutures of choice and an extramucosal but otherwise full thickness suture exploits the strength of the submucosa but allows mucosa to regenerate across the suture line.

The bowel is carefully prepared so that there is no extraneous fat such as appendices epiploicae and there is a 5 mm naked margin at the mesenteric border; as a consequence every stitch is precisely inserted through bowel wall. Stay sutures are next placed (Fig. 22.39) so that gentle tension permits unequal lumens to be brought into opposition. If the terminal ileum is the proximal opening then an oblique division is essential to avoid a major discrepancy between ileum and colon. Next, sutures are placed precisely with 1–1.5 mm bites through all layers except the mucosa. With a fully serosa-covered mobile bowel the knots are placed externally (Fig. 22.40) but there need be little hesitation in tying towards the lumen if this is more convenient. All sutures are best placed on each aspect before any is tied. The end result is a 'butt-ended' extramucosal apposition

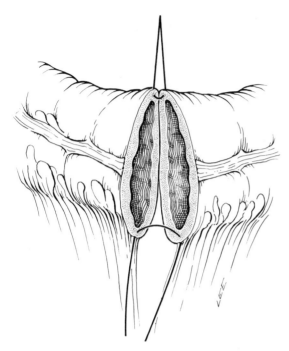

Fig. 22.39 Stay sutures placed for single layer anastomosis

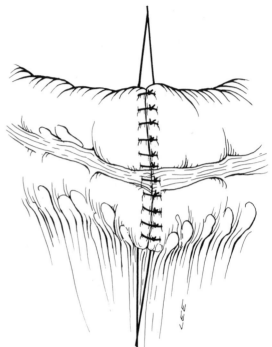

Fig. 22.41

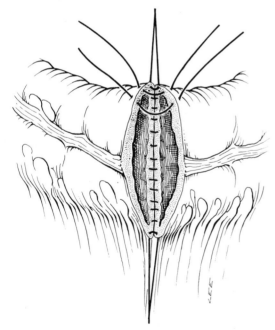

Fig. 22.40 Principles of single layer extramucosal anastomosis

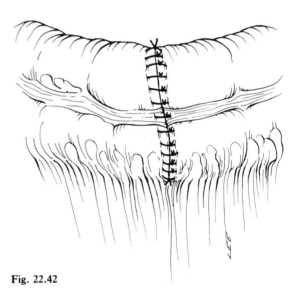

Fig. 22.42

Figs. 22.41 & 22.42 The anastomosis completed

(Fig. 22.41). The stay sutures are finally tied and any mesenteric defect closed (Fig. 22.42).

For those who still feel more comfortable—albeit without any evidence—with a two layer anastomosis, an inner layer of continuous 3/0 polyglycolic acid (Dexon or Vicryl) is gently inserted either after the posterior all coats row or, if the anastomosis can be turned round to expose either face, before the outer layer is done.

Stapling. Since the dawn of modern surgical time, surgeons have sought alternative, more precise techniques of co-apting tissues, particularly hollow tubes. The initial devices everted tissue edges but more

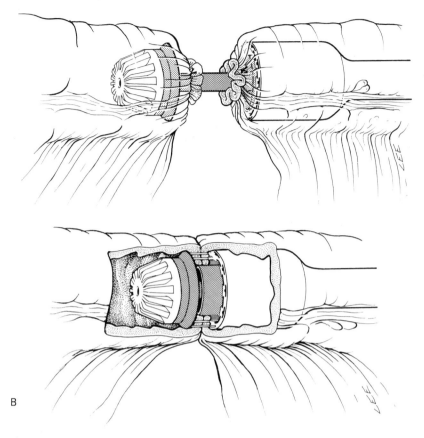

Figs. 22.43 The principles of a stapled anastomosis

recently inverting techniques which closely approach tried and established hand sutured methods have been introduced. Numerous rechargeable or disposable devices are available, all working on the principle of bringing the two ends of bowel together over an 'anvil' and then inserting staples through the full thickness of the bowel wall, while at the same time cutting a central core with a circular knife (Fig. 22.43A, B). The result is a full thickness but single layer interrupted anastomosis either with a row or a staggered double row of staples. The anastomosis heals as does a single layer suture procedure but there may be delay in mucosal apposition.

Stapling devices do not provide an easy alternative to hand suturing for the beginner. They are precision instruments which exact the same need for care in the preparation of the bowel and precise insertion of the purse string (Fig. 22.44). A fine sense of tissue apposition is needed before the device is fired though recently new aids are becoming available to assess tissue thickness (Fig. 22.45). There is no doubt that stapling can achieve a sound anastomosis. Its exact role in colonic surgery is yet to be defined, though many surgeons currently regard it as the appropriate technique for a low

sigmoid tumour which after adequate distal resection requires anastomosis of the descending colon or splenic flexure below the peritoneal reflexion. The device is inserted from below and purse string applied to proximal and distal bowel, tightened and the instrument fired. It can then be withdrawn per anum. For details of technical problems and practical advice the reader is referred to the recent publications (see p. 456).

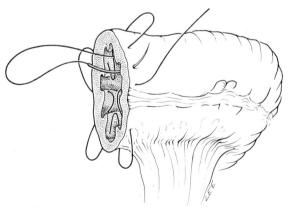

Fig. 22.44 The preferred purse string for a stapled anastomosis. Very small bites should be taken

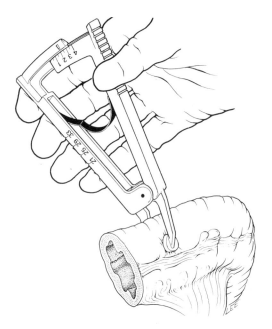

Fig. 22.45 Method of assessment of tissue thickness

The obstructed case

Left sided tumours in particular tend to narrow the bowel lumen; the patient presents as an emergency with acute colonic obstruction or with subacute obstruction so that there is banked up faeces and gas behind a narrow lumen. The one situation merges into the other.

In acute or acute-on-chronic obstruction the danger lies in progressive caecal dilatation with the development of a gangrenous patch and ultimate rupture. A profound degree of gaseous distension of the colon and/or right iliac fossa tenderness are the only indications for really urgent surgery. Otherwise most patients can be tided over a day or two for more leisurely assessment and an operation at a more convenient time. Nevertheless, it is unusual before operation to be able to empty the colon proximal to the lesion to the high standard now deemed mandatory for definitive colonic surgery.

The conventional answer to this situation has been to establish a proximal defunctioning colostomy (Fig. 22.46A) and then after a variable interval to resect the tumour, either eliminating the colostomy (Fig. 22.46B) or leaving it for closure at a later stage. The disadvantages of this safe approach are logistic and humanitarian: the long expenditure of hospital time and resources; and the inconvenience of a temporary colostomy. Some patients do not reach the second or third stage because of complications or progression of their disease.

The alternatives are three. Immediate resection with an end colostomy followed by second stage reconstruction (Fig. 22.47); as a variant on this immediate resec-

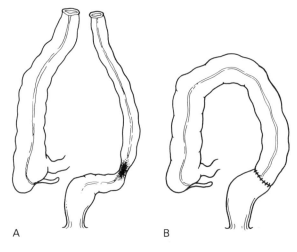

Figs. 22.46 Conventional management of the obstructed case

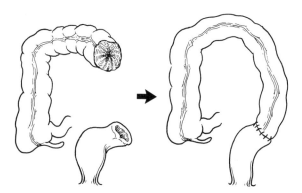

Fig. 22.47 Immediate resection and mucous fistula followed by reconstruction

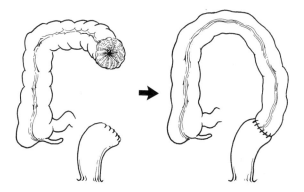

Fig. 22.48 Hartmann's resection followed by reconstruction

tion, end colostomy and closure of the distal stump (Hartmann's procedure) again followed by later reconstruction (Fig. 22.48); an immediate resection and primary anastomosis. The first two are safe procedures when the bowel is unprepared. The last has great attraction in terms of short hospital stay, particularly if there are circumstances which make the patient's life expectancy short (e.g. a locally advanced tumour or hepatic metastases).

Laparotomy in obstruction

The major cause of colonic distension is gas which contrasts with the usually liquid content of small bowel. It follows that fine needle aspiration of the colon will deflate the bowel and permit safer and easier exploration. This is achieved by attaching a 21 SWG needle to a suitable adaptor and so to the suction line. The moment the abdomen is opened and distended transverse colon presents, the needle is inserted obliquely through a taenia (Fig. 22.49). Firm pressure is exerted in the flanks to drive the air up into the transverse colon. Within a few moments a tense, friable and awkward colon is collapsed and exploration and subsequent action much facilitated. The following situations are encountered:

Caecal gangrene

The presence of this potentially lethal complication rests on the competence of the ileocaecal valve. Thus the ileum is of normal diameter. Consequently, if the tumour is right sided, right hemicolectomy and primary anastomosis can be done. In a left sided tumour there are three options: an extended right hemicolectomy and primary anastomosis; the same with a terminal ileostomy and mucous fistula; or exteriorization of the gangrenous patch as a caecostomy. Circumstance and experience dictate the most appropriate choice, but it cannot be too strongly emphasized that the only appropriate caecostomy is one which brings the caecal wall to the surface. After laparotomy, decompression and assessment, a small *muscle cutting* incision is made in the right iliac fossa, the caecum brought to the surface and healthy bowel wall beyond the gangrenous patch stitched with carefully placed nonabsorbable seromuscular sutures to the parietal peritoneum. The patch is next excised and a submucosa to subcutaneous tissue junction fashioned (see below). Though the result may appear somewhat untidy, it is usually possible to apply a stoma bag and control the effluent quite satisfactorily. Tube caecostomies do not work and should not be done.

Caecal devitalization not present

In the absence of caecal gangrene but the presence of obstruction and a loaded bowel, a right or proximal left sided tumour may still be subjected to primary resection. The alternatives already discussed are appropriate to more distal lesions.

It remains only to consider in more detail the possibility of primary anastomosis. The contraindications have always been the loaded, unprepared bowel. Some years ago Muir proposed that this might be emptied by retrograde lavage. We have now modified his technique to combine it with the desirable features of preoperative whole gut irrigation. The procedure is illustrated in Figure 22.50. The tumour is mobilized in the usual

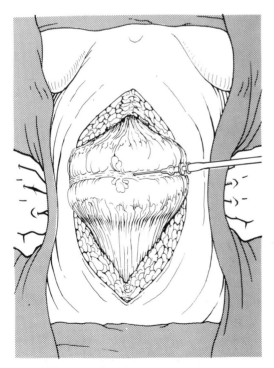

Fig. 22.49 Technique for colonic decompression in obstruction

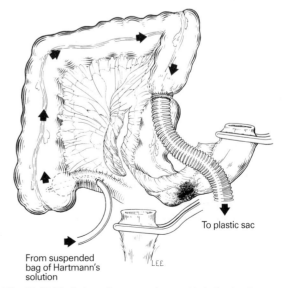

From suspended bag of Hartmann's solution

To plastic sac

Fig. 22.50 Technique for antegrade on table irrigation in obstruction

manner. The bowel is intubated proximal to the tumour but distal to the proposed site of resection with semirigid corrugated tubing and a wide bore Foley catheter is inserted into the caecum via a small ileotomy. Antegrade irrigation is now undertaken with warm Hartmann's solution, breaking up faecal masses by gentle finger pressure. Irrigation is continued until the effluent is clear. The bowel is then amputated at the site of election. It is our experience that though distended before on table irrigation, it will now have come down to normal size and is suitable for primary anastomosis either by suture or staples. The ileal catheter can be removed or preferably left to permit an antegrade radiological study of the colocolonic suture line on the 6th to 8th day.

Temporary stomata

Indications for these in colonic surgery have already been discussed and the technique of caecostomy described.

Transverse colostomy is made on the right side and if possible the hepatic flexure is mobilized so that there is not a redundant proximal loop which can subsequently prolapse. The usual circumstance is when a laparotomy incision has already been made. Then the temptation to make a large hole for the colostomy should be resisted, as should the urge to bring it out through the same incision. A two finger vertical or transverse opening suffices and avoids the problems of prolapse, paracolostomy hernia and infection. The cut is taken directly through all layers in the abdominal wall, haemostasis attained and the size of the opening tested by passing the fingers through it. A convenient 6 cm length of transverse colon is stripped of greater omentum and drawn out through the wound either with a Babcock's forceps or by passing a loop of soft rubber tubing around it (Fig. 22.51). The bowel is best attached to the parietal peritoneum internally by four sutures of synthetic absorbable (Vicryl: Dexon) and to the anterior rectus sheath or external oblique aponeurosis similarly. A rod may now be inserted beneath the loop but is rarely necessary and the old fashioned glass rod and looped rubber tubing is obsolete. More complex devices with subcutaneous plastic inserts are described but in the writer's opinion are quite unnecessary. A soft clamp is applied across the loop so as to prevent any inflammable gasses from being ignited by the diathermy and the colostomy opened forthwith by a longitudinal incision made with that device. Its margins are stitched to the parieties. In all instances this is best done with an absorbable suture passing extramucosally in the bowel and subcuticularly in the skin (Fig. 22.52) (the illustration demonstrates the suture on an end colostomy as might be required after resection without anastomosis).

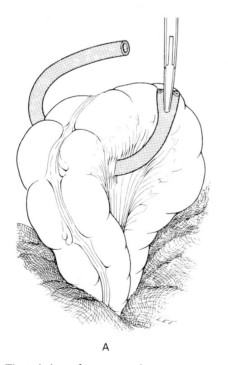

A

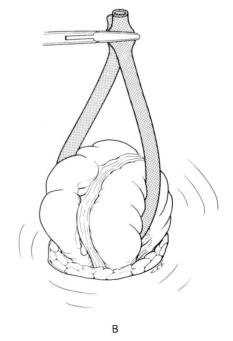

B

Fig. 22.51 The technique of transverse colostomy

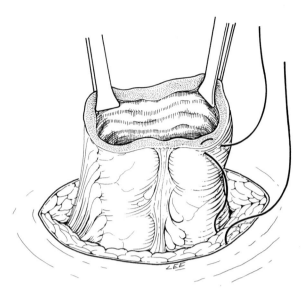

Fig. 22.52 Suturing the colon to the skin

OPERATIONS FOR OTHER INTESTINAL CONDITIONS

Meckel's diverticulum

In 2% of the population the segment of vitello intestinal duct joining the ileum persists on the antimesenteric border as a diverticulum within 80 cm of the caecum. The diverticulum may contain ectopic gastric and pancreatic tissue and gastric secretion may cause peptic ulceration in adjacent ileal mucosa. The clinical problems associated with a diverticulum are gastro-intestinal haemorrhage, obstruction, acute abdominal pain and intussusception. Rarely the entire vitello intestinal duct may persist, establishing a fistula between the ileum and the umbilicus. Preoperative diagnosis of Meckel's diverticulum is difficult but in some patients labelled technetium pertechnate will demonstrate ectopic gastric mucosa. When discovered incidentally at laparotomy, it should probably be removed because of the high risk of associated pathology (Hutchinson, 1981).

Haemorrhage is most common in children under 3 years of age and it is usually accompanied by abdominal pain. Blood loss is variable; it may be insidious, resulting in iron deficiency anaemia, or sufficiently severe to cause melaena or the loss of fresh blood from the rectum.

Intestinal obstruction may result from volvulus of ileum round a persistent band that runs from the apex of the diverticulum to the umbilicus or internal herniation of small bowel caught under an adhesion between the diverticulum and adjacent mesentery. Obstruction

may occur in any age group including the neonate.

Acute inflammation of the diverticulum may resemble appendicitis. For this reason the distal ileum must be carefully inspected when a normal appendix is found at laparotomy. On rare occasions the diverticulum will be found at the apex of an *intussusception* and is presumed to have been the cause.

Operation

A choice must be made between either diverticulectomy or excision of that segment of ileum carrying the diverticulum followed by end-to-end anastomosis. The latter is favoured when the bowel adjacent to the diverticulum is oedematous or the site of a peptic ulcer, or when the ileum is of small calibre so as to ensure complete excision of ectopic tissue.

A *diverticulectomy* is performed by applying light occlusion clamps to the ileum after ligation of any supplying vessels. The diverticulum is then excised at its base and the bowel wall closed transversely in two layers (Fig. 22.53).

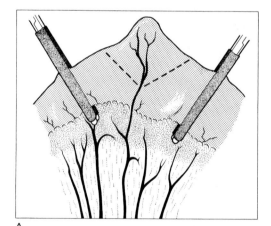

A

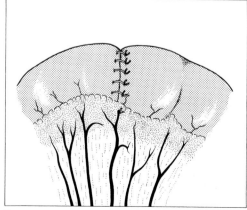

B

Figs. 22.53 Excision of Meckel's diverticulum

Ileocaecal tuberculosis

The belief is now widely held that most cases described in the past as examples of ileocaecal tuberculosis were, in fact, forms of nonspecific ileocolitis. Anand (1956), however, has shown that in India at least the tubercle bacillus can undoubtedly be responsible, since he succeeded in culturing it from a large proportion of the lesions encountered. The treatment of choice is a right hemicolectomy, with a simple short-circuiting operation as a second-best alternative. If a tuberculous lesion is suspected before operation, the patient should be prepared by a course of specific chemotherapy. When the diagnosis is made or confirmed at operation, such therapy should, of course, be employed postoperatively.

Crohn's disease

Regional ileitis

The acute form of this disease is indistinguishable clinically from acute appendicitis, and as a rule it is diagnosed only when the abdomen has been opened for the purpose of appendicectomy. The terminal segment of the ileum is found to be deeply congested, sodden and oedematous. Its mesentery is usually much thickened and contains enlarged glands. As a rule the inflammatory process ceases abruptly at the ileocaecal junction, but the caecum also may be involved (*ileocolitis*). Abscess formation may result from perforation of the gut, or from the breaking down of mesenteric glands, but owing to adhesions general peritonitis is rare.

There is now general agreement that, when the disease in its acute phase is encountered at operation for appendicectomy, no definitive procedure should be undertaken, but the appendix may be removed unless the caecum is heavily involved. About 80% of cases resolve spontaneously (Williams, 1972; Brooke, 1973).

The chronic form of regional ileitis may be a legacy of one or more acute attacks, but not infrequently it appears to develop insidiously. It is characterized by mucosal ulceration, accompanied by great thickening of the submucous and muscular layers owing to granulomatous and fibro-fatty infiltration. Similar changes are found in the mesentery, and the caecum may frequently be involved in continuity with the ileum. The clinical features are those of sub-acute or intermittent obstruction, resulting from reduction in the lumen of the gut, and also diarrhoea of intermittent type. An abdominal mass may be present or the patient is noted to have suffered weight loss, malabsorption and anaemia. Fistula formation may occur—either to the exterior, or to adjacent organs such as the bladder.

Operation. Since Crohn's disease affects the whole gastro-intestinal tract, surgical excision can not effect a cure (Irving, 1981; Kyle, 1982). When the ileum alone is involved the affected part may be excised and bowel continuity restored. When the caecum is involved, a right-sided hemicolectomy may be carried out, all the diseased ileum being removed. Bypass procedures, such as ileotransverse anastomosis, are less satisfactory than resection but may be required if the bowel mass is fixed. There is always a tendency, whatever operation is employed, for the disease to recur at a higher level in the small bowel, so that further operation may be required at a later date.

Surgery is not undertaken lightly if a large part of the small bowel is involved, but it may be necessitated by complications such as obstruction or fistula formation, or if the patient's condition is deteriorating. Massive resection of nearly the whole of the small bowel may be required as a life-saving measure, and it is remarkable how, after such resections, a good state of nutrition may be maintained.

Regional ileocolitis

It is now well recognized that the changes described as being characteristic of regional ileitis (Crohn's disease) can affect the colon as well. When they involve the terminal ileum and the caecum together as a confluent lesion, the term *granulomatous ileocolitis* can be applied. The condition may give rise to a painful mass in the right iliac fossa, associated with a variety of intestinal symptoms.

At operation the findings suggest an inflammatory lesion, rather than a carcinoma. The caecum is grossly thickened, shrunken and often elevated as the result of retroperitoneal fibrosis, the changes tailing-off gradually into the ascending colon; the terminal part of the ileum is likely to be thickened and rigid, and may enter the elevated caecum in an almost vertical line.

The treatment of choice is by right-sided hemicolectomy. If, however, fixation of the mass is present to a degree which materially increases the risks of resection, and if malignancy can be excluded, a simple short-circuiting operation may be preferred.

Segmental colitis (Crohn's disease of the colon)

This designation is most applicable to cases where long or short segments of colon become involved by a *granulomatous* process, the changes of which are again very similar to those of Crohn's disease as it affects the ileum or the ileocaecum. There is gross thickening and rigidity of all coats of the bowel, leading to a 'hosepipe' appearance, with uniform constriction of the lumen although obstructive symptoms develop less frequently than in the small bowel. It tends to involve the right side of the colon in the first instance, and to spread distally towards the rectum, so that the whole colon may eventually become affected. It is frequently associated with peri-anal suppuration (Lockhart-Mummery, 1972) or the disease may be confined to the rectum and anal canal (Williams, 1979).

The treatment is by excisional surgery, and this should not be delayed, since in the early stages limited resections may suffice. If surgery is withheld until the distal colon has become extensively involved, either a three-quarter colectomy with ileorectal anastomosis, or a total proctocolectomy with permanent ileostomy, will be required. In the case of localized lesions, a further reason for advising early surgical intervention lies in the fact that it may be difficult or impossible to exclude carcinoma.

The *ulcerative* type of segmental colitis is considered in the section on ulcerative colitis (p. 451).

Ulcerative colitis

The last three decades have seen great advances in the understanding of this disabling condition. Medical treatment alone is of value when the disease is mild or is localized to the rectum but it is now generally accepted that in a severe or established case the changes in the colon are irreversible; thus there is little prospect of cure unless the diseased bowel is removed. Apart from the general ill-health caused by the mere presence of the infected and ulcerated bowel, operation may be required for stricture or fistula formation, or because of the risk of carcinoma (Johnson, 1983; Schofield, 1981). This is a very real risk in patients with a history of 10 years or more and in those with extensive colitis, particularly if it developed during childhood. Such patients, who do not otherwise agree to surgical treatment, should have sigmoidoscopic biopsy twice each year and barium examination or colonoscopy every 2 years.

Steroid therapy, while it has not proved to be curative, is of undoubted value in tiding the patient over an acute phase of the disease, and in improving his general condition to an extent where radical surgery becomes a relatively safe procedure. Such treatment should be combined with replacement of protein, which may have been lost in large quantities from the ulcerated bowel. It should be noted that some surgeons have blamed steroid therapy for causing extreme friability and even perforation of bowel, and advise against its use for longer than 2 weeks if no remission occurs. This suspicion is not confirmed by Goligher (1984).

The present aim of surgery in ulcerative colitis is to remove all the affected bowel before cancer can develop. The choice lies between complete excision of both colon and rectum (*total proctocolectomy*), and excision of the colon alone, continuity of the alimentary tract being re-established by *ileorectal anastomosis*. Ileostomy alone has no place in the treatment of ulcerative colitis—even as a first-stage procedure in the acute or fulminating case, for it leaves the diseased bowel *in situ* as a toxic reservoir. Furthermore, when performed on an ill patient,

it carries a very high mortality. It is now agreed that in such cases the patient is better served, and is more likely to be made fit for radical surgery, by intensive medical treatment, which should include steroid therapy and protein replacement.

Total proctocolectomy with permanent ileostomy

This is the procedure favoured by the majority of surgeons at present (Parks, 1980). The rectum is usually involved by the disease to a greater or lesser extent, and, if the changes which have occurred are accepted as being irreversible, its normal function (including that of reservoir action) cannot be restored. If the colon alone is removed, and the rectum retained, the patient may continue to suffer from intractable diarrhoea, and may therefore be little benefited by the operation; furthermore, there is the risk of cancer. With total proctocolectomy, the patient must necessarily accept a permanent ileostomy, but this may be regarded as the price which he has to pay for health, if not for life itself. An ileostomy is not as grievous an affliction as might be supposed. With modern appliances to collect the ileostomy efflux, the majority of patients adapt themselves well to their disability and lead a normal life, the ileostomy interfering little with business, social or sporting activities.

The operation of total proctocolectomy was formerly carried out in two or more stages, and this may still be the best procedure in seriously ill patients, leaving the rectum to be excised at a later date. Multiple operations, however, increase the risk of complications, and introduce additional hazards from wound infection. It is now generally agreed that, in selected cases and after suitable preparation, a one-stage operation is the procedure of choice.

The technique of total proctocolectomy starts with excision of the rectum, usually by the synchronous combined method, but, because of the nonmalignant nature of the condition, a more restricted dissection is permissible; there is therefore less risk of interference with sexual function. The entire colon is then mobilized and its mesentery divided. The site of the ileal division is selected by careful attention to its blood supply, usually about 15 cm from the ileocaecal junction. The proximal cut-end, occluded by a clamp, is laid aside while the ileostomy site is prepared. The ileostomy is then fashioned.

Technique of ileostomy. Ileostomy is most commonly performed as part of a one-stage proctocolectomy. It may be performed also in combination with a 'three-quarter colectomy' (Fig. 22.54), as the first stage of a total proctocolectomy. Great care should be taken with the siting and fashioning of the ileostomy stoma, since it is largely upon the accurate fitting of a collecting appliance that the success of the operation will depend.

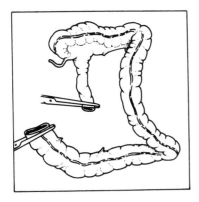

Fig. 22.54 Subtotal colectomy as performed for ulcerative colitis or for diffuse polyposis of the colon

Following excision of the colon, the proximal end of ileum is brought to the surface in the right iliac fossa, through a small incision separate from the main wound, and at such a distance from it that the skin for 3–4 cm around will be free from scarring. The ideal position for the stoma is equidistant from the umbilicus, the anterior superior spine and the fold of the groin but it is advisable to confirm this in each patient by applying an ileostomy bag prior to operation, adjusting the site if necessary. A *circular* incision, 2 cm in diameter, is recommended, since it reduces the likelihood of subsequent stenosis from contraction of the scar. For the same reason, the external oblique aponeurosis, or the anterior rectus sheath, is incised in cruciate manner. The ileum, held by a clamp, is brought out so that at least 5 cm projects above the skin surface (Fig. 22.55), and is anchored by a stitch between its mesentery and the external oblique aponeurosis. The peritoneal space to the right of the emerging ileum (*the para-ileal gutter*)is closed by a running suture, which unites the cut edge of the

mesentery to the peritoneum of the floor and lateral side of the right iliac fossa. Alternatively, the terminal ileum is passed along an *extraperitoneal tunnel* fashioned by the surgeon's fingers, starting within the abdomen (Goligher, 198?). Finally, the terminal half of the projecting ileum is turned back as a cuff, and the cut edge of mucosa is joined to the skin margin with 6 to 8 interrupted sutures (Fig. 22.55). As a result the ileostomy stoma takes the form of a completely epithelialised nipple or 'bud'; this fits accurately into the aperture of an ileostomy bag, so that the risk of leakage is diminished and skin damage is avoided.

The ideal of a reservoir or continent ileostomy can only be achieved at the risk of complications and the need for several operations. The operation for its construction is thus restricted to those centres where continuing experience in its use can be obtained (Kock, 1976, 1981).

Ileostomy in children. The indications for emergency ileostomy and the method of construction in infants is described on p. 432. The procedure for a permanent spout ileostomy in an older child with ulcerative colitis is the same as that used in the adult.

Complications of ileostomy. Difficulties of control are common, especially in less intelligent patients who cannot manage to fit their appliances correctly. They may well result, however, from an unsatisfactory ileostomy. Ideally, the efflux should drop directly into the bag, without contaminating the flange or disturbing its adherence to the skin—hence the necessity of an ileostomy which projects outwards from the skin surface. An ileostomy which is flush with the skin is very difficult to control. Excoriation of the skin around the stoma should not occur unless the ileostomy or the appliance are unsatisfactory. Relief may be obtained by changing to an alternative bag or one which is retained in position by a belt. Intestinal obstruction may occur from failure to close the para-ileal gutter, in which a loop of small bowel may become entrapped. Stenosis of the stoma, which may develop insidiously, is a frequent cause of ileostomy dysfunction. Because of the degree of obstruction produced, normal evacuation ceases, and is replaced by the continual passage of wind and watery fluid; associated with this there may be vomiting, colicky pains and abdominal distension.

Remaking of the ileostomy should at once be undertaken in cases where, because of stenosis or difficulties of control, the existing stoma is in any way unsatisfactory. It is usually best to perform laparotomy, and to bring out the ileum anew, through a new circular incision in a part of the abdominal wall where the surrounding skin is smooth and healthy.

Colectomy with ileorectal anastomosis

This operation is, of course, designed to preserve nor-

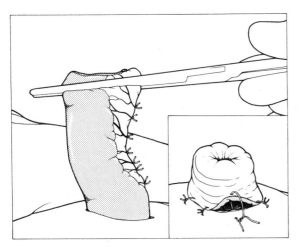

Fig. 22.55 Technique of ileostomy

mal sphincter control. Its use is restricted to cases where the rectum is either healthy or shows minimal involvement by the disease—and such cases are in a considerable minority. Unfortunately, the good results obtained by Aylett (1970, 1981) have not been repeated by other authors. Not more than half the patients seem to obtain a good result; about a quarter eventually require an excision of the rectum, with permanent ileostomy, because of the continuation of their diarrhoea. A not inconsiderable proportion of the patients develop carcinoma in the rectal stump; because of this risk, they must be kept under careful supervision, and regular sigmoidoscopy carried out.

The technique of ileorectal anastomosis is very similar to that described for restorative resection of the rectum except that it is often possible to preserve the whole or the greater part of the rectum, and that it is the ileum, instead of the left colon, that is brought down for the anastomosis. If there appears to be a risk of the anastomosis breaking down, with possibly disastrous results, it may be protected by a loop ileostomy.

Restorative proctocolectomy with ileal reservoir may be carried out on selected patients in specialized centres (Parks, 1978). A pouch of ileum is constructed from adjacent loops in a similar fashion to the Kock ileostomy and ileo-anal anastomosis is carried out (Cranley, 1983).

Segmental type of ulcerative colitis

This type of ulcerative colitis is stated to occur in about 10% of cases (Watkinson, 1960). The changes closely resemble those of the classical or generalized form of the disease, except that they tend to involve the proximal part of the colon (and possibly also the ileum), the distal colon and the rectum being spared in the first instance; the complications are similar, and there is the same tendency towards malignant change. The distinction between this condition and Crohn's colitis may not always be a clearcut one.

Treatment. As in the case of generalized ulcerative colitis, medical treatment has not a great deal to offer, and excisional surgery provides the best prospect of cure. This should not be too long delayed, since in the early stages of the disease limited resections may suffice. If surgery is withheld until the greater part of the colon is involved, radical excision must be carried out on the lines described for the generalized form of the disease.

Diverticulitis

This degenerative and inflammatory condition affects mainly the left side of the colon, the changes being maximal in the pelvic loop. It can give rise to symptoms and signs closely resembling those of carcinoma, and both radiological and sigmoidoscopic examination may fail to establish the diagnosis. On this account surgical intervention may be required.

At operation, often the first sign to be noted is an obvious increase in the mesenteric and pericolic fat of the pelvic colon. The bowel wall itself is thickened (from fibro-fatty infiltration), and, according to the extent of *peridiverticulitis*, the changes vary from slight induration to an enormous mass involving the greater part of the pelvic colon. Even at operation the condition may be difficult to distinguish from carcinoma. Owing to surrounding reaction, a peridiverticular mass is usually more fixed than a carcinoma, except when this is very far advanced. It involves a longer segment of gut, tapering-off gradually; it tends therefore to be sausage-like or spindle-shaped, and its limits are less clearly defined.

Treatment

With increasing experience of bowel resection for carcinoma, treatment of diverticulitis has become much more radical, and resection can often be considered—especially if, as is frequently the case, malignancy cannot be excluded. A one-stage operation is now generally favoured (Charnock, 1977) although symptoms are most often relieved in patients undergoing surgery for complicated diverticular disease. Resection is carried out on lines very similar to those described for carcinoma of the colon, except that, when malignancy can be excluded, clearance of the glandular fields need not be so extensive. In the presence of obstruction or other complications, the initial treatment should usually be by a defunctioning transverse colostomy; resection may be undertaken at a later date after the bowel has been suitably prepared. The incidence of complications is greater when surgery is undertaken in stages (Underwood, 1984).

Not infrequently certain *complications* of diverticulitis, such as intestinal obstruction, paracolic abscess, perforation or fistula formation, bring the patient to urgent surgery.

Intestinal obstruction is dealt with as described on pages 420 & 433, usually by a defunctioning transverse colostomy.

Paracolic abscess. This usually comes to lie in contact with the abdominal wall, and may present as a visible swelling. In such cases, it can be evacuated safely through a small stab incision placed over its most prominent part.

Perforation is a most serious complication, since its very occurrence indicates that the infection is not walled-off by adhesions, and a degree of generalized peritonitis therefore results. The condition is likely to be diagnosed preoperatively as an appendix peritonitis. At operation, this diagnosis seems at first to be confirmed by the putrid smell of bowel organisms in the peritoneal cavity, but the appendix is found to be normal; further search may then disclose either a peridiverticular mass in relation to the pelvic colon, or merely some congestion and thickening of its wall, together with an increase in pericolic fat. The perforation itself may be difficult to find (Bolt, 1973), but if identified should be closed by a plug of omentum or any other available tissue. When the bowel shows gross disease, the best treatment is to perform a defunctioning transverse colostomy, and to wash out the peritoneal cavity with 1% tetracycline solution (see p. 333) and to combine this with drainage. Frequently, however, the changes in the colon may be comparatively slight, and the diagnosis of a perforated diverticulitis may be reached only because no other cause can be found to account for the presence of malodorous pus in the pelvis. Such cases may be treated by peritoneal lavage and drainage alone, for the perforation will often heal spontaneously, and there may be no recurrence. This is specially to be remembered in the case of the aged, in whom perforated diverticulitis is comparatively common. Such patients are unlikely to come to resection, and should not therefore be burdened with a colostomy, unless this is necessary as a life-saving measure, or because a faecal fistula develops and persists after the drainage operation.

Colovesical fistula is a not uncommon complication of diverticulitis of the colon. Its treatment is discussed on page 589.

Haemorrhage occurs more often from diverticulosis than from diverticulitis and does not usually require operation—mainly because of the difficulty in locating the site of bleeding and hence the segment of colon which should be removed.

Polypoid disease of the colon

Two main types of polypoid tumours are recognized—*adenomata* (90%) and *villous papillomata* (10%). An adenoma may produce bleeding, prolapse or discharge. A villous papilloma more commonly results in profuse mucus discharge which may sometimes result in electrolyte depletion—particularly of potassium. Although essentially benign, each type has a risk of developing invasive cancer. This risk is much greater in the villous group whereas, the larger the adenoma, the greater the risk. All polypi should therefore be treated energetically, with the possible exception of an adenoma less than 1 cm in diameter. If they occur singly or in small numbers they are likely to be of the acquired type rather than inherited.

Single or isolated polypi

These are found most commonly in the pelvic colon or rectum (80%), but any part of the large bowel may be involved. If they can be viewed through a sigmoidoscope they may be destroyed by fulguration or removed by diathermy snare. In clinics where a colonoscope is available, endoscopic removal of polypi can be extended to

all parts of the colon should the necessary expertise be available (Williams, 1974). Sessile polyps *above the peritoneal reflection* should not be treated in this way for fear of perforating the gut. Should such polypi be identified or suspected they should be subjected to colonoscopic inspection before a decision is made on treatment. A much less satisfactory alternative is laparotomy with systematic examination of the whole colon by palpation. If a polypus (detected as a mass, which does not appear to be faecal, within the bowel lumen) is milked by the fingers in either direction, the serous surface may show a dimple at the site of attachment (unless this lies on the mesenteric border), and a local excision of the tumour-bearing area can then be carried out. If the attachment of the polypus cannot be clearly identified it is better to open the bowel through an incision placed in a longitudinal band near the antimesenteric border, and to perform an excision. Larger polypi, or multiple ones confined to one segment of bowel, are treated by partial colectomy. After the removal of polypi whether locally or by partial colectomy, review of the patient should include 6-monthly sigmoidoscopy and yearly colonoscopy (Fairbairn, 1981) or double contrast barium enema. This is necessary for several years after operation—if not for the rest of the patient's life.

Diffuse (inherited) polyposis

In this rare condition (which, although inherited, does not appear usually until late childhood or early adult life) the development of carcinoma is practically certain, unless surgical treatment is carried out in the early and benign stage. Since the greater part of the colon is likely to be involved with many hundreds of polyps, a very radical excision is required, and is justified by the almost hopeless prognosis if the disease is not completely eradicated. Sub-total colectomy with anastomosis of the ileum to the rectum (Fig. 22.56) has been carried out in those cases (the minority) where the rectum is not seriously involved, and where it is thought that existing polypi or others developing in this part can be controlled by fulguration; the results, however, have been most discouraging since recurrences and malignant change almost invariably take place. The treatment of choice is a *total proctocolectomy with permanent ileostomy*.

Hirschsprung's disease

Pathology

In this condition the autonomic innervation of the distal bowel is abnormal and causes partial or complete obstruction to the normal passage of faeces. It is thought that the normal craniocaudal migration of neuroblasts in the bowel wall is incomplete; hence the abnormal segment always includes the distal rectum and extends proximally for a variable distance. The classical histo-

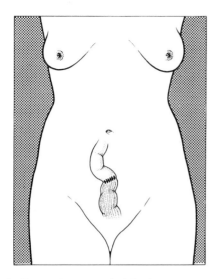

Fig. 22.56 Ileorectal anastomosis following subtotal colectomy

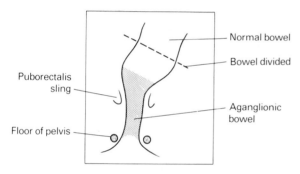

Normal bowel

Bowel divided

Puborectalis sling

Aganglionic bowel

Floor of pelvis

Fig. 22.57 Hirschsprung's disease—longitudinal section of rectum showing the abnormality and level of bowel division

logical feature of the condition is the absence of ganglion cells from Auerbach's and Meissner's plexus but, in addition, the nerve fibres in the myenteric plexus are increased both in number and size. The normal bowel proximal to the aganglionic segment is secondarily hypertrophied and dilated whilst the abnormal segment is relatively narrowed (Fig. 22.57). Hirschsprung's disease is arbitrarily divided into short or long segment according to whether the aganglionic segment is confined to the rectum and sigmoid colon or extends proximal to the junction between the descending and sigmoid colon.

Clinical presentation
The incidence of the condition is one in 5000 births and the male to female ratio is 4 to 1. Babies with the condition are of normal birth weight and, with the possible exception of Down's syndrome, associated anomalies are rare. The clinical presentation varies from complete or

partial obstruction in the new born to chronic constipation in the older child. Necrotising enterocolitis is a dangerous complication of the condition, presenting paradoxically with diarrhoea and, unless recognized and treated appropriately, it may be fatal. The diagnosis of Hirschsprung's disease is confirmed by demonstrating the histological features on either a punch rectal biopsy of mucosa and sub-mucosa taken 2 cm above the dentate line or a longitudinal full thickness strip, 0.5 by 1.5 cm long taken from the posterior rectal wall. A barium enema may outline a 'coned' segment between the dilated normal segment of bowel and the relatively narrowed distal aganglionic segment. Rectal manometry can be used to demonstrate the absence of normal relaxation of the internal sphincter in response to rectal dilatation.

Operation
The surgical management of the condition depends on the clinical presentation. In a baby with obstruction it may be possible to clear the bowel content by gentle rectal irrigation with warm saline; alternatively an emergency colostomy should be performed. In the absence of acute obstruction the diagnosis can first be established by investigation and a colostomy then fashioned prior to the definitive operation. According to preference, either a right transverse colostomy is made or a left iliac colostomy using the distal part of normal bowel. The definitive operation follows after an interval of 3 to 6 months. When the condition presents in the newborn, it is customary to delay the procedure until the baby is 9 months or reaches 10 kg in weight.

Excision of the aganglionic segment in Hirschsprung's disease presents two problems, first the technical difficulties of a low anastomosis close to the anorectal junction, and second the risk of damage to the pelvic splanchnic nerves. The different techniques designed to overcome these problems are important and have relevance to sphincter conserving operations in adult surgery. In Swenson's operation (1948), the bowel is divided above the aganglionic segment and the two ends oversewn (Fig. 22.58). The aganglionic bowel is then drawn inside-out through to the perineum by forceps introduced through the anal canal. Normal bowel is pulled down through the invaginated abnormal segment and anastomosed 2 cm from the mucocutaneous junction. The anastomosis is then pushed back through the anal opening to its normal position. In Duhamel's operation (1960) normal bowel is once again divided (Fig. 22.59). A tunnel is made from the pelvic floor posterior and lateral to the rectum within the puborectalis sling and opened into the posterior wall of the upper part of the anal canal. Normal bowel is drawn down through the tunnel so that it lies alongside the rectum. The adjacent walls of rectum and small bowel are sta-

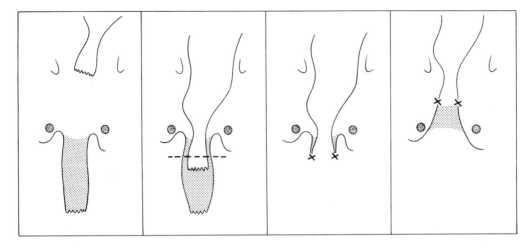

Fig. 22.58 Swenson's pull-through operation

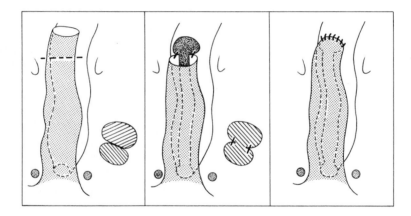

Fig. 22.59 Duhamel's operation

pled and divided longitudinally so as to form a common cavity. Rectal sensation is thus preserved within the cavity and the normal bowel provides peristalsis. In Soave's endorectal pull through (1960), the muscle wall of the rectum is left in situ. This is achieved by circular myotomy of the pelvic floor so that the distal dissection to the anal canal can be performed in a sub-mucosal plane. Normal bowel is drawn down through the muscle cuff and left with a stump projecting beyond the anal opening. After an interval, during which the normal bowel becomes fixed in position by adhesions, the stump can be excised. In a modification of this procedure, which eliminates the need for a second operation, normal bowel is anastomosed to anal mucosa. This can be achieved using a technique similar to that used by Swen-son but only the rectal mucosa is pulled inside-out.

An alternative to rectosigmoidectomy is to reduce the outlet resistance of the aganglionic segment by anorectal myectomy. This was first used for older children with ultra short segment Hirschsprung's disease. More recently myectomy has been used in combination with anterior resection in children with more extensive aganglionosis (Orr & Scobie, 1979). Anorectal myectomy is performed with the child in the lithotomy position. An incision is made at the mucocutaneous junction on the posterior wall of the anal canal and a plane dissected between mucosa and underlying muscle. The strip of muscle, 0.5 to 1.0 cm in width, including the internal sphincter is excised along the length of the aganglionic segment.

REFERENCES

Anand S S 1956 Hypertrophic ileo-caecal tuberculosis in India with a record fifty hemicolectomies. Annals of the Royal College of Surgeons of England 19: 205

Aylett S O 1970 Delayed ileo-rectal anastomosis in the surgery of ulcerative colitis. British Journal of Surgery 57: 812

Aylett S O 1981 Total colectomy and ileorectal anastomosis. Journal of the Royal College of Surgeons of Edinburgh 26: 86

Baker J W 1959 A long jejunostomy tube for decompressing intestinal obstruction. Surgery Gynaecology and Obstetrics 109: 519

Bland Sutton J 1889 Imperforate ileum. American Journal of Medical Science 98: 457

Bolt D E 1973 Diverticular disease of the large intestine. Annals of the Royal College of Surgeons of England 53: 237

Brooke B N 1973 The relation of aetiology to treatment in non specific inflammatory disease of the gut. Journal of the Royal College of Surgeons of Edinburgh 18: 144

Charnock F M L, Rennie J R, Wellwood J M, Todd I P 1977 Results of colectomy for diverticular disease of the colon. British Journal of Surgery 64: 417

Childs W A, Phillips R B 1960 Experience with intestinal plication and a proposed modification. Annals of Surgery 152: 258

Cranley B 1983 The Kock reservoir ileostomy: a review of its development, problems and role in modern surgical practice. British Journal of Surgery 70: 94

Dudley H A F 1977 Operative dispositions and ergonomics. In: Rob C, Smith R Operative surgery—General principles, breast and hernia. Butterworths, Sevenoaks, p 17

Duhamel B 1960 A new operation for the treatment of Hirschsprung's disease. Archives of Diseases of Childhood 35: 38

El-Katib Y 1973 Volvulus of the caecum: caecopexy by polyvinyl alcohol sponge. British Journal of Surgery 60: 475

Fairbairn R D, Dean A C B, McNair T J 1981 Colonoscopy in the detection of polyps of the large bowel. Journal of the Royal College of Surgeons of Edinburgh 26: 150

Goligher J C 1984 Surgery of the anus, rectum and colon, 5th edn. Bailliere Tindall, London, p 497, 828

Hutchinson G H, Randall P E 1981 Meckel's diverticulum. Journal of the Royal College of Surgeons of Edinburgh 26: 86

Irving M 1981 Inflammatory bowel disease 1: with special reference to the small bowel. In: Lumley J S P, Craven J L (eds) Surgical review 2 Pitman Medical, London, p 134

Johnson W R, McDermott F T, Hughes E S R, Pihl E A, Milne B J, Price A B 1983 Carcinoma of the colon and rectum in inflammatory disease of the intestine. Surgery Gynaecology and Obstetrics 156: 193

Kock N G 1976 Present status of the continent ileostomy; surgical revision of the malfunctioning ileostomy. Diseases of the Colon and Rectum 19: 200

Kock N G, Myrvold H E, Nilsson L O, Philipson B M 1981 Continent ileostomy. An account of 314 patients. Acta Chirurgica Scandinavica 147: 67

Kyle J 1982 Inflammatory bowel disease—surgery for Crohn's disease. British Journal of Hospital Medicine 27: 482

Lockhart-Mummery H E 1972 Crohn's disease of the large bowel. British Journal of Surgery 59: 823

Louw J H, Barnard C N 1955 Congenital intestinal atresia. Observations on its origin. Lancet 2: 1065

Munro A, Jones P F 1978 Operative intubation in the treatment of complicated small bowel obstruction. British Journal of Surgery 65: 123

Nanni G, Garbini A, Luchetti P, Nanni G, Ronconi P, Castagneto M 1982 Ogilvie's syndrome (Acute colonic pseudo-obstruction): Review of the literature (October 1948 to March 1980) and report of four additional cases. Diseases of the Colon and Rectum 25: 157

Neely J, Catchpole B 1971 Ileus: the restoration of alimentary-tract motility by pharmacological means. British Journal of Surgery 58: 21

Nixon H H 1955 Intestinal obstruction in the new born. Archives of Diseases of Childhood 30: 13

Noble T B 1937 Plication of small intestine as prophylaxis against adhesions. American Journal of Surgery 35: 41

Ogilvie H 1948 Large intestine colic due to sympathetic deprivation: a new clinical syndrome. British Medical Journal 2: 671

Orr J D, Scobie W G 1979 Anterior resection continued with anorectal myectomy in the treatment of Hirschsprung's disease. Journal of Paediatric Surgery 14: 58

Parks A G, Nicholls R J 1978 Proctocolectomy without ileostomy for ulcerative colitis. British Medical Journal 2: 85

Parks A G, Nicholls R J, Belliveau E 1980 Proctocolectomy with ileo-reservoir and anal anastomosis. British Journal of Surgery 67: 533

Schofield P F 1981 Inflammatory bowel disease 2: with special reference to the colon In: Lumley J S P, Craven J L (eds) Surgical Review 2 Pitman Medical, London, p 157

Shatila A H, Chamberlain B E, Webb W R 1976 Current status of diagnosis and management of strangulation obstruction of the small bowel. American Journal of Surgery 132: 299

Soave F 1966 Hirschsprung's disease: Clinical evaluation and details of a personal technique. Zeitschrift fur Kinderchirurgie Suppl. 66

Swenson O, Bill A H 1948 Resection of rectum and recto-sigmoid with preservation of the sphincter for benign spastic lesions producing megacolon. Surgery 24: 212

Underwood J W, Marks C G 1984 The septic complications of sigmoid diverticular disease. British Journal of Surgery 71: 209

Watkinson G, Thompson H, Goligher J C 1960 Right-sided or segmental ulcerative colitis. British Journal of Surgery 47: 337

Welch G H, Azmy A F, Ziervogel M A 1983 The surgery of malrotation and mid gut volvulus: a nine year experience in neonates. Annals of the Royal College of Surgeons of England 65: 244

Wilkinson A W 1973 Body fluids in surgery, 4th edn. Churchill Livingstone, Edinburgh

Williams C B, Hunt R H, Loose H, Riddell R H, Sakai Y, Swarbrick E T 1974 Colonoscopy in the management of colon polyps. British Journal of Surgery 61: 673

Williams J A 1972 Surgery and the management of Crohn's disease. Clinics in Gastroenterology 1: 469

Williams N S, Dixon M F, Johnston D 1983 Re-appraisal of the 5 cm rule of distal excision for carcinoma of the rectum: a study of distal intramural spread and of patients' survival. British Journal of Surgery 70: 150

Williams N S, Macfie J, Celestin L R 1979 Anorectal Crohn's disease. British Journal of Surgery 66: 743

FURTHER READING

Colon resection
Sepsis control

Dudley H A F, Fielding L P 1980 Management of patients undergoing colorectal surgery with particular reference to sepsis. In: Karran S J (ed) Controversies in surgical sepsis, Praeger, New York

Keighley M R B, Burden D W (eds) 1979 Antimicrobial prophylaxis in surgery. Pitman Medical, London

Stewart D J, Matheson N A 1978 Peritoneal lavage in appendicular peritonitis. British Journal of Surgery 65: 54

Willis A T, Ferguson I R, Jones P H (and 14 others)1977 Metronidazole in prevention and treatment of bacteroides infections in elective colonic surgery. British Medical Journal 1: 607

Stapling devices

Goligher J C, Lee P W, Macfie J, Simpkins J C, Lintoff D J 1979 Experience with the Russian model 249 suture gun for anastomosis of the rectum. Surgery, Gynaecology and Obstetrics 148: 516

Heald R J 1980 Towards fewer colostomies—the impact of circular stapling devices on the surgery of rectal cancer in a district hospital. British Journal of Surgery 67: 198

Waxman B P 1983 Large bowel anastomoses. II The circular staplers: a review. British Journal of Surgery 70: 64

Medio-lateral dissection

Turnbull R B, Kyle K, Spratt J, Watson J 1967 Cancer of the colon: the influence of the 'no touch' isolation technique on survival rates. Annals of Surgery 166: 420

Sutured anastomoses

Irvin T T, Goligher J C 1973 Aetiology of disruption of intestinal anastomoses. British Journal of Surgery 60: 461

Matheson N A, Irving A D 1975 Single layer anastomosis after rectosigmoid excision. British Journal of Surgery 62: 239

Inflammatory bowel disease and colonoscopy

Alexander-Williams J 1976 Crohn's disease and the surgeon. In: Hadfield J, Hobsley M (eds) Current surgical practice, Vol. 1. Arnold, London, ch 14

Goligher J C 1980 Surgery of the anus, rectum and colon, 4th edn. Bailliere Tindall, London

British Journal of Hospital Medicine 1982 27: 448–487 Inflammatory bowel disease:
Ansell I D Inflammatory bowel disease and malignancy
Jewell D P Diagnosis and treatment of ulcerative colitis
Walker F C Surgery for ulcerative colitis
Chadwick V S Diagnosis and management of Crohn's disease
Kyle J Surgery for Crohn's disease

Brooke B N, Wilkinson A W 1980 Inflammatory disease of the bowel. Pitman Medical, Tunbridge Wells

Hunt R, Waye J D 1981 Colonoscopy, techniques, clinical practice and colour atlas. Chapman and Hall, London

Kyle J 1972 Crohn's disease. Heinemann, London

23

Operations on the rectum and anal canal

H. A. F. DUDLEY, J. M. S. JOHNSTONE & R. F. RINTOUL

Anatomy

The rectum

This is the direct continuation of the pelvic colon, and, when straightened out, is about 12 cm in length. It begins opposite the third piece of the sacrum, and follows the curvature of the sacrum and coccyx; it ends 2.5 cm beyond the tip of the coccyx by making an acute angle concave backwards with the anal canal.

The rectum has three lateral curvatures or *flexures*— the upper and lower being convex to the right, and the middle convex to the left. Corresponding to the flexures, *horizontal folds*, consisting of mucous and circular muscle coats, project into the lumen of the gut (Fig. 23.1). The lower third of the rectum is somewhat dilated, and is termed the *ampulla*.

Relations. The upper third of the rectum is clothed with peritoneum anteriorly and on each side; the middle third is covered only in front, while the lower third is entirely devoid of peritoneal covering because it lies below the peritoneum of the pelvic floor. The upper two-thirds is related anteriorly to the recto-vesical (or recto-uterine) pouch and to its contents (a coil of ileum or pelvic colon and the retroverted uterus that is normal in 20% of females). The lower third is related in the male to the base of the bladder, with the seminal vesicles and vasa deferentia intervening, and, below this, to the prostate; in the female it is related to the posterior vaginal wall. Posteriorly, the rectum lies first in front of the sacrum and coccyx, and then the raphe of the levatores ani, which converge on it from the side walls of the pelvis.

Blood supply (Fig. 23.2). Arteries supplying the rectum are the *superior, middle and inferior rectal*, and the *middle sacral*. The superior rectal, a single vessel formed as the continuation of the inferior mesenteric, divides into two branches, which run down the posterior wall of the rectum. The middle and inferior rectal arteries are bilateral; the middle arises from the internal iliac artery in the pelvis and the inferior is a branch of the pudendal artery in the perineum. The middle sacral is a single twig branching directly from the aorta. The veins drain partly into the portal system by the superior

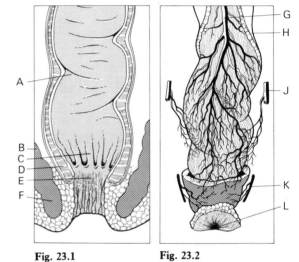

Fig. 23.1   Fig. 23.2

Fig. 23.1 Musculature and internal structure of rectum and anal canal (coronal section)
Fig. 23.2 Blood supply of rectum and anal canal (posterior view)
Annotations for Figures 23.1 and 23.2 (A) Horizontal fold; (B) Levator ani; (C) Anal columns; (D) Internal sphincter; (E) Pectinate line; (F) External sphincter; (G) Superior rectal vessels; (H) Peritoneum; (J) Middle rectal vessels; (K) Inferior rectal vessels; (L) Anus

rectal vein and partly into the systemic veins through the middle and inferior rectal and middle sacral veins. Thickened bands in the investing fascia accompany the middle rectal vessels, stretching between the rectum and the side walls of the pelvis and are termed *lateral ligaments*.

Lymph drainage. Lymph vessels of the rectum drain first to glands lying alongside the viscus and within its fascial sheath (*pararectal glands*). From the pararectal glands related to the upper two-thirds of the rectum further drainage occurs mainly to glands in the pelvic mesocolon, along the course of the superior rectal and inferior mesenteric vessels. From the lowermost pararectal glands efferents pass laterally across both surfaces of levator ani to glands alongside the internal iliac and common iliac vessels.

The anal canal

This is 4 cm in length, and passes downwards and backwards from the lower end of the rectum to the anal orifice which is defined arbitrally as the point where the anal canal begins to increase in diameter. The upper two-thirds of the canal is surrounded by the internal sphincter, a condensation of the lowermost circular fibres of the rectum. The physiological external sphincter, composed of striated muscle, is in effect the levator ani fibres as they encircle the anal canal. The important feature is the puborectalis sling—those fibres of levator which, arising from the pubis, pass backwards and around the canal just distal to the internal sphincter but fused with it. The levatores ani are inserted into the sides of the canal between the overlapping internal and external sphincters.

The mucous membrane of the anal canal is loosely attached, and in the upper part presents a number of longitudinal folds, called *anal columns*; these are joined at their lower ends by crescentic folds termed *anal valves*. The level of the valves is marked by a white wavy line—the line of Hilton or *pectinate line*. The part of the canal above this line is lined by columnar epithelium, the part below by modified stratified epithelium, which at the anal orifice takes on the character of true skin. The skin around the anal orifice contains numerous sebaceous and sweat glands.

Relations. Anteriorly the anal canal is related in the male to the apex of the prostate and to the membranous and bulbous parts of the urethra; in the female it is related to the lower third of the vagina. On each side the levator ani separates the canal from the ischiorectal fossa. Posteriorly the canal is related to the tip of the coccyx and to the anococcygeal raphe.

Blood supply is derived from descending branches of all three rectal arteries. Corresponding veins communicate with each other in a plexus (*haemorrhoidal plexus*) lying in the anal cushions which are analagous to erectile tissue and complete the closure of the anal canal.

Lymph drainage. Lymphatics from the upper part of the anal canal accompany the inferior rectal vessels across the ischiorectal fossa, and pass to internal iliac (*hypogastric*) glands. Lymphatics from the lower part of the canal and from the anal margin drain to the superficial inguinal glands on both sides.

The ischiorectal fossa is a wedge-shaped space filled with fat, lying on each side of the anal canal. Its base lies downwards at the skin surface, and its thin edge, which is directed upwards, lies along the attachment of levator ani to the fascia covering obturator internus. It is bounded medially by the levator and anal canal, and laterally by the ischium covered by obturator internus. The *internal pudendal vessels* run forward in the substance of its lateral wall; they give off the *inferior rectal vessesl*, which cross the fossa to reach the bowel.

PROCTOSCOPY AND SIGMOIDOSCOPY

For proctoscopy in the average patient, whose bowels have already moved on the day of examination, no special preparation is required. This may apply equally well to sigmoidoscopy, since small masses of solid faeces do not materially interfere with the examination. If, however, constipation has been present, an aperient should be given 1 or 2 days before the examination and only fluids are allowed until the examination has been completed. An enema may be necessary on the evening prior to sigmoidoscopy if the bowel cannot be cleared by suppositories.

A male patient may be examined in the knee-elbow position, but the left lateral position, with the buttocks over the edge of the table (see Fig. 23.3) is preferred by most patients. Unless the patient is excessively nervous, an anaesthetic is unnecessary and should be avoided, since, in the unconscious patient, there is an inescapably greater risk of damage to the bowel. Both proctoscope and sigmoidoscope should be well lubricated before use. If they are also warmed in hot water, their introduction causes less discomfort to the patient.

Proctoscopy

The proctoscope (or anal speculum) enables a visual examination to be made of the lower part of the rectum and the anal canal. With the obturator in situ, the instrument is introduced gently and with due regard to the direction of the anal canal, i.e. in a line pointing forwards towards the umbilicus. When its point is felt to have passed the resistance offered by the sphincters and to have entered the rectum, its direction is altered so that it points posteriorly towards the hollow of the sacrum, and in this line it is inserted to its fullest extent. The obturator is removed and a light is directed into the speculum. The mucous membrane of the rectum is examined, and any abnormalities such as inflammation, ulceration or new growth are noted. The speculum is now slowly withdrawn, when the internal end of the anal canal will be seen to close over it. If internal haemorrhoids are present they will project into the speculum at this stage, and their number, size and position should be noted.

If the proctoscope requires to be reinserted, it should be completely withdrawn and the obturator refitted.

Sigmoidoscopy

By the use of the rigid sigmoidoscope, which is about 30 cm in length, the whole of the rectum and a large part of the pelvic colon can be examined. The instru-

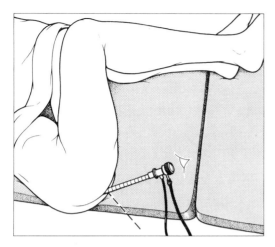

Fig. 23.3 Technique of sigmoidoscopy. The sigmoidoscope is introduced through the anal canal in the direction shown by the broken line. It is then advanced, under direct vision, around the hollow of the sacrum

ment is passed through the anal canal in a direction towards the umbilicus (Fig. 23.3). *As soon as its point is felt to have entered the rectum all further introduction must be carried out under direct vision.* The obturator is therefore withdrawn; the glass eye-piece and light-carrier are fitted, and the bellows is attached. The sigmoidoscope is now directed posteriorly (Fig. 23.3), so that it lies in the line of the rectum, and by circumduction of the instrument the rectal wall is thoroughly examined. The horizontal folds are encountered and are easily circumvented as the sigmoidoscope is passed upwards. As it follows the sacral curve its point must gradually be directed more anteriorly towards the pelvirectal junction, which often lies a little to one side, usually the left. As the bowel is sharply kinked at this level, the introduction of the instrument into the pelvic colon is the most difficult part of the operation, but, by careful manipulation always under direct vision, and by gentle inflation of the bowel, the lumen can usually be made to open out in advance of the instrument. By continuing in the same manner the sigmoidoscope can, in favourable cases, be passed up to its full extent, so that the greater part of the pelvic colon can be examined.

During the introduction of the sigmoidoscope, and again during its withdrawal, the condition of the bowel wall and the presence of any tumour formation are noted. The colour of a tumour is almost invariably a brighter red than that of the surrounding mucosa. The proliferative type of carcinoma has an irregular nodular surface which is friable and bleeds easily; in a growth of the ulcerative type the appearance of the raised everted margin is characteristic. A simple tumour is usually pedunculated; if it is smooth and lobulated it is probably an adenoma. Simple growths of sessile type

may be difficult to distinguish from carcinoma, and in such cases a portion should be removed for biopsy, by means of special long forceps introduced through the sigmoidoscope. Various inflammatory conditions have their own characteristic appearance which usually involve the entire bowel under inspection whereas a tumour tends to be localized. Thus, if *no normal mucosa* can be seen, the condition is probably inflammatory.

When a tumour is encountered, and if it does not obstruct the passage of the instrument, it is an advantage to examine the bowel above, in order to ascertain the extent of the growth, and to ensure that a second tumour at a higher level is not missed.

Flexible fibreoptic sigmoidoscope
Greater skill is required for the use of this expensive instrument but it is superior to barium enema in detecting growths in the sigmoid colon (Vellacott, 1982).

WOUNDS AND INJURIES

Injuries of the anal canal and rectum are commonly caused by the patient sitting or falling astride on some sharp object such as a spiked railing. Penetration of the rectal wall, or even of the mucosa alone, is liable to give rise to a severe pelvic cellulitis, to which both streptococci and anaerobic organisms contribute. Where the peritoneum has been entered peritonitis may result.

It is important to note that such injuries may occur in the absence of any external damage. A slender object may pass into the anal canal or rectum before penetrating its wall, and rupture of the rectum may occur simply as the result of a blow on the anal region. In such cases of suspected internal damage the bowel should be carefully examined under an anaesthetic. The sphincter is stretched, and the examination is carried out both by the finger and by the aid of a proctoscope.

Lacerations of the anal canal are best left open and packed with gauze. If a penetrating wound of the rectum is found, it is rarely possible or desirable to repair it by primary suture. It is wiser to be content with providing free drainage through the anal canal. This is done by leaving a corrugated drain or a wick of petroleum gauze in contact with the damaged area, and by bringing it out through the anus. Drainage may be further improved by division of the sphincter in the midline posteriorly. If the damage to the rectum is severe it may be advisable to provide complete rest to the part by means of a temporary colostomy. Broad spectrum antibiotics are given in full dosage.

In all cases a careful watch must be kept for the development of pelvic cellulitis, and a secondary operation for drainage of the perirectal tissues may be required.

In wounds of the buttocks and perineal region the

wound should be enlarged if necessary to permit of careful exploration, in order that penetration to the rectum does not pass undetected. If the rectal wall is seen to be torn no attempt should be made to suture it, but free drainage of the peri-rectal tissues is provided, by enlarging the wound as necessary and by the insertion of a gauze pack. If the tear is a large one the advisability of a colostomy should be considered. At the same time an opportunity is taken to examine for, and to exclude, any intraperitoneal injury.

Intraperitoneal injuries. Penetration to the peritoneal cavity may be suspected, either at the initial clinical examination, or after the condition of the rectum has been more fully investigated in the operating theatre. In either case an immediate laparotomy should be carried out *as the first step in operative treatment.* If an intraperitoneal rupture is found it is repaired in two layers, and a drain is left in the pelvis. Unless the rupture is a comparatively small one a pelvic colostomy should be performed.

Gunshot wounds of the rectum are particularly serious, owing to their inaccessibility, the frequency of damage to other structures, and especially because of the risks of a virulent infection of the retroperitoneal tissues. Early exploration of the wound is therefore most essential; devitalized tissues are excised, and free posterior drainage of the perirectal space is provided through a curved incision in front of the coccyx. In nearly all cases a colostomy should be performed.

BENIGN TUMOURS AND STRICTURES OF THE RECTUM

Benign tumours of the rectum and of the colon
These have the same pathology and frequently co-exist. Their great importance lies in the tendency which they show towards malignant change. The classification of such tumours (polypoid disease) of the colon has already been described (p. 452).

Tumours of the lower half of the rectum can be detected easily by the examining finger, and, if pedunculated, may be delivered through the anus. Tumours at a higher level in the rectum are diagnosed by sigmoidoscopy. If the tumour is sessile and of large size, or shows any evidence of induration, biopsy should be performed in view of the serious suspicion of malignancy. When an apparently benign tumour is found in the rectum, careful search by sigmoidoscopy and barium enema, or by colonoscopy, should be made for another lesion, especially a carcinoma, at a higher level, for the association of such lesions is a very common one.

Benign tumours in the lower rectum
If the tumour is pedunculated and can be delivered at

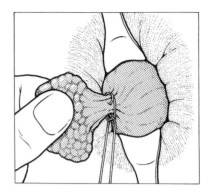

Fig. 23.4 Method of removing a pedunculated rectal polyp which can be delivered at the anus

the anus, its removal presents no difficulty (Fig. 23.4). Sessile (papillomatous) tumours, when small, may be excised also per anum. When the rectal wall is lax, the part bearing the tumour may be drawn through the anus; the affected area of mucosa is then excised with the diathermy knife, and the defect is closed by suture. Otherwise the sphincter must be stretched and subsequently held open by retractors to allow access. Sometimes, when the tumour is small, an artificial pedicle may be created by traction, and this can be dealt with by a transfixing ligature, prior to division.

Benign tumours in the upper rectum
These may be dealt with, through a short operating sigmoidoscope, by fulguration with a diathermy electrode, or by removal with the diathermy snare. Such methods should not be used when the tumour is above the peritoneal reflection (unless it is pedunculated), because of the risk of perforating the bowel; in such cases it is safer to approach it by laparotomy.

In view of the inescapable risks of malignant change—either in further tumours developing or in undetected tumours already present, systematic re-examination of the patient is essential for many years after operation—if not for the duration of his life. For the first two years after operation sigmoidoscopy and double contrast barium enema or colonoscopy are advised every 6 to 12 months; in the absence of recurrence the interval between examinations may be progressively lengthened, but the patient is told to report at once if bleeding recurs.

Large tumours and those suspected of malignancy
If the tumour is too large for local excision, or if there is evidence that it has undergone malignant change, one of the operations described for carcinoma of the rectum must be undertaken. If the tumour is situated in the upper part of the rectum, and *if tumours elsewhere in the*

bowel have been excluded, a sphincter-conserving resection is ideal.

Benign strictures of the rectum

These result most commonly from injuries, from chronic inflammatory conditions such as proctitis or Crohn's disease, or from infections such as lymphogranuloma inguinale. Occasionally they may be due to excessive fibrosis following irradiation treatment of carcinoma of the cervix uteri. When the stricture is not too far advanced, and is sufficiently low for the finger to reach above it, regular dilatation with bougies may suffice in treatment. Low-level ring strictures, such as may result from postoperative scarring, may be treated first by *internal proctotomy*, i.e. division of the constriction from within with a probe-pointed knife. A finger passed upwards through the stricture is used as a guide, and several shallow incisions are made in the posterior half of the circumference of the constricting ring. Dilatation with bougies is immediately carried out; this is repeated daily for several days, and thereafter at longer intervals.

Localized strictures which cannot be dilated satisfactorily may, provided no active inflammation is present, be treated by one of the methods of sphincter-conserving resection described for carcinoma or by using the circular stapling device alone (Ross, 1980).

Tubular strictures and those associated with severe inflammatory reaction can be treated only by colostomy. When the inflammation has subsided it may be possible to restore evacuation through normal channels, or to perform a sphincter-conserving resection. More often, however, the colostomy will be permanent. In some cases the inflammatory condition is progressive and causes chronic invalidism from continued pain, fever and rectal discharge; radical excision of the rectum should then be advocated.

PROLAPSE OF THE RECTUM

In the less severe varieties of this condition—*partial prolapse*, the everted tissue consists of mucosa alone which is both lax and redundant. A mild degree of partial prolapse occurs in association with prolapsing haemorrhoids and effective treatment of the haemorrhoids is usually curative. *Complete prolapse*, in which the entire thickness of the rectal wall is extruded, is essentially a sliding hernia of the anterior rectal wall through the anal canal. If the protusion is longer that 5 cm, it is probable that a peritoneal sac prolonged downwards from the rectovesical or recto-uterine pouch lies between the two layers of rectal wall forming the anterior part of the protrusion (Fig. 23.5).

Minor degrees of partial prolapse, especially when

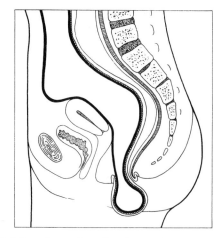

Fig. 23.5 Drawing to show the relation of the peritoneum to a complete prolapse of the rectum

they occur in children or in old people, are treated by conservative measures including the avoidance of constipation and straining at stool.

Injection therapy
Suitable for cases of partial prolapse. Its objective is to secure fixation of the lax mucosa to the underlying muscular coat. This may be achieved by the injection of 5% phenol in almond oil into the submucous layer, as in the 'high injection' treatment of haemorrhoids (p. 469). Through a proctoscope, five or six injections, each of 2 ml are given at the first treatment; these are spaced around the circumference of the bowel at as high a level as posssible. The results are at best uncertain.

Radical operations

The difficulty of cure in cases of complete prolapse is evidenced by the large number of operations which have been described.

Amputation of the prolapse from below
This operation, first described by Mikulicz and practised by Miles under the name of *rectosigmoidectomy*, is no longer popular in UK. It involves excision of as much lax bowel as can be withdrawn through the anal canal followed by reanastomosis, reattachment of peritoneum and suture of levator ani muscles anteriorly. The results are disappointing in that about half the patients so treated suffer either from a recurrence of the prolapse or from anal incontinence, this latter complication resulting probably from the fact that the short anorectal stump is inadequate for sensory purposes.

Anterior resection of the rectum
As performed for carcinoma, this has been advocated as an effective method of treating rectal prolapse, since the

bowel usually becomes firmly adherent to the sacrum at the level of the anastomosis. This, however, is a formidable operation for a nonmalignant condition.

Repair of the defect from above, without resection of bowel

This is designed to deal directly with what are believed to be the essential factors in its causation—the abnormally deep rectovesical or recto-uterine pouch which is a constant feature in all cases, and the lax or atonic condition of the pelvic floor. In Goligher's (1958) modification of Graham's operation, there are three essential steps—thorough mobilization of the rectum, suture of the puborectales muscles in front of the rectum in order to provide support for the bowel, and excision or exclusion of the abnormally deep peritoneal pouch. Mobilization of the rectum is carried out as for anterior resection, except that the inferior mesenteric pedicle is not divided, and that the dissection is kept close to the bowel wall. When the bowel has been mobilized down to the level of the anorectal ring, and the lateral ligaments divided, it is drawn upwards and forwards, whereupon the puborectalis sling can be defined by scissors dissection close to the gut. The rectum is now pushed firmly backwards, and the puborectales muscles, lying laterally, are drawn together in front of it by three or four sutures of unabsorbable material. When, because of tension, it is impracticable to do this, the puborectales muscles may be approximated behind the rectum, thus accentuating the normal angulation at the anorectal junction. Finally, the peritoneal flaps are sutured to the rectum at a high level, so that the deep pouch in the pelvis is eliminated. Goligher has reported good results from this operation in curing the prolapse, but admits that varying degrees of incontinence may persist.

Implantation of plastic sponge material (Fig. 23.6)

This operation, devised by Wells in 1959, is simpler than any hitherto described, and is successful in a high proportion of cases (Morgan, 1972; Anderson, 1981). The technique is relatively straightforward, and the operation is well tolerated by elderly patients. The rectum is mobilized as for anterior resection, and, with its vascular pedicle intact, is lifted forwards from the hollow of the sacrum. A sheet of polyvinyl alcohol sponge, 3 mm thick and 8 to 10 cm square, is attached to the fascia in front of the sacrum, from the promontory down to the 3rd or 4th segment inserting all sutures into the presacral fascia before passing them through the sponge. The rectum is then drawn firmly upwards; the sheet of sponge is folded around it, to cover all except the anterior one-quarter or one-fifth of its circumference, and is secured by three or four stitches uniting its lateral margins to the bowel wall. Finally the peritoneal flaps are sutured in front of the bowel or against its sides, so

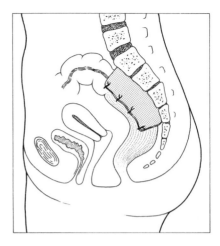

Fig. 23.6 Wells's operation for rectal prolapse

that the sponge is completely buried. The effect of the plastic sponge is to provoke a vigorous fibrotic response, so that the rectum becomes anchored against the sacral hollow by firm adhesions. In most cases, this effectively cures the prolapse, and although incontinence cannot always be abolished it is usually much improved. Marlex mesh is an alternative material which may be used (Keighley, 1983). A method of inserting a mersilene mesh sheet through a perineal approach posterior to the anus has recently been devised (Wyatt, 1981) for those patients who are particularly frail.

The Thiersch operation

Of limited use in the palliation of rectal prolapse. A ring of silver wire or nylon suture, or a band of silicone rubber (Jackaman, 1980) is inserted within the fibres of the weakened external sphincter to deter the prolapse of rectum through the anus. It may be inserted under local anaesthesia and is tied sufficiently tightly to admit one finger.

CARCINOMA OF THE RECTUM

The principles of surgery for rectal carcinoma are similar to those for colonic carcinoma, as described on page 435. The approach to operation will, to some extent, be influenced by the findings at sigmoidoscopy and the degree of fixity of the growth as assessed by rectal examination.

Biopsy

It is essential that histological confirmation of tumour is obtained since the finding of an anaplastic carcinoma, with poor prognosis, will influence the choice of operation. Although it may be technically possible to restore bowel continuity, this is not usually advisable for a tumour of Dukes' Stage C (often anaplastic) where local massive recurrence of tumour would lead to recurrence of bowel symptoms. The presence of liver metastases, detected by ultrasound or CAT scan and confirmed at laparotomy, is an indication for conservative surgery and the avoidance of a colostomy in a patient whose life expectancy is limited.

Choice of operation

In 60 to 70% of patients suffering from carcinoma of the rectum, radical removal of the tumour can be carried out with a reasonable prospect of cure. In such cases the operation is designed to remove the growth in its entirety, along with any regional extensions or metastases. If continuity cannot be re-established, a permanent colostomy must be performed.

Three main types of operation are carried out at the present time for carcinoma of the rectum:
1. Abdominoperineal excision is the operation of choice for all tumours in the lower half of the rectum. Classically it implies the removal of the entire anorectum together with the lower pelvic colon, and the establishment of a permanent colostomy. Where facilities exist, it is usually carried out by the *synchronous combined method* (Fig. 23.7).
2. Conservative resection with preservation of the anal sphincters is the operation of choice for all early growths involving the upper rectum or pelvirectal junction (*rectosigmoid*). The advent of the EEA (end to end anastomosis) stapling gun allows for restoration of bowel continuity after excision of virtually the whole rectum, although it may not always be advisable that this is attempted.
3. Abdominal excision alone (Hartmann's operation) is a valuable procedure in old or debilitated patients, in whom abdominoperineal dissection is too formidable, or in whom, because of general or local conditions, restorative resection is impracticable. It does not obviate a permanent colostomy, but, the anal canal being left in situ, the patient is spared the additional strain and recovery entailed by a perineal dissection.

It is generally agreed that no final choice of operation can be made until the situation and extent of the growth have been investigated by laparotomy. This is necessary in order to confirm that the growth itself is removable, and that there are no metastases in other organs or inaccessible lymph glands, such as might invalidate the operation. Furthermore, it is seldom possible before laparotomy to determine the type of operation best suited to the individual case.

Preoperative treatment

Preparation along the lines described for bowel preparation is essential (p. 436), and the policy of perioperative antibiosis (p. 437) also applies.

Abdominoperineal excision

Restorative resection or complete removal of the rectum?
Until relatively recently and with a few notable exceptions, tumours of the extraperitoneal rectum have been managed by total removal of that organ and permanent colostomy. As indicated on page 435, the pathological and physiological basis for this irreversible ablative procedure is not now regarded as well found and, provided the rectum and its enveloping fascia are carefully dissected en bloc, and provided also the operator is confident about reconstruction, tumours as low as 5–6 cm from the dentate line can be treated by restorative resection. The exception must be those in which there is a high risk of early recurrence—extensive pararectal infiltration and clinically involved nodes. Here palliation is better achieved by abdominoperineal resection. In addition, there will always remain some tumours in which adequate surgical clearance cannot be achieved without removal of the tissues and associated lymph nodes as shown in Figure 23.8.

Abdominal dissection
The standard operation in the United Kingdom is done synchronously by two teams with the patient in the Lloyd Davis position and a urethral catheter in situ. (Fig. 23.9) The colostomy position is determined the day before, preferably with the co-operation of a stoma therapist. The abdominal mobilization proceeds as described (p. 439) to separate the rectum, down to the levator ani and puborectalis, from its surrounding structures — behind in the hollow of the sacrum, laterally in relation to the rectal ligaments and in front. Anteriorly in the male this involves careful blunt dissection in the retrovesical and retroprostatic space, displacing the seminal vesicles forward. The whole fibrofatty mass en-

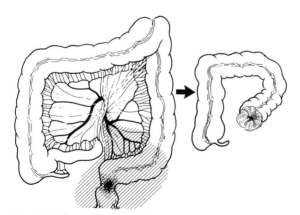
Fig. 23.7 The extent of resection in abdominoperineal excision of the rectum

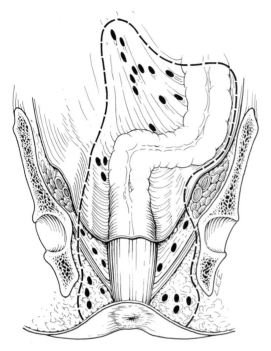

Fig. 23.8 Drawing to show the tissues removed with a tumour in the distal rectum. Wide removal of the pelvic mesocolon with its contained glands can be carried out

circling the rectum is thus freed and the rest of the dissection must be completed from below, though the abdominal operator can and should assist the perineal worker by identifying the planes.

Perineal dissection

The anus is closed with a subcutaneous purse string— 0 nylon on a half circle needle is suitable (Fig. 23.10). A transverse incision is made in the perineum half way between vaginal orifice and anus in the female or just posterior to the perineal raphe in the male. From the centre of this, encircling incisions are carried back around the anus at a distance from it of about 2 cm to meet at the tip of the coccyx. The transverse incision is deepened to expose the transverse perinei muscle and its posterior fibres split, allowing access to the retro- prostatic space in the male (Fig. 23.11). The urethral catheter is a useful guide at this point and should be felt only distantly through the soft tissues surrounding the urethral bulb. As this dissection is carried upwards the fibres of puborectalis are encountered to either side as they pass anteroposteriorly. At this point the encircling incisions are deepened through the fat of the ischiorectal fossa. Posteriorly the coccyx is encountered with, on either side, the firm fibrous origin of the levator ani. Either the coccyx is detached from the sacrum by cut-

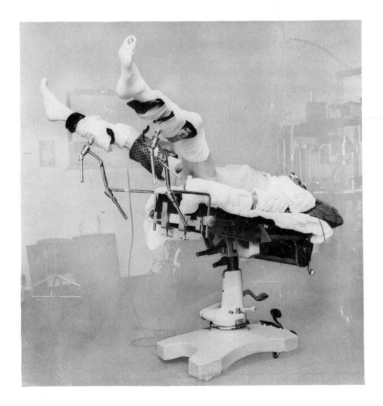

Fig. 23.9 Position of the patient for synchronous combined abdomino perineal excision of the rectum

ting through the sacroccocygeal joint with a knife or, as the writer prefers, the levator insertion is cut in the midline at the coccygeal tip. Either manoeuvre permits the blades of a scissors to be inserted into the gap in the midline which is so produced and the levators to be divided forwards close to the pelvic wall (Fig. 23.12). Entry is thus made into the retrorectal space where the abdominal operator is encountered.

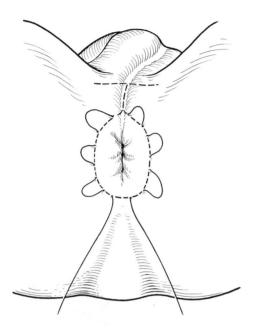

Fig. 23.10 The anal purse string

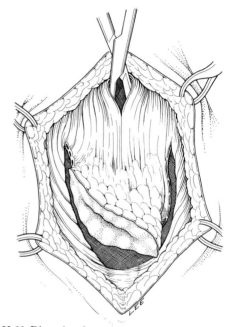

Fig. 23.11 Dissecting the perineum

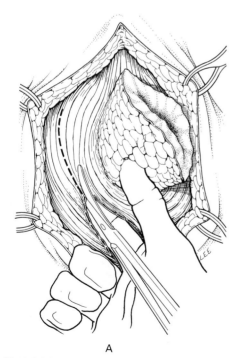

A

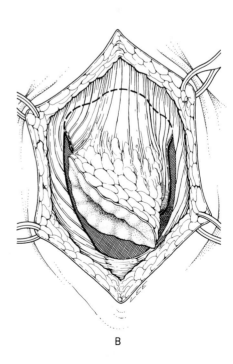

B

Fig. 23.12 Dividing the levators

Division of the levators is next carried forward to meet the point where the puborectalis fibres have been identified anteriorly. By a combination of sharp and blunt dissection the musculofibrous tissue here is divided off the back of the prostate and dissection then carried up behind the bladder to meet the abdominal operator. The latter then divides the colon at an appropriate place to permit it to be passed through the abdominal wall at the colostomy site and the specimen is delivered per anum. In the female it is permissible, but not desirable, to remove the posterior vaginal wall, in which case the perineal and abdominal dissections join in the posterior vaginal fornix. Healing of the vagina is said to be satisfactory but there is little objective evidence on this point.

Establishing the colostomy
Either an extraperitoneal or intraperitoneal method can be used. If the former, the edge of parietal peritoneum, formed when the sigmoid is mobilized, is raised and a blunt dissection made outside it round the lateral aspect of the abdominal wall to the colostomy site. A disc of skin is excised and the abdominal wall cut through in all layers in two directions at right angles; the resulting gap must easily take two fingers without any feeling of grip. The colon is then drawn through behind the peritoneum and stitched to the skin (Fig. 22.52 p. 447).

If the colostomy is established intraperitoneally, there is a danger of herniation lateral to the colon in the old paracolic gutter. This gap must be obliterated by either a running or a close series of interrupted sutures of silk or braided nylon passed from the lateral aspect of the colon wall to the parietal peritoneum (Fig. 23.13).

Closure of the pelvic floor and perineum
No attempt should be made to close the pelvic peritoneal cavity. A few absorbable sutures (catgut, dexon, vicryl or polydioxanone) are inserted to draw the fatty margins of the ischiorectal fossa together and the skin closed with soft nonabsorbables, with a suction drain led out through a stab incision. If there has been contamination or if there is tension, it is better to leave the wound open and lightly packed with dry gauze. At four to five days, the pack is removed under general anaesthesia and the wound will usually rapidly contract to heal by second intention in two to three weeks.

It has been suggested that there is less likelihood of adhesion of small bowel to the pelvic floor if the omentum is pedicled on one gastroepiploic vessel and brought down into the pelvis. This manoeuvre is recommended if the perineal wound is to be left open.

Anterior resection of the rectum
The technique for mobilization of the upper rectum has already been described in the section on colonic carcinoma (p. 438). Dissection within the pelvis proceeds on the lines of the abdominal dissection in the synchronous combined operation. Continuity of bowel is most safely established by the stapling gun (Fig. 23.14) although suturing is preferred by many surgeons. For a sutured anastomosis deep in the pelvis, the posterior row of sutures must be inserted *prior to* approximation of the gut ends if accuracy of apposition is to be achieved. In skilled hands, sutured colo-anal anastomosis can be achieved by the perineal approach (Parks, 1982), with only minor deficiencies in bowel function.

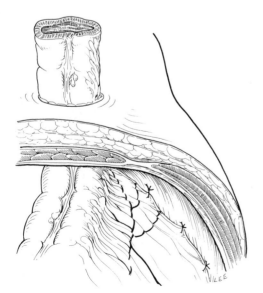

Fig. 23.13 Closure of the lateral paracolic gutter (exposure through transverse abdominal incision)

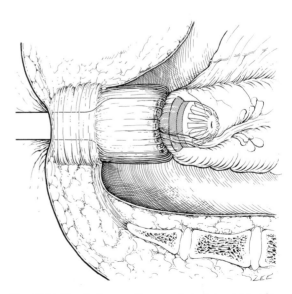

Fig. 23.14 The final stage of transanal stapled anastomosis

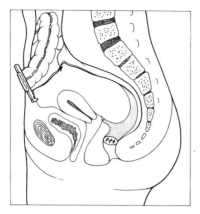

Fig. 23.15 Anterior (transabdominal) resection of the rectum with permanent colostomy—Hartmann's operation

Abdominal excision alone with permanent colostomy

This method may be preferred in selected patients (p. 463) or as a first stage procedure in the presence of obstruction (p. 444). *Abdominal dissection* is carried out as already described and a terminal colostomy is made. The distal stump of rectum is closed by sutures (Fig. 23.15) and the peritoneum of the pelvic floor is repaired above it. An alternative method of dealing with the rectal stump is to close it around a tube drain which is brought out through the anus.

Palliative procedures

Removal of the primary growth, where this is practicable, is the best method of palliation. The presence of metastases in the liver or elsewhere should not therefore preclude an excision, provided, of course, that the growth is not fixed by malignant infiltration to surrounding tissues. It is obvious that, when the excision is considered to be purely palliative, extensive clearance of the glandular fields is unnecessary, and that sphincter-conserving resections have a special application.

Fulguration of the tumour
When the patient is too enfeebled to stand an excision, and when the main symptom is bleeding, this may sometimes be arrested by fulguration with the diathermy electrode, carried out if necessary at several sessions (Madden, 1983). Considerable shrinkage of the growth may result, and symptomatic relief may be obtained for many months (Gingold, 1983).

Colostomy alone
This should be considered when the growth appears to be irremovable, but it should not be advised as routine in all such cases. When obstruction exists or threatens to develop at an early date, or when the patient's life is made miserable by tenesmus or continual discharge,

colostomy may provide a considerable measure of relief during the time that is left to him. Occasionally after colostomy there is an astounding improvement in both general and local conditions. Fixation of the growth may be due mainly to inflammatory reaction; it may diminish or even disappear with free drainage of the bowel above, so that radical removal may become practicable. Even in apparently fixed growths, therefore, the possibility of radical cure at a later date should not be entirely discounted. Colostomy is contraindicated in advanced malignancy with widespread metastases or carcinomatosis peritonei. Unless obstruction is present the patient will be made more miserable by a colostomy, and he is unlikely to live long enough to derive any benefit from it. In such cases *there is no evidence to show that colostomy prolongs life.*

ANAL FISSURE

The fissure is most commonly situated in the midline posteriorly. It varies in appearance from a superficial crack in the mucosa to a long oval-shaped ulcer, with indurated or undermined edges, and in the base of which plain muscle fibres may be exposed. At its external end there is usually a hypertrophied and oedematous tag of skin, the *sentinel pile*. The fissure is invariably associated with sphincteric spasm, which is not only the main cause of pain, but which also keeps up the irritation and delays healing.

Treatment directed towards correction of constipation will, in many cases, lead to healing of a recent fissure. The application of analgesic ointments will result in pain relief and relaxation of sphincteric spasm. In some cases, daily use of an anal dilator will be found helpful but its use may be required over a prolonged period (Lock, 1977).

Sphincter injection

This method of treatment is now infrequently employed but may be of value where urgent relief of pain is required. With the patient in the *right* lateral position, a wheal of local anaesthetic is raised 2.5 cm posterior to the anus in the mid line. A larger needle is then introduced into the sphincteric muscle for injection of aqueous or oil-soluble local anaesthetic, the site of injection being guided by the surgeon's left index finger which has been inserted through the anal canal.

Operation

General anaesthesia is usually necessary to achieve adequate anal dilatation.

Simple stretching of the sphincter
In many cases this is successful in effecting a cure. It

should be noted that it is the *internal*, rather than the external sphincter which requires to be stretched, since it is this muscle which underlies the fissure. Stretching is carried out slowly and gently until the orifice admits three or four fingers without difficulty.

Sphincterotomy consists in division of the fibres of the internal sphincter, this muscle being identified by palpation after the anal canal has been stretched and everted. Relief of pain is usually quite dramatic and is almost certainly due to the abolition of spasm. A bivalve speculum is introduced into the anal canal, and is gradually opened to expose the fissure and to put the fibres of the internal sphincter on the stretch. These fibres are then completely divided to just above the dentate line, to expose the smooth conjoined longitudinal muscle lying underneath. The wound is prolonged outwards on to the peri-anal skin, so that a 'sentinel' pile, if present, can be excised. Any well developed commissural fibres of the subcutaneous external sphincter are divided also, in order to avoid a ridge.

Excision

When the fissure is a chronic one, or shows much induration, it is probable that complete excision is the operation of choice. After the sphincter has been stretched two pairs of light tissue forceps are placed on the mucocutaneous junction well to each side of the fissure, and are drawn downwards until the entire fissure comes into view. With a sharp knife, the fissure and its fibrous tissue covering is then cleanly excised by an elliptical incision which is deepened down to the fibres of the internal sphincter. To ensure free drainage the ellipse, which includes the sentinel pile, should be carried well out on to the peri-anal skin, where it should be at least 1 cm in breadth (Fig. 23.16). The sphincteric fibres immediately deep to the fissure may be divided at the same time. Thereafter the floor of the wound should be completely smooth and free from ridges or hollows (Fig. 23.17).

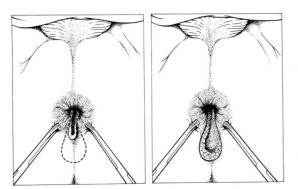

Figs. 23.16 & 23.17 Excision of an anal fissure

After-treatment

After either sphincterotomy or excision, bleeding is arrested by the application of a gauze swab, a corner of which may be tucked into the anal canal. It is covered with wool and secured with a T-bandage. The dressings are changed daily, but subsequent repacking of the wound should not be required. Hot sitz-baths are instituted as early as possible, and gentle cleansing with soap and water is carried out after each evacuation. There is usually almost complete relief of pain immediately after operation, and healing may be expected to be complete in from 10 days to 3 weeks. The bowel motions should be kept soft for several months after operation, since, if constipation is allowed to exist, there is a considerable risk that the fissure may recur.

HAEMORRHOIDS

External haemorrhoids

True external haemorrhoids (i.e. covered with skin alone) are not very common. Usually they are no more than small skin tags, which require no treatment unless they become irritated or inflamed. In such cases they may, when quiescent, be snipped off with scissors or treated with the Cryoprobe, so that a flat surface results. Frequently they co-exist with internal haemorrhoids or fissure, and their removal should then be included in the operation for the more troublesome condition.

Peri-anal haematoma. This is often incorrectly referred to as a 'thrombosed external pile', but it is in reality a small haematoma due to the rupture of an anal venule. It is usually 4 or 5 days before the patient seeks advice; by this time the period of maximum discomfort has passed, and, unless the haematoma is a large one, no treatment is required, as the clot will shrink and disappear in a further few days. When the condition is seen soon after its onset, a small incision may be made under local anaesthesia, and the clot evacuated.

Internal haemorrhoids

Internal haemorrhoids, or intero-external haemorrhoids (which lie at the mucocutaneous junction, and have a covering partly of mucosa and partly of skin) are much more common. In those cases which are not relieved by adjustment of the dietary fibre, aperients or suppositories, the choices of treatment are injection, rubber banding, cryosurgery, anal dilatation or excision.

Conservative treatment

Injection therapy

This gives satisfactory results in selected cases of internal haemorrhoids. It has the advantage over operation that the patient can be treated as an outpatient but a course of several injections is frequently required. Injection treatment is most satisfactory when the piles are small and cause no symptoms other than bleeding at defaecation. Prolapse of the haemorrhoids during defaecation is not necessarily a contraindication to injection, provided that they can be replaced.

Injection treatment must not be employed in cases of external piles, or of internal piles which tend to remain prolapsed outside the anal sphincter, in view of the danger that sloughing may result. It is contraindicated also in the presence of infection.

The patient is placed in the knee elbow or in the lateral position. A well lubricated anal speculum is introduced, and the number, size and arrangement of the haemorrhoids are carefully noted. Frequently they present in three distinct groups, with one or more in each group—left lateral, right anterior and right posterior being a common arrangement. This is due to the anatomical arrangement of the blood vessels supplying the anal cushions (Thomson, 1975).

The method of *high injection* is now generally employed. The term denotes an injection made into the submucous coat of the bowel *above* a group of piles (Fig. 23.18). Its object is to cause thrombosis of the vessels draining the piles and to promote a localized fibrosis which will lead to retraction of the lax mucosa. Where possible a special syringe and needle should be used; the latter is long enough to use through a proctoscope, and is bent at an obtuse angle; it has a shoulder about 1 cm from its point, so that too deep penetration is avoided. The solution advocated is 5% phenol in almond oil, and up to 5 ml may be injected in each situation. It is best to make the first injection in the quadrant which presents the largest pile mass. The injection should be carried out slowly, and the fluid should be seen to raise a pale swelling which spreads immediately deep to the mucosa. A white wheal appearing at the site of puncture indicates that the solution is being injected into the mucosa with consequent risk of local necrosis; the needle should be withdrawn immediately and another site selected. Similar injections may be made above other pile masses in the remaining quadrants, or this may be postponed until another session. It is probably not advisable that more than three injections should be made at any one treatment.

After treatment

The patient is instructed to avoid prolonged standing or strenuous exercise for a few days, and to keep the bowel motions soft by the regular taking of liquid paraffin. If a pile prolapses during defaecation it should be replaced immediately. Further injections are carried out if required at fortnightly intervals. They are given normally in those quadrants which have not already been injected, and in which piles are present.

Rubber band ligature of the pedicle of each haemorrhoid may be carried out without anaesthesia in the manner of injection described above but using a special applicator. The results of each method are similar (Greca, 1981).

Cryosurgery of haemorrhoids is an alternative procedure and is done using a fenestrated proctoscope or bivalve speculum. The cryoprobe is applied to the haemorrhoidal mass until freezing reaches the mucocutaneous junction (Kaufmann, 1977). Liquefaction of frozen tissue over the ensuing 2 or 3 weeks necessitates the wearing of an absorbent pad.

Manual dilatation of the anus, as advocated by Lord (1969), aims to dilate the sphincter to accept 4 fingers of each hand and to maintain sphincter laxity by regular use of a specially designed dilator. General anaesthesia is required but the patient need not be detained in hospital.

Operation

Operative removal of haemorrhoids is indicated when they are of significant size, and especially if they tend to remain prolapsed outside the anal sphincter.

Preparation

The bowel should be thoroughly cleared out before operation, in order to minimize faecal contamination, and to promote quiescence of the colon for the first few days of the postoperative period. As a rule an aperient is given 36 to 48 hours before operation, and thereafter the patient is kept on a fluid or nonresidue diet. An enema is administered on the evening before operation, and a low washout (of the rectum alone) may be given early

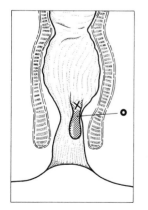 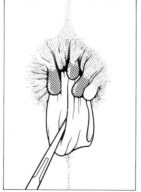

Fig. 23.18 Internal haemorrhoids—site for high and low injections

Fig. 23.19 Method of withdrawing internal haemorrhoids by the use of a dry gauze swab

on the morning of operation. It is customary to employ general or low spinal anaesthesia, and to operate with the patient in the lithotomy position.

Dissection-ligature operation

This is the most widely practised operation at the present time (Hawley, 1973). The anal sphincter is gently stretched between the two index fingers. A dry swab is pushed into the rectum, and is then partially withdrawn, when the haemorrhoids will appear alongside it (Fig. 23.19). They are picked up individually with artery forceps, and each is then dealt with in turn. In the case of intero-external piles two forceps are applied; one to the mucous part and one to the cutaneous part. The pile is drawn downwards, and with a pair of scissors, a V-shaped cut is made through the overlying mucosa at its junction with the skin. If the pile is intero-external in type, the cut is commenced in the skin just at its external border (Fig. 23.20). By blunt dissection with the scissor points the submucous space is opened up until the pile is entirely stripped from its bed, and is attached only by its vascular pedicle, and by a narrow strip of mucous membrane. Care is taken not to elevate any of the fibres of the external sphincter in the dissection. A ligature of strong thread or catgut is used to transfix and tie the pedicle as high up as possible (Fig. 23.21), and the distal part is cut off. The ends of the ligature may be used as a mattress suture to unite the stump of the pedicle to the skin edge, thus covering the raw area which would otherwise remain. After all the piles have been dealt with, two fingers are introduced into the anal canal, to ensure that no stenosis has been caused. A large pad of gauze liberally smeared with sterile vaseline

is applied to the anus. This is secured with a T-bandage, which is firmly tied, so that the pressure exerted will tend to prevent oedema of the part. Some surgeons leave a rubber tube within the anal canal; this gives warning of haemorrhage but, although it allows the passage of flatus, it may increase the patient's discomfort.

Submucosal haemorrhoidectomy is a modification of the ligature operation which avoids suture of anal mucosa with the pedicle and does not result in any raw areas to cause fibrosis. It is, however, technically difficult and may result in some blood loss.

Clamp and cautery operation

This method is now frequently described as obsolete, but it has certain advantages over the dissection-ligature operation, in that it involves no opening up of the tissue planes by dissection—a factor of some importance in view of the potentially septic character of the operative field. A special clamp is employed; its blades are guarded with ivory or plastic plates which protect the skin from burning. Additional protection is provided by pads of moist wool or gauze placed around the clamp, between it and the skin. The clamp must always be applied radially to the anal orifice, and both an external and an internal pile may therefore be clamped together (Fig. 23.22). The greater part of the pile mass is then cut away with scissors, only a little of its substance being left projecting beyond the clamp. The copper cautery specially designed for the operation is heated over a gas ring; it is applied at a black heat, so that the pile stump

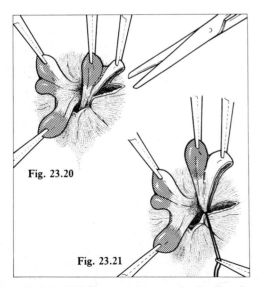

Figs. 23.20 & 23.21 Haemorrhoidectomy by the dissection-ligature technique

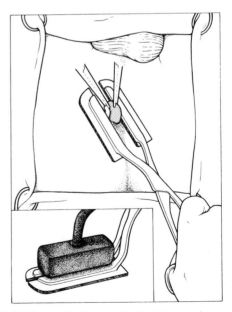

Fig. 23.22 Haemorrhoidectomy by the 'clamp-and-cautery' method. Inset shows copper cautery block applied to the Smith's pile clamp

projecting beyond the clamp is *slowly* burned away. The surface area of the cautery is sufficiently large to heat up the blades of the clamp; in this way the tissue grasped by the clamp is thoroughly seared, so that the haemorrhage is effectively arrested. The only objection to this old-fashioned cautery is that a gas ring is seldom readily available in a modern operating theatre. The electric cautery or the diathermy knife are unsatisfactory substitutes, since they are ineffective in arresting haemorrhage, while the coagulating current penetrates too deeply into the tissues (Chamberlain, 1970).

After-treatment
The foot of the bed is elevated for 24 to 48 hours after operation, in order to reduce congestion of the part. Retention of urine is a fairly common complication, especially in older men, and may require attention. The bowels are kept confined if possible for several days, and to assist in this a fluid diet only is allowed. Small doses of liquid paraffin or of magnesia emulsion may be given daily after the first day. Pain from defaecation can be relieved by the introduction of local anaesthetic ointment into the anal canal. Twice-daily sitz baths are very comforting and promote rapid healing. Recurrence of the piles is rare, except in the chronically constipated.

Thrombosed or strangulated piles
It is generally taught that removal of haemorrhoids in the 'acute' stage is contraindicated, in view of the risk of spreading infection, especially to the portal tract (*pylephlebitis*); also, because the haemorrhoids are very friable, they bleed readily, and ligatures tend to cut through.

Conservative treatment, therefore, is commonly employed until the acute condition has subsided. The patient is confined to bed with its foot raised on blocks. Pain is relieved by moist compresses and by sedatives as required. In cases seen early, it may be possible, under an anaesthetic, to reduce the prolapsed piles after stretching the sphincter. Surgery is then undertaken later in the quiescent stage.

The results of such treatment are not impressive. Ten days or more may elapse before the protruding mass shrinks within the anus and this is a painful and distressing time for the patient. When he has recovered from the attack, he still has to face operation at a later date. Even when the prolapse can be successfully reduced, it frequently recurs within a few hours.

It now appears that the dangers of operation in the acute stage have been exaggerated (Smith, 1967). Dissection should obviously be reduced to the minimum, but crushing clamps can safely be applied to the pile pedicles which are relatively normal, and the protruding masses cut off. The stumps are then ligatured or over-sewn. The 'clamp-and-cautery' method is particularly suitable for use in such conditions.

ANORECTAL ABSCESSES

Peri-anal abscess

A subcutaneous abscess
This lies under the skin at the anal margin (Fig. 23.23A). It results usually from inflammation of a sebaceous follicle, or from infection through some superficial abrasion. It should be opened by a cruciate incision, and any undermined edges are cut away. The injection of a small quantity of local anaesthetic into the skin renders the operation quite painless.

A submucous abscess is less common. It is located under the mucosa of the anal canal (Fig. 23.23B), and is due frequently to infection which has entered an anal gland through an anal crypt. It usually bursts spontaneously, but if necessary it should be opened by incision, access having been obtained by stretching of the anal sphincter.

Ischio-rectal abscess
The presence of brawny induration to one or other side of the anus, accompanied by throbbing pain, justifies the diagnosis of ischiorectal abscess (Fig. 23.23C). Drainage should always be provided without delay. If redness of the overlying skin or signs of fluctuation are awaited, the abscess is very liable to rupture into the bowel, in which case a fistula is almost certain to result.

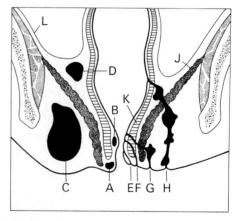

Fig. 23.23 Diagram to show the situation of the various anorectal abscesses and fistulae.
Abscesses: (A) subcutaneous; (B) submucous; (C) ischiorectal; (D) pelvirectal
Fistulae (E) superficial or extra-sphincteric; (F) inter-sphincteric; (G) trans-sphincteric; (H) extrasphincteric
Normal anatomy (J) levator ani; (K) internal sphincter; (L) peritoneum

If early incision is carried out this sequel can usually be prevented. Spread to the ischiorectal fossa of the opposite side is not uncommon; this complication also is avoided by early incision.

Operation

It is most essential that the incision should be a large one. Not only must it provide free drainage, but it should also be sufficiently large to ensure that the wound will heal from its deepest part outwards. It is no kindness to the patient to employ a small incision, for satisfactory healing is then unlikely to be obtained unless the surface wound is kept open by continual repacking which is always an uncomfortable and tedious procedure. A large cruciate incision is recommended, one limb of which radiates towards the anus; it is deepened through skin and fascia, and the corners are then cut away, so that the final opening represents the entire floor of the abscess cavity (Figs. 23.24 & 23.25). Fibrous septa are broken down with the finger or by further incisions, and the whole cavity is then carefully packed with gauze. In some series, satisfactory healing has followed suture of the abscess cavity after curettage (Ellis, 1960; Macfie, 1977; Wilson, 1964).

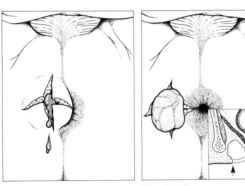

Fig. 23.24 **Fig. 23.25**

Figs. 23.24 & 23.25 Method of opening an ischiorectal abscess by cruciate incision. Inset shows how the entire floor of the abscess cavity is removed

After-treatment

The packing is normally removed after about 48 hours. When the external opening has been made sufficiently large repacking can be dispensed with, but sitz baths should be commenced as early as possible. Healing should occur steadily from the depths outwards, the time taken depending, of course, upon the size of the cavity. The wound must be inspected regularly, and, if there is any sign that surface healing is progressing too rapidly, gauze packing should at once be reinstituted, the pack being renewed each day.

A *chronic ischiorectal abscess* may be tuberculous. The fat normally occupying the ischiorectal fossa is replaced by tuberculous granulation tissue and caseous material. Local treatment is on similar lines to that described for an acute abscess. All caseous material should be removed, and the wall of the fossa gently curetted with a sharp spoon and sent for histological examination, bacteriological culture and sensitivities. Antituberculous chemotherapy is instituted on confirmation of the disease.

Pelvi-rectal abscess

This type of abscess is situated above the levator ani muscle, between it and the rectum (see Fig. 23.23D). It originates from some septic process in the pelvis, e.g. pelvic cellulitis. It may track downwards through the levator ani to become ischiorectal in location, or it may burst directly into the rectum. The treatment consists in providing drainage by the most accessible route— usually through the ischiorectal fossa. At operation it will be evident that pus is tracking downwards through an opening in the levator ani muscle; this opening should be enlarged to provide adequate drainage.

FISTULA-IN-ANO

The condition is usually a sequel to some variety of anorectal abscess, the infection arising within an anal gland and most frequently involving the intersphincteric plane. It is most likely to occur in cases where incision has been too long delayed, or where the drainage has been inadequate. The external opening of the fistula lies at the skin surface, usually to one or other side of the anus, and at a varying distance away. From this the fistulous track passes towards the mucous membrane of the bowel. The majority of fistulae are comparatively superficial, in that the track lies immediately deep to the skin and mucous membrane (*superficial or extrasphincteric*, 16%) or traverses the fibres of the internal sphincter to involve the intersphincteric plane to a variable extent (*intersphincteric*, 54%). Fistulae passing through both sphincters (*trans-sphincteric*, 21%) are less common (Marks, 1977). If the external opening is in front of the transverse line bisecting the anus the track is usually more or less straight, and opens therefore into the corresponding quadrant of the anal canal. If the external opening is behind that line the fistula can be expected to pursue a curved course and to enter the anal canal in the midline posteriorly.

A high level fistula (*extrasphincteric*, 3%), which is a sequel usually to pelvirectal abscess, passes deep to both sphincters and traverses the levator ani, to enter the rectum at a high level.

The different types of fistula are shown diagramatically in Figure 23.23.

Operation

The essential aim in treatment is to lay the fistulous track widely open or to excise it completely, and to ensure that the wound heals from the depths outwards.

The preoperative treatment is similar to that described for haemorrhoidectomy. A general or low spinal anaesthetic is employed, and the patient is placed in the lithotomy position. After gentle stretching of the sphincter the fistulous track is explored with a grooved probe or director, which should be either curved or easily bendable. Frequently the probe passes without difficulty by way of the fistula into the anal canal. By the aid of a finger introduced into the bowel, it is then bent round or manipulated in such a way that its tip can be brought out at the anus. When the probe cannot be made to locate the internal opening, its tip can usually be felt by the finger to lie just below the mucous membrane. In such cases the probe should be thrust through the mucous membrane into the lumen of the bowel, after which its tip is brought out at the anus.

The fistula may now be laid widely open by division of all tissue between it and the skin surface, i.e. by cutting down on the probe. If possible, however, it is better to excise the track completely with the probe in situ (Fig. 23.26). The wound should be piriform or triangular in shape with its wider part externally. In the case of trans-sphincteric fistulae, the superficial fibres of the external and internal sphincters are included in the excision. Any ramifications of the main track are dealt with in the same way. Irregularities on the floor of the wound and any overhanging skin edges are cut away, so that there can be no interference with free drainage (Fig. 23.27) and the wound is packed with gauze. Even if the fistulous track is believed to have been cleanly and completely excised, it is seldom advisable to attempt to close it by suture.

For a trans-sphincteric fistula, in which the greater part of both sphincters must be divided, a two-stage operation was formerly advised in order to reduce the risk of anal incontinence. However, this is no longer considered necessary provided that the puborectalis is preserved (Hawley, 1978).

A two-stage operation may be advisable when the track pursues a curved course ('horse-shoe fistula'). In such cases, a ligature of stout silk is passed on a probe or aneurysm needle through the deep part of the track and is loosely tied. At the first operation the external and lateral part of the track, which is usually subcutaneous, is excised (Figs. 23.28 & 23.29). The silk ligature serves to identify the residual track so that, when the first wound has healed (except for the new external opening of the fistula at its medial end) the remainder of

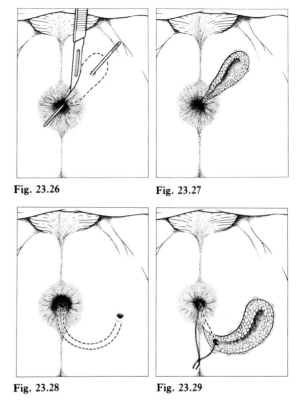

Fig. 23.26   **Fig. 23.27**

Fig. 23.28   **Fig. 23.29**

Figs. 23.26 & 23.27 Excision of a superficial anal fistula passing directly into the anal canal
Figs. 23.28 & 23.29 First part of a two-stage operation for a deep fistula pursuing a curved course into the bowel, excision of the superficial and lateral part of the track. A silk ligature identifies the residual fistula to be excised at the second stage

the track entering the bowel is dealt with by a further excision.

Multiple fistulae

In longstanding fistulae it is common to find several external openings scattered around the anus particularly in the suprasphincteric or extrasphincteric type. They are likely to be connected to each other by subcutaneous tracks, but to share a common track by which they communicate with the bowel. Operative treatment should be carried out in two or more stages, the subcutaneous or communicating tracks being excised in the first instance. It is not advisable to divide sphincteric fibres in more than one place at the same operation. Excised tissue is examined for Crohn's disease if this has not already been suspected.

High level fistula

The track in this type of fistula cannot be laid open into the bowel, nor can it be completely excised, since it extends to too high a level in the rectum. A circular incision is made round the external opening, and the fistulous track is cored out along with a generous margin of surrounding tissue, including the levator ani muscle, to as high a level as possible. The large wound is carefully packed with gauze and allowed to granulate outwards. The internal opening in the rectal wall may then close spontaneously. If not, a temporary pelvic colostomy, preferably of defunctioning type (p. 433), should be advised. As the result of complete rest to the bowel, healing may occur.

Tuberculous fistulae are characterized by multiple tracks with widespread undermining of skin. In general, treatment is carried out on the lines described. All tracks are laid open as far as possible, and undermined skin is excised; unhealthy wound surfaces are cauterized with the diathermy electrode. Complete division of the external sphincter is contraindicated, since, owing to impaired healing power, incontinence may result. Antituberculous chemotherapy should be instituted.

After-treatment is very similar to that described for abscesses. The necessity for repacking the wound depends upon the type of fistula. In superficial fistulae the excision wound is comparatively shallow, so that packing is both unnecessary and difficult to retain. When, however, the track has been deeply situated, a narrow and relatively deep cleft is inevitable, and in such cases careful cleansing and repacking should be carried out after each bowel movement. Otherwise, superficial healing is liable to occur, with stagnation of pus in the depths of the wound; in such cases recurrence of the fistula is a probable result.

OTHER CONDITIONS AFFECTING THE ANUS

Carcinoma of the anus or anal canal

Some 3% of rectal carcinomata are of squamous type arising either at the anal margin or at a higher level within the canal, the latter being three times commoner than the former (Morson, 1979). There are two varieties, those involving the peri-anal skin or anal margin, and those arising within the anal canal above the dentate line, each carrying a very different prognosis. In the first type, the upper margin of the growth is often visible on everting the anus, and a finger detects no abnormality within the canal; this type is of relatively low malignancy, and can be treated by local excision (Madden, 1981). In the second variety, the growth may not be visible at all on inspection, but is at once detected within the canal by the examining finger; such growths are much more malignant, and should be treated by radical excision of the anorectum.

Columnar epitheliomata are sometimes encountered;

they arise immediately above the dentate line or represent the downward extension of a rectal tumour. Basal celled carcinomata are occasionally reported; they may be superficial, locally aggressive or metastasising (Nielsen, 1981).

Local excision by diathermy is suitable for early marginal growths confined to one quadrant of the anus and arising below the dentate line. The growth is excised with the diathermy knife, together with a generous margin of surrounding skin and with the underlying fibres of the external sphincter aiming for a clearance of 2.5 cm; the wound is left open to granulate. Provided that the puborectalis sling remains intact, incontinence does not normally result.

Radical excision of the rectum

More advanced growths and those involving the anal canal rather than the peri-anal skin should be treated by radical excision of the rectum by the abdominoperineal method. An extra wide excision of the peri-anal tissues must be undertaken.

Irradiation therapy

Some encouraging successes have been obtained by this method of treatment alone, but in general the results are less satisfactory than those of excisional surgery. Certain cases may be dealt with by a combination of radiotherapy (which causes the growth to shrink) and subsequent excision.

Treatment of the inguinal glands

It should be noted that glandular swellings may be due simply to infection, and may subside rapidly after effective treatment of the primary growth. If, however, the swellings persist for more than 2 or 3 weeks, or if their hardness suggests that they are metastatic in nature, a block dissection of the glands should be carried out in one or both groins, according to conditions present (p. 620).

In inoperable cases the severe pain and anal incontinence of the terminal stages may be relieved by a palliative colostomy.

Anal incontinence

Most cases of incontinence of the anal sphincter are due to accidental or obstetrical injuries, or are the result of operations in the anorectal region. Some may result from congenital abnormalities or their treatment.

Many types of repair have been described, but no one has proved entirely satisfactory, for by any method failures are common, owing to the high incidence of infection with dehiscence of the wound. It is, therefore, advisable to establish a defunctioning colostomy prior to repair.

Direct repair of the sphincter

If the sphincter has not been too extensively damaged, an attempt should be made to reconstitute it by suturing together its divided ends. Probably the most promising methods are those which depend on the use of stainless steel wire as suture material. This does not predispose to infection, and engenders a minimal tissue reaction. A crescentic incision is made just lateral to and centred over the defect, excising all underlying scar tissue. A fringe of mucosa is mobilized and sutured to restore the mucosal tube. The cut or torn ends of the sphincter muscle are identified and brought together with some overlap using mattress sutures of No. 40 SWG stainless steel wire (Browning, 1984). The residual wound is allowed to heal by granulation.

Plastic methods of repair

These may be undertaken as a preferable alternative to a colostomy, in cases where the sphincter is considered to be irreparable. In Thiersch's operation a ring of silver wire or nylon (Baker, 1970) is passed round the anus, and is tied sufficiently tightly to admit one finger. It will allow motions to be passed, but at the same time will give considerable support to the anus. Alternative procedures using muscle grafts or fascial slings have been generally abandoned.

Pruritus ani

In cases where no treatable cause can be discovered, or where local applications have failed to bring relief, recourse may be had to injection treatment.

Injection of alcohol

Under general or lowspinal anaesthesia, the affected area may be 'stippled' by multiple subcutaneous injections of 95% alcohol. The needle punctures are made about 1 cm apart; the needle is thrust vertically through the skin, and usually not more than 0.25 ml is injected at each site. There is some danger of the skin sloughing if these quantities are exceeded. If successful this treatment may give complete relief of symptoms for several months or even years (Stone, 1926).

Cryosurgery

Of value in the elimination of unhealthy skin tags which aggravate pruritis ani. Several applications may be required before a smooth moisture-free anal margin is obtained.

Anorectal malformations

The incidence of this relatively common and important condition is 1 in 3000 births. The malformation develops in the foetus between 4 and 10 weeks. During this period, the cloaca is divided into a urogenital chamber anteriorly and rectum posteriorly by a septum that grows caudally to the cloacal membrane. On the surface, the ectodermal pit overlying the rectum becomes the lower part of the anal canal. The more severe malformations form at an earlier stage of development. 33 different types were described at an international conference in Melbourne in 1970 which illustrates the complex nature of the problem. However, the important practical distinction is between the high and low types. In a high anomaly, the bowel ends above the levator ani but in the low anomaly the bowel passes down through the limbs of the puborectalis sling.

Classification

The more common malformations are best understood in relation to development. High anomalies (Fig. 23.30), which include rectal atresia with or without fistula, develop at a relatively early stage as a result of incomplete division of the cloaca. In rectal atresia the normal bowel ends above the levator ani, occasionally blind, but more

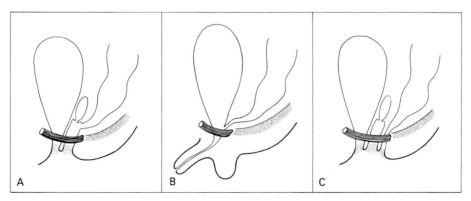

Fig. 23.30 High anorectal anomalies
A. Rectal atresia with recto-vaginal fistula
B. Rectal atresia with recto-urethral fistula
C. Rectal atresia with rectovestibular fistula

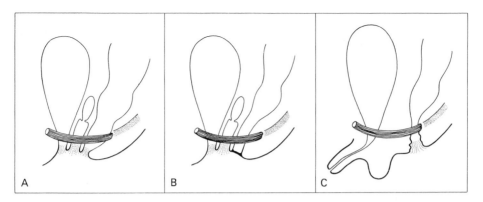

Fig. 23.31 Low anorectal anomalies
A. Vulva ectopic anus
B. Covered anus
C. Anorectal stenosis

commonly connected by a fistula to the prostatic urethra in the male and to the posterior wall of the vagina or vestibule in the female. In contrast the low anomalies (Fig. 23.31), which include ectopic anus, covered anus and anal stenosis, develop at a later stage. It is suggested that an ectopic anus results from incomplete migration of the anus back across the perineum. The opening may be perineal in the male or perineal, vulval or vestibular in the female. The covered anus probably results from overgrowth of the anal folds and as a result the underlying rectum and anal canal are normal. The covered anus appears either as a membrane which may be crossed by a median bar or as a fine superficial fistulous tract running forward in the midline of the perineum. Anorectal fibrosis may be caused by incomplete involution of the cloacal membrane. Normally a narrow rigid fibrous ring can be felt but occasionally fibrosis may extend along the length of the canal.

The uncommon high anomaly of atresia of the middle third of the rectum in which the proximal rectum and anal canal are normally formed but are joined by a fibrous band is difficult to explain by the sequence of events described above.

Clinical presentation
The clinical diagnosis is normally made during examination of the newborn baby. However, anorectal fibrosis and marginal displacement of an ectopic anus may be missed and present later in life with chronic constipation. In a baby with a high anomaly, no bowel opening is seen but meconium may stain the urine of a male or may be passed from the vagina in a female. In a baby with a low anomaly the opening is visible when the perineum is examined. Care must be taken to differentiate between rectal atresia with a rectovestibular fistula and a vestibular ectopic anus. The

former runs deep in close relation to the vagina and is supported by the puborectalis whereas the latter runs backwards in a superficial plane (Figs. 23.30C and 23.31A).

The distinction between high and low anomalies is not always clear. The value of radiology in this respect is debatable; the position of gas in the distal bowel in relation to the puborectalis can be demonstrated on a lateral X-ray taken at the level of the greater trochanter with the baby inverted and the hips flexed (Stephens & Smith, 1971) but the result must be interpreted with caution. An X-ray of the sacrum, however, is important as sacral agenesis may be associated with abnormal pelvic innervation. An intravenous pyelogram should also be performed in the first month of life to exclude an associated urinary tract abnormality.

Operation
A high type of malformation is treated by a transverse or left iliac colostomy according to preference and a definitive operation performed when the baby is 9 months or 10 kg. The operation is approached through a transverse lower abdominal incision. The distal bowel is mobilized by careful dissection to preserve the pelvic splanchnic nerves and the fistula is divided. The puborectalis sling can be felt with the tip of a finger pushed down into the pelvis in the midline immediately behind the posterior wall of the urethra or vagina. A perineal incision is then made over the anal dimple which can be recognized by stimulating the underlying fibres of the superficial external sphincter. Forceps are passed through the perineal opening to the abdominal cavity and are directed through the limbs of the puborectalis by a finger placed deep in the pelvis. The bowel is then drawn down through the tunnel and anastomosed to perineal skin. An initial sacral approach to safeguard the

puborectalis sling may be preferred (Stephens & Smith, 1971). The tip of the coccyx is separated from the sacrum to provide access to the front of the levator ani. The sling can then be identified under direct vision and marked. An endorectal dissection may be used to preserve the pelvic splanchnic nerves which are closely related to the fistula (Rehbein, 1959). The distal dissection of the rectum from the peritoneal reflection is continued at a submucosal plane. The muscle wall of the rectum is thus left in position and an opening made in the distal part so that the bowel can be pulled down through the muscle cuff toward the perineum.

The low type of malformation should be treated within 48 hours of birth if the bowel is obstructed. An ectopic anus is treated by a cutback operation. The anal mucosa and overlying skin are divided with scissors in a posterior direction. The cut edges of mucosa and skin are then sewn together. If the blade is allowed to pass too deeply, the puborectalis may be damaged. Although a cutback operation is described for treatment of a vestibular ectopic anus, some surgeons consider it undesirable in view of the proximity of the vagina. Instead, the vestibular opening can be circumcised, the distal bowel freed by dissection and then transposed to the normal position. A covered anus may be treated either by excision of the membranous covering or by tracing proximally the fine fistulous tract; the mucosa of the anal canal is then stitched to skin. In anorectal stenosis the rigid band should be divided using a longitudinal incision and mucosa and skin stitched together in a transverse plane. It is essential that, after the initial treatment of a low anomaly, anal dilatation is continued daily for three months to ensure an adequate and supple opening. Failure to do this may result in constipation and secondary rectal inertia which can be extremely difficult to manage.

Results

Continence can be described as excellent, meaning no accidents; good, meaning occasional accidents; and unsatisfactory. In children with low type malformations continence should be excellent in the majority and good in the rest; in those with high malformations approximately one third have an excellent result, one third are good and the remainder are unsatisfactory. In expert hands, however, the unsatisfactory group can be as low as 10% (Nixon, 1978).

PILONIDAL SINUS

Pilonidal sinuses are found in the midline of the natal cleft overlying the coccyx or lower part of the sacrum. They were formerly ascribed to a defect in development, leading to subcutaneous inclusion of epidermal structures, but it now seems more likely that they are acquired lesions, due to penetration of the skin by hairs. There are often two or more sinus openings, leading to tracks of varying depth; these are lined by squamous epithelium and not infrequently contain hairs (hence the name, *pilonidal sinus*).

Most patients come first to treatment on account of suppuration related to the sinuses, and abscesses commonly form either in the natal cleft or to one or other side; such abscesses may discharge spontaneously through an existing sinus, or may require to be opened. Thereafter, the infection may clear up completely, and no further trouble is experienced. More often, however, the discharge persists; either continuously, or after periodic abscess formation.

Surgical treatment should usually be advised when there have been two or more infective episodes, or when the discharge shows no sign of clearing up. It should be carried out at a time when the infection is quiescent. Although several conservative procedures have been described (Lord, 1965; Edwards, 1977; Mansoory 1982), the usual treatment—and probably the most effective one—is complete excision of the sinus tracks, together with all their ramifications.

Technique of excision

The operation is carried out with the patient in the left lateral or in the inverted-V position. An elliptical incision is made to include all sinus openings, and is deepened vertically down to the fascia covering the sacrum and coccyx. Coloured dye injected into the sinus track for identification during operation does not always reach the smaller sinuses and it is preferable to look carefully for granulation tissue during the dissection. If it is apparent that one of the ramifications of the sinus have been opened, a wider line of excision must be followed. By sharp dissection, the tissue enclosed by the incision is separated from the sacrococcygeal fascia and is removed.

Primary wound suture

When there has been no recent infection, it may be justifiable to suture the wound in an attempt to obtain healing by first intention. This offers the prospect of rapid cure, *but the possibilities of failure are considerable*, since, if the slightest infection develops, a discharging sinus is likely to persist or to recur. If the method is adopted, every effort must be made to avoid leaving dead space in the wound, for such will undoubtedly predispose to infection. Various methods of closure may be employed. The tissues on each side of the wound may be mobilized by undercutting, so that they can be approximated without undue tension. Thereafter, several deep sutures may be placed to pick up the sacrococcygeal fascia on the floor of the wound, and are tied firmly over a large roll

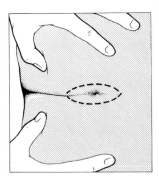

Fig. 23.32 Pilonidal sinus before operation. The opening of the sinus is seen between the index fingers

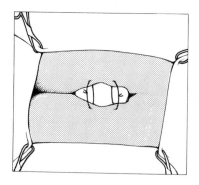

Fig 23.33 Excision completed and wound packed with gauze. (The stitches serve only to retain the pack in position)

of gauze, so that continual pressure is exerted on the wound. Alternatively, the wound may be closed in layers, with a large number of buried thread sutures. By both of these methods however, some tension on the wound is inevitable. To obviate this, numerous plastic procedures have been described (Bose, 1970; Rainsbury, 1982), but their value has not yet been established.

Gauze packing without suture
This entails a somewhat tedious convalescence, but has the advantage of effecting a permanent cure in nearly every case. No sutures whatever are inserted for closure; the wound is left widely open, and is packed either with dry gauze or with gauze impregnated with petroleum jelly, the dressing being held in place by sutures (Figs. 23.32 & 23.33). The pack is removed in 5 days. The large cavity which is present at this stage may occasion some misgivings but it is virtually painless and heals with amazing rapidity by granulation from the depths outwards. After the initial pack has been removed only a flat dressing secured by a T-bandage (or later, by tight fitting pants) is required. For cleansing and irrigation of the wound sitz baths are taken twice daily. Dressings are simplified and wound healing encouraged by the use of silicone foam sponge dressing (Wood, 1975). The sponge is renewed weekly, and is changed daily by the patient himself.

Healing is rarely complete before 4 or 5 weeks, but the patient can be discharged from hospital in 14 to 21 days. He is instructed to continue with daily baths and requires no treatment other than the simple dressings which he himself can apply.

The author agrees with those who believe that, because of the almost complete certainty of cure, open treatment of the wound has great advantages over primary suture, and should be the method of choice in most cases. Halfway measures—*partial* closure of the wound with drainage or packing—are not recommended.

COCCYGECTOMY

Removal of the coccyx is indicated occasionally when it is the seat of pain due to dislocation or mal-alignment of the bone in relation to the sacrum, or to arthritic changes at the intervening joint. Such conditions may result from childbirth or from other forms of local trauma. The lesion may be at the articulation between the 1st and 2nd coccygeal segments, and not at the sacrococcygeal articulation; in such case the distal segments alone are removed.

Before any operation is contemplated there should be *definite* evidence of deformity, or of arthritis (indicated by acute pain when the coccyx is moved on the sacrum by a finger in the rectum and a thumb externally). Pain in the coccygeal region, *coccydynia*, is common in young women, and frequently follows a fall on the buttocks. It may persist for months or even years, but definite evidence of deformity or arthritis is usually lacking, and there is likely to be a functional element in the complaints. In these cases coccygectomy is contraindicated, since the pain persists after operation. Relief can often be obtained by injection of local anaesthetic on both surfaces of the coccyx.

The operation of coccygectomy is a simple one. Through a longitudinal incision the coccyx is freed first at its tip and on each side, and disarticulation is carried out with a scalpel at the joint affected. The coccyx is then drawn backwards and is dissected off the underlying fascia. The knife is kept close to the bone in order to avoid injury to the fascia or to the middle sacral artery.

REFERENCES

Anderson J R, Kinninmonth A W G, Smith A N 1981 Polyvinyl alcohol sponge rectopexy for complete rectal prolapse. Journal of the Royal College of Surgeons of Edinburgh 26: 292

Baker W N W 1970 Results of using monofilament nylon in Thiersch's operation for rectal prolapse. British Journal of Surgery 57: 37

Bose B, Candy J 1970 Radical cure of pilonidal sinus by Z-plasty. American Journal of Surgery 120: 783

Browning G G P, Motson R W 1984 Anal sphincter injury. Management and results of Parks' sphincter repair. Annals of Surgery 199: 351

Chamberlain J, Johnstone J M S 1970 The results of haemorrhoidectomy by clamp and cautery. Surgery Gynaecology and Obstetrics 131: 745

Edwards M H 1977 Pilonidal sinus: A five year appraisal of the Millar-Lord treatment. British Journal of Surgery 64: 867

Ellis M 1960 Incision and primary suture of abscesses of the anal region. Proceedings Royal Society of Medicine 53: 652

Gingold B S, Mitty W F, Tadros M 1983 Importance of patient selection in local treatment of carcinoma of the rectum. American Journal of Surgery 145: 293

Goligher J C 1958 The treatment of complete prolapse of the rectum by the Roscoe Graham operation. British Journal of Surgery 45: 323

Greca F, Hares M M, Nevah E, Alexander-Williams J, Keighley M R B 1981 A randomised trial to compare rubber band ligation with Phenol injection for treatment of haemorrhoids. British Journal of Surgery 68: 250

Hawley P R 1973 Haemorrhoids. In: Taylor S (ed) Recent advances in surgery 8th edn. Churchill Livingstone, Edinburgh p 244

Hawley P R 1978 Common anal conditions. In: Hadfield J, Hobsley M (eds) Current surgical practice, Vol. 2. Arnold, London, p 108

Jackaman F R, Francis J N, Hopkinson B R 1980 Silicone rubber band treatment of rectal prolapse. Annals of the Royal College of Surgeons of England 62: 386

Kaufman H D 1977 Haemorrhoids—an 'out-patient package'. Journal of the Royal College of Surgeons of Edinburgh 23: 40

Keighley M R B, Fielding J W, Alexander-Williams J 1983 Results of Marlex mesh abdominal rectopexy for rectal prolapse in 100 consecutive patients. British Journal of Surgery 70: 229

Lock M R, Thomson J P S 1977 Fissure in ano: The initial management and prognosis. British Journal of Surgery 64: 355

Lord P H, Millar D M 1965 Pilonidal sinus: A simple treatment. British Journal of Surgery 52: 298

Lord P H 1969 A day case procedure for the cure of third degree haemorrhoids. British Journal of Surgery 56: 747

Macfie J, Harvey J 1977 The treatment of acute superficial abscesses: A prospective clinical trial. British Journal of Surgery 64: 264

Madden J L, Kandalaft S I 1983 Electocoagulation as a primary curative method in the treatment of carcinoma of the rectum. Surgery Gynaecology and Obstetrics 157: 164

Madden M V, Elliot M S, Botha J B C, Louw J H 1981 The management of anal carcinoma. British Journal of Surgery 68: 287

Mansoory A, Dickson D 1982 Z-plasty for treatment of disease of the pilonidal sinus: Surgery Gynaecology and Obstetrics 155: 409

Marks C G, Ritchie J K 1977 Anal fistulas at St Mark's Hospital. British Journal of Surgery 64: 84

Morgan C N, Porter N H, Klugman D J 1972 Ivalon (polyvinyl alcohol) sponge in the repair of complete rectal prolapse. British Journal of Surgery 59: 841

Morson B C, Dawson I M P 1979 Gastro-intestinal pathology, 2nd edn. Blackwell, Oxford, p 741

Nielsen O V, Jensen S L 1981 Basal cell carcinoma of the anus—a clinical study of 34 cases. British Journal of Surgery 68: 856

Nixon H H 1978 Surgical conditions in paediatrics. Butterworth & Co, London, p 93

Parks A G, Percy J P 1982 Resection and sutured colo-anal anastomosis for rectal carcinoma. British Journal of Surgery 69: 301

Rainsbury R M, Southam J A 1982 Radical surgery for pilonidal sinus. Annals of the Royal College of Surgeons of England 64: 339

Rehbein F 1959 Operation for anal and rectal atresia with recto-urethral fistula. Chirurgia 30: 417 (Year book medical publishers, Chicago)

Ross A H M 1980 Rectal stricture resection using the EEA auto stapler. British Journal of Surgery 67: 281

Smith M 1967 Early operation for acute haemorrhoids. British Journal of Surgery 54: 141

Stephens F D, Smith E D (eds) 1971 Anorectal malformations in children, Year book medical publishers, Chicago

Stone H B 1926 Pruritus ani, treatment by alcohol injection. Surgery Gynaecology and Obstetrics 42: 565

Thomson W H F 1975 The nature of haemorrhoids. British Journal of Surgery 62: 542

Vellacott K D, Amar S S, Hardcastle J D 1982 Comparison of rigid and flexible fibreoptic sigmoidoscopy with double contrast barium enemas. British Journal of Surgery 69: 399

Wells C 1959 New operation for rectal prolapse. Proceedings Royal Society Medicine 52: 602

Wilson D H 1964 The late results of anorectal abscesses treated by incision, curettage and primary suture under antibiotic cover. British Journal of Surgery 51: 328

Wood R A B, Hughes L E 1975 Silicone foam sponge for pilonidal sinus: A new technique for dressing open granulating wounds. British Medical Journal 3: 131

Wyatt A P 1981 Perineal rectopexy for rectal prolapse. British Journal of Surgery 68: 717

FURTHER READING

Goligher J C 1985 Surgery of the anus, rectum and colon, 5th edn. Bailliere Tindall, London

Parks A G, Gordon P H, Hardcastle J D 1976 A classification of fistula in ano. British Journal of Surgery 63: 1

Parks A G, Stitz R W 1976 The treatment of high fistula in ano: Diseases of the colon and rectum 19: 487

24
Operations for hernia

J. M. S. JOHNSTONE & R. F. RINTOUL

OBLIQUE INGUINAL HERNIA

Anatomy

The inguinal canal, which is about 4 cm in length, runs obliquely between the muscles, aponeuroses and fasciae of the abdominal wall above the medial part of the inguinal ligament. Its internal end is the *deep inguinal ring*, an opening in the transversalis fascia 1 cm above the midinguinal point, and immediately lateral to the inferior epigastric vessels. Its external end is the *superficial inguinal ring*, a triangular aperture in the aponeurosis of external oblique situated immediately above the pubic tubercle. The base of the ring is formed by the inguinal ligament; its margins (*crura*) are sewn together at the apex, which points laterally and upwards, by the *intercrural fibres*.

Boundaries. The *anterior wall* is formed in its whole length, by the aponeurosis of external oblique, and in its lateral third by the lowest fibres of internal oblique arising from the inguinal ligament. The *posterior wall* is formed in its whole length by the transversalis fascia, and in its medial half by the conjoined tendon. The *roof* is formed by the lower borders of internal oblique and transversus, which arch over the canal before fusing together to form the conjoined tendon. The *floor* is the grooved upper surface of the inguinal ligament, and of its reflection on to the superior ramus of the pubis.

Contents. In the male, the main contents of the canal are the *spermatic cord* and the vestigial remnant of the *processus vaginalis*, the fetal prolongation of peritoneum which accompanies the testis in its descent into the scrotum. In the female, the canal transmits the *ligamentum teres uteri* (*round ligament*). The *ilio-inguinal nerve* lies in the medial part of the canal and emerges through the superficial ring. The *iliohypogastric nerve*, which is not strictly a content of the canal, but which is displayed when the canal is opened, lies on the front of internal oblique a little above its lower border.

The spermatic cord consists of the vas deferens with its artery, the testicular artery, the pampiniform plexus of veins (its bulkiest constituent), lymph vessels and sympathetic nerves. The cord has three *coverings*: (1) the internal spermatic fascia derived from fascia transversalis at the deep ring, (2) the cremasteric muscle and fascia derived from internal oblique, and (3) the external spermatic fascia derived from external oblique aponeurois at the superficial ring.

Oblique inguinal hernia

The *sac*, or peritoneal tube through which the abdominal contents protrude, accompanies the spermatic cord in its oblique course, and is enclosed within its coverings usually lying anterior to the structures of the cord proper. The neck of the sac, which is often constricted, lies at the deep inguinal ring, lateral to the inferior epigastric vessels. The *coverings* of the sac, from within outwards, are those of the cord *plus* deep fascia, superficial fascia and skin.

Aetiology and types of sac. It has long been taught that, even in the adult, most oblique inguinal herniae are of congenital origin, the sac being formed by the processus vaginalis, which either wholly or in part has failed to become obliterated, and that, although the sac is present from birth, the hernia may not appear until adult life. The sac is usually of the *funicular* type, terminating below in a blind end or *fundus*: this is attributed to the fact that only the upper part of the processus has remained open, while the rest has become obliterated. The evidence in favour of such a congenital origin for adult herniae is not, however, convincing, and many surgeons now believe that most of these herniae are acquired, the sac being formed as a true protusion of the parietal peritoneum through the inguinal canal. In support of this belief, there is the important finding that when operation for oblique inguinal hernia is followed by a recurrence, the sac is noted in over 75% of cases to be again an oblique one; this proves conclusively that an oblique hernia *can* be acquired. In infants and young children there is no doubt that the hernia is congenital: in males the entire processus vaginalis may have remained patent, in which case the sac is of the *vaginal* type, extending down to the testis to become continuous with the tunica vaginalis; in females the sac is necessarily funicular, being developed from a blind process of peritoneum accompanying the round ligament.

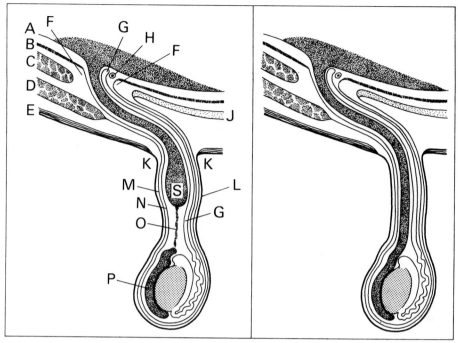

Fig. 24.1   **Fig. 24.2**

Figs. 24.1 & 24.2 Schematic drawing to show the relations and coverings of an oblique inguinal hernia; also the two common types of sac—*funicular* in Figure 24.1, *vaginal* in Figure 24.2. A—peritoneum; B—transversalis fascia; C—transversus; D—internal oblique; E—external oblique; F—margins of deep ring; G—vas deferens; H—inf. epigastric art.; J—conjoined tendon; K—margins of superf. ring; L—ext. spermatic fascia; M—cremasteric fascia; N—int. spermatic fascia; O—processus vaginalis; P—tunica vaginalis; S—sac

Selection of patients

Oblique inguinal hernia should as a rule be treated by operation. This advice is given in spite of the fact that, in many surgeon's hands, the end-results of surgical treatment are disappointing, in that the recurrence rate is in the region of 10–15%. This is to a large extent avoidable if a careful technique is followed, despite the fact that the inguinal canal has to be left open in order to transmit the spermatic cord. The aim should be to have a recurrent rate of around 1% (Devlin, 1979).

The smaller the hernia, and the shorter its duration, the more certain are the prospects of operative cure. Surgical intervention should be advised therefore even although the hernia is small and is causing no symptoms, for there is an invariable tendency for it to increase in size and for symptoms to develop. With modern anaesthesia (local, regional or general) there are few contraindications to operation. In general, a truss should be prescribed only when the patient refuses surgery; it is at best an unpleasant encumbrance, and its use for any length of time causes pressure atrophy of the muscles around the hernial orifice, thus reducing the chances of a successful operation, should this be desired at a later date. Whether a truss is worn or not (for there are few

trusses which do not slip occasionally and allow the hernia to protrude), the danger of strangulation is always present, and is one of the most cogent arguments in favour of operation. This danger is greatest when the orifice is narrow, or when the hernia is partly irreducible. If there have been temporary attacks of incarceration, or of threatened strangulation, operation should not be delayed.

Preparation for operation

If the patient is to have an elective operation, the arrangement should allow this to be done when his general health is at its optimum. Any chest affliction should be treated, if necessary, by physiotherapy or operation postponed until the season of the year when his respiratory function is at its best. This will minimise postoperative problems and reduce the strain placed on the repair by an explosive cough. The general considerations outlined on pages 309 and 310 also apply.

Choice of operation

While there is almost universal agreement as to the advisability of surgery, there is a considerable divergence of opinion regarding the best method of operative repair.

In the truly congenital herniae of infancy or childhood, where a preformed sac is undoubtedly present, removal of the sac alone—*simple herniotomy*—is all that is required. In adult cases of hernia the same operation may be considered adequate by those surgeons who believe that the aetiological concept of a congenitally preformed sac applies. Its use should be restricted, however, to younger patients, in whom the deep ring is unstretched and the musculature of the canal appears to be sound. It is probable that the majority of surgeons at the present time prefer to carry out some form of reconstructive operation in *all* adult cases. Thus, in patients over the age of 16 years, the operation has two parts: (1) removal of the sac, (2) repair of the defect.

Inguinal herniotomy in children

Inguinal herniae in children are of congenital origin and associated with a patent processus vaginalis which extends partly or completely along the spermatic cord in boys and the round ligament in girls. Such herniae are common, the incidence being 10 per 1000 live births. Boys are affected 10 times more frequently than girls and, in approximately 1 in 5 of such children, the condition is bilateral.

The presenting sign is that of an intermittent or persistant swelling which appears over the pubic tubercle and may extend down towards the scrotum. The swelling, if present, can be reduced with a characteristic gurgling sensation. Alternatively, thickening of the spermatic cord can be felt when the cord is under light traction and rolled between finger and thumb. A hernia which appears in early infancy is at risk of becoming strangulated and operation should be carried out as soon as possible.

Operation

Inguinal herniotomy is a safe and effective operation which can, under normal circumstances, be performed as a day case procedure. In most children under 7 years of age the internal inguinal ring lies deep to the external ring and the foreshortened inguinal canal can be explored without opening the external oblique aponeurosis.

A skin crease incison 2–3 cm in length is made just above the pubic tubercle (Fig. 24.3) and the superficial and deep abdominal fascia divided. The external spermatic fascia is then split in the line of the cord, exposing the bluish coverings of the cord. Using blunt dissecting forceps, both the spermatic cord and testis are cleared of adherent tissue and delivered through the wound (Fig. 24.4). With the cord under light traction the coverings over the proximal half are divided longitudinally. In order to secure the correct plane, it is helpful to make a small incision over a spermatic vein so that the vessel stands proud when the opening is complete; the incision can then be extended with ease (Fig. 24.5). The cut

Figs. 24.3–24.6 *Inguinal herniotomy in children.*

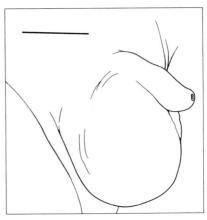

Fig. 24.3 Skin crease incision above pubic tubercle

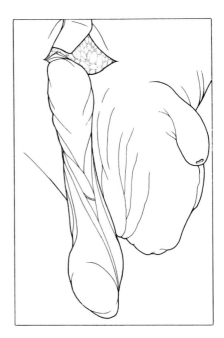

Fig. 24.4 Cord and testis delivered through wound

edges of the cord coverings are gripped with forceps and held aside so as to expose the content of the cord. The hernial sac, which may have an opaque appearance, will be found lying in front of the vas deferens and the testicular vessels (Fig. 24.6).

When the processus vaginalis is complete the hernial sac is lifted at a point in the proximal part of the cord and cleared circumferentially of adherent tissue, particular care being taken with the closely adherent vas and vessels. Artery forceps can then be placed across the hernial sac. The sac is divided distal to the forceps and the open fundus left in situ. With gentle traction on the for-

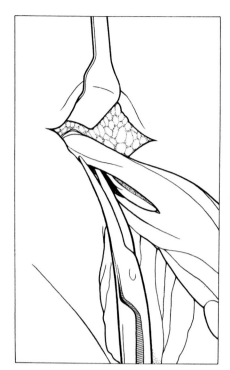

Fig. 24.5 Coverings incised over a spermatic vein which bulges out

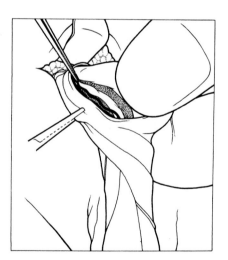

Fig. 24.6 Sac cleared circumferentially and vas and vessels lying underneath

ceps, the proximal part of the sac is traced towards the inguinal ring. The dissection is complete when the neck of the sac is reached as indicated by the presence of extraperitoneal fat. The sac is twisted to exclude intra-peritoneal content (Fig. 24.7), the neck of the sac is ligated and the sac distal to the neck excised. When the processus vaginalis is incomplete the fundus of the sac

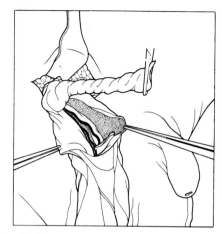

Fig. 24.7 Divided sac traced proximally and twisted

will be seen and the dissection started from that point. It is important that the testis be replaced and manipu-lated well down into the scrotum and the alignment of the spermatic vessels checked to exclude torsion. The wound is then closed with a single absorbable suture in the deep fascia and a subcuticular absorbable skin suture. The treatment of imperfect descent of the testis associ-ated with hernia is discussed on pages 624–628.

Inguinal herniotomy prior to reconstruction

Technique
The classical incision is made 2.5 cm above and parallel to the medial three-fifths of the inguinal ligament, but a more horizontally placed skin-crease incision will be found to produce a more acceptable scar. The superficial epigastric and superficial external pudendal vessels are secured. The incision is deepened until the aponeurosis of external oblique is exposed, and the superficial inguinal ring, through which the cord emerges, is ident-ified. (At this stage in the operation, it is advisable to check for the presence of a femoral hernia emerging below the inguinal ligament.) The external oblique apo-neurosis is divided in the line of its fibres, the incision being placed so that it opens into the ring in its upper medial part if a satisfactory overlapping is to be achieved later in the operation. Forceps are applied to the two cut edges; the upper leaf is retracted to expose the conjoined muscles arching over the cord, and the lower to expose the upper surface of the inguinal ligament. The ilio-inguinal and iliohypogastric nerves are identified and safeguarded. The cord, with which is included the her-nial sac, is lifted up from the medial part of the incision, and is spread out on the finger. Its coverings are incised longitudinally, and are further separated by blunt dis-section, care being taken to avoid injuring the spermatic veins. If the hernia is recent and is completely reducible,

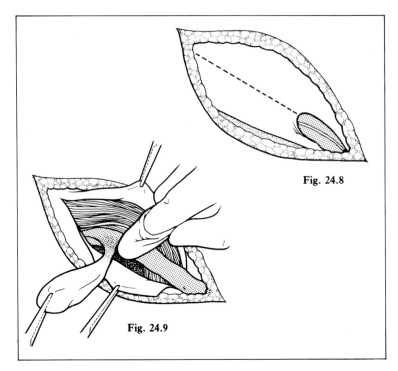

Figs. 24.8 & 24.9 Simple herniotomy for oblique inguinal hernia. Line of incision in external oblique aponeurosis, and separation of the sac by gauze dissection

recognition of the sac may be a matter of some difficulty. It appears as a pearly-white structure, lying as a rule anterior to the components of the cord proper. In adults it is almost invariably of the *funicular* type, and is more easily isolated if its fundus, the crescentic border of which lies transversely across the cord, is defined first and is held in artery forceps. Further separation of the sac is then effected by gauze stripping. Care must be taken that the vas deferens, which is palpable as a firm cord, is not detached along with the sac in the process of stripping. As the separation proceeds, traction is applied to the sac and the stripping is continued until the neck comes into view. This is identified from the presence of an adherent pad or collar of fat. The inferior epigastric vessels lie to its medial side, and care should be taken that they are not injured. When separation is complete the sac is opened at some distance from its neck, and a finger is introduced into its interior to ensure that it is empty of contents. In general it is better that the sac should be completely separated before it is opened, for otherwise during the process of separation, the opening may become extended as a split proximally beyond the neck of the sac—a complication to be avoided if possible. When, however, the sac is very adherent, it can often be more easily separated if it is opened and a finger introduced at an early stage. Glassow (1973, 1976),

with an experience of 50 000 such herniae, stresses the importance of freeing the sac right up to the deep ring. Adherent contents are freed from the sac and returned to the abdomen.

The sac is now drawn strongly downwards, and a transfixion ligature is applied immediately above its neck. When the neck is wide, care must be taken that underlying bowel is not transfixed or caught up in the ligature. In such cases it is an advantage to twist the sac at its neck, in order to occlude it before the ligature is applied. The sac is amputated 1 cm below the ligature *prior* to cutting the ligature so that there is adequate control of the stump in the event of bleeding. If the ligature has been applied at a sufficiently high level, the stump will immediately retract well above the deep inguinal ring to lie flush with the general peritoneum.

In the case of *scrotal* herniae, where the fundus of the sac may not come easily into view, there is no objection to leaving the distal part of the sac in situ. The sac is first separated for a short distance from the cord structures, and is then divided transversely. The distal part is dropped back, while the proximal part is cleared up to its neck and removed in the usual way. This method obviates the dissection required to deliver the sac from the depths of the scrotum, and greatly reduces the risk of subsequent haematoma formation.

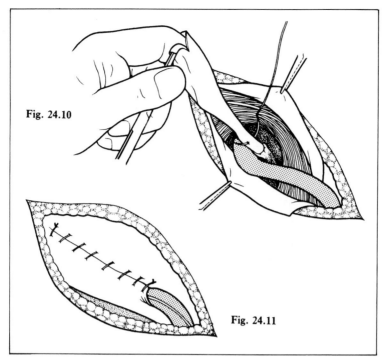

Figs. 24.10 & 24.11 Simple herniotomy for oblique inguinal hernia. Transfixion-ligature of the sac as its neck, and repair of external oblique aponeurosis

Reconstructive procedures

The Bassini method of repair

This classical operation was first described by Bassini in 1888. Although it has been frequently criticised, it may be said to have stood the test of time, and has probably cured more inguinal herniae than has any other method. It consists essentially in strengthening the posterior wall of the inguinal canal in its lateral part, by stitching the lower border of the conjoined muscles and tendon down to the inguinal ligament *behind the cord*.

After the sac has been removed, the cord together with the ilio-inguinal nerve, is held out of the way by drawing the lower leaf of the external oblique aponeurosis downwards superficial to it (Fig. 24.12). The lower border of the conjoined muscles and tendon and the upper surface of the inguinal ligament are carefully cleared of fat and areolar tissue. The muscles and tendons are lifted forwards with dissecting forceps and five or six stitches are inserted at about 1 cm intervals between them and the inguinal ligament. The most lateral suture is inserted first, picking up tissue at the margins of the deep ring and narrowing the ring around the emerging cord. In placing these initial stitches, great care must be taken not to injure the external iliac vessels which lie immediately deep to the inguinal ligament. To avoid such an accident the actual ligament alone should be lifted forwards on the point of the needle, before the stitch is passed. The most medial suture is placed under the periosteum overlying the pubic tubercle. All stitches should be introduced at different depths into the inguinal ligament, in order that they may not cause splitting of the ligament along the line of sutures.

It is particularly important that the stitches should not be tied too tightly or they will cause strangulation of the muscular fibres, which then become replaced by weak scar tissue. Care must be taken that the iliohypogastric nerve is not included in any suture. The conjoined muscles should lie snugly around the cord in the lateral part of the wound, thus giving support to the deep inguinal ring. In the approximation of the muscles to the inguinal ligament, *it is essential that there should be no tension on the sutures*, for this may determine the failure of the operation. If the approximation cannot be made without tension, the case is unsuitable for simple Bassini repair, and some other method of reconstruction should be considered.

Finally, the cord is allowed to fall back on the strengthened posterior wall of the canal. The aponeurosis of external oblique is repaired, either by simple suture, or preferably by overlapping (Figs 24.14 and 24.15). The reconstituted superficial ring should fit snugly around the cord, but it must not be too tight or atrophy of the testis may result; it should admit the tip of the little finger

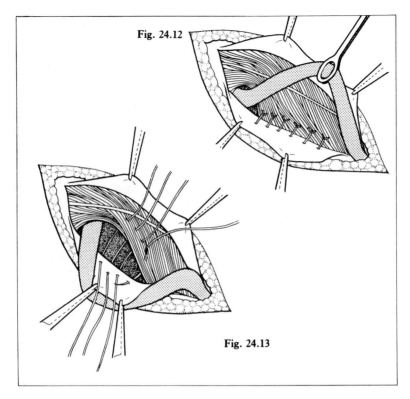

Figs. 24.12 & 24.13 The Bassini method of repair in inguinal hernia—approximation of the conjoined muscles and tendon to the inguinal ligament, behind the spermatic cord; this is held out of the way, under cover of the lower flap of external oblique

without difficulty, in addition to the cord. After careful haemostasis the wound is closed by suture of the superficial fascia and skin.

Suture material. The type of suture material to be used is a matter of choice, and many conflicting views have been expressed. Dexon, nylon, linen and silk thread, and stainless steel and tantalum wire have all been advocated, but the results have not determined the superiority of any one method. The choice must therefore depend upon individual preference.

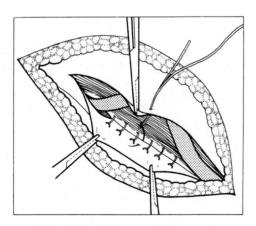

Fig. 24.14 Inguinal herniorrhaphy—third stage. The upper leaf of the external oblique aponeurosis is mobilized and drawn down *in front of the cord* to be stitched to the deep surface of the inguinal ligament

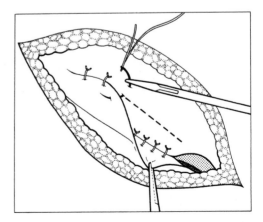

Fig. 24.15 Inguinal herniorrhaphy—fourth stage. The lower leaf of the external oblique is stitched against the upper leaf thus overlapping it, so that a strong anterior wall to the canal is constructed

Modifications of the Bassini repair and alternative methods
Most other methods of inguinal herniorrhaphy are based essentially upon the Bassini operation, but are designed to avoid such tension as may be inseparable from this method. In general they serve to occlude the gap between the conjoined muscles and the inguinal ligament, by methods other than that of simply stitching these structures together.

The Shouldice operation. The essential steps in this method of repair of the posterior wall are (1) double breasting of fascia transversalis in order to tighten and narrow the deep ring, (2) approximation of conjoined tendon to inguinal ligament in two layers. The operation depends on removal of the cremaster muscle from that portion of spermatic cord which lies within the inguinal canal so that clear identification can be made of transversalis fascia as it is reflected on to the cord at the deep ring.

Relaxation incisions, designed to relieve tension at a Bassini repair, may be made either before or after the repair has been carried out. In the 'muscle-slide' operation described by Tanner (1942) the upper leaf of the external oblique aponeurosis is elevated and retracted upwards, so that a curved incision can be made in the aponeuroses of the internal oblique and transversus where they form the anterior rectus sheath. This incision begins over the pubic crest, passes vertically upwards about 4 cm from the mid line, and then turns laterally to end 2 cm from the lateral border of the rectus muscle a handsbreadth above the pubis. The lateral leaf of this incision at once retracts downwards owing to the tone of the conjoined muscles, which are now found to lie without tension alongside the inguinal ligament (Fig. 24.17).

Repair by nylon darn A monofilament nylon suture has inherent strength and produces no tissue reaction. The advantage of a nylon darn lies in the continuous suture which does not result in any localised areas of tension. The posterior wall is repaired in two layers with particular care to support the deep ring.

Repair by fascial suture. This method of suture, introduced by Gallie in 1924, need no longer be used, unless modern sutures are unavailable. Strips of fascia are obtained from the lateral aspect of the thigh and threaded on to a special fascial needle.

Repair by skin ribbon suture. This method, described by Gosset (1949), consists in the use of a long strip of skin as suture material. The customary incision is made, and one extremity of this is rounded by excision of a tiny segment of skin (Fig. 24.18). A strip of skin, 0.5 cm wide, is then cut from the entire margin of the wound, continuous around one end (the rounded one), so that its total length equals twice that of the wound (Fig. 24.19). The skin ribbon is threaded on a Gallie's needle, and is used to approximate the margins of the defect, or (if tension is present) to construct a lattice-work or 'darn'. Since a skin ribbon, employed as suture material, is made to pass through the tissues at some distance from the defect, a very good hold is obtained, and the repair does not depend for its strength upon surrounding stitches of foreign material. Sebaceous glands and hair follicles completely disappear and there is no tendency for the ribbon to become infected. When such a suture is used in the repair of a large incisional hernia, the incision can be prolonged indefinitely to provide a strip of adequate length, and the defect is not noticeable even when two or more strips have been taken. No complications attributable to the buried skin have been observed in over 300 cases of hernia treated by this method.

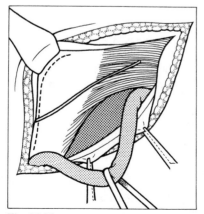
Fig. 24.16

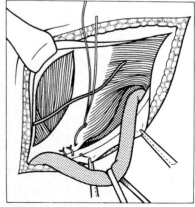
Fig. 24.17

Figs. 24.16 & 24.17 The 'muscle-slide' operation in inguinal herniorrhaphy. An incision is made in the aponeuroses of internal oblique and transversus near the medial border of the rectus muscle, where they form its anterior sheath. This relaxes the lower border of these muscles, which now lie alongside the inguinal ligament without tension (After Tanner.)

Figs. 24.18 & 24.19 *Method of preparing skin ribbon suture*

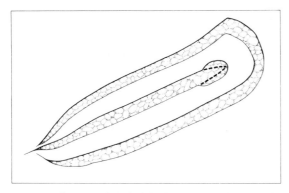

Fig. 24.18 One end of the incision is rounded and a strip of skin is outlined with a scalpel

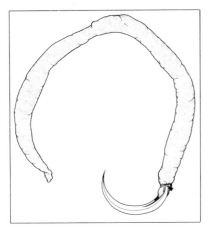

Fig. 24.19 Skin strip threaded on a Gallie's needle

Implantation of foreign material Gauzes or meshes made of tantalum wire or nylon, or materials such as polyvinyl alcohol sponge or marlex mesh, have been implanted with success in cases where there is a large defect as in a recurrent hernia.

Overlapping of the external oblique aponeurosis
In the author's opinion this is a most important part of any operation for inguinal hernia. The strength of the inguinal canal lies in its obliquity, and for this a strong external oblique is indispensable (Fig. 24.20). In nearly all inguinal herniae the external oblique aponeurosis is weak and bulging over the greater part of the canal, the degree of weakness being directly proportional to the size of the protrusion. It is not enough to narrow the deep ring and to strengthen the posterior wall of the canal, for the hernia will recur if the deep ring lacks the support

which it can derive from a strong anterior wall to the canal. This can readily be provided by overlapping the external oblique oponeurosis *in front of the cord* (Figs 24.14 and 24.15). Since the aponeurosis is invariably lax, the overlapping can be effected with ease and without any undue tension.

Preperitoneal approach
This method of approach to inguinal herniae has been advocated by certain workers, notably in America. The incision is made through the muscles *above* the inguinal canal; it is deepened as far as the peritoneum, and it is in this plane that the hernia is approached. The sac is identified at its neck, i.e. where it enters the canal, and is withdrawn inwards before being removed. The posterior wall of the canal is then repaired by stitching the aponeurosis of transversus to the deep surface of the inguinal ligament.

The operation is more difficult and more time-consuming than the standard approach through the inguinal canal. It does not allow any reconstruction of the anterior wall of the canal, and this, in the author's opinion, is an important factor in preventing recurrence.

After-treatment
Surgeons who believe in the benefits of early ambulation (p. 325) may allow their patients to get up within a few hours of operation, or may even operate on them as out-patients (Farquharson, 1955; Ruckley, 1978). It seems certain that there is nothing to be gained in the average case of inguinal hernia by postoperative rest in bed. Unrestricted mobilisation should be encouraged but the patient should refrain from heavy lifting for two to three months depending on his occupation.

Operation in the female
The inguinal canal is opened as in the male. The sac is separated from the round ligament and is amputated at its neck. Should the separation prove difficult the ligament may be removed along with the sac. If the inguinal canal is weak it is completely obliterated with sutures, the round ligament being disregarded.

DIRECT INGUINAL HERNIA

Anatomy
A direct inguinal hernia traverses only the medial part of the inguinal canal, and does not, therefore, pursue the oblique course taken by the spermatic cord. It protrudes

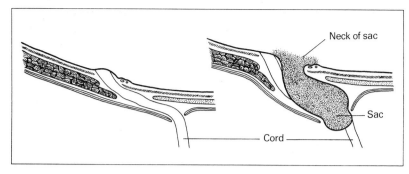

Figs. 24.20 Obliquity of the inguinal canal—one of the most important factors in its strength—requires a strong anterior wall as well as a strong posterior wall. Unless the external oblique is repaired strongly *in its normal relationship to the cord*, much of this obliquity is lost, and recurrent herniation is more liable to take place

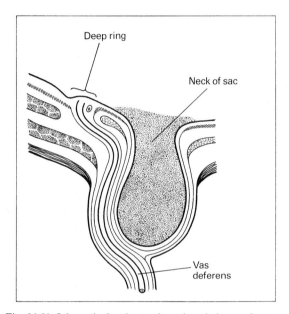

Fig. 24.21 Schematic drawing to show the relations and coverings of a *direct* inguinal hernia

from the abdominal cavity through the inguinal triangle (triangle of Hesselbach), which is bounded medially by the rectus muscle, laterally by the inferior epigastric vessels, and below by the inguinal ligament. It passes forwards, either below the arch of the conjoined muscles or through a weak area in the conjoined tendon, and finally emerges through the superficial inguinal ring. It seldom descends completely into the scrotum, but exceptions occur.

The sac, which is often wider at its neck than at its fundus, and which may be no more than a bulging of the peritoneum, is usually found lying posterior to the spermatic cord. Its coverings are the same as in oblique hernia, except that the covering it receives from transversalis fascia is not derived from the margins of the deep ring.

If the sac passes through a weak area in the conjoined tendon, it receives a fascial covering from this structure instead of from internal oblique.

Selection of patients

Direct inguinal hernia occurs most commonly in patients of the obese or flabby type, or in those of asthenic build with poor muscular development or a chronic cough. It differs from oblique hernia in that it is never congenital, and in the fact that it invariably results from, or is associated with, weakness of the abdominal muscles—particularly those which form the conjoined tendon. Operative cure is, therefore, a matter of greater difficulty than in the oblique hernia and the key to success lies in a careful reconstructive operation.

Direct inguinal herniae, as compared with oblique herniae, do not show the same tendency to increase in size, and, since the sac is wide-necked, there is seldom any risk of strangulation. It is unnecessary, therefore, to advise operation where the hernia is small, symptomless, and showing no increase in size. An unsuccessful operation with recurrence increases the risk of strangulation since the resultant defect is smaller, and has more rigid margins, than the initial hernia.

Operation

An incision is made as for oblique inguinal hernia and the external oblique is divided. The sac is sought for behind the cord, and is easily separated from it. It is freed up to its neck by blunt dissection and by gauze stripping. This must be done gently, or the inferior epigastric vessels which lie to the lateral side of the neck may be wounded (Fig. 24.22). Care must be taken also not to injure the bladder which lies in the extraperitoneal fat at the medial side of the sac, and may be adherent to it. If there is difficulty in separating the sac, or if bleeding is caused, close proximity of the bladder should at once be suspected.

The sac is opened and any contents are returned to the

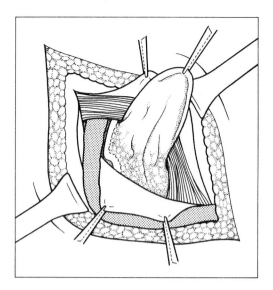

Fig. 24.22 Direct inguinal hernia—appearances at operation. Note the inferior epigastric artery lying lateral to the neck of the sac

abdomen. If it is a wide-necked one, it is impracticable to deal with it by the method of transfixion-ligature; it is better to cut away the redundant part, and to repair the peritoneum at its base by continuous suture as in laparotomy. If the patient is obese and access is difficult, this suture may be inserted in mattress fashion *before* cutting away the excess tissue. Additional coverings of the sac are dealt with in the same manner. When the sac is no more than a slight bulging of the peritoneum, it should be ignored, and the treatment directed solely towards repair of the muscular defect. The cord should be carefully examined to exclude the presence of an oblique sac which sometimes coexists. If such a sac is found it is dealt with in the usual manner, and any lipoma of the cord is removed in order to reduce cord bulk.

Reconstructive measures
Owing to weakness of the conjoined muscles, and to the large gap which is usually present between these and the inguinal ligament, a simple Bassini repair is unlikely to be successful. The choice of operation is largely a matter of individual preference. Probably the majority of surgeons at the present time will choose to repair the defect by 'darning' with some material such as monofilament nylon; if modern sutures are not available a strip of skin taken from the margins of the wound may be used (p. 487). If the defect is particularly large, marlex mesh or similar sheet of foreign material may be inserted.

When, as is frequently the case, the patient is an old or elderly man, with very poor muscles, no hesitation should be felt in removing the testis, since this allows complete obliteration of the inguinal canal to be carried out, and almost entirely obviates the risk of recurrence. In all cases where the advisability of orchidectomy might be considered, permission should if possible be obtained before operation.

SLIDING HERNIA

This condition may present both in indirect and in direct inguinal herniae. The term 'sliding' hernia denotes that some or all of the hernial contents lie *outside* the peritoneal sac. A part of the colon which is devoid of mesentery (the caecum on the right side and the pelvic colon on the left side), or a portion of the bladder, is found to be incorporated in the posterior wall of the sac, and is therefore not reducible in the ordinary way, owing to the fact that the sac forms part of its peritoneal coverings. If the condition is not recognized, and an attempt is made to clear the sac in the customary manner, the vessels of the colon or bladder are very liable to be torn. When the neck of the sac is unusually bulky, when it does not separate easily, or when bleeding is induced, a sliding hernia should at once be suspected.

Ordinary ligature and removal of the sac at its neck are impossible and the following method of repair has been recommended. A U-shaped incision is made in the peritoneum at a distance of about 2 cm from the bowel, so that a fringe of peritoneum remains on each side (Fig. 24.23), and is carried upwards beyond the neck of the sac. The bowel is then elevated; its retroperitoneal surface is covered by stitching together the peritoneal fringes on each side, and the gap in the posterior wall of the sac is closed by suture (Fig. 24.24). The bowel which has been freed from the sac and reperitonized is replaced within the abdominal cavity. The neck of the sac is closed securely by a purse-string suture and the rest of the sac cut away.

Many surgeons believe, however, that such elaborate methods are unnecessary, and are content with removing the free portion of the sac below the attached viscus. The peritoneum is then repaired and the whole is returned to the abdomen. Whatever method is adopted, special attention must be paid to a sound reconstruction of the canal, since this is always weak, and the chances of recurrence are considerable.

FEMORAL HERNIA

Anatomy
The femoral canal is the medial of the three compartments of the femoral sheath; this is formed by a prolongation into the thigh of the fascia transversalis and of the fascia iliaca, which line respectively the anterior and posterior

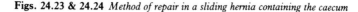

Figs. 24.23 & 24.24 *Method of repair in a sliding hernia containing the caecum*

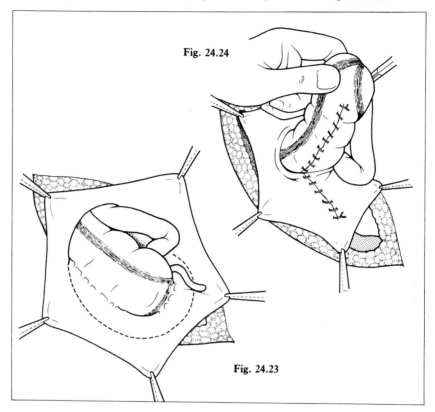

Fig. 24.23 Line of incision in peritoneum forming posterior wall of sac
Fig. 24.24 Caecum peritonised posteriorly and defect in sac sutured

abdominal walls. The lateral compartment of the sheath contains the femoral artery, and the intermediate one, the femoral vein. The femoral canal is about 2 cm in length, and is funnel-shaped. It lies on pectineus under cover of the cribriform fascia and the upper margin of the saphenous opening.

The femoral ring, which is the name given to the internal orifice of the canal, is relatively rigid. It is bounded anteriorly by the inguinal ligament and posteriorly by the pectineal line of the pubis. Laterally, it is related to the femoral vein, and medially to the free edge of the *lacunar ligament. The pectineal ligament* (of *Cooper*), a thickened band running along the pectineal line of the pubis, incorporated in its periosteum, forms an additional posterior boundary to the femoral ring. The ring is normally occluded by a pad of fatty tissue containing a lymph gland, and know as the femoral septum. The inferior epigastric artery crosses the upper lateral margin of the ring; a branch of this, constituting an *abnormal obturator artery*, may descend along the lateral (or less commonly medial) margin of the ring (McMinn, 1977) and is in danger of being wounded in an operation for strangulated femoral hernia.

Femoral hernia
The sac descends through the femoral canal, and turns forwards through the saphenous opening, the cribriform fascia, which covers the opening, being thinned-out in front of it. It may then turn upwards and laterally for a short distance in front of the inguinal ligament.

The *coverings* of the sac are (1) fat and lymphoid tissue derived from the femoral septum (2) transversalis fascia derived from the anterior wall of the canal, (3) cribriform fascia and (4) superficial fascia and skin.

Indication for operation
Femoral hernia occurs most commonly in women, especially those who have borne children. There are few contraindications to surgical intervention, and operative treatment should almost invariably be advised since, owing to the narrowness of the orifice, there is an ever-present danger of strangulation. The hernia may be approached either from below or from above the inguinal ligament.

The 'low' operation
This was for many years the standard operation, and in

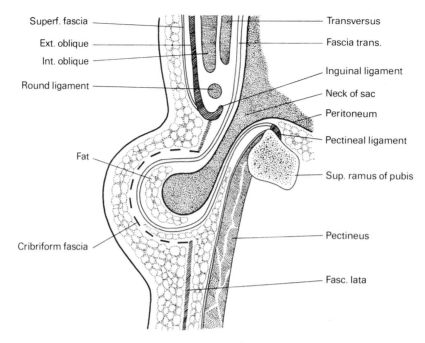

Fig. 24.25 Schematic drawing to show the relations and coverings of a femoral hernia

the writer's opinion, should still be regarded as the procedure of choice, unless strangulation is present.

Removal of the sac
The incision is made 1 cm below and parallel to the inguinal ligament. If the hernia is irreducible, it will present as a swelling which emerges through the saphenous opening. The actual sac is often surprisingly small. It is covered by the thinned-out cribriform fascia, and is deeply embedded in condensed fatty tissue; these structures must therefore be incised and separated before it can be isolated. It is freed by gauze dissection up to its neck, which is seen to emerge through the femoral canal, and is then opened at its fundus. Any contents are returned to the abdominal cavity; omentum is often adherent and requires to be separated, but if it is free at the neck the adherent part may be removed. When the neck of the sac is constricted by a tight femoral ring, so that the return of contents is difficult, the ring may be gently dilated by a finger passed upwards outside the sac. The neck of the sac is freed from the margins of the canal, if necessary by a few touches of the knife. It is drawn down so that it can be ligatured by transfixion at the highest possible point, and is cut off. The stump should then retract, or should be pushed upwards, well above the canal. Suture of the coverings over the stump helps to achieve this objective.

Closure of the canal?
It is held by some that this is an important part of the

operation, and that it can be done effectively only at the level of the femoral ring. The fact that the ring is inaccessible from the 'low' approach has been used as an argument against this operation. In cases where the canal is narrow, it will be effectively blocked by the remnants of the sac coverings sutured over the stump of the sac. When the femoral canal is wide and the inguinal ligament lax, it may be possible to place sutures between the pectineal ligament and inguinal ligament from below.

Alternatively, sutures may be inserted between the inguinal ligament and fascia over pectineus muscle, inserting *all* sutures before tying any (Fig. 24.28). Many surgeons are content with a still lesser procedure—merely to obliterate the space formerly occupied by the hernial protrusion, by two or three stitches which pick up the fasciae forming the floor and the lateral margin of the saphenous opening. Care must be taken not to injure the femoral vein, which lies immediately posterolateral to the saphenous opening; the vein should, therefore, be protected by a finger placed upon it while the stitches are being introduced.

The 'high' operation
This operation was first performed by Annandale in 1876, but is usually associated with the name of Lotheisen. It gives more generous access than does the 'low' approach, and is considered to be the better procedure when strangulation has occurred. It allows the sac to be dealt with more easily at its highest point, and provides direct access to the femoral ring, should it be desired to

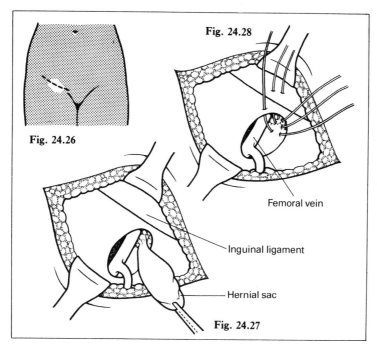

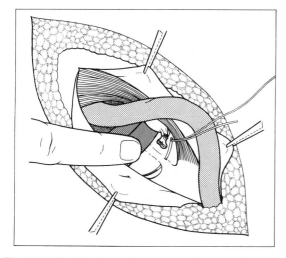

Figs. 24.26–24.28 The 'low' approach to a femoral hernia. Drawings to show the incision employed, the relationship of the sac to the inguinal ligament and saphenous opening, and the method of obliterating the femoral canal

Fig. 24.29 The 'high' operation for femoral hernia. The sac is exposed at its neck through an approach made above the inguinal ligament. It is drawn upwards through the canal and removed at its neck. The femoral ring is then obliterated by stitches which draw down either the inguinal ligament (as shown here), or the conjoined tendon, to the pectineal ligament, the femoral vein being protected by the finger

Method of approach

The incision is similar to that used for inguinal hernia, but it may be placed a little nearer to the inguinal ligament. The inguinal canal is opened by division of the external oblique aponeurosis; the cord or round ligament is displaced, and the conjoined muscles are drawn upwards. The transversalis fascia is divided in the line of the incision, care being taken to avoid injury to the inferior epigastric vessels which ascend from the mid-inguinal point. Extraperitoneal fat is wiped aside by gauze stripping until the sac can be seen entering the femoral canal. The bladder is sometimes adherent on the medial side, and must be carefully safeguarded. If the sac is empty and if it is not too adherent to its surroundings, it can often be withdrawn without difficulty from above, by gentle traction on a pair of forceps applied to its neck. If not, the lower margin of the wound is retracted, and the sac is isolated from below as in the 'low' operation; it is then opened at its fundus and any contents dealt with, after which it is manoeuvred upwards through the canal and is delivered above the inguinal ligament. Finally, the sac is removed flush with the general peritoneum.

Closure of the canal

The lower leaf of the external oblique aponeurosis is drawn downwards, and the deep surface of the inguinal ligament is cleared of fatty and areolar tissue. The femoral ring is now obliterated by stitching either the con-

attempt closure of this. Its main disadvantage is that it involves very wide opening (and therefore weakening) of the inguinal canal. It is an operation of greater magnitude than that required by the low approach, and in an elderly patient this is a point worthy of consideration.

joined tendon or the inguinal ligament down to the pectineal ligament. Two or at the most three sutures of unabsorbable material should be used. While the sutures are being placed the external iliac vein must be protected by the finger, and care should be taken that it is not compressed when they are tightened.

The inguinal canal is repaired in the usual way, care being taken to reconstruct the posterior wall where this has been weakened by the exposure.

McEvedy's approach

This approach, which was first described in 1950, has all the advantages of the transinguinal approach, and gives better access—but without weakening the inguinal canal.

In the original description of the operation (McEvedy, 1950), a vertical incision was employed, but an oblique incision, placed in a skin crease above the medial part of the inguinal ligament, gives equally good access and is now preferred. The anterior rectus sheath in its lower part is incised 2 cm medial to the *linea semilunaris*, and the rectus muscle is displaced towards the midline. The transversalis fascia is divided to expose the peritoneum, on which the inferior epigastric vessels are displayed as they run upwards on its surface (Fig. 24.30). The hernial sac is identified where it enters the femoral canal, and in most cases which are reducible can be drawn up without difficulty; it is then ligatured and removed. In irreducible or strangulated herniae, it is necessary first to clear the sac below the inguinal ligament, and, to enable this to be done, the lower margin of the wound is retracted strongly downwards; the sac is then opened at the fundus and its contents dealt with, after which it is withdrawn upwards through the canal. The femoral ring may now

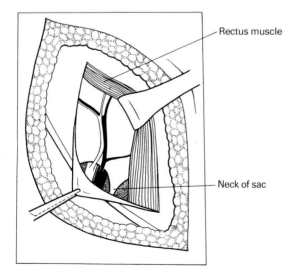

Fig. 24.30 McEvedy's approach to a femoral hernia. (For description, see text)

Rectus muscle

Neck of sac

be obliterated by one of the methods already described, after which the wound is repaired by allowing the rectus muscle to fall back into place, and by suture of its anterior sheath.

UMBILICAL HERNIA

Umbilical hernia in children

This is discussed with anomalies of the umbilicus on page 496.

Umbilical hernia in adults

This occurs most commonly in middle-aged or elderly women. The contributory causes are obesity and repeated child-bearing, which result in stretching and thinning-out of the linea alba, together with wide separation of the recti. The hernia normally occurs through a weak area in the linea alba either above or below the actual umbilicus, so that it is strictly *para-umbilical* in type. The deeper layers of the aponeurosis form a well-defined margin to the aperture, which is as a rule roughly circular in outline. The superficial layer becomes stretched out over the protruding peritoneal sac; since it stretches unevenly, it becomes split and forms fibrous septa, which cause the sac to be divided up into loculi. The fundus of the sac is often adherent to the skin of the umbilical cicatrix. The most frequent contents are portions of large and small intestine, together with omentum; these contents tend to become adherent both to the fundus of the sac and to each other.

Owing to the loculation of the sac and to the presence of adhesions the hernia is usually irreducible, and there is a very real danger of intestinal obstruction, with or without strangulation of the bowel—a complication in which the mortality may be high.

Even in reducible cases any form of belt or appliance is unlikely to be effective in controlling the hernia or in preventing its enlargement. Operation therefore should almost invariably be advised.

Preoperative treatment
Since many of the patients are in poor condition, careful preparation is essential. Gross obesity should be treated by dietetic measures. Cardiac and renal functions are investigated, and regular action of the bowels is secured. Careful skin preparation is especially important, for the crease below the protuberance is frequently ulcerated or infected.

Mayo's operation
In this operation, after the hernial sac and contents have been dealt with, the defective linea alba is repaired by overlapping across a transverse axis. This has definite advantages over any repair in a vertical line, since a sat-

isfactory degree of overlapping can be obtained without tension, and the sutures are subject to less strain in the postoperative period.

Treatment of the hernial sac and contents. A transverse elliptical incision is made enclosing the umbilicus and the skin covering the hernia. It should extend laterally on each side for at least 5 cm beyond the protuberance. It is deepened through the subcutaneous fat until the glistening surface of the aponeurosis is exposed. *The neck of the sac is generally free from adhesions, and should always be opened first.* To enable this to be done the aponeurosis is cleared centrally from all directions, until the neck of the hernia is exposed at the level where it emerges through the linea alba. A small incision is made in the fibrous coverings of the neck at any convenient point on its circumference, and is carefully deepened until the sac itself has been opened. A finger is now introduced and is passed round the inside of the sac to determine the presence of any adhesions. The remaining circumference of the neck of the sac is then divided with scissors, the finger being used to protect the contents from injury. The central 'island' comprising the sac together with the attached ellipse of skin and fat is now joined to the abdomen only by the contents passing into the sac. These contents are carefully examined. If they consist of omentum alone, this may at once be clamped and divided in small sections at a time, after which each segment of tissue is transfixed and ligatured. If, as is frequently the case, bowel is seen entering the sac, a finger is introduced

alongside, and is passed towards the fundus; a segment of the sac wall free from adhesions is sought for, and is opened up as far as possible. The sac is now gradually turned inside-out, so that the contents come freely into view, and can be gently peeled off its interior. Dense adhesions within the loculi of the sac are frequently present; their separation rarely presents much difficulty, but it must be carried out carefully and without undue haste. Adherent omentum may be removed along with the sac. Adhesions between adjacent coils of bowel—such as might give rise to subsequent obstruction—are separated as far as is practicable, and the hernial contents are returned to the abdominal cavity.

Repair of the abdominal wall. No attempt is made to separate the peritoneum from the margins of the defect in the linea alba, or to suture it as a separate layer unless this can be achieved with ease. The opening is enlarged laterally on each side by a transverse incision so that comfortable overlapping of the aponeurosis can be obtained. The recti are usually so widely separated that their sheaths are not normally opened. The two leaves of the aponeurosis together with the peritoneum are then sutured in the overlapping position, it being a matter of convenience which flap is placed anteriorly. The suture material used (nylon, silk, wire, etc.) will depend upon the surgeon's preference. For the first stage of the overlap a series of four or five mattress sutures is employed. These are introduced so that they will draw the free edge of one flap for a distance of 4 cm under cover of the other

Figs. 24.31 & 24.32 *Mayo's operation for umbilical hernia—treatment of the sac*

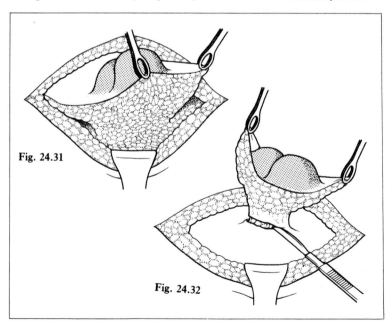

Fig. 24.31

Fig. 24.32

Fig. 24.31 Clearance of the aponeurosis centrally towards the neck of the sac
Fig. 24.32 Circular division of the neck of the sac and its fibrous covering

Figs. 24.33 & 24.34 *Mayo's operation for umbilical hernia—repair by overlapping*

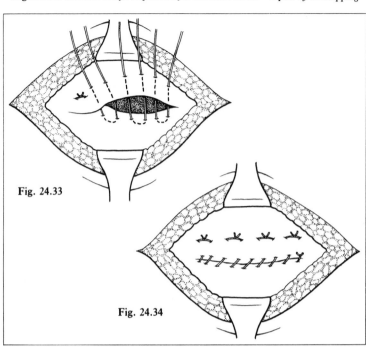

Fig. 24.33

Fig. 24.34

Fig. 24.33 Mattress sutures inserted to draw one flap under cover of the other
Fig. 24.34 Overlapping completed by suturing down free edge of superficial flap

flap. In order to promote more ready adhesion between the two flaps, the aponeurosis of the deeper flap is carefully cleared of all fatty tissue. The overlapping is then completed by suturing the free edge of the superficial flap against the deep flap. Details of the technique are shown in Figures 24.31 to 24.34. All dead space in the wound is obliterated by suture if possible. Open drainage should be avoided since it may predispose to infection, but the use of a vacuum drain (p. 2) for a large wound can be recommended.

After treatment. The method of transverse repair has the great advantage that it allows the patient to be nursed from the outset in the fully propped-up position. This not only brings about relaxation of the sutured aponeurosis but is also much more comfortable for the patient, who is often prone to cardiac or respiratory embarrassment.

ANOMALIES OF THE UMBILICUS IN CHILDREN

Umbilical hernia

This condition is relatively common and is due to incomplete closure of the umbilical ring. Since this process may continue during the first three or four years of life, it is possible that the condition will resolve spontaneously.

The hernia is seen as a forward protrusion of the umbilicus which becomes tense with straining and is easily reduced when the child is relaxed. A hernia that persists after three or four years should be treated by operation as the same condition in an adult may be complicated by strangulation or obstruction.

Operation
The operation is performed through a curved skin incision below and parallel to the inferior margin of the umbilicus (Fig. 24.35). The subcutaneous fat is divided to expose the linea alba and the medial margin of the rectus sheath on either side. The hernial sac protrudes through a circular opening in the midline towards the apex of the umbilicus and is covered by a condensation of fascia that is continuous with the linea alba. The junction of fascia and linea alba is defined and forceps passed round above the hernia to provide traction. The hernial sac rarely contains viscera but should, nevertheless, be opened with care. To achieve this, the fascia over the inferior half of the neck of the sac is first divided to expose the underlying peritoneum which is opened and the interior of the sac inspected. The neck of the sac is then transected leaving a circular defect in the linea alba and peritoneum which can be closed in one layer in a transverse manner with nonabsorbable sutures. To aid this, it is helpful to lift the margins of the defect with

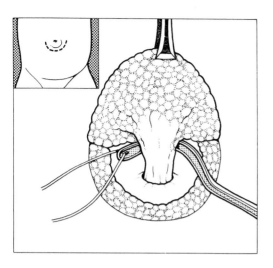

Fig. 31.35 Repair of umbilical hernia in an infant—isolation and ligature of neck of sac. *Inset* shows incision

forceps. During closure, the apex of the umbilicus should be fixed to the linea alba with a subcutaneous stitch and the skin edges then sewn together. For appearances sake the umbilicus should never be excised.

Exomphalos
This is a congenital abnormality in which viscera protrude through a defect in the abdominal wall into the base of the umbilical cord. The viscera are contained by a semi-transparent covering made up of amniotic membrane and peritoneum separated by Wharton's jelly. The umbilical cord is attached either to the apex or to the side of the lesion near the base. The condition is arbitrarily divided into minor and major depending on whether the defect is smaller or larger than 5 cm. The content of an exomphalos varies from a few coils of ileum to most of the abdominal viscera including liver, spleen, stomach, small bowel and colon. Malrotation is common (p. 426), remnants of the vitello-intestinal duct may persist (p. 498) and a diaphragmatic hernia may be present (p. 305). In two-thirds of babies there is an associated congenital abnormality. Of particular interest is the relationship between exomphalos, macroglossia and gigantism (EMG), the Beckwith Wiedman Syndrome.

The diagnosis of exomphalos is obvious at birth. There may be a history of maternal hydramnios and amniotic alpha fetoprotein may be raised (Brock, 1976). Surprisingly, the membranous covering is rarely ruptured during delivery. A baby with exomphalos should be carefully examined to exclude associated congenital anomalies. In the immediate management, a nasogastric tube is passed to empty the stomach and an intravenous infusion is started. The blood sugar should be monitored as hypoglycaemia is a feature of EMG.

Treatment
In the past, exomphalos has been successfully treated by painting the membranous sac with mercurochrome. An eschar forms which is later sloughed and the underlying granulation tissue is gradually epithelialised. The disadvantages of this method are that underlying visceral anomalies remain undetected and, because the process of epithelialisation is slow, the baby may remain in hospital for several months. However, the technique remains suitable for babies unfit for operation although antiseptics other than mercurochrome are used to avoid the danger of mercury poisoning.

Operation
Where possible an exomphalos should be treated by operation. The sac is excised with a circumferential incision at the junction of membrane and skin. The umbilical vessels and urachus are identified and ligated. After the bowel has been carefully inspected an attempt is made to return the viscera to the abdominal cavity. If successful, the defect in the abdominal wall is closed in two layers. However, a large lesion is not easily reduced and forcing prolapsed viscera back into a relatively small abdominal cavity may restrict respiration by splinting the diaphragm and impair venous return by pressure on the inferior vena cava. In this situation an attempt can be made to increase the capacity of the abdominal cavity by stretching the abdominal wall from within. Failing this a choice can be made between closing the defect in a single layer with the skin or a staged repair using a temporary prosthesis. In the former, skin flaps are generously mobilized over the abdominal wall and brought together in the midline in a single layer; an incisional hernia is inevitable and can be repaired if necessary at a later date. In the latter, a pouch of Dacron reinforced silastic sheet is sutured to the margin of the defect and after an interval of seven to ten days a further attempt is made at a formal two layer closure of the abdominal wall (Allen & Wrenn, 1969).

The postoperative care includes nasogastric suction and intravenous infusion until the baby feeds normally. When the defect has been closed with difficulty, ventilatory support may be needed for the first 24–48 hours. If delay in normal feeding is anticipated, feeding by the intravenous route should be started.

Gastroschisis
In many respects gastroschisis is similar to exomphalos and only the important differences need to be considered below.

In gastroschisis the gut is eviscerated through a defect in the abdominal wall immediately adjacent and usually to the right of the umbilicus but the bowel lies free as there is no covering membrane. The embryogenesis is uncertain; it may be similar to that of exomphalos but an alternative view is that the lateral ectodermal fold of the abdominal wall is unsupported by underlying meso-derm and breaks down. The prolapse is limited to mid-gut which is oedematous, often short and covered with a fibrinous exudate. A degree of malrotation is inevitable and adhesions may be present. Curiously the incidence of associated congenital anomalies is small. The diag-nosis, as with exomphalos, is obvious at birth.

Treatment

The immediate management is to place the lower half of the baby, including the lesion, in a polythene bag—the intestinal bag used in abdominal surgery is suitable. The bag serves to protect the bowel, limits fluid and heat loss and allows inspection of the abdominal wall. It may be necessary to support the viscera with moist packs to avoid drag on the mesenteric vessels. In the early man-agement a nasogastric tube is passed and plasma should be given intravenously to replace the loss of protein rich fluid from the exposed serosal surface. There is no alter-native but to treat gastroschisis by operation as there is no membranous covering, and it is an advantage if primary closure can be achieved (Filston, 1983).

Operation

The viscera are carefully examined before being returned to the abdominal cavity and loose matter is removed. The abdominal defect is relatively small and is normally extended by a longitudinal midline incision. Because there is often delay in gastric emptying in the postop-erative period some surgeons perform a gastrostomy. The technique of closure of the abdominal wall is the same as for exomphalos.

In the *postoperative management*, early oral feeding is often unsuccessful because of the oedematous condition of the bowel and intravenous feeding should be started.

Patent vitello-intestinal duct

Incomplete involution of the vitello-intestinal duct may result in a persistent fistulous communication between the distal ileum and umbilicus. The patent duct is seen as a mucosal lined opening at the umbilicus which may discharge small amounts of meconium and flatus. The duct itself is of little consequence but there is a danger of prolapse and of volvulus, and early operation is there-fore advisable. The prolapse of ileum through the duct may give the lesion a curious T-shaped or horned appearance.

Operation

The abdomen is opened through a 2 cm transverse incision lateral to the umbilicus. The umbilicus is excised in continuity with the duct, care being taken to identify and ligate the umbilical vessels and the urachus.

A short segment of ileum bearing the proximal end of the duct is then excised.

Urachus

A patent urachus may be suspected when there is a clear discharge from the umbilicus. A fleshy swelling may be present or the umbilicus may appear normal. Outlet obstruction of the bladder can co-exist and a cystogram is therefore performed, the contrast being introduced through a catheter inserted at the umbilicus.

Operation

A patent urachus should be closed by operation. The approach is similar to that used for a patent vitello-intestinal duct. The umbilicus is first mobilized with the urachus in continuity and the umbilical vessels ligated and divided. The urachus is traced to the fundus of the bladder where it is divided and the bladder repaired in two layers.

EPIGASTRIC HERNIA

This term is applied to herniae occurring in or near the mid line between the umbilicus and the xiphisternum. There is usually no more than a small protrusion of extraperitoneal fat through a defect in the linea alba, but a slender peritoneal sac may also be present.

Operation is indicated for the relief of local discomfort or of the 'dyspepsia' which is commonly present as a result of increased pressure within the hernia following a large meal.

A vertical or transverse incision is employed. The fatty protrusion, and sac if present, are ligatured and removed; the defect in the linea alba is then closed by simple suture or by overlapping.

INCISIONAL HERNIA

A hernia developing in the site of a previous operation occurs most commonly as the result of wound infection which has led to healing by weak scar tissue. Inadequate wound repair following abdominal surgery may also be responsible (Ellis, 1983). Other causes are injury at oper-ation to the nerves supplying the abdominal wall, and severe bouts of coughing in the postoperative period. Part of the abdominal wall, with the exception of skin, becom-es unable to support the intraperitoneal structures and this results in an abnormal protrusion or hernia. The peritoneal sac is often covered by little more than a thin layer of unhealthy skin.

Clinical types

Two distinct types of incisional hernia require to be considered for they present rather different problems in treatment.

In the first type, there is a wide defect in the aponeurotic or muscular layer of the abdominal wall with smooth and regular margins which are easily defined. The hernia takes the form of a diffuse bulge through the defect; it reduces spontaneously as soon as the patient lies down, and there appears to be no risk of strangulation. There is no urgency about operation except for the patient's comfort since an abdominal support may prove equally helpful. One of the considerations in advising operation is that there is adequate space within the reconstructed abdomen to accept the hernial contents and that the patient's breathing will not thereby be compromised.

In the second type of incisional hernia, conditions are different. The defect is often relatively small and irregular, and two or more such defects may be present in the same scar. The contents, which are normally both bowel and omentum, are matted together and are often adherent to a loculated peritoneal sac, so that the hernia is partially or wholly irreducible. The hazard lies in the narrow neck of the defect. No form of support is likely to be effective, and may increase the risk of strangulation, which is a particularly serious complication. Every effort should be made, therefore, to persuade such patients to accept surgery.

Operation

An elliptical incision is made enclosing the area of unhealthy skin, and is prolonged sufficiently to give adequate access. The outer edges are undercut, and are reflected beyond the limits of the hernial protuberance; since they are often adherent to the sac, the reflection must be carried out with great care. The incision is then deepened to the aponeurosis, and the dissection is continued inwards towards the margins of the defect. If the sac is no more than a redundancy of peritoneum, and if it is not too adherent to the skin, it may be possible to free it and to replace it unopened within the abdominal wall. More often, however, it is loculated and very adherent. It is then better to open it around its neck, and to free the contents by turning it inside out, in the manner described for umbilical hernia. Adherent omentum may be ligatured and removed along with the sac. Any adhesions involving bowel should be separated as far as practicable, before the hernial contents are returned to the abdomen.

The type of repair to be adopted depends on the size and situation of the hernia, and on the amount of scar tissue present. The following methods may be considered.

Anatomical restoration. This is the ideal method of repair, and is suited to small herniae where scarring is minimal. The edges of the defect are excised, and by careful dissection the surrounding abdominal wall is separated into its constituent layers—usually peritoneum, fleshy muscle and aponeurosis. Each layer is freed sufficiently to allow it to be sutured individually and without tension.

Closure of the defect using nylon. This method is applicable to any hernia where there are rigid margins capable of holding suture. It is important to use a continuous suture with bites in the abdominal wall up to 2.5 cm from the edges to be sutured so that a generous suture-length to wound-length ratio results. The suture must allow for the increase in wound length which results from abdominal distension and a suture length four times greater than the wound is advised (Jenkins, 1980).

Onlay graft of foreign material, such as tantalum gauze or polypropylene mesh (Drainer, 1972) may be used where the defect is large.

OBTURATOR HERNIA

Obturator hernia is very uncommon. It is encountered most frequently in elderly women who have lost weight. The herniation occurs through the obturator foramen—usually along the narrow canal traversed by the obturator vessels and nerve. Strangulation is therefore liable to ensue.

The abdominal approach

The condition is usually discovered only after laparotomy has been performed for intestinal obstruction, a coil of small bowel being found passing into the obturator foramen. In such circumstances the patient is tilted into the Trendelenburg position, and the general peritoneal cavity is carefully packed off in order to avoid contamination by toxic exudate escaping from the sac. It may be possible to extricate the imprisoned bowel by drawing it back into the general peritoneal cavity, but no more than the gentlest traction must be employed. If necessary the fibres of the obturator membrane which constrict the neck of the sac are carefully incised. The obturator vessels have no constant relationship to the sac, and are therefore liable to be injured in whatever direction the incision is made. After the bowel has been released the sac may be withdrawn into the abdomen and removed; if this presents any difficulty, it is sufficient to close its neck by suture.

The femoral approach must be employed if the bowel cannot be freed from the abdominal aspect, and it is the method of choice when the condition is diagnosed before operation. A vertical incision is made extending downwards from the inguinal ligament 2 cm medial to the femoral vessels. The adductor longus is retracted medially, and the fibres of the pectineus are separated or divided, so that the obturator externus is exposed. The sac is usually found lying on the surface of this muscle, having emerged at its upper border or between its fibres. The sac and contents are dealt with in the usual manner, and the space which was occupied by them is obliterated by suture.

STRANGULATED HERNIA

A hernia is said to be strangulated when the contents are constricted in such a way that interference with their blood supply results. When a loop of bowel is involved in the constriction, intestinal obstruction is also present—except possibly in the case of *Richter's hernia* (Fig. 24.36), where only part of the circumference of the gut is affected.

Preparation

Operations for strangulated hernia are among the most urgent in surgery. Not only is acute obstruction usually present, but the patient suffers from additional toxaemia due to absorption of toxic products arising from devitalisation of the imprisoned bowel. The high mortality in this condition results from failure to appreciate its potential seriousness and is clearly linked with the duration of symptoms (Andrews, 1981). Nevertheless, despite the urgency for operation, preoperative treatment should not be neglected (p. 420).

When there has been much vomiting, or when the patient is in poor condition, local anaesthesia may with advantage by employed. This occupies more time, but it causes less shock and reduces the risk of postoperative complications.

Operation

In general the operation is very similar to that described for non-strangulated cases, but certain important differences should be noted.

1. The hernial sac contains a varying quantity of dark-coloured fluid derived from devitalised bowel or omentum. When the vitality of bowel is seriously impaired this fluid is highly toxic and is swarming with organisms. If possible the sac should always be opened at its fundus and the fluid evacuated before the constriction is relieved, as otherwise there is a serious risk of contaminating the peritoneal cavity.

2. After the constriction has been divided, the hernial contents must be carefully examined before they are returned to the abdominal cavity. They should be drawn down well out of the wound, so that the constricted areas, which often sustain the greatest damage, can be inspected and healthy tissue identified beyond. Sometimes the contents slip back before the constriction has been divided, or even before the sac has been opened. In such cases it is essential that the affected parts should

be sought from within the peritoneal cavity and brought out for examination; fortunately they usually remain in the vicinity of the sac.

3. It should be remembered that the operation has been undertaken not to cure the hernia but to save life, and that its essential part has been completed as soon as the hernial contents have been returned to the abdomen. The defect in the abdominal wall is dealt with as effectively as possible, but the simpler methods only should be employed.

Viability of the bowel

When a loop of bowel has been damaged by the strangulation, the question of its viability must at once be decided. The damage may affect only localised areas of the bowel wall, either at the convexity of the loop or at the *constriction rings*, or it may involve the entire loop which has been imprisoned within the hernia.

The decision is one of supreme importance, especially if the circumference of the bowel is affected. The inexperienced surgeon is probably apt to decide too hastily that the damage is irreparable, and to proceed at once to resection and anastomosis. Even though the bowel is deeply congested and oedematous, with haemorrhages into its wall, and possibly with some loss of its normal lustre, it may still be capable of recovery. The affected loop should be covered with a hot moist towel, in order to stimulate any possible circulation within it, and the anaesthetist is asked to flood the lungs with oxygen. After an interval the bowel is carefully re-examined. Frequently the discoloration will be found to have become noticeably less, and there may be a return of the normal lustre. The stimulus of the heat applied may induce a peristaltic wave of contraction, and, if this can be seen to pass uninterruptedly along the damaged segment, it is irrefutable evidence of its viability. Such a contraction may be induced also by gentle flicking with the finger of the healthy bowel on the proximal side. If doubt still exists as to the viability of the loop, it is justifiable to wait for 4 to 5 minutes, applying fresh towels at intervals.

When the vitality of the bowel is more seriously impaired, the fluid within the sac is likely to have been turbid and foul-smelling. The bowel is ashen-grey or even black in colour, and is completely lustreless; its wall is flaccid and sodden to the touch—its consistence being compared to that of wet blotting paper. In addition there is likely to be thrombosis of the associated mesenteric vessels. In such cases the bowel is almost certain to be non-viable, but if the slightest doubt exists it should be treated in the manner described, in order that any possibility of its recovery should not be overlooked.

Treatment of devitalised bowel

In the great majority of cases it is the small bowel which is affected. The choice of procedure then varies accord-

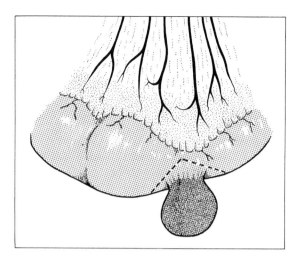

Fig. 24.36 Richter's hernia—suitable for *partial* resection, by the method indicated

area. The line of sutures should lie in the transverse axis of the gut, so that narrowing of the lumen will not be produced.

Partial resection is preferable when localized gangrene is present. Light occlusion clamps are applied to the healthy bowel on each side, and after careful packing-off the gangrenous area is cleanly excised. Repair is effected in the transverse axis by two layers of suture. The method is especially suited to cases of *Richter's hernia* (Fig. 24.36).

Resection and anastomosis. Under modern conditions of anaesthesia and of pre- and postoperative care, the dangers of this operation have been considerably reduced. Even in very old or seriously ill patients the operation is often surprisingly well tolerated, and there are a gratifying number of unexpected recoveries. The technique of resection prior to end-to-end anastomosis is shown in Figure 24.37. This is the procedure of choice when there is no great disparity in the size of the bowel above and below the segment to be resected (see also p. 430). When such disparity exists, the narrow segment of bowel is divided obliquely, opening up the anti-mesenteric border or incising along it.

In the rare cases where a segment of colon has been devitalised by inclusion in a strangulated hernia, it should be excised between clamps and the ends left on the surface, as in the Mikulicz operation (p. 429). Only when obstruction is minimal, and the operating conditions ideal, should a primary anastomosis be attempted.

ing to the severity and extent of the damage. *Localised* areas of impaired vitality (or even of frank gangrene), not involving the entire circumference of the gut, can be treated satisfactorily by the relatively simple procedures of infolding or partial resection. If, however, the damage extends over a wider area, the only practicable treatment is by resection and anastomosis.

Infolding is obtained by Lembert sutures which take up the seromuscular coat on each side of the damaged

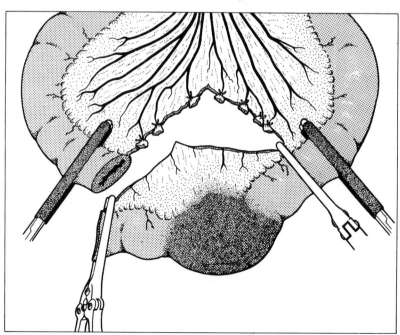

Fig. 24.37 Strangulated hernia of small bowel. Technique of resection prior to end-to-end anastomosis (see also Figs. 22.15 & 22.16, p. 430)

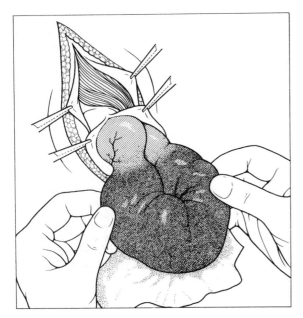

Fig. 24.38 Strangulated inguinal hernia. The sac has been opened to expose the site of constriction (After Hamilton Bailey.)

Treatment of strangulated omentum
Even if viable, strangulated omentum should always be excised, since if returned to the peritoneal cavity it may set up adhesions. The pedicle is clamped and divided in small sections at a time, after which each segment is transfixed and ligatured.

Strangulated inguinal hernia
The constriction is usually caused by the narrow neck of the sac, and is situated therefore at the level of the deep ring. When skin and fascia have been divided the tense sac is at once seen emerging through the superficial ring; this ring is divided and the inguinal canal is opened up in the usual manner. The sac is gently separated from surrounding structures, and is delivered at the wound. A small fold of it is picked up with forceps, and is opened so that the contained fluid is evacuated externally. The sac is now drawn downwards, and is slit up beyond the level of any constriction, a grooved director being used if necessary to protect the contents from injury. Should the constriction appear to be at the level of the superficial ring, it is better that the sac should be opened and the fluid evacuated before this ring is divided. When the sac is a large one it may be left in situ, its neck being cut across and the opening into the general peritoneal cavity is closed by suture.

Strangulated femoral hernia
One of the 'high' approaches (*Lotheisen* or *McEvedy*) is generally advised since it allows the constriction at the level of the femoral ring to be divided under the guidance of the eye; furthermore, it provides better access for the investigation and treatment of damaged bowel. As soon as the skin and fascia have been divided, the lower part of the wound is retracted, and the sac is cleared and opened at its fundus. The femoral ring is now exposed above the inguinal ligament, and the constriction is investigated. This may be due to narrowness of the neck of the sac itself, or to pressure from the pectineal part of the inguinal ligament (*lacunar ligament*). In the latter case the ligament is incised sufficiently to allow the sac to be freed. If an abnormal obturator artery is present it can, from the 'high' approach, be seen and avoided, or at least secured without difficulty. The neck of the sac is now divided against a grooved director, which has been slipped upwards from the fundus. The contents are then drawn out above the inguinal ligament, and are dealt with as their condition demands. If the hernia is of the *Richter's* type, the imprisoned bowel is very apt to slip back into the abdomen as soon as the constriction has been relieved, but in every case it must be sought for and its condition carefully investigated.

If difficulty is experienced in freeing the hernial contents, as may occur in obese subjects, it may be justifiable in a very ill patient to divide the inguinal ligament, or to detach its medial end from the pubic tubercle. When the hernial contents and sac have been dealt with, the free end of the ligament is sutured against the pectineal ligament, thus obliterating the femoral ring. Such a drastic step, however, should seldom be required. If, for any reason such as that of infection in the wound, the repair gives way, a most unpleasant type of inguinofemoral herniation results. This is extremely difficult to repair, since the integrity of the inguinal ligament—a structure which is vital to the whole anatomy of the groin—has been destroyed. An attempt may be made to reattach it to the pubis by means of wire or nylon sutures passed through drill holes in the bone.

Strangulated umbilical hernia
As a rule the strangulation occurs not at the neck of the sac, but in one of the loculi. Operation is carried out on the same lines as described for non-strangulation cases. When the patient is in poor condition, it may be advisable to repair the defect by simple suture, rather than by overlapping.

Strangulated incisional hernia is most likely to occur when the hernia has developed in a lower abdominal scar when multiple small defects may be present. It is a particularly serious condition, since the early symptoms of strangulation may be masked, and gangrene of the bowel will often be found to have occurred. Operation is carried out as described on page 499.

REFERENCES

Allen R G, Wrenn E L 1969 Silan as a sac in the treatment of omphalocoele and gastroschisis. Journal of Paediatric Surgery 4: 5

Andrews N J 1981 Presentation and outcome of strangulated external hernia in a District General Hospital. British Journal of Surgery 68: 329

Brock D J H 1976 Mechanisms by which amniotic-fluid alpha-fetoprotein may be increased in fetal abnormalities. Lancet 2: 345

Devlin H B 1979 Inguinal hernia. Short stay surgery and the Shouldice technique. In: Lumley J, Craven J (eds) Surgical review 1. Pitman Medical, London, p 328

Drainer I K, Reid D K 1972 Recurrence-free ventral herniorrhaphy using a polypropylene mesh prosthesis. Journal of the Royal College of Surgeons of Edinburgh 17: 253

Ellis H, Gajraj H, George C D 1983 Incisional hernias: when do they occur? British Journal of Surgery 70: 290

Farquharson E L 1955 Early ambulation with special reference to herniorrhaphy as an out-patient procedure. Lancet 2: 517

Farquharson E L 1955 Some problems in the treatment of hernia. Annals of the Royal College of Surgeons of England 17: 386

Filston H C 1983 Gastroschisis – primary fascial closure. Annals of Surgery 197: 260.

Glassow F 1973 The surgical repair of inguinal and femoral hernias. Canadian Medical Association Journal 108: 308

Glassow F 1976 Short-stay surgery (Shouldice technique) for repair of inguinal hernia. Annals of the Royal College of Surgeons of England 58: 133

Gosset M J 1949 L'usage des bandes de peau totale comme matériel de suture auto-plastique en chirurgie. Mémoires de L'Académie de chirurgie 75: 277

Jenkins T P N 1980 Incisional hernia repair: A mechanical approach. British Journal of Surgery 67: 335

McEvedy P G 1950 Femoral hernia. Annals of the Royal College of Surgeons of England 7: 484

McMinn R M H, Hutchings R T 1977 Colour atlas of human anatomy. Year Book Medical Publishers, Chicago, p 249

Ruckley C V 1978 Day care and short stay surgery for hernia. British Journal of Surgery, 65: 1

Tanner N C 1942 A 'slide' operation for inguinal and femoral hernia. British Journal of Surgery 29: 285

25
Operations on the urinary tract

J. E. NEWSAM

INVESTIGATIONS

Urological surgery is concerned with diseases and injuries of the kidneys, ureters, bladder, urethra and the male genital tract. The morphology and function of these structures, the site, nature and extent of disease involving them, and the effects these diseases have on other parts of the urinary tract and on the patient's general health, can be so accurately assessed, that in most cases the appropriate operation can be predetermined, the patient properly prepared, and difficulties (during and after operation) anticipated. Nevertheless, the surgeon must always be prepared to modify the operation if unexpected anatomical or pathological features are encountered. Operation is now much more a means of treating disease, and much less a method of investigation.

Advances in other branches of medicine, such as radiation and medical oncology, nutrition, antibiotics, blood transfusion and anaesthesia enable us to operate more safely and more effectively, to operate on patients who would previously have been regarded as unfit for surgery, and to do operations which would otherwise be impossible.

In investigating patients with diseases of the urological or male genital tract, I need not remind you of the importance of taking a full history of the patient's present problems, previous health, family, occupation, social life, and of the medicines he or she takes or has taken; to carry out a thorough physical examination, and to do routine examinations of the urine and blood. In some patients enough information can be derived from these investigations alone to determine the appropriate treatment, but usually more detailed tests are required.

Straight X-ray (Fig. 25.1)

In the straight X-ray, which must extend from the 9th rib above and include both ischial tuberosities and the whole of the pubic symphysis below, the renal outlines, the psoas shadows, abnormal opacities and bony lesions are looked for. Its value can be enhanced in some cases by taking oblique films, which should distinguish opaci-

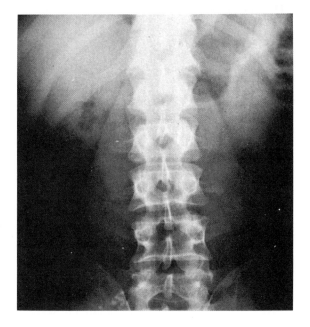

Fig. 25.1 Straight X–ray of the renal tract

ties in the gall bladder, costal cartilages or lymph nodes from those in the urinary tract.

Intravenous excretory urography

Intravenous or excretory urography has replaced the term intravenous pyelography because the procedure reveals the morphology, not only of the pelvis and calices of the kidney, but also of the renal parenchyma, ureters and bladder, and, furthermore, gives much information about the excretory functions of the kidney.

The *contrast media* presently used for intravenous urography are sodium or meglumine diatrizoate, iothalamate or metrizoate which are water soluble salts derived from triiodinated benzoic acid. In the kidneys they are all treated like Inulin which is excreted by glomerular filtration and neither absorbed nor excreted by the tubules. As side effects, which are rare and usually mild, seem unrelated to the dose, large volumes of the contrast media can be given and repeated if desired. Usually about 60 ml of a 50% solution (equivalent to 20 g of iodine) is given and repeated once or even twice if the early films are unsatisfactory. Some radiologists give a much larger initial dose, especially if renal function is subnormal.

Three phases can be recognized

1. The nephrographic phase (Fig. 25.2) is seen in films made immediately the injection finishes, while the contrast medium is in the glomeruli and tubules and rapidly being concentrated, as 80% of the water is reabsorbed in the proximal tubule. It shows the size, position and contours of the kidneys, and the ability of the glomeruli to filter plasma, and of the proximal tubules to reabsorb water. The quality of the nephrograms can be enhanced by taking tomograms (nephrotomography) although a second injection of contrast medium will be required.

2. The pyelographic phase (Fig. 25.3). The pelvicaliceal systems are seen in films made 5, 10, 15 and 20 minutes after injection. The clarity of the pictures depends on the amount of water reabsorbed in the distal tubule (under the influence of antidiuretic hormone) and is enhanced if the patient is dehydrated for some hours before the examination is started. It can be further enhanced if we prevent the dye escaping too quickly from the pelvis into the ureter and bladder, by tilting the patient into the Trendelenberg position or applying

pressure to the anterior abdominal wall with a pneumatic cushion.

The ureters are seen best in films made after the compression is released. However, peristalsis interferes with the visualization of some parts of the ureters and their whole lengths can usually be seen only in retrograde ureterogram (p. 507). In patients with nephroptosis, stone or obstruction, erect, oblique or late films or tomograms, or films taken after the intravenous injection of Frusemide, are useful.

3. Cystogram (Fig. 25.4). The quality of the cystogram can be improved if the patient empties his bladder before the examination, and its value enhanced with oblique films. A post micturition cystogram should always be taken (Fig. 25.5). Although it is not a reliable means of measuring the amount of residual urine, it may reveal filling defects, the true size of acquired diverticula which fill as the bladder empties or early ureteric obstruction.

Ultrasound

Ultrasound waves cannot be appreciated by the human ear because they have frequencies above 20 000 cycles (20 000 herz) per second. For ultrasonography, waves with frequencies of 1 to 5×10^6 cycles (1–5 megaherz) per second produced by ultrasound transducers are used. They are directed onto the object being studied and are reflected back by the interfaces separating tissues of different densities and different sound velocities. The echoes are analysed, displayed and stored. The de-

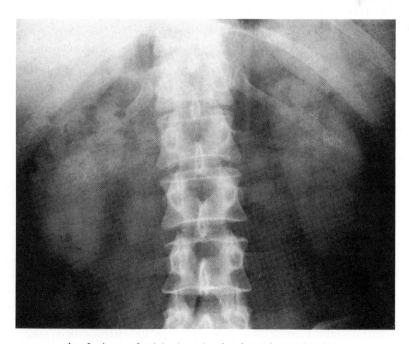

Fig. 25.2 Intravenous urogram taken 3 minutes after injection, showing the nephrographic phase

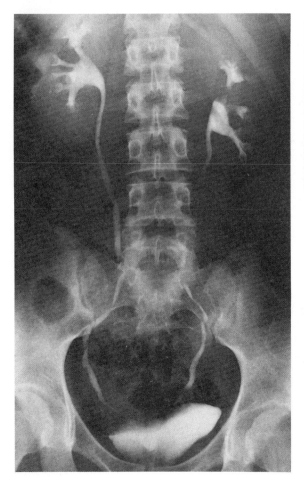

Fig. 25.3 Intravenous urogram taken 10 minutes after the injection, showing the pelvicaliceal system of the kidney and the ureters

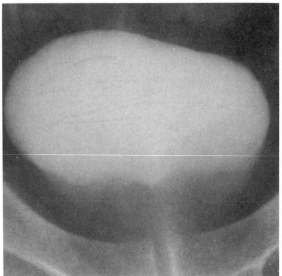

Fig. 25.4 Cystogram. Premicturition film showing the normal bladder

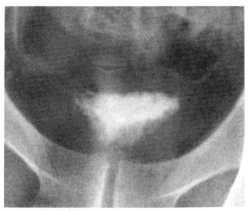

Fig 25.5 Cystogram. Post micturition film

lay between the transmission of the wave and the return of the echo reveals the depth of the object from the surface and the amplitude of the wave, its nature. The kidneys (Fig. 25.6) are easily recognizable by ultrasound, even if they are not functioning and their size, position, contours and the nature of any space occupying lesions can be appreciated. Furthermore, under ultrasound control, a needle can be inserted into the kidney to obtain a biopsy, into the pelvis to provide a percutaneous nephrostomy or an antegrade pyelo-ureterogram or into a cyst. Ultrasound is also of value in some diseases of the bladder and prostate.

Angiography
Main stream aortography and selective renal angiography are carried out by the Seldinger technique in which the catheter is passed directly, using a needle and guide wire, into a femoral artery. Main stream aortography

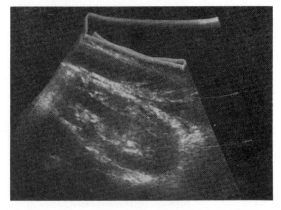

Fig. 25.6 Ultrasound scan of the kidney demonstrating a normal kidney with a normal collecting system

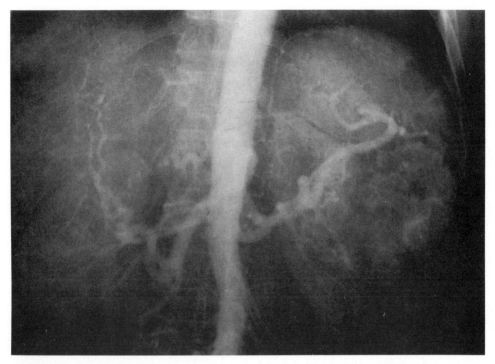

Fig. 25.7 Main stream aortogram showing a large tumour in the left kidney and a normal right kidney

(Fig. 25.7) shows the number, position and distribution of the renal arteries. Selective renal angiography has three phases: the arterial (Fig. 25.8); the nephrographic

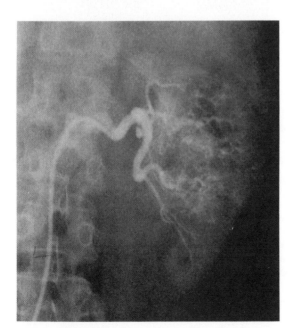

Fig. 25.8 Selective left renal angiogram showing a large tumour in the left kidney

and the venous. Angiography is valuable for the investigation of patients with hypertension, or with injuries, arteriovenous anomalies, or tumours of the kidney. Its value can be enhanced by the injection of adrenaline which constricts normal vessels, but not tumour ones. In patients with tumour or vascular abnormalities, the 'feeding' or main artery can be embolized by the injection through the catheter of absorbable gelatin foam or occluding springs, or by the distension of a ballooned catheter (Fig. 25.9).

Retrograde pyelography

Retrograde pyelography began in 1906 using, at first, aqueous solutions of colloidal silver and later sodium iodide, and was the only means of examining the upper urinary tract until the early 1930s when the synthesis of the water soluble organic iodine compounds made intravenous urography a safe and efficient procedure. The author now uses the same contrast media for retrograde pyelography as for intravenous urography, but in a lower concentration of 20 to 30%.

Nowadays, we carry out retrograde pyelography much less often than we used to, partly because it involves cystoscopy and ureteric catheterization (p. 522) (which can so easily induce or exacerbate infection, particularly in obstructed kidneys) but predominantly because intravenous urography, ultrasonography and radionuclide and CAT scanning provide, with less trouble and danger,

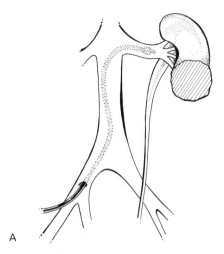

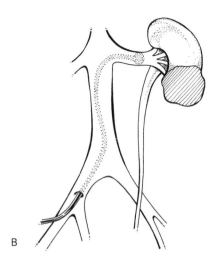

Fig. 25.9 Renal artery embolisation

good pictures of the anatomy of the kidneys. Further-more, they tell us much about function. However, retro-grade pyelograms may still be required to show the pelvicaliceal systems of obstructed or otherwise poorly or nonfunctioning kidneys; to clarify the exact relation-ship of opacities to the urinary tract, or the size and nature of filling defects in the ureters or pelvicaliceal system and to reveal the whole length of a ureter. (The whole length of a ureter is rarely seen in an intravenous urogram) (Fig. 25.10). The normal renal pelvis has a

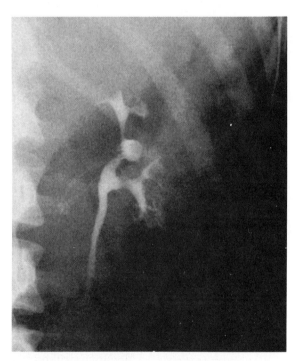

Fig. 25.11 Pyelovenous and pyelotubular backflow

capacity of about 5 or 6 ml. If too much contrast medium is injected into the ureteric catheter, backflow or extra-vasation (Fig. 25.11) can easily be produced and not only makes interpretation of the films difficult or even impossible, but may cause septicaemia.

Ureteric catherization, though not necessarily pyelo-graphy, is also necessary if we want to collect separate specimens from each kidney, for biochemical or cytolog-ical examination. Retrograde pyelo-ureterograms are best made under a screen and image intensifier, but, if carried

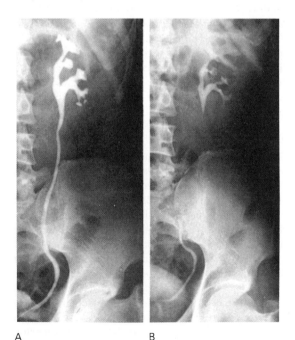

Fig. 25.10 (A) Retrograde pyelo-ureterogram, using a Braasch catheter, revealing the whole length of the ureter. (B) IVU, in same patient, for comparison

out using Braasch or Chevasseur catheters (p. 526), have to be made on the endoscopic table.

It is vital to fill the ureteric catheter with the contrast medium before it is introduced so that air bubbles are not injected, because they may be confused with tumours or stones.

Antegrade pyelo-ureterography
Dye can be injected through a needle inserted into the renal pelvis under X–ray or ultrasonic control, if pictures of the ureter or pelvicaliceal system are needed and cannot be obtained by other means.

Ascending or retrograde urethrocystography
(Fig. 25.12)
This procedure is carried out by inserting a 14F catheter into the external meatus and inflating the balloon with 2–3 ml of water.

A 10–25% solution of one of the water soluble contrast media is injected slowly and carefully so that the dye does not extravasate into the corpora or cause oedema. Anteroposterior and oblique films are taken and show the urethra clearly as far as the external sphincter. Considerable pressure is usually required to force the dye through the external sphincter into the bladder, and the membranous and prostatic parts appear narrow because they only open when the bladder contracts.

It is important to fill the catheter with the contrast medium otherwise air bubbles will be introduced and spoil the films.

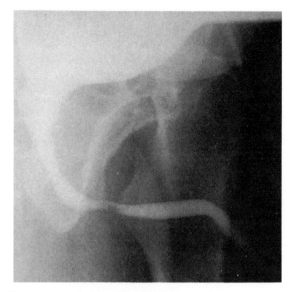

Fig. 25.13 Micturating cystogram

Cystogram
Adequate cystograms are often obtained during intravenous urography, especially if the patient empties his bladder just before the examination commences. Nevertheless, to demonstrate diverticula, vesico-ureteric reflux and bladder injuries, or to obtain micturating (voiding) cystograms with pictures of the bladder neck, the prostate, and membranous parts of the urethra, cystograms (Fig. 25.13) are best done by injecting a 10% or 20% solution of one of the water soluble contrast media directly into a catheter passed through the urethra into the bladder.

Pedal Lymphangiography (Fig. 25.14)
This is best carried out by injecting indigocarmine mixed with 1% lignocaine hydrochloride into the skin and subcutaneous tissues of a webbed space on the dorsum of the foot. A 27 g needle can be inserted into one of the lymphatic channels when they become visible some 5–10 minutes later and 5–6 ml of ethiodized oil containing 37% of iodine is then injected. X-rays show lymph vessels 1 hour and lymph nodes 12–24 hours after the injection. The lymph nodes seen are the inguinal ones and those along the common and external iliac vessels and the aorta. The lymph nodes alongside the internal iliac vessels are not shown, so the procedure is of limited use in patients with prostatic or bladder tumours.

Some of the fat soluble contrast leaks into veins, especially if the lymphatics are obstructed and can cause pulmonary embolism. The procedure is particularly dangerous in patients with lung disease and must always be preceded by a chest X–ray.

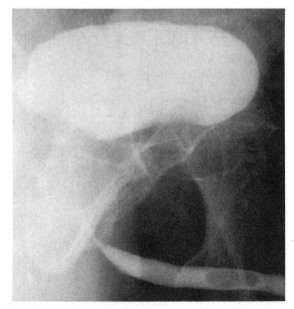

Fig. 25.12 Ascending urethrogram

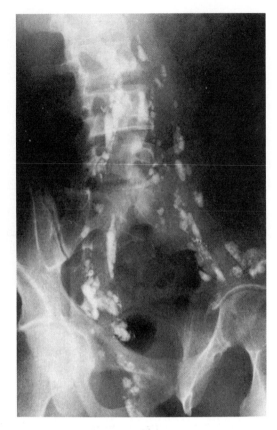

Fig. 25.14 Lymphangiogram showing normal lymph nodes along the common and external iliac vessels and aorta

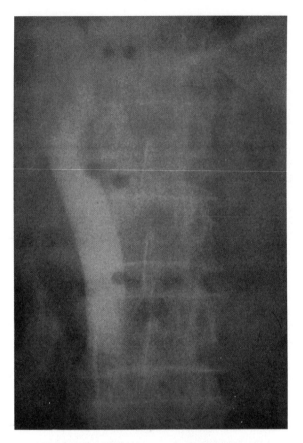

Fig. 25.15 Inferior vena cavogram revealing a filling defect in the left side of the vena cava at the level of the renal vein. The defect is caused by an extension of the renal cell carcinoma seen in the intravenous urogram (which is a feature of all inferior vena cavograms) of the left kidney

Venography (Fig. 25.15)

Radiographs of the inferior vena cava and the renal veins can be obtained by applying the Seldinger technique through the femoral vein and are of value in patients with renal cell carcinoma or renal vein thrombosis. The technique can be used to collect venous blood from the vena cava and each renal vein for the estimation of rennin production in patients with hypertension.

Nuclear medicine

The procedures used in nuclear medicine are noninvasive, require little if any preparation, cause few side effects and are unaffected by bowel or gas shadows.

Renography (Fig. 25.16)

A renogram can be made using either [131]iodine-or [123]iodine-labelled iodohippurate, or [99m]technetium labelled diethylene tetramine pentacetic acid (DTPA). The curves obtained have three components: A vascular phase, which lasts about 20 seconds, is a steep rise and depends on the arterial supply to the kidneys; a secretory phase, which lasts up to 5 minutes, depends on the amount of dye filtered at the glomerulus and excreted by

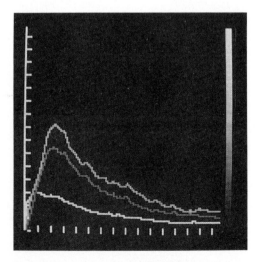

Fig. 25.16 Renogram showing normal curves from both left and right kidney (the lower curve represents the blood level of the isotope)

the tubules; and an excretory phase which falls rapidly as the dye drains out of the kidney into the pelvis and ureter. Obstruction hinders the third phase and can be shown more easily if the patient is given Frusemide.

Renal scan (Fig. 25.17)

The ^{99m}technetium-labelled chelates diethylene tetramine pentacetic acid (DTPA) and dimercapto succinic acid (DMSA) are used and the images recorded by gamma cameras. For dynamic imaging DTPA is used; it is excreted by glomerular filtration and the scan provides in picture form the same information that the renogram does in graphic form. For static imaging DMSA is used; it is taken up by normally functioning parenchyma and tells us more about morphology than function.

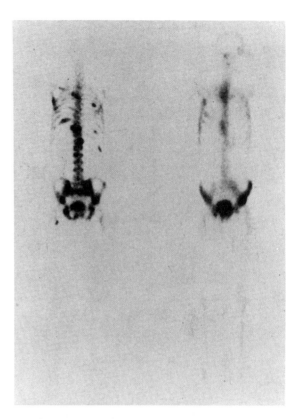

Fig. 25.18 Bone scan revealing multiple hot spots in the pelvis, lumbar and thoracic spine. As X-rays of these areas were normal, hot spots were considered to be caused by metastatic disease

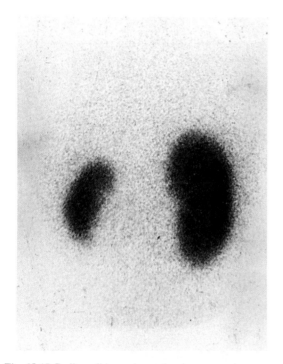

Fig. 25.17 Radionuclide renal scan showing a normal right kidney and a small left one. (The detector camera is applied posteriorly)

Bone scan (Fig. 25.18)

This is carried out using ^{99m}technetium-labelled phosphate or diphosphonate compounds. Scans can show metastases at an earlier stage than X–rays, particularly in patients with prostatic carcinoma; however, the changes are non specific and must be compared with the appropriate conventional X–rays. If the scan is positive and the X–ray negative, metastases are the likeliest cause.

Urodynamics (Fig. 25.19)

For many years cysto-urethroscopy and cysto-urethrography have proved to be satisfactory means of studying the structure of the bladder and the urethra. Now urodynamics provides a means of studying their function, and helps to elucidate the causes of incontinence, frequency, urgency and the severity of obstruction. The most useful measurements are the residual urine, the bladder capacity, the bladder pressures and the urine flow rates, but much else can be measured with the sophisticated apparatus now available.

A two way catheter is passed into the bladder. The bladder is emptied and the amount of urine recovered is the residual. One limb of the catheter is connected to a fluid reservoir and the other to a pressure recorder. The pressure recorded from the bladder is a combination of the detruser pressure and the general intra-abdominal pressure. The latter can be measured with a rectal catheter, and when subtracted from the bladder pressure, gives us the intrinsic bladder or detrusor pressure. The flow rate is measured with a flow meter; and if apparatus is available, a micturating cystogram (p. 509) can be done at the same time. The bladder only contracts prop-

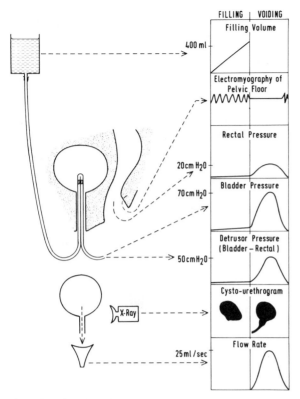

Fig. 25.19 Urodynamics

Computerized axial tomography (CAT scanning)

In CAT scans many X–rays are taken, from all angles, of one thin section of the body by rotating the tube through 360°. The X–rays are received by a scintillator detector which integrates and transforms the images into one picture. As each picture shows only one thin section of the body a large number of pictures are needed to show the whole of the abdomen or chest. The size, shape and position of the kidneys, and the size and nature of space occupying lesions is revealed (Fig. 25.20). CAT scans also show calcification or stones too small to be revealed in conventional X–rays. Retroperitoneal swellings like para-aortic glands are also clearly demonstrated, so that the precedure is particularly valuable in a patient with a testicular tumour.

URETHRAL CATHETERIZATION

Although the complications of urethral catheterization occur less often now than they used to, and can be better treated, they can still be serious or long lasting when they do occur, and catheterization should only be used as an investigative procedure, if the information required cannot be obtained by noninvasive and safer methods.

Indications

Urethral catheterization is employed:
1. To empty the bladder in most patients with acute and clot retention and in many with chronic retention.
2. To empty the bladder before operating on pelvic viscera like the rectum or uterus and to fill the bladder

erly when it is full (300 ml +) and flow rates and residual urine should only be measured when the patient passes urine because he wants to, not because he's told to.

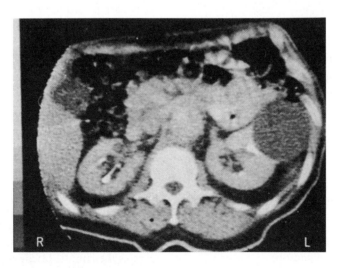

Fig. 25.20 CAT scan. This reveals that the right kidney, or at least the thin section revealed in this picture, is normal. The left kidney contains a large cyst (Reproduced from Sutton D 1980 A textbook of radiology, 3rd edn Churchill Livingstone, Edinburgh by kind permission of the author)

before some operations on the bladder and prostate.

3. To instil antiseptics like Noxythiolin (Noxyflex) or Chlorhexidine 1/5000 into the infected bladder, or tumour inhibitors like Ethoglucid (Epodyl) into the neoplastic bladder.

4. To measure residual urine, bladder capacity and other urodynamic parameters.

5. To carry out cysto-urethrography in the investigation of bladder, vesico-ureteric, vesico-urethral and urethral disease.

6. In patients with, or liable to develop, acute renal failure so that the urinary output can be measured hourly.

7. In the treatment of neuropathic bladder disorders following diseases or injuries of the nervous system and other causes of urinary incontinence.

8. As a means of draining, and keeping empty, the bladder after operations on the bladder, prostate and urethra and after some gynaecological and rectal operations.

9. To determine the nature and extent of urethral and bladder injuries.

Catheter type

If the catheter is to be removed as soon as the bladder is emptied or filled or fluid is injected, a non-ballooned catheter of the Nelaton, Harris or Jacques type made of polyvinyl chloride (PVC)(Fig. 25.21) can be used; on the other hand, if the catheter is to be left in, a ballooned (Foley) or Gibbon catheter (Fig. 25.22) should be used.

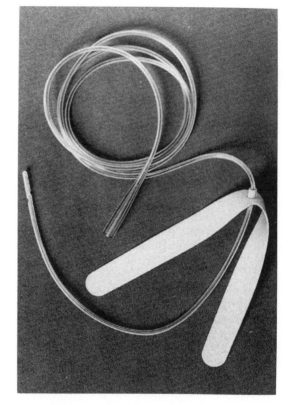

Fig. 25.22 Gibbon catheter (Courtesy of Eschmann)

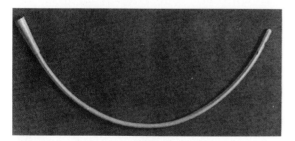

Fig. 25.21 Jacques catheter (Courtesy of Eschmann)

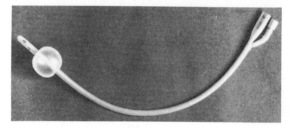

Fig. 25.23 Foley catheter two way (Courtesy of Eschmann)

Ballooned catheter

a. Two way Foley (Fig. 25.23). This is called two way because it has two channels, one for urine drainage, the other, which is much smaller, for inflating the balloon which retains the catheter in the bladder. Sterile water or saline should be used to distend the balloon. If air is used, the balloon floats on the surface of the urine and the bladder does not drain properly.

b. Three way Foley (irrigating catheter) (Fig. 25.24). This has three channels: one for urine drainage, one for inflating the balloon, and one, which opens just below

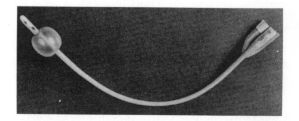

Fig. 25.24 Foley catheter three way (Courtesy of Eschmann)

the tip of the catheter, for continuous irrigation. The three way Foley is predominantly used after endoscopic and open operations on the bladder or prostate (with a closed drainage system) to prevent clot retention. It can also be used for the continuous irrigation of a very infected bladder.

Foley catheters are made of latex, which is elastic and strong, and has a low toxicity. However, after 9 or 10 days, encrustations form around the drainage holes which progressively restrict urinary flow. Some latex catheters are coated on the inside or the outside (or both inside and outside) with silicone or teflon. Such coated catheters are smoother and less likely to encrust, but they are expensive.

Early ones were liable to delaminate, when the outer coating broke away from the latex and remained in the bladder after the catheter was removed, but this is not likely to happen with the present day ones. Some Foley catheters are constructed entirely of silicone. They are less irritant than latex or coated latex, but expensive, and generally only for people who require longterm catheterization.

c. 'Haematuria' Foley catheters (Fig. 25.25) are latex catheters whose walls are reinforced with nylon thread. They can withstand, without collapsing, the strong suction necessary for the removal of blood clots, and the three way ones are often used after prostatic surgery.

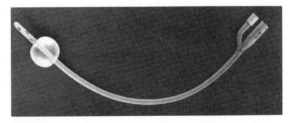

Fig. 25.25 Foley catheter—haematuric type (Courtesy of Eschmann)

Catheter size

If the catheter is too small, urine leaks around its sides; if too large, it can irritate the urethra. The French (F)— often called Charriere (CH)—gauge is used for sizing catheters, endoscopes, and many other tubes used in medicine. Dividing the French gauge by 3 gives the outside diameter of the tube in mm, i.e. an 18F catheter has an outside diameter of 6 mm. In adults, a 12–16F or CH catheter is adequate if the urine is clear, but a 20 or 22F should be used if the urine is turbid or blood stained. The balloon sizes of the Foley catheter range from 3–5 ml.; 5–10 ml.; 30 ml and 75–100 ml.; the smallest is used with 8 or 10F catheters; in adults a 30 ml is used although often no more than 10 ml is introduced. The full 30 ml should be used after prostatectomy

otherwise the balloon may be displaced into the prostatic cavity, especially if traction is applied to the catheter to control venous bleeding (p. 602).

The inflated balloon of a Foley catheter provides a large surface area for the deposition of calcium phosphate and the formation of stones. As little fluid as necessary should be inserted into the balloon and it is good practice, although not always possible, to deflate the balloon for a few minutes each day or week in patients requiring prolonged catheterization. Some catheters are made for females only. The commonest are two way catheters with a shorter shaft length than the male ones. A double ballooned catheter (Fig. 25.26) is also available; the distal balloon (below the eyes) retains the catheter in the bladder; the other balloon is inflated outside the external meatus and prevents the shaft moving within the urethra, reducing, some believe, the risk of infection.

Various tips are available with two and three way Foley catheters; some have a terminal eye as well as side ones (Whistle tip) (Fig. 25.27), others only side eyes and a solid end (Fig. 25.28) which can be used with an introducer (Fig. 25.30).

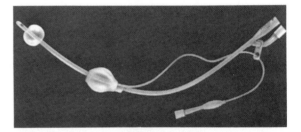

Fig. 25.26 Catheter with two balloons (Courtesy of Eschmann)

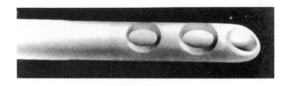

Fig. 25.27 Whistle tip catheter (Courtesy of Eschmann)

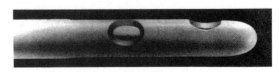

Fig. 25.28 Catheter with solid end and side eyes (Courtesy of Eschmann)

Procedure

The procedure of urethral catheterization must be carried out with the most rigorous aseptic precautions and gentleness, otherwise infection can easily be introduced or exacerbated, or the urethra damaged, and the patient discomforted. If the patient is excessively apprehensive he can be given pethidine or diazepam intravenously before the procedure starts. The procedure, often done in the patient's bed in the ward, is best done in a dressing room or theatre, and the operator should wear sterile gloves. The patient is placed supine; in males, the legs are separated; in females, the knees are bent then separated with the feet together. The genitalia are cleaned with an aqueous antiseptic solution (spirit irritates the skin). In males, the penis is held in a sterile swab, the prepuce retracted and all smegma removed; in females, the labia should be separated with one hand while the meatus is cleaned (from before backwards) and only released after the catheter has been inserted. Sterile towels are used to prevent the catheter or operator's hands touching the skin or bedclothes. The urethra is filled with an antiseptic anaesthetic gel (Lignocaine hydrochloride 1 or 2% with chlorhexidine 0.25%) using the nozzle supplied with the tube (both nozzle and tube are supplied sterile). Two minutes are allowed for the local anaesthetic to become effective while the catheter is prepared.

Most catheters are now supplied sterile and are often double-wrapped. When the outer pack is carefully removed by an assistant, the operator can handle the sterile inner pack. This is opened to expose the distal end of the catheter which is then well lubricated. (Petroleum products like liquid paraffin dissolve latex, and must not be used). The catheter is then slowly fed into the urethra out of the inner tube, elevating the penis in the male, and keeping the labia separated in the female. When the catheter reaches the bladder, urine drains through it. If a balloon catheter is being used the catheter is advanced a little further into the bladder before the balloon is inflated. The catheter is then connected to a drainage bag

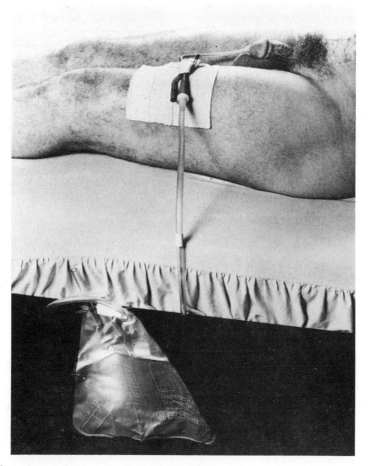

Fig. 25.29 A method of securing a catheter at the thigh with strapping

providing a closed drainage system. The bag should have a one way valve which will prevent urine returning to the bladder if the bag is lifted or sat upon.

Difficulties

In women catheterization is usually easy because the urethra is short, wide and straight, although sometimes the external meatus is hidden within the vaginal introitus.

In males catheterization may obviously be difficult if the patient has a urethral stricture or enlarged prostate, but may also be difficult if the external meatus is narrow (attempts to force a catheter through the meatus can cause a fissure and later a stricture). The patient may be apprehensive and his muscles in spasm, but, gentleness, patience and appreciation of the sensitivity of the urethra and the value of using plenty of lubricating gel and rotating movements, usually succeed in guiding the catheter safely into the bladder.

The catheter should be anchored securely to the thigh with elastoplast (Fig. 25.29).

A catheter introducer can be inserted into a Foley catheter to facilitate introduction, but great care must be taken because false passages can easily be made. The *Maryfield* introducer is of value to those experienced in the use of urethral dilators. If a catheter cannot be passed, the procedure should be abandoned until the urethra can be further investigated, and, if the patient has retention, the bladder can be drained by a suprapubic cystostomy (p. 575). Sometimes the balloon of a Foley catheter cannot be deflated when we wish to remove it. The first thing to do is to cut the valve off the balloon channel and try to deflate the balloon by applying a syringe directly to the channel. If this is unsuccessful, wait 12 hours, because the balloon may gradually and spontaneously deflate. If still unsuccessful, injecting liquid paraffin down the main drainage channel may dissolve part of the balloon. Over inflation is not recommended because it often leaves pieces of latex in the bladder. A stylet from a ureteric catheter can be passed down the balloon channel and used to puncture the balloon. If all else fails, or if inability to deflate the balloon is associated with retention and instant relief required, the balloon can be punctured with a 19 g spinal needle passed suprapubically, transvaginally or transrectally, after first ensuring that the bladder is partially distended.

ENDOSCOPY (CYSTO-URETHROSCOPY)

Mainly due to the work of Professor H H Hopkins,

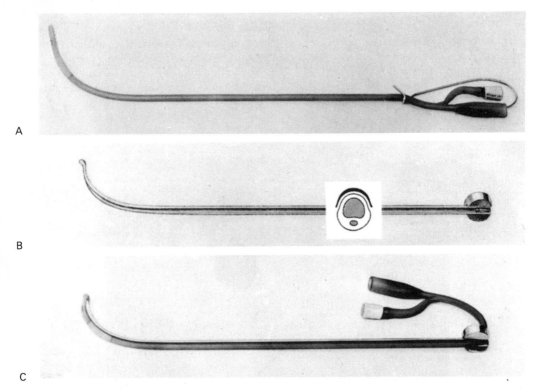

Fig. 25.30 A. Foley catheter mounted on a wire stretcher. B. The *Maryfield* introducer for Foley catheters. C. The catheter is stretched along a groove on the convex surface of the instrument as shown on the inset in B.

endoscopy has improved enormously over the past two decades, for the following reasons:

1. Fibre illumination (which has replaced the small delicate, unreliable terminal incandescent bulb previously used in urology) provides a powerful safe and reliable lighting system, suitable not only for endoscopic procedures, but also for still and cine photography, and the use of teaching attachments. The light is produced by a large quartz iodine lamp housed in the light source box. It is transmitted to the fibre light pillar of the telescope by a flexible cable made up of glass fibre bundles wrapped in a protective sheath of coiled metal wadding and coated with rubber or plastic. The light is then transmitted down the telescope by another set of glass fibre bundles which are incorporated in the wall of telescope.

Glass tubes can transmit not only light, but also images (fibre optics) and are widely used for this purpose by gastro-enterologists. Although we use rigid telescopes for cysto-urethroscopy, flexible ones, using fibre optics, have been developed for the inspection of the ureter and pelvicaliceal systems with a larger one for the bladder.

2. The invention of the rod lens telescope. In the conventional telescope, the lenses were made of glass and the spaces between them filled with air; in the rod lens telescope the lenses are narrow spaces of air and the spaces between them are filled with glass rods. This change augments the amount of light transmitted from object to viewer, the optical resolution and the field of view.

3. The improved methods of coating the fibre optics reduces the amount of light lost by reflection.

The basic endoscopic examination system (Fig. 25.31) consists of a sheath which is a straight hollow metal tube from 17F to 24F for adults, but as small as 8F for infants. The end of the sheath may be straight or slightly bent, but is always made with little if any beak or curvature, so that it can be used for examining the urethra with a fore-oblique telescope, as well as the bladder. The proximal end of the sheath has one or usually two side channels, each controlled by a small tap, for the supply of fluid. Sometimes these channels are on a rotating collar and sometimes they are fixed. Although sheaths of 17F–18F upwards accept the standard telescopes, and can be used for inspection, the sheath size determines the size of ureteric catheters, electrodes, or biopsy forceps that can be used, and for adults a 21F sheath is probably best. The latter will accept the pinch biopsy forceps and one 9F electrode or two 6F catheters, but a larger sheath is needed for stone crushing forceps.

An obturator inserted into the sheath prevents the open end of the sheath damaging the urethra as it is passed into the bladder.

Nowadays the obturator is often not used and the sheath is passed with the fore-oblique or direct view telescope so that the urethra can be visualized from the external meatus to bladder neck as the instrument is slowly passed. (Some manufacturers supply a special hollow obturator for this purpose, but it is not necessary). Urethroscopy can be done after the bladder has been examined, but it is better done first. To examine the urethra requires a steady flow of irrigating fluid, otherwise the urethral walls collapse onto the end of the telescope and only a red haze will be seen.

When the tip of the sheath is in the bladder, the obturator or telescope is removed and the bladder

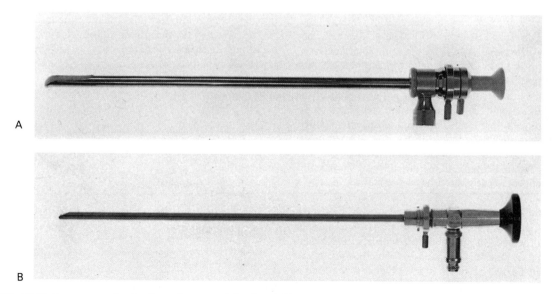

A

B

Fig. 25.31 Cystoscope—the sheath, a telescope and the short bridge

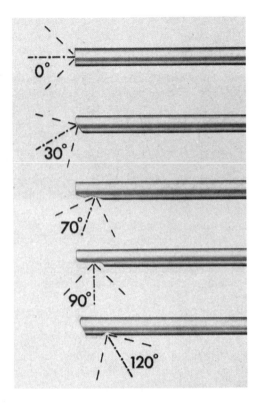

Fig. 25.32 The angle of the view provided by different telescopes

emptied. The bladder is then filled with sterile water or saline, and fully examined.

Telescopes (Fig. 25.32)

The rigid telescopes used in cysto-urethroscopy are classified by the angle of view they provide into fore-oblique, lateral, direct and retrograde. The fore-oblique telescope usually provides a 30° angle, but with some manufacturers, it is 12° or 20°. This telescope can be used with the inspecting sheath to examine the urethra, prostate, bladder neck and the trigone and posterior wall of the bladder; and with biopsy forceps, stone crushing forceps, catheter deflecting mechanisms and most resectoscopes. Telescopes are the most expensive items of urological endoscopes and if the surgeon can afford only one telescope, the fore-oblique is the one to buy. To examine the bladder properly, however, a lateral 70° telescope is needed. It can also be used with the catheter deflecting mechanism (Albarran lever) but not with biopsy or stone crushing forceps or resectoscepes. The anterior wall of the bladder, and in patients with prostatic hypertrophy, the base can be best seen with the retrograde (120°) telescope; however, in most patients, the fundus can be seen well enough with the 70° telescope if the abdomen is compressed, the patient tilted or the bladder

only partly filled, so that the purchase of a retrograde telescope, which is rarely used, may be unnecessary.

The direct viewing telescope (0°) is used with some models of resectoscopes and is perhaps the best for urethroscopy or visual urethrotomy; but most surgeons use a resectoscope with a fore-oblique (30°) telescope which can also be used for urethroscopy and visual urethrotomy.

The fibre light sources and fibre light cables of one manufacturer can be used with the endoscopes of another, using adapters that are freely available. Unfortunately, interchangeability finishes there, and so far as the rest of the endoscopy set is concerned, it is advisable to buy a matched set from one maker, because the telescopes, sheaths, forceps etc., of one maker, are, sadly, not interchangeable with those of another.

Urethroscopy should be done in all male patients, but is essential when carrying out endoscopy on patients with benign or malignant prostatic disease, bladder tumours, and urethral diverticula or strictures.

Deflecting mechanism

The telescopes are longer than the inspection sheath and, when used for observation, are connected to the sheath by a short bridge. In order to catheterize the ureters, diathermize a bladder tumour or take biopsies from the bladder, the telescope and the short bridge are removed, and a single or double catheterizing deflecting mechanism (Albarran Bridge) (Fig. 25.33) or pinch biopsy forceps are inserted into the sheath.

The catheter deflecting mechanism has, at its distal end, a platform on which the ureteric catheter or electrode rests. This platform can be raised or lowered by rotating a wheel at the proximal end of the instrument (Albarran lever) and the catheter thus guided visually into the ureter or the electrode onto the tumour. The one or two openings at the proximal end of the catheter deflecting mechanism can be kept closed by taps. However, if catheters or electrodes are being passed, these taps have to be left open.

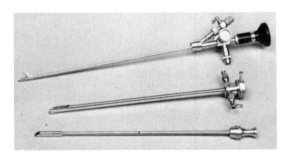

Fig. 25.33 Catheter deflecting mechanism (Albarran bridge) with sheath and obturator (Courtesy of Key Med.)

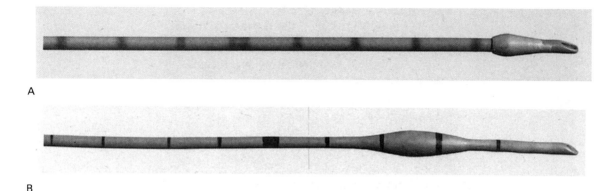

A

B

Fig. 25.34 A & B Ureteric catheters. (A) Braasch; (B) Chevasseur

In these circumstances the openings are occluded with perforated rubber nipples which grip the catheter or electrode and prevent the irrigating fluid from leaking out. Ureteric catheters are made of plastic or dacron and vary in size from 3F to 12F. (Size 5F is normally used). They are usually radio-opaque and, therefore, visible in straight X–rays. They have various tips, plain, whistle tip or with bulbs (Braasch or Chevasseur) (Fig. 25.34). They are about 70 cm in length and calibrated by rings in cm (the adult ureter is 25 to 30 cm long) with additional rings each 5 cm, so 2 rings can be seen when 10 cm of the catheter has passed into the ureter, 3 at 15 cm, 4 at 20 cm and 5 at 25 cm.

The calibre of the catheter or electrode that can be used depends on the calibre of the inspection sheath. A 21 F sheath takes $2 \times 6F$ or $1 \times 8F$; and a 17F sheath $2 \times 4F$ or $1 \times 5F$.

Mucosal biopsies can be accurately and safely taken under direct vision with the pinch biopsy forceps used with a fore-oblique telescope (Fig. 25.35), but biopsies of bladder tumours and the prostate are best and most easily taken with a resectoscope.

Resectoscope
Many feel that only a urologist should use a resectoscope, and use of this instrument in urethral, prostatic and bladder surgery requires some general comment. Transurethral resection of the prostate or a bladder tumour by untrained, inexperienced surgeons, especially if they are using poor or poorly maintained equipment can cause serious complications, but so can the performance of any open or endoscopic procedure in similar circumstances. The general surgeon who can easily refer his patients to a urologist, may well decide to do no resections or any other urology, for that matter; but the general surgeon who has to do his own urology must learn to use a resectoscope, at least, for patients with bladder tumours and with fibrous, malignant, and the smaller hypertrophied

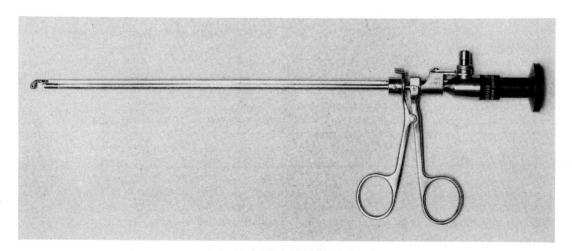

Fig. 25.35 Pinch biopsy forceps. These are used with a fore-oblique telescope through a cystoscope or resectoscope sheath (Courtesy of A C M I Ltd.)

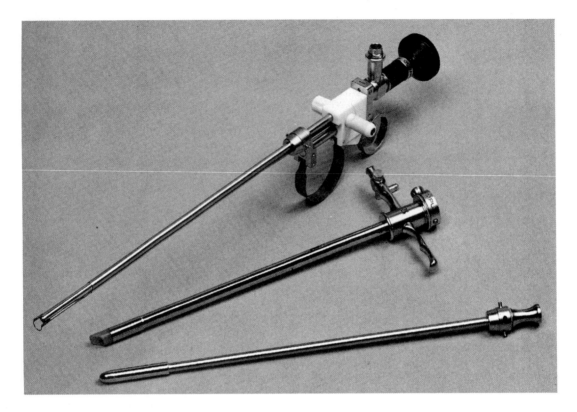

Fig. 25.36 Resectoscope—the resectoscope working element (with telescope), sheath and obturator (Courtesy of Key Med.)

prostates, because it is the best way to treat these conditions.

There are many types of resectoscopes, but they all consist of an outer sheath, a working element which moves the diathermy loop backwards and forwards; a telescope which is usually a fore-oblique but sometimes a direct viewing one (Fig. 25.36).

The sheath is made of fibre glass or stainless steel with a fibre glass tip so that the diathermy current is not transmitted down the sheath as the loop is withdrawn into the sheath at the conclusion of a cut. However, fears that transmission of the current down the sheath in this way would burn the urethra, and even the operator, seem exaggerated, and some surgeons use an all metal noninsulated sheath.

The sheath sizes vary from 24F to 28F, but, since the larger sheaths are much more likely to damage the urethra and leave strictures, most surgeons use a 26F sheath.

The end of the sheath can have a long or short beak, and those used with direct vision telescopes have no beak at all. The long beak covers the whole journey of the loop and is perhaps safer, but most urologists prefer the short beak. The fluid inlet tap on the sheath is usually fixed, but on some sheaths rotates. The sheath can be passed blindly into the bladder with an appropriate obturator, but is best passed under vision using the appropriate telescope, 30° or 0° depending on the make of the instrument.

The working element

This carries and moves the loop and fits into the sheath, the telescope fitting into it. There are many different types of working elements, but each can be used with any adult sized sheath and with each the loop moves about 2.5 cm. They fall into 3 groups including two spring loaded groups. (1) The Baumrucker type in which the spring aids the return of the loop to the extended position, and in the resting state, the loop projects out of the sheath; (2) the Iglesias type in which the spring aids the cutting action of the loop and in the resting state the loop is inside the tip of the sheath; and (3) a group without spring assistance at all. Of these, the Iglesias type is the safest because the patient will not be burnt if someone accidentially treads on the diathermy pedal.

The resection is carried out while fluid flows into the bladder, and the working element and telescope have to be removed from the sheath at regular intervals to empty the bladder. A continuous flow resectoscope was introduced in 1975 by Iglesias, but balancing the inflow and

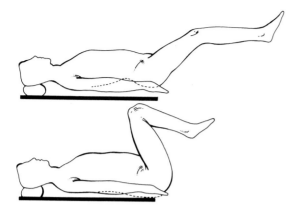

Fig. 25.37 Position of the patient for urological endoscopic procedures is shown in the upper figure. The lower figure shows the lithotomy position which is unsuitable for endoscopy

outflow is not easy, and most urologists still prefer the conventional resectoscope.

Various loops can be fitted. The loop electrode is used for cutting and vessel coagulation; but roller and ball electrodes are available for vessel coagulation and a knife electrode for incising a bladder neck or ureteric orifice.

Technique of endoscopy

Position (Fig. 25.37)

The patient's legs should be separated and the thighs flexed to 45°. This is a half lithotomy position; the full one makes endoscopy difficult.

Anaesthesia

General anaesthesia is preferred because it facilitates the examination and allows for painfree biopsies, electro coagulation or resection and a satisfactory bimanual examination. An adequate endoscopic examination, however, can be done using intravenous diazepam and injecting lignocaine gel 1% antiseptic (which contains lignocaine hydrochloride 1% and chlorhexidine gluconate solution 0.25%) into the urethra.

Procedure (Fig. 25.38)

The instrument sheath and obturator are well lubricated (liquid paraffin, K. Y. jelly or lignocaine gel) and allowed to fall down the urethra and into the bladder under its own weight, depressing the instrument in the male to allow the beak to traverse the membranous and prostatic parts of the urethra. Once the instrument is in the bladder the obturator is removed and the bladder emptied. However, most urologists now prefer to pass the instrument under direct vision, so that they can view the entire length of the urethra before it is affected by instrumentation. For this purpose the foreoblique or direct telescope is inserted into the sheath using the short

bridge; the instrument is then passed slowly down the urethra continuously irrigating in order to prevent the urethra collapsing on to the end of the telescope and obscuring the view. In this way, the spongy, membranous and prostatic parts of the urethra are seen in turn. Once in the bladder, the bladder neck, trigone and posterior wall of the bladder are examined before removing the telescope and emptying the bladder. The bladder is then filled with 250 to 300 ml of sterile water or saline and carefully examined with the 70° telescope. Vision may be obscured by a number of factors and can often be improved if the bladder is washed out a few times (Fig. 25.39).

The bladder

All parts of the bladder are carefully examined by moving the cystoscope in and out and gradually rotating it. It is probably easier to start at the bladder neck at 6 o'clock viewing the bladder as the cystoscope is moved in as far as it will go and then out again, rotating it a few times and repeating the movement (Fig. 25.40) and continuing this way until the instrument has rotated 360° and all the bladder has been inspected. If the cystoscope is moved closer to any suspicious areas, they will be magnified and seen more clearly. The anterior wall of the bladder or the bladder pouch that forms behind an enlarged middle prostatic lobe may not be seen even with the 70° telescope, but can be seen with the retrograde telescope (120°). If a retrograde telescope is not available, these parts may still be visualized with the 70° telescope if pressure is applied to the anterior abdominal wall or the anterior rectal wall or if the patient is tilted into a Trendelenberg position. The trigone of the bladder is always redder than the rest of the bladder and failure to appreciate this accounts for the apparent epidemics of trigonitis that occur whenever a new surgeon starts doing cystoscopies.

Both ureteric orifices should next be examined (Fig. 25.53); they are situated some 2 or 3 cm above the posterior bladder neck at 4 and 8 o'clock at the lateral angles of the interureteric bar. The easiest way to find the ureteric orifices (which may be difficult or even impossible to locate if the bladder is inflamed or trabeculated, or the middle prostatic lobe much enlarged) is to find the interureteric bar in the midline posteriorly then follow it to the left and right. Sometimes the intravenous injection of indigocarmine (with frusemide, if the examination is done under general anaesthesia, and the patient is dehydrated) may help to locate an orifice if one can see the dye emerging from the ureter, although the dye rapidly diffuses and mixes with the fluid in the bladder, and obscures the view (Fig. 25.39). The air bubble is seen in the highest part of the bladder (the fundus) and obscures the mucosa underlying it. This mucosa can be examined if the air

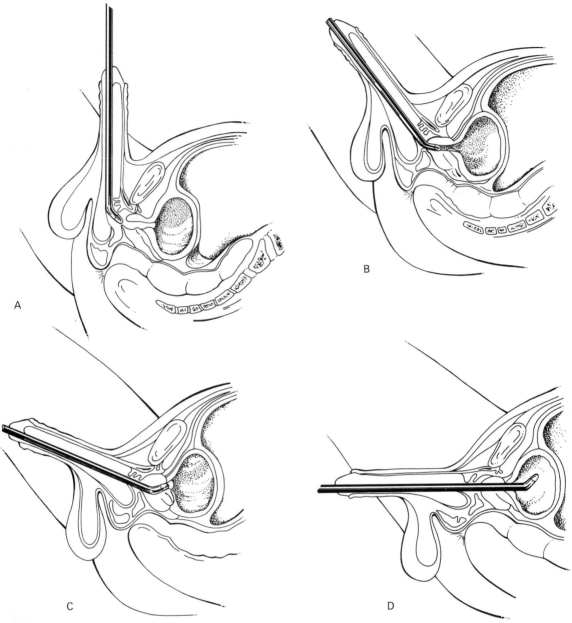

Fig. 25.38 A–D The method of passing cystoscope

bubble is moved by tilting the patient. (If a large air bubble enters the bladder as it is being filled, the patient may complain of pneumaturia, the first or second time he passes urine after the examination).

Although the bladder neck and posterior urethra were examined with the 30° fore-oblique telescope, they should be examined a second time with the 70° telescope. The bladder neck cannot all be seen in one view, but successive views seen as the instrument is rotated through 360° reveal its shape. Common conditions seen at GU endoscopy are shown in Figs. 25.41 to 25.52.

Retrograde catheterization

The indications for this procedure (p. 507) and apparatus required (p. 518) have been discussed. At one time retrograde pyelograms were made often instead of intravenous ones as a means of determining whether or not the upper urinary tract was normal. Nowadays, they are done, if at all, to elucidate an abnormality seen in IVU, ultrasound or other investigation, and it is safest to do one side at a time.

With the inspection sheath catheter deflecting mechanism (Albarran lever) and telescope (either 70° or fore-

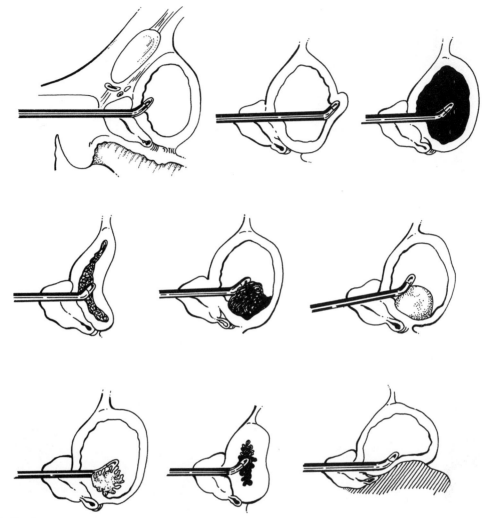

Fig. 25.39 The factors which may obscure the view obtained through an endoscope

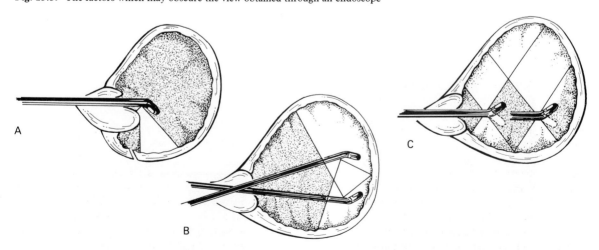

Fig. 25.40 A–C The fields of view obtained with various positions of the telescope and the means by which the whole bladder can be examined by moving the cystoscope

Figs. 25.41–25.52 *Cystoscopic photographs*

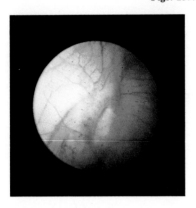

Fig. 25.41 Normal ureteric orifice

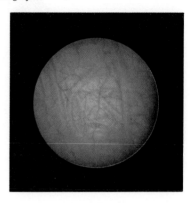

Fig. 25.42 Bladder trabeculation

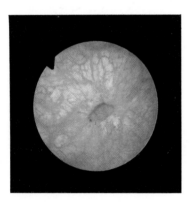

Fig. 25.43 Bladder diverticulum

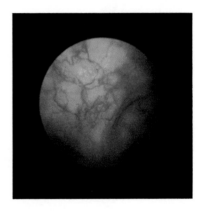

Fig. 25.44 Simple patchy cystitis

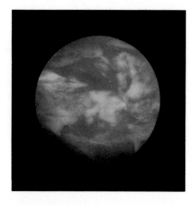

Fig. 25.45 Tuberculous ulcer

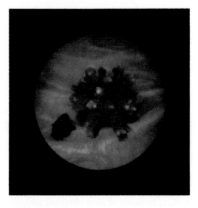

Fig. 25.46 Bladder calculi

Figs. 25.41–25.52 *Cystoscopic photographs*

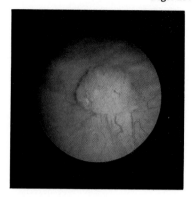

Fig. 25.47 Papillary bladder tumour

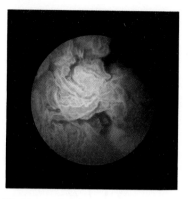

Fig. 25.48 Bladder carcinoma

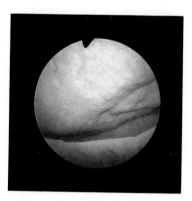

Fig. 25.49 Bladder neck and beyond

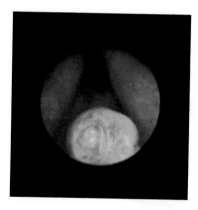

Fig. 25.50 Normal verumontanum and lateral lobes

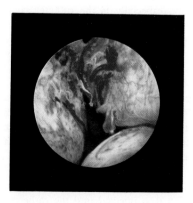

Fig. 25.51 The three lobes of prostate

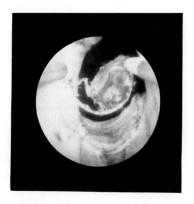

Fig. 25.52 Resection of the prostate

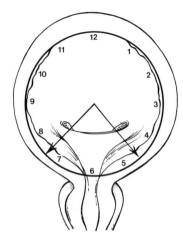

Fig. 25.53 The ureteric orifices

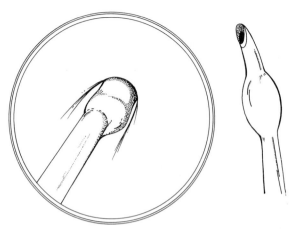

Fig. 25.55 Method of using Braasch or Chevasseur ureteric catheters

oblique can be used), the catheter is threaded through until its tip can be seen emerging into the bladder from the end of the instrument. By moving the endoscope the ureteric orifice can be located and the catheter tip approximated to it (Fig. 25.54). The tip of the catheter can then be pushed into the orifice by moving the whole endoscope or only the Albarran lever; once the catheter is in the ureter the stylet should be removed, either completely, or 1 cm or 2 cm at a time, as the catheter is pushed 25 to 30 cm up the ureter.

At this stage some 10 cm of catheter still projects out of the cystoscope; this is pushed down the cystoscope and into the bladder until the end of the catheter is flush with the rubber nipple. The cystoscope is then carefully removed, making sure the platform is first lowered, leaving the 10 cm of ureteric catheter sticking out of the external meatus. Its end is inserted into some collection appliance like a small bottle with a rubber cap. Once X–rays have been made or collections completed, the catheter is removed. In many units the patient is transferred from the theatre to an X–ray department before the retrograde films are taken. It is important to do this expeditiously, especially if the catheter could not be passed up the whole length of the ureter; otherwise, the catheter may be found coiled up in the bladder and no longer in the ureter because of extrusion by ureteric peristalsis. Failure to pass a catheter does not mean the ureter is obstructed, nor does success mean it is not.

Ureteric catheterisation may introduce or aggravate infection, it may also aggravate obstruction by causing oedema. For this reason, retrograde pyelograms and ureterograms are often made using a bulb catheter of Braasch or Chevasseur (Fig. 25.55) type. The tip of the catheter is inserted into the ureter and the bulb impacted in or against the orifice to prevent dye effluxing into the bladder when it is injected into the catheter. Contrast medium 25% is slowly injected into the catheter, and

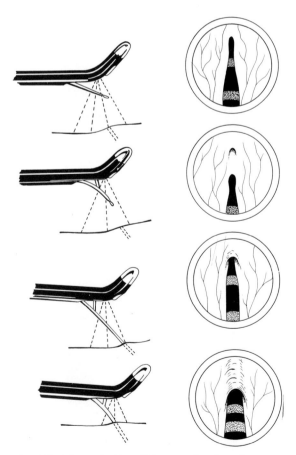

Fig. 25.54 The method by which a ureteric catheter is inserted into the ureter

ascends to fill the ureter and pelvicaliceal system, and X–rays can be taken. As only 1 or 2 cm of the catheter are inserted, the procedure is done with the cystoscope tip in the bladder, and with the operator viewing the ureteric orifice to ensure that the catheter does not dislodge during the injection.

Bimanual examination

Once the endoscopy is completed, the bladder emptied and the instruments removed, a bimanual examination should always be done. Under general anaesthesia with an empty bladder, bimanual examination can determine the local extent of bladder and prostatic tumours, or detect lesions of vagina, cervix, uterus, rectum, colon or pelvis that are associated with or indeed the cause of urinary problems.

FURTHER READING

Gow J G, Hopkins H H 1978 Handbook of Urological Endoscopy Churchill Livingstone, Edinburgh
Lees W R 1984 Abdominal Ultrasonography. Blackwell, Oxford.
Lloyd-Davies R W, Gow J G, Davies D R 1983 A colour atlas of Urology. Wolfe Medical, London
Mitchell J P 1981 Endoscopic Operative Urology. John Wright & Son, Bristol
Sherwood T 1980 Uroradiology. Blackwell, Oxford.
Turner-Warwick R, Whiteside C G 1982 Urodynamic Studies. In:Chisholm G D, Williams D I (eds) Scientific Foundations of Urology, 2nd ed. Heinemann, London, p 442
Uszler J M, Holmes J H, Boswell W D 1983 Radionuclear and Radiographic Techniques. In:Massry S G, Glassock R J (eds) Textbook of Urology. Williams & Wilkins, Baltimore, London, p 12.3
Whitfield H N, Hendry W F (eds) 1985 Textbook of Genito-urinary Surgery. Churchill Livingstone, Edinburgh, Vol 1

26

The kidney, the adrenal glands and the ureters

J. E. NEWSAM & R. F. RINTOUL

Anatomy of the kidney

The kidneys have a characteristic shape and measure about 11 by 6 by 4 cm. They lie on the posterior abdominal wall opposite the 12th thoracic and first three lumbar vertebrae (Fig. 26.1). Their long axes are slightly oblique, so that the upper poles are nearer one another than the lower. The right kidney is pushed down by the liver and lies at a lower level than the left one. *The hilum* is a vertical slit on the medial border of the kidney. It opens into a space called the renal sinus, lies about the level of the 1st lumbar vertebra some 4 cm from the midline and transmits the ureter, blood vessels, sympathetic nerves and lymphatics (Smith, 1983).

Structure of the kidney

The kidney is enveloped by a *fibrous capsule* and consists of the parenchyma and the collecting system. The *parenchyma* has an outer cortex which is pale and granular and

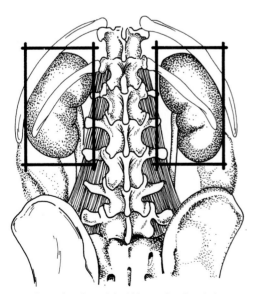

Fig. 26.1 Posterior view of the kidneys showing their relationships with the thoracic and lumbar vertebrae and the ribs

composed of glomeruli and proximal and distal tubules, and an inner medulla which is striated and composed of the loops of Henle and the collecting tubules. The medulla is divided into a number of pyramids, the apices of which are called papillae and invaginate the minor calices. The *collecting system* comprises the 8 to 10 minor calices which embrace the papillae and which unite to form 2 to 4 major calices. These in turn unite to form the pelvis which is funnel shaped and tapers to become the ureter.

The *renal fascia* encloses the kidney, the adrenal gland and the perinephric fat. It consists of anterior and posterior layers which blend laterally with the retroperitoneal tissues, superiorly with the diaphragmatic fascia and medially invest the blood vessels and renal pelvis. The extraperitoneal fat lies outside the renal fascia and is sometimes called *pararenal fat*.

Relations

Posteriorly the upper part of the kidney lies on the diaphragm which separates it from the 11th intercostal space, the 12th rib and the pleura (Fig. 26.2); the lower part on the psoas major, quadratus and transversus muscles, the subcostal vessels and the subcostal, iliohypogastric and ilio-inguinal nerves (Fig. 26.3). *Anteriorly* the right kidney is related to the 2nd part of the duodenum and the right colic flexure; the left, to the pancreas and splenic vessels. *Laterally* the right kidney is related to the hepatic flexure and the ascending colon; the left, to the left colic flexure and the descending colon (Fig. 26.4).

The pedicle of the kidney

This consists of the vein, artery and ureter or renal pelvis (from before backwards) the sympathetic nerves and the lymph vessels. The right renal vein is short and, therefore, more difficult to deal with at operation than the left one and more likely to be invaded by a renal cell carcinoma. The renal artery often has two main branches. Sometimes accessory or aberrant arteries enter the kidney above or below the hilum and may pass behind or in front of the ureter.

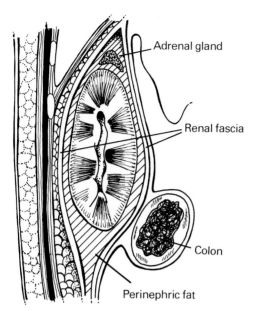

Fig. 26.2 A sagittal section of the kidney showing its relationships to the pleura, adrenal gland and colon

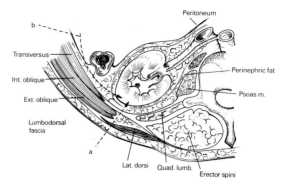

Fig. 26.4 A transverse section of the body at the level of the first lumbar vertebra showing the relationships of the left kidney and the renal pedicle. The lumbar approach (a) and the transperitoneal anterior approach(b) are indicated

SURGICAL APPROACHES TO THE KIDNEY

Position of the patient for posterolateral incisions
The patient is placed on his sound side, with his back, at which the surgeons stands, brought over towards the edge of the table. The leg next to the table is fully flexed at the hip and knee; the upper leg is extended (Fig. 26.5). The patient is maintained in this position by a back support or strapping. To increase access, the trunk should be flexed laterally by raising the 'kidney bridge' if the table has one, or 'breaking' the table to lower the feet and the head. A support for the upper arm prevents the shoulder from sagging forwards and makes the arm and hand easily accessible to the anaesthetist.

Lumbar subcostal approach
This approach can be used for some operations on the kidney and the renal pelvis and for most operations on the upper ureter. In fat patients, and for operations on high kidneys for large tumours and for reoperations, it provides a poor exposure and cannot easily be extended and most surgeons prefer the lateral approaches made through or above the 12th or 11th rib. The subcostal incision can be extended anteriorly, but it is not easy to extend it posteriorly and superiorly by excising or mobilizing the 12th rib if access is restricted. Investigations can image the kidney and assess disease so accurately that the surgeon should know what incision is best before starting the operation.

Incision (Fig. 26.6)
This begins below the angle between the 12th rib and the lateral border of sacrospinalis and is carried downwards and forwards in a curved line between the 12th rib and the iliac crest.

It usually stops 4 to 5 cm above the anterior superior spine, but can be extended forwards to the lateral border

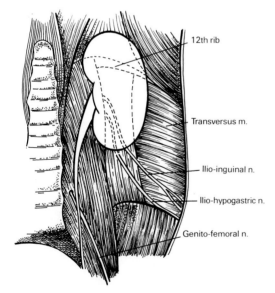

Fig. 26.3 The posterior relations of the left kidney which are the diaphragm above and the psoas, quadratus lumborum and transversus muscles, separated by the iliohypogastric and ilioinguinal nerves, below

The adrenal glands
These are small yellow bodies which lie on the superomedial aspect of the kidneys. They are enclosed within the renal fascia, but separated from the kidney by a fascial septum (see also p. 556).

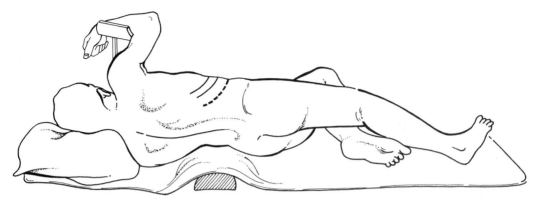

Fig. 26.5 Position of patient on the operating table for posterolateral approaches to the kidney. Note the flexed lower limb and the extended upper one

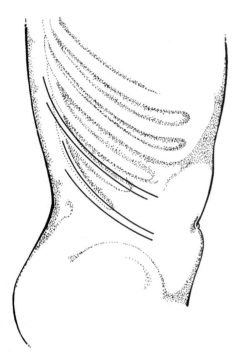

Figs. 26.7–26.9 *The lumbar exposure of the left kidney*

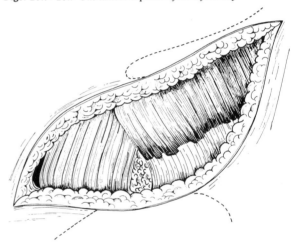

Fig. 26.7 The skin incision exposes the external oblique muscle anteriorly and the latissimus dorsi posteriorly. Between them is the lumbar triangle

Fig. 26.6 The skin incisions for the various posterolateral exposures of the kidney. From below upwards, the subcostal approach, the twelfth rib approach, the eleventh rib approach and the thoraco-abdominal incision through the tenth intercostal space

of the rectus muscle or beyond. The skin incision exposes the muscle fibres of latissimus dorsi and serratus posterior inferior posteriorly, and of the external oblique anteriorly. They are incised in the same line as the skin incision to expose the quadratus lumborum posteriorly, the internal oblique anteriorly and the three fused layers of lumbodorsal fascia, which form a strip of fibrous tissue about 3 cm wide between them. The lumbodorsal fascia is incised or split transversely in front of the lateral

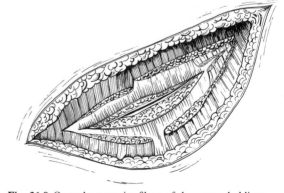

Fig. 26.8 Once the posterior fibres of the external oblique and the anterior fibres of the latissimus dorsi are divided in the line of the skin incision, the serratus posterior inferior posteriorly, and the internal oblique muscle anteriorly, are exposed. They are divided to expose the renal fascia. A self retaining retractor can now be inserted

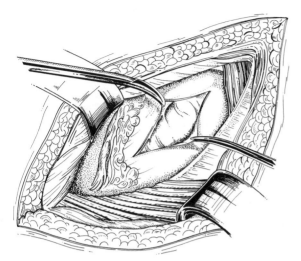

Fig. 26.9 The renal fascia is picked up well posteriorly so that it is not confused with the peritoneum. It is incised exposing perinephric fat and the kidney which can then be mobilized

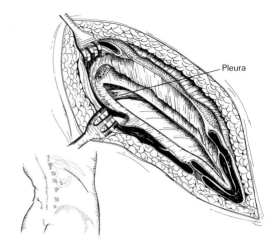

Fig. 26.10 Twelfth rib approach. The skin incision is made along the line of the twelfth rib starting at the angle posteriorly and continued into the abdomen as far as necessary. The rib is resected subperiosteally taking care to avoid, if possible, the pleura which descends below the level of the twelfth rib

border of the quadratus lumborum exposing extraperitoneal fat (Figs. 26.7–26.9). Two fingers or a swab on forceps can be inserted into this space and used to separate the peritoneum from the deep surface of transversus and to protect it as the transversus and internal oblique are divided in the line of the incision. The subcostal nerve and vessels passing downwards and forwards within the deep layers of internal oblique can often be retracted. If they are in the way the vein and artery can be divided between ligatures, but every effort should be made to preserve the nerve.

Closure of the incision
The patient is straightened by lowering the kidney bridge or straightening the table so that the wound margins fall together. The retroperitoneal space should be drained with a tube, a strip of corrugated plastic, or a Redivac drain (p. 2). The muscles are repaired in three layers; the author uses number 1 chromic catgut for each layer.

12th Rib approach
This approach provides better access to the kidney and is little, if any, more difficult than the subcostal incision (Fig. 26.10).

The incision starts a little medial to the lateral border of sacrospinalis, directly over the angle of 12th rib and is continued forwards along the rib and carried beyond its tip as far as required, depending on the build of the patient and how complex the operation is expected to be. The latissimus dorsi and the serratus posterior inferior muscles are divided. The periosteum over the 12th rib is incised in the line of the incision and the rib freed

subperiostally using a periosteal elevator. If the lower border is freed first, a finger can be introduced behind the rib to protect the pleura (which extends below the 12th rib) while the rest of the rib is freed; the rib is divided near its angle and the anterior part removed. The bed of the rib, consisting of the periosteum on the inner surface of the rib and some fibres of the diaphragm, is incised and the extraperitoneal fat exposed. Two fingers or a swab on forceps can now be inserted anteriorly to push the peritoneum forwards off the deep aspect of the transversus muscle and kept there to protect the peritoneum as the incision is extended forwards by cutting the external and internal oblique and the transversus muscles. The incision can be extended anteriorly if necessary by dividing the rectus sheath and muscle. The pleura can be identified in the medial part of the rib bed and safeguarded as the incision is extended medially. If the 12th rib is absent or very short, the incision can be made along the 11th rib. In other words, it is the last palpable rib that is excised, usually the 12th but maybe the 11th. The renal fascia is then incised and the kidney exposed.

Supracostal incision (see Turner-Warwick, 1980)
This incision is usually made above the 12th rib, but if the 12th rib is short or absent it can be made above the 11th rib. It provides as good an exposure as resecting the rib but has advantages, as the rib provides a sound foundation for retracting the lower part of the incision and adds strength to the final wound. The skin incision, like that used for rib resection, is made over the rib but for the supracostal approach it starts some 4 or 5 cm further

back over the rib. The upper and medial aspects of the rib are mobilized extraperiostally if possible, (subperiostally if not) aiming to avoid the pleura because this is meant to be an extrapleural approach. Once fully mobilized, the rib can be easily rotated downwards on its single articulation with the 12th thoracic vertebra. Mobilization must extend back as far as this joint and include division of the costovertebral ligament, otherwise the rib may be fractured as it is retracted. If the rib is fractured it should be removed because it may sequestrate. The incision is extended forwards through the muscles of the anterior abdominal wall as described for the incision resecting the 12th rib.

Lumbotomy

This exposure is used by many surgeons for simple operations on the renal pelvis or upper ureter. It gives less access than the lumbar incision, especially in fat people, but can be extended upwards by resecting a small segment of the 12th or even 11th rib.

The patient is placed in a lateral position, but as this is a posterior incision the upper shoulder and buttock are allowed to roll forward, exposing more of the back than for the posterolateral incision (Figs. 26.11).

A vertical skin incision is made downwards from the 12th or 11th rib to the iliac crest along the lateral border of the sacrospinalis, and the latissimus dorsi is incised or split in the same line. Retracting forwards the free posterior border of the external oblique exposes the 3 cm wide strip of fused lumbodorsal fascia at the lateral edge of the quadratus lumborum. This fascia is incised vertically and the retroperitoneal space entered (Fig. 26.12).

Thoraco-abdominal approach

This approach is made through the bed of the 10th rib or through the 10th intercostal space, and affords an excellent exposure of the renal pedicle and kidney. A long incision is made over the 10th intercostal space and continued across the costal margin downwards and forwards to the midline or even across the midline to the lateral edge of the opposite rectus. The thoracic component of the incision is deepened through the muscles of the space and the pleura is opened. The abdominal component is deepened through the oblique abdominal muscles and one or both recti and the peritoneum opened. The diaphragm is incised in the line of the incision. On the left the colon and on the right the colon and duodenum are reflected medially and the kidney and its pedicle exposed.

Nagamatsu incision

This is an extrapleural extension of the incision excising the 12th rib. It is used by some surgeons for the exposure of large renal tumours and certainly provides a wide exposure. The incision is the same as the one used for

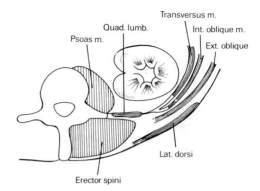

Fig. 26.11

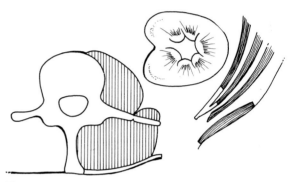

Fig. 26.12

Figs 26.11 & 26.12 Lumbotomy incision. The skin incision is a vertical one along the lateral edge of the sacrospinalis exposing the latissimus dorsi. Incising the latissimus dorsi in the same line the free posterior edge of the external oblique is seen and retracted forwards exposing the fused layers of lumber dorsal fascia and the external and transversus muscles taking origin from them. The fused layers of lumbar dorsal fascia are incised vertically exposing the renal fascia which is then opened

12th rib resection. The 12th rib is resected and the incision extended anteriorly as described, but the posterior end is extended vertically upwards across the angles of the 11th and 10th ribs, incising the latissimus dorsi and serratus posterior inferior and excising a 2.5 cm segment from the angles of the 11th and 12th ribs. It provides a large anterosuperior flap of skin, muscles and ribs which when retracted gives an extensive exposure.

Exploratory technique for posterior approach

Pleura

No matter how much care is taken, it is inevitable that the pleura will occasionally be opened when the kidney is exposed by resecting the 12th or 11th rib, or by a supracostal incision. Little disturbance results at the time because most patients are on some form of positive pressure anaesthesia; but if air remains in or can be sucked into the pleural cavity postoperatively, the patient may develop respiratory difficulties.

Some surgeons suture the pleura (more easily done with the supracostal than the rib resection exposures) while the anaesthetist hyperinflates the lungs; some leave in a tube, one end in the pleura and the other in a basin of water, removing it when the wound is sutured and the anaesthetist hyperinflates the lungs; it is preferable to close the pleura, but leave in a water seal drain which is removed 24 or 48 hours after operation when a chest X-ray shows that the lung is reinflated.

Exposure and delivery of the kidney

The muscles are retracted and the loose retroperitoneal fatty tissue exposed. The renal fascia is identified in the posterior part of the wound behind the peritoneum. It is opened between forceps and the opening is enlarged by cutting with scissors or scalpel or stretching with the fingers. The smooth glistening surface of the renal capsule may be seen, but is usually hidden amid perinephric fat. With fingers, forceps or scissors the kidney in its capsule is carefully separated from the perinephric fat and from the peritoneum which may be adherent anteriorly. The upper pole of the kidney is anchored to the diaphragm by strong fibrofatty bands which should be divided and ligated. The adrenal gland is separated from the kidney by fascia and unlikely to be disturbed if the dissection is kept close to the kidney. Equally easily separated are the colon and duodenum on the right side and the colon and pancreas on the left side. The kidney can be mobilized and brought out of the wound without difficulty when there are no surrounding adhesions. In many patients, however, because of infection, stones or previous operations, the kidney is densely adherent to surrounding structures and the posterior abdominal wall and can be mobilized only with great difficulty. In some circumstances the dissection must be patiently pursued with great care to avoid damaging pleura, diaphragm, renal pedicle, duodenum and even the liver, the spleen, the pancreas and the vena cava.

Anterior approach

This approach is often preferred for the removal of a large renal cell carcinoma, for the exploration of an injured kidney and the treatment of hydronephrosis, but it is not very suitable for the removal of stones or for operations on an infected kidney. It is, however, ideal for most operations on the pelves of horseshoe or ectopic kidneys or of other kidneys which have failed to rotate because in such kidneys the pelvis and pelvi-ureteric junctions lie anteriorly, not medially.

A subcostal or a paramedian incision, depending on the build of the patient, can be used for benign disease but for renal cell carcinoma a larger incision is essential (Fig. 26.13). A useful one starts at the tip of

Figs. 26.13 & 26.14 *Anterior approach to the kidney*

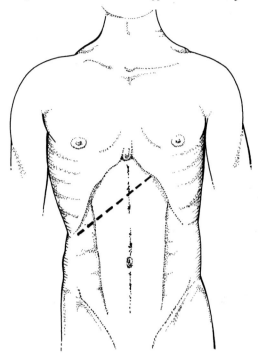

Fig. 26.13 The skin incision starts at the tip of the twelfth rib and is carried below and more or less parallel to the costal margin across the midline to the opposite costal margin

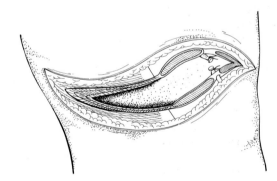

Fig. 26.14 The incision is deepened through the oblique muscles of the abdomen laterally and the rectus medially to expose the peritoneum, and can be extended anteriorly by dividing the opposite rectus muscle or posteriorly through or above the twelfth rib

the 12th rib on the affected side and extends transversely and slightly upwards across the midline to the opposite costal margin, dividing both recti (Fig. 26.14). It can be extended backwards along or above the 12th rib if necessary. The peritoneum is opened and the falciform ligament is divided between forceps and ligated. Small bowel is packed into the opposite side of the abdomen. The peritoneum of the posterior wall is incised along the lateral aspect of the ascending colon, hepatic flexure and 2nd part of the duodenum on the right side, or descending colon and splenic flexure on the left side and the colon is mobilized and displaced medially to expose the anterior surface of the kidney and its pedicle.

NEPHRECTOMY

The surgery of the kidney has become increasingly conservative and far fewer nephrectomies are done for hydronephrosis, stones, infection, trauma or vascular disease than used to be the case. Even for malignant disease some surgeons now favour more conservative operations than nephrectomy, particularly in patients with impaired renal function or low grade tumours.

Indications
Nephrectomy is indicated in:
1. Patients having renal transplants or chronic dialysis if their own kidneys are infected or considered the cause of uncontrollable hypertension.
2. Patients with a nonfunctioning or very poorly functioning hydronephrotic, infected, ischaemic or stone containing kidney on one side and a normal kidney on the other.
3. Patients with unilateral renal hypertension, when it is thought better to remove the kidney rather than reconstruct the artery.
4. Patients with renal tuberculosis in whom the organisms are resistant to chemotherapy, or chemotherapy is otherwise considered inappropriate.
5. Some patients with a severely traumatized kidney or renal pedicle on one side and a normal kidney on the other.
6. Patients with malignant disease of the kidney. For renal cell carcinoma a radical nephrectomy is considered better than a simple nephrectomy and for transitional cell tumours, a nephro-ureterectomy better than a nephrectomy.

Nephrectomy
The kidney is exposed and mobilized. By gentle dissection with scissors or gauze the pedicle is cleared on both aspects and the major vessels separately identified. The main renal artery lies behind the vein in front of the renal pelvis, but there may be other blood vessels passing to or from the upper or lower poles of the kidney, arteries that arise from the renal artery or aorta or veins which join the renal vein or vena cava.

All vessels should be dealt with separately if at all possible to reduce the risks of a ligature slipping and of an arteriovenous anomaly forming.

Whether the vessels should be ligatured in continuity before being divided, or clamped and divided before ligation, is a matter for personal preference and expediency although the first method is safer. The artery is separated from investing fat, which is often firm and fibrous, and nerve fibres. Two ligatures are placed on the aortic side and one on the kidney side using a right angled forceps like an O'Shaughnessy and the artery divided between them (Fig. 26.15, 26.16). The renal vein is similarly dealt with. Be careful not to pull too hard on the kidney while placing the ligatures around the vein, otherwise you may tear the vein off the inferior vena cava, and have some anxious minutes wondering why you ever took up surgery!

The right renal vein is short and may be difficult to ligate in the way described; if so, apply a Satinsky clamp laterally on the vena cava where the vein enters. Divide the vein distal to the clamp and suture the cava with a 5/0 arterial suture before the clamp is removed.

If the kidney has been operated on before or is infected and there are dense adhesions, it may be impossible to identify, isolate and ligate the vessels in the way described. In such cases the pedicle can be clamped en masse and the kidney removed, leaving sufficient tissue beyond the clamp that can be picked up, with forceps, separately ligating the stumps of the main vessels before removing the clamp. If even this procedure is impossible, the pedicle may be ligated en masse. To do this the pedicle is divided on the distal side of two heavy kidney clamps. The deeper clamp is slowly removed as a ligature is tied on the proximal side; a second ligature is then applied and tightened as the superficial clamp is removed. It is tempting to use No. 1 silk or nylon to ligate the vessels of the renal pedicle. To use nonabsorbable materials, however, when removing an infected kidney often causes a persistent sinus or recurrent infection, which only heals when the suture material is extruded or removed, and removing it by operation is not easy. The author uses No. 1 chromic catgut whether the kidney is infected or not. The kidney, attached now only by the ureter, is drawn forwards; the ureter is freed downwards to a convenient level and divided between ligatures (Fig. 26.17, 26.18). Dense adhesions, likely to be found if the kidney is infected, or has been previously operated on, add greatly to the difficulties of the operation. Some can be anticipated by making an incision that provides a generous exposure and by cross matching the patient for several more units of blood than is usual for a simple nephrectomy. It is often useful to open deliberately the peritoneum at an early stage of the operation to free the liver and duodenum on the right side or the spleen and colon on the left side, as these structures may not be seen easily if an extraperitoneal exposure alone is attempted. If it proves impossible to mobilize the kidney in the plane between capsule and fat, a subca-

Figs. 26.15–26.18 *Left nephrectomy*

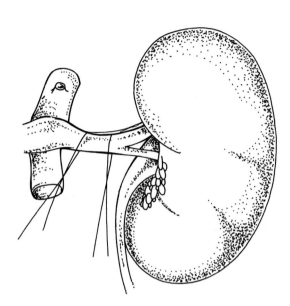

Fig. 26.15 The renal vein is exposed and gently separated from the artery. Two ligatures are placed around the vein

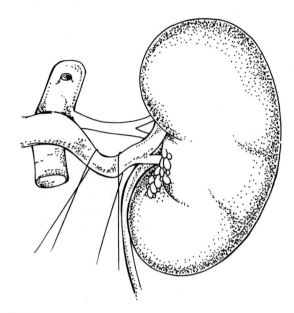

Fig. 26.16 The artery is displayed by gentle downwards traction on the ligatures around the vein. (Because the vein lies anterior to the artery it may seem easier to ligate it first. This is a mistake because it congests the kidney)

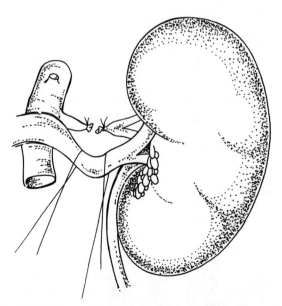

Fig. 26.17 The artery has been ligated and divided prior to ligation of the vein. Two ligatures can be placed on the aortic side and one on the renal side for safety. (It is important at this stage to look carefully for aberrant or accessory vessels)

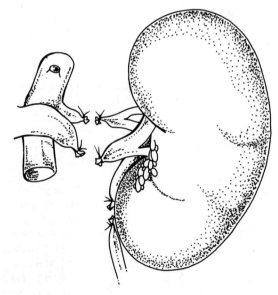

Fig. 26.18 The ureter is divided between ligatures at a convenient level and the kidney is then removed

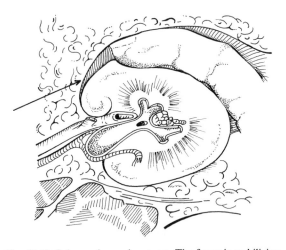

Fig. 26.19 Subcapsular nephrectomy. The finger is mobilizing the kidney in the plane between parenchyma and renal capsule. Once the front and back and lateral aspects of the kidney have been mobilized in this way it is essential to divide by sharp dissection the capsule of the kidney anteriorly (arrowed) to expose the renal pedicle

psular nephrectomy can be done. An incision is made through the renal capsule on the lateral aspect of the kidney and by finger and gauze dissection, the plane of cleavage between it and the kidney is opened up. The separation is continued on all surfaces as far as the pedicle, where the everted capsule must be incised (Fig. 26.19) so that the vessels of the pedicle can be dissected out. This can be very difficult and the procedure should only be done when a careful and patient effort to mobilise the kidney in its capsule proves impossible.

Nephrectomy for renal cell carcinoma

Nephrectomy for renal cell carcinoma (sometimes known as hypernephroma or adenocarcinoma) differs in several ways from nephrectomy for nonmalignant disease. Firstly it is more radical and involves the removal of all the perinephric fat and the adrenal gland; secondly it involves ligation of the veins at an early stage in the procedure so that malignant cells are not disseminated to other parts of the body as the kidney is handled and

Figs. 26.20 & 26.21 *Renal artery embolization*

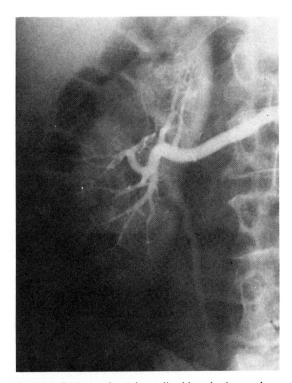

Fig. 26.20 Right renal arteries outlined by selective renal angiography

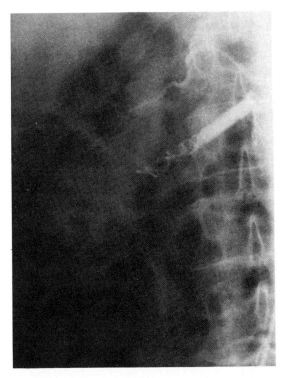

Fig. 26.21 Several occluding springs have been inserted into the renal artery. The springs carry thrombogenic tails of Dacron strands which cannot be seen on the X-ray

manipulated and thirdly the tumour, especially when it involves the right kidney, often grows along the renal vein and into the inferior vena cava and in these circumstances it is essential to open the vena cava and remove the tumour within, but considerable care has to be exercised otherwise a tumour embolus can be caused. Fourthly many surgeons now embolize the renal artery with a balloon catheter, occluding spring or gelatin foam, some days before operation. This procedure obviously facilitates the operation by reducing the amount of bleeding, and it may also have some beneficial immunological effects. Embolization is done by selective renal angiography (Fig. 26.20) and the main renal artery is occluded with a balloon catheter (see Fig. 25.9) which has to be left in place until operation, or by the insertion of a spring with thrombogenic tails of dacron strands or pieces of soluble gelatin foam (Fig. 26.21). The second of these is best. The procedure usually causes pain and fever, which resolves within a day or two. It is by no means certain how long to wait after embolization before carrying out nephrectomy, but 2 or 3 days is usual. At that time oedema around the kidney aids mobilization; later oedematous tissue becomes fibrous and operation more difficult. Angiography and inferior caval venography carried out before operation suggest the size, position and extent of the tumour (Fig. 26.22).

Although a large posterolateral incision through or above the rib, a Nagamatsu or a thoraco-abdominal incision can and often are used, an anterior incision is preferred. This can be a long paramedian or transverse incision, or a subcostal one (see p. 533) The patient is placed supine and elevated on the affected side with sandbags to an angle of 45°, i.e. halfway to a lateral position and an anterior incision is made.

First the renal vein is gently mobilized using a right angled clamp. A ligature is passed round the vein, but it is not tied at this stage unless the artery has been embolized pre-operatively, otherwise the kidney swells, congests and bleeds. Next the artery is located behind the vein in fibrofatty tissue. It is mobilized, ligated and divided. If the right renal vein or the inferior vena cava contain tumour, special care must be exercised to avoid dislodging a tumour embolus, and an attempt must be made to remove tumour from the vein.

In these circumstances the right renal artery is best ligated at its origin from the aorta medial to the vena cava. Occlusion clamps should be applied to the inferior vena cava above and below the renal veins, and to the left renal vein, and any lumbar veins entering the vena cava between them ligated. The inferior vena cava is opened and the tumour removed by suction. The incision in the vena cava is closed with a 5/0 arterial suture and the renal vein ligated.

Once the pedicle has been dealt with the kidney can be mobilized and removed with its perinephric fat, the

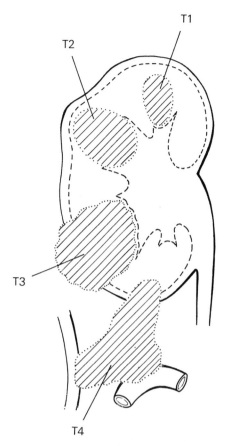

Fig. 26.22 The local extent of renal cell carcinoma. This can be expressed as its T stage.

T1. The tumour is confined to the parenchyma of the kidney and neither disturbs the outline of the cortex nor invades the collecting system.

T2. The tumour is confined to the parenchyma of the kidney but distorts the outline of the kidney and invades or distorts the collecting system.

T3. The tumour extends through the capsule into perinephric fat

T4. The tumour extends through the perinephric fat and involves adjacent viscera or muscles

adrenal gland and as much renal fascia as possible. Haemostasis is secured and the wound is closed with drainage.

Renal cell carcinomas are relatively radioresistant and much controversy surrounds the place of radiotherapy. Few regard routine preoperative or postoperative radiotherapy of much value, but postoperative radiotherapy is worth considering if tumour is found in the regional lymph nodes at the time of operation. These nodes are involved in as many as 20% of patients with renal cell carcinoma. Some patients have abnormal blood findings such as an elevated ESR and less often polycythaemia, hypercalcaemia or other abnormalities. Such changes can be used as tumour markers to assess the progress of the disease after treatment.

How should we treat patients who have metastases when first seen?. If a metastasis seems solitary and is in a site amenable to surgery, both it and the primary can be treated. If the metastases are multiple the problem is much more difficult and filled with unanswerable questions; should we do a nephrectomy? should we just embolize the kidney? should we do neither? Well, no one knows, but it is obviously sensible to remove the kidney if the patient has pain or bleeding, and probably sensible to remove it if the patient has bony or pulmonary metastasis because there is evidence that such metastases may regress when the primary tumour is removed.

Hormone therapy using either Medroxyprogesterone acetate (Provera) 100 mg t.d.s. or androgens may be useful and without side effects. No other chemotherapeutic agent or combination of agents offers much at the present time although several are on trial.

Haemorrhage from the renal pedicle

This may occur if a mass ligature has been applied and slips, if the pedicle is inadvertently divided while mobilizing an adherent kidney, or if the clamps slip or are pulled off the pedicle before the ligatures are applied. Profuse haemorrhage obscures all structures.

On the right side profuse bleeding often comes from a hole in the inferior vena cava. No attempt should be made to secure the bleeding vessels by plunging forceps into a pool of blood in the hope that the vessels and nothing else will be picked up. Instead two or more gauze packs are pressed into the wound for at least 10 minutes. When the gauze packing is slowly removed the haemorrhage should have slowed enough for the severed vessels to be seen and secured. A tear in the inferior vena cava may be controlled by a Satinsky clamp and repaired with a continuous suture of 5/0 arterial silk.

Large hydronephrotic kidney

The removal of a large hydronephrotic kidney is facilitated if the fluid is first aspirated through a large bore needle inserted into the posterior surface of the hydronephrotic sac. The collapsed sac is then easily mobilized and removed.

NEPHRO-URETERECTOMY

In nephrectomy for nonmalignant disease or renal cell carcinoma the ureter is divided at a convenient level, only a small part being removed. If the ureter is dilated, tuberculous or one in which reflux has been demonstrated, it should all be removed with the kidney. Similarly, in patients with transitional cell tumours of the calices or pelvis of the kidney or the ureter, the whole

length of the ureter, including the intramural part should be removed with the kidney, unless a conservative approach is needed because the kidney is solitary, the disease bilateral, renal function poor or the tumour small and of low grade. The operation can sometimes be done through one incision, but it is best and most easily done through two. Firstly the kidney is mobilized through an appropriate posterolateral or anterior incision removing perinephric fat and renal fascia if the operation is being done for malignant disease. The vessels of the pedicle are separately ligated. The ureter, which is all that now holds the kidney, is mobilized as far down as possible, but not divided. The kidney is then dropped back into the retroperitoneal space and the incision closed over it. The patient is transferred to the supine position and a transverse suprapubic incision is made through skin and rectus sheath with retraction of the recti or a low oblique muscle cutting incision through the oblique muscles and transversus is made (Fig. 26.23). The transversalis fascia is incised and the peritoneum retracted medially. The mobilized kidney is located in the retroperitoneal tissues and lifted out of the wound. The ureter can then be easily traced down to the bladder. In nonmalignant cases to open the bladder is unnecessary and the lower ureter can be pulled up and ligated flush with the bladder wall. In malignant cases the whole ureter, including the intramural part and the ureteric orifice must be removed together with a cuff of bladder, and to do this means opening the bladder. The bladder, thereafter, is closed in two layers with plain catgut and kept empty with a catheter for a week. The wound is drained through the lower incision.

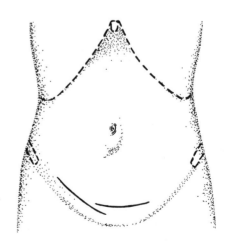

Fig. 26.23 The position on the anterior abdominal wall of the suprapubic or oblique incision used to mobilize and remove the lower end of the ureter in the operation of nephroureterectomy

PARTIAL NEPHRECTOMY

This operation, once popular for the treatment of patients with calculus or tuberculosis of the kidney, was particularly recommended for patients who had a stone or stones in one calix, in the belief that removing the calix would prevent recurrence of stone. However, it is no longer considered justifiable to remove a large piece of normally functioning kidney because the cause of stone formation is hardly confined to one calix and there is now much evidence to show that stones recur no more frequently after nephrolithotomy than they do after partial nephrectomy. In stone disease, therefore, a partial nephrectomy would now be considered appropriate treatment only if the pole containing the stone was seriously fibrosed or infected and has been shown to contribute little, if anything, to overall renal function.

In tuberculosis, too, partial nephrectomy is rarely, if ever done now, because if the disease is localized enough to be curable by partial nephrectomy, it should respond to chemotherapy alone. Partial nephrectomy nowadays, therefore, is mostly carried out for renal cell or transitional cell tumours of the kidney when the more radical procedures are inappropriate because the kidney is solitary, the disease bilateral, renal function poor, or the tumour small and of low grade; or for some renal injuries.

Operation

The kidney is exposed by the appropriate posterolateral incision and fully mobilized. The vessels of the pedicle are cleared of all fat and displayed. If a branch of the renal artery appears to be supplying the area or part of the area of the kidney to be removed it can be ligated but only after temporary occlusion confirms that it does not also supply some part of the kidney that is to be left; the capsule is incised in the coronal plane over the pole to be removed and reflected back as two flaps, one anterior and one posterior (Fig. 26.24).

Next the pedicle needs to be occluded while the kidney is resected. At normal temperature the kidney can withstand complete ischaemia without permanent damage for only about 15 minutes. This time can be extended by using inosine or by cooling. Inosine is a purine nucleotide and 30 to 60 mg/kilo is injected into a peripheral vein 10 minutes before operation or into the renal artery just before the occlusion clamp is applied. It protects the kidney from the effects of total ischaemia for 1 hour (provided preoperative renal function was satisfactory). Cooling the kidney to 15° or 20°C can provide up to 2 to 3 hours protection against complete ischaemia and can be achieved by packing 2 to 3 kg of crushed ice around the mobilized kidney for about 10 minutes, by irrigating the outside and the inside of the kidney and the pelvi-

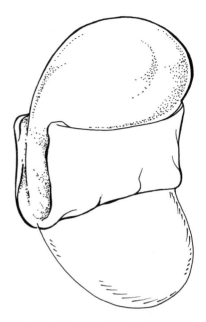

Fig. 26.24 Partial nephrectomy. The capsule is incised in the coronal plane and reflected upwards

caliceal system with ice cold water, or by circulating cold water through two heat exchange coils applied to the surface of the kidney. With all methods of cooling the temperature inside the kidney must be measured with a telethermometer probe and not allowed to fall below 15°C. A vascular occlusion clamp is applied across the pedicle. The kidney is divided transversely at the level of raised capsular flaps or with short anterior and posterior flaps at the appropriate plane, taking great care to avoid the main vessels and the renal pelvis (Fig. 26.25). Further slices can be removed if the initial resection was inadequate. The opened vessels and calix are closed with fine catgut sutures and the occlusion clamp then removed, and any other bleeding vessels are controlled with sutures; the capsule is folded back over the raw surface of the kidney and loosely sutured with catgut (Fig. 26.26). The wound should be drained. Some renal cell carcinomas are so well encapsulated that they can almost be enucleated if it is thought best to treat them conservatively.

Transitional cell tumours of the pelvicaliceal system present special problems if they are unsuitable for the radical treatment described; some in the renal pelvis can be removed locally if they are pedunculated or by resecting part of the pelvis (like a pyeloplasty); tumours in the calix can be treated by partial nephrectomy. However, transitional cell tumours are often much more extensive than the X-rays suggest and it is necessary to examine the whole pelvicaliceal system before proceeding with a conservative operation thought suitable after inspecting the X-rays. This can be done with a nephro-

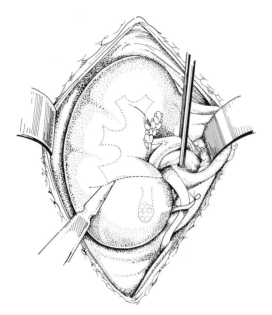

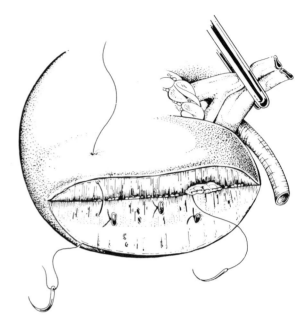

Fig. 26.25 Partial nephrectomy. The renal vein and artery have been temporarily occluded with a vascular occlusion clamp. A small vessel to the lower pole of the kidney has been ligated. The incision made to remove the lower pole of the kidney passes through the neck of the lower calyx which contains stones

Fig. 26.26 Partial nephrectomy. The excision exposes the neck of the calix and opens a number of blood vessels. The neck of the calix can be closed with 4/0 catgut sutures although this is not absolutely necessary. The opened vessels are stitched or ligated and this can be difficult because renal parenchyma is friable. Once haemostasis has been secured the flaps of renal capsule are folded back over the divided lower pole of the kidney and loosely secured with sutures. It is probably unwise and unnecessary to suture the parenchyma of the kidney with mattress sutures as some advise, provided haemostasis has been satisfactorily secured by ligating or suturing the open vessels themselves

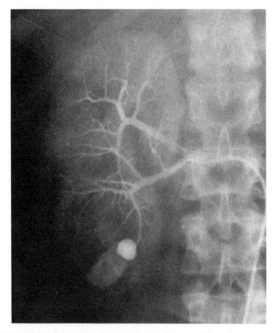

Fig. 26.27 Secondary haemorrhage after partial nephrectomy. Selective angiogram of a patient with severe secondary haemorrhage 10 days after a right nephrolithotomy. It demonstrates that the haemorrhage was due to the formation of an aneurysm which was cured by embolizing its feeding artery with gelatin foam

scope passed through a small incision in the renal pelvis, but if one is not available, a cystoscope can be used.

The major complication of partial nephrectomy is secondary haemorrhage which may be due to vascular abnormality rather than infection and can often be stopped by embolizing the feeding artery at selective renal angiography (Fig. 26.27).

STONES

The condition of stones in the bladder has been known since 4800 B.C. Lithotomy is one of the earliest operations and was practised by the ancient Greeks and Romans. Even in the 19th century it was still the most commonly performed of all operations. Primary bladder stones form almost exclusively in males, especially male children below 5 years of age, and are still endemic in such parts of the world as India, Turkey, Thailand, China, Egypt and Sudan but are now unknown in Western Europe and North America.

In affluent countries upper urinary tract stones, almost unmentioned in medical literature before 1900, are becoming commoner, and now affect about 2 to 4% of the population at some time during their lives. Not only do they occur in affluent societies, but in the most affluent parts of such societies; thus professional workers are 10 times more likely to develop them than unskilled workers.

Diagnosis

The signs and symptoms of stones in the upper urinary tract will not be discussed here; the diagnosis can only be confirmed if the stone is passed or demonstrated radiologically.

About 90% of upper urinary stones contain calcium usually as calcium oxalate or calcium phosphate and, with infection, magnesium ammonium phosphate. Calcium stones are more opaque than soft tissues like muscle and kidney and can be seen in straight X–rays if they overlie soft tissue, but if they overlie the bone of the ribs, transverse processes or sacrum, they may not be visualized. Nor may they be seen, even though overlying soft tissue, if they are small. Calcium stones tend to be about the same density as the contrast media used for urography and, in urograms, are either not seen at all or appear as filling defects and may, like uric acid stones, be confused with tumours or air bubbles. Of the stones that do not contain calcium, about 5% are made of uric acid; 1 or 2% of cystine and the few remaining ones of Xanthine or matrix.

Uric acid stones are no more opaque than soft tissues and can only be seen in pyelo-ureterograms as filling defects; cystine stones contain sulphur, but although slightly more opaque than soft tissues appear in straight X–rays only if the patient is thin and the X–ray of high quality. It follows that many stones, even ones containing calcium, do not show up in a straight X–ray and if the patient's complaints suggest a renal or ureteric stone, further investigations are necessary.

Indications for operation

Once the diagnosis is made and confirmed radiologically treatment can be considered under various headings.

1. Urgent symptoms such as severe pain, severe infection or acute renal failure require urgent treatment.

2. Investigations to identify risk factors that predispose to stone are desirable in most stone patients and essential in those with recurrent or bilateral stones. For calcium stones, the major risk factors are metabolic and include the excretion of excessive quantities of calcium, phosphate or oxalate; low urinary volumes; a low urinary pH and a reduction in the urinary agents such as uric acid and the acid mucopolysaccharides which inhibit crystallization. Other risk factors include anatomical

abnormalities which interfere with the free flow of urine by causing obstruction, reflux or stasis and infection. Cystine stones only occur in patients with cystinuria who can be easily identified by estimating the amount of cystine in a 24 hour specimen of urine. Uric acid stones tend to occur in patients with gout, or with excessive amounts of uric acid in the blood or urine for other reasons (Robertson, 1982).

3. Treatment of the stones:

Renal calculi

Renal calculi less than 1 cm in diameter may pass themselves, and should be observed; larger ones should be removed if they are responsible for recurrent pain, obstruction, progressive hydronephrosis or hydrocalicosis, persistent infection or bleeding; if they are increasing in size or if the kidney is solitary. If they are larger than 1 cm, but causing no symptoms it is tempting to wait and see what happens. This is sensible if the stone is in a calix, but if it is in the pelvis further trouble is inevitable and it should be dealt with.

Pyelolithotomy

In this procedure the stone is removed through an incision in the renal pelvis and it is an ideal operation also for the removal of stones from the calices if they are accessible. For stones in an intrarenal pelvis and for staghorn stones an extended pyelolithotomy of Gil-Vernet type can be done (p. 542). Stone fragments may be removed by coagulation pyelolithotomy (p. 543).

Nephrolithotomy

The stone, usually one in a calix, is removed with an incision through the parenchyma of the kidney. A radial incision damages the kidney less than other incisions. Stones in two or more calices are best removed through separate small radial incisions rather than one big coronal incision. Nephrolithotomy can be combined with pyelolithotomy for the removal of multiple or staghorn calculi.

Partial nephrectomy (p. 539)

Formerly a popular method for treating stones in one calix (usually a lower calix) as a means not only of removing the stone but also of preventing others forming; it is no longer popular and nowadays such stones would be treated by pyelolithotomy or nephrolithotomy. The pole containing the stone would only be removed if it was very scarred or infected.

Nephrectomy

A nephrectomy may be the appropriate operation if one kidney contains multiple stones or a staghorn stone, and has little function or much infection and the other kidney is normal, especially if the patient is elderly.

Percutaneous pyelolithotomy

This procedure has developed because of the ease with which needles can now be inserted percutaneously into the collecting system of a kidney under radiological or ultrasound control. The track made by the needle is progressively dilated with special dilators until it will admit a cystoscope or nephroscope. (This takes some days). The stone can then be removed from the pelvis or calix with biopsy forceps or a stone dislodger of the Dormia type (p. 561) or fragmented with an ultrasound lithotriptor.

Pyelolithotomy

The kidney is exposed by a subcostal or lumbotomy incision if the pelvis is extrarenal, the stone solitary and not large, the patient thin and the kidney neither too high nor previously operated upon; otherwise it should be exposed through or above a rib.

Before mobilization is started the upper ureter should be found and secured with a tape or plastic or silicone tube. This serves two purposes, it prevents stone fragments falling into the ureter if the stone crumbles while it being removed, and secondly, it acts as a guide to find the pelvis. As the renal pelvis is covered anteriorly by the renal vein and artery, it is best approached posteriorly. The operation can often be done without fully mobilizing the kidney if the stone is medium sized and lies in an extrarenal pelvis not previously operated on.

The upper ureter and posterior aspect of the bluish coloured pelvis are exposed by dissecting off perinephric fat which is often very adherent to the pelvis and separated with difficulty. The pelvis is incised transversely or longitudinally between stay sutures of 3/0 silk and the stone is gently removed (Fig. 26.28).

Usually, however, it is easier, once the ureter is controlled by a tape, to mobilize fully the kidney which can then be supported by a netelast sling while the

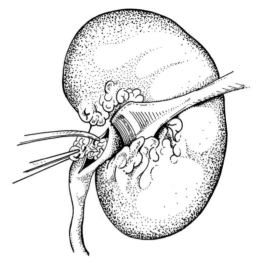

Fig. 26.28 Pyelolithotomy. The renal pelvis has been opened longitudinally and the stone is being removed. A transverse incision, if there is room, is favoured by many surgeons

posterior aspect of the pelvis is freed of fat and opened between stay sutures.

Extended Pyelolithotomy (see Gil-Vernet 1983)

For stones in an intrarenal pelvis and for staghorn stones the procedure is extended to demonstrate the pelvis within the renal sinus. The kidney is fully mobilized after the ureter is secured, and the posterior aspect of the renal pelvis or upper ureter is exposed. The thin connective tissue which passes from the renal capsule to the pelvis and seals the entry into the renal sinus is opened by blunt dissection (Fig. 26.29). The dissection is continued into the sinus between muscle and the pelvis and its adventitial tissue using blunt dissection with scissors or wet pledgets aided by Gil-Vernet retractors which

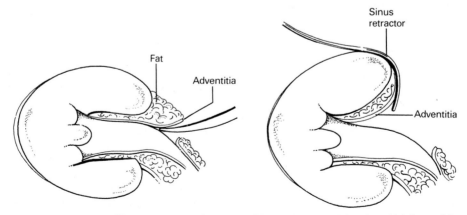

Fig. 26.29 Extended pyelolithotomy. The plane between the muscle of the renal pelvis and the adventitial tissue of the renal sinus must be developed to expose the intrarenal part of the renal pelvis without damaging arteries or veins

Figs. 26.30 & 26.31 *Extended pyelolithotomy*

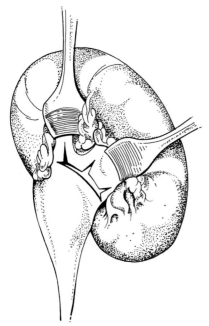

Fig. 26.30 Retractors of the Gil-Vernet type are used to retract the fat of the renal sinus and expose the intrarenal pelvis which has been incised transversely. The incision can be extended into the neck of one or more calices if necessary

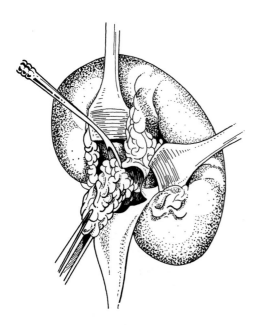

Fig. 26.31 The stone is being gently removed from the pelvis and the calices, often easier done using a dissector as illustrated rather than stone holding forceps

are specially designed for the purpose, when the whole pelvis and caliceal necks can be exposed without damaging any retropelvic arteries or veins. The pelvis is opened transversely and the incision can be extended into the necks of the calices if the stone is a staghorn one (Fig. 26.30).

Large stones are often partly adherent to the mucosa and best removed by gently easing them out using a Macdonald or Watson-Cheyne dissector rather than grasping them with forceps which may crush the stone and make the procedure more difficult than it need be (Fig. 26.31).

If the caliceal extensions of a staghorn calculus are bigger than the necks of the calices containing them, they can be cut from the pelvic part of the stone with heavy scissors or bone cutters, and removed through separate nephrolithotomy incisions as attempts to drag them into the pelvis will only damage the caliceal necks. Once the stone or stones have been removed the pelvis should be thoroughly washed out with sterile water or saline and a contact X-ray taken to ensure that the kidney has been cleared of all stones or stone fragments. The author sutures the pelvis incision loosely with 4/0 dexon or catgut suture, though this is not necessary for small incisions. The wound must be drained for 3 or 4 days because some urine leaks out after operation, no matter how well the pelvis is closed.

Coagulum pyelolithotomy (see Dees, 1981)
This procedure is complementary to one of the other forms of pyelolithotomy and is one method of removing tiny stones and gravel from the pelvicaliceal systems after the main stone has been removed. The pelvic incision is tightly sutured around a 14 or 16F Malecot or De Pezzer catheter and the upper ureter is occluded by a tape. The pelvis is emptied by aspiration and its capacity determined by injecting sterile water or saline. Human or bovine albumin in liquid form, equal in volume to about 90% of the pelvic capacity is injected through the catheter; at the same time thrombin solution equal in volume to 10% of the pelvic capacity is injected through a needle inserted into the pelvis or catheter. The two substances mix and rapidly form a clot or coagulum. Five minutes later the pelvis is reopened and the coagulum, together with the gravel and small stones entrapped in its meshes, is removed.

Nephrolithotomy
This is the appropriate procedure for removing caliceal stones too large to be extracted through the caliceal neck by a pyelolithotomy; the expanded caliceal portions of staghorn calculi and other caliceal stones that cannot be removed by pyelolithotomy or extended pyelolithotomy because of adhesions from previous operations or an abnormal distribution of vessels in the renal sinus. If the

stone is large, is lying in a middle or lower calix and is
palpable on the external surface of the kidney, it may be
tempting to proceed with nephrolithotomy without fully
mobilizing the kidney or opening the renal pelvis, but
this is not advisable. The kidney is exposed through or
above the 12th rib, the ureter is secured, the kidney fully
mobilized and the vessels of the pedicle fully displayed.
The pelvis is opened, as in the operation of pyelolithotomy, and the pelvic stones or pelvic component of
a staghorn stone, if any, removed. The caliceal stone can
sometimes be palpated on the external surface of the
kidney, but its exact position within the kidney can
usually only be determined by palpating it through the
open pelvis with forceps, probe or finger (if the calix is
dilated) or by probing through the exterior of the kidney
with a 19 g needle. The pedicle should always be
clamped in order to reduce blood loss. This can be done
without special precautions if the calyx can be cleared
within 15 minutes; otherwise the patient should be given
Inosine or the kidney should be cooled (p. 539)
(Fig. 26.32).

The pelvicaliceal system is thoroughly irrigated with
sterile water or saline before the incisions in the kidney
and pelvis are closed with 4/0 catgut. When multiple
stones or large soft stones have been removed, an X-ray
should be made before completing the operation to
ensure that stones or stone fragments have not been left
in the kidney, because they will inevitably grow and
cause trouble later. Small flexible X-ray films in equally
flexible sterile plastic cassettes are available. They are
applied directly to one surface of the mobilized kidney
so that the kidney lies between film and the tube of a
portable machine. A detachable cone, previously sterilized, can be attached to the X-ray tube and its wider
distal end placed on or around the kidney. If metal clips
are applied to the netelast sling supporting the kidney
the position of stones can be accurately plotted from the
X-ray. Many surgeons routinely make an X-ray before
and after removal of stones and this should certainly be
done if the stones are large or multiple.

Drainage
The site of operation should always be drained after
pyelolithotomy and nephrolithotomy no matter how
straightforward the operation and how well the pelvis
was sutured, because urine almost invariably leaks out
for a few days. The drain used must be one that leaves
a track so that any urine that leaks after the drain is
removed can escape and does not accumulate. For this
reason a Redivac drain should not be used alone. A
persistent fistula occurs if a stone is inadvertently left and
obstructs the pelvis or ureter, but otherwise a urinary
leak should stop, and may be assisted to do so by passing
a ureteric catheter up the ureter and leaving it in place
for a day or two.

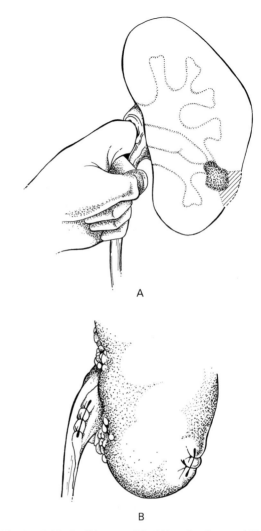

Fig. 26.32 Nephrolithotomy. The kidney has been mobilized
and the renal pelvis opened. The stone is located in its calix
using, in this case, finger. (If a finger is used in this way it
must be used gently and carefully, and can be used safely
only if the pelvis and necks of the calices have become dilated
by obstruction. Otherwise it is much safer to use a probe or
forceps, or to locate the stone by inserting a fine needle
through the outer cortex). Once the stone is located it can be
removed by a transverse incision made through the
parenchyma of the kidney into the calix

Haemorrhage
Primary haemorrhage should be controlled at the time
of the operation; secondary haemorrhage, which occurs
7 to 10 days after operation may still be a problem. It is
as often due to some vascular abnormality at the site of
the nephrolithotomy incision as to infection (p. 540).
At one time a nephrectomy was often the only means of
stopping the bleeding from secondary haemorrhage, but
now the responsible vessel can usually be detected and
occluded by selective renal angiography (p. 506).

Infection

Since many kidneys operated on for stone are already infected, wound infections are not uncommon and should be treated with the appropriate antibiotic. It is sensible to give patients with urinary tract infection an antibiotic before operation.

Renal function

Pyelolithotomy preserves or improves the function of the kidney. Nephrolithotomy, on the other hand, may reduce it because the incision or incisions are made through parenchyma, some at least of which is normal.

Multiple radial nephrotomies, however, seem to do less damage than longitudinal incisions, especially the lateral longitudinal incision (through Brodel's line) that splits open the kidney. The removal of staghorn calculi, even from infected scarred kidneys, generally improves function.

ACUTE RENAL FAILURE

Acute renal failure is a sudden and severe reduction in renal function which causes serious defects in the regulation of the body's internal environment. It is usually associated with anuria or oliguria, but can occur when the urinary output is normal. The causes may be prerenal, renal or postrenal in origin (Newsam, 1981).

Prerenal acute renal failure

Prerenal acute renal failure is caused by impairment in renal perfusion. The reduced blood flow lowers the glomerular filtration rate and filtration stops altogether if the renal artery pressure falls below 35 mm Hg. Impaired perfusion may result from (1) a low blood volume caused by the loss of blood, or plasma, or of fluid and electrolytes or (2) from conditions like myocardial infarction, pulmonary embolism, or septicaemic shock, when the blood pressure falls despite a normal blood volume.

In prerenal acute renal failure, renal function usually recovers if the blood pressure and blood volume are restored to normal. If impaired renal perfusion persists, however, acute tubular necrosis or (less often) renal cortical necrosis occurs.

Renal causes of acute renal failure

Any cause of prerenal acute renal failure or nephrotoxic agents can lead to acute tubular necrosis (which is reversible) or to renal cortical necrosis (which is not). Acute glomerulonephritis, malignant hypertension, polyarteritis, leptospirosis, fat embolism, Goodpasture's syndrome and disseminated intravascular coagulation can all present as acute renal failure and such parenchymal

diseases of the kidney must be kept in mind, when there is no definite history of hypotension.

Chronic renal disease usually progresses insidiously, but an intercurrent infection, a gastro-intestinal upset, causing dehydration or even Tetracycline ingestion (which produces a hypercatabolic state) can precipitate patients into acute renal failure. Acute or chronic renal failure of this kind is suggested by a history of ill-health and the presence of a normocytic anaemia. Plain X–rays of the abdomen or high dose urography may reveal the outlines of scarred and contracted kidneys.

Postrenal acute renal failure

Obstruction in the urinary tract causes back pressure which reduces glomerular filtration and may stop it completely. If obstruction involves both kidneys or a solitary kidney, acute renal failure occurs. Relief of the obstruction restores renal function, unless back pressure and infection have destroyed a considerable amount of renal paranchyma. A postrenal cause should be suspected if the patient has complete anuria, periods of anuria alternating with periods of polyuria, renal colic with analgesic abuse or diabetes, necrosed papillae or cancer of the bladder, cervix or prostate, which can all spread to involve both ureters.

Early diagnosis and early treatment are important in postrenal failure, and it is essential to exclude obstruction when the cause of impaired renal function is not obvious. In the early stages of obstruction before much structural damage has occurred, intravenous urography or renography provides the diagnosis but the only way to be certain whether or not obstruction is present is to carry out cystoscopy and attempt ureteric catheterization and ureteropyelography. An antegrade pyelogram, if the necessary skill is available, will provide diagnosis *and* treatment at a single procedure.

Treatment of postrenal acute renal failure

This consists of relieving obstruction by removing or bypassing the cause as soon as possible and only in the most exceptional circumstances is it advisable to dialyse the patient first.

Retrograde ureteric-catheterization

This is usually carried out to confirm that obstruction is the cause of the acute renal failure, and to relieve it if the catheters can be negotiated beyond the obstruction into the renal pelvis, where they are left. Although ureteric peristalsis pushes them down into the bladder within a few days, the procedure provides time to plan and carry out an elective procedure. However, ureteric catheterization often fails and may introduce or exacerbate infection in an obstructed kidney, and must be carried out with scrupulous attention to asepsis. If ureteric catheterization fails the cause of the obstruction can be removed

Figs. 26.33–26.38 *Percutaneous nephrostomy*

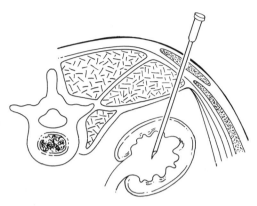

Fig. 26.33 A needle is inserted into the renal pelvis under ultrasound control

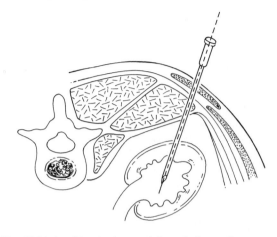

Fig. 26.34 A guide wire is passed through the needle

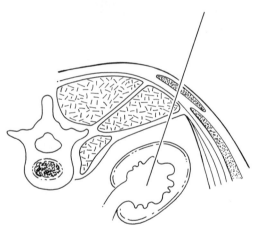

Fig. 26.35 The needle is removed

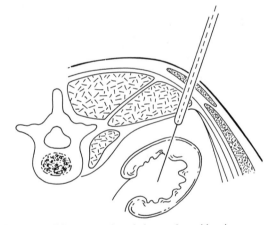

Fig. 26.36 Dilators are threaded over the guide wire to enlarge the tract

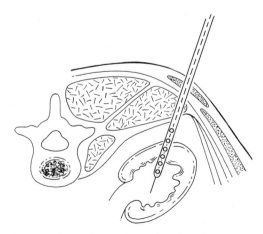

Fig. 26.37 The stent is passed over the guide wire

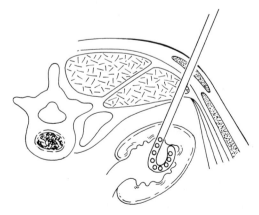

Fig. 26.38 The end of the stent curls in a pigtail fashion when the guide is removed

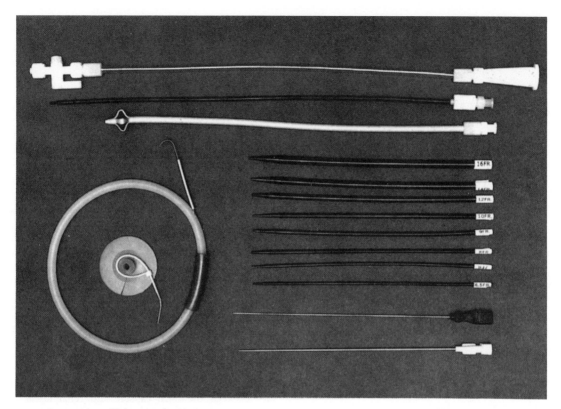

Fig. 26.39 Percutaneous Malecot nephrostomy set

if the patient is reasonably fit and the operation appears straightforward, for instance a stone in a renal pelvis. Otherwise, temporary diversion by nephrostomy, pyelostomy or ureterostomy is required.

Nephrostomy (Figs. 26.33–26.37)

This operation diverts urine from the ureter by draining it to the exterior and is often done as part of some other procedure like pyeloplasty. On its own it is indicated in patients with pyelonephrosis or obstructive acute renal failure who are unrelieved by ureteric catheterization and considered unfit or unsuitable for a more extensive procedure. The operation is now usually carried out by inserting a needle into the kidney percutaneously under radiographic or ultrasonic control, threading a guide wire through it and hence placing a stent in the pelvis of the kidney (Fig. 26.38). The tip of the stent curls up once it is in the pelvis in order to retain it in position. Most stents are small (5F) and liable to become blocked. However, instruments are now available to dilate the track to a size that will admit a large Malecot catheter (Fig. 26.39) or even a cystoscope. An open nephrostomy may still be needed for pyonephrosis or an infected hydronephrosis although it can make later conservative renal operations like pyeloplasty very difficult. A lumbotomy or posterolateral incision is required. It is

tempting, once the kidney is exposed, to stretch a Malecot or De Pezzer catheter tightly onto an introducer and push it blindly through a small incision on the lateral aspect of the kidney in the hope that it will go into a calix or the renal pelvis. It is better and safer to expose and open the renal pelvis, to pass a probe through the pelvis and lower calix and out through the lower pole of the kidney after tying a De Pezzer or Malecot catheter to the distal end (Cabot's method) (Fig. 26.40).

The wound is closed round the tube which can be brought out through a separate stab incision inferiorly. A loop nephrostomy can be used instead of a De Pezzer or Malecot catheter (Fig. 26.41).

Pyelostomy

The pelvis can be drained by a tube which is inserted into the pelvis at open operation. The procedure is less satisfactory than nephrostomy and not recommended.

Ureterostomy

Temporary ureterostomy is sometimes an easier procedure than nephrostomy for the urgent relief of obstructions involving the lower end of a ureter. The upper third of the ureter is exposed by a muscle cutting incision. There is no advantage in using a T tube; it is preferable to pass a simple tube through a small incision in the

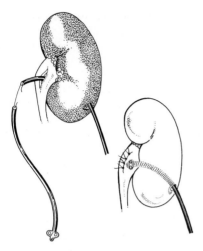

Fig. 26.40 Nephrostomy. The kidney has been mobilized and the pelvis opened. A probe is passed through the pelvis, lower calix and out through the lower pole of the kidney. A Malecot catheter is tied to the end of the probe and withdrawn through the lower pole of the kidney so that the bulb of the catheter lies in the renal pelvis. The tube can then be brought out through a separate stab incision below the wound

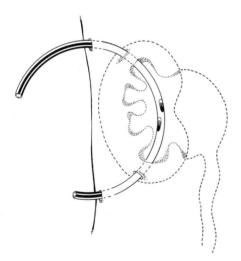

Fig. 26.41 Method of making a loop nephrostomy. The two open ends of the tube are connected to a single tube by a Y connection and thus drawn into one appliance. The probe has to be passed through the pelvis, calix and parenchyma of the kidney twice, once through the upper pole and once through the lower pole. Positioning the tube so that the holes lie in the calices or the renal pelvis is not easy. Many tubes, however, are radio-opaque and the position of the tube can be adjusted if it fails to drain properly. The advantage of the loop nephrostomy is the ease with which the tube can be changed

ureter up to the renal pelvis and bring the other end out through a separate stab incision. A Gibbon catheter (see Fig. 25.22), with the solid tip removed, is useful because the flanges on this catheter can be secured to the skin with sutures or tape.

When the patient's renal function has recovered, the cause of the obstruction can be assessed and appropriate elective treatment decided. This may just involve the removal of pelvic or ureteric stones, but calculus anuria is not common and most patients with obstructive acute renal failure have a disease like retroperitoneal fibrosis (p. 572) or malignant disease of cervix, prostate or bladder and pose much greater problems. The former will be explored in the appropriate way unless the kidney is solitary, but the latter can pose many problems, of which the surgical ones may be the least. In the presence of incurable or recurrent malignancy obstructing the ureters, it might be kinder to let the patient die of renal failure. If the disease causes acute renal failure before it has been treated, it is usually worth bypassing the obstruction by nephrostomy or ureterostomy.

PERINEPHRIC ABSCESS

A perinephric abscess forms in the perinephric fat, which lies between the renal capsule and renal fascia. The infection, usually staphylococcal, originates in a small abscess or carbuncle in the cortex of the kidney or spreads from a distant infection by the blood stream and the kidney itself is usually remarkably normal. Severe gram negative infections of the kidney, particularly those associated with staghorn calculi, do extend into perinephric fat, but tend to cause low grade inflammation with fibrous adhesions rather than an abscess. The problem with perinephric abscess is not the treatment, which is straightforward, but the diagnosis, which can be difficult because the lesion, like subphrenic abscess, is deeply situated and produces few, if any, local signs until it is very advanced. In the early stages the features are those of a nonspecific febrile illness with malaise, anorexia, myalgia, intermittent fever and gradual loss of weight with leucocytosis and an elevated ESR. A swelling does not appear in the loin for some time, or may be undetected by an inadequate examination. The swelling renders the normally concave loin, first flat, later convex and can only be appreciated if we look down the back of the sitting patient.

In a straight X-ray the abscess often reveals itself because it obliterates the psoas shadow, displaces the colonic flexure and kidney, elevates the diaphragm and sometimes causes a small effusion on the base of the lung. Intravenous urography may reveal the displacement of the kidney most clearly, but is often of little more help than the straight X-ray unless the abscess is secondary to gross renal disease. Ultrasonography should reveal the mass around the kidney.

By the time a perinephric abscess is diagnosed it is usually beyond cure by chemotherapy alone and should be exposed and drained through a subcostal posterolateral incision. The incision is made below and parallel to the 12th rib dividing muscles in the same line. A finger can then be inserted into the retroperitoneal space and the abscess drained.

HYDRONEPHROSIS

Hydronephrosis means dilatation of the pelvis and calices of the kidney and implies, unless the word hydroureter is added, that the ureter is normal. When it is not secondary to stone, stricture, tumour or other obvious disease it is called idiopathic or congenital and it is the congenital type which is treated by pyeloplasty or, if little useful function remains, by nephrectomy.

The cause of *congenital* hydronephrosis is still not known. The kinks, adhesions and high insertion of the ureter are regarded as effects and not causes. Although all surgeons regard an aberrant artery to the lower pole of the kidney (found in 70% of patients with congenital hydronephrosis) an aggravating factor, few consider it the cause. The obstruction is probably functional rather than physical and caused by some defect of the musculature of the pelvi-ureteric junction that prevents contraction waves, and therefore urine from passing through, but no less amenable to pyeloplasty because of that. Although it has been recognised for many years that not all hydroureters are obstructed (some for instance are dilated because of vesico-ureteric reflux) only recently has it been widely appreciated that not all hydronephrotic kidneys are obstructed. The best example of this is seen in the kidney after pyeloplasty, which, no matter how successfully it relieves symptoms and obstruction, leaves the calices and sometimes the pelvis as dilated as before. Kidneys may also be hydronephrotic, but not obstructed after vesico-ureteric reflux is cured, or in the condition of hydrocalicosis.

Before pyeloplasty, therefore, it is essential to demonstrate not only hydronephrosis, but also obstruction. This can be done most easily by taking late films at the time of intravenous urography, by renography, radionuclide scanning, or in doubtful cases by Whitaker's test. In Whitaker's test, a needle is inserted into the renal pelvis percutaneously or at open operation and used to measure pressures in the renal pelvis while perfusing it at a flow rate of 10 ml/min. The renal pelvis pressure minus the bladder pressure (measured simultaneously) gives the relative pressure (RP). An elevated RP (> 15 cm water) indicates obstruction. The assessment of hydronephrosis is further complicated because the

obstructed type (and it is the commonest) may be chronic or intermittent (Whitaker, 1977).

In the chronic type, the pelvis and calices are permanently dilated as seen on X-ray whether the patient has pain or not. In the intermittent type, the dilatation comes and goes and can be detected only if the X-rays are taken when the patient has pain or is given intravenous Frusemide; at other times the kidney may appear normal or nearly normal. Hence there are kidneys that are obstructed, but not always dilated, and others which are dilated, but not obstructed. Pyeloplasty is an operation which relieves obstruction enabling the kidney to drain better; it should only be done if the hydronephrotic kidney is obstructed; on the other hand, it should not be denied to those patients whose symptoms suggest renal obstruction, but whose pyelogram is relatively normal, until the X-rays or renograms have been repeated during an episode of pain or diuresis. If, in cases of obstructive hydronephrosis, the *ureter* is also dilated the cause and treatment of the disease will be entirely different. If the upper ureter is seen in the intravenous urograms the distinction is easy; if not, its normality must not be assumed and it should be demonstrated by retrograde ureterogram. Doing this with a Braasch or Chevasseur catheter is less likely to cause oedema and infect the obstructed kidney, but even then is best done immediately before operation and under the same anaesthetic. If the findings are unexpected, operation is avoided. The *principles* of the operation of pyeloplasty are to excise the pelvi-ureteric junction and remake a new one that is wide, dependant and spouted; to excise the redundant part of the renal pelvis and to preserve the aberrant vessels especially those that cross anterior to the pelviureteric junction, by displacing them behind the new pelvi-ureteric junction (Fig. 26.42).

Many methods of pyeloplasty fulfil these requirements, but none perhaps so well as the Anderson Hynes pyeloplasty (called the dismembered Foley pyeloplasty in America) which is suitable for all types of congenital hydronephrosis.

Pyeloplasty

The kidney is exposed through or above the 12th rib although some surgeons use an anterior subcostal or paramedian approach. The redundant pelvis is excised. The pelvi-ureteric junction is reformed by suturing, with 4/0 catgut or dexon, the spatulated ureter to the lower part of the pelvis providing a new pelvi-ureteric junction that is wide spouted and dependant. If an aberrant vessel is present the anastomosis is made in front of it. The upper part of the pelvis is closed with the same suture material. Many surgeons use a Cummings catheter (Fig. 26.43) which acts both as a splint across the anastomosis and a nephrostomy tube, and is removed some 7 days after operation; others use two separate tubes so

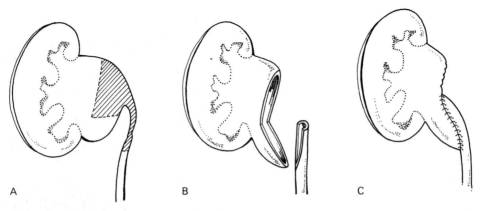

Fig. 26.42 Anderson-Hynes pyeloplasty for congenital hydronephrosis: (A) the amount of renal pelvis and upper ureter to be excised. (B) the means by which the upper end of the ureter is spatulated thus facilitating reconstruction of a wide pelvi-ureteric junction. (C) the anastomosis completed, the ureter being sutured to the lower cut half of the pelvis forming a dependant, wide and spouted anastomosis. The upper part of the cut pelvis is sutured (the operation resembles and is derived from the Billroth 1 gastrectomy)

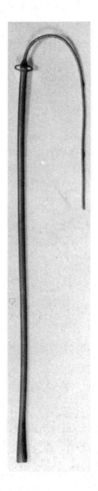

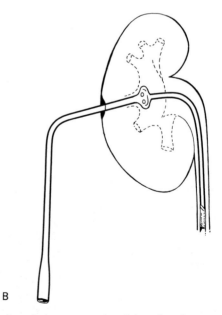

that the splint can be removed a day or two before the nephrostomy tube.

CONGENITAL ANOMALIES OF THE KIDNEY

Congenital hydronephrosis is one congenital anomaly of the kidney that often requires surgical treatment, solitary cyst is another, but few of the many other anomalies

Fig. 26.43 Cummings catheter. The narrow part of the catheter passes through the anastomosis and down into the ureter. The expanded part of the catheter with the Malecot wings lies in the renal pelvis and the wider tube is brought out through the calix and parenchyma, and acts as a nephrostomy. Thus one tube is used as both splint and nephrostomy. (Courtesy of G U Manufacturing Co)

require operation unless affected by secondary disease processes such as stone, infection, obstruction (to all of which anomalous kidneys are more liable than normal) injury or tumour. Nevertheless, surgeons must be familiar with all common and many of the uncommon congenital anomalies, otherwise they may mistake the images they produce in X–rays, ultrasonic, radionuclide and CAT scans for disease, and be confused by their abnormal site, morphology and blood supply during operations for secondary disease processes.

Details of congenital abnormalities of the kidney need not be described here although the problems they may present before and during surgery should be anticipated.

Intrarenal pelvis

Most kidneys have an extrarenal pelvis which can be exposed easily because most of it lies outside the renal sinus. Some kidneys have an intrarenal pelvis. The latter is small, lies wholly within the renal sinus and appears as if the upper ureter enters the renal sinus and breaks up into major calices without first forming a pelvis. Operations, such as pyelolithotomy, are more difficult on intrarenal than extrarenal pelves. The presence of an intrarenal pelvis can usually be recognised in the preoperative X-rays.

Unrotated kidney (sometimes called malrotated) (Fig. 26.44)

The metanephros, which becomes the adult kidney, develops in the caudal part of the embryo. At first the renal pelvis lies anterior to the kidney and some calices lie posteromedially and some posterolaterally. As the kidney ascends to its adult position in the loin it also

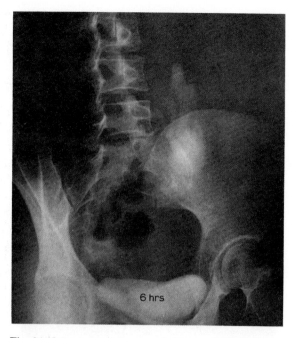

Fig. 26.45 i.v.u. showing an ectopic kidney which is also hydronephrotic

rotates through 90%, the left one clockwise, the right one anticlockwise so that the pelvis comes to lie medial to the kidney and the calices all lie laterally. If the kidney fails to rotate the pelvis remains anterior to the kidney and some calices point medially. The kidney looks abnormal but usually functions normally.

Ectopic kidney (Fig. 26.45)

An ectopic kidney is one that has neither ascended nor rotated. It lies in the pelvis on or below the brim with an anterior pelvis and receives its blood from a number of small arteries; a renal artery develops only if and when the kidney ascends. Despite its appearance it usually functions satisfactorily unless secondarily diseased.

If an i.v.u. fails to reveal a kidney the pelvic films must be inspected carefully for an ectopic kidney.

Fused kidneys

Of the several ways in which kidneys may be joined to each other, the commonest is the horseshoe anomaly in which the kidneys lie on their own side of the midline, but are joined together at their lower poles by a bridge made of renal fibrous tissue (Fig. 26.46). The horseshoe kidney like other fused kidneys is unrotated and usually lies at a lower level than normal. Each requires treatment only if it is secondarily involved by disease, and there is no point in dividing the bridge joining the kidneys in the hope that they will assume the positions they should have attained during the fourth month of intrauterine life.

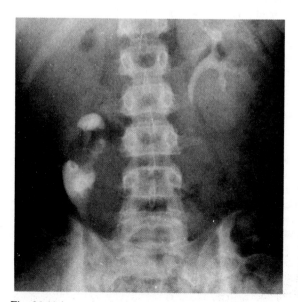

Fig. 26.44 i.v.u. showing an unrotated right kidney

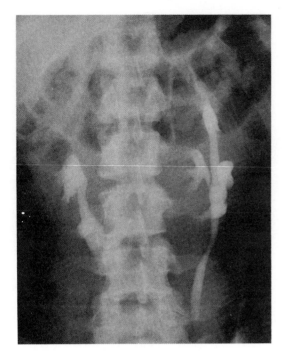

Fig. 26.46 i.v.u. showing a horseshoe kidney

Operations on horseshoe, ectopic and unrotated kidneys are often easier than expected because they lie at a low level and have anterior pelves.

Duplication

Duplication of the renal pelvis with partial or complete duplication of the ureter is probably the commonest congenital anomaly of the urinary tract. Secondary disease processes often involve only one moiety or half of a duplex kidney and a heminephrectomy is often the appropriate treatment. Heminephrectomy is easier than the operation of partial nephrectomy on a normal kidney because each moiety has its own pedicle and is often clearly demarcated from the other.

The two pelves of a duplex kidney are unusual; the upper one rarely has more than 2 calices and in the lower the calices tend to be short and crowded together. If both moieties are functioning the condition can easily be recognized. If only one moiety is working, however, the abnormal appearance may be confused with gross disease of the pelvis of a normal kidney.

RENAL INJURIES

The kidneys are small, mobile and well protected by muscles, ribs, other viscera and the spine; nevertheless, they may be damaged by the perforating injuries of knives or gunshot wounds, by the blunt trauma or by the deceleration of road traffic accidents, sports injuries or falls. Perforating injuries, often complicated by infection or vascular problems like arteriovenous fistulae, are uncommon in the UK and most renal injuries are caused by blunt trauma or deceleration when the kidney is crushed between ribs and spine, impaled by a fractured rib or transverse process or torn from its pedicle. 80% of perforating injuries of the kidneys are associated with injuries to other viscera, whereas the injuries caused by blunt trauma or deceleration are either solitary or associated with skeletal injuries to the ribs, transverse processes or spine (Guerriero, 1982).

Classification

Injuries of the kidney can be classified into 4 groups: (1) Contusion (2) Laceration (3) Fragmentation or (4) Major vessel injury: (Fig. 26.47). Haematuria is the commonest finding but the amount of bleeding does not necessarily correlate with the severity of the injury; with severe injuries to major vessels haematuria may be slight and transient. Despite the large renal blood flow, severe shock is not a feature of renal injury and its presence suggests that other viscera are also damaged. Once the patient has been resuscitated and injuries to other structures assessed (and treated if they are lifethreatening) attention can be focussed on the renal injury.

A straight X–ray may reveal injuries to ribs, transverse processes or spine, and a soft tissue mass obliterating the outline of the kidney and the psoas shadow. An intravenous urogram is essential; it reveals the presence and function of the uninjured kidney and gives some information about the injured kidney. Bruised kidneys often look surprisingly normal, lacerated ones can be recognized by their depressed function and by the extravasation of contrast medium into perirenal tissues. Nonfunction implies that the kidney is fragmented or the major vessels severely damaged and arteriography should be carried out. Ultrasonography and radionuclide scanning are useful in following the progress of the patient, but of limited help in establishing the extent of the injury when the patient is first seen. Patients with *contusions* (Group 1) and *lacerations* (Group 2) can be treated conservatively (unless there are associated injuries).

Many patients with a *fragmented kidney* can also be treated conservatively unless bleeding is persistent and severe, when the kidney should be explored and an attempt made to suture the lacerations or remove only part of the kidney. But nephrectomy is often the only solution, provided the other kidney is normal. *Injury of the renal vessels* usually involves intimal tears with secondary spasm and thrombosis, or partial or complete transection of the renal artery, and can only be distinguished from a fragmented kidney by angiography because the kidney is nonfunctioning on the intravenous urogram. Haematuria is often transient in patients with

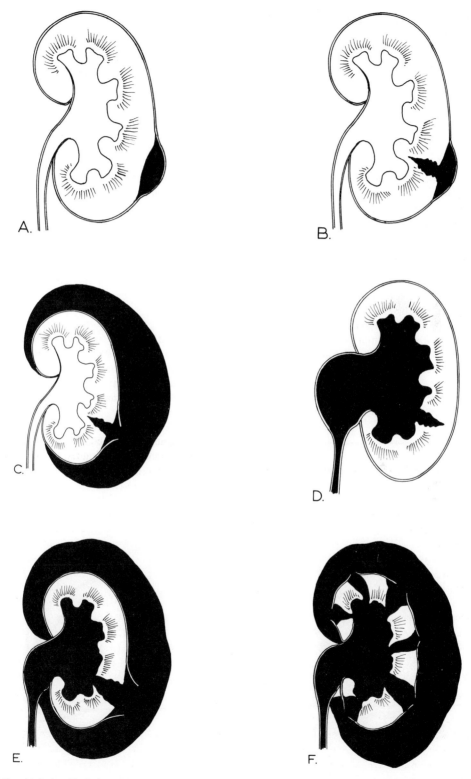

Fig. 26.47 Renal injuries. (A) Subcortical haematoma. (B) and (C) Lacerations involving the cortex but not the collecting system. (D) Laceration involving the collecting system but not the cortex. (E) Laceration involving both collecting system and cortex. (F) Fragmentation of the kidney

injuries of the renal artery, but retroperitoneal bleeding can be extensive with transection, particularly partial transection, when contraction of the vessel widens the hole.

As the kidneys can withstand ischaemia for only 15 minutes little is to be gained by exploring injuries of the pedicle, but careful follow up is essential as many develop hypertension.

A fragmented kidney or injured pedicle can be explored through a posterolateral incision, but is best explored through an anterior one, which allows examination of other viscera and an easier approach to the renal pedicle. Sometimes (especially in patients with perforating wounds) a renal injury is suspected only when a retroperitoneal haematoma is found during the course of a laparotomy for the exploration of other injuries. It is tempting just to explore and deal surgically with the kidney. However, an intravenous urogram should be done on the table as it is impossible to assess the functional state and integrity of the other kidney by palpating or even looking at it. All patients should be followed up for some time after injury, especially those who had lacerations, fragmentation or injuries of the renal artery because complications such as vascular abnormalities or hypertension can develop silently.

OTHER RENAL CONDITIONS AND OPERATIONS

Renal cysts
Solitary cysts are rare. They are usually situated in the cortex especially towards the lower pole, and communicate with neither the pelvis nor the calices. Their importance lies in the fact that they may be difficult to distinguish from neoplasms, but 95% are detectable by ultrasound scanning. Percutaneous puncture of the cyst under X–ray or ultrasonic control may be attempted; if clear or straw-coloured fluid is obtained, the cyst is outlined with radio-opaque medium. Simple aspiration is curative in 30 to 40% of cases. If operation is undertaken, it is wise to excise only the projecting part of the cyst (Fig. 26.48).

Polycystic disease is not amenable to surgery, since the cysts are scattered throughout the substance of both kidneys. Complications such as pain, bleeding or infection may be relieved (even if only temporarily) by Rovsing's operation, in which the kidney is exposed and all the larger cysts projecting on the surface are punctured or incised, but the correct treatment of polycystic disease is the treatment of the chronic renal failure it causes.

Nephropexy
Operative fixation of an abnormally mobile kidney is seldom performed since the undue mobility is often part of a generalized visceroptosis. Symptoms vary greatly and often bear little relationship to the degree of mobility and in many cases a considerable psychological element is present.

Nephropexy should, however, be considered (1) when symptoms appear to be related to the excessive mobility of the kidney, and are not relieved by an abdominal support (2) if intravenous urography or radionuclide scan

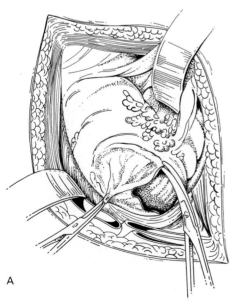
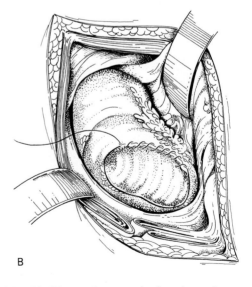

A   B

Fig. 26.48 Excision of solitary renal cyst. (A) The cyst has been deroofed and in (B) a running suture has been inserted around the cut edge of the cyst to control bleeding

demonstrate obstruction to the outflow of urine, (especially if there is also infection or hydronephrosis) or (3) if variations in urinary output occur because the renal artery is stretched and the kidney made ischaemic when the patient is erect.

When the patient is erect and the kidney ischaemic less sodium and therefore less water is excreted; when supine, the sodium and therefore water is excreted. Such patients complain that they pass little urine during the day, but much at night.

Technique
Probably the most effective method of anchoring the kidney is to stitch it to the quadratus lumborum. The kidney is exposed through a subcostal or lumbotomy approach and is delivered at the wound. The pelvis and ureter are carefully examined to exclude any organic obstruction to the urinary outflow. In order that the kidney may adhere to its muscular bed its posterior surface is cleared of all fatty tissue and is denuded of capsule except for a small strip near the convex border. The kidney is placed as high as possible with its upper pole under cover of the 12th rib and with the denuded area on its posterior surface in direct contact with quadratus lumborum. It is anchored to the lateral part of the muscle by three or four stitches. In order to promote adhesions, a sheet of polyvinyl alcohol sponge may be placed between kidney and the muscle, but is usually unnecessary.

Percutaneous operations on the kidney
Rapid progress is being made in the development of percutaneous renal operations, which now include the long established needle biopsy, the insertion of nephrostomy tubes (Fig. 26.38), the aspiration of renal cysts and procedures such as removal or ultrasonic destruction of calyceal or pelvic calculi. Biopsy, electrocoagulation or resection of transitional cell tumours of the collecting system, and the dilatation and even incision of a narrowed pelvi-ureteric junction are also being accomplished, all of which require special endoscopic instruments or other apparatus.

The first three procedures are relatively commonplace and can be done in most hospitals with standard X-ray and ultrasonic facilities. The others are still experimental and are presently being done only on selected patients in a few specialized centres.

Renal ischaemia and hypertension
Renal ischaemia is now well recognized as a cause of hypertension. The two conditions most commonly encountered are atheroma of the renal artery, usually causing stenosis near its origin, and fibromuscular hyper-

trophy of the arterial wall, causing a more generalized constriction. The diagnosis is best made by *selective renal arteriography* (p. 506).

Surgery may be advised in otherwise fit patients who do not respond to medical treatment. The operations commonly employed are *thrombo-endarterectomy, splenic artery to renal artery anastomosis* and *bypass grafting*. If, however, the kidney is shrunken and atrophic, and frozen section examination of a biopsy section shows gross tubular atrophy and fibrosis, nephrectomy is indicated, provided that the other kidney is healthy.

Renal transplantation
The technique of renal transplantation is now well established although its use is confined to those centres with facilities for haemodialysis and with a surgeon experienced in the problems which may arise. In carefully selected cases of homotransplantation, with transfer of a kidney from a related donor or from a cadaver, success can be expected in well over 50%. While the operative technique has been largely standardized, there remains the problem of rejection whereby the body's defence mechanisms attempt to discard the transplanted organ in much the same way as any foreign body or infective organism is rejected. Control of rejection has allowed transplantation of liver and heart to be carried out with increasing success. The complex mechanism of rejection can be controlled with immunosuppressive therapy but more major advances can be expected in the field of tissue typing (a more detailed method of blood grouping) so that the cells of the donated kidney can be more accurately matched to the recipient patient.

The main indication for renal transplantation is in the treatment of chronic irreversible renal failure, as an alternative to chronic intermittent haemodialysis or in addition to it (Morris, 1979). The recipient must be fit enough to withstand a major surgical procedure, he should be free from systemic infection and should possess a normal lower urinary tract. The kidney itself must be free from disease and capable of good function. Its vessels should be of sufficient length to allow for a satisfactory anastomosis and it is preferable for it to have a single renal artery.

Technique
It is now standard practice to transplant a kidney to an extraperitoneal site in the contralateral iliac fossa. This makes it possible to re-establish the circulation in the kidney with the minimum of delay since the ureter lies anteriorly and can be dealt with after suture of the blood vessels. The renal vein is joined end-to-side to the external or common iliac vein and the artery is anastomosed end-to-end to the divided internal iliac artery. Finally, the ureter is implanted into the bladder.

OPERATIONS ON THE ADRENAL GLANDS

Partial or complete removal of the adrenal glands is a relatively safe procedure, linked to the availability of cortisone and its synthetic substitutes. The operation may be curative in cases of adrenal dysfunction (adrenogenital or Cushing's syndrome), and also of tumour formation, whether this involves the cortex or the medulla of the gland. It is no longer used in the treatment of metastatic carcinoma of the breast and rarely for prostatic carcinoma.

Except in the case of a tumour which has been clearly localised by radiography (p. 512) to one or other side, both adrenal glands will require at least to be exposed and examined. In most cases, therefore, the operation will be a bilateral one.

Anatomy

The right adrenal gland
Triangular in shape, it lies partly on the diaphragm, and partly capping the upper pole of the kidney; anteromedially it is in contact with the vena cava, and anterolaterally, with the liver.

The left adrenal gland
Semilunar in shape, it also caps the kidney, but extends further down its medial border towards the hilum. Its anterior surface is closely applied to the pancreas and the splenic artery.

Each gland is embedded in fat and enclosed within the renal fascia, but is separated from the kidney by an incomplete fascial septum. It is attached lightly to the kidney below by loose connective tissue, and more firmly, to the diaphragm above by thickened fascial bands.

Arterial supply is derived from the aorta, the inferior phrenic and the renal arteries, but the individual branches from these vessels are seldom encountered at operation, for they divide before reaching the gland into a number of smaller vessels; these may be difficult to identify before division, but bleeding is seldom troublesome.

Venous drainage is usually by one large vein, which may however be duplicated; this is very easily torn, and the bleeding may be dangerous. On the right side the vein, which is very short, emerges on the anteromedial surface of the gland near the apex, and immediately enters the vena cava with which the gland is in contact. The left vein is longer; it emerges from the anterior surface of the gland near the lower pole, and joins either the inferior phrenic or the renal vein.

Surgical approach
The adrenal glands, like the kidneys, may be approached by the lumbar route, by the anterior (transperitoneal) route, or by the transthoracic route. The anterior route has many advantages, and is now generally regarded as the best method of approach. Both adrenal glands can be exposed at the same time; their condition can be compared, and a bilateral removal carried out if desired. It thus greatly facilitates a one-stage operation, with much less disturbance to the patient than if each adrenal were exposed separately by one of the other routes. In the ectopic ACTH syndrome, it allows for exploration for a possible intra-abdominal primary tumour. These advantages, together with the ease with which the left adrenal gland can be exposed from the front, compensate for the greater difficulties of access to the right adrenal.

Technique of bilateral adrenalectomy by the anterior approach
The patient is placed in the dorsal position with the thoracolumbar region slightly arched over the raised bridge. A curved transverse incision, convex upwards and with its centre 5 cm above the umbilicus, may be employed. This provides much better access than a straight incision of the same length. Surgeons with experience in this field may use a midline incision (Welbourn, 1980).

The left adrenal gland is approached first, by incision of the posterior layer of the lienorenal ligament (Fig. 18.2 p. 368). This incision should not be made too close to the spleen, since the peritoneum may then tear back on to the organ, with consequent bleeding. The spleen is turned forwards and to the patient's right, together with the tail and body of the pancreas and the splenic vessels, thus bringing the left kidney and adrenal gland into view. The gland is recognized from its orange colour which distinguishes it clearly from fat or pancreatic tissue. It is cleared first along its lateral border, and a finger is inserted behind it; it is then dissected free, all vessels—especially the large veins at its medial border—being secured as they are displayed. A search is made in the surrounding retroperitoneum for any islands of accessory adrenal tissue, and these, if present, are removed. The spleen and pancreas are then replaced in their original position.

The right adrenal gland is now sought for deeply in the subhepatic pouch, in the area bounded by the lower border of the liver, the right side of the vena cava and the renal vessels. A small gauze pack is laid deeply on the inferior surface of the liver, and by the use of a retractor placed against this the liver is gently drawn upwards. The kidney is then drawn downwards by pressure with the fingers and the posterior-wall peritoneum is incised around the upper pole and about 2.5 cm

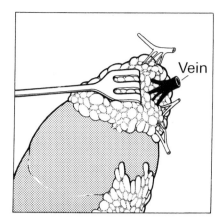

Fig. 26.49 Blood supply of right adrenal gland which is rotated laterally to expose medial surface. Note that there are considerable variations in the vascular pattern, but the veins are always much larger than the arteries which may divide into a large number of small branches before entering the glands

above it. Elevation of this curved peritoneal flap should now display the adrenal gland, which can be brought better into view by a finger inserted above it into the space between the two fascial layers enclosing it. By the use of a small rake retractor, the gland is gently rotated laterally, so that the vessels related to its medial surface (Fig. 26.49), especially the large and dangerously short vein which joins the vena cava, can be cleared. Once this vessel has been safely secured, removal of the gland should present no serious difficulty, all other vessels being dealt with *seriatim*. The fascial connections between the gland and the kidney should be divided last, since otherwise the gland may become retracted upwards to a less accessible level.

Finally, all haemorrhage having been arrested as far as possible, the incision is repaired, drains from the adrenal fossae being brought out at each end, or through separate stab wounds.

Adrenalectomy by the lumbar or transthoracic approach

This may be through the bed of the 10th, 11th or 12th rib (pp. 529–534), and may be either subpleural or transpleural. The upper pole of the kidney is delivered, and adrenalectomy is carried out as described above.

Adrenalectomy for cortical tumours

Cushing's syndrome is believed to result from excessive secretions of adreno-cortical hormones, due to hyperplasia of the adrenal cortex, an adenoma or an occasional carcinoma. *Primary hyperaldosteronism* due to a solitary adenoma or nodular hyperplasia causes hypertension (Bledsoe, 1974).

In cases where the glands are hyperplastic, due to pituitary or ectopic ACTH stimulation, the usual policy in surgical treatment is to control the source of ACTH. If this is not possible, removal of the whole of each gland is required. When a unilateral tumour is present, the affected gland only is removed; if there are bilateral tumours, total adrenalectomy must necessarily be performed. If the tumour is still encapsulated on removal, the prognosis is reasonably good.

Adrenalectomy for medullary tumours

These tumours (*chromaffinomata or phaeochromocytomata*) are associated with paroxysmal or sustained hypertension. Since they are usually unilateral and larger than cortical tumours, they can usually be localized by ultra sound scanning, selective venous sampling or by selective angiography (Fig. 25.8).

An anterior (transperitoneal) approach is advised, since this enables the main veins to be ligated before any manipulation of the tumour can release adrenaline into the circulation, thereby causing a dangerous rise in blood pressure. Alpha adrenergic blocking agents should be administered preoperatively to control blood pressure and to minimize the effect of paroxysmal release of catecholamines. *Phenoxybenzamine* (10–20 mg twice daily) is usually given orally until several days before operation (Welbourne, 1980), when *phentolamine*, by intravenous infusion (5–30 mg in 5% dextrose 500 ml in 4 hours) should be substituted, the dose being carefully titrated against blood pressure. Arrhythmias during operation require intravenous lignocaine or practolol.

Substitution therapy. In order to combat possible hormone insufficiency, all operations on the adrenal glands should be carried out under cortisone control, and after total adrenalectomy administration of this hormone must be continued throughout life. After partial or unilateral adrenalectomy, the majority of patients eventually become independent of steroid therapy. The cortisone may therefore be withdrawn gradually, the length of time during which it is required varying from one patient to another. The dosage of steroids and the duration of such therapy are determined by the absence of signs of adrenal insufficiency when trial reductions are made. A suggested scheme of therapy is as follows:

On the 2 days before operation	100 mg of cortisone acetate by intramuscular injection.
1 to 2 hours before operation	100 mg of hydrocortisone hemisuccinate intravenously.
At the end of the operation	Repeat i.v. injection of hydrocortisone, unless BP has returned to preoperative level.

| Until 5th postoperative day | 100 mg of cortisone acetate daily—by mouth or intramuscularly. |
| After 5th postoperative day | Reduce oral dosage gradually to maintenance dose of 37.5 mg daily. |

The maintenance dose of 37.5 mg of cortisone daily should at once be increased to 100 mg during any conditions of stress—illness, accident or emotional disturbance, or if signs of adrenocortical deficiency appear—apathy, weakness, nausea, vomiting, etc.

Fludrocortisone in a daily dose of 0.1 mg has greater salt-retaining powers and may be employed to supplement cortisone during the first few days after operation.

Complications of adrenalectomy. Acute circulatory failure may be the first sign of adrenocortical insufficiency and may not be prevented by routine substitution therapy. It may occur with dramatic suddenness, usually within 48 hours of operation, and may terminate fatally. Treatment consists in the intravenous administration of 200 mg of hydrocortisone hemisuccinate, every 2 hours if necessary. If profound shock is present, a simultaneous infusion of noradrenaline should be given.

Salt deficiency is likely to be mistaken for cortisone deficiency, for the clinical features are very similar. In the early postoperative period it may be prevented by fludrocortisone, or by daily estimations of serum electrolytes so that sodium chloride may be given—by intravenous infusion if necessary. Symptoms which develop later may be treated by giving salt by mouth. Alternatively, a maintenance dose of fludrocortisone may be preferred.

Every patient who has undergone adrenalectomy should, on discharge from hospital, be issued with a printed card which he should carry with him at all times. This should contain advice on the indications for increasing the dosage of cortisone, and there should be an instruction that, if he is found in a state of collapse, hydrocortisone should be administered intravenously.

OPERATIONS ON THE URETER

Anatomy (see Gosling, 1982)
The ureter is a muscular tube 24 to 30 cm long and about 4 mm (12F) in diameter. Starting at the pelvic-ureteric junction it passes down the posterior abdominal wall, crosses the pelvic brim and then runs medially and forward to the bladder. It is lined throughout by transitional cell epithelium and enclosed in a firm sheath of adventitial tissue derived from the retroperitoneal fascia.

Relations
The abdominal part of the ureter, accompanied by the testicular or ovarian vessels, is separated from the tips of the lumbar transverse processes by the psoas muscle. Anteriorly, peritoneum separates the right ureter from the third part of the duodenum, the right colic and the ileocolic vessels and the root of the mesentery; and the left ureter from the left colic vessels. However, as these structures are reflected medially with the peritoneum they are not usually seen in the extraperitoneal approaches to the ureter. The ureter is loosely attached to, and lifted forwards with, the peritoneum and usually therefore found in the loose fat behind the peritoneum rather than on the psoas major muscle.

In the pelvis the ureter runs down the side wall, below the internal iliac artery to the level of the ischial spine, then forwards and medially in the fat above the levator ani muscle to the bladder, where it is surrounded by a plexus of veins. In males it is crossed anteriorly near the bladder by the vas deferens and overlapped by the upper end of the seminal vesicle. In females it is crossed by the uterine artery and vein in the broad ligament and runs immediately above the lateral fornix of the vagina at the side of the cervix uteri to reach the bladder.

The intramural portion of the ureter is about 1 cm long. It passes obliquely through the muscular wall of the bladder so that 5 cm separate the ureters as they enter the bladder but only 2.5 cm separate them as they open into the bladder at the upper angles of the trigone.

Blood supply
The ureters receive blood by transverse branches from various arteries in the abdomen and pelvis which feed a freely anastomosing plexus in the adventitial sheath. If this sheath is undisturbed a considerable length of the ureter can be mobilized without fear of ischaemic damage.

Exposure of the ureter
The upper third of the ureter, including the pelvi-ureteric junction, can be exposed through a posterolateral subcostal or lumbotomy incision as described for exposure of the kidney (p. 529).

The middle third of the ureter lies in the iliac fossa and is usually exposed through a muscle cutting incision. The patient lies supine or has the shoulder and buttock of the affected side slightly elevated by a pillow or sandbag. The incision, centred on McBurney's point, extends from the midaxillary line posteriorly to the lateral edge of the rectus sheath anteriorly. The incision can be extended forwards or backwards depending on the extent of the operation and the build of the patient. The muscles of the anterior abdominal wall and transversalis fascia are divided in the same line as the incision and retracted. The unopened peritoneum is gently swept forwards and medially off the fascia covering the iliacus muscle with gauze or fingers. The ureter may be identified as it crosses the bifurcation of the common iliac vessels but more often is elevated along with the peritoneum and found in the loose fatty tissue alongside the spermatic or ovarian vessels. The ureter can be recognized by its white colour, by the blood vessels that run longitudinally in its adventitial coat, by its lack of branches and by its peristaltic contractions (which can be stimulated if they are not obvious by pinching or tapping the ureter). However a dilated ureter may have a bluish colour or look too wide to be a ureter; furthermore peristalsis may not be obvious nor easily provoked.

If doubt exists, it is advisable to aspirate its contents with a fine needle and syringe before proceding with mobilization. A normal ureter can usually be mobilized without great difficulty and secured with a sling of tape, a silicone tube or a piece of Paul's tubing. Difficulty may arise if it is bound down by firm adhesions from previous operations or infection. Mobilization is always facilitated by first securing the ureter above and below the lesion with slings before proceeding further.

The pelvic part of the ureter can be exposed through a low paramedian incision, a low oblique incision above and parallel to the inguinal ligament or a transverse suprapubic incision like that used for exposing the bladder or prostate (p. 575) (Fig. 26.50). The patient lies supine with the head of the table lowered. The incision is made through transversalis fascia but not through peritoneum (although some urologists consider that stones can be more easily removed from the pelvic part of the ureter if it is exposed transperitoneally). The peritoneum is reflected medially and the ureter found as it crosses the iliac vessels and enters the pelvis. The ureter is secured with tape or tube and the pelvic ureter can then be mobilized as far as the bladder. Apart from

some vesical vessels, it is crossed anteriorly by the vas deferens in males; by the broad ligament and the uterine arteries and veins (which can be very large) in females.

The ureters are approached *transperitoneally* for such operations as ileal loop ureterostomy, or ureterocolic anastomosis and by some surgeons for the removal of stones from the ureter.

Transvaginal approach to the pelvic ureter through the lateral fornix of the vagina has been described for the removal of stones from the lower part of the ureter in women. It can only be done if the stone is easily palpable and even then is not very satisfactory because it is impossible to control the ureter with slings before incising it and the stone can easily be displaced upwards.

Ureteric stones

Stones do not form in the ureter, but pass from the kidney while they are still small. Some pass silently through the ureter and into the bladder; stones that pass through the ureter, which has a diameter of 10 F or less can easily pass through the normal urethra which has a diameter of 26 F or more. Even small stones may arrest temporarily in the ureter, producing renal or ureteric colic and sometimes infection, haematuria or acute renal failure (p. 545). All stones with a diameter less than 5 mm, and many with a diameter between 5 and 7 mm, pass spontaneously into the bladder and it is wise to treat such patients conservatively unless there are good reasons for interfering. However, urgent relief is required for the patient with acute renal failure or severe infection. Less urgent operation is necessary if the patient has a ureterocele or stricture below the stone, persistent pain or progressive hydronephrosis. Stones tend to increase in size as they remain in the ureter and those more than 7 mm in diameter which are unlikely to pass without help should probably be given only about 3 months to do so. Smaller ones can be left much longer provided they are doing no harm. The patient should be followed up by straight X-rays and renography at 3-monthly intervals or earlier if symptoms or signs appear.

Stones that do not pass unaided have to be removed by an endoscopic or open operation. Those in the lower third of the ureter can often be removed by endoscopic methods or alternatively by the open operation of ureter-olithotomy which is the best operation for stones in the middle and upper thirds of the ureter where endoscopic methods are dangerous.

Ureterolithotomy (Fig. 26.51–26.54)

It is essential to X–ray the patient on the operating table to confirm that the stone has not moved since the previous examination before making the incision. The ureter is exposed, and secured with a sling of tape, Paul's tubing or silastic tube above the level of the calculus. This facilitates mobilization of the ureter and prevents

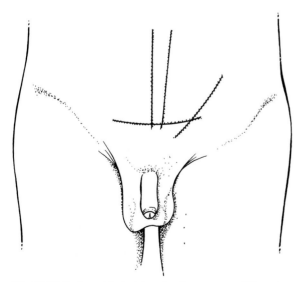

Fig. 26.50 Various skin incisions for the exposure of the lower third of the left ureter

Figs. 26.51–26.54 *Ureterolithotomy*

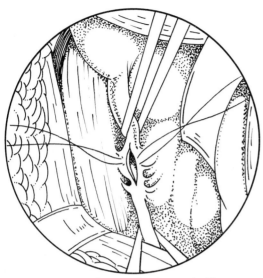

Fig. 26.51 The ureter is exposed and secured with a tape sling above the stone. The ureter has been opened between stay sutures over the stone

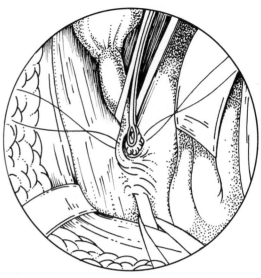

Fig. 26.52 The stone has been dislocated with a dissector and is now being removed with the stone-holding forceps

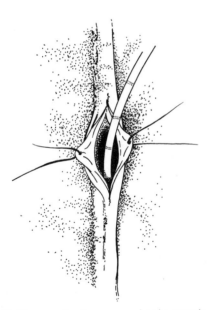

Fig. 26.53 The stone has been removed and a ureteric catheter is being passed down the ureter to ensure its patency

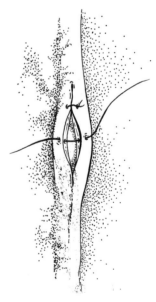

Fig. 26.54 The ureteric incison is being loosely sutured with stitches that do not pass through the mucosa

the stone slipping upwards to a level where it may be inaccessible from the approach employed—most likely if the ureter is dilated. After the ureter has been secured, the patient may be tilted into a Trendelenberg position which facilitates exposure, especially of the lower part of the ureter. The ureter is gently mobilized downwards as far as the stone which may be recognized by the fusiform swelling of the ureter it produces or by palpation. A

second sling or a tissue forceps is applied across the ureter below the stone to prevent the stone or small fragments slipping downwards. The stone is steadied between the slings or between a finger and thumb and a longitudinal incision is made through the ureter directly over it. This incision begins over the thickest part of the stone and extends upwards to a level just above its upper end. The stone can then be partly dislocated out of the ureter with a Watson-Cheyne or a Macdonald dissector and carefully removed with forceps, avoiding fragmentation. It is essential to mobilize the ureter as described, no matter how difficult this may be. Do not be tempted to open the ureter somewhere above the stone and hope to remove it by passing forceps down the ureter. It is not usually possible to dislodge the stone upwards and remove it through healthy ureter, although this is often described. However if you attempt to do this it is essential to have firm control of the ureter above the stone otherwise the stone might slip upwards to an inaccessible part of the ureter, even to the pelvis or calyces of the kidney. After removing the stone, insert a fine tube or ureteric catheter into the incision and wash out the ureter before and after removing the slings. Then pass a ureteric catheter upwards and downwards to make sure nothing has been missed. The incision in the ureter may be repaired with 3/0 or 4/0 absorbable sutures which do not penetrate the mucosa, although many urologists feel that it is unnecessary and leave the incision open (Fig. 26.54). Sometimes urine does not leak from an unsutured ureteric incision; more usually there is leakage for a few days whether or not the ureter is sutured and the area must be drained.

Transperitoneal ureterolithotomy

This is a safe procedure unlikely to be followed by intraperitoneal complications and is sometimes an easier way of removing stones in the lower third of the ureter than the more usual extraperitoneal approach. Some urologists favour this approach for all stones in the lower third of the ureter. An oblique or paramedian incision is made and deepened into the peritoneal cavity. The bowel is reflected and the ureter exposed by incising the peritoneum overlying it. The stone is removed in the way already described.

Transvaginal ureterolithotomy

In women some stones in the lower third of the ureter can be palpated vaginally and in such patients some surgeons recommend removing them through an incision in the lateral fornix of the vagina. With the patient in the lithotomy position an incision is made in the lateral fornix after appropriate retraction. The ureter is secured above the stone, which must be easily palpable for this procedure to be successful, and opened. The stone is removed, the ureter is sutured and the vaginal fornix loosely closed around a drain. There seems little risk of producing a ureterovaginal fistula but the procedure is not as easy as it sounds. The ureter can only be identified by palpating the stone within and it is usually impossible to secure and control the ureter above the stone before incising it. It is not difficult therefore to displace the stone upwards inadvertently and the patient must be advised before a transvaginal ureterolithotomy is attempted that it may be unsuccessful and an abdominal procedure may be required.

Endoscopic methods

Stones in the intra-mural part of the ureter. Few stones that have travelled as far down the ureter as its intramural part have difficulty travelling the last few mm into the bladder; those that do can usually be removed endoscopically (Ford, 1983).

At cystoscopy, an oedematous ureteric orifice is usually seen, sometimes with the lower end of the stone visible within it. The ureteric orifice and the intramural part of the ureter over the stone can be incised with a Lane or Bee Sting meatome (Fig. 26.55). The stone then falls into the bladder or can be persuaded to do so by gently nudging it with the closed meatome (Fig. 26.56). The stone can be removed by irrigating the bladder through the cystoscope sheath with an Ellik evacuator (p. 602). Some surgeons prefer to incise the intramural part of the ureter over the stone leaving the ureteric orifice itself intact, believing that this procedure is less likely than the others to cause vesico-ureteric reflux. However this is a more difficult procedure because the incision can only be made with a diathermy knife passed through a resectoscope.

Stones in the lower third of the ureter

Most stones that progress to the lower third of the ureter pass without interference into the bladder; those that do not can be removed by ureterolithotomy but, for stones smaller than 7 mm in diameter, it is worth attempting endoscopic methods, bearing in mind what damage can be inflicted on the ureter by some of the instruments available for the removal of stones from its lower third, especially when they are used in ways other than those recommended. Some surgeons pass one or two ureteric catheters up the ureter beyond the stone and leave them in for a few days. Others use stone dislodgers of one sort or another; the author favours the Dormia type (Fig. 26.57). The Dormia stone dislodger is a size 5 French ureteric catheter, the interior of which is occupied by four pliable stainless steel threads which project from the proximal end: when the threads are pushed forward a basket of spiral wires emerges from the distal end of the catheter; when the threads are pulled backwards the basket retracts into the catheter. The dislodger is passed through the catheterizing part of the cystoscope and into the ureter with the basket retracted. If it cannot be negotiated past the stone no more can be done although some surgeons dilate the ureter by opening the basket before it is withdrawn. If it passes beyond the stone the basket is opened and the dislodger slowly and gently withdrawn (Fig. 26.58) until its tip and the open basket are safely back in the bladder. No

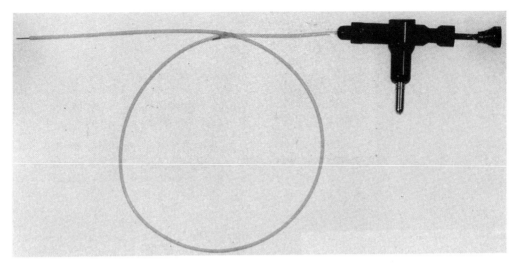

Fig. 26.55 Lane meatome. The handle of the instrument is connected to diathermy; the handle also contains a mechanism for extruding or retracting a small length of bare wire at the end of the instrument, which is insulated

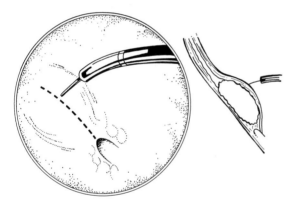

Fig. 26.56 Use of meatome. The bare wire is extruded and can be used for incision of the ureteric orifice. The incision can be made in the way illustrated from the outside but is often more easily accomplished if the wire is inserted into the ureteric orifice and pulled forward into the bladder as it cuts

attempt must be made to close the basket while it is still in the ureter. If the stone is trapped in the basket it may be difficult to pull the dislodger and the trapped stone downwards into the bladder. In such circumstances, steady firm even traction should be applied for half an hour or more if necessary. If this still fails to dislodge the stone into the bladder the ureteric orifice can be split using the Lane meatome.

If endoscopic measures fail it is worth waiting a few days before doing an open operation. X–ray is essential before proceeding with another operation since the stone may have been pushed upwards as far even as the pelvis or calices of the kidney.

Injuries of the ureter and methods of repair
(see Asmussen, 1983)

The ureter is more likely to be injured during pelvic operations, especially those on the uterus, than by road traffic accidents, falls or perforating wounds. It is important that the ureter should be identified and safeguarded at an early stage of such operations. When damaged, the ureter may be partially or completely divided, crushed by a clamp or occluded by a ligature or suture. If the accident is recognized at the time immediate steps should be taken to rectify matters. Removal of the constricting agent may be all that is required if the ureter has been clamped or occluded by ligature or suture but not divided, although there is some risk that a stricture or fistula may develop later. Incomplete tears may be loosely sutured with fine absorbable sutures that do not penetrate the mucosa and complete tears are treated if possible by an end to end anastomosis using absorbable sutures, diminishing the risk of stricture by spatulating the cut ends of the ureter before suturing (Fig. 26.59). Some surgeons make the anastomosis over a fine portex or silastic tube, leaving the lower end of the tube projecting into the bladder. The tube is removed some 7 or 10 days later with biopsy forceps through a cystoscope. If the injury involved the lower 5 or 6 cms of the ureter the most satisfactory procedure is to ligate the lower stump and reimplant the upper cut end into the bladder (p. 564). If the ureter can be neither repaired nor reimplanted into the bladder without tension even after hitching the bladder up to the psoas muscle (Fig. 26.60), a temporary cutaneous ureterostomy can be done by stitching a portex or silastic tube into the ureter and bringing the other end of the tube out of the skin through a separate stab incision, being careful to leave a reason-

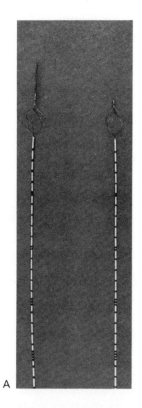

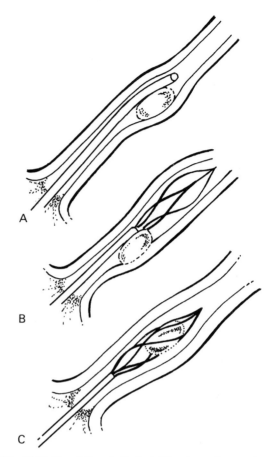

Fig. 26.58 Use of Dormia 'basket' (A) catheter tip passed beyond calculus (B) 'basket' opened (C) catheter and 'basket' withdrawn

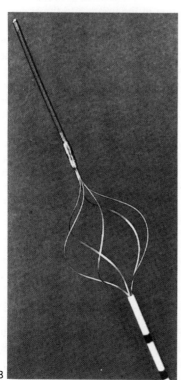

Fig. 26.57 Dormia stone dislodger (A) long and short tips (B) long tip

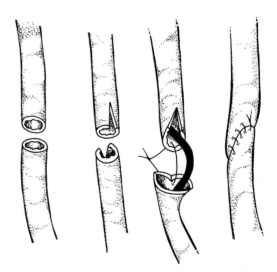

Fig. 26.59 End-to-end anastomosis of ureter. Each end of the ureter is spatulated. This results in a wide oblique anastomosis which is carried out with interrupted sutures over a ureteric splint

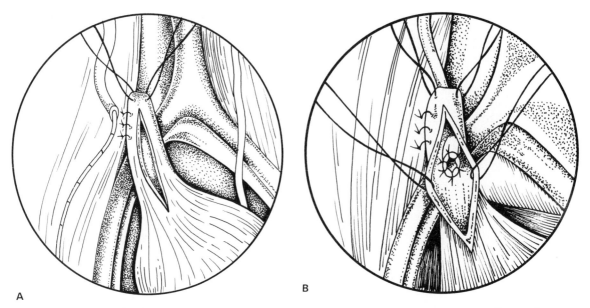

A   B

Fig. 26.60 The psoas hitch operation. (A) The right side of the bladder has been pulled up above the common iliac vessels and secured to the psoas muscle by three stitches. (B) These stitches are not tied until the reimplantation has been completed

able length of tube within the patient so that the ureter is not dislodged too far from its anatomical position. The ureter can then be repaired by a second operation at a later date using a Boari pouch (p. 565) or by replacing the damaged segment of ureter with an isolated loop of ileum. Uretero-ureteric anastomosis i.e. anastomosing the cut end of one ureter into the side of the other ureter is not recommended because it then endangers the integrity of the opposite urinary tract.

In patients who are poor risks and whose opposite kidney is known to be healthy, the ureter may be ligated but renal atrophy by no means always ensues and about 35% of patients so treated develop fistula or hydronephrosis and require nephrectomy. In many patients the ureteric injury remains unsuspected until some days after the operation when the patient develops renal pain, infection, or anuria (if the injury involves a solitary ureter or both ureters); or urine extravasates into the peritoneum or extra peritoneal tissues; or a fistula develops between ureter and vagina or skin. Sometimes the injury is never discovered because the obstructed kidney progresses silently to renal atrophy.

The elective repair of a damaged ureter (discovered some days after operation) should be delayed until the wound is fully healed and the patient fit. In the meantime an attempt can be made to introduce a ureteric catheter or stent endoscopically and if this fails a temporary ureterostomy or nephrostomy is necessary.

If the ureter has not been completely divided and a ureteric catheter can be passed, no more need be done and the ureter may heal. Otherwise the pelvis should be explored and the damaged ureter treated by reimplantation using a Boari pouch or end-to-end anastomosis.

Reimplantation of the ureter into the bladder (ureterocystostomy)

This procedure is used for *injuries* of the lower ureter and it is often the best means of treating lower ureteric *strictures*. It is the operation of choice for restoring continuity of the urinary tract following excision of the ureteric orifice and intramural ureter during removal of a bladder diverticulum or partial cystectomy, of preventing vesicoureteric reflux and of treating megaureter. It is also part of the operation for renal transplantation. The method of approach and the technique of reimplantation vary according to the conditions present. *Transperitoneal approach* is likely to be employed if the ureter has been accidently divided during an abdominal operation, otherwise an extraperitoneal approach is normally preferred since it obviates the risk of peritoneal complications. The ureter is exposed and divided as low down as conditions permit, ligating or excising the lower segment. The remaining part of the ureter is mobilized so that it pursues a fairly straight course to the bladder and lies without tension. Provided that its adventitial sheath remains intact there is little risk of ischaemic necrosis. Each side of the cut end of the ureter is split longitudinally for a distance of about 2 cm so that anterior and posterior flaps are formed for anchoring the ureter inside the bladder. A small incision is made in the posterior wall of the bladder above the normal ureteric orifice. The cut end of the ureter is then brought

THE KIDNEY, THE ADRENAL GLANDS AND THE URETERS 565

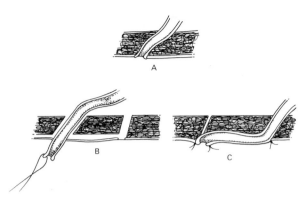

Fig. 26.61 The Politano-Leadbetter method of ureteric reimplantation. (A) shows the normal anatomy. (B) the intramural ureter has been mobilized and freed from the surrounding bladder and an incision has been made through the bladder above the ureteric orifice. (C) the ureter has been removed from the bladder, reinserted through the recently made incison, brought down through a subcutaneous tunnel and sutured to the margins of the old ureteric orifice

through this incision into the bladder and secured by suturing the ureteric flaps to the mucosa of the bladder with absorbable material. Fine sutures are then used to join the fibrous sheath of the ureter to the outside of the bladder. This method is the simplest one of reimplanting the ureter but has to be modified or replaced by a different operation in most patients because it offers little if any protection against vesico-ureteric reflux, particularly if the ureter is dilated (Johnson, 1984).

If the operation is being carried out to cure vesico-ureteric reflux, the *Politano-Leadbetter* operation is appropriate (Fig. 26.61). The bladder is exposed through a transverse suprapubic incision and opened between stay sutures. The ureter is catheterized (Fig. 26.62) with a plastic or silastic tube (about 5F in size) which is tied to the edge of the ureteric orifice with a fine catgut suture. A circular incision is made around the ureteric orifice and, by sharp dissection (Fig. 26.63) aided by traction on the tube, the intramural ureter is freed and drawn into the bladder. A right angled clamp of the O'Shaugnessy type is passed out of the bladder alongside the freed ureter and used to invaginate the posterior bladder wall some 5 or 6 cm above the ureteric orifice (Fig. 26.64). A small incision is made through the bladder wall onto the tip of the clamp which then appears inside the bladder. A suture is passed, by means of the clamp, between the two openings in the bladder and tied to the tube previously inserted into the ureter. Traction on the other end of the suture takes the ureter out of the bladder and in again through the newly made opening (Fig. 26.65). The ureter is drawn down through a submucosal tunnel (made by blunt dissection with scissors or forceps between this new opening and the old ureteric orifice) spatulated and sutured to the margins of

the ureteric orifice using interrupted 4/0 absorbable material. The hole in the mucosa is closed with similar material (Fig. 26.66).

The Politano-Leadbetter procedure is not suitable for adults nor is it suitable if the ureter is dilated and has to be tapered as well as reimplanted. In these circumstances the ureter is exposed by an extraperitoneal approach and freed down to the bladder. This is facilitated if the superior vesical vessels, and in women the uterine vessels also, are ligated and divided. The ureter is divided at the bladder and its lower end is ligated. The bladder is opened anteriorly and the proximal end of the ureter is brought into the bladder through a small stab incision in the posterolateral wall. A submucosal tunnel is fashioned downwards from this incision for some 5 cm and the mucosa (some distance above the ureteric orifice) is incised. The ureter is brought through the submucosal tunnel and sutured to the edges of the second incision.

If the ureter is very dilated (e.g. in patients with megaureter or reflux) the lower end should be tapered before it is brought through the submucosa tunnel. The ureter is tapered by excising a 'dart' from each side and suturing the defects with 4/0 catgut. The 'darts' must be longer than the length of the ureter incorporated into the submucosal tunnel. A splint can be left in if desired and removed later with cystoscopic biopsy forceps.

When the ureter is too short to be reimplanted into the bladder by these methods, a pedicled flap may be fashioned from the bladder wall (Boari), the intact bladder may be hitched up by stitching it to the psoas, an isolated segment of ileum may be used to bridge the gap, or (if the other kidney is normal) the kidney can be removed.

Boari flap (Figs. 26.67–26.71)
This is used to bridge a long gap between ureter and bladder when treating strictures or injuries of the lower third of the ureter. The bladder has a good blood supply which is not compromised when the length of the flap is much longer than the base.

The ureter is mobilized and the superior vesical pedicle is divided. The flap is marked on the distended bladder with sutures or clips, cut with its base superolaterally, and folded upwards and backwards. A small incision is made through the posterior aspect of the flap about 2 cm from its cut edge and the ureter brought through it (Fig. 26.69). A submucosal tunnel is fashioned downwards for some 2 to 3 cm, opening the mucosa at its distal end. The cut end of the ureter is pulled through the submucosal tunnel into the lumen of the pouch with about 1 cm projecting. The projecting ureter can be spatulated and sutured to the margins of the opening or fliped and left projecting into the lumen like a nipple. It is best to splint the ureter with a 6–8F portex tube leaving the distal end in the bladder so that

Figs. 26.62–26.66 *Politano-Leadbetter method of ureteric reimplantation*

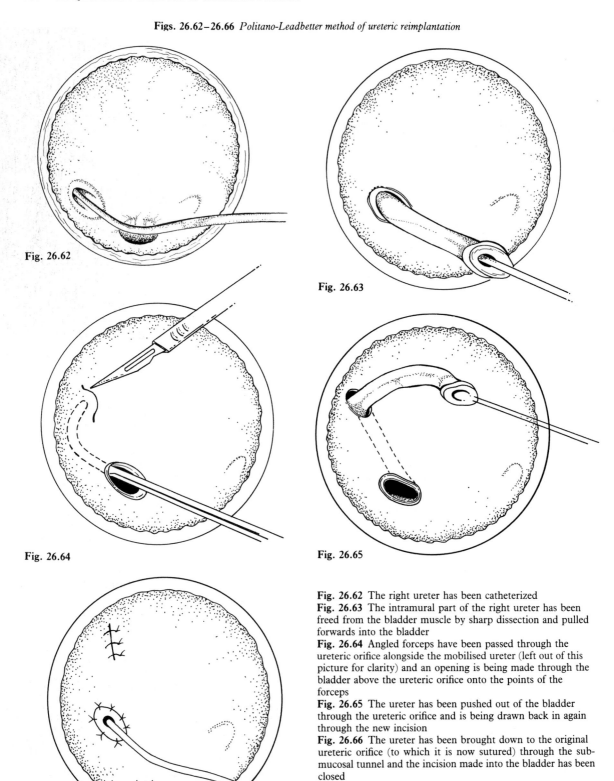

Fig. 26.62

Fig. 26.63

Fig. 26.64

Fig. 26.65

Fig. 26.66

Fig. 26.62 The right ureter has been catheterized

Fig. 26.63 The intramural part of the right ureter has been freed from the bladder muscle by sharp dissection and pulled forwards into the bladder

Fig. 26.64 Angled forceps have been passed through the ureteric orifice alongside the mobilised ureter (left out of this picture for clarity) and an opening is being made through the bladder above the ureteric orifice onto the points of the forceps

Fig. 26.65 The ureter has been pushed out of the bladder through the ureteric orifice and is being drawn back in again through the new incision

Fig. 26.66 The ureter has been brought down to the original ureteric orifice (to which it is now sutured) through the submucosal tunnel and the incision made into the bladder has been closed

Figs. 26.67–26.71 *The Boari pouch*

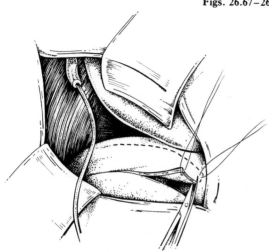

Fig. 26.67

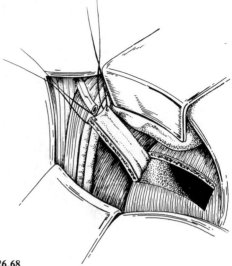

Fig. 26.68

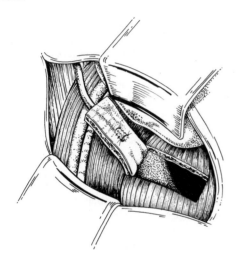

Fig. 26.69

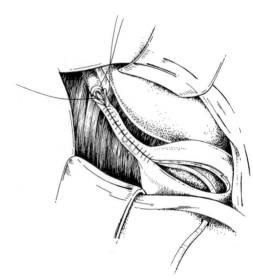

Fig. 26.70

Fig. 26.67 A long flap has been cut from the bladder with its base superolaterally and the ureter has been intubated
Fig. 26.68 The flap is raised
Fig. 26.69 The ureter has been anastomosed to the flap using a submucosal tunnel
Fig. 26.70 Alternatively, the ureter can be anastomosed to the edge of the flap
Fig. 26.71 The flap is closed

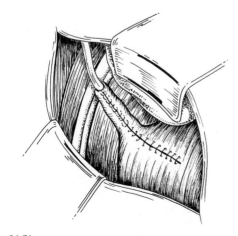

Fig. 26.71

it can be removed later. The flap and the bladder are closed with two layers of catgut and the site drained.

Urinary diversion operations (see Ashken, 1982)

Permanent diversion of urine is necessary in patients with malignant disease of the bladder either as part of the operation of total cystectomy or as a palliative measure when the growth is irremovable but causing severe symptoms; in patients with a contracted bladder due to tuberculosis, radiation or chronic interstitial cystitis (if conservative measures fail and bladder expanding operations are thought inappropriate); in some patients with vesicovaginal fistulae (particularly when caused by X–ray therapy or malignant disease and irreparable by operation); in patients with congenital extroversion of the bladder and in some patients with neurological disturbance of bladder function.

Transplantation of the ureters into the colon (Ureterosigmoidostomy)

This operation, evolved from techniques originally described by Stiles and Coffey, is now considered an unsatisfactory means of urinary diversion. Its complications include (1) disruption and leakage from one or both anastomoses especially in patients who have had radiotherapy (2) renal infection caused by an obstruction at the anastomosis or reflux of colonic content into the ureter (3) hyperchloraemic acidosis (because colonic mucosa absorbs hydrogen and chloride from the urine) and (4) hypokakaemia from excesive loss of potassium-containing mucus.

Despite the external fistula and the need to wear an appliance permanently, diversion of urine to the skin using an ileal loop is the best and safest form of permanent diversion. A ureterosigmoidostomy may still be done however if a patient requires a diversion and refuses to have an external fistula. Before operation it is essential to determine the condition of the ureters and the function of the kidneys. Thickened or dilated ureters increase the hazards of the operation, but are not necessarily a contraindication.

The ultimate success of the operation depends on the ability of the anal sphincter to preserve continence when the colon is the receptacle, not only for faeces, but also for the entire urinary output. Assessment of the tone and contractility of the anal sphincter by rectal examination is not enough. If 250 or 300 ml of water can be retained in the colon for some hours during normal activities, the sphincters may be considered satisfactory.

The colon should be prepared as for colonic surgery (p. 436) and both ureters (if there are two) are transplanted at the same procedure, which can be done trans or extra peritoneally.

Trans-peritoneal approach. With the patient in the Trendelenberg position the lower abdomen is opened through a left paramedian or transverse incision and the small bowel is packed upwards. The right ureter is usually dealt with first. It is identified on the medial side of the caecum as it crosses the iliac vessels and delivered through an incision in the overlying peritoneum. It is mobilized with its adventitial coat down to the bladder and divided above a ligature applied as closely to the bladder as possible. The upper cut end is trimmed obliquely, and stay sutures are inserted (Fig. 26.72). It is laid alongside the lower part of the pelvic colon just above the pelvirectal junction, and a seromuscular incision 2 to 3 cm long is made in the bowel wall along the line in which the ureter lies comfortably without tension or kinking. The upper end of this incision is extended a little on either side, converting the linear into a T incision through serous and muscular coats only in the first instance. Flaps are carefully undermined with sharp and blunt dissection to separate them from the underlying mucosa at the lower end of the seromuscular incision, compatible in size with the obliquely cut end of the ureter. The mucous membrane of the colon is anastomosed to all coats of the ureter with interrupted 3/0 absorbable sutures (Fig. 26.73). When this has been completed, the edges of the seromuscular incision are sutured together over the ureter to provide protection and a valve, taking great care to avoid constriction of the lumen of the ureter especially at the upper end.

The peritoneum on the left side of the pelvic colon is incised along the 'white line' and the left ureter found. It is mobilized, like the right one, into the pelvis, divided above a ligature close to the bladder and transplanted into the colon in a similar manner to the right one, but usually at a slightly higher level (Fig. 26.74). Finally, the posterior peritoneal flaps are stitched to the bowel wall in front of the anastomosis which thus becomes extraperitoneal.

Extraperitoneal approach. This method has the advantage that the consequences of anastomotic leaks are less serious. It can be done through a single central incision or two oblique ones. The peritoneum is displaced medially, but unopened. The ureter is identified and freed downwards as far as possible to the bladder and divided above a ligature. An incision is made in the peritoneum, medial to the genital vessels and a loop of pelvic colon withdrawn. The edges of this peritoneal incision are stitched around the area of bowel selected for the anastomosis which is carried out by the technique already described. A similar operation is then undertaken on the opposite side. The site must be drained.

Many surgeons use splints of 5F plastic or silastic tube; one end is inserted into the ureter for 10 cm and the other end is brought into the rectum and pulled out through the anus using a sigmoidoscope. Whether or not splints are used, the colon and the rectum should be kept

Figs. 26.72–26.74 *Ureterosigmoidostomy*

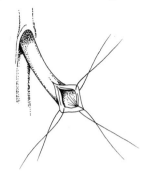

Fig. 26.72 The mobilized ureter spatulated and secured with stay sutures

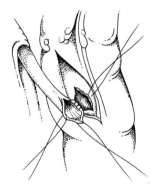

Fig. 26.73 Shows the colon illustrating the submucosal tunnel, intact mucosa above and an opening into the mucosa below. The full thickness of the ureteric wall is being sutured to the mucosa of the colon

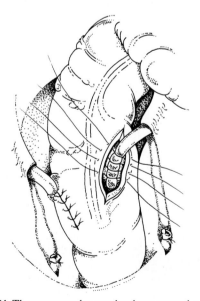

Fig. 26.74 The seromuscular coat has been sutured over the anastomosis of the right ureter. The left ureter has also been anastomosed and the sutures covering the anastomosis with seromuscular flaps have been inserted but not yet tied

empty for some days by inserting a rectal tube or a large (30F) Foley catheter.

Ileal conduit

The ileal conduit introduced by Bricker in 1958 has become the most popular method of permanent urinary diversion. The ultimate success of the operation depends upon the patients adjusting psychologically to the change in their way of life and of tolerating the appliance and managing it well enough to keep dry.

Before operation, time must be spent explaining the procedure to the patient and trying out the appliance (partly filled with water) on the intact skin. It is very helpful to introduce the patient to others who have had the same operation and who may answer questions the patient hesitates to ask of his medical advisers.

Operation. The bowel is prepared in the same way as for any small bowel resection. The best position for the stoma, predetermined by wearing the appliance on intact skin, is marked indelibly.

The abdomen is opened through a long left lower paramedian incision (Fig. 26.75). The appendix is removed, and the caecum is mobilized so that an isolated ileal loop will lie comfortably on the side wall of the abdomen, below or behind the caecum. Select a loop of terminal ileum which is not too near the ileocaecal junction (because of vitamin B_{12} absorbtion) which is healthy, which has not suffered radiation damage and which has a mesentery undistorted by calcified glands or adhesions. The loop must have a good blood supply; appropriate vessels are ligated after holding the bowel up and illuminating its mesentery with a powerful spot light while the loop is being prepared (Fig. 26.76). The loop must be long enough to extend without tension from the midline to some 5 cm beyond the site chosen on the skin for the stoma. The mesenteric incision can be much shorter on the left end of the loop, which will remain at or near the promontory of the sacrum, than on the right which has to emerge through the skin and form the stoma. The loop is then isolated, by cutting the bowel across at each end, and washed out with water or saline (Fig. 26.77). The continuity of the small bowel is restored in front of the isolated loop by an end-to-end anastomosis (p. 429). If the patient has previously had radiotherapy to the pelvis, the author does a one layered anastomosis using interrupted Nuralon sutures, inserted through all coats of the bowel except the mucosa. The ureters are then found (the right one by incising the posterior peritoneum on the medial aspect of the caecum, the left one by mobilizing the pelvic colon after dividing the peritoneum on its lateral aspect) mobilized and divided at a convenient level above the bladder. The left ureter is brought medially under the pelvic mesocolon to lie alongside the right one, both then emerging side by side through the incision in the posterior peritoneum,

Figs. 26.75–26.79 *Cutaneous ileo-ureterostomy*

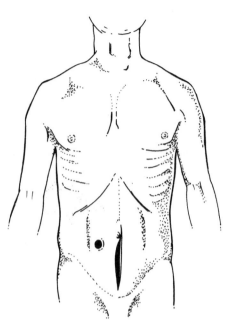

Fig. 26.75 Shows the incision, which can be a long midline or a left paramedian, and also the marking on the right side of the abdomen where the stoma will be

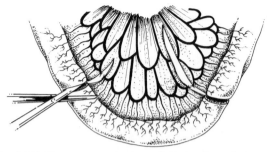

Fig. 26.76 The mesentery has been divided and vessels ligated on each side of the loop which is just being fashioned

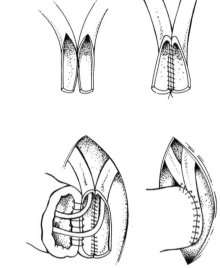

Fig. 26.78 The Wallace method of anastomosing the ureters to the open left end of the ileal loop. The lower ends of each ureter are approximated and spatulated. The medial aspects are sutured together to form one oval stoma. Each ureter has been separately intubed with a splint brought through the ileal loop from left to right and the oval stoma formed by the two ureters is being sutured to the left end of the ileum

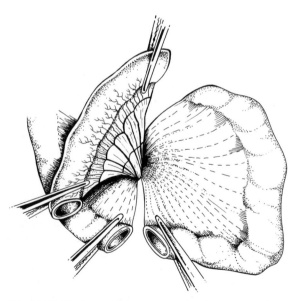

Fig. 26.77 The loop with its mesentery has been separated from the rest of the small bowel and ends of the ileum have been prepared for anastomosis (shown posterior to the loop for clarity)

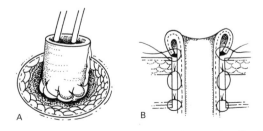

Fig. 26.79 The stoma has been constructed, everted or fliped and then sutured to the skin. Although many surgeons sutur the stoma to deeper tissues as well, as illustrated here, the author tends not to do so

making sure that the left ureter does not form an acute angle, as it passes medially under the mesocolon, by mobilizing it well upwards. Various methods are available for implanting ureters into the loop, including the Wallace method or the Stiles method for patients who have previously had radiotherapy. In the *Wallace method* the ends of the ureter are spatulated by making a short slit anteriorly in each and their medial walls are sutured together to form one oval shaped stoma (Fig. 26.78). Each ureter is intubated for a distance of about 10 cm with 6 or 8F (depending on the calibre of the ureters) polyvinyl or silastic tube, secured to the ureter with a stitch. A pair of forceps is passed down the ileal loop from the right to left and the tubes drawn through it. The oval stoma constructed from the lower ends of the ureters is stitched to the open left end of the loop with interrupted 3/0 catgut or dexon. The left end of the loop is then fixed by stitching it to the margins of the peritoneal opening. In the *Stiles procedure* (Fig. 26.80), the left end of the loop is closed with sutures or staples and the ureters are inserted separately into the loop. A splint is passed into each ureter and secured with a stitch. An Allis forceps is passed into the loop through the right end and a small incision made onto its opened jaws on the antimesenteric border some 2.5 cm from the left end of the loop. The ureteric splint is drawn through. A 2/0 catgut stitch is inserted into the loop about 2 cm to the right of the small incision made on the tips of the Allis forceps and brought out of the incision. It is then passed through one wall of the ureter (which can be spatulated) then passed back through the incision and out of the loop close to the entering thread. The ureter is pushed into the ileal loop and firmly secured by tying the suture. The right ureter is similarly inserted one cm or so to the right of the left one. The site for the stoma is prepared by excising a disc of skin and external oblique aponeurosis and incising the underlying muscles and peritoneum, making sure that

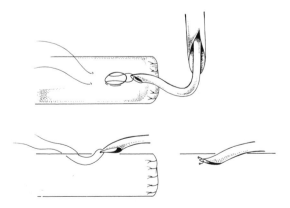

Fig. 26.80 Stiles method. The splint and forceps have been left out to improve clarity

the opening is wide enough to avoid narrowing the stoma. The stoma, with protruding ends of the splints, is slowly and very carefully withdrawn through the opening until about 5 cm projects. Any attempt to force it through may tear its mesentery and imperil its blood supply. The peritoneal aspect of the stoma is lightly scarified with a scalpel then everted or fliped so that some 2.5 cm projects beyond the skin (Fig. 26.79). The edge is sutured to the skin margin with dexon or catgut sutures. Finally the mesenteric defect is closed and the space lateral to the mesentery of the loop obliterated with a few sutures before the wound is closed with drainage. The splints are cut short so that 3 or 4 cm project from the stoma and an adhesive bag is applied.

Early complications include ileus, urinary leakage from the ureteric anastomosis or intestinal leakage from the small bowel anastomosis; later ones include stenosis of the stoma, parastomal hernia, ureteric obstruction, pyelonephritis, stone formation or intestinal obstruction. Reflux from loop to one or both ureters can often be demonstrated by X-rays made after the injection of radio-opaque media into the stoma (loopogram) but causes little problem because it is a low pressure system.

Transplantation of the ureter to the skin surface (cutaneous ureterostomy)

This operation, performed bilaterally as an elective procedure, was formally employed as an alternative to ureterocolic anastomosis but has been replaced by uretero-ileostomy which has many advantages. The operation may still be useful however in patients who have only one ureter.

The middle third of the ureter is mobilized and divided as far down as possible, the lower end is ligated and the upper end is brought out through a small stab incision below the main incision (which should be much higher than usual so that it does not interfere with the positioning of the appliance). Its fascial sheath is sutured to the wound margin, so that it projects 2 to 3 cm beyond the surface. The protruding segment often sloughs away, leaving a meatus which tends to stenose. If the ureter is dilated it can sometimes be fliped or everted like the stoma of an ileal loop (Fig. 26.81). The procedure is obviously much simpler than an ileal loop, but much less satisfactory because the stoma stenoses and retracts, cannot easily be reconstructed and often has to be kept open with a small indwelling tube which has to be changed regularly. Nevertheless, it can be a useful operation if the aim is palliation and the patient's prognosis poor. Attempts to form a satisfactory stoma by incorporating the ureter into a pedicle skin flap, enclosing it in the flaps of a Z incision or constructing a nipple ureterostomy by drawing the exteriorized part of the ureter into a cutaneous pedicle tube, are not always successful.

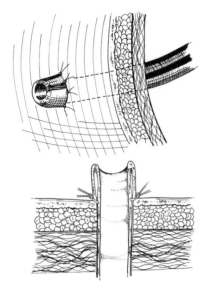

Fig. 26.81 Cutaneous ureterostomy. The ureter is brought through a separate stab incision away from the main wound used to expose it and is everted or fliped, if that is possible, and sutured to the skin margin

Ureterolysis

Retroperitoneal fibrosis

This reveals itself when it envelops and obstructs one or both ureters. It may also involve the aorta, the inferior vena cava or the common iliac vessels and it sometimes extends upwards to surround the heart and become one form of constrictive pericarditis (Ormond, 1981).

In some patients the fibrosis results from radiation therapy or the organization of a retroperitoneal haematoma from a leaking aortic aneurysm or other cause; in others it is the fibrous tissue of a scirrhous carcinoma containing so few malignant cells that they cannot easily be detected. The idiopathic form of the disease is the one requiring surgical correction and, as its name implies, the cause is unknown. Although it has been thought to be a neoplasm or autoimmune disease or a side effect of drugs like Methysergide (sometimes used in treatment of migraine), as little is known about the cause of idiopathic retroperitoneal fibrosis as about Peyronie's disease (p. 621) or Dupuytren's contracture (p. 147).

Patients with idiopathic retroperitoneal fibrosis present with renal failure, usually chronic but sometimes acute, or with other features of obstruction like pain or infection. The renal symptoms may be associated with, and sometimes overshadowed by, symptoms and signs of arterial or venous obstruction.

Treatment. If the disease is diagnozed early it is worth attempting treatment with glucocorticoids or drugs with glucocorticoid effects, but the patient must be carefully observed because, although retroperitoneal fibrosis is considered an insidious disease, it can advance very rapidly.

If the patient has acute or severe chronic renal failure, elective operation is deferred until renal function is improved by draining one or both kidneys by ureteric catheterization or percutaneous nephrostomy although glucocorticoids can be given in the meantime. Both ureters are usually involved, although one side is worse than the other. If the disease is not too extensive, the patient fit and renal function satisfactory, it is tempting to deal with both ureters at one operation through an anterior incision; otherwise it is better to do one side at a time using a postero-lateral approach and freeing the ureter of what appears to be the best kidney.

Operation. After dissection enters the retroperitoneal space, the normal parts of the ureter, above and below the level of the fibrous plaque, are secured with tapes. The ureter is next separated and displaced from the fibrous tissue encasing and obstructing it. Fortunately this is often not difficult and the ureter can be lifted out intact after the fibrous tissue overlying it is cut or split. Sometimes however separation can be difficult and fraught with the risk of splitting open the ureter which is then very difficult to repair. Once the ureter is freed it is important to protect it from subsequent involvement in fibrous tissue, which may continue to increase. Some surgeons displace it laterally, securing it loosely to the quadratus lumborum muscle; others invaginate it into the peritoneum on the posterior abdominal wall with a few loose sutures.

If a small opening is inadvertently made into the ureter while it is being freed, it can be left or loosely sutured; if a large opening or split is made it is probably better to insert a splint rather than attempt repair. The splint can be a plastic or silicone tube, 6 or 7F in diameter, 25 to 30 cm in length. One end is passed up the ureter so that its tip lies in the renal pelvis; the other end is passed down the ureter so that its terminal few cm lie in the bladder. The splint can be removed some time after the operation using a cystoscope and biopsy forceps. If the patient also has features of arterial or venous obstruction, an attempt should be made to free the affected vessels.

The operation does nothing for the cause, whatever that may be, of the disease. The fibrosis may later extend to involve blood vessels and even the ureters again no matter how well they are protected and patients must be followed up for a long time.

REFERENCES

Ashken M H 1982 Clinical Practice in Urology — Urinary Diversion. Springer Verlag, Heidelberg

Asmussen M, Miller A 1983 Clinical Gynaecological Urology. Blackwell, Oxford

Bledsoe T 1974 Surgery and the adrenal cortex. Surgical Clinics of North America 54: 449

Dees J E, Anderson E E 1981 Coagulum pyelolithotomy. Urological Clinics of North America 8: 313

Ford T F, Watson G M, Wickham J E A 1983 Transurethral ureteroscopic retrieval of ureteric stones. British Journal of Urology 55: 626

Gil-Vernet J M 1983 Pyelolithotomy. In: Glenn J F (ed) Urological Surgery, 3rd edn. Lippincott, Philadelphia, p 159

Gosling J A, Dixon J S, Humpherson J R 1982 Functional anatomy of the urinary tract. Churchill Livingstone, Edinburgh

Guerriero W G 1982 Trauma to the kidneys, ureters, bladder and urethra. Surgical Clinics of North America 62: 1047

Johnson J H 1984 Reimplantation of the ureter. Williams & Wilkins, London

Morris P J 1979 Renal Transplantation. In: Black D, Jones N F (eds) Renal disease, 4th edn, Blackwell Scientific Publications, Oxford, ch. 18

Newsam J E, Petrie J J B 1981 Urology and Renal Medicine. 3rd edn. Churchill Livingstone, Edinburgh, p. 82

Ormond J K 1981 Idiopathic retroperitoneal fibrosis. In: Bergman H (ed) The Ureter, 2nd edn. Springer Verlag, Heidelberg

Robertson W G, Peacock M 1982 Risk factors in the formation of urinary stones. In: Chisholm G D, Williams D I (eds) Scientific Foundations of Urology. 2nd edn. Heinemann, London, p 267

Smith J W, Murphy T R, Blair J S G, Lowe K G 1983 Regional Anatomy Illustrated. Churchill Livingstone, Edinburgh

Turner-Warwick R 1980 Surgical access. In: Chisholm G D (ed) Urology. Heinemann, London, p 402

Welbourne R B 1980 Some aspects of adrenal surgery. British Journal of Surgery 67: 723

Whitaker R H 1977 Hydronephrosis. Annals of the Royal College of Surgeons of England 59: 388

FURTHER READING

Blandy J P 1984 Operative Urology, 2nd edn. Blackwell, Oxford

McDougal W S (ed) 1984 Urology. In: Dudley H, Pories W J Rob and Smith's Operative Surgery, 4th edn. Butterworth, London

Whitfield H N, Hendry W F (eds) 1985 Textbook of Genito-urinary Surgery. Churchill Livingstone, Edinburgh, Vol 2

Wickham J E A, Miller R A 1983 Percutaneous Renal Surgery. Churchill Livingstone, Edinburgh.

27

Operations on the bladder and prostate

J. E. NEWSAM

Anatomy of bladder

The normal bladder has a capacity of 300 to 500 ml and lies in the pelvis. Its wall consists of smooth muscle separated from the internal lining of transitional cell epithelium by the lamina propria. When empty it is pyramidal in shape, with *an apex, a base, a superior surface, two inferolateral surfaces* and *a neck* which tapers to become continuous with the urethra. Only the superior surface and a small part of the base are covered with peritoneum (Fig. 27.1). As the bladder fills it becomes globular and the demarcation between its various surfaces is lost but its neck and base remain unaltered. When overdistended the bladder rises out of the pelvis into the abdomen pushing the peritoneum upwards. In infants, the bladder is an abdominal organ even when empty (Gosling, 1982).

The transitional cell epithelium is smooth and flat in the full bladder, but falls into transverse folds in the empty one. The *trigone* forms the base of the bladder. It is more vascular than the rest of the bladder, is firmly attached to the underlying muscle and smooth whether the bladder is full or empty. The ureteric orifices are found at the upper lateral angles of the trigone, and the bladder neck at its lower angle.

Relations

The *apex* of the bladder lies behind the symphysis pubis and is connected to the umbilicus by the median umbilical

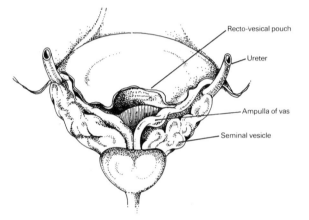

Fig. 27.2 A posterior view of the bladder

ligament (the fibrous remnant of the allantois). The *base* faces downwards and backwards and is separated from the rectum by the vasa deferentia and the seminal vesicles in the male (Fig. 27.2) and is closely related to the cervix uteri and the vagina in the female.

The *superior surface* is covered by peritoneum and related to ileum and pelvic colon and in the female to the body of the uterus. The *inferolateral surfaces* are separated from the pubis and from the floor and side walls of the pelvis by fat, and from each other by an ill defined border which disappears as the bladder fills. They lie below the peritoneum and are the parts of the bladder exposed by the suprapubic approach. The bladder is supported by thickenings of the pelvic fascia called the puboprostatic or pubovesical ligaments and by its attachments to the urethra and in the male to the prostate also.

The *retropubic space* (of Retzius) lies between the bladder and the pubis and contains fatty and areolar tissue. Below it is bounded by the puboprostatic or pubovesical ligaments, laterally by the side walls of the pelvis and superiorly it becomes continuous with the space between peritoneum and transversalis fascia.

Blood supply

The bladder receives blood from the superior and inferior vesical, the middle rectal, the obturator and the

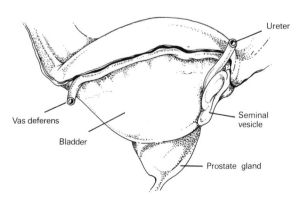

Fig. 27.1 A lateral view of the bladder

pudendal arteries (all branches of the internal iliac artery). The vesical veins drain into the prevesical plexus or join the prostatic plexus which lies in the sulcus between bladder and prostate (plexus of Santorini). Both plexuses drain into the internal iliac veins.

Lymphatic drainage
Lymph from the bladder and the prostate goes first to nodes alongside the internal and common iliac and the obturator vessels, thence to the para-aortic nodes.

SURGICAL APPROACH TO THE BLADDER

The bladder can be approached endoscopically (p. 516), or openly by a suprapubic incision.

The suprapubic route is generally used for the treatment of bladder stones, diverticula, trauma and some tumours, for ureteric reimplantation or for access to the prostate gland. The operation is entirely extraperitoneal and usually through a transverse incision; for cystectomy the approach is intraperitoneal and usually through a vertical incision.

Technique
The operation is easier, particularly if the patient has had previous operations on the bladder or lower abdomen, if the bladder is filled with sterile water or saline through a catheter before operation. The table is tilted into a slight Trendelenberg position and illumination arranged so that light can be directed into the interior of the bladder. Although a vertical paramedian or midline incision can be used, the best approach is by a transverse one, because it heals better and is less liable to herniate. A transverse incision is made (Fig. 27.36) in a skin fold about 2.5 cm above the pubis, opening the anterior rectus sheath with a transverse or U-shaped incision and freeing it from the underlying rectus and pyramidalis muscles by sharp dissection in the midline and by blunt dissection laterally. The lower flap of the rectus sheath can be split vertically in the midline down to the pubis to improve exposure of the retropubic space (Fig. 27.37). (The U incision is useful because one or both limbs can be extended upwards to expose the lower ends of the ureters and even the lower pole of the kidney.) The recti and pyramidalis muscles are separated in the midline and retracted laterally although it is often better to divide the pyramidalis muscles transversely and reflect them with the rectus sheath.

The extraperitoneal fat and peritoneum are stripped upwards to expose the bladder wall which is easily recognized by its fasciculated appearance and by the many thin walled veins that course over its surface. The bladder wall is picked up at two points with tissue forceps or with stay sutures, opened vertically or transversely, and emptied by suction.

Difficulties and closure
The peritoneum may be inadvertently opened while exposing or opening the bladder especially if the two structures are adherent to each other after previous bladder or pelvic operations, but complications are unlikely if the peritoneum is repaired. The bladder is closed with continuous or interrupted absorbable stitches which should probably not penetrate the mucosa, although absorbable suture material rarely forms a nucleus for stone formation. A second layer of sutures can be inserted to invaginate the first layer, or to close the prevesical fascia over it. The rest of the wound is closed in layers and the retropubic or prevesical space is drained for 48 hours or sometimes longer.

SUPRAPUBIC CYSTOSTOMY

In this operation, a tube is placed in the bladder for drainage or as part of an operation on the bladder, prostate or urethra. As an operation on its own, when no more is done than drainage, it is much less frequently performed than formerly, and then only when urethral drainage is impracticable or is considered inadequate or unwise. When used in these circumstances, the operation can be performed openly or percutaneously under local anaesthesia.

Suprapubic cystostomy by open operation
This allows correct positioning of the tube, exploration of the bladder and the placement of the tube at a higher level on the abdominal wall than is possible by percutaneous methods; any future operations on the bladder are thus facilitated.

Technique
The bladder is exposed and a small incision is made into it as high as possible between two forceps or stay sutures. The bladder is emptied by suction and its interior explored with a finger to exclude calculi, diverticula and tumour. A self-retaining catheter of the De Pezzer, Malecot or Foley type (Fig. 27.3) is introduced and the bladder wall is sutured around it with one or two catgut stitches. The catheter is brought through a stab

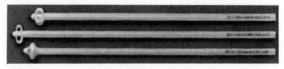

Fig. 27.3 Suprapubic catheters. Two Malecot above, and a De Pezzer below

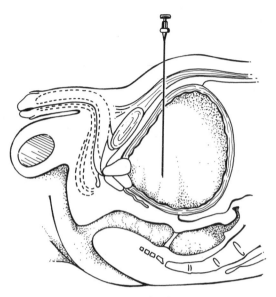

Fig. 27.4 Suprapubic cystostomy by the percutaneous method

wound in the upper skin flap and anchored with a stitch prior to wound closure.

Suprapubic cystostomy by the percutaneous method (Fig. 27.4)

This method causes little discomfort to the patient and little scarring, but can only be done safely if the bladder is distended. It is the method of choice unless there are compelling reasons for exploring the bladder or for bringing the tube out at a high level.

Technique

Local anaesthetic (1 or 2% Lignocaine solution) is injected into the midline skin some 5 cm above the pubis. As the needle is advanced anaesthetic is injected into subcutaneous tissue, linea alba, extraperitoneal fat and bladder wall. The position and depth of the needle tip required to enter the bladder is recognized when urine can be aspirated. After a 5 minute interval for anaesthesia to develop, a 2 cm incision is made through skin and linea alba, and the suprapubic trocar and cannula are introduced into the bladder with a quick stabbing movement. It is best to introduce the needle— and later the trocar, cannula and catheter—directly backwards. To introduce them backwards and downwards is hazardous because they may pass below the bladder into the prostate.

The patient may experience momentary discomfort, but should have no pain if the anaesthetic has been correctly introduced. The trocar is withdrawn and the cannula is closed with a finger. A well lubricated Malecot or De Pezzer catheter stretched on an introducer is inserted and the cannula and introducer removed. The catheter is anchored to the skin margin with a stitch. Some 10 cm of catheter is left below skin level so that it is not forced out when the bladder contracts. One of the proprietary suprapubic cystostomy kits (Fig. 27.5) can be used, instead of a trocar and cannula with a Malecot or De Pezzer catheter.

INJURIES OF THE BLADDER

The bladder may be damaged by blows or crushing

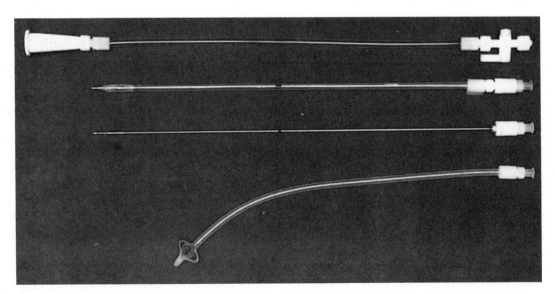

Fig. 27.5 Stamey suprapubic catheter set

injuries to the lower abdomen or pelvis, by penetrating wounds from sharp weapons or gunshot wounds (which are likely to be associated with damage to adjacent structures such as the rectum) or by fractures of the pelvis when the posterior urethra is also often injured. The bladder may be damaged during almost any major pelvic operation, especially hysterectomy, and during endoscopic resections of bladder tumours or the prostate. If recognized at the time, such injuries can be treated by simply keeping the bladder empty for some days after operation with a urethral catheter, although, if injured at an open operation, the bladder can be repaired with absorbable sutures as well. If not recognized at the time, urine or irrigating fluids extravasate into the extraperitoneal tissues and fistulae may develop between bladder and vagina or rectum. Intraperitoneal rupture, when urine extravasates into the peritoneal cavity, is uncommon and only occurs if the bladder is distended at the moment of injury.

The diagnosis should be made from the patient's history and inability to pass urine. The bladder distends if the urethra is injured, but a palpable suprapubic swelling may not be a distended bladder but a haematoma from a ruptured bladder, which will always be empty or contain only a small quantity of bloodstained urine.

If bladder rupture is suspected, a catheter should be passed and a cystogram made. If a catheter cannot be passed, the posterior urethra is probably injured and only operation will determine if the bladder is also injured. A ruptured bladder should be explored once adequate resuscitation has been achieved. If the tear is extraperitoneal, blood stained urine wells up from the retropubic space. An anterior tear is usually located without difficulty and can be closed. A posterior tear may not be seen until the bladder has been opened and even then may be difficult to repair. If the tear cannot be repaired satisfactorily, it is essential to drain the bladder by suprapubic cystostomy. In all cases the extravesical tissues must also be drained. If there is no evidence of extraperitoneal rupture, the peritoneum is opened, the intestines packed upwards and the upper surface of the bladder examined. If a tear is found it is repaired with two layers of stitches.

Both the peritoneal cavity and the bladder are carefully dried out and each is drained. After both extra and intraperitoneal ruptures the bladder may be kept empty with a urethral catheter, but it is wise to leave a suprapubic tube as well, if bladder repair was difficult.

DIVERTICULA OF THE BLADDER

Nearly all bladder diverticula are acquired as a result of increased intravesical pressure caused by obstruction to the urinary outflow. Congenital diverticula may occur at the vault (site of the urachus) or near the ureteric orifices where the part of the bladder derived from the cloaca joins the part derived from the mesonephric duct. The walls of congenital diverticula have the same structure as the bladder, whereas the walls of acquired diverticula have little if any muscle, and therefore little if any contractility. They fill and expand when the bladder contracts and empty when it relaxes. The urine within them stagnates predisposing to infection, stones, metaplasia and tumour. Most diverticula arise from the inferolateral or posterior wall of the bladder close to a ureteric orifice. The opening of the diverticulum into the bladder (called the neck of the diverticulum) is smaller than the cavity of the diverticulum. Diverticula can be seen in the cystographic phase of an intravenous urogram, but their size, shape, position and relationship to the ureteric orifices can only be determined by cystoscopy and by cystography (Fig. 27.6), which must include micturating and postmicturition views (Fig. 27.7). Many diverticula cause little if any trouble after the associated obstruction has been dealt with, and excision is indicated only for those that are large or infected, that contain stone or tumour (Fig. 27.8), that obstruct a ureter or distort a ureteric orifice or cause vesico-ureteric reflux.

Methods of diverticulectomy
At operation, the diverticulum is completely excised leaving the bladder wall smooth. Small diverticula may be exposed through an intravesical approach. The bladder is opened by a suprapubic incision and the depth of the diverticulum is ascertained with finger or probe. The wall of the diverticulum is seized with tissue forceps (Fig. 27.9) and invaginated into the bladder (Fig. 27.10) to allow excision at its neck and closure of the defect in the bladder wall with catgut sutures. If this is considered unsafe, two or more pairs of tissue forceps are applied to the margin of the opening and a circular incision is made through the mucosa and muscular coats of the bladder wall around it. The severed neck of the diverticulum is drawn into the bladder and dissection is continued closely around the diverticulum with curved scissors until it can be removed. As the ureter lies close to the diverticulum, it is wise to insert a ureteric catheter into the ureter as soon as the bladder is opened and before any attempt is made to mobilize or remove the diverticulum. It is best to mobilize large diverticula extravesically (Figs. 27.11–27.13), preserving the ureter which is often adherent to the wall of the diverticulum. The procedure is facilitated if the bladder is opened and a finger or pack placed in the diverticulum so as to combine intra- and extravesical dissection (Fig. 27.12).

Once the diverticulum is freed it is removed flush with the bladder wall and the bladder is repaired. Both bladder and extravesical space must be drained. Some-

Fig. 27.6–27.8 *Bladder diverticulum on contrast X-rays*

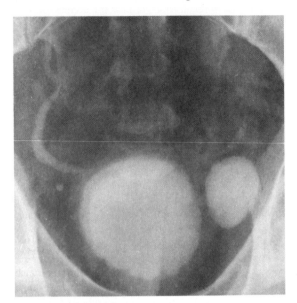

Fig. 27.6 Prevoiding phase

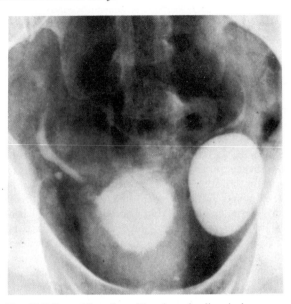

Fig. 27.7 Postvoiding phase. Note how the diverticulum expands as the bladder contracts

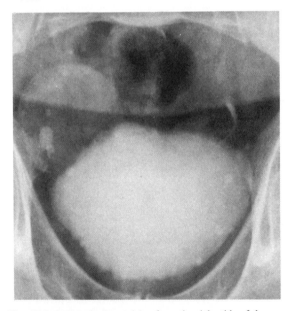

Fig. 27.8 A diverticulum arising from the right side of the bladder and filled with tumour

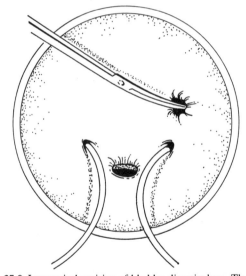

Fig. 27.9 Intravesical excision of bladder diverticulum. The ureters are 'protected' by ureteric catheters. The wall of the diverticulum is grasped with tissue forceps

times a ureter opens into the diverticulum or is so close to the diverticulum that it has to be divided and reimplanted into the bladder after the diverticulum has been excised. When the fundus of the diverticulum lies posteriorly between bladder and rectum, and is densely adherent to rectum, it is best to leave some of the diverticulum rather than risk making a rectal fistula.

STONES IN THE BLADDER (See Husain, 1984)

Operations for the removal of stones from the bladder (lithotomy) were carried out before the time of Hippocrates, but only in the early part of this century were instruments constructed for treating bladder stones endoscopically. Primary bladder stones were very

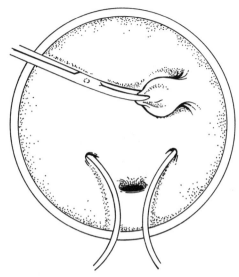

Fig. 27.10 Intravesical excision of bladder diverticulum. The diverticulum has been invaginated into the bladder

Fig. 27.11–27.13 *Extravesical excision of bladder diverticulum*

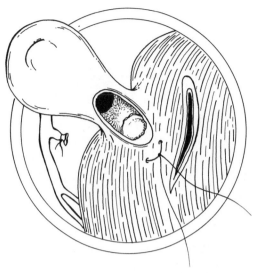

Fig. 27.12 The diverticulum is gradually and carefully mobilized and freed from colon, pelvis, ureter and bladder until only attached to the bladder by its neck. This procedure can be facilitated by inserting a finger or pack into the diverticulum through an incision in the anterior bladder wall

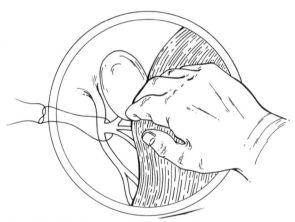

Fig. 27.11 The diverticulum is partially displayed and the superior vesical pedicle is ligated and divided

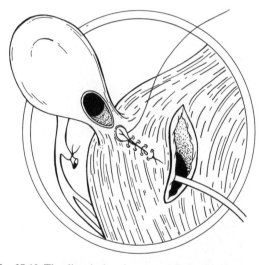

Fig. 27.13 The diverticulum is removed flush with the bladder wall, and the defect closed with absorbable sutures. Some of the fundus can be left behind to fibrose if densely adherent to rectum or colon

common in Britain until the end of the 19th century, but although still common in such developing parts of the world as Egypt, Thailand and Sudan, they are now all but unknown in Britain and other affluent parts of Western Europe and North America. Instead renal stones have become increasingly common and bladder stones (Fig. 27.14, 27.15) now only form in an infected or obstructed bladder or in one containing foreign material. The treatment of bladder stone depends as much on the primary disease as it does on the stone itself, and many stones eminently suitable for endoscopic removal are removed by open operation when the primary disease can be treated at the same time.

Stones smaller than 8 mm in diameter are usually passed spontaneously because the normal urethra measures 26F or more (i.e. 8.6 mm); if not, they can be washed out or gently removed intact with biopsy forceps through a resectoscope sheath.

Do not attempt to crush a stone, however small or soft it may appear, with biopsy forceps otherwise you can break the delicate hinge mechanism of the instrument and find the cups of the instrument fixed immobile in the open position.

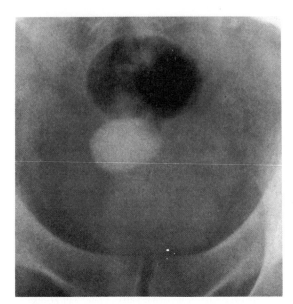

Fig. 27.14 Plain X–ray showing a large smooth bladder stone

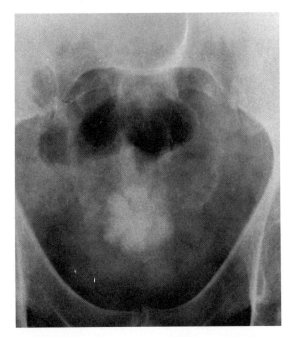

Fig. 27.15 Plain X–ray showing a bladder stone of Jackstone type

Stones larger than 8 mm can be treated by litholapaxy or open operation.

Litholapaxy (see Mitchell, 1981)

In this procedure, a 'blind' or an optical lithotrite is passed through the urethra into the bladder and used to crush the stone into fragments small enough to be washed out of the bladder through a resectoscope sheath using an Ellik or similar syringe. Lithotrites are all large instruments (26F) which can easily damage the urethra, prostate or bladder while being passed, manipulated or rotated as the stone is grasped or crushed. There are several contraindications to their use:

1. Stones larger than 2 cm cannot be grasped between the jaws of a visualizing lithotrite and although stones up to 3 cm diameter can be crushed with a blind lithotrite by experienced hands, they are usually best removed by open operation.

2. Stones inside bladder diverticula, even ones smaller than 2 cm, cannot be safely grasped and crushed with a lithotrite and should be treated by open operation when the diverticula can also be removed.

3. Attempts to crush bladder stones in patients with large prostates are often unsuccessful and frequently followed by urinary retention or septicaemia or both. It is usually best to remove both stone and prostate by open operation, although if the prostate can be resected a lithotrite can be passed and the stone crushed when the resection is completed or at a second operation some weeks later.

4. Some bladder stones, particularly those with a high content of urate, are too hard to crush and best removed by open operation.

5. Attempts to crush stones in a very infected, congested bladder are frequently followed by severe bleeding or septicaemia and should only be made if the infection can be controlled by treatment with antibiotics.

6. In young boys the urethra is always too narrow to accomodate even a small lithrotrite. In adults, a narrow, strictured urethra can be enlarged by dilatation or urethrotomy before litholapaxy but the procedure may well aggravate the stricture.

7. Stones that form around the balloon of a Foley catheter or the end of a suprapubic catheter can usually be crushed after the catheter has been removed; ones that form on fragments of catheters left behind in the bladder, or other foreign bodies inserted into the bladder by the patient, are best removed by open operation when the foreign material can also be removed.

8. Phosphatic encrustations on the surface of bladder tumours may be mistaken for stones. They can usually be easily crushed and washed out even though attached to the bladder wall but the underlying mucosa must be carefully inspected and biopsied even if it looks reasonably normal.

Stones may form on nonabsorbable suture material—'a hanging stone'. Such material is never used for suturing the bladder but may be inserted inadvertently through the bladder during operations on women for stress incontinence. Both stone and suture can usually be removed endoscopically.

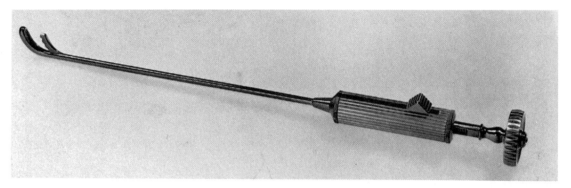

Fig. 27.16 The Miller Lithotrite (Courtesy of GU Manufacturing Co Ltd)

Technique

The patient is prepared and placed in the same position as he would be for cystoscopy or transurethral resection and the X–rays should be reviewed. The urethra, prostate and bladder are examined endoscopically and a decision madè about the appropriate procedure for removing the stones, remembering that strictures, infection and bleeding complicate litholapaxy more often than open operations.

'Blind' lithotrite

This instrument is safe if the operator knows what he is doing, unsafe otherwise (Fig. 27.16). After the preliminary endoscopic inspection, the whole cystoscope is removed leaving 100 to 150 ml of fluid in the bladder. With the jaws of the lithotrite closed and the instrument well lubricated, it is passed through the urethra into the bladder in the same way as a bougie or a cystoscope. Once its tip lies in the bladder the jaws are opened so that they face towards the centre of the bladder.

The instrument is gently moved, rotated from side to side and shaken as the jaws are gently opened and closed until the stone is felt between them. The stone is gripped but not yet crushed, by partially tightening the jaws and the instrument is advanced into the bladder and rotated through 180° to make sure that mucosa is not also gripped. The stone is crushed by screwing the jaws of the instrument together. The procedure is repeated until all the stone appears crushed; the lithotrite is removed and replaced with a 24 or 26F resectoscope sheath, through which the fragments can be evacuated with an Ellik syringe. The bladder is then examined by inserting a telescope and short bridge into the resectoscope sheath. If any fragments remain they can be lifted out with biopsy forceps if they are small, or crushed by reinserting the lithotrite (after removing the resectoscope sheath and telescope) if they are large.

The greatest care and gentleness must be exercised when passing and repassing the resectoscope sheath and lithotrite.

The visualizing lithotrite

Visualizing or optical lithotrites tend to be smaller and less strong than 'blind' ones and should only be used for stones less than 2 cm in diameter.

Some visualizing lithotrites are inserted directly into the urethra (Fig. 27.17) while others are passed through a 26 or 27F resectoscope sheath (Fig. 27.18).

With each type, a direct view or fore-oblique telescope is passed through the centre of the instrument. The author prefers those that are passed through a sheath because the same sheath can be used for washing out the fragments and inspecting the bladder and the repassing of different instruments down the urethra is avoided. With modern lithotrites it is not usually difficult to see, grasp and crush the stone. Small fragments and dust may obscure vision, but can be removed by frequent irrigation. A urethral Foley catheter is retained for 2 or 3 days after litholapaxy.

The ultrasonic lithotriptor

This instrument fragments stones by ultrasonic waves applied directly to the stone with an ultrasonic transducer which is passed through a specially designed endoscope. The instrument incorporates a powerful suction system which prevents the stone moving out of contact with the vibrating transducer when it is being used. The instrument is no larger than an ordinary visual lithotrite and the ultrasonic waves do no damage to the bladder wall, thus distinguishing it from the electronic lithotriptor which generates explosive discharges and which can damage the bladder wall. However, the ultrasonic lithotriptor is very expensive and not yet in general use.

Vesicolithotomy

This is the name given to the open operation for the removal of bladder stone. The bladder is exposed and opened as already described and the stone is removed. The bladder is drained with a urethral Foley catheter for at least 3 days.

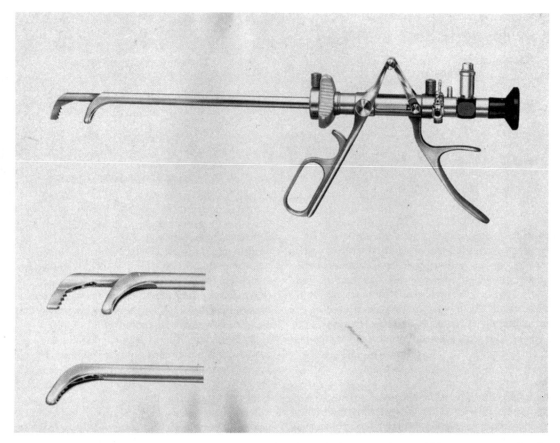

Fig. 27.17 Visualizing Lithotrite. The jaws are closed and lubricated and the instrument is passed like a cystoscope or bougie (Courtesy of Storz Ltd)

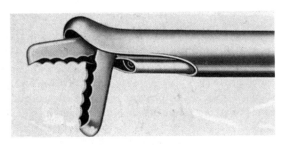

Fig. 27.18 Vizualising Lithotrite. This instrument is passed through a resectoscope sheath. Detail shows the end of the instrument with the jaws opened (Courtesy of Storz Ltd)

BLADDER TUMOURS

Most patients with a bladder tumour complain of painless haematuria; however, those with carcinoma insitu or squamous carcinoma often present with frequency, urgency and dysuria and may be thought to be suffering only from chronic cystitis and indeed they may have secondary infection. Many tumours reveal themselves as filling defects in the cystographic phase of the intravenous urogram (Fig. 27.19) and all can be seen at cysto-urethroscopy.

Only when the *stage of the tumour* has been assessed and been put into its correct TNMG category, can the appropriate treatment be decided. The *T category* represents the local state of the tumour and is assessed by clinical examination, urography, cystoscopy, bimanual examination under anaesthesia and by biopsy or transurethral resection of the tumour. The *N category* represents the state of the regional and juxtaregional lymph glands and is assessed by clinical examination and radiography including lymphography and urography. The *M category* represents the presence or absence of metastases and is assessed by clinical examination, radiography and isotope studies. *The G category* represents histological grading (UICC, 1978).

The T categories (Fig. 27.20)

Tis   A preinvasive carcinoma, carcinoma in situ or flat tumour

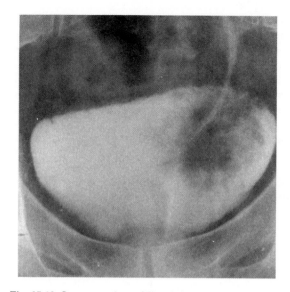

Fig. 27.19 Cystogram shows filling defect caused by a tumour in left side of the bladder

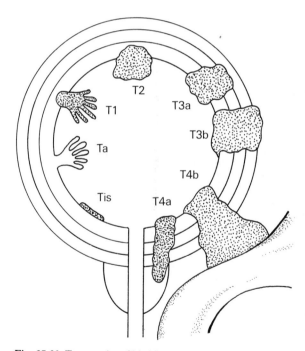

Fig. 27.20 T categories of bladder tumour

Ta   A papillary noninvasive carcinoma (confined to mucosa)

T1   A T1 tumour is often impalpable on bimanual examination but if it is palpable it is a freely mobile mass that can no longer be felt after complete transurethral resection. Microscopically the tumour does not invade beyond the lamina propria.

T2   On bimanual examination there is induration of the bladder wall which is mobile. There is no residual induration after complete transurethral resection of the lesion and/or there is microscopic invasion of superficial muscle.

T3   On bimanual examination a nodular mobile mass is palpable in the bladder wall and persists after transurethral resection of the exophytic portion of the lesion and/or there is microscopic invasion of deep muscle (T3a) or of extension through the bladder wall (T3b).

As attempts to resect too much of a T3 tumour can cause serious complications it is mainly on the results of bimanual examination that the decision is made whether the lesion is T3a or T3b.

T4   A T4 tumour is fixed or extends to neighbouring structures.

T4a   The tumour infiltrates the prostate, uterus or vagina.

T4b   The tumour is fixed to the pelvic wall or abdominal wall or both.

The suffix (m) may be added to the appropriate T category to indicate multiple tumours, e.g. T2(m)

N category
N0 No evidence of regional lymph node involvement
N1 Evidence of involvement of a single homolateral regional lymph node
N2 Evidence of involvement of contralateral or bilateral or multiple regional lymph nodes
N3 Evidence of involvement of fixed regional lymph nodes or there is a fixed mass on the pelvic wall with a free space between this and the tumour.
N4 Evidence of involvement of juxtaregional nodes
NX The minimum requirements to assess the regional and/or juxtaregional lymph nodes cannot be met.

As pedal lymphangiography does not show the internal iliac nodes which are the regional glands of the bladder the N category is usually expressed as NX, meaning that the condition of the lymph nodes is unknown.

M category
M0 No evidence of distant metastases
M1 Evidence of distant metastases

G—histopathological grading
G0 Papilloma i.e. no evidence of anaplasia
G1 High degree of differentiation
G2 Medium degree of differentiation
G3 Low degree of differentiation or undifferentiated
GX Grade cannot be assessed.

Endoscopy
A careful endoscopy is carried out and must include

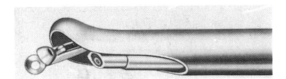

Fig. 27.21 Pinch biopsy forceps (Courtesy of Storz Ltd)

urethroscopy because secondary tumours are frequently present in the urethra, particularly in the prostatic part. Assessment of the tumour includes its size, site appearance and number; the bladder is emptied, noting its capacity, the cystoscope is withdrawn and a bimanual examination carried out to determine the T category (which may be changed following the histologist's report).

After the bimanual examination, the endoscope is reintroduced and biopsies obtained using a resectoscope for proliferative tumours and pinch biopsy forceps (Fig. 27.21) for flat tumours. Three or four random mucosal pinch biopsies must be taken from other parts of the bladder because dysplastic mucosa or areas of carcinoma in situ may look normal when viewed through a cystoscope. Tumours of the bladder can be much more extensive than at first appears. Transurethral resection of the tumour provides a good biopsy which helps to assess the T category of the tumour and is a means of treating Ta, T1 and some T2 tumours, which can often be completely resected. (The specimen obtained should be submitted to pathology in two containers; the bulk of the tumour in one, the base in the other, so that the depth of the tumour invasion can be determined).

Tis (carcinoma in situ)

The description suggests a very early stage of malignant disease and indeed, the changes are initially confined to mucosa and do not even extend into the lamina propria. However, in situ tumours of the bladder are frequently anaplastic (G3), much more widespread in the bladder than first appears, and often also involve the transitional epithelium of the urethra, ureters and pelvicaliceal systems. The bladder capacity is often reduced. In situ areas are flat and red, sometimes messy and often look infective rather than neoplastic. Furthermore, biopsies taken from mucosa that looks normal often reveal in situ or dysplastic changes and pinch biopsies must be taken from not only the suspicious areas, but also from selected normal areas in the bladder and prostatic urethra. To confuse in situ tumours with infection is particularly easy, because patients often complain, not of haematuria, but of frequency and dysuria, and it is, perhaps, not surprising that many are treated with antibiotics.

It is tempting to treat this stage of disease by resection or by electrocoagulation using an electrode through a cystoscope or a ball or roller loop through a resectoscope.

But the change from dysplasia to in situ carcinoma and then to infiltrative carcinoma can be rapid, and patients treated in these ways must be carefully followed up by cytology, endoscopy and biopsy and treated more radically if the disease progresses or fails to respond. If the prostatic urethra or ducts are not involved, intravesical instillations of Epodyl (p. 585), Thio-tepa or Methotrexate can be tried; radiotherapy has little to offer, and many patients with in situ carcinoma of the bladder require cystectomy. When cystectomy is carried out, the cut ends of the ureters should be examined for in situ change by frozen section before the diversion procedure starts. If in situ changes are so extensive that healthy ureter is not available for the diversion, parenteral chemotherapy with Cyclophosphamide or Methotrexate may be considered postoperatively.

Ta tumours

These tumours are usually 3 cm or less in diameter, pedunculated and papillary. They can be resected easily and completely with one or two sweeps of the cutting loop of a resectoscope (Fig. 27.22) and the base can be coagulated with the cutting or ball loop. Larger ones can be excised by resecting the proliferative part of the tumour first and then the base which should be kept separate from the proliferative part of the tumour when the specimen is sent to the pathologist.

T1 tumours

These tumours can also be completely resected and are

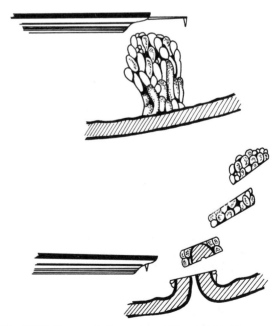

Fig. 27.22 Transurethral resection of Ta or T1 bladder tumour

often only recognized to be T1 rather than Ta ones when the pathologist reports that they involve the lamina propria.

Multiple tumours (Tam, T1m)
Ta or T1 tumours can be resected if they are solitary or few in number. If there are too many to resect and they do not involve the urethra, they can be treated by bladder instillations. Of the various substances available for this purpose, Ethoglucid (Triethyleneglycol Diglycidyl, Epodyl) is as useful as any. 100 ml of a 1% solution is instilled into the bladder through a catheter which is then removed; the patient empties the bladder 1 hour later. This process is repeated weekly for 12 weeks then monthly for an indefinite period (Soloway, 1982). More radical treatment by X–ray therapy or cystectomy needs to be considered if multiple tumours do not respond, if the tumours are large or the prostatic urethra is involved.

Large T0 or T1 tumours
To resect large T0 or T1 tumours is possible but requires much time and patience and is often accompanied by severe haemorrhage which can be difficult to control. Bleeding vessels are best coagulated before more cuts are made into the tumour and resecting part of the prostate or the bladder neck often facilitates the procedure, by rendering the base more accessible. The size of the tumour can often be reduced before resection by suction using a Wardill syringe through a resectoscope sheath or by the Helmstein distention method. Open diathermy is a poor alternative to resection as it seems to spread the tumour throughout the bladder or worse, into the suprapubic wound. Many large tumours considered to be T0 or T1 before resection prove to be T2 or worse when examined by the pathologist.

T2 tumours
T2 tumours involve the superficial muscle and are usually palpable on bimanual examination although some are considered T1 until the resected base of the tumour is examined under a microscope. They can be resected if the tumour is well or moderately differentiated (G1 or G2) (Fig. 27.23), but if the tumour is anaplastic (G3) it is wise to treat them like T3 tumours.

T3 tumours
T3 tumours have infiltrated the deep muscle of the bladder (T3a) or right through the bladder wall into the perivesical tissues (T3b), but remain mobile and are easily palpable. All of the tumour cannot be resected and attempts to do so will only perforate the bladder (Fig. 27.24). Although such perforations are usually extraperitoneal and heal if the bladder is kept empty for some time, they delay the radical treatment necessary to

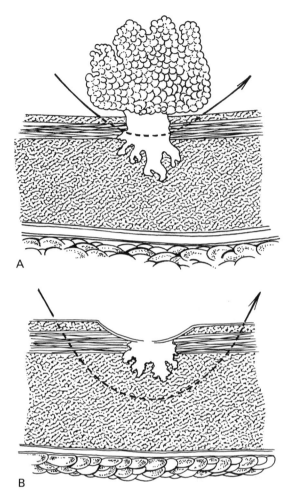

Fig. 27.23 Resection of T2 tumour

cure the tumour and it is necessary to resect only sufficient of the tumour for biopsy purposes. The treatment of T3 tumours, which causes much discussion and controversy, can be by X–ray therapy or by cystectomy or by cystectomy and X–ray therapy. Which treatment is offered depends upon the facilities available and the views of the surgeon and radiotherapist; although many believe that cystectomy preceded by a modified course of X–ray therapy gives better results than X–ray therapy or cystectomy alone, especially in patients under 65 years. The author treats patients with T3 tumours by a full course of X–ray therapy and carries out cystectomy later, if the tumour fails to respond. This decision is made only after some 3 to 6 months have elapsed since X–ray treatment has been completed.

T4 tumours
T4a tumours involve the prostate but are amenable to the same sort of treatment given to patients with T3 tumours because the prostate gland can be included in the X–ray

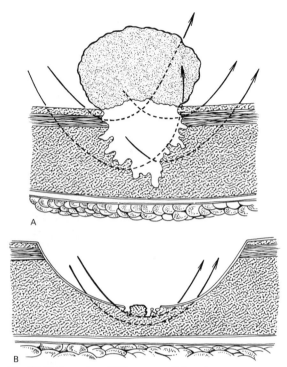

Fig. 27.24 Resection of T3 tumour. Although complete resection of T3a tumours is theoretically possible it is very unwise to attempt it

field and is invariably removed at cystectomy. In women T4b tumours involving the vagina or uterus (which can be removed along with the bladder) can be radically treated by surgery, but most T4b tumours are incurable because they are too large or too fixed and suitable only for palliative treatment.

Tumours in bladder diverticula

Tumours in bladder diverticula present special problems. Firstly, the extent or even the presence of the tumour may not be appreciated by endoscopy or on the pre- and postmicturition cystograms. These must be interpreted carefully because blood clot can produce filling defects indistinguishable from those of tumour. Secondly, since acquired diverticula have little, if any, muscle in their walls, a tumour becomes T3b as soon as it spreads through the lamina propria.

In diverticula, Ta, T1 or T3b tumours cannot be resected endoscopically and are best treated by excising the diverticulum together with a margin of bladder at its neck (p. 577); more serious tumours are treated by X–ray therapy or cystectomy.

PARTIAL CYSTECTOMY

This was once a popular operation for the treatment of

bladder tumours that could be excised together with a 2.5 cm margin of healthy bladder, even if this included one ureteric orifice or part of the bladder neck. It is now only used to treat some tumours in the vault of the bladder which may be primary or secondary to rectal or colonic tumours, when the partial cystectomy is part (often a small part) of an operation which includes resection of rectum or colon.

Technique

For primary vault tumours, a transverse suprapubic incision is made and the peritoneum opened. The peritoneum is incised transversely over the back of the bladder so that the peritoneum on the vault will be excised with the tumour. The bladder is mobilized from peritoneum posteriorly by blunt dissection, except in the midline where it has to be cut away from peritoneum. Next the bladder is mobilized on each side by dividing the superior vesical pedicles and the bladder is opened anteriorly well away from the tumour. The tumour, with a 2.5 cm margin of healthy bladder, is excised together with the overlying peritoneum (Fig. 27.25). The bladder is closed in two layers with plain catgut and the wound closed in layers with drainage. The bladder should be kept empty for at least 7 or 8 days with a Foley catheter.

For the resection of bladder adherent to or infiltrated by rectal or colonic tumours, the technique varies with each case. In all it is important to find and secure both ureters at an early stage in the dissection; one or even both, may have to be reimplanted into the bladder once the procedure is completed. The bladder is sutured in two layers and kept empty with a Foley catheter.

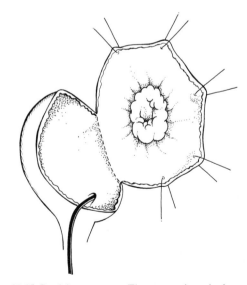

Fig. 27.25 Partial cystectomy. The tumour is excised together with a wide margin all round it of healthy bladder, without disturbing ureters or bladder neck

TOTAL CYSTECTOMY (see Paulson, 1983)

The major indication for total cystectomy is malignant disease of the bladder which has not responded to or is unsuitable for less radical treatment. Thus the operation for malignant disease will be described although cystectomy may also be required for patients (fortunately now few) with severe haemorrhage from radiation cystitis or for patients with a neurogenic bladder who have previously had a urinary diversion and develop a *pyocystis* (a bladder filled with pus).

Preparation

The type of urinary diversion to be done will have been decided when the operation was discussed with the patient and this determines the preoperative preparation. Despite the disadvantages of an external fistula the author prefers an ileal loop diversion and will only do a ureterosigmoidostomy if the patient refuses to have an external opening.

Operation

A long lower left paramedian incision rather than a transverse one is recommended because it provides adequate exposure and does not interfere with the siting of the ileostomy opening in the right iliac fossa, nor with the wearing of the appliance. On opening the peritoneum, the bladder is examined to ensure that it can be removed, and the iliac, obturator and abdominal lymph glands and the liver are assessed for metastatic spread. In men an elliptical incision is made in the peritoneum behind the bladder so that the peritoneum on its vault can be removed with the bladder and the posterior aspect of the bladder is freed from peritoneum by a combination of blunt and sharp dissection. In women the uterus, cervix uteri and upper part of the vagina are removed together with the bladder and, in them, the posterior layer of the broad ligament is incised behind the uterus. Next the lateral aspects of the bladder are mobilized close to the side walls of the pelvis, dividing first the superior vesical pedicles and next the inferior vesical pedicles. In women, the round and the falciform ligaments are also divided. It should now be possible to demonstrate and secure the ureters with slings of tape or tube. These are divided about 2.5 cm above the bladder and the distal ends ligated. To prevent contamination of the wound with urine some surgeons temporarily put the proximal ends of the ureters into plastic bags. A long 6 or 8F polythene or silastic tube (a wider one if the ureter is very dilated) may be inserted some 10 cm into each ureter and secured to the cut end of the ureter with a suture, inserted in such a way that it does not interfere later with the ileo-ureteric anastomosis (p. 569). These tubes will eventually be brought through the ileal loop and out of the stoma (or put into the bowel if a ureterocolic anastomosis is done) and left some days, but meantime they are drained into a plastic bag.

The steps of the operation can be modified by exposing and ligating the internal iliac arteries at an early stage of the operation as follows: once the peritoneum has been incised transversely behind the bladder in men (behind the uterus in women) the peritoneum (that is to remain) is incised upwards on each side along the line of the ureter as far as the brim of the pelvis and the ureters are secured with slings at or below the brim of the pelvis. Then the internal iliac arteries are mobilized and their anterior divisions are ligated and divided. Mobilization is continued down the lateral walls of the pelvis removing as much fascia and as many lymph glands as possible, dividing and ligating the deep vesical vessels and finally dividing the ureters. If doing the operation for carcinoma in situ, sections from the proximal cut ends of the ureters are sent for frozen biopsy examination. If these sections show carcinoma in situ or severe dysplasia, the ureter is sectioned at a higher level and further sections are sent, continuing until normal ureter is obtained. Of course it may not be possible to do this, yet leave enough ureter for the diversion procedure. In men once the lateral aspects of the bladder are fully mobilized and the posterior aspect partly mobilized, the anterior prostatic capsule is cleared of fat and veins and the puboprostatic ligaments are divided between right angled forceps, thus mobilizing the prostate gland which can now be pulled upwards to expose the membranous urethra. If the whole urethra is not being removed the membranous urethra is divided below the prostate. By dissecting from above and below the prostate and seminal vesicles can be peeled safely off the anterior wall of the rectum and the specimen removed. If this is difficult, it is prudent to leave some of the seminal vesicles rather than remove some of the anterior rectal wall and produce a rectal fistula. In women the posterior part of the dissection is completed by incising the lateral and posterior vaginal fornices around the cervix. The specimen is now held only by the urethra, the anterior vaginal wall and the connective tissue and veins around the bladder neck. Once these are divided the specimen can be removed and one or two large packs are put into the pelvic cavity and left there while the diversion procedure (p. 568) is carried out. The packs are then removed, haemostasis secured and the wound closed in layers with drainage.

Urethrectomy

Some surgeons routinely excise the whole length of the urethra when removing the bladder for malignant disease. Others think it preferable only to do so if there is evidence of tumour within the urethra at the time of cystectomy. If tumour develops in the urethra later, a urethrectomy can be done then.

Operation

In women the entire urethra with a strip of vagina can be removed through two parallel vertical incisions 1 cm apart in the anterior wall of the vagina. In men the whole of the spongy part of the urethra can be mobilized through a transverse perineal incision. The bulbous part is mobilized and secured with a tape or tube. Applying traction to the tape or tube, the entire penile urethra can be mobilized by sharp dissection as the penis invaginates, without separately incising the penile skin. Once the urethra is freed it can be pushed upwards into the pelvis and removed with the specimen if urethrectomy is being done at the same time as cystectomy, otherwise it is just removed.

OPERATIONS TO EXPAND OR REDUCE THE CAPACITY OF THE BLADDER

Expansion operations

The problem of the contracted bladder is encountered much less frequently now than it was some years ago, but there are still patients whose bladder has been contracted by Hunner's ulcer (interstitial cystitis), radiotherapy, tuberculosis or bilharziasis and whose bladder capacity is so reduced that their lives are miserable. If their symptoms cannot be relieved by medical treatment, bladder instillation or hydrodistension, urinary diversion or some operation to increase bladder capacity has to be considered. The capacity of the bladder can be increased using an isolated ileal loop (made in the same way as for urinary diversion). The loop is opened along its antimesenteric border and sutured to the margin of the bladder after the vault of the bladder has been excised. In tuberculosis and bilharziasis the ureteric orifices and lower ureters are often stenosed and are best reimplanted into the isolated ileal loop before it is sutured to the cut margins of the bladder.

The expansion operation should not be considered until the patient has been given an extensive trial with conservative measures and the advantages of a diversion operation have been discussed, since the operations used to expand the bladder are by no means always successful.

Reduction procedures (see Gow, 1980)

Patients with an atonic bladder must be assessed very carefully to decide if the cause is obstructive or neurological. With prolonged obstruction to the outflow of urine from the bladder, chronic retention occurs and the bladder loses contractility because its muscle fibres are overstretched. Its contractility recovers if it is kept empty for some time after the cause of the obstruction is treated. Parasympathomimetic drugs like Dystigmine bromide or myotonine chloride may accelerate this recovery.

With neurological causes of bladder atony, attempts

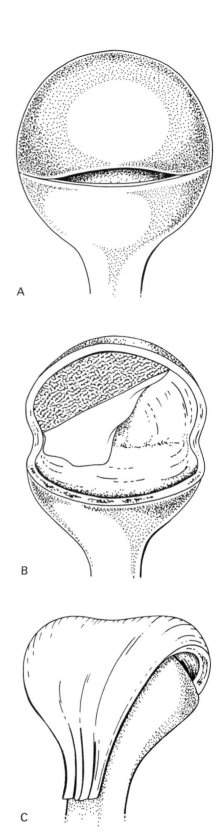

Fig. 27.26 Vanwelkenhuyzen's operation

to restore contractility by prolonged bladder drainage or drugs are often unsuccessful and permanent, intermittent or continuous drainage of the bladder by a urethral or suprapubic catheter is necessary; alternatively diversion or a bladder reduction operation is considered. Bladder reduction operations not only reduce bladder capacity but also improve contractility and the best of them is the one described by Vanwelkenhuyzen in which the bladder is double breasted (Fig. 27.26). The bladder is exposed through a generous transverse incision and mobilised extraperitoneally as far down as the bladder neck anteriorly and laterally and the interureteric bar posteriorly. A transverse incision is made through the front half of the bladder (a hemitransection) about 6 cm above the bladder neck. The upper part of the bladder is stripped of its mucosa by sharp dissection. The lower cut surface of the bladder is sutured to the posterior wall of the bladder some 5 cm above the interureteric bar and some 5 cm below the upper cut margin in two layers, mucosa to mucosa, muscle to muscle. The posterior wall of the bladder already deprived of mucosa is now folded over the lower anterior wall and sutured to the bladder neck. The bladder is drained with a urethral catheter and the wound drained.

VESICAL FISTULAE

Colovesical fistula

This may occur in advanced diverticulitis of the pelvic colon—less frequently in carcinoma. A classical sign of the condition is the passage of faecal-smelling urine, accompanied by pneumaturia. The fistulous opening may show on cystoscopy, with gas or intestinal material occasionally visible.

Depending upon the extent of the diverticulitis, and the amount of healthy bowel below the lesion, it may be possible to resect the affected segment of colon and to repair the bladder. In poor risk patients, with gross infection, it is better to perform a defunctioning transverse colostomy in the first instance, in order to divert the faecal contents proximal to the fistula, and in the hope that reparative surgery can be undertaken later. If the primary condition is a carcinoma, it is likely to be irremovable, and in such cases the only available treatment may be a palliative colostomy.

Vesico-vaginal fistula

This may result from pressure necrosis affecting the contiguous walls of the bladder and vagina during prolonged labour, from injury to the bladder during a difficult hysterectomy, from advancing carcinoma of the cervix or from post-irradiation necrosis.

Sometimes a recent fistula of small size will heal if the bladder is kept empty by an indwelling urethral catheter.

As a rule operative treatment is necessary, but this should be delayed until infection has been overcome by vaginal lavage and by antibiotics.

The operation consists in excision of the fistulous opening with surrounding scar tissue, and in separation of the vagina and bladder sufficiently to permit separate closure of each without tension.

Smaller fistulae are approached usually through the vagina, but when there is much scarring in the vagina or when the cervix has been removed a transvesical approach is more satisfactory. Often a combination of the two methods is employed. After operation the bladder should be drained by an indwelling urethral catheter, in order to ensure that it does not become distended.

In cases where a fistula has recurred after local methods of repair, a more determined attempt at cure may be made through an abdominal approach. After the viscera have been separated from above, a pedicled flap of omentum may be packed into the space between them (Turner-Warwick, 1973).

Irreparable fistulae

In a proportion of cases vesicovaginal fistula results from radiation necrosis sustained during treatment of carcinoma of the cervix. This type of fistula is not amenable to any form of local repair. Such cases together with those in which operative repair has proved unsuccessful, should be treated by transplantation of the ureters to an ileal loop.

OPERATIONS ON THE PROSTATE GLAND

Anatomy

The prostate consists of glandular tissue in a fibromuscular stroma and surrounds the beginning of the male urethra (Fig. 27.48). It lies below the bladder, behind the pubis and in front of the rectum, through which some parts of it can be readily palpated. Its *base*, directed upwards, embraces the bladder neck; its *apex*, directed downwards, rests on the deep aspect of the external sphincter; its *posterior surface* is separated from the rectum by the two layers of the rectovesical fascia (Denonvillier) and divided by the ejaculatory ducts into an upper *middle lobe* and a lower *posterior lobe* which lies in the shallow median furrow separating the posterior aspects of the right and left lateral lobes (Fig. 27.27). The lateral lobes comprise most of the 6 or 7 g of the normal prostate and in front they are joined together by the anterior lobe which contains few, if any, glands. Only the posterior parts of the lateral lobes and the posterior lobe, in the median furrow between them, can be palpated through the rectum. The prostate contains two kinds of glands, an inner zone which surrounds the urethra and an outer zone which surrounds the inner

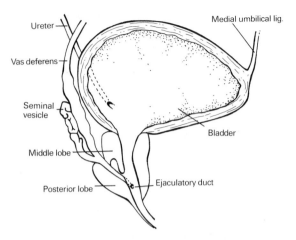

Fig. 27.27 A sagittal section of the bladder, urethra and prostate. It shows the relationships of the middle and posterior prostatic lobes to the ejaculatory duct and to each other

available for those patients who require treatment, and not all patients with the disease do require treatment. Benign hypertrophy begins in inner zone glands and consists of an increase in the number of glands (*adenosis*) some of which form small cysts because their ducts are blocked and their secretions retained, an increase in the number of cells forming the glands (*epitheliosis*) and an increase in the amount of fibrous tissue. If adenosis is the predominant change, the lobe or lobes affected enlarge and acquire the elastic consistence associated with benign hypertrophy. If *fibrosis* predominates, the prostate may be no bigger than normal, yet can obstruct the outflow of urine from the bladder as much as the largest gland. The changes of benign hypertrophy may involve one or more lobes of the prostate (Fig. 27.29). Involvement of the lateral lobes can be appreciated by rectal examination (unless fibrosis predominates) whereas involvement of the middle lobe cannot, no matter how extensive the change becomes. When the middle lobe enlarges it

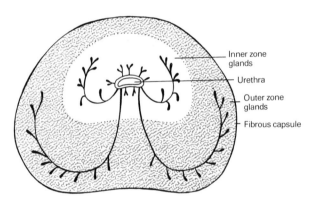

Fig. 27.28 Transverse section of the prostate

zone, and which is separated from the loose pelvic fascia, containing the prostatic plexus of veins, by the thick fibrous capsule (Fig. 27.28). *Blood supply* to the prostate is from the internal iliac artery and *venous drainage* into the plexus around the front of the gland and thence into the internal iliac veins. *Lymph drains* first to nodes alongside the internal iliac or obturator vessels.

Benign simple prostatic hypertrophy
This disease is most frequently seen in men in the 7th, 8th or 9th decades of life, but also occurs in the 6th and even 5th decades. It is obviously related to, and probably caused by, changes that occur in hormone activity with increasing age, but the precise cause has not yet been identified. Although medical treatment may alleviate symptoms by curing superadded infection, oedema or congestion, it does not prevent the disease nor alter the basic pathological changes; however, many safe and effective surgical methods of dealing with the disease are

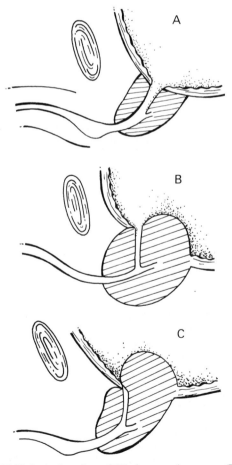

Fig. 27.29 Sagittal sections of (A) the normal prostate; (B) the hypertrophied prostate in which both lateral and middle lobes are involved; and (C) the hypertrophied prostate in which only the middle lobe is involved

Figs. 27.30–27.33 *Effects of obstruction upon the bladder (diagram of cystoscopic appearance and cross section)*

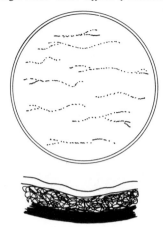

Fig. 27.30 Normal bladder

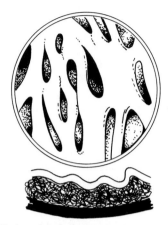

Fig. 27.31 Early trabeculation

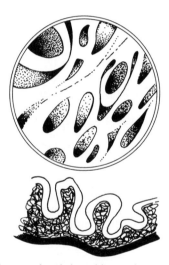

Fig. 27.32 Severe trabeculation with saccules

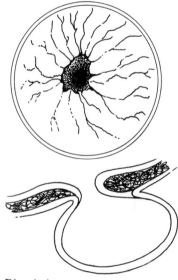

Fig. 27.33 Diverticulum

bulges forwards into the bladder, not backwards into the rectum, yet can severely obstruct the outflow of urine by impacting in the bladder neck like a ball valve when the bladder contracts. Benign prostatic hypertrophy obstructs the outflow of urine from the bladder by narrowing, distorting and elongating the urethra or narrowing the bladder neck. The bladder responds to obstruction (Figs. 27.30–27.33) by hypertrophy called *trabeculation*, and saccules and sometimes *diverticula* develop between the bundles of hypertrophied muscle fibres (Fig. 27.32). In the early stages the increased contractility of the hypertrophied bladder compensates for the increased resistance in the urethra and the bladder is still able to empty. Later, however, the bladder fails to empty completely so that residual urine remains in it after micturition and gradually and progressively increases in

quantity. Later still the flow of urine from the kidney to the bladder through the ureters is hindered by a combination of factors, which include obstruction and vesico-ureteric reflux, and hydroureter, hydronephrosis and chronic renal failure ensue.

Treatment

Treatment is not required because the gland is large or fibrous, but because it is obstructing the outflow of urine from the bladder. In the early stages of obstruction the patient may have no complaints, but later he finds that micturition is slow to start, and difficult to stop so that terminal dribbling occurs; that the urinary stream is poor in force and calibre and the need to micturate is frequent, especially at night and often urgent. The symptoms usually become gradually worse and in time the patient develops chronic or acute retention. In *chronic retention* the residual urine has slowly, progressively and insidiously increased over some time; the patient presents with increased frequency, overflow incontinence and sometimes enuresis, and is often quite unaware that his bladder is very distended and still contains a litre or more of urine after micturition. Most patients with chronic urinary retention have dilated upper urinary tracts and some degree of chronic renal failure. *Acute retention* may be the culmination of increasing difficulties with micturition or superimposed on chronic retention, but often occurs in patients who have had little, if any, previous trouble. The sudden increase in prostatic size that causes acute retention in such patients may be due to infection or to oedema and congestion such as occurs in cardiac failure and in some patients who suppress the need to micturate rather than interrupt a meal or journey. As obstruction interferes with the free flow of urine, it inhibits the ability of the urinary tract to decontaminate itself of organisms and thus some patients have, and may indeed present with, recurrent or chronic bladder infections or stones.

In some patients the history and physical examination provide overwhelming evidence of obstruction, and it is apparent without any further investigations that treatment is needed; in others, it is less obvious and obstruction must be confirmed before proceeding with treatment. The author is not convinced that prostatectomy is a good prophylactic operation, even though many patients say 'surely it is better to have the operation now while I'm fairly young and fit, rather than in 10 years time, when I'll not be so young and may not be so fit'. What objective evidence of obstruction should be sought?

Rectal examination

The normal prostate is felt as a low lying elevation in the anterior wall of the rectum just within the anal orifice. It is smooth in outline, elastic in consistence and its lateral edges and upper limit are clearly defined. The shallow furrow, easily felt in the midline between the two lateral lobes, is the posterior lobe. Neither anterior nor middle lobes can be felt, even if they are abnormal. The rectal mucosa over the gland is mobile. In benign enlargement the prostate is enlarged, smooth and bulges backwards into the rectum on either side of the median furrow if the lateral lobes are involved, but feels normal if the middle lobe alone is involved. A fibrous prostate is not normally enlarged and, though it may be firmer than the healthy gland, often feels surprisingly normal in consistence and morphology. A malignant prostate becomes hard, nodular, irregular, fixed and infiltrates the surrounding structures, obliterating the median furrow, but in its early stages may feel normal (p. 604). In benign enlargement there is no correlation between the

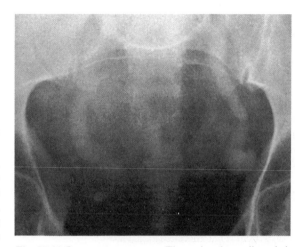

Fig. 27.34 Intravenous urogram. The patient has a distended bladder but it is not clearly seen because the dye entering it has been diluted by the large amount of urine within. Both ureters are dilated and their lower ends show the characteristic 'hooking' associated with a large prostate and distended bladder

size of the gland assessed rectally, and the degree of obstruction, since a small prostate may cause severe obstruction, and a large one little, if any.

Intravenous urography (Fig. 27.34)

This provides a good assessment of renal function, and will reveal dilatation of the ureters and pelvicaliceal system (if such exist), trabeculation, sacculation, diverticula of the bladder and the amount of residual urine. It may also reveal problems unrelated to the prostate such as a space occupying lesion in the kidney, and thus suggest the need for further investigations.

Residual urine

Inability to empty the bladder completely is an important sign of bladder outflow obstruction, and the measurement of residual urine (i.e. the volume of urine that remains in the bladder after micturition) can be useful if carried out after the patient has passed urine because he needed to; it is useless if done when the patient tries to pass urine, because he is told to do so. The intravenous post micturition cystogram is not a reliable means of assessing residual urine because the patient is dehydrated, has usually emptied the bladder before the examination, and has difficulty attempting to pass completely the small volume of urine the bladder usually contains when a cystogram is being done.

Cystourethroscopy

This may reveal evidence of obstruction, trabeculation, sacculation, diverticula or stones, and provides a satisfactory way of determining the size of the prostate including the middle lobe, and its effect upon the urethra. However, the procedure may make the prostate oedematous and aggravate urinary symptoms, or even cause acute urinary retention in patients with a large prostate.

Urodynamics

The measurement of flow by uroflowmeter is a useful test provided the rate is measured when the patient's bladder is filled to the extent that he wants to pass urine. In outflow obstruction the flow rate is reduced. Diseases other than obstruction may cause a low flow rate, but only in obstruction is it associated with a high detrusor pressure.

In summary, then, patients with prostatic hypertrophy only require treatment if they have bladder outflow obstruction. That there exists such obstruction may be obvious from the patient's history and the findings on physical examination; if not, further evidence of obstruction should be sought in the intravenous urogram or by measuring residual urine, flow rates or bladder pressures or by cysto-urethroscopy. If there is no evidence of obstruction, or the evidence is slight, some other cause of the patient's symptoms should be suspected.

Choice of operation

It is not easy to describe operations on the prostate gland in a manner which will find general acceptance, because widely divergent views are held on the choice of operation and on pre and post operative treatment.

Three methods of prostatectomy—suprapubic, retropubic, and transurethral will be considered, and the detailed technique of each described. With all three methods of prostatectomy the same end result is produced, but the approach is different. In all operations the hypertrophied part of the prostate together with the prostatic urethra is removed leaving a cavity which is lined by the compressed outer group glands and the fibrous capsule (Fig. 27.35). The cavity contracts and its raw surface is gradually covered by epithelium growing downwards from the bladder and upwards from the urethra. In open prostatectomy, the plane between the hypertrophied part of the gland and the compressed

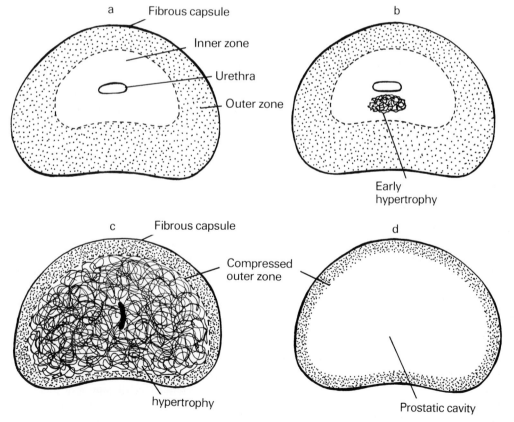

Fig. 27.35 Transverse sections of the prostate. (a) The normal prostate. (b) Early benign prostatic hypertrophy, the change beginning in the inner zone glands. (c) Marked benign prostatic hypertrophy. The prostatic urethra is squashed and displaced. The hypertrophied gland has compressed the outer zone glands into a false capsule. (d) After prostatectomy the cavity is lined by the compressed outer zone glands and the true fibrous capsule of the prostate

outer glands is easily felt and can be extended with a finger (like separating an orange from its skin) until the hypertrophied part is all freed or enucleated and can be removed. In transurethral prostatectomy the plane between the hypertrophied part of the gland, which is being removed, and the capsule, which must be left, can be clearly seen. In the suprapubic prostatectomy, popularized by Freyer in 1901, the prostate is approached through the bladder and it is the simplest and safest method. In the retropubic prostatectomy which attained considerable popularity with the work of Millin, a suprapubic incision is made, but the bladder is not opened. Instead the prostate is approached behind the pubis and removed through the anterior aspect of the prostatic capsule. In the transurethral operation a resectoscope (or less often a cold punch) is used to remove the prostate in a series of small pieces or chips through the urethra, thus avoiding some of the hazards of an open operation, though bleeding, infection and strictures can still occur.

Ligation or division of the vas deferens

Epididymitis caused by the direct spread of infection from the prostatic bed down the vas used to be a common postoperative complication of any form of prostatectomy. Many urologists considered bilateral vasectomy a part of the operation of prostatectomy. It inflicts no additional disability, since after prostatectomy the ejaculate, if any, refluxes into the bladder. This operation is described on page 633 but is now rarely, if ever, done as part of prostatectomy.

TREATMENT OF PROSTATIC RETENTION OF URINE

About 20% of patients needing prostatectomy have acute or chronic retention of urine. The need to carry out a preliminary suprapubic cystostomy has long since been abandoned. The treatment of choice now, for patients in good general health without serious infection or renal insufficiency, is urethral catheterization followed a day or two later by prostatectomy if they have acute retention. If they have chronic retention they are catheterized before operation only if they have a serious degree of chronic renal failure.

TRANSVESICAL PROSTATECTOMY

The patient is placed in the supine position on the operating table with a slight Trendelenburg tilt. Suitable illumination is arranged and the surgeon stands at the patient's left side. The external genitals and the abdominal wall are thoroughly washed. Towels are arranged so that the penis is accessible as well as the suprapubic area. The bladder is exposed through a transverse incision as described for the operation of suprapubic cystotomy (p. 575) and opened between stay sutures. A self retaining retractor is introduced. The bladder interior and the prostate gland are carefully inspected and the presence of calculi, diverticula or tumour determined. The self retaining retractor is then removed, and the margins of the bladder wall are held up by the sutures.

Technique of enucleation

The simplest method of finding the correct plane of cleavage between the hypertrophied part of the gland and false capsule is to introduce the index finger into the bladder neck and prostatic urethra and then to split the anterior commissure (the junction between the two lateral lobes) forwards until an obvious plane of cleavage is reached. The index finger is now swept round the prostate first on one side and then on the other, until the gland has been freed on both sides; enucleation continues on the anterior aspect, until the gland has been completely freed anteriorly and on each side. The urethra is now torn across from before backwards at the distal level of the plane of cleavage obtained, which is at the apex of the prostate. The tear occurs obliquely upwards and backwards above the verumontanum, so that the posterior lobe, the ejaculatory ducts, and much more importantly, the external sphincter, are undisturbed. The enucleation is completed by separating the posterior surface of the gland from the fibrous capsule which should also remain intact. Great care must be taken to keep the correct plane of cleavage within the false capsule, otherwise considerable venous bleeding may be encountered and the seminal vesicles, ejaculatory ducts or sphincter damaged. If the mucosa of the bladder neck remains adherent to the prostate and is liable to be stripped upwards from the trigone as the gland is removed, it should be divided close to the gland with scissors or a diathermy knife. It enucleation is difficult posteriorly due to fibrosis it can be completed under vision. For this purpose the self-retaining retractor is reinserted, the partially separated lobes are pulled into the bladder with tissue forceps and held apart to display the floor of the prostatic urethra, which can be divided immediately above the verumontanum with diathermy or scissors, when enucleation can usually be completed without difficulty. If access is difficult, the operation can be facilitated if an assistant introduces an index finger into the rectum to steady and push forward the gland against the enucleating finger of the surgeon. This manoeuvre however, is seldom necessary.

Although it is usually possible to assess the size and determine the pathology of the prostate gland accurately before operation and to decide that enucleation at open operation rather than transurethral resection is the best treatment, sometimes no plane of cleavage is found at operation because the prostate is smaller and more fibrous than anticipated or even malignant. It is usually better to do something than abandon the procedure in favour of a resection at a later date. For the fibrous prostate careful enucleation can be attempted but it is safer to dilate the prostatic urethra and excise a wedge from the back of the bladder neck. For some malignant prostates enucleation is possible because the malignant process is confined to the interior of a benignly hypertrophied gland; for others enucleation is impossible because the malignancy has extended through the capsule and no more than a wedge resection should be attempted.

Haemostasis

As soon as enucleation has been completed, one or more packs are packed tightly into the prostatic bed for 5 minutes. A self retaining retractor is then reinserted and the bladder cavity is dried out with suction and swabs. The pack in the prostatic bed is cautiously withdrawn, the cavity inspected and tags of mucosa or remnants of prostatic tissue are carefully removed.

Bleeding vessels are secured with long artery forceps and sealed by diathermy coagulation or underrun with sutures. With care, patience and good illumination (preferably from a lighted retractor) major blood vessels can be secured and the haemorrhage reduced to an ooze. A Foley catheter is passed through the urethra into the bladder. Its balloon is inflated in the bladder or within the prostatic cavity, where it acts like the gauze pack which used to be left in the prostatic bed for some days after operation.

Removal of a posterior wedge from the bladder neck (trigonectomy)

A wedge of mucosa and muscle can be cut from the posterior aspect of the bladder neck with a diathermy electrode or scissors if it overhangs the prostatic cavity. The apex of the wedge extends up between the ureteric orifices which must first be identified and carefully safeguarded. The wedge resection also facilitates inspection of the prostatic cavity and identification of bleeding points.

Suprapubic drainage of the bladder is now thought to be unnecessary and most urologists insert a three-way Foley catheter, close the bladder, and continuously irrigate it for a day or two after operation, but if you are doubtful about haemostasis and fearful of clot retention, even while irrigating the bladder through the three-way Foley, you can leave a suprapubic tube in the bladder for a few days. A drain is brought out from the prevesical space. Usually normal micturition is restored following

catheter removal about the sixth day and the suprapubic wound has healed within 7 to 10 days of operation.

Second stage prostatectomy

This means prostatectomy after a previous suprapubic cystostomy and nowadays is a rare procedure. As the first step in the operation the suprapubic fistula and scar tissue are excised, safeguarding if possible the peritoneum; the bladder is separated from the abdominal wall to which it is usually adherent, and opened downwards from the cystostomy opening. The prostate is enucleated as described. If, as is frequently the case, the bladder is contracted and immobile, it may be difficult to introduce a self retaining retractor, and impossible, therefore, to arrest haemorrhage by securing individual vessels but the latter can usually be controlled by inflating the balloon of the three way Foley catheter in the prostatic cavity and applying traction to it.

RETROPUBIC PROSTATECTOMY

This operation provides direct access to the prostatic cavity, facilitates haemostasis, is followed by a relatively short convalescence, restores micturition early and has a low incidence of complications, but is more difficult to do than the suprapubic operation.

Technique

Cystourethroscopy is essential at some stage before operation otherwise associated bladder conditions such as stone, neoplasm or diverticula can be missed. It can be done immediately before operation or some days previously. The bladder, which is emptied before operation, is exposed by the usual suprapubic approach (Fig. 27.36). A transverse approach is used and the lower rectus sheath flap split vertically to the pubis (Fig. 27.37). The prevesical fat and the peritoneum are

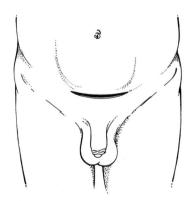

Fig. 27.36 Retropubic prostatectomy. The transverse suprapubic incision is made in a skin crease

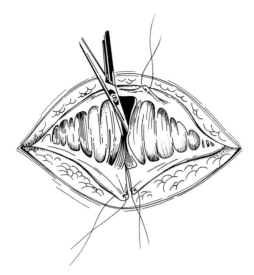

Fig. 27.37 Retropubic prostatectomy. The anterior rectus sheath has been divided in the line of the skin incision and separated from the underlying rectus and pyramidalis muscles. The lower flap has been split vertically to the pubic bone

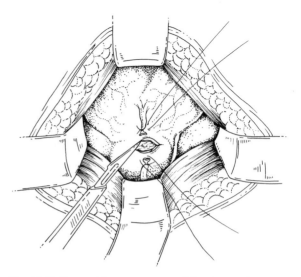

Fig. 27.38 Retropubic prostatectomy. After the anterior prostatic capsule has been completely cleared of fat and veins it is incised transversely between stay sutures

gently stripped upwards. A Millin self retaining retractor is inserted, the lateral blades spreading the recti, and the upper blade depressing the bladder neck which is protected by a folded gauze pack or two swabs. This opens up the retropubic space but the prostate is obscured by fat and veins. By gentle dissection the anterior surface of the prostatic capsule is completely cleared of fat and veins which are displaced laterally or divided, coagulated, ligated or clipped and divided. The later stages of the operation are very difficult unless the anterior prostatic capsule is properly exposed but considerable care is needed when dealing with the pre-prostatic veins which are often large and which can retract out of the field unless they are firmly secured before they are divided. Small gauze packs can be introduced into each lateral recess, but are not usually necessary. Using a long handled scalpel, a 2.5 cm incision is made through the anterior fibrous and false capsule of the prostate about 1 to 2 cm below its junction with the bladder, between two stay sutures one inserted at the lower part of the exposed prostatic capsule and the other at the bladder neck (Fig. 27.38). The incision is deepened through the capsule, which is often surprisingly thick, until the typical white colour of the 'adenoma' is seen (Fig. 27.39). The capsular flaps are undermined with curved scissors, freeing the anterior and lateral parts of the hypertrophied gland. The lower limits of the lateral lobes are defined by retracting the lower capsular flap and the urethra is divided at the apex of the prostate as close to the lateral lobes as possible with blunt ended scissors (Fig. 27.40). All packs and

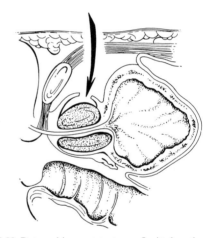

Fig. 27.39 Retropubic prostatectomy. Sagittal section of bladder and prostate. The incision in the anterior prostatic capsule goes through fibrous and false capsules to expose the adenoma which has a whiter colour than the surrounding tissues

the retractor are now removed. While the assistant holds and elevates the proximal stay suture with his left hand and uses the sucker or a swab on a forceps with his right hand, the surgeon holds and elevates the distal stay suture with his left hand and, using the index finger on his right hand, frees the adenomatous mass posteriorly, and finally removes it by dividing the mucosal cuff connecting it to the bladder, with scissors (Fig. 27.41).

A gauze pack is placed temporarily into the prostatic bed to control haemorrhage and the Millin retractor is reinserted. The pack is gently withdrawn and any remaining nodules of prostatic tissue or loose tags of

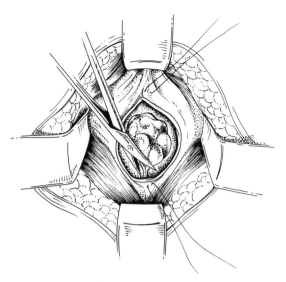

Fig. 27.40 Retropubic prostatectomy. The hypertrophied part of the prostate has been mobilized anteriorly and at both sides. It is pulled up by the fingers of the left hand (which have omitted from the diagram) while the urethra at its apex is divided by scissors

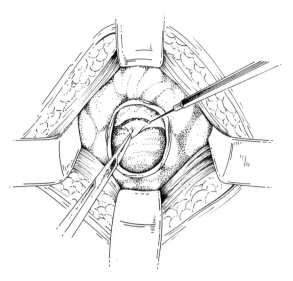

Fig. 27.42 Retropubic prostatectomy. The bladder neck has been grasped with tissue forceps and a V shape wedge with its apex superiorly is being excised; cutting diathermy is being used in this case although scissors may be used

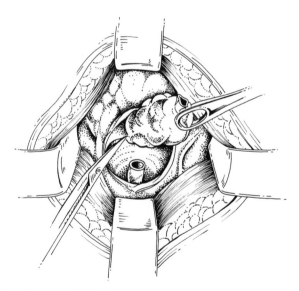

Fig. 27.41 Retropubic prostatectomy. The hypertrophied prostate has now been freed posteriorly and is being separated from the mucosa of the bladder neck by sharp dissection, thereafter it will be completely removed

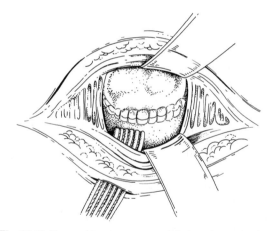

Fig. 27.43 Retropubic prostatectomy. The anterior prostatic capsule has been closed with a continuous catgut suture and a drain inserted into the retropubic space

capsule are removed. The bladder neck spreader is inserted into the bladder neck and held open by the assistant. The ureteric orifices are identified and protected while a generous wedge is excised from the back of the bladder neck (Fig. 27.42). Four or five interrupted sutures of No. 1 plain catgut are inserted into the cut edges of the wedge pinning down the bladder neck mucosa to the back of the prostatic capsule. A 22F three-

way Haematuric Foley catheter is introduced into the urethra, and guided through the prostatic bed into the bladder. About 5 ml water is injected into the balloon at this stage (a further 15 ml is injected after the capsule is closed). After a final inspection to ensure that haemorrhage has been arrested, the capsular incision is closed with a continuous catgut suture (Fig. 27.43) placing the stitches close enough together to arrest haemorrhage especially at the lateral angles. Although this suture and the stay sutures used at an earlier stage can be inserted with a boomerang needle, the author prefers to use No 1 plain catgut on an ordinary needle with a Stratte needle holder. A drain is left in the retropubic space and the wound is repaired in layers. As soon as the operation has been completed, the bladder is washed out with water and some is left in the bladder until irrigation can be started. Irrigation is maintained as long as there is significant bleeding and the urethral catheter is removed on the third to fifth day after operation.

TRANSURETHRAL PROSTATECTOMY

Although for the large benign prostates a retropubic or transvesical prostatectomy is a satisfactory alternative to a transurethral resection, the latter is preferable for the smaller benign prostates, for the fibrous or malignant prostates and for bladder neck contractures. Any surgeon who practices urological surgery must learn to use a resectoscope for these procedures and for the treatment and assessment of bladder tumours (p. 582). The largest prostates he can remove by open operation and, the more experienced he is with the resectoscope, the larger the prostates he will resect. Any surgeon, reasonably experi-

enced in endoscopy, can learn to use a resectoscope from the many books, pictures, videos, and films about it, although of course instruction from an experienced resectionist is invaluable.

Position
The patient is placed in the appropriate position for endoscopy. A 'steridrape' or similar drape is applied. This is a plastic sheet one edge of which is adherent and sticks to the abdominal wall. The penis is brought through a hole in the centre of the sheet; below this hole is a finger cot which is lubricated and inserted into the rectum. The drape enables the surgeon to use the rectum to examine the prostate and facilitate resection without becoming unsterile. First the urethra, prostate and bladder are examined by cysto-urethroscopy, looking for strictures, diverticula, stones or tumours, which may have been unsuspected from the clinical examination. Next prostatic size is assessed and a decision made whether to proceed with a transurethral or an open procedure.

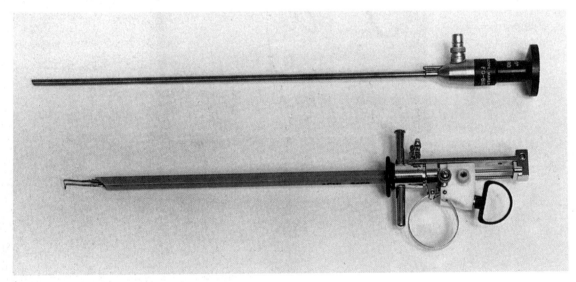

A

B

Fig. 27.44 Resectoscope. (A) Telescope and resectoscope sheath with loop extruded. (B) Sheath with loop retracted

Assessment

The assessment of prostatic size is made partly by endoscopy, and partly by bimanual examination, which is best done while the cystoscope is in the bladder. Endoscopically the size of the middle lobe is estimated by the extent to which it bulges into the bladder and the size of the lateral lobes by the amount they encroach into the urethra, the length of contact between them and the length of the prostatic urethra from the bladder neck to the verumontanum. This length is about 2.5 cm (1 field of the cystoscope using a 70° telescope) for the normal prostate; it increases to about 5.0 cm (2 fields) with the 25 gm prostate and to about 7.5 cm (3 fields) with the 50 gm prostate. This endoscopy should be done in a theatre, where transurethral or open prostatectomy can be done so that operation need not be deferred until another day. Two units of blood should be available, but are rarely used.

Resectoscope

A resectoscope sheath with its obturator is passed into the bladder choosing a 26F or 24F sheath depending on the ease with which it will pass. The sheath may be all fibreglass or metal with a fibreglass beak and the obturator is either straight or has a flexible tip (Timberlake obturator), which can be bent to facilitate introduction of the sheath into the bladder. If it proves difficult to pass even a 24F resectoscope sheath the urethra must first be enlarged by dilating with bougies, or better, by carrying out an internal urethrotomy with an Otis urethrotome. Once the sheath has passed into the bladder, the obturator is removed and replaced by the working element of the resectoscope, which has a channel for the fore-oblique or direct view telescope, (a 0° or 12° or 30°, depending upon the make of the instrument) and one for the loop electrode. Different working elements have different mechanisms for moving the loop backwards and forwards but most are now one handed, i.e. the instrument is held with the fingers and the loop is manipulated with the thumb of the same hand and most have a spring which assists either the cutting action or the return of the loop after cutting (cutting is done as the loop is drawn towards the operator) (Fig. 27.44). Cutting loops vary in size and are colour coded. One uses a 24F loop with the 24F sheath, because a loop will obviously not move freely in a sheath which is smaller. The larger the loop, the larger the chips or piece of prostate that can be resected in one cut, and for this reason most urologists prefer a 26 or 27F sheath to a 24 or 25F one, but only if it can be passed easily without damaging the urethra. The loop consists of the cutting wire, supported on an insulated stem by an insulated fork, which often incorporates a stabilising device. The proximal end of the loop fits into the insulated block of the working element, which is attached to the diathermy

machine by the diathermy cable. Loops, other than the cutting ones, are available; some have balls or rollers for coagulating, and others have knives for incising the bladder neck or ureteric orifice. The tap on the resectoscope sheath is connected to the source of the irrigating fluid, which is usually in plastic containers. If two bags are connected to the resectoscope via a Y connection (Fig. 27.45) there need be no delay in changing over when one bag is empty. Sterile saline cannot be used for transurethral resection because it forms an electroconductive solution which interferes with the electrocutting coagulation current. During resection large volumes (10 or more litres) of irrigating fluid are used and consider-

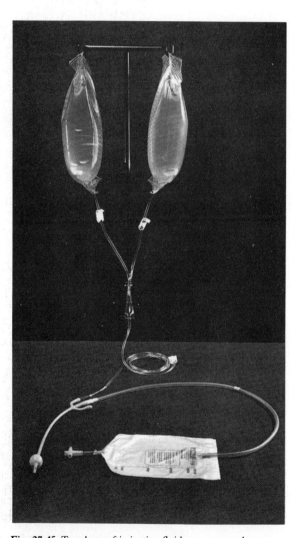

Fig. 27.45 Two bags of irrigating fluid are connected to a single tube by a Y connection. The single tube can then be attached to either resectoscope or, as in the illustration, to a catheter. The irrigation is carried out from only one bag at a time but, as soon as that bag is empty, irrigation can be continued from the other without delay

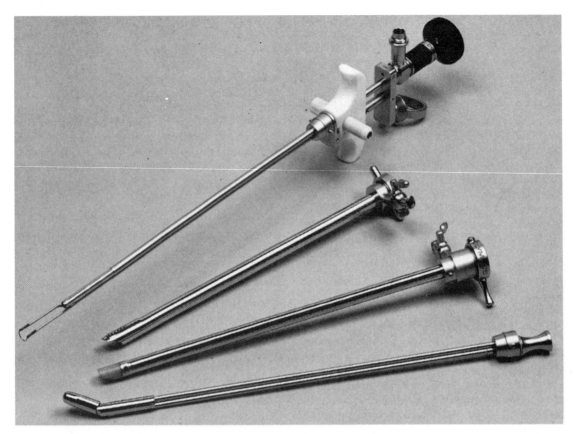

Fig. 27.46 Continuous irrigating resectoscope. The instruments shown are (from above downwards) the working element with loop and fore-oblique telescope, the inner sheath (24F), the outer sheath (26F), and the deflecting or Timberlake obturator (Courtesy of Key Med)

able amounts may be absorbed into the veins opened during resection. Since water reduces osmotic pressure and causes haemolysis it should not be used. Of the various isotonic or near isotonic fluids available, 1.5% glycine is as good as any. The irrigating fluid is allowed to run into the bladder as cutting takes place and washes blood and the resected chips into the bladder.

Irrigation
The working element has to be removed from the sheath at regular intervals to empty the bladder. Cystoscopes with continuous irrigation are available (Fig. 27.46). They have a double sheath; the fluid flowing in through one by gravity is sucked out of the other by a suction pump, but many urologists still prefer the conventional nonirrigating resectoscopes. The author uses a diathermy machine (Fig. 27.47) with separate cutting and coagulating circuits with a separate pedal for each, although cutting can be done with high coagulation current from older machines. The appropriate machine settings can only be worked out by practice. The blending of cutting and coagulating currents is probably best avoided.

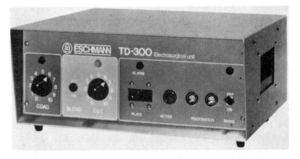

Fig. 27.47 Electrosurgical unit. This unit has two circuits, one for coagulating and one for cutting each activated by its own pedal. The machine also has a facility for blending (Courtesy of Eschmann Co.)

Cutting
The loop moves about 2.5 cm and this is the maximum length of the chip if the sheath is not moved apart from tilting it while the cut is made. It is possible to cut larger chips by moving the resectoscope as well as the loop, but this can only be done with experience. It is far safer to

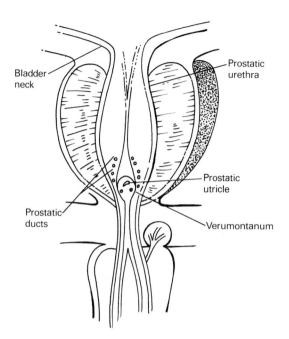

Fig. 27.48 Anatomy of prostatic urethra

keep the sheath steady while making the cut. The knack of cutting and the strength of diathermy needed can be estimated and practised by cutting soap and meat.

Before resection begins it is essential to recognise the two vital landmarks, the bladder neck above, the verumontanum below. No cuts must be made below the verumontanum (Fig. 27.48) which marks the level of the external sphincter, and no cuts must be made higher than the bladder neck. At the start of the procedure the muscle fibres of the bladder neck are exposed by resecting the middle lobe from 5 o'clock to 7 o'clock (Fig. 27.49). Next the lateral lobes are resected, exposing the bladder neck muscle fibres and the reticulate pattern of the inner aspect of the prostatic capsule. Of the many ways in which this can be done, it is best to finish one lobe before starting on the other, and to commence cutting about 1 o'clock for the left lobe and 11 o'clock for the right (Fig. 27.50). Enough chips are cut in each position to expose the muscle of the bladder neck and capsule, and haemostasis is secured before rotating the instrument and making the next move; this is repeated until one is back at 5 o'clock or 7 o'clock depending which lobe is tackled first. Resection is continued until only apical tissue remains (Fig. 27.51) before proceeding to the other lateral lobe (Fig. 27.52). Finally the apical tissue is resected on both sides (being extremely careful not to go beyond the verumontanum and so damage the external sphincter) and the anterior lobe between 11 o'clock and 1 o'clock (where the wall is very thin and easily perforated). Although it is tempting to keep cutting if the bleeding does not hinder vision it is

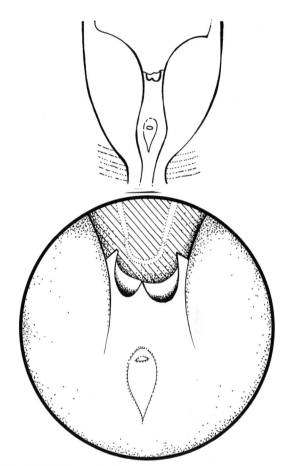

Fig. 27.49 Transurethral resection of prostate. The procedure starts by exposing the muscle fibres of the bladder neck by resecting the middle lobe from 5 to 7 o'clock

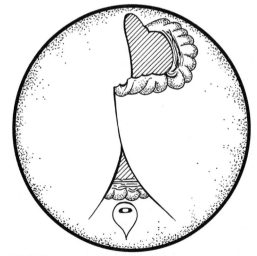

Fig. 27.50 Transurethral resection of prostate. A trench is dug into the left lateral lobe at 1 o'clock until the muscle fibres of the bladder neck and the criss-cross pattern of the prostatic capsule are exposed.

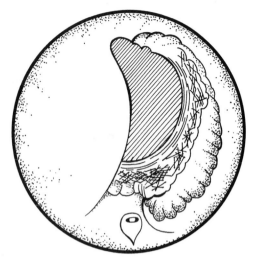

Fig. 27.51 Transurethral resection of prostate. The left lateral lobe has all been resected apart from apical tissue

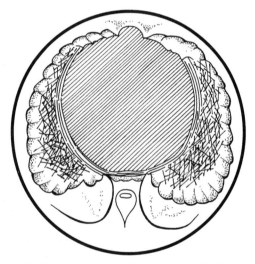

Fig. 27.52 Transurethral resection of prostate. The final stage consists of resection of the apical tissue seen on either side of the verumontanum. It is during this stage that great care must be taken to avoid damage to the external sphincter

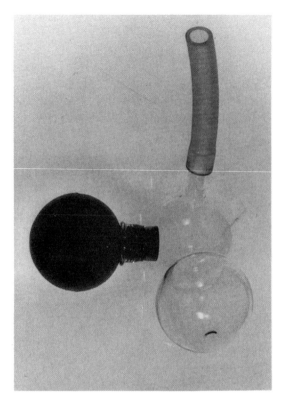

Fig. 27.53 Ellik evacuator (Courtesy of GU Manufacturing Co Ltd)

better, though slower, to secure haemostasis after each cut or after the cuts needed to form a trench deep enough to expose the muscle of the bladder neck and the prostatic capsule. Do not leave haemostasis to the end, when rebound bleeding can make recognition of the source and site of bleeding extremely difficult. Once the resection is complete, the chips which have not escaped when the working element was removed and the bladder emptied, are removed by washing the bladder out with an Ellik evacuator (Fig. 27.53). The working element is then reinserted and haemostasis secured, although of course many bleeding vessels will have

already been dealt with during the resection; any remaining ones can often be coagulated more easily with a ball or roller electrode. Bleeding from veins opened when cuts are made close to, or even through, the prostatic capsule are more easily controlled by the Foley catheter than diathermy. Once all chips have been removed and bleeding reasonably controlled, a three-way 22 or 24F Foley catheter of haematuric type is introduced on a curved introducer to prevent the catheter passing behind the trigone of the bladder into the perivesical tissues. Its entry into the bladder can be readily confirmed if some fluid is left in the bladder when the resectoscope sheath is removed. The bladder is then continuously irrigated through the catheter with sterile water or saline. Haemostasis is often improved if the catheter, with 30 ml in the balloon, is pulled down so that the balloon compresses the bladder neck by traction (Fig. 27.54).

Precautions

1. Do not resect below the verumontanum nor above the muscle fibres of the bladder neck (exposed by resecting the middle lobe from 5 to 7 o'clock at the start of the operation).

2. Hold the resectoscope sheath still while resecting,

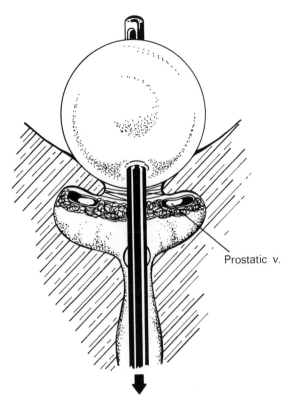

Fig. 27.54 Transurethral resection of prostate. A Foley catheter has been passed and its balloon inflated in the bladder. When traction is applied to the catheter, the prostatic cavity is squashed and open veins compressed

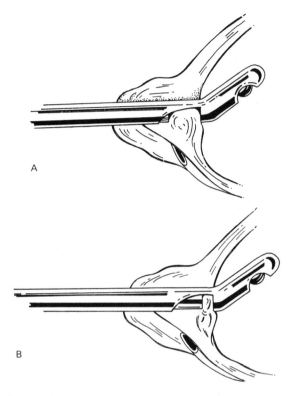

Fig. 27.55 Punch prostatectomy. In (A) the fenestra of the sheath is open and hypertrophied prostatic tissue is projecting through it into the lumen of the sheath. In (B) the hypertrophied tissue is being cut as the circular knife is pushed down the sheath

so that only the loop moves and all cutting is done under vision.

3. Achieve haemostasis after each cut, or at least before rotating the sheath to dig another trench.

4. Do not cut unless you can see clearly; abandon the procedure, if you can not. One can always go back later and resect more, or do open procedure. You can not go back later and replace bits of the external sphincter or ureteric orifices.

Continuous irrigation is maintained through the threeway Foley catheter for 24 to 48 hours, depending how much bleeding occurs. The catheter is removed a day or two later. In patients with chronic retention, the bladder is usually hypotonic or even atonic and the catheter should be left in longer.

Punch prostatectomy
This operation is carried out by an instrument often referred to as a 'cold punch' resectoscope. The sheath is straight and close to its distal end, which is open, is a large fenestra.

This sheath with its obturator is introduced into the bladder, and the obturator removed. Under direct vision,

the sheath is slowly withdrawn until prostatic tissue in the quadrant selected projects into the fenestra (Fig. 27.55). A tubular knife is now inserted into the sheath and it shears off the projecting tissue when it is pressed home with a punching movement. Partial withdrawal of the knife allows more glandular tissue to project into the sheath, and this in turn is sheared off. The process is repeated until all obstructing tissue has been removed. As with diathermy loop resection, great care is taken to cut only above the verumontanum and below the bladder neck. Bleeding is arrested by means of a diathermy electrode passed together with a telescope through a separate channel in the sheath. The after treatment is similar to that described for diathermy loop resection.

The protagonists of the 'cold' punch method hold that, since cutting is carried out with a sharp knife rather than by diathermy there is no devitalization of tissue and less risk of sepsis; furthermore since the cuts are made in an upward direction away from the verumontanum, the external sphincter is less likely to be damaged. Few urologists now however would consider it as good or as useful as the diathermy loop methods.

Complications of prostatic surgery

Clot retention
This is one of the most serious immediate complications of any prostatectomy and may occur if the catheter or other drainage tube becomes blocked by blood clot and is not expeditiously dealt with. It is unlikely to occur while the bladder is being irrigated through a three-way Foley catheter, provided that any blockage is detected and treated early. Small clots can be cleared by using a bladder syringe or just milking the catheter and these measures may be adequate to empty the bladder and restore drainage even if the bladder is distended by clot and fluid (irrigating fluid may continue to run in even if it is not running out).

If these measures are unsuccessful the patient should be taken to theatre and a large bore catheter or resectoscope sheath passed under general anaesthesia to allow evacuation of the clot by vigorous irrigation with a Wardill's all-glass or Ellik syringe. If even this fails, the bladder must be opened or reopened, although that is rarely necessary. *Secondary haemorrhage* may occur on the 7th to the 10th day after any form of prostatectomy, but is perhaps more common after transurethral procedures; if the patient goes home before the 10th postoperative day, he should be warned that it might happen. In some patients secondary haemorrhage is enough to cause clot retention.

Stricture
Strictures, especially those at the external meatus, often result from forcing a catheter or resectoscope through the meatus. A smaller catheter or resectoscope sheath is tried, and if that will not pass easily, carry out a meatotomy or a urethrotomy with the Otis urethrotome first. The patient who has difficulty passing urine after prostatectomy, is not likely to be helped when told that it is no longer the prostate causing his trouble, but a stricture (and strictures may be more difficult to treat).

Incontinence
Some patients have stress or urge incontinence for some days after operation, but permanent incontinence is very uncommon unless the external sphincter has been damaged and this should not happen. Prostatectomy can cure the overflow incontinence of chronic retention once bladder contractility is restored, but is not advised for patients who have other sorts of incontinence unless it is certain that their problems are obstructive and not neurological.

Infection
Epididymitis is now an uncommon complication and few surgeons do a vasectomy to prevent it. Bladder infection may ascend to the kidneys causing pyelonephritis and even endotoxaemia and, with open prostatectomies, wound infection still occurs and should be treated appropriately. There is some evidence that prophylactic antibiotics given before or at the time of operation speed recovery.

Perforation of the prostatic capsule
It is easy to make a small perforation during prostatic resection and expose veins and sometimes fat. If a large perforation occurs the irrigating fluid leaks into the extravesical space; fluid fails to return through the resectoscope, the patient's abdomen swells and becomes cold (unless the irrigating fluid is warmed) and the anaesthetist appears concerned. The resection must be abandoned, a urethral catheter passed and the retropubic space drained through a transverse suprapubic incision, opening the peritoneum if intraperitoneal extravasation is suspected.

Transurethral resection (tur) syndrome
Large volumes of irrigating fluid may be absorbed into the general circulation through open veins. If water has been used, severe haemolysis with acute renal failure can occur. Even isotonic fluids like Glycine may cause problems by expanding the blood volume which causes hypertension, and reduces electrolyte concentration, with resultant neuromuscular disturbances such as fits and temporary paralysis.

CARCINOMA OF THE PROSTATE

At one time, nearly all patients with prostatic carcinoma were treated by hormone manipulation. Nowadays, the treatment depends on the category of the disease according to the TNMG system. The *T category* represents the local extent and is assessed by clinical examination, urography, endoscopy and biopsy (UICC, 1978).

Tis Preinvasive carcinoma (carcinoma in situ)

T0 No tumour palpable (includes the incidental finding of carcinoma in an operative or biopsy specimen)

T1 Tumour intracapsular surrounded by palpably normal gland

T2 Tumour confined to the gland. Smooth nodule deforming contour but lateral sulci and seminal vesicles not involved

T3 Tumour extending beyond the capsule with or without involvement of the lateral sulci or seminal vesicles or both

T4 Tumour fixed or infiltrating neighbouring structures (Fig. 27.56)

The *N category* represents the state of regional and

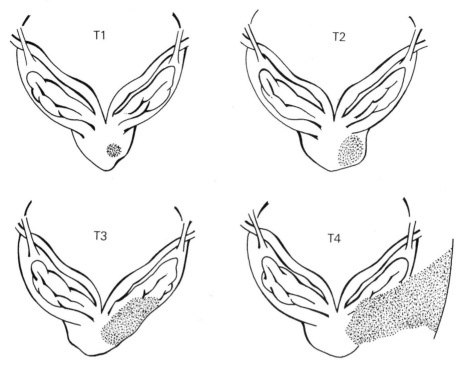

Fig. 27.56 Carcinoma of the prostate. The T categories

juxtaregional lymph nodes and is assessed by clinical examination and radiography.

N0 No evidence of regional lymph node involvement.

N1 Evidence of involvement of a single homolateral regional lymph node.

N2 Evidence of involvement of contralateral or bilateral or multiple regional lymph nodes

N3 Evidence of involvement of fixed regional lymph nodes (there is a fixed mass on the pelvic wall with a free space between this and the tumour)

N4 Evidence of involvement of juxta-regional nodes

NX The minimum requirements to assess the regional and/or juxtaregional lymph nodes cannot be met.

The *M category* represents the presence or absence of distant metastases and is assessed by bone scan, radiography and at least two estimations of the serum acid phosphatase

M0 No evidence of distant metastases

M1 Evidence of distant metastases or raised serum acid phosphatase or both (Fig. 27.57)

The *G category* represents histopathological grading

G1 High degree of differentiation

G2 Medium degree of differentiation

G3 Low degree of differentiation or undifferentiated.

As lymphagiography is of no value in demonstrating

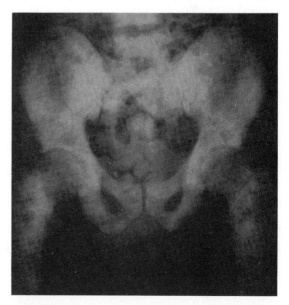

Fig. 27.57 Carcinoma of prostate. An X-ray showing widespread osteosclerotic prostatic metastases in femora, pelvis and lumbar spine

internal iliac glands most carcinomas of prostate are categorised NX.

Treatment

In all patients a biopsy is taken, either transperineally or transrectally with a Trucut needle or by transurethral resection. A transurethral resection is done in nearly all patients, not only to obtain a biopsy but also to create or enlarge the channel through the tumour and allow the patient to pass urine more easily.

So little is known about the natural history of the very early localized tumours (TO and T1) that the Medical Research Council have organized a controlled trial in which patients with T0, T1, M0 tumours are either treated with radiotherapy or have treatment deferred until or unless symptoms develop or the disease progresses. The author treats locally advanced tumours (T2, 3 or 4 M0) with radiotherapy, although many treat them like M1 patients. Patients with metastases or raised serum acid phosphatase levels or both (M1) are treated by methods which limit the production of androgens or neutralize their effects, and some 80 to 90% of patients respond (for a time anyway) to this treatment. It consists of giving Stilboestrol 1 to 3 mg daily for ever. For those who cannot tolerate oestrogens, have cardiovascular or thromboembolic disease, or who do not respond a subcapsular orchidectomy is carried out (p. 630). However, some urologists start treatment with orchidectomy or with both orchidectomy and oestrogens (Chisholm, 1982).

What of patients whose tumour is not controlled by hormone manipulation after an initial response or who do not respond at all? To change the oestrogen helps little although Tetrasodium Fosfestrol (Honvan) and others can be tried. Cyproterone Acetate (Androcur) in-hibits the binding of testosterone to its receptors but offers little more than oestrogens although it does not have their side effects. Hypophysectomy or adrenalectomy are sometimes done to suppress adrenal secretions and the former is well worth considering for patients with bone pain unrelieved by other measures and too diffuse for local X–ray therapy. Non hormonal treatment of advanced prostatic cancer using a variety of chemotherapeutic agents, including cyclophosphamide, 5 fluorouracil, estramustine (a drug combining an oestrogen and an alkylating agent) and more recent Cis-platinum have been tried but results await evaluation before the treatment can be recommended.

PROSTATIC CALCULI

True prostatic calculi develop in stagnant or infected acini by the deposition of calcareous material on the corpora amylacea (small bodies of amorphous debris and desquamated epithelium which lie in the acini of the prostatic glands), and are usually found in men between the ages of 50 and 65. They are generally small and multiple, and found in infected glands or in the compressed outer zone or capsule of a hypertrophied gland.

Calculi themselves rarely cause symptoms, and are detected only on X–ray examination or during prostatectomy for benign hypertrophy. The clinical features of prostatic calculi are those of the associated simple hypertrophy or chronic infection although on rectal examination a gland containing calculi is hard and irregular and crepitus may be elicited.

Prostatic stones can be removed transurethrally, or at the time of prostatectomy. They are usually small enough to wash out without first crushing them.

REFERENCES

Chisholm G D, Beynon L L 1982 The response of the malignant prostate to endocrine treatment. In: Ghanadian R(ed) The Endocrinology of Prostate Tumours. MTP Press, Lancaster, p 241
Gosling J A, Dixon J S, Humpherson J R 1982 Functional Anatomy of the Urinary Tract. Churchill Livingstone, Edinburgh
Gow J G 1980 Bladder too small/too large. In: Chisholm G D (ed) Urology Heinemann, London, p 434
Husain I 1984 Tropical Urology and renal disease. Churchill Livingstone, Edinburgh
Mitchell J 1981 Endoscopic Operative Urology. John Wright, Bristol
Paulson D F 1983 Radical Cystectomy. In: Glenn J F (ed) Urological Surgery. 3rd edn, Lippincott, Philadelphia, p 583
Soloway M S 1982 Intravesical Chemotherapy for Superficial Bladder Tumours. In: Spiers A S D (ed) Chemotherapy and Urological Malignancy. Springer Verlag, Heidelberg, p 50
Turner-Warwick R 1973 Observations on the treatment of traumatic urethral injuries and the value of the fenestrated urethral catheter. British Journal of Urology 60 : 775
UICC 1978 TNM Classification of Malignant Tumours. 3rd edn, International Union against Cancer, Geneva

FURTHER READING

Blandy J P 1978 Handbook of Urological Endoscopy. Pitman-Medical, Tunbridge Wells
Blandy J P 1984 Operative Urology, 2nd edn. Blackwell, Oxford
Clark P 1985 Operations in Urology. Churchill Livingstone, Edinburgh
Mauermayer W 1983 Transurethral Surgery. Springer Verlag, Berlin/Heidelberg
Paulson D F 1984 Genitourinary Surgery. Churchill Livingstone, Edinburgh

28

Operations on the male urethra and genital organs

J. M. S. JOHNSTONE & J. E. NEWSAM

OPERATIONS ON THE URETHRA

Anatomy of the urethra

The male urethra is about 20 cm long and is divided into prostatic, membranous and spongy parts (Fig. 28.1). *The prostatic part* is about 3 cm long and is the widest part of the urethra. It is surrounded by the prostate gland. The prostatic ducts (10 to 15 in number) open onto its posterior wall on either side of a longitudinal ridge called the urethral crest. At the lower end of this crest there is a rounded elevation called the verumontanum, on which lie the openings of the prostatic utricle and the ejaculatory ducts. The verumontanum marks the position of the external sphincter and it is a most important landmark when resecting the prostate.

The membranous part, 1 cm in length, is surrounded by

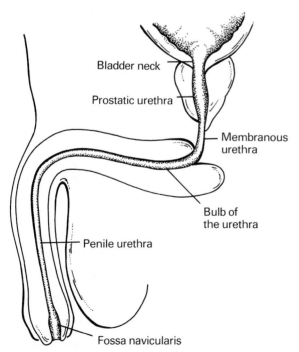

Fig. 28.1 A sagittal section of the male urethra

Bladder neck

Prostatic urethra

Membranous urethra

Bulb of the urethra

Penile urethra

Fossa navicularis

fibres of the external sphincter and passes through the perineal membrane to become continuous with the spongy part.

The spongy part is about 15 cm long and traverses the corpus spongiosum from the bulb (where it is wide) to the external meatus (which is the narrowest part of the whole male urethra). The ducts from the bulbo-urethral glands, which lie behind the membranous urethra, pierce the perineal membrane and open into the spongy urethra.

Injuries of the urethra: general considerations

The early signs of urethral injury are urethral bleeding, bruising and swelling in the perineum and an inability to pass water. Later the bladder distends and later still urine extravasates into the extraperitoneal tissues or the superficial perineal pouch depending upon the site of injury. The general principles of treatment are to prevent extravasation of urine by draining the bladder with a urethral or suprapubic catheter and to allow or encourage the urethra to heal with as little fibrosis and deformity as possible.

Injuries of the anterior urethra (see Newsam, 1980)

Injuries of the anterior urethra usually involve the bulbous part of the urethra in the perineum and are caused by blows or kicks or falling astride a hard object, such as a wooden plank. After such an injury blood leaks out of the external urinary meatus, and into the perineum. Spasm of the sphincter prevents the patient passing urine and urine only extravasates when the bladder distends and overflows. For that reason the patient can be left safely for some 24 hours after injury to see whether or not he can pass urine. If he is able to do so the injury probably consists of no more than a bruise and requires no active treatment. If he is unable to do so the injury is probably more serious and a complete or partial tear of the urethra is suspected. One cautious attempt is made to pass a *soft* 12 or 14F catheter through the urethra into the bladder with the strictest of aseptic techniques. If successful, the catheter is left in situ; if not, a suprapubic cystostomy is required. On no account should

attempts be made to pass a stiff plastic or metal catheter
or a catheter on an introducer for fear of damaging the
urethra further by converting a partial tear into a complete one. If there are obvious signs of extravasation in
the superficial perineal pouch the extravasated urine
must be drained. After 10 to 12 days the catheter is removed or the suprapubic tube clipped. If the patient
passes urine satisfactorily no more need be done for 3
months when urethroscopy and urethrography will reveal any stricture. If the patient cannot pass urine satisfactorily these investigations are done earlier and the
stricture, which is usually short, treated appropriately.

Injuries of the membranous urethra

Injuries of the membranous urethra are usually associated with a fractured pelvis and occur at the junction of
prostatic and membranous parts. Tears are often
complete because the urethra is damaged by the splint-
ered rami. If the perineal membrane and the puboprostatic ligaments are also torn, the prostate and the neck
of the bladder dislocate upwards and backwards and
continuity of the urethra is completely lost (Fig. 28.2).
About 10% of patients with injuries of the membranous
urethra also have injuries of the bladder. The internal
sphincter goes into spasm and urine extravasates into
the extraperitoneal tissues only when the bladder
becomes distended, unless of course the bladder is also
injured. Many patients require blood transfusion and
other resuscitative measures and have serious other injuries to abdomen, chest or pelvis that take precedence
over the urethral injury. Fortunately, there is no urgency
in treating the urethra. One attempt is made to pass a
small soft catheter through the urethra; if it passes into
the bladder and clear urine emerges, it is certain
that little damage has occurred to either urethra or
bladder. Nevertheless, it may be useful to leave the catheter in for a few days to measure the urinary output if
the patient has serious other injuries. If the catheter
appears to pass into the bladder but nothing more than
blood or a little blood stained urine emerges, a cystogram
is done to see if there is an extraperitoneal rupture of the
bladder. If the catheter does not pass into the bladder a
partial or complete tear of the urethra must be suspected.
The bladder is drained by a suprapubic cystostomy if the
patient is ill but more can be attempted if the patient is
fit.

Operation

A transverse suprapubic incision is made although a
midline or paramedian one is better if it is necessary to
inspect the peritoneal cavity also. The prevesical and
retropubic spaces are gently cleared of blood and urine,
taking great care not to open or reopen any of the pelvic
veins. If the bladder is empty the injury is probably
vesical although the urethra may also be damaged. If the

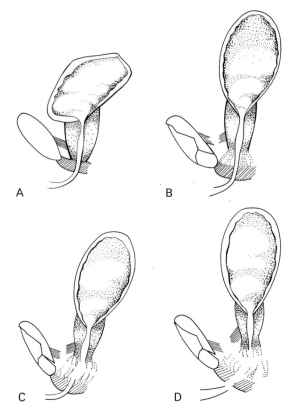

Fig. 28.2 Injuries of the urethra (A) The normal anatomy of
the bladder, prostate, perineal membrane and puboprostatic
ligaments. (B) The pelvis is fractured and the puboprostatic
ligament ruptured but the urethra is only stretched and
bruised. (C) The pelvis is fractured, the puboprostatic
ligament disrupted and there is a complete tear through the
membranous part of the urethra but the perineal ligament is
intact. (D) The pelvis is fractured, both puboprostatic and
perineal ligaments are disrupted and there is a complete tear
which involves the membranous and bulbous part of the
urethra with an upward and backward dislocation of the
prostate and bladder

membranous urethra is injured it is necessary to realign
the ruptured ends, which may be widely separated from
each other, and maintain them in a satisfactory position
until healing occurs. To suture the cut ends together or
to suture the upper cut end to the perineal membrane is
seldom possible and reliance must be placed on the
splinting effect of an indwelling catheter. To achieve this
the bladder is opened and a soft 12 or 14F catheter passed
through the bladder neck and down the urethra until it
emerges at the site of injury. A silastic Foley catheter is
then passed up the urethra from the external meatus.
When its tip emerges from the site of injury it is tied to
the tip of the catheter passed from above. By withdrawing the upper one out of the urethra and out of the
bladder the Foley catheter is negotiated into the bladder
and its balloon inflated. By applying traction to the cath-

eter the balloon pulls the prostate down to the perineal membrane apposing the cut ends of the urethra. The procedure can also be accomplished by using two bougies instead of two catheters. One is passed down the urethra from within the open bladder to the injury. The second is passed retrogradely to the injury through the external urinary meatus. By preserving contact between the tips of the two bougies the second one is manoeuvred into the bladder by withdrawing the first. A catheter is attached to the tip of the second bougie as it lies in the bladder and manoeuvred through the whole length of the urethra by withdrawing the bougie out of the external meatus. A Foley catheter can then be attached to the tip of this catheter and withdrawn back into the bladder. With both procedures it is wise to drain the bladder with a suprapubic tube.

Urethral strictures (see Turner-Warwick, 1983)

Congenital strictures are found at the external urethral meatus in boys, often secondary to hypospadias, but are uncommon elsewhere in the urethra. (Congenital lesions causing obstruction consist of either bladder neck contracture or posterior urethral valves.) Malignant strictures are uncommon but can occur in patients who have a urethral tumour secondary to tumour of the bladder or prostate. They usually occur in the spongy part of the male urethra and are often palpable or even visible. Most urethral strictures are post inflammatory or post traumatic.

Post inflammatory strictures

Non specific urethritis is caused by Chlamydia trachomatis, ureaplasma urealyticum, candida species, trichomonas or herpes and rarely causes strictures because the infection never extends more deeply into the urethral wall than the mucosa. Gonorrhoea on the other hand involves not only the mucosa of the urethra but also the submucosa and corpora spongiosa, and, unless effectively and rapidly treated, causes strictures in the bulbous part of the spongy urethra. Post gonococcal strictures are often multiple and complicated by sinuses, fistulae and false passages.

Post traumatic strictures

Injuries in the perineum may cause strictures of the bulbous part of the spongy urethra which are usually short, straight and uncomplicated unless previously maltreated. Fractures of the bony pelvis can cause strictures of the membranous urethra which can be severe and complicated; endoscopic procedures and open operations on the rectum, colon, prostate and bladder may injure the urethra and cause or aggravate strictures. Even catheterization may cause a stricture of the external meatus.

Assessment

Strictures obstruct the outflow of urine from the bladder causing symptoms similar to those of prostatic diseases

Figs. 28.3 & 28.4 *False urethral passages*

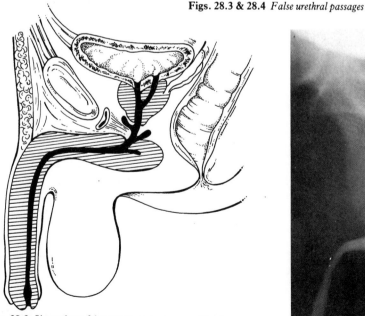

Fig. 28.3 Sites where false passages may occur. The lower three are sinuses, the upper one is a fistual forming an abnormal communication between bladder and prostatic urethra.

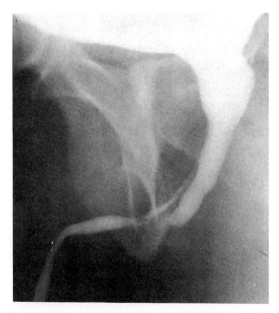

Fig. 28.4 Descending urethrogram showing false passage between prostatic urethra (which is dilated) and spongy urethra.

(p. 590); furthermore there may be local complications such as sinuses, abscesses, fistulae and false passages (Figs. 28.3 & 28.4).

The diagnosis is sometimes made from the patient's history especially if the stricture is of traumatic origin, but confirmation of its extent and effects on the urinary tract requires investigation such as *urethroscopy*, ascending and descending *urethrography* and *intravenous urography*. The methods available for treating urethral strictures consist of:
1. Urethral dilatation
2. External urethrostomy
3. Internal urethrotomy—Blind or optical
4. Excision and suture
5. Urethroplasty
6. Urinary diversion

Urethral dilatation by graduated bougies (Figs. 28.5–28.7)
This used to be the standard treatment and there were few strictures to which it was not applied. Metal bougies

Figs. 28.5–28.7 *Urethral bougies* (Courtesy of G U Manufacturing Co Ltd).

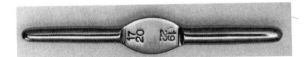

Fig. 28.5 Canny-Ryall bougie. This is used for dilatating structures of the anterior part of the urethra but is also a useful instrument for dilating perineal urethrostomies or nephrostomies

can be more easily controlled than plastic ones and if used carefully and gently do no more damage. The procedure can usually be accomplished by anaesthetising the urethra with 1 or 2% *Lignocaine gel*. If general anaesthesia is used, dilatation must be carried out even more carefully and gently. If records of previous urethral dilatations are available it is wise to choose a bougie three or four sizes smaller than the largest one passed on the previous occasion, remembering that false passages are more likely to be made by small bougies. The bougie is introduced by the following technique. Its tip is kept on the floor of the anterior urethra until the bulb is reached; then, the instrument is rotated, depressed and very gently pushed upwards towards the bladder with its tip in contact with the roof. If the first bougie arrests and cannot be passed, smaller ones are tried successively until the stricture is negotiated. Thereafter the scale of bougies is ascended until the patient complains of discomfort or dilatation is considered adequate. The last bougie, usually 26 or 28F, should be left in place for a few minutes if the maximum benefit is to be obtained from the dilatation. To overstretch the urethra causes bleeding and stimulates fibrosis. No stricture is cured by dilatation and it has to be repeated at intervals which vary from three weeks to a year or more. Nevertheless, urethral dilatation remains a sensible means of treating strictures if the patient is old; the procedure easily accomplished, and unassociated with haemorrhage, infection, or other reaction; the intervals between treatments at least 6 months and the patient content. Strictures at the external meatus are usually caused by an endoscope or catheter and can often be cured by one or two dilatations; if not, they should be treated by *meatotomy*.

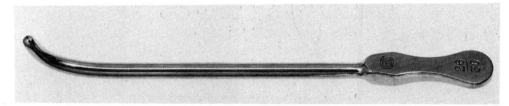

Fig. 28.6 Clutton bougie

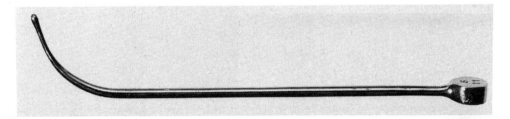

Fig. 28.7 Lister bougie

Acute retention of urine due to stricture

A urethral stricture should be suspected as the cause of acute retention if the patient is young, has a normal prostate, or has had previous operations on the urethra or prostate; it is confirmed as the cause when a small catheter is arrested in the region of the bulb or membranous urethra. An attempt is made to negotiate the stricture with a metal bougie, and thereafter introduce a catheter. If this is not easily possible, the bladder is drained suprapubically, and the stricture treated in the appropriate way later.

Urethrostomy

External urethrostomy means entering the urethra through an incision in the skin. On the rare occasions when this is done, the patient is more likely to be suffering from urethral stone than stricture. However, in an elaborate form, it is the first part of a two stage urethroplasty.

Internal urethrotomy

This can be done blindly or optically.

Blind urethrotomy

Of the several urethrotomes available, the Otis (Fig. 28.8) or one of its several modifications is the most popular. The Otis urethrotome is a 13F instrument which can be expanded from 13F to 43F by rotating the wheel at its proximal end. The instrument is passed beyond the stricture, which is usually possible only if the tip of the urethrotome has been modified to screw on to a filiform bougie which is passed first. Once beyond the stricture, the wheel of the urethrotome is rotated and the stricture dilated. Then the knife, hidden within the instrument, is withdrawn cutting the narrowed parts of the urethra lineally to a depth of 3 mm. (This instrument is also used before transurethral prostatic resections if the urethra does not easily accept the 26F resectoscope sheath and some surgeons use it routinely before all prostatic resections).

Visual urethrotomy

Most firms now make an optical urethrotome (Fig. 28.9). It consists of a straight metal sheath with a side opening through which a ureteric catheter can be passed. An Iglesias resectoscope working element, modified to take and move a long knife instead of a loop electrode, is passed into the sheath, and vision obtained with a fore-oblique or direct view telescope. Under vision, the instrument is passed into the urethra, which is continuously, but slowly, irrigated through the side tap to separate the walls of the urethra. The stricture can be seen clearly. A ureteric catheter is passed through the side opening of the sheath, and on through the stricture into the bladder and acts as a guide for the knife which is then used to incise the stricture at 12 o'clock. Thereafter, a silastic

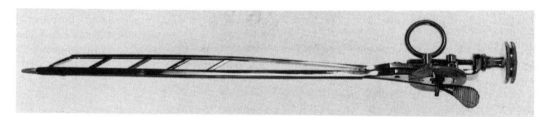

Fig. 28.8 The Otis urethrotome (Courtesy of G U Manufacturing Co Ltd

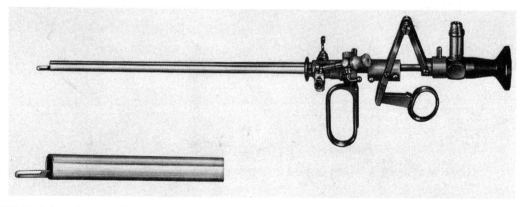

Fig. 28.9 Optical urethrotome (Courtesy of Stortz Ltd)

Foley catheter is passed into the bladder and left for at least 2 weeks, although some surgeons leave it longer. Only the fibrous tissue of the stricture is cut but if the cut is made too deeply the corpora spongiosa is opened and much bleeding and bruising occurs. The optical urethrotome is proving of considerable value in the treatment of urethral strictures, and seems destined to replace urethral dilatation and many types of urethroplasty as the standard method of treatment (Chilton, 1983).

Excision of the stricture and reanastomosis

Short uncomplicated strictures of the bulbar part of the urethra often respond to dilatation or optical urethrotomy; if not, they can be excised and the cut urethral ends anastomosed (Fig. 28.10). The patient is placed in the semilithotomy position, and a vertical or ∩-shaped incision is made in the perineum. The bulbous part of the urethra is exposed and opened just in front of the stricture by cutting against the tip of a bougie passed from the external meatus. The urethra is opened again just behind the stricture. The whole procedure can often be accomplished through the perineal incision; if not, the bladder is exposed through a suprapubic incision and a second bougie passed through the bladder neck and down the urethra. The stricture and the fibrosed corpora spongiosum, which may extend beyond the stricture, are excised. The anterior segment of urethra is mobilised and displaced backwards to permit a tension free end-to-end anastomosis with the proximal segment. The ends should be spatulated and sutured with 3/0 catgut. A small silastic Foley catheter is passed into the bladder and the wound is sutured.

Strictures of the membranous urethra are usually short in length, but difficult to treat because they are S shaped. They can often be managed by dilatation or by internal visual urethrotomy, which may be done more safely and effectively if the bladder is first opened and a cystoscope or bougie is passed down the urethra to the proximal level of the stricture.

Pull through operation (Badenoch)

This operation was described for strictures of the membranous urethra. The urethra is exposed by a perineal incision and divided transversely just below the stricture. The bladder is opened and the bladder neck and the prostatic and membranous parts of the urethra are dilated from above. A catheter is passed down the urethra from the bladder until its tip appears in the perineal wound. The tip of this catheter is sutured to the cut end of the distal urethra, which is pulled up to the bladder neck through the dilated prostatic and membranous urethra as the catheter is withdrawn into the bladder. By suturing the catheter to the suprapubic wound, the urethra is retained in its new position. The catheter is removed after 2 weeks.

Urethroplasty

One stage skin patch operation

This operation can be used for strictures of the bulbar part of the urethra which are unsuitable for dilatation, internal urethrotomy or excision and are uncomplicated by fistulae or sinuses. The stricture and the healthy urethra and corpora spongiosum proximal and distal to it are exposed through a vertical or ∩ incision. The stricture is widely opened and the urethral defect is covered by a full thickness skin graft (Fig. 28.11) (the epidermis on the inside forming urethral lumen) secured all round with 4/0 absorbable sutures (Fig. 28.12). The skin patch can be a free one taken from the prepuce or penis or a pedicled one attached by the dartos muscle and taken from the side of a vertical skin incision or from the front of an ∩ one. A small silastic catheter is passed through the urethra into the bladder at the conclusion of the operation.

Two stage urethroplasty

A number of two stage operations have been described and perhaps the best of these is the scrotal flap proce-

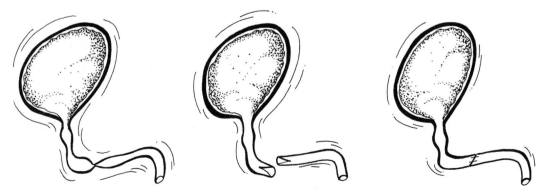

Fig. 28.10 Excision of urethral stricture and end-to-end anastomosis

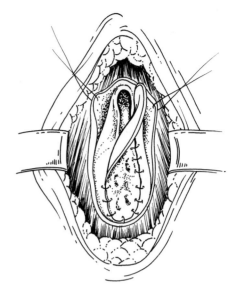

Fig. 28.12 Urethral stricture. Graft almost completed

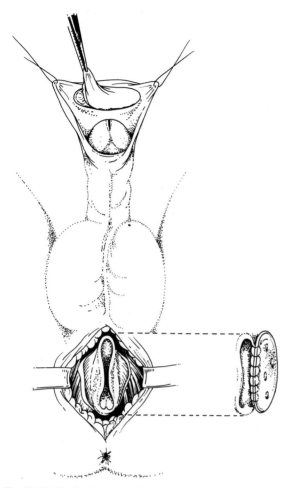

Fig. 28.11 Urethral stricture. A free full thickness graft taken from the prepuce is applied and sutured to the urethra, which has been laid open throughout the length of the stricture

dure. This is indicated for strictures of the bulbar urethra complicated by fistulae, sinuses, or excessive scar tissue from infection or previous operations.

First stage (Figs. 28.13–28.15). An ∩ incision is made in the perineum and extended vertically forwards between the two halves of the scrotum. The perineal flap of skin and fat is separated and allowed to fall backwards. The bulbospongiosum muscle is split in the midline and carefully separated from the spongy tissue and the underlying urethra. The urethra is incised vertically onto a bougie passed down from the external meatus. The incision into the urethra is continued forwards and backwards until the stricture is completely divided and healthy corpora spongiosum exposed. The front edge of the scrotal flap is then stitched to the proximal edge of the healthy urethra using 3 or 4/0 nylon sutures. The urethra is sutured to the skin edges and a catheter is passed through the exposed part of the urethra into the bladder.

Second stage (Figs. 28.16 & 28.17). A bougie or catheter is passed through the urethra into the bladder. An incision is made around the exposed part of the urethra forming a skin tube which is loosely sutured over the bougie or catheter to reform the urethra. The skin edges are then undermined and closed over the skin tube.

Diversion

Urine is temporarily diverted from the urethra by perineal urethrostomy or suprapubic cystostomy for some of the repair operations just described; a permanent diversion by perineal urethrostomy, suprapubic cystostomy, ileal loop or ureterocolic anastomosis should rarely if ever be necessary.

Other urethral conditions

Urethral fistulae
Urethral fistulae may develop from peri-urethral abscesses, which can complicate urethral trauma or infection. They occur most commonly at the penoscrotal angle or in the perineum and are usually associated with strictures. If the stricture is treated and the urethral obstruction relieved the fistula often heals. If it does not, the fistulous tract can be excised together with surrounding scar tissue down to the urethral wall, and the defect closed in layers or covered with a full thickness skin graft.

Urethral stones
Stones that pass through the bladder neck into the urethra usually pass right through without difficulty.

Figs. 28.13–28.17 *Two stage urethroplasty*

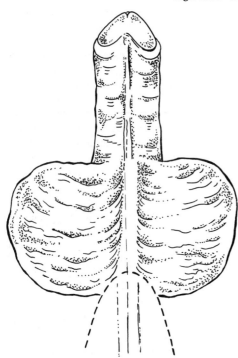

First stage

Fig. 28.13 An ∩ incision is made in the perineum and extended forwards in the midline along the urethra

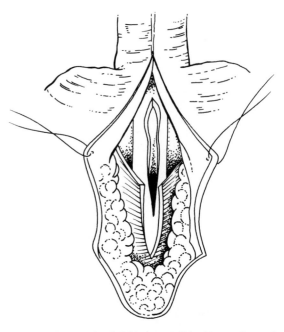

Fig. 28.14 The urethra is laid open until healthy urethra and healthy corpus spongiosum are demonstrated distally and proximally

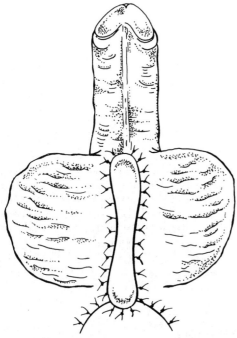

Fig. 28.15 The proximal end of the laid open urethra is sutured to the apex of the flap, the rest to the skin margin

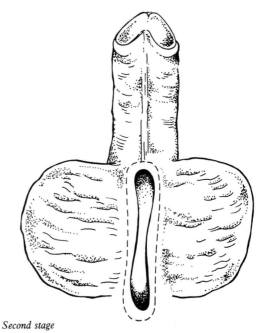

Second stage

Fig. 28.16 An incision is made around the exposed open urethra

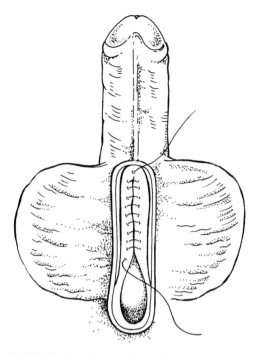

Fig. 28.17 The skin tube thus formed is loosely sutured over a bougie or a catheter to reform the urethra. The skin edges are then undermined and closed over the skin tube

Occasionally they impact at the external meatus or behind a stricture more proximally in the urethra. Stones that impact immediately proximal to the external urinary meatus can usually be removed after a meatotomy (Fig. 28.18) has been carried out. Stones that impact in the urethra proximal to a stricture are more difficult to manage. It is probably best to push them back into the bladder with an endoscope or bougie and treat them appropriately (p. 578).

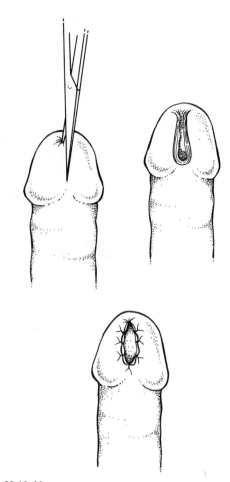

Fig. 28.18 Meatotomy

OPERATIONS ON THE PENIS

Anatomy

The penis has three parts, the glans, the body and the root. The *glans* is the enlarged conical extremity which bears the external urinary meatus. It has a basal oblique rim called the *corona* and it is covered to a variable extent by the *prepuce*. The prepuce has two layers: the outer layer is an extension of the hairless skin of the penis; the inner layer is thin and delicate and fuses at the corona with the epithelium covering the glans. The *frenulum* is a thin median fold of skin connecting the inner layer of the prepuce with the glans immediately below the external urinary meatus and it contains the main artery. The rest of the mobile part of the penis is called the *body*. The *root* of the penis is fixed and buried in the perineum. The penis consists of three longitudinal columns of cavernous erectile tissue, the two corpora cavernosa and the corpus spongiosum, bound together by fibrous tissue (Buck's Fascia) and covered with skin. The *corpora cavernosa* lie dorsally side by side in the body of the penis and diverge posteriorly to become the *crura* which are firmly adherent to the inferior rami of the pubis. The *corpus spongiosum* contains the urethra and lies anteriorly in a groove formed by the corpora cavernosa: inferiorly it expands to form the glans, posteriorly it expands to form the *bulb of the penis* which lies on the perineal membrane. The *suspensory ligament* holds the posterior part of the body of the penis against the front of the symphysis pubis.

Blood supply

The penis is supplied by three *arteries*, all derived from the internal pudendal artery; the artery of the bulb runs within the corpus spongiosum, the deep arteries run within the corpora cavernosa and the dorsal artery runs superficially. The *veins* correspond to the arteries except that the dorsal veins are superficial and deep not right and left. The superficial dorsal vein divides into right and left branches which drain by the external pudendal veins into the long saphenous vein; the deep dorsal vein joins the prostatic venous plexus. *Lymph vessels* follow superficial veins to the inguinal lymph nodes.

Circumcision

The common indications for circumcision are the presence of phimosis and recurrent balanitis; the former is a narrowing of the opening of the prepuce and the latter an infection in the subprepucial space. These two conditions are often related and are both associated with incomplete retraction of the prepuce. Phimosis makes hygiene difficult, may cause discomfort during coitus and predisposes to balanitis and carcinoma. Following an erection, which can be painful, paraphimosis may occur. Circumcision is still performed extensively for cultural reasons although the removal of a normal prepuce is of no medical benefit.

Phimosis in the child may impede micturition with spraying of urine and ballooning of the foreskin but repeated retraction of the prepuce probably aggraves the situation and parents should not be encouraged to do this. In the infant, adhesions between the prepuce and the glans may prevent retraction of the prepuce and give the appearance of a phimosis. However, the difference becomes apparent when the prepuce is pulled forward from the glans rather than retracted and an adequate opening can then be seen. Prepucial adhesions rarely persist after 3 years of age but are physiological in infancy, protecting the sensitive glans from the irritation of sodden napkins. Balanitis is usually caused by staphylococcal infection of smegma or debris trapped under the prepuce. Infection is often recurrent but in some children adhesions retaining smegma can be broken down and, in the absence of phimosis, the condition will then resolve. Balanitis must be distinguished from ammoniacal dermatitis as both may present with inflammation of the prepuce. In the latter, however, the prepuce serves to protect the glans and a circumcision is therefore contraindicated.

In *children* the surgical management of phimosis and recurrent balanitis is by circumcision. Occasionally minor adhesions causing pain or recurrent infection may be successfully freed under general anaesthetic but a dorsal slit operation should rarely be necessary. In *adults*, circumcision is advisable if the phimosis is so marked that little more than the external meatus can be exposed, particularly if it is complicated by balanitis or paraphimosis, or hinders sexual function. Circumcision or a dorsal slit is also required in the assessment and treatment of patients with carcinoma of the penis.

Circumcision in the child
The operation is performed under general anaesthesia

with the child supine. The prepuce is first fully retracted to expose the coronal sulcus and retained smegma removed. To allow retraction it may be necessary to stretch the opening of the prepuce and to free adhesions by sweeping back the inner layer of the prepuce from the glans with a blunt probe. The prepuce is then returned to its normal position and the skin marked at the level of the corona, to serve as a guide to the line of dissection. Excessive suprapubic fat may carry abdominal skin onto the shaft of the penis and, before marking, this should be pushed firmly down onto the pubic symphysis so that the shaft is covered only by penile skin (Fig. 28.19). The tip of the prepuce is then grasped with two forceps and pulled forward with light traction. A narrow clamp is placed obliquely across the prepuce distal to the glans and parallel to the corona and the prepuce then divided immediately distal to the clamp (Fig. 28.20). As the clamp is released the outer layer will retract, leaving the inner layer partly covering the glans. The inner layer is then trimmed back so as to leave a cuff approximately 0.5 cm long which just covers the corona of the glans. This is most easily done by making a dorsal incision from the free margin of the inner layer to the level of the corona (Fig. 28.21); from that point the dissection is carried round both sides of the glans (Fig. 28.22) to the frenulum. Haemostasis is then secured with care, particular attention being paid to the dorsal vein and the artery within the frenulum. Finally the inner and outer layer of the prepuce are closed with fine interrupted absorbable sutures (Fig. 28.23).

A number of devices, of which the Hollister Plastibell is the best known, are available for circumcising the small infant and they make the operation simpler and quicker. The Plastibell is pushed into the space between glans and prepuce and the ligature, supplied with the kit, is applied around the lip of the bell. The prepuce is cut off with scissors and the plastic device extruded.

Circumcision in the adult
Although the operation can be done under local anaesthesia by injecting 1% Lignocaine solution subcutaneously around the body of the penis and into the sensitive region near the frenulum, it is best done under general anaesthesia. Since the prepuce is seldom as long in the adult as in the child, and is much more vascular, the clamp method is unsuitable. Three small artery forceps are applied to the edge of the prepuce, one in the midline ventrally, two (side by side) in the midline dorsally. Adhesions between the prepuce and the underlying glans are separated and the prepuce in the mid dorsal line is slit between the two dorsally placed artery forceps as far as the corona, taking great care not to enter the urethra. After smegma has been removed the redundant part of the prepuce is cut off parallel to the corona. The underlying inner layer of the prepuce is trimmed in the same

Figs. 28.19–28.23 *Circumcision in the child (see text)*

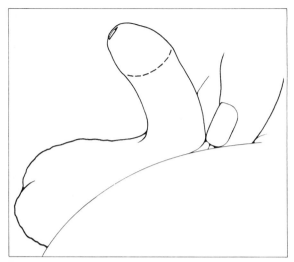

Fig. 28.19

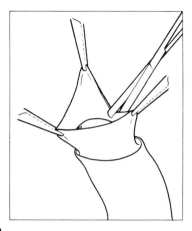

Fig. 28.21

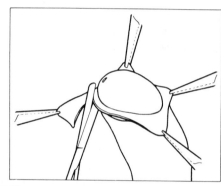

Fig. 28.22

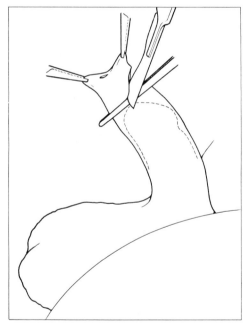

Fig. 28.20

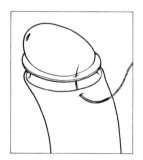

Fig. 28.23

way leaving it about 0.5 cm longer than the skin. All bleeding vessels are ligated with 4/0 absorbable sutures and the cut edge of the skin is sutured to the cut edge of the inner layer of the prepuce with the same material (Fig. 28.24). Painful erections are rarely a problem during convalescence but can be prevented with Chlorpromazine.

Paraphimosis

Paraphimosis occurs when a tight prepuce has been forcibly retracted behind the corona and remains there as a constricting ring beyond which the inner layer of the prepuce swells rapidly to form an oedematous collar which prevents reduction. In most cases manipulative reduction should be attempted before operation is considered. An attempt is made to dispel some of the oedematous fluid by squeezing; then the glans is compressed and elongated with the thumb and first two fingers of the right hand and an attempt is made to draw the prepuce down over it with the fingers and thumb of

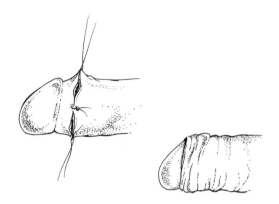

Fig. 28.24 End result of circumcision in the adult

the other hand. It is a mistake to try and push the glans upwards through the constricting ring. If manipulation fails, the constricting ring should be divided with a short longitudinal dorsal incision after which the prepuce can easily be drawn down. The incision is left unsutured. Circumcision should be carried out at a later date when all oedema and reaction has disappeared because a paraphimosis often recurs.

Tumours of the penis (see Lloyd-Davies, 1983)

Of the benign tumours the venereal wart (condyloma acuminatum), coronal papillae and the Buschke-Loewenstein tumour are the commonest. The common wart is viral in origin and found most frequently on the glans penis around the corona or at or just within the urethral meatus. Cases have been described however in which the warts have involved the whole of the urethra and even the bladder when it may be difficult to distinguish them from transitional cell tumours. Warts can be treated with 10% podophyllin or electrocoagulation although those inside the meatus may have to be exposed by a meatotomy. Coronal papillae appear as tiny pale papillary processes along the edge of the corona and they can be disregarded. Buschke-Loewenstein tumours look like enormous common warts but tend to infiltrate deeper tissues. They are not considered to be malignant because they never metastasize and they can be treated by electrocoagulation or local excision.

The malignant tumours consist of in situ carcinoma called Paget's Disease, Bowen's Disease and the Erythroplasia of Queyrat and can only be distinguished from benign skin disorders by biopsy: epithelial carcinoma of which the vast majority are squamous; connective tissue tumours like sarcomas and lymphomas are rare as are secondary tumours which have metastasized from prostate or bladder. Squamous cell carcinoma usually begins near the corona and is easily overlooked in the early

stages because it is usually hidden beneath the prepuce (which is often phimotic) or obscured by secondary infection. Many patients only seek advice when the tumour has spread down the body of the penis or to the inguinal glands. Penile carcinoma must be suspected when an elderly male patient presents with an offensive or blood stained discharge from the preputial orifice. In such cases a biopsy must be taken from the glans and the corona although it may be possible to do this only after a dorsal slit or a circumcision. The latter procedures also facilitate treatment of the local infection which is often severe.

Of the various ways of *staging* carcinoma of the penis clinically, the TNM system is probably the best although it is little used. It considers the local extent of the tumour (*T category*) separately from the state of the regional lymph nodes which are the inguinal ones (*N category*). With the other methods, the stage is decided after considering the local extent of the tumour and the state of the regional lymph nodes together. The treatment depends upon the local extent of the disease.

Carcinoma in situ

Carcinoma in situ can be treated by radiotherapy, by excision or by chemotherapy. Most surgeons would treat it first by radiotherapy because it can always be excised later if it fails to respond. If the lesion is excised the defect has usually to be covered with a skin graft. For chemotherapy 5-fluorouracil is applied locally but the treatments have to be continued for a long time and local reactions may be severe.

Carcinoma of the penis

If the growth is confined to the prepuce it may all be removed by circumcision. More often the tumour involves the glans as well as the prepuce and can be treated by X–ray therapy or partial amputation of the penis. It is worth considering X–ray therapy because amputation can still be carried out at a later date if the tumour fails to respond. If the tumour has extended to the shaft of the penis, X–ray therapy can still be considered but is likely to be less successful than it is with the earlier tumours. Partial amputation may be possible if enough healthy tissue can be left between the edge of the tumour and the incision otherwise a total amputation should be carried out particularly if the tumour has recurred after a previous partial resection.

Amputation of the penis

Before partial or total amputation of the penis the patient will already have had a dorsal slit or circumcision and biopsy and some treatment to ameliorate the local infection.

Figs. 28.25–28.28 *The operation of partial amputation of the penis for carcinoma by the flap method*

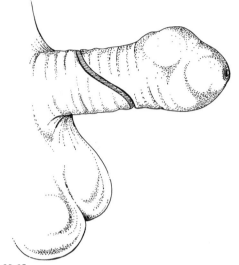

Fig. 28.25

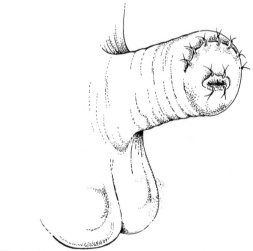

Fig. 28.26

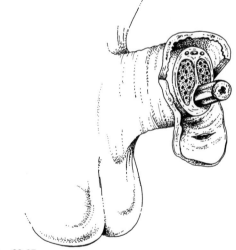

Fig. 28.27

Fig. 28.28

Partial amputation (Figs. 28.25–28.28)

A *flap* method (Fig. 28.25) is commonly employed. A fine catheter, a piece of soft rubber tubing or a non crushing intestinal clamp is applied around the base of the penis as a tourniquet. The combined lengths of the two flaps, the cut edges of which must be at least 2.5 cm clear of the growth, should be a little more than the diameter of the penis. The inferior flap should be longer than the superior one so that the suture line is at a higher level than the urethra which is brought out through a stab incision in the inferior flap. The flaps are fashioned by incising skin and subcutaneous tissue down to Buck's fascia which covers the corpora cavernosa and the corpus spongiosum and reflecting them back to their bases. The corpora cavernosa are divided at this level but the corpus spongiosum and the urethra are divided some 1.5 to 2 cm more distally. The tourniquet is now removed and all bleeding vessels secured. The stump of the urethra is brought through a suitably placed stab wound in the inferior skin flap. The end of the emerging urethra is split into two halves by short lateral incisions and each half is sutured beyond the margin of the stab wound so that the urethra protrudes slightly beyond the skin. If haemostasis proves difficult the wound can be drained. A selfretaining catheter is introduced into the bladder and removed some 4 or 5 days later. The new external urinary meatus may have to be dilated periodically with bougies but, unless the stump of the penis is very short, the patient should experience no difficulty with micturition.

Total amputation of the penis
The patient is placed in the lithotomy-Trendelenberg position and the penis is enclosed in a polythene or rubber glove to allow cleaning of the whole area. A racquet incision is made encircling the base of the penis and is carried backwards in the midline of the scrotum and perineum to a point some 2–3 cm in front of the anus. Alternatively, an inverted U scrotal flap is used extending the incision forwards to encircle the base of the penis. By dissection exactly in the midline towards a bougie which has been placed in the urethra, the scrotum is split into two halves which are retracted laterally. The penis is then mobilized anteriorly by dividing the suspensory ligament and ligating the dorsal vessels. The penis is further separated from the pubic arch, and the deep vessels (especially the deep dorsal vein of the penis) ligated. The perineal part of the incision is deepened to expose the bulb of the penis (covered by the bulbospongiosus muscle) and the crura (each covered by the ischiocavernosus muscle). The bulb is separated from the anterior part of the perineal membrane, and the crura are detached from the margins of the pubic arch and divided, leaving a thin rim of tissue which is secured with sutures to control bleeding. The bougie is now removed; the urethra is dissected out of the muscular fibres surrounding the bulb and is divided about 5 cm below the perineal membrane.

The anterior part of the wound is repaired by suturing the skin flaps together in the midline; the posterior part is sutured around the stump of the urethra so that this now pursues a direct course from the bladder neck to the perineum and protudes some 5 cm beyond the skin. The protuding part of the urethral stump is split into two halves by making short anterior and posterior incisions; these are then separated and loosely sutured to overlap the surrounding skin edges. A catheter is left in the bladder for some days. The perineal urethral meatus functions well and seldom becomes stenosed.

In the operation described, the scrotum and testes are retained. Many patients find that the perineal urethrostomy is difficult to manage so long as the scrotum remains, because it tends to get in the way of the urinary stream and becomes wet and excoriated. It may be preferable, therefore, to remove the scrotum and testes as part of the procedure.

Treatment of the inguinal lymph nodes in penile carcinoma
Few surgeons remove the inguinal lymph nodes at the time of amputation of the penis because lymph node enlargement is often due to secondary infection and subsides after the primary growth is removed. If the glands remain enlarged for some weeks after the operation—particularly if they feel hard—biopsy is advisable. If this confirms metastatic disease and if there is no reason to suppose from pedal lymphangiography or CAT scan that deeper glands are also involved, a block dissection of the inguinal glands can be carried out or they can be treated by X–ray therapy.

Anatomy of the inguinal lymph nodes
The *superficial nodes*, which are numerous and large, are often palpable even when healthy. They form two chains forming the letter T; a horizontal chain immediately below the inguinal ligament, and a vertical one along the upper 5–8 cm of the long saphenous vein. They receive lymph from the superficial tissues of the greater part of the abdominal wall and lower limb, from the external genitalia, the buttocks and the anal canal. The *deep nodes*, 4 or 5 in number, lie alongside the proximal end of the femoral vein, the uppermost one being within the femoral canal. They receive lymph from the superficial glands and from the deep tissues of the lower limb and drain to nodes around the external and common iliac vessels.

Biopsy of the inguinal lymph nodes
Biopsy from enlarged inguinal lymph nodes or from clinically normal nodes should be taken from the superficial nodes which lie superomedially and can be carried out through an incision or by percutaneous aspiration.

Inguinal gland dissection
An incision is made 2 cm above and parallel to the whole length of the inguinal ligament. The upper skin flap is reflected and the incision is deepened through the fat to expose the external oblique aponeurosis some 5 cm above the ligament. All fascial and glandular tissue is then stripped cleanly off the aponeurosis down to the level of the inguinal ligament, securing three small arteries, the superficial circumflex iliac, the superficial epigastric and the superficial external pudendal together with their accompanying veins. The lower margin of the wound is strongly retracted; the long saphenous vein is divided between ligatures at least 10 cm below the ligament, and its stump is turned upwards together with all surrounding fat and lymph glands. The partially separated tissue is now stripped off the inguinal ligament from lateral to medial side. As this dissection proceeds, the small arteries already secured and the long saphenous

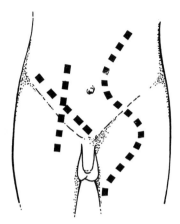

Fig. 28.29 The incisions used for inguinal lymph node dissection. On the patient's right side is shown the oblique incision just above the inguinal ligament and the vertical incision. On the left is shown the flap incision which heals better because the blood supply to the medial flap is preserved

vein are divided again at their junctions with the femoral vessels, which are now left clearly exposed. All fatty and glandular tissue is cleared away from the medial side of the femoral vein and from the femoral canal.

There is usually profuse discharge of lymph after operation and free drainage of the wound should always be provided. Sepsis often occurs and lymphoedema of one or even both legs is common. Healing of the wound is facilitated if the skin incision is not a simple linear one above and parallel to the inguinal ligament, but a flap incision (Fig. 28.29), which leaves intact the superficial inguinal, the superficial external pudendal and the superficial circumflex iliac arteries.

Curvature of the penis

Curvature of the penis may be congenital or acquired. The congenital forms are often associated with epispadias or hypospadias (see p. 622). The most common acquired form is Peyronie's disease which is an inflammatory process with fibrotic changes in the elastic connective tissue of the corpora cavernosa of unknown aetiology. 10% of patients with Peyronie's disease also have Dupuytren's contracture and some 3% of patients with Dupuytren's contracture also have Peyronie's disease. The disease usually begins in middle life but is sometimes found in younger men. Most patients present complaining of angulated and painful erection but some complain of a lump in the penis. The lump consists of a plaque of fibrous tissue which replaces some of the elastic tissue of the corpora cavernosa. This plaque of fibrous tissue does not elongate as the penis expands with erection. The penis therefore becomes angulated and

painful when erect. Although impotence is not a feature of Peyronie's disease, the penis beyond the plaque does not become as erect as the rest of the penis and some patients develop psychological impotence if they have had the disease a long time.

The patient must be reassured that the disease is not cancer and that there is every reason to believe that it will improve although it may take a long time in doing so. It is doubtful if the disease should be treated unless it is causing pain or interfering with intercouse. If treatment is required a number of drugs are available including Alpha Tocopheryl Acetate (Vitamin E), Potassium Amino Benzoate (Potaba), Phenylbutazone and Corticosteroids which can be injected locally or given parenterally and they should probably be tried in that order. Operation should only be considered in patients who remain incapacitated a year or more after the condition was first diagnosed, because the disease has not resolved or has failed to respond to medical treatment.

Operations aimed at removing the fibrous plaque and replacing it with a skin graft are nearly always unsuccessful and frequently make the condition worse. The best operation is the Nesbit procedure in which a wedge of Buck's fascia is excised from the convex aspect of the curve without damaging the corpora cavernosa or corpus spongiosum and without touching the fibrous plaque, the effect being like that of an osteotomy (Pryor, 1979).

Operation

A Foley catheter is first passed into the bladder along the urethra. A circumferential incision is made through the penile skin 1 cm proximal to the corona and the prepuce is excised unless the patient has already been circumcised. The skin can now be drawn back easily, like a sleeve, to the base of the penis exposing Buck's fascia, which is the extension into the penis of the membranous layer of superficial fascia. Buck's fascia is incised longitudinally to expose the corpus spongiosum (which contains the urethra) and the thick fibrous tissue of the tunica albuginea which surrounds and binds together the corpora cavernosa. The corpus spongiosum is separated from the corpora cavernosa for some 5 cm by sharp dissection, avoiding damage to the erectile tissue and the urethra. The corpus spongiosum can now be secured with tapes or Paul's tubing and retracted. To determine precisely the site and size of the wedge, it is now necessary to produce an artificial erection by injecting or infusing into the corpora carvenosa about 100 ml or more of sterile saline after temporarily excluding the venous return from the penis by applying a light occlusion clamp across its base or by compressing the crura against the under surfaces of the pubic rami. The most convex aspect of the artificially erected penis is marked with a stitch in the tunica albuginea. Two parallel incisions, 0.5 cm to 1 cm apart depending on the degree of angulation, are made through the tunica albuginea for about half the circumference of the penis centred on the point of greatest convexity. The tunica is excised between the incisions and the cut edges are sutured together using polyglycolic acid, catgut or polydioxanone sutures in such a way that the knots lie deeply. Alternatively the intervening tunica can be buried and not excised. The skin is drawn back to the tip of the penis and sutured as after a circumcision. The urethral catheter is removed 24 hours later.

Hypospadias

Hypospadias is a congenital malformation in which incomplete fusion of the urethral folds results in an ectopic urethral meatus on the ventral aspect of the penis proximal to the normal opening. Depending on the position of the meatus the condition may be described as *glandular*, *coronal*, *penile*, *penoscrotal*, *scrotal* or *perineal*. The meatus is often stenosed though it may be of normal size. The prepuce fails to fuse along the ventral aspect and has a characteristic hooded appearance. The penis may be bowed (*chordee*) by a fibrous band running forward from the ectopic meatus to the corona; this appearance may be exaggerated or indeed only apparent when the penis is erect. There is an increased incidence of upper urinary tract abnormality in boys with hypospadias and those with urinary tract symptoms should have an intravenous urogram performed early. Problems of intersex must be considered in boys with scrotal or perineal hypospadias and the scrotum must be carefully examined to confirm that normal testes are present.

A glandular or coronal hypospadias may cause no problem. However, when the malformation is more severe urine may be sprayed downwards and backwards during micturition and bowing of the penis may prevent normal coitus.

Depending on the severity of the lesion, three stages may be necessary to correct the malformation; meatotomy for meatal stenosis, straightening of the penis by release of chordee, and urethroplasty. The procedures can conveniently be performed in the first, second and fourth years of life respectively.

Meatotomy

This can easily be performed by introducing the point of a blade or scissors into the urethra and cutting back in the midline through the ventral wall of the urethra and the overlying skin. The cut margins of urethral mucosa and skin are then sewn together with a fine absorbable suture.

Straightening of the penis

Chordee is corrected by excising the fibrous cord lying between the ectopic meatus and the corona. A transverse skin incision is made over the ventral aspect of the penis just proximal to the corona and extended on either side into the prepuce. The skin flaps are generously undermined and the underlying fibrous cord completely excised. As the penis is straightened it will be noted that the ectopic meatus falls back into a more proximal position. The skin incision is then closed longitudinally with a fine absorbable suture.

Reconstruction of the urethra

Most techniques of urethroplasty depend on the concept that a buried skin strip forms an epithelial tube by proliferation from the edges. Thus, a distal urethra can be created by fashioning a 1 cm strip that runs from the ectopic meatus to the end of the glans and by covering that strip with skin taken from elsewhere on the penis. In Van der Meulen's operation (1977) use is made of excessive skin from the dorsum of the prepuce whilst in the Denis Browne operation (1949) skin is mobilized from the shaft of the penis.

Van der Meulen's operation is particularly suitable when the meatus lies in the distal half of the penis. A circumferential skin incision is made starting just proximal to the ectopic meatus, running distally on either side of the midline towards the corona so as to leave a strip of skin 1 cm wide and then extended along the free margin of the prepuce (Fig. 28.30). The skin is undermined along the length of the shaft of the penis and rotated so that the skin from the dorsal aspect of the prepuce comes to cover the ventral surface of the glans (Fig. 28.31, 28.32). An oblique incision on the dorsum of the penis allows the flap to be rotated more freely. The skin strip from the ectopic meatus is then extended along the length of the glans by excising two triangular areas of skin from the ventral surface on either side of the midline. Using fine absorbable sutures the skin flap is then sewn to the outer margin of the triangles (Fig. 28.33). The rotation creates a deficiency on the dorsum of the penis which is filled by folding back the inner layer of the prepuce. The skin margins around the remaining circumference of the penis can then be sewn together with ease.

Denis Browne's operation may be preferred when the ectopic meatus lies in the proximal half of the shaft of the penis. As a preliminary to the procedure, suprapubic bladder drainage can be established with a 12F Malecot catheter. A U-shaped skin incision including the ectopic meatus is made to fashion a skin strip 1 cm in width on the ventral surface of the penis from the meatus to the glans. Lateral flaps are then created by extensively undermining the remaining skin round the shaft of the

Figs. 28.30–28.33 *Van der Meulen's operation for hypospadias (see text)*

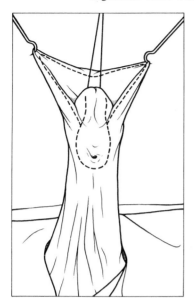

Fig. 28.30

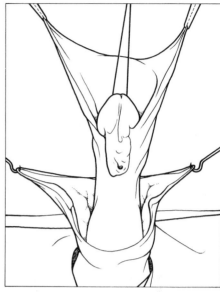

Fig. 28.31

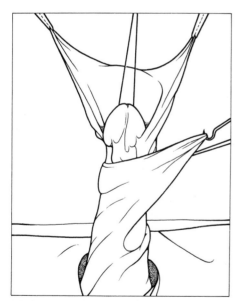

Fig. 28.32

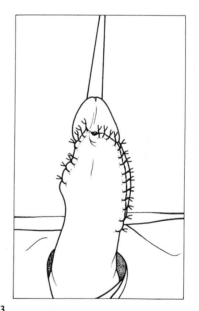

Fig. 28.33

penis. A releasing incision along the full length of the dorsum of the penis enables the lateral flaps to be brought together in the midline along the ventral aspect so as to cover the skin strip. The flaps are then sutured with fine absorbable stitches. Denis Browne used tension sutures supported by beads to protect the tissues. The tension sutures are removed after 7 days and the suprapubic catheter after 10. The raw area on the dorsum of the penis gradually epithelialises.

THE TESTES, THE SPERMATIC CORD AND THE SCROTUM

Anatomy

The testis is oval in shape and measures about 4 cm by 2.0 cm by 2.5 cm. Dense fibrous tissue, the *tunica albuginea*, encloses the testis and projects posteriorly into it as the *mediastinum testis* which is pierced by the efferent ducts of the testis and by blood vessels and lymphatics

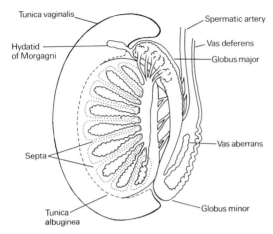

Fig. 28.34 A sagittal section of the testis and epididymis

(Fig. 28.34). *The epididymis*, crescentic in shape and attached to the posterior border of the testis, has a head, body and tail. The tail becomes the vas deferens which runs upwards behind the testis to join the spermatic cord. The *tunica vaginalis*, which is derived from peritoneum, surrounds the testis and epididymis and extends upwards for a short distance into the spermatic cord. It has a *parietal* layer that lines the scrotal cavity and a *visceral* layer that covers the testis and epididymis. The two layers become continuous posteriorly forming a broad ligament called the *mesorchium* that attaches the testis and epididymis to the posterior wall of the scrotum. The testis is covered by the external spermatic fascia, the cremasteric muscle and fascia and the internal spermatic fascia, all of which are derived from the abdominal wall.

Blood supply
The testis is supplied not only by the testicular artery, which arises from the aorta at the level of the first lumbar vertebra, but also by the cremasteric artery, the artery to the vas deferens, and the posterior scrotal arteries. Veins from the testis form the *pampiniform plexus* which drains into the testicular vein. The right testicular vein joins the inferior vena cava, the left one joins the left renal vein. *Lymphatic vessels* from the testis run upwards in the spermatic cord alongside the veins and end in the para-aortic lymph nodes at the level of the first lumbar vertebra (Smith, 1983).

The spermatic cord and its coverings (which are those of the testis also) have been described on page 480.

The scrotum is composed of skin, muscle and fascia. It is divided by a median septum into two compartments. The superficial fascia is devoid of fat, and is largely replaced by a thin sheet of unstriped muscle, the *dartos*.

The wall of each scrotal chamber consists from without inwards of skin, dartos muscle, the three coverings of the testis and the parietal layer of the tunica vaginalis. These structures are traversed in aspiration of a hydrocele, or in exposure of the testis through the scrotum.

Lymphatic drainage of the scrotum takes place to the inguinal glands.

Imperfect descent of the testes
Imperfect descent of one or both testes in boys is relatively common, the incidence being approximately 0.3% of the male population. Several problems are associated with the condition of which the two most important are impaired spermatogenesis and an increased incidence of testicular tumour. Because of these problems, such children should undergo orchidopexy, an operation in which the testis is transferred from the abnormal site to the scrotum.

Embryology. The testis develops in the embryo from the genital ridge in the germinal epithelium and can be recognized in the upper lumbar region and in front of the mesonephros at 6 weeks. The testis then migrates caudally and comes to lie in the iliac fossa at 3 months. Little further movement takes place until the 7th and 8th months when the testis, preceded by the tunica vaginalis and following the line of the gubernaculum, passes through the inguinal canal to the scrotum. The factors responsible for descent are not understood but placental chorionic gonadatrophins and interstitial cell function influence the final stages.

Classification. The testis may be absent from the scrotum because of imperfect descent or because of retraction into the abdominal wall by cremaster muscle. The distinction is important since the retractile testis will come to lie in the scrotum in due course and should be regarded as a variant of normal. The imperfectly descended testis is abnormal and may be either incompletely descended or ectopic. The *incompletely descended testis* lies along the line of normal descent and may therefore be found in the abdomen, the inguinal canal, the superficial inguinal tissues or immediately above the neck of the scrotum. The *ectopic testis* is said to have deviated from the normal line of descent; it is usually found in the superficial inguinal pouch, above and lateral to the external inguinal ring, but may occasionally lie in the femoral or perineal tissue or at the base of the penis.

Associated problems. A number of problems are associated with imperfect descent of the testes. Spermatogenesis is impaired, there is an increased incidence of testicular tumour, the risk of both torsion and trauma are greater, inguinal herniae are more common and, finally, the appearance may be the cause of severe embarrassment.

Impaired spermatogenesis in a male with bilateral imperfect descent of the testes is likely to be the cause of infertility. Early changes indicating impaired development are present by 5 years of age and become increasingly evident with time. Failure of maturation may be related to the temperature differential between the abdomen and the scrotum or to primary tissue dysplasia. The value of orchidopexy with regard to spermatogenesis is difficult to assess; it is doubtful that established changes in the testis are reversed but it is quite probable that further deterioration is prevented.

The association of malignant change and imperfect descent of the testis is well established; the incidence of tumour developing in an abnormal testis is thirty times greater than normal and it is interesting to note that the abdominal testis is particularly at risk. Curiously, the incidence of malignant change in the normal testis of a man with unilateral descent is also greater than normal. The advantage of orchidopexy in averting malignancy is difficult to assess; it is doubtful that the operation carried out after puberty alters the prognosis but it is suggested that the procedure carried out in a younger child may be of value.

Clinical evaluation. The condition usually presents in childhood but surprisingly often remains unnoticed until the first school medical examination. Less often the patient presents for the first time in adult life and this may be because of infertility. The clinical assessment of a child needs to be carried out with great care. Questions should be asked about torsion, trauma, orchitis and mumps. Both the weight and height should be recorded on percentile charts. The child should be warm and relaxed and placed supine on an examination couch with the legs slightly apart. It is important to note the development of the penis and scrotum as bilateral impalpable testes in association with microgenitalia raises the possibility of endocrine or chromosome abnormality. The scrotum should be examined next as, not infrequently, two normal testes are found.

An attempt is then made to locate the testis and to push it down into the scrotum so that a distinction can be made between imperfect descent and retraction. First the superficial inguinal and prepubic tissue is palpated. If no testis is found, as is particularly common in the obese child, an attempt is made to displace the gonad from the superficial inguinal pouch or the inguinal canal towards the neck of the scrotum where it can be felt more easily. This is achieved by sweeping fingers of one hand firmly across the inguinal region from the anterior superior iliac spine towards the pubic tubercle and placing the fingers of the other hand at the neck of the scrotum. If the testis can be pushed through the neck of the scrotum it should be lightly grasped and pulled down towards the normal position. The testis which remains impalpable may either lie in one of the less common ectopic positions or it may be intra-abdominal, hypoplastic or absent.

The typical ectopic testis lies above and lateral to the external inguinal ring; it can be felt with relative ease both with abdominal muscles relaxed and tense and,

when pushed towards the scrotum, will run down and lateral to the neck of the sac. The incompletely descended testis often lies in the inguinal canal; it may be difficult to feel initially but, with manipulation, may be pushed through the external ring towards the neck of the scrotum. The retractile testis lies in the superficial inguinal tissues and can be drawn down into the middle or lower thirds of the scrotum; the testis remains temporarily within the scrotum when pressure is released but is promptly withdrawn into the abdominal wall when the cremaster reflex is stimulated by touching the inner aspect of the thigh. When there is doubt it is helpful to ask the child to squat down as, in this position, the cremaster reflex is diminished and the testis may move spontaneously into the scrotum. In some children the testis lies in the superficial inguinal tissues, can be manipulated into the upper third of the scrotum but retracts when pressure is released. In this group it is difficult to distinguish between imperfect descent and a retractile testis; if the latter seems more probable the child can safely be reviewed at a later date.

Management

Investigation of a child with imperfect descent of testes is rarely necessary unless a chromosome or endocrine abnormality is suspected. Hormonal therapy using intramuscular testosterone to provoke testicular descent has some advocates but doubtful efficacy; side effects and the discomfort of the injections have discouraged more general acceptance. More recently luteinizing hormone releasing hormone, which stimulates pituitary gonadotrophins, has become available as a nasal spray and this may prove more acceptable. Orchidopexy should, under normal circumstances, be recommended for all children with incomplete descent of the testis. Orchidectomy should not be considered before puberty as interstitial cell function remains although spermatogenesis is impaired. It is an ideal to achieve orchidopexy before the child is 5 years old (Ashby, 1980), although many boys have not been diagnosed at this age.

The object of orchidopexy is that the testis should be mobilized and placed in the scrotum without tension on the testicular vessels. Occasionally mobilization may be inadequate to allow the testis to be placed in the scrotum; the testis should then be fixed at a point in the normal line of descent and a second operation may be performed at a later date. If at operation no testicle is found a search should be made of the inguinal canal for a structure resembling a vas deferens which may lead distally to a hypoplastic gonad that can be excised. In the absence of a vas deferens it can be assumed that the testis is intraabdominal or absent. It is then prudent to continue the search in the extraperitoneal tissues (Jones, 1979) through an incision two cm above the deep ring as described in the operation for varicocoele on p. 633.

Orchidopexy

A skin crease incision is made 1 cm above and parallel to the medial two thirds of the inguinal ligament. The subcutaneous tissue is explored with care as the testis may lie in the superficial inguinal pouch immediately deep to Scarpa's fascia. Once found, the tunica of the testis is cleared of adherent tissue and the gubernaculum at the lower pole divided. Artery forceps are then applied to the tunica and, with gentle traction, the spermatic cord will be seen emerging from the external inguinal ring. The inguinal canal is then opened by dividing external oblique aponeurosis in the line of its fibres. Cremasteric fascia is cleared from the spermatic cord by blunt gauze dissection so that the cord lies free up to the internal ring (Fig. 28.35).

The covering of the cord is then divided longitudinally and the free margins held apart with forceps so as to expose the contents. A hernial sac will usually be found and, using the technique described on p. 482, an inguinal herniotomy is performed. In the proximal part of the cord the vas deferens and testicular vessels are dissected free from surrounding tissue. The vas and vessels are then held to one side and the remaining tissue divided transversely (Fig. 28.36).

At this stage the testis is suspended from the internal ring only by the vas and vessels and can usually be placed within the scrotum. However, if needed, greater length can be provided by retroperitoneal dissection of the vessels and by releasing the fascia restricting the vas at the medial margin of the internal ring. The vessels are tethered by the overlying peritoneum and by fascial bands that run laterally in a retroperitoneal plane. The peritoneum is lifted free by blunt dissection using a finger or gauze pledget and the bands, which are clearly seen when the vessels are under traction, are divided (Fig. 28.37)

The testis should only be placed in the scrotum when it lies without tension on the vessels. To prevent accidental displacement, it is usual to *fix* the testis in place and a dartos pouch (Figs. 28.38–28.42) provides a convenient method. First a finger is pushed through the inguinal wound to break down fascia occluding the neck

Figs. 28.35–28.37 *Mobilization of the testis and spermatic cord for orchidopexy*

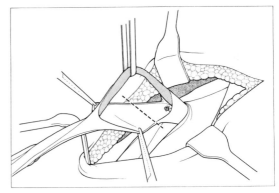

Fig. 28.36

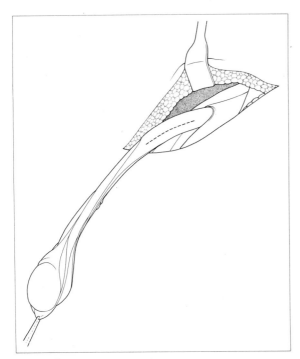

Fig. 28.35

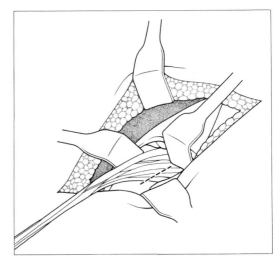

Fig. 28.37

Figs. 28.38–28.42 *Dartos pouch method of fixation*

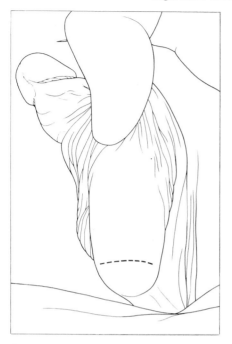

Fig. 28.38

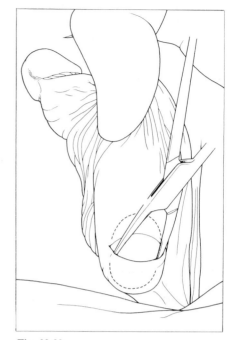

Fig. 28.39

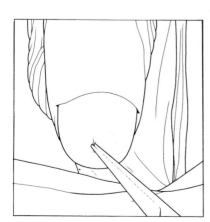

Fig. 28.40

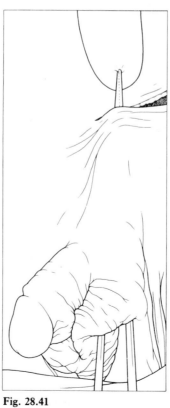

Fig. 28.41

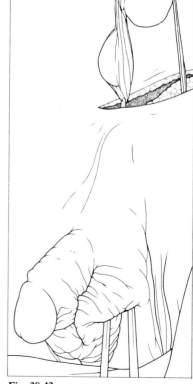

Fig. 28.42

of the scrotum and to stretch the corrugated skin. With the finger still in place, the skin over the lower part of the scrotum is incised and a pouch made between the skin and dartos fascia. An artery forceps is then pushed through the dartos fascia, through the scrotum and up to the inguinal wound where the testis is grasped. By withdrawing the forceps, the testis is pulled down through the dartos fascia into the pouch and is retained in position by the narrow opening in the fascia. The scrotal skin is then closed over the testis with absorbable interrupted sutures.

A final check is made of the testicular vessels and vas in the inguinal canal to exclude tension or torsion and the inguinal wound is closed in layers.

Torsion of the testis (or torsion of the spermatic cord)

The testis and epididymis are suspended in the scrotum by the spermatic cord which passes through the mesorchium. If the mesorchium is abnormally long or narrow (bell-clapper type of testis) torsion can occur within the tunica vaginalis and this is called *intravaginal* torsion (Fig. 28.43). *Extravaginal* torsion occurs when the cord twists above the mesorchium and the whole tunica (including the parietal layer) rotates within the scrotum but is rare. Torsion occurs most commonly in adolescents between the ages of 12 and 16 and in a distressingly large proportion of cases is misdiagnosed. It is often considered to be epididymitis, because the signs are similar to those of acute inflammation, but infarction and atrophy of the testis inevitably results if it is treated as such. The age of the patient distinguishes torsion from epididymitis because epididymitis is rare before the age of 20. The onset of torsion is sudden with pain, often referred to the iliac fossa, and swelling in the scrotum associated with nausea. The affected side becomes tender and red with oedematous and sometimes bruised skin. Because the cord is twisted and shortened, both epididymis and testis lie at a high level in the scrotum but it is usually impossible to distinguish by palpation one from the other. It is a good rule that *a swollen and painful testis in a boy in his 'teens is a torsion until proved otherwise by operation.* Torsion is much less common in adults but may be suspected if an acute scrotal condition develops without obvious cause. Torsion of an undescended testis may be mistaken for a strangulated inguinal hernia but the true diagnosis should be reached by operation.

Immediate operation should be undertaken on *suspicion* alone, since the testis cannot survive more than 6 hours ischaemia. As the torsion is usually intravaginal, it is best approached through a scrotal incision and is untwisted. The direction of torsion is usually obvious at operation and generally anticlockwise on the left and clockwise on the right. If the testis seems viable it is returned to the scrotum and anchored to the scrotal wall with two or three sutures to prevent recurrence. If the testis is obviously nonviable, it should probably still be replaced in the scrotum, even though it will atrophy because sufficient interstitial cells may survive to produce some testosterone. The anomaly that predisposes to torsion is usually bilateral and, if torsion occurs in one testis, it is very likely to occur at a later date in the other which must also be fixed. Fixation of both testes should of course be advised if the torsion reduced spontaneously without operation.

Technique

To fix a testis in these circumstances, an incision 1 cm long is made through skin, scrotal coverings and into the tunica albuginea. A few 3/0 catgut sutures are then inserted through skin and tunica albuginea, and tied, so that the testis is secured to the skin of the scrotum.

Torsion of the appendix testis

The appendix testis, or Hydatid of Morgagni (Fig. 28.34) is a small pedunculated structure attached to the tunica albuginea on the anterior aspect of the testis and it is a remnant of the Müllerian or paramesonephric duct. The clinical features of torsion of the appendix testis are similar to, but less severe than, those of torsion of the testis. The pain is severe, but localized and the twisted appendix can usually be palpated, or even seen through the scrotal skin. The testis and epididymis can be recognized as normal, unless a hydrocele forms. The lesion is treated by excising the twisted appendix testis through a small scrotal incision.

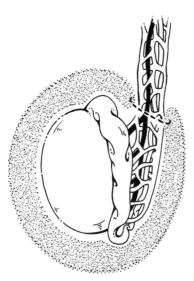

Fig. 28.43 Intravaginal torsion of the testis. Note the narrow mesorchium compared with Fig. 28.34

Orchidectomy

There are a number of indications for the removal of a testis, but malignant disease is the principal one. Orchidopexy (p. 626) is the operation of choice for the ectopic or undescended testis before puberty, but orchidectomy is best after puberty unless the condition is bilateral, when orchidopexy should still be attempted. The repair of large indirect or direct inguinal herniae in elderly men is often facilitated if the testis is removed and the inguinal canal obliterated. Orchidectomy is the operation of choice in the rare granulomatous disease of the testis, and, in carcinoma of the prostate, orchidectomy is frequently advocated but usually done by the subcapsular method (p. 630).

Malignant disease (see Einhorn, 1979)

Most patients with a testicular tumour present with a painless lump in the testis. Lumps in the testis should always be explored if doubt exists as to their nature. Apart from malignant disease only syphilis, granulomatous lesions and mumps produce lumps in the testis and only the last of these can be confidently diagnosed without operation (and then only if the patient has or has recently had mumps in one or more salivary glands). It is important not to be misled by a history of trauma, of variations in the size of the lump and of its response to tablets. Before operation, the tumour markers, Human chorionic gonadotrophin (HCG), Alphafetoprotein (AFP), and Lactic dehydrogenase (LDH) must be estimated in the blood, since changes in their levels after orchidectomy can be a useful means of monitoring the progress of the disease. Chest X-ray, intravenous urography, CAT scans and lymphangiography can all be deferred until after operation unless it is proposed that the para-aortic lymph nodes should be removed at the

time of orchidectomy. Orchidectomy for nonmalignant disease can be carried out through a scrotal or an inguinal incision, but for malignant disease a more radical procedure is done through an inguinal incision.

Orchidectomy for malignant disease (see Hendry, 1981)

Through an incision (Fig. 28.44) above the appropriate inguinal ligament, the inguinal canal is opened. (Fig. 28.45). The spermatic cord is freed from the internal spermatic fascia and mobilized to the deep inguinal ring where it is divided between ligatures (Fig. 28.46). The cord and testis are then mobilized and removed. If the tumour is large, removal is facilitated by

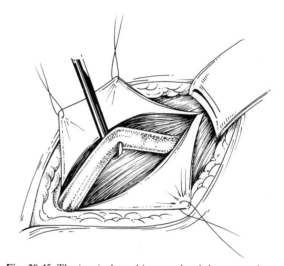

Fig. 28.45 The inguinal canal is opened and the spermatic cord is gently mobilized upwards to the deep inguinal ring

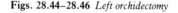

Figs. 28.44–28.46 *Left orchidectomy*

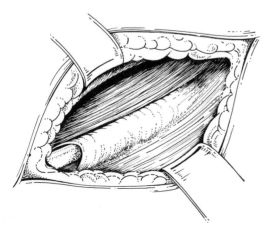

Fig. 28.44 The skin is incised parallel to the inguinal ligament and the external oblique aponeurosis exposed

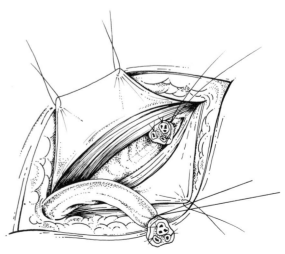

Fig. 28.46 The cord is ligated at the deep inguinal ring and divided

extending the skin incision into the neck of the scrotum, but scrotal skin need only be excised with the tumour if it is adherent.

If the nature of the swelling is uncertain, the testis may be examined and a frozen section taken before proceeding to orchidectomy. Instead of dividing the spermatic cord between ligatures, the vessels are occluded with a Potts or Craaford arterial occlusion clamp. The cord and the testis can then be mobilized and delivered through the wound. Unless the diagnosis is obvious, a biopsy can be taken, making sure that no cells spill into the wound. If the lesion is malignant it is easy to ligate and divide the cord. The wound is sutured in layers and not usually drained. Some surgeons have reported dysplasia or carcinoma in situ of the normal (contralateral) testis in a significant proportion of patients with testicular tumour. However, it is not yet common practice to take a biopsy from the normal testis unless it feels abnormal.

Subcapsular orchidectomy
Removal of testicular substance from within the tunica vaginalis is frequently carried out in patients with M1 category carcinoma of the prostate instead of (and sometimes as well as) giving oestrogens and is now generally regarded to be as satisfactory a method of treating this disease as a formal orchidectomy.

It can be carried out through a scrotal incision. The tunica albuginea is exposed and incised anteriorly from top to bottom revealing the seminiferous tubules (Fig. 28.47). These are easily freed from the inside of the tunica with a swab or pledget except posteriorly, where the vessels enter. The vessels are clamped and the tubules severed from their attachments. The tunica is

plicated with a catgut stitch (Fig. 28.48), and the wound is closed. The same procedure is carried out on the other testis through another scrotal incision.

Epididymectomy
This operation is rarely if ever done now but it may be indicated for a tuberculous infection of the epididymis when no other active focus can be discovered, and when it shows no response to the appropriate chemotherapy. The testis is exposed through an inguinal or a scrotal incision. The tunica vaginalis is opened and it is confirmed that the disease is confined to the epididymis. Separation of the epididymis from the body of the testis and from the tunica vaginalis is commenced at its lower pole taking care not to damage the testicular vessels entering the mesorchium. The vas deferens may be divided at the upper pole of the epididymis, but if it also is involved it should be divided as close to the deep inguinal ring as possible.

Hydrocele
A hydrocele is a collection of clear fluid within the tunica vaginalis. Hydroceles can be classified as congenital, encysted, infantile or vaginal (idiopathic). The vaginal or idiopathic hydrocele occurs in a normally formed tunica vaginalis and is by far the commonest. The other varieties occur when the tunica is abnormal and the processus vaginalis fails to close in whole or in part. In the congenital hydrocele the tunica communicates with the peritoneal cavity, and the fluid disappears into the abdomen when the scrotum is elevated (indeed the fluid in the hydrocele may be ascitic fluid). The emptied congenital hydrocele forms a smooth oval swelling associated with the spermatic cord, and is often mistaken for

Figs. 28.47 & 28.48 *Subcapsular orchidectomy*

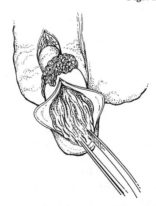

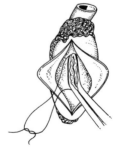

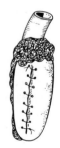

Fig. 28.47 The testis has been exposed through a scrotal incision and the tunica albuginea incised vertically (to expose the seminiferous tubules). The seminiferous tubules are separated from the inside of the tunica with a swab or pledget.

Fig. 28.48 The seminiferous tubules are removed and their blood vessels clamped and ligated. The tunica albuginea is then repaired with a catgut stitch

a hernia. An infantile hydrocele extends as far as the deep inguinal ring but does not communicate with the peritoneal cavity. In the child, excision of the processus vaginalis within the inguinal canal resolves *congenital hydrocoele* or *hydrocoele of the cord* (p. 482).

Vaginal hydrocele

The condition is called idiopathic because the pathogenesis is obscure, but it may be associated with disease of the testis or epididymis, or follow an operation for hernia or varicocele. Many patients with small hydroceles seek reassurance that the condition is not serious, rather than treatment; others require treatment. Cure of an adult hydrocele by operation is usually advised but aspiration (tapping) with or without injection treatment may be preferred. Aspiration is painless, can be carried out in an ambulant patient and rarely causes haematoma, but gives only temporary relief because the fluid inevitably reaccumulates.

Aspiration. The position of the testis, which usually lies posteriorly, is confirmed by palpation and transillumination. The scrotum is grasped so that the fluid is pressed towards the lower anterior part of sac, rendering it tense. A small wheal of local anaesthetic solution is raised in an area of the scrotal skin that is free of visible vessels, and well clear of the testis. A fine trocar and cannula (or needle cannula, Fig. 3.30) is thrust through it into the sac. After all fluid has been evacuated and the cannula withdrawn, the testis is carefully examined to ensure that it is healthy.

Injection treatment. The solution most commonly employed is made up to the following formula:

Quinine hydrochloride	4 g
Urethane	2 g
Water for injection	30 ml

10 ml of this solution is injected through the cannula into the cavity of the tunica vaginalis when all the hydrocele fluid has been evacuated. Gentle massage is employed to disperse the solution throughout the cavity of the tunica, and the scrotum is supported for some days with a suspensory bandage. The procedure may be repeated at a later date if necessary, using 5 ml of the solution. An alternative solution is 2 ml sodium tetradecyl (see p. 48) used for sclerotherapy.

Inguinal approach

The incision is placed over the superficial inguinal ring. A finger is passed downwards and swept around the hydrocele sac to separate it from the inside of the scrotum. The sac together with the testis and epididymis is pushed out of the scrotum into the wound. If the sac is very large, its fluid content can be aspirated before it is pushed out of the scrotum. After the coverings have been stripped aside an opening is made into the tunica vaginalis and the testis is carefully examined. If it is

healthy the hydrocele alone requires treatment. If the hydrocele is small and the sac thin walled the Jaboulay procedure is the operation of choice. It consists simply of turning the sac inside out (*eversion*) so that it lies entirely behind the testis and inserting a few sutures to retain it in position. These sutures must not pull the margins of the sac too tightly around the cord otherwise the blood supply to the testis may be impaired. If the hydrocele is large or the sac thick walled, the sac is better *excised* by cutting it off closely around its attachment to the testis. The bleeding points on the small remaining fringe of sac must be secured by ligatures or a running stitch, otherwise a haematoma will form. After both these operations haemostasis is secured, and the testis is returned to the scrotum from which a drain is brought out through the wound. As a further precaution against haematoma formation, the scrotum should be well supported with a compression bandage.

Scrotal approach

A scrotal approach can be used instead of an inguinal one for either of these two operations and is preferable. For the operation described by Lord, a scrotal approach must be used. Lord's procedure is virtually bloodless, and considerably reduces the risk of a scrotal haematoma, which is, unfortunately, very common after the other operations. The hydrocele is grasped in the left hand and the anterior scrotal skin stretched. An incision, about 4 cm in length, is made through the skin and dartos muscle avoiding, as far as possible, the superficial vessels, which are easily seen through the stretched skin. The tunica vaginalis is opened by an incision of the same length, but neither mobilized nor separated from the inside of the scrotum and the hydrocele fluid is evacuated. The testis is then lifted out through the incision in the tunica vaginalis. Five or six 'gathering' stitches are now inserted into the evaginated tunica, radiating outwards from its attachment to the testis towards its cut edge (Fig. 28.49). When these are tied, the tunica is plicated and forms a collar around the junction of testis and epididymis. Finally, the testis is returned to the scrotum, and the dartos muscle and skin are closed as one layer by stitches or clips.

Haematocele

A haematocele (an effusion of blood into the tunica vaginalis) results from direct injury or follows an operation on the scrotum such as vasectomy. Operation is probably advisable in all but the mildest cases if the condition is recognized at an early stage before the clot has organized. A haematocele is best evacuated by a direct approach through the anterior wall of the scrotum, but it is often disappointing how little clot one is able to remove. The lower part of the scrotal wound should be drained.

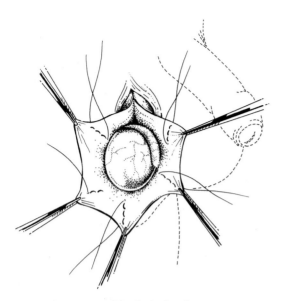

Fig. 28.49 Lord's procedure for hydrocele

Figs. 28.50–28.52 *Excision of spermatocele*

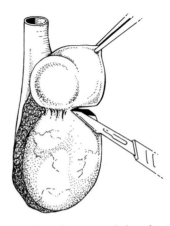

Fig. 28.50 The testis and spermatocele have been exposed through a scrotal incision and removal of the spermatocele begun

Spermatocele

A spermatocele is a retention cyst arising from either the vasa efferentia of the testis or from the epididymis and when large it is frequently mistaken by the patient for a third testis. If is normally situated above and behind the testis, and contains white opalescent fluid and spermatazoa. Small spermatoceles are usually symptomless and do not require treatment. Larger ones, and those which cause symptoms, may be dealt with by injection (on the same lines described for hydrocele) or by operation. At operation the sac is excised through a scrotal incision (Figs. 28.50–28.52).

Varicocele

This is the name given to varicosity of the pampiniform plexus. It is usually idiopathic and occurs almost exclusively on the left side, doubtlessly due to the anatomical differences in the venous drainage of the testis on the two sides (p. 624).

Some left sided varicoceles are secondary to an obstructed renal vein in patients with carcinoma of the kidney. Secondary varicoceles are usually obvious even when the patient lies down, whereas idiopathic ones can only be recognized while the patient is standing. Some fullness of the pampiniform plexus is normal in healthy men and the diagnosis of a small varicocele is not easy. The symptoms of slight aching or dragging pain, are usually relieved by the wearing of a suspensory bandage, although operation may fail to relieve the symptoms in some patients. The operative treatment of varicocele does have a definite place in the treatment of some subfertile men (Nilsson, 1983). Otherwise operation should only be

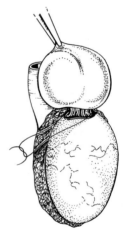

Fig. 28.51 The vessels supplying the spermatocele are ligated and excision continues

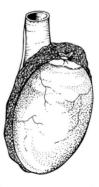

Fig. 28.52 The final result

advised if gross varicosity is present, or if the patient is convinced that his symptoms are due to the varicocele and unlikely to be relieved by conservative treatment and reassurance.

The classical operation for varicocele is carried out through an inguinal approach, the inguinal canal being opened and the spermatic cord delivered. The coverings are incised and the vas deferens, the arteries and two or three veins, are carefully separated from the main mass of dilated vessels. The latter are freed for a short distance upwards and downwards, and excised between ligatures placed some 5 cm apart. Approximation of these ligatures shortens the cord so that the testis is suspended at a higher level. An alternative method is to dissect out the selected veins right down to the level of the testis, but it is doubtful whether this confers any additional advantage, because bleeding is more troublesome and a scrotal haematoma is more liable to complicate convalescence. Some surgeons open and evert the tunica vaginalis (Jaboulay) to prevent subsequent hydrocele formation.

Paloma described an operation carried out *above* the inguinal canal for the cure of varicocele. A transverse or oblique incision is made 3 cm above the level of the deep ring, the external oblique aponeurosis is incised in the line of the incision, and the lateral edge of the rectus sheath nicked to expose the underlying transversalis fascia. The internal oblique and transversus muscles and transversalis fascia are then split as in the classical gridiron incision. Extraperitoneal fat and peritoneum are swept forwards to expose the psoas major muscle on the posterior abdominal wall. The testicular veins, usually two in number, are found as they lie on the posterior abdominal wall, lateral to the external iliac artery. They are usually lifted forward with the peritoneum, but can generally be identified in the extraperitoneal fat, even in a fat person. (The ureter lies more medially and is not usually seen). The testicular veins are identified and divided between ligatures, preserving the testicular artery which at this level is usually well separated from the veins (Fig. 28.53). Care must be taken not to ligate the inferior epigastric vein instead of the testicular vein.

Ligation or division of the vas deferens (Vasectomy)

Vasectomy is carried out to effect sterilization, and is rarely performed now to prevent infection spreading from the posterior urethra to the epididymis along the vas or its lymphatics after prostatectomy.

Technique

The operation is usually done under local anaesthesia; general anaesthesia is preferable if the patient has had a previous scrotal or inguinal operation or when the vas cannot be easily distinguished by touch from the other cord structures. The vas is identified, then grasped and steadied under the skin with the thumb and index finger

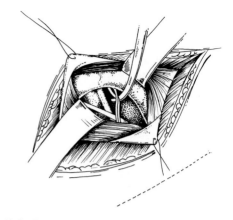

Fig. 28.53 The Paloma operation for varicocele. A gridiron incision has been made and the peritoneum retracted medially exposing the testicular artery and the testicular veins which are being held up with an artery forceps

of one hand. A small bleb is raised in the skin over the vas by injecting 1 or 2 ml 1% Lignocaine; the needle is then passed through the bleb and a further 2 or 3 ml of local anaesthetic injected into the cord. A 1 cm transverse incision is made through the bleb overlying the cord, and the cord enclosed in its fibrous sheath is picked up with an Allis or Poirier tissue forceps and released from its grip by thumb and index finger. (If holding the vas for this time proves difficult, the needle used for injecting the local anaesthetic can be passed underneath the vas and out through the skin beyond, while injecting the local anaesthetic.) The fibrous sheath of the cord is incised and the vas itself grasped with small artery forceps and lifted out. A window is made in the 'mesentery' of the vas and the proximal end is ligated and divided (the author uses 2/0 absorbable material). The distal end is ligated about $1\frac{1}{2}$ cm away and the intervening section excised. If the distal ligature is now tied around the point of an artery forceps applied to the dartos muscle, the proximal end is buried underneath the dartos and the distal end kept between it and the skin. The same procedure is then done on the otherside. It is important to separate the cut and ligated ends of the vas by a gap and a tissue plane in the way described because regeneration, either directly or through a granuloma, can occur. After haemostasis has been secured, the skin is loosely sutured with a catgut stitch. The operation can be done through one anterior median incision or two lateral incisions, one for each vas. It is important to tell patients requesting vasectomy that they must regard themselves fertile, and take other contraceptive precautions until two negative seminal analyses have been obtained (the first at least 3 months after the operation and the second at least 3 weeks after the first); that occasionally the fluids do not become negative, and the operation has to be redone, and that 1 or 2% of patients get more bruising than others and may be uncomfortable for some time.

Reversal of vasectomy

A reversal of vasectomy is occasionally requested. The presence of antisperm antibodies in serum or seminal plasma are not a contraindication to operation but make its success less likely. The operation is usually done under general anaesthetic, but is possible under local. The vas is easily palpable after vasectomy because the cut ends are buried in a granuloma (which varies in size) and closer together than might be expected. An incision is made over the vas and the granuloma picked up with Allis forceps and excised to expose normal vas above and below. An end-to-end or side-to-side anastomosis is made using interrupted 6/0 nylon or prolene sutures. As the lumen of the vas is small, anastomosis is facilitated if a splint, such as a piece of No. 1 nylon, is used and left in for some days after operation. The author passes one end of the splint some 5 cm into the distal end of the vas and passes the other end on a needle, into the proximal lumen, bringing it out through the side wall of the vas and the skin, to which it is secured with a button or bead. The skin incision is closed with catgut and the splint removed after 7 days.

Vaso-epididymostomy

In patients with azoospermia, the cause is either testicular dysfunction or a congenital obstruction situated usually at the tail of the epididymis as it becomes continuous with the beginning of the vas. If the history, the physical examination and the results of hormone assays and testicular biopsy suggest that the cause of azoos-

permia is obstruction, it is worth exploring the scrotum and carrying out the operation of vaso-epididymostomy. The patient should be told that the chances of success are not high. The operation is carried out through two scrotal incisions, one for each side. The vas is exposed and mobilized so that it can be brought alongside the head of the epididymis without tension. A deep incision is made into the head of the epididymis until creamy fluid, which usually contains spermatozoa, appears. An incision of similar length is made in the side wall of the vas and a side-to-side anastomosis carried out between the head of the epididymis (Fig. 28.54) and the vas using 5 or 6/0 prolene sutures (Fig. 28.55, 28.56).

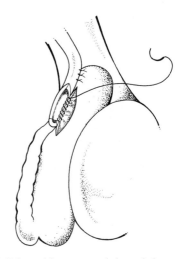

Fig. 28.55 Side-to-side anastomosis is carried out using 6/0 prolene sutures

Figs. 28.54–28.56 *Vaso-epididymostomy*

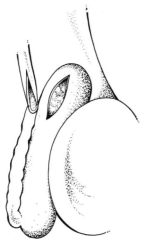

Fig. 28.54 The vas has been mobilized, incised and offered to a deep incision in the head of the epididymis

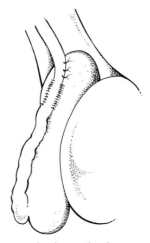

Fig. 28.56 The operation is completed

Operations on the scrotum

Avulsion of the scrotal skin, a not uncommon accident, requires careful treatment, especially if the testes are exposed. All available fragments of scrotal skin should be utilized to cover the testis and split skin grafts can be applied where deficiencies remain. *Carcinoma of the scrotum* is treated by radical excision of the local lesion and block dissection of the inguinal glands if they are involved. *Elephantiasis of the scrotum* is caused by filariasis and surgery is the only treatment of avail. The greater part of the oedematous scrotum is excised, preserving the penis, the urethra and the testes. Flaps of scrotal skin are preserved to form a pocket for the testes, and a covering for the penis. Deficiencies are covered with split skin grafts.

Fournier's gangrene (idiopathic gangrene of the scrotum)

This is an acute fulminating cellulitis of the scrotum which develops suddenly and often without any apparent cause. Infection is usually mixed, with haemolytic streptococci and clostridium welchii predominating. Gangrene probably due to thrombosis of cutaneous vessels of the scrotal skin occurs early and, if uncontrolled, the infection spreads upwards into the abdominal wall. Early cases can be aborted by intensive chemotherapy but if gangrene develops, no time should be lost before excising the necrotic tissue. One or both testes may be exposed by the excision of scrotal tissues, but seldom suffer damage. As soon as the wound is clean and the patient's condition is satisfactory, the scrotum is repaired by secondary suture and skin grafting.

REFERENCES

Ashby E C 1980 Maldescended testis. In: Taylor S(ed) Recent advances in surgery, No. 10. Churchill Livingstone, Edinburgh, Ch 15
Browne D 1949 An operation for hypospadias. Proceedings of the Royal Society of Medicine 42:466
Chilton C P, Shah P J R, Fowler C G, Tiptaft R C, Blandy J P 1983 The impact of optical urethrotomy on the management of urethral strictures. British Journal of Urology 55:705
Einhorn L H 1979 Platinum combination chemotherapy in disseminated testicular cancer. In: Johnson D E, Samuels M L (eds) Cancer of the Genitourinary Tract. Raven Press, New York, p 181
Hendry W F 1981 The diagnosis and management of the Primary Testicular Tumour. In: Peckham M (ed) The Management of Testicular Tumours. Edward Arnold, London, p 83
Jones P F, Bagley F H 1979 An abdominal extraperitoneal approach for the difficult orchidopexy. British Journal of Surgery 66:14
Lloyd-Davies R W, Gow J G, Davies D R 1983 A Colour Atlas of Urology. Wolfe, London, ch 11
Meulen J C M Van der 1971 Hypospadias and cryptospadias. British Journal of Plastic Surgery 24: 101
Newsam J E, Buist T A S 1980 Trauma. In: Chisholm G D (ed) Urology. Heinemann, London p 389

Nilsson S 1983 Varicocele. In: Hargreave T B (ed) Male Infertility. Springer Verlag, Heidelberg, p 199
Pryor J P, Fitzpatrick J M 1979 New approach to correction of penile deformity in Peyronie's disease. Journal of Urology 122:622
Smith J W, Murphy T R, Blair J S G, Lowe K G 1983 Regional Anatomy Illustrated. Churchill Livingstone, Edinburgh
Turner-Warwick R 1983 Urethral Stricture Surgery. In: Glenn J F (ed) Urological Surgery, 3rd edn. Lippincott, Philadelphia, p 689

FURTHER READING

Blandy J P 1984 Operative Urology, 2nd edn. Blackwell, Oxford
Clark P 1985 Operations in Urology. Churchill Livingstone, Edinburgh
Mitchell J P 1984 Urinary Tract Trauma. Wright, Bristol
Paulson D F 1984 Genitourinary Surgery. Churchill Livingstone, Edinburgh
Whitaker R H, Woodward J R (eds) 1984 Paediatric Urology. Butterworth, London

29

Gynaecological encounters in general surgery

J. R. B. LIVINGSTONE

Not infrequently the general surgeon, when performing a laparotomy, encounters an unexpected gynaecological condition, the correct management of which may cause him some doubt and anxiety. In a large hospital, he can usually call upon the assistance of a gynaecological colleague and should do so if at all possible. Unfortunately, there have been many occasions when an essentially normal ovary has been removed by an inexperienced surgeon, who has mistaken follicular or luteal cysts for disease. Furthermore, in cases of suspected or unsuspected ovarian malignancy, surgery has very often been incorrect or incomplete in inexperienced hands. However, in a small hospital without access to gynaecological opinion, the general surgeon himself has to accept responsibility for deciding what, if any, operative procedure is indicated and of mastering the techniques required. It is for his guidance that this chapter is written.

Anatomy

The uterus is a thick-walled muscular organ, situated between the bladder and the rectum; in its normal position of anteversion it lies obliquely overhanging the bladder. It is piriform in shape and flattened anteroposteriorly. It is about 7.5 cm long, 5 cm broad, and 2.5 cm thick. Its upper part or *body* projects upwards into the pelvic cavity and has a complete peritoneal covering. Anteriorly, the peritoneum is reflected on to the upper surface of the bladder, with the shallow *uterovesical pouch* between; posteriorly, it sweeps downwards to form the *rectouterine pouch* (of Douglas); laterally on each side, it forms the broad ligament. The rounded upper end of the uterus is called the *fundus*; this is demarcated from the body by the entrance of the uterine tube at each side. The lower part of the uterus or *cervix* lies mainly below the peritoneum, and is invaginated into the vaginal vault, so that it is divided into supra- and intravaginal parts. The

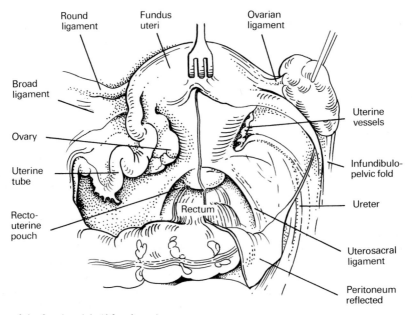

Fig. 29.1 Anatomy of the female pelvis (After Anson)

body and cervix are separated by a circular constriction called the *isthmus*. The supravaginal part of the cervix is related anteriorly to the bladder, to which it is connected by some loose fibrous strands, the *uterovesical fascia*. Laterally, it is related to the *transverse cervical ligament*, which runs to the side wall of the pelvis; posteriorly, it is joined to the sacral fascia by the *uterosacral ligaments*, which pass backwards on each side of the rectum, raising folds in the peritoneum of the pelvic floor.

The broad ligament is a double fold of peritoneum stretching from the lateral border of the uterus to the side wall of the pelvis. The ovary is attached to the lateral part of its posterior surface. Its upper free border contains the uterine tube in its medial four-fifths; its lateral one-fifth, containing the ovarian vessels, constitutes the *infundibulopelvic ligament*. The uterine vessels lie between the layers of the ligament, first at its base, and then close to its attachment to the uterus. Other contents of the broad ligament, beside lymph vessels and glands, are the *round ligament* of the uterus, which raises a ridge on its anterior surface as it passes towards the inguinal canal, and the *ovarian ligament*, which joins the ovary to the uterus, and raises a small ridge on its posterior surface. Some vestigial tubules, remnants of the Wolffian body, may also be present within the ligament. The part of the broad ligament between the uterine tube and the ovary is termed the *mesosalpinx*.

The vagina (intrapelvic part)

The space between the intravaginal part of the cervix and the vaginal wall is divided into *fornices*—anterior, posterior, right and left lateral. The posterior fornix is in direct contact with the peritoneum of the pelvic floor. The ureter passes forwards immediately above the lateral fornix.

The ovary

Each ovary is about the size and shape of a very large almond, measuring 3–5 cm in its long axis. It is greyish-white in colour but its size, shape and surface can vary considerably depending on whether the patient is pre- or postmenopausal, and on the time of the menstrual cycle. In prepubertal girls the surface is smooth but following puberty the surface becomes wrinkled and scarred, and it may contain several or single cysts. (Failure to recognise that these changes may be physiological has led to countless ovaries being sacrificed needlessly.) It lies against the posterior surface of the broad ligament, part of which is drawn outwards to form the *mesovarium* containing the ovarian vessels. It is connected to the side wall of the pelvis by the infundibulopelvic ligament, and to the uterus by the ovarian ligament. The open end of the uterine tube overlaps its medial surface.

The uterine tube

Each tube is about 10 cm long, and 6–7 mm in diameter. It lies along the upper free border of the broad ligament in its medial four-fifths. Medially, it traverses the lateral wall of the uterus between body and fundus, to open into the upper angle of the uterine cavity. Laterally, it emerges through the posterior layer of the broad ligament, and opens into the peritoneal cavity, where it overlaps and is attached to the medial surface of the ovary. Its medial part is narrow and is called the *isthmus*; its lateral part is wider and is called the *ampulla*. Its open lateral end or *infundibulum* is divided into several finger-like processes termed *fimbriae*, the largest of which is attached to the ovary.

Vessels

The uterine artery arises from the anterior division of the internal iliac; it runs forwards to the base of the broad ligament, and then medially within it above the lateral fornix of the vagina, where it crosses the ureter 1–2 cm lateral to the supravaginal part of the cervix; finally, it runs upwards along the lateral margin of the uterus, to which it gives numerous branches, including one to the uterine tube. *The ovarian artery* arises from the aorta, a little below the renal, and runs down the posterior abdominal wall; it then passes forwards and medially to reach the ovary via the infundibulopelvic ligament. There is an anastomosis between the uterine and ovarian arteries in the mesosalpinx at the lower border of the tube, and this anastomosis is important because it allows an alternative blood supply to the uterus when internal iliac artery ligation is required to control uterine haemorrhage.

Veins correspond to the arteries, but the right ovarian vein enters the inferior vena cava, and the left, the left renal vein.

CONDITIONS AFFECTING THE UTERINE TUBE

Ruptured ectopic pregnancy

The rupture occurs commonly between the 6th and the 10th week, although it may occur earlier or later. There is usually a history of at least one missed period, but this is not necessarily the case, and in 30% of patients a clear history of amenorrhoea is absent. Classically, the patient shows signs of internal haemorrhage with shock, but much more commonly the development of symptoms and signs is more insidious, due to the fact that most ectopic pregnancies end in tubal abortion with less bleeding than that associated with tubal rupture. Thus these signs may be absent, and not infrequently the case is diagnosed as one of acute appendicitis or of some other general surgical emergency. However, if the possibility of ectopic pregnancy is seriously entertained (and this diagnosis can frequently be confused with salpingitis which should be treated conservatively) then it can be confirmed or excluded by laparoscopy—a relatively simple procedure which may save the patient from laparotomy.

Laparoscopy

This is usually carried out under general but may be performed under local anaesthesia.

The patient is catheterised and is then placed in the Trendelenburg position and a site is selected at the lower margin of the umbilicus if this can be sterilised adequately. At this point a Verey's needle with the cannula retracted is thrust obliquely through the skin, superficial fascia and rectus sheath. Once the rectus sheath has been penetrated, the spring on the cannula is released and it is then thrust boldly through the parietal peritoneum towards the midpoint of the pelvic brim and into the peritoneal cavity. A gas source is then connected to the cannula and either carbon dioxide or nitrous oxide is passed into the peritoneal cavity at a pressure of no more than 60 cm water and a rate of approximately 1 litre per minute. About 3 litres of gas are usually required to distend the abdomen and to lift the anterior abdominal wall from the intestinal contents. The abdominal distension should be even, but if it is asymmetric then insufflation of the extraperitoneal space or even of bowel must be suspected. The Verey's needle is then withdrawn, and a small transverse incision 1.5 cm long is made along the lower margin of the umbilicus and carried obliquely down to the rectus sheath where a similar small transverse incision is made. This allows the subsequent easy and less traumatic passage of the trocar and cannula. Some surgeons prefer to make the skin incision before introducing the Verey's needle but others find that the 'feel' which is experienced on passing the needle through the skin and layers of the abdominal wall allows better appreciation of entry into the peritoneal cavity. The trocar is then withdrawn and the laparoscope, connected to a fibre-optic light source, is passed through the cannula. This allows very accurate inspection of the pelvic cavity but if vision is obscured by omentum or adhesions, the uterus, tubes and ovaries may be manipulated by passing a pair of Palmer's biopsy forceps through a trocar and cannula inserted through a separate 1 cm incision made in the lower abdomen. Preferably this should be made near the mid-line so as to avoid the inferior epigastric artery.

Once the diagnosis of ectopic pregnancy has been confirmed then the instruments are withdrawn and laparotomy is performed.

Laparotomy (see p. 332)

Sometimes the diagnosis of ectopic pregnancy can be

made clinically with such certainty that laparoscopy can be omitted and at operation, if profuse bleeding has occurred into the peritoneal cavity, this will be apparent from the blueish tinge of the peritoneum as soon as the muscles have been separated. After the peritoneal cavity has been entered, it may be difficult, because of the amount of blood in the pelvis, to identify the affected tube, unless much time is wasted in scooping out blood clot. It is better to insert the hand, to seize the fundus of the uterus, and to draw it up to and out of the wound. The affected tube is now readily identified. The broad ligament is compressed with the fingers in order to arrest haemorrhage; forceps are then applied, first to the uterine end of the affected tube, along which passes its main arterial supply derived from the uterine artery, and then to that part of the broad ligament connecting the tube to the ovary, i.e. the *mesosalpinx* (Fig. 29.2). The tube is now removed, the pedicles are tied off, and the stumps invaginated. If the ovary is healthy, it is not necessary to remove it, but consideration should be given to doing so if there has been a history of subfertility. By removing the ovary on the affected side the patient is left with a normal tube and ovary on the other side so that ovulation subsequently will always take place from the ovary adjacent to the remaining tube. This must only be considered when the remaining tube and ovary appear perfectly normal. If the ovary is unhealthy on the affected side, e.g. involved in endometriosis, then again it should be removed together with the tube.

Preservation of the tube is not normally recommended, because there is a considerable risk of a further ectopic pregnancy in the already abnormal tube. If, however, the opposite tube is hopelessly diseased, or has been removed, and if the patient is very anxious for a further pregnancy, an attempt may be made to conserve the tube. In such cases, the gestation is evacuated either

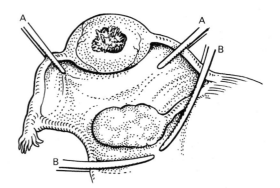

Fig. 29.2 Salpingectomy for ectopic gestation. Clamps are placed on the mesosalpinx and on the uterine end of the tube (AA). The infundibulopelvic ligament, carrying the ovarian vessels, is preserved. If the decision is made to remove the ovary along with the tube, then the tissue between clamps BB would be excised

through a longitudinal incision in the wall of the tube (which is thereafter repaired by 4/0 Dexon interrupted sutures, taking care to exclude the mucosa), or by milking it through the ampulla and inducing a tubal abortion. Continued bleeding thereafter, however, can be a problem.

Provided that the patient's condition allows, an effort should be made to remove all blood within the peritoneal cavity. Before the abdomen is closed, therefore, the patient should be tilted into the feet-down position so that any blood in the upper abdomen will gravitate into the pelvis from which it can be removed by swabbing or by suction. In some parts of the world where facilities for blood transfusion are scarce this blood can be returned to the patient by means of the autotransfusion pump.

Occasionally, the rupture of an ectopic pregnancy takes place within the broad ligament, leading to the development of a haematoma between its layers. In such cases, the tube should first be removed; thereafter, the haematoma may be evacuated by incising either the anterior or the posterior layer of the broad ligament. Sometimes placental tissue will be found to be adherent and serious bleeding can be provoked by injudicious attempts at removal. In these cases the remaining placental tissue should be left undisturbed.

Salpingitis

When this is found at laparotomy, conservation is usually called for, especially since the infection is likely to be bilateral. Unless peritonitis has developed, it is usually sufficient to take a swab from the abdominal osteum of the tube and from any pelvic exudate for bacteriological examination (Cameron, 1976). The wound is closed without drainage and antibiotic therapy is instituted. If, however, a spreading peritonitis is present, and if only one tube is involved, its removal may be considered. The ovary, if healthy, should be preserved.

CONDITIONS AFFECTING THE OVARY

Simple ovarian cysts

A normal healthy ovary, during the childbearing period, contains Graafian follicles and corpora lutea. Both of these may become cystic and may project from the surface of the ovary. Such cysts may be single or multiple, very small or as large as the ovary itself. They are common in women who have no symptoms referable to them, and are in no way pathological. Corpus luteum cysts are often associated with menstrual disturbances, and contain blood. If they rupture, a quantity of blood may be present in the peritoneal cavity, and the symptoms may be taken for those of acute appendicitis. No treatment of such cysts is required, unless bleeding is still taking

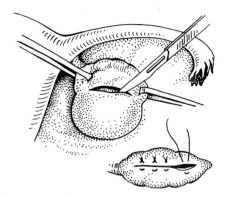

Fig. 29.3 Ovarian cystectomy, the cyst being shelled out through an incision in the ovarian cortex around its base. The ovary is then repaired by suture

place from a ruptured cyst, when it may be arrested by one or two sutures placed in the ovarian substance.

When a cyst is of significant size, i.e. more than 5 cm in diameter, it is in the patient's interests that it should be removed. If the ovary itself is healthy, and if the patient is under 45, as much of it as possible should be preserved. In the operation of *ovarian cystectomy*, an incision is made through the ovarian cortex around the base of the cyst, which is then shelled out by sharp dissection, after which the wound in the ovary is sutured either by interrupted or continuous 2/0 catgut taking care to abolish the dead space (Fig. 29.3). In the case of larger cysts, where it is thought that little functioning ovarian tissue remains, *oophorectomy* should normally be performed—that is, provided that the other ovary is healthy. Clamps are applied as shown in Figure 29.4. In still larger cysts, the uterine tube is often stretched out over the surface of the cyst so that it is best removed. The incision should be enlarged, or a fresh incision made, so that the cyst can be brought out of the wound and removed intact by division of its pedicle. The lateral part of the pedicle is formed by the infundibulopelvic ligament containing the ovarian vessels, which in the case of a large cyst are likely to be much dilated; the medial

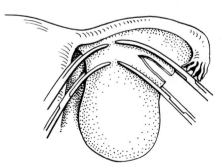

Fig. 29.4 Oophorectomy for a cystic ovary containing little functioning tissue. The infundibulopelvic fold and the ovarian ligament are divided between clamps

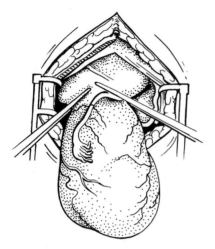

Fig. 29.5 Salpingo-oophorectomy for large ovarian cyst. On the lateral side of the pedicle, the infundibulopelvic fold, containing the dilated ovarian vessels, is divided between clamps, two being placed on the proximal side. On the uterine side a clamp has been placed across the ovarian ligament and the uterine tube, which is usually stretched out over the surface of the cyst

or uterine part contains the uterine tube and the ovarian ligament (Fig. 29.5). These structures are divided between clamps. For the lateral part of the pedicle (containing the vessels) it is advised that two clamps should be placed proximal to the level of division, and that a transfixing ligature should be employed. This is advised because, if the clamp or ligature slips, the cut ovarian artery may retract behind the peritoneum, causing very troublesome haemorrhage.

Torsion of an ovarian cyst may well be misdiagnosed as a case of acute appendicitis, especially in stout women. The incision should be enlarged sufficiently, or a fresh incision made, so that the cyst can be untwisted under vision and removed intact. Rarely in prepubertal girls and teenagers, torsion of a normal tube and ovary may occur. In such cases the affected tube and ovary may be untwisted and infarcted blood can be removed from the ovary by incising the cortex which is then repaired. If, thereafter, the tube and ovary recover viability, they may safely be left in situ and function may be preserved.

Endometrial cysts of the ovary are essentially benign but come into a special category. The cyst rarely exceeds 10 cm in diameter, its capsule is thick, firm and white in colour frequently mottled with brown, and adhesions bind it to adjacent structures. Often the cyst bursts while adhesions are being separated, and the escape of chocolate-coloured or tarry fluid establishes the diagnosis. Additional confirmation may be obtained from the presence of vascular adhesions on the surface of the ovary or of endometrial deposits in other parts of the pelvis (p. 643).

Tumours of the ovary

Serous cystadenoma is the commonest tumour or pathological cyst of the ovary. It is usually unilateral and unilocular and is thin walled and pearly white in colour. Pseudomucinous cystadenoma is the next commonest; as a rule it is mainly cystic, containing pseudomucinous material. It is pearly white in colour, bossed or loculated, and may reach very large dimensions. Sometimes there is little functioning ovarian tissue on the affected side and oophorectomy should then be performed together with salpingectomy if the tube has been unduly stretched over the surface of the cyst. Every effort should be made, however, to determine whether the cyst is simple or malignant, and for this reason it should be cut open immediately after removal.

Pseudomyxoma peritonei may result from intraperitoneal rupture of a pseudomucinous cyst of the ovary, and the whole of the peritoneal cavity may then be filled with pseudomucinous material. The treatment advised is bilateral oophorectomy, and (if the operator has the necessary experience) total hysterectomy.

Ovarian carcinoma

The classical picture of malignant disease is that the ovarian swellings are bilateral—one being much larger than the other. They are mainly solid, but may contain cystic spaces; their internal structure is necrotic in appearance and consistency. When malignancy is suspected a careful exploration of the pelvis and abdominal cavity should be made and the observations noted so that a base-line may be established on which to plan, monitor and evaluate appropriate adjuvant therapy. If the disease appears to be unilateral in Stage I A(i) and the patient desires to maintain reproductive function then a salpingo-oophorectomy can be carried out on the affected side and no further treatment is required if a biopsy from the contralateral ovary taken at the same time is normal. If reproductive function is no longer desired or if the ovarian cancer is more advanced a bilateral salpingo-oophorectomy and total hysterectomy should be performed if at all possible. Omentectomy and removal of any bulk disease should also be carried out and any spread to the undersurface of the diaphragm, pelvic or para-aortic lymph nodes or elsewhere in the peritoneal cavity together with an estimate of the maximum volume of any remaining bulk disease should be carefully noted. There is no doubt that the effect of chemotherapy is considerably enhanced if residual disease can be kept to a minimum. In many cases, however, the ovarian tumours may be so densely adherent to surrounding structures that their removal is fraught with such hazards that they are inoperable. In such cases a biopsy should be taken and, depending on the type of tumour, treatment with radiotherapy or chemotherapy can be instituted and a significant number may then become operable.

HYSTERECTOMY

The general surgeon will seldom be called upon to perform a hysterectomy, but the unexpected necessity or indication may occasionally arise. In an operation for excision of the rectum (especially with conservation of the sphincter) an unusually bulky uterus, or one that is the seat of fibroids, may so obstruct the operative field that its removal is imperative. A carcinoma of some neighbouring organ, such as the rectum, the pelvic colon or the bladder, may involve the uterus, so that this may require to be removed as part of any operation which aims at radical cure. Endometriosis also is an occasional indication for hysterectomy—but not in the hands of the inexperienced.

Total hysterectomy has now almost entirely replaced the older subtotal operation. As a rule there is nothing to be gained by leaving the cervix, and indeed some risk is incurred, for it may be the seat of existing or subsequent disease, e.g. carcinoma. The total operation involves a deeper dissection into the pelvis, and entails a greater risk of damage to the ureter, but, unless the dissection is rendered unusually difficult by the presence of dense adhesions, the risk is not a serious one, provided that reasonable care is taken.

Technique
The incision is enlarged if necessary or a fresh incision made. The patient is placed in the Trendeleburg position (p. 641), small bowel is packed off into the upper abdomen, and self-retaining retractors are inserted. If the ovaries are healthy, and if the patient is under 45, it is best to leave them; otherwise, they are removed. The fundus of the uterus is grasped with a vulsellum forceps, and is drawn upwards and to the left, so that the right appendages come into view. When the ovaries are to be preserved, the upper part of the broad ligament, containing the uterine tube, the round ligament, the ovarian ligament and anastomoses between ovarian and uterine arteries, is divided between clamps close to the uterus, the round ligament being clamped separately from the uterine tube and ovarian ligament. The clamps are at once tied-off, since they would get in the way of the rest of the operation. The peritoneal incision in the anterior leaf of the broad ligament is carried downwards close to the uterus towards the base of the ligament, and is then continued towards the left across the utero-vesical pouch at the level of the isthmus, where the peritoneum

is loose. The anterior peritoneal flap is raised to expose the bladder, which is joined to the cervix by fascial strands (uterovesical fascia). This fascia is divided (Fig. 29.6) in order to open up the plane of cleavage between bladder and cervix. The bladder is now pushed downwards off the cervix and upper part of the vagina. This carries the ureter downwards with the bladder to below the level of the uterine artery, and should safeguard it when this vessel is clamped. The stripping, however, must be done gently, especially on the lateral side of the cervix, where the parametrial venous plexuses may be torn; injudicious clamping of these veins may result in damage to the ureter. It is advisable, therefore, that, before the stripping is carried too far, the ureter should be identified, as it runs forwards and medially above the lateral fornix of the vagina to enter the bladder. As soon as this has been done, the uterine artery should be clamped close to the uterus (Fig. 29.7).

A similar dissection is now carried out on the left side of the uterus, the uterine artery being clamped and divided after the ureter has been safeguarded. At this stage after dividing the pedicle right to the points of the forceps, the clamps containing the uterine vessels may be pushed downwards and laterally on each side for a distance of about 1 cm. This maneouvre exposes the

Figs. 29.6–29.11 *Hysterectomy (after Shaw)*

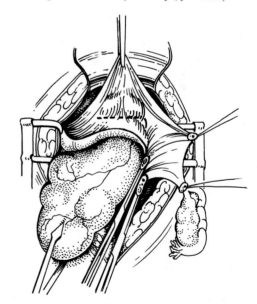

Fig. 29.6 The uterus has been siezed with a vulsellum and drawn upwards to expose the appendages on the right side. The uterine tube and the ovarian ligament have been divided between one pair of clamps, and the round ligament between another; the laterally placed clamps have been tied-off. The incision in the broad ligament has been extended across the peritoneum of the uterovesical pouch at the level of the isthmus. The uterovesical fascia (shown by broken line) must next be divided

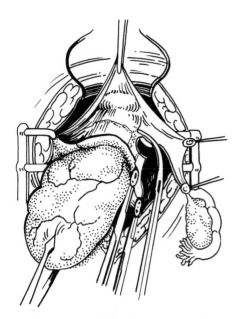

Fig. 29.7 The uterovesical fascia has been divided, to open up the plane of cleavage between the bladder and cervix. The bladder has been mobilized and displaced downwards, first from the cervix and then from the vagina. This carries the ureter downwards, clear of the uterine artery, which is then clamped as shown—*close to the uterine wall*. Before the clamp is applied, it is usually advised that the ureter should be identified as it passes forwards and medially to the bladder at a lower level

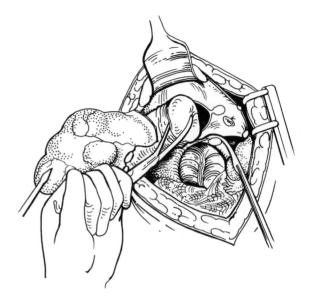

Fig. 29.8 A similar dissection has been carried out on the left side, and the uterine artery secured. The vagina is now opened posterolaterally on the right side, after cutting through the transverse cervical and uterosacral ligaments (to which a clamp is shown attached), and the incision is carried round to the front of the vaginal vault close to the cervix. A vulsellum forceps has been applied to the cervix for traction so that division of the vagina can be completed on the opposite side. The uterus may then be lifted out

transverse cervical ligament and uterosacral ligament which may be clamped (either together or separately depending on the size) by curved Kocher's forceps which are applied so that the ends of the forceps reach the lateral fornix of the vagina on each side. A long handled knife is then used to divide these pedicles and this incision is carried across the vault of the vagina, thus removing the uterus together with the cervix. Care must be taken at this stage to avoid injuring the rectum which may be adherent to the back of the posterior fornix. The vault of the vagina is then closed with a continuous No. 1 Dexon suture to reduce the risk of postoperative vault granulations developing and thereafter the parametrial and uterine pedicles are ligated. Careful haemostasis is secured and the pelvic peritoneum is reconstituted with a continuous stitch taking care not to damage or kink the ureter.

Sub-total hysterectomy

In this operation, the dissection is not carried so deeply into the pelvis, and the bladder is not separated from the vaginal vault. The uterine artery is secured as in total hysterectomy, the ureter being safeguarded. The cervix is then divided just below the isthmus; its remaining part is closed by two or three interrupted sutures, and the stump is buried below the peritoneal flaps.

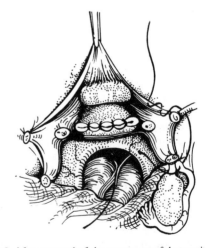

Fig. 29.9 After removal of the uterus, careful attention is paid to haemostasis, vessels in the vaginal wall and in the parametrial tissues around the uterosacral ligaments being secured. The vagina is now closed by suture, and the peritoneum of the pelvic floor is reconstituted, the several ligatured stumps being invaginated beneath the flaps. If complete haemostasis has not been secured, it is better *not* to suture the vagina, but to bring out a gauze pack through it from below the sutured peritoneum

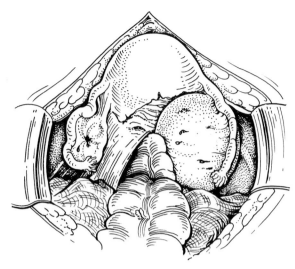

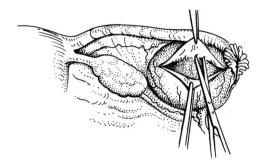

Fig. 29.11 Removal of a broad ligament cyst after incision of the peritoneum of the ligament

Fig. 29.10 Typical appearances of endometriosis. Dense adhesions, obliterating the recto-uterine pouch and binding the uterus to the rectosigmoid, have been separated, leaving extensive raw areas on these structures. The left ovary shows a puckered scar, the right ovary an endometrial cyst. Scattered nodules are present elsewhere over a wide area in the pelvis

OTHER GYNAECOLOGICAL CONDITIONS

Endometriosis is a term used to denote the presence of ectopic endometrial tissue in various organs within the pelvis. The ovaries, the uterine tubes, the uterosacral ligaments and the peritoneum of the recto-uterine pouch are areas commonly affected. The condition occurs also on the posterior surface of the uterus and within its muscular wall. The endometrial tissue presents in the early stages of the condition in the form of dark brown or purplish nodules, which are characteristically the size of lead shot. Around each nodule the peritoneum may be drawn into a series of puckers. In more advanced cases, there may be an inextricable mass of adhesions, completely obliterating the recto-uterine pouch and binding together all the pelvic structures; bowel and omentum may also be involved. The ovaries are white and opaque, and may show puckered scars on their surface; alternatively they may be cystic, containing altered blood—the so-called 'chocolate' or 'tarry' cysts.

Fortunately, endometriosis can often be cured by abolishing ovarian function. It is essentially a benign non-neoplastic condition, but malignant degeneration

has occasionally been reported. In women near the menopause, bilateral oophorectomy can be performed. Hysterectomy may be carried out at the same time, provided that the operator is experienced in gynaecological surgery, but, if dense adhesions are present, the uterus is best left alone, since there is a serious risk of damaging adherent bowel. In young women, bilateral oophorectomy is obviously undesirable but, if one ovary is extensively diseased, it may be removed and the other left. At the same time, obvious and readily removed areas of disease may be excised and their beds cauterised.

The general surgeon, who unexpectedly discovers the condition of endometriosis at laparotomy, should suffer no reproaches if he simply closes the abdomen for the condition can often be improved if not cured by hormone therapy. A further operation can then be undertaken if necessary.

Parovarian (broad ligament) cysts
These cysts, which are probably derived from vestigial remnants of the Wolffian body, lie within the broad ligament, usually between the uterine tube and the ovary. They contain clear watery fluid and are usually unilocular. They never attain any great size and are of little clinical significance. Owing to their situation within the broad ligament, they cannot be delivered at the wound.

If such a cyst is found at laparotomy, and appears to be reasonably accessible, it may be removed. The broad ligament is incised over the cyst, which is then shelled out by dissection close to its wall, with due regard to the proximity of the ureter and the ovarian vessels (Fig. 29.11). Haemorrhage is arrested, and the broad ligament is repaired by suture.

REFERENCE AND FURTHER READING

Cameron M D 1976 Gynaecological problems and the general surgeon. In: Hadfield J, Hobsley M (eds) Current surgical practice, vol. 1. Arnold, London, ch 15

Index

Abdomen
  burst, 327
  distension, post-operative, 326
  incisions
    children, 317–19
    gridiron, 316
    Kocher's, 317
    Lanz, 316
    midline, 314
    muscle-cutting iliac, 316
    paramedian, 314
    Pfannenstiel's, 317
    Rutherford-Morison, 316
    transverse, 317
  operations on
    anastomosis of gut, 322
    complications, 326
    fluid and electrolyte balance, 310, 325
    general technique, 319
    infection in, prevention, 319, 320, 322, 386, 413, 437
    position for, 312
    post-operative care, 325
    preparation for, 309
    repositioning of viscera, 321
    see also Laparotomy
  penetrating wounds, 329, 330, 332
  wall of, anatomy, 312
  see also specific parts of abdomen
Abscesses
  amoebic, 377
  anorectal, 471
  appendix, 412, 414
  brain, 210
  breast, 279
  dental, 223
  hand, 142, 143, 145
  liver, 376
  lung, 290
  muscle, 17
  neck, 238
  osteomyelitis, 113, 223
  pancreas, 404
  paracolic, 451
  pelvic, 413
  perinephric, 548
  salivary glands, 263
  subphrenic, 375, 413
  tuberculous
    anal canal, 472

neck, 256
spine, 217
Achilles tendon *see* Tendo Achilles
Acidosis, 311
Acrocyanosis, 80
Acromioclavicular joint, 90
Adenoidectomy, 244
Adenomata, colon, 452
Adrenal glands
  anatomy, 529, 556
  removal, 556–8
    complications, 558
    surgical approach, 556
  tumours, 557
Albumin solutions, 61
Alkalosis, 311, 422
Amputations
  surgical
    at ankle, 183–6
    at elbow, 178
    at knee, 190
    at shoulder, 178
    at wrist, 177
    below knee, 186–90
    bone division, 169
    children, 166
    Chopart's, 183
    fingers, 172–7
    in foot, 182
    Gritti-Stokes, 194
    guillotine, 167, 172
    hands, 172–7
    indications for, 163–5
    inter-innomino-abdominal, 195
    inter-scapulo-thoracic, 180
    Krukenberg, 178
    management of soft tissues, 168
    methods, 167–71, 172
    optimum levels, 165–7, 172
    penis, 618–20
    phantom pain, 169
    Pirogoff's, 186
    post-operative management, 171
    in presence of sepsis, 171
    Symes, 166, 167, 183–6
    through forearm, 177
    through leg, 186–90
    through thigh, 191–4
    through upper arm, 178
    thumb, 176
    toes, 180–2

traumatic
  arm, 168
  finger, 137
  hand, 139
Anaemia
  blood transfusions for, 59, 60
  haemolytic
    post-operative, 353
    splenectomy in, 367
  iron deficiency, post-operative, 353
Anaesthesia
  field block, 6
  hand, 131
  infiltration, 5
  local, 5
  neck operations, 236
  paravertebral block, 80
  scalp injuries, 197, 199
  skin operations, 5–6
Anal
  canal
    abscesses, 471
    anatomy, 458
    carcinoma, 474
    congenital anomalies, 475
    examination, 458
    fistulae, 472–4
    injuries, 459
    pruritus ani, 475
  fissure, 467
  incontinence, 474
Anastomosis
  gall-bladder to gastro-intestinal tract, 398, 403
  intestines, 322, 429–31, 441–3
  portal vein, 371
  ureter, 562
  vascular, 27, 35
Aneurysmal varix, 43
Aneurysms
  aorta, 42
  arterial, 41–4
  arteriovenous, 43
  varicose, 43
Angiography
  adrenal, 557
  cerebral, 207
  renal-selective, 506, 555
  see also Arteriography
Ankle
  amputation at, 183–6

Ankle (*cont'd*)
  anatomy, 183
  arthrodesis, 106
  arthroplasty, 106
  exposure, 106
  fractures, 127
Annuloplasty, 297
Antibiotics
  biliary surgery, 386
  bowel surgery, 413, 437
  joint surgery, 85
Anticoagulant therapy, 38–40
Anticoagulants
  oral, 39
  see also Heparin
Anus
  covered, 476, 477
  ectopic, 476, 477
Aorta
  aneurysms, 41
  coarctation (stenosis), 298
  embolectomy, 45
  rupture of, 285
Aortic valve disease, 298
Aortography, 40
  transbrachial (transaxillary), 41
  transfemoral, 41, 506
  translumbar, 40
Appendicitis
  acute, 408
    with perforation, 412
  chronic, 409
Appendix
  abscess, 412, 414
  anatomy, 408
  carcinoid, 409
  carcinoma, 409
  removal
    children, 409
    complications, 413
    elderly, 409
    elective, 409
    emergency, 411
    indications for, 408
    retrograde, 412
Apudomas, pancreatic, 403
Arm
  forearm
    amputation through, 177
    anatomy, 177
    fractures, 121
    operations on, 90–2
  upper
    amputation through, 178
    anatomy, 178
    fractures, 120
    operations on, 85–90
Arteries
  anatomy, 26
    see also specific arteries
  aneurysms, 41–4
  basic surgical techniques, 26–8
  contracted and empty, 35
  dilatation, 38
  exposure of, 26
    see also specific arteries
  femoral

aneurysm, 43
  bypass, 37
  forceps, use of, 1
  grafts, 36, 37, 43
  haematoma, 34, 41
  injury, 43
  innominate, aneurysm, 43
  ligatures, 1
  obliterative disease, 36, 38
  occlusion of, 44
  pulmonary, embolectomy, 45
  reconstruction, 36, 41, 44
  repair, 35
  wounds, 34
  see also Aorta
Arteriography, 18, 40
  peripheral, 41
Arteriotomy, 27
Arteriovenous fistulae, 43
Arthritis
  septic, 144
  see also Osteoarthritis; Rheumatoid
    arthritis
Arthrodesis
  ankle, 106
  compression, 104, 106
  elbow, 91
  foot
    forefoot, 107, 108
    toes, 109, 110, 111
  hand, 141, 149
  hip, 96
    ischiofemoral (V-), 96
    with osteotomy, 97
  knee, 103
  shoulder, 90
  wrist, 92
Arthroplasty
  ankle, 106
  elbow, 91
  forefoot, 110, 111, 112
  hand, 152
  hip, 98
  Keller's, 110, 111
  knee, 100
Atherosclerosis, 80
Athletes *see* Sports injuries
Axial tomography *see* Computerized
    axial tomography
Axillary
  arteries, 179
  anatomy, 29
  aneurysm, 43
  exposure, 30
  vein, 179
Axonotmesis, 68

Balanitis, 616
Bankhart operation, 89
Barium
  meal, 339
  swallow, 339
Bassini repair of inguinal hernia, 485
Beckwith Wiedman syndrome, 497
Bile ducts
  anatomy, 381
  anomalies, 382

atresia, 399
  drainage, 399
  fistulae, 398
  hypoplastic, 399
  injuries, 332, 396
  obstruction, 384
  operations on, 389, 392–8
    choice of, 388
    general technique, 385–8
    indications for, 383–4
    surgical examination, 387
  reconstruction, 397
  stones, 384
    impacted, 394
    removal, 393–6
    retained, 395
  strictures, 397
  tumours, 384, 399, 400
Billroth I partial gastrectomy, 351
Bites, 138, 155, 158
Bladder
  anatomy, 574
  carcinoma, 526, 641
  cystectomy, 586–8
  cystostomy, 575
  diverticula, 525, 577, 591
    tumours, 586
  endoscopy, 521–2
  fistulae, 589
  injuries, 332, 576
  investigation of, 509–27
  outflow obstruction, 591–3
  reconstruction of, 588
  stones, 525, 578
  surgical approach, 575
  trabeculation, 525, 591
  trigonectomy, 595
  tumours, 526, 582–6
    classification, 582
    operations for, 586–8
Bleeding *see* Haemorrhage
Blisters, septic, 142
Blood
  collection, 57
    emergency, 63
  components, 60
  group systems, 57
  loss *see* Haemorrhage
  pre-operative tests, 309
  storage, 57
  transfusion, 57–66
    in acute loss, 59
    compatibility in, 58, 63–6
    emergency, 63
    hazards, 62
    immunology, 57
    side effects, 62
    in surgery, 59
    typing, 58, 63–6
  whole, 60
Blood vessels
  anastomoses, 27
    see also Arteries; Veins; Vascular
Blunt instruments, wounds from, 154
Boari flap, 565, 567
Bones
  cysts, 113, 116

Bones (*cont'd*)
  division at amputation, 169
  fractures *see* Fractures
  grafts, 128
    cancellous strip, 129
    onlay, 92
    tumour treatment, 115
  osteomyelitis, 112
  scans, 272, 511
  surgery,84–130
    infection and,84
    techniques, 84
  tumours, 113–16
    biopsy, 115
  see also names of specific bones and
    specific operations
Bougies
  oesophageal, 300, 304
  urethral, 610
Boutonniere deformity, 22, 151
Bowel preparation for surgery, 436
Bowel *see* Colon; Intestines
Brachial
  arteries
    anatomy, 30
    exposure, 30
    upper arm, 178
  plexus
    anatomy, 71
    traction lesions, 72
Brain
  abscesses, 210
  diagnostic procedures, 206
  gunshot wounds, 201
  haemorrhage, 202–5, 211
  injuries, treatment, 201
  intracranial aneurysms, 211
  oedema, 205
  operative access to, 208
  tumours, 209
Branchial
  cysts, 240
  fistulae, 240
Breast
  abscesses, 279
  anatomy, 270
  carcinoma
    clinical staging, 271
    mode of spread, 271
    operations for, 274–7
    operative diagnosis, 274
    prognostic factors, 272
    treatment, 272–7
  cysts, 277
  lactiferous ducts
    excision, 280
    papilloma, 278
  operations on, 274–81
    Gaillard Thomas method, 278
    plastic, 280
  reconstruction, 280
  simple tumours, 277–8
Bronchiectasis, 290
Bronchus, division of, 291, 292
Burns
  protein replacement, 61
  skin grafting, 9

Burr hole exploration, 203, 205, 212
Buschke-Loewenstein tumours, 618
Butler operation, 111
By-pass
  bilary, 398, 399, 403
  carcinoma
    intestines, 431
    oesophagus, 303
    stomach, 346
  cardiopulmonary, 296–8
  grafts, vascular, 37

Caecopexy, 429
Caecostomy, 433
Caecum
  anatomy, 417
  gangrene, 445
  inspection of, 423
  tuberculosis, 448
  volvulus, 429
Calcaneum, osteotomy, 107
Calculi
  parotid, 264
  salivary, 226
  submandibular, 267
  see also Stones
Cancer *see* Tumours *and specific of cancer*
Cannulae, insertion of, 54
Cantor's tube, 421
Carbuncles, 142
Carcinoma
  adenoid cystic, 266
  adrenal glands, 557
  anal canal, 474
  appendix, 409
  basal cell, skin, 8
  bile ducts, 384, 399, 400
  bladder, 526, 582–4, 587, 641
  breast, 271–7
  bronchial, 290, 291
  colon, 420, 435–47, 452
  ear, 232
  gall-bladder, 378, 379, 384, 392
  larynx, 248
  lip, 227
  lymph glands, 267
  oesophagus, 300–3
  ovaries, 640
  pancreas, 384, 388, 400
  penis, 618–22
  pharynx, 245
  prostate, 604–6
  rectum, 459, 462–7, 641
  renal cell, 510, 533, 536–8, 539
  salivary glands, 264, 266
  scrotum, 635
  squamous cell
    hand, 153
    oesophagus, 299
    penis, 618
    skin, 8
    stomach, 359
  stomach, 339, 354, 358–61
  testes, 630
  thyroid gland, 257, 261
  tongue, 228, 245
  tonsil, 245

Cardiac
  arrest, 293
  resuscitation, 293
  tamponade, 294
Cardioplegia, cold, 295
Cardiopulmonary bypass, operations
    under, 296–8
Cardiospasm, 305
Carotid arteries
  anatomy, 28
  exposure, 28
  external, 263
  fistulae, 211
  rupture, 255
Carpal tunnel syndrome, 73
Cast syndrome, 420
CAT scanning, 203, 207, 210, 401, 512,
    620, 629
Catheterization
  suprapubic, 575
  ureter, 524, 545
  urethra, 512–16
    male, 608
Catheters
  Cummings, 550
  de Pezzer, 575
  Foley, 513, 514
  Gibbon, 513
  Jacques, 513
  Malecot, 286, 547, 575
  sizes, 514
  Stamey, 576
  types, 513
  ureteric, 519, 561
Causalgia, 79, 80
Cavitation, 155
Celestin's tube, 300
Cellulitis
  anaerobic, 161, 162
  hand, 145
Cephalic vein, shoulder, 179
Cerebrospinal fluid, rhinorrhoea, 201,
    202
Cervical rib, 243
Cervicothoracic block, 80
Charnley
  compression arthrodesis, 104, 106
  hip prosthesis, 95
Cheilitis, actinic, 225
Chest
  injuries, 283–5
  operations on, 286–307
  wall, defects, 285
Cholangiography, 384, 386, 388
Cholecystectomy, 383, 388, 390, 398
Cholecystitis
  acute, 383, 388, 389
  chronic, 384
Cholecystoduodenostomy, 399
Cholecystogastrostomy, 398
Cholecystojejunostomy, 399, 403
Cholecystostomy, 383, 388, 389, 398
Choledochoduodenostomy, 394, 398
Choledochotomy, 392, 398
Chondromas, 114
Chondrosarcomas, 114, 116
Chopart's amputation, 183

Chromaffinomata, 557
Circulation
    collateral, 26
    extracorporeal, 295
    limbs, disorders, 79
Circumcision, 616–18
Cisternal pucture, 213
Clamps
    Pott's multi-point, 298
    vascular, 26
Clawing
    foot, 107, 108
    toes, 108, 109, 182
        hallux, 111
Cleft
    lip, 232
    palate, 233
Club foot, 107, 108
Coagulation factors, replacement, 61–2
Coccygectomy, 478
Colectomy, 449–51, 452
Colitis
    segmental, 448
    ulcerative, 449
        segmental, 451
Colon
    anatomy, 417
    carcinoma, 420, 435, 452, 641
        obstruction in, 444–7
        operative techniques, 437–47
        preparation for surgery, 436, 445
    Crohn's disease, 448
    decompression, 424, 425
    diverticulitis, 451
    examination, 423
    injuries, 331
    irrigation, peroperative, 445
    mobilization, 438–41
    obstruction, 419, 422, 444
    polypoid disease, 452
    strangulation, 422, 501
    suture, 441–3
    volvulus, 420, 428
Colostomy, 432
    carcinoma of rectum, 466, 467
    in children, 434
    closure, 434
    Hirschsprung's disease, 452
    pelvis, 433
    transverse, 433, 446
Colovesical fistulae, 452, 589
Commando Operation, 245
Compression plates, 119
    mandible fractures, 222
    use of, 120
Computerized axial tomography (CAT
    scanning), 401, 512, 620, 629
    brain, 203, 207, 210
Connel suture, 320, 430
Cordotomy, spinothalamic, 218
Costotransversectomy, 217
Courvoisier's law, 388
Cricoid ring, 250
Cricopharyngeus muscle, division of,
    248
Crohn's disease, 448
Cushing's syndrome, 557

Cut-throat, 237
Cylindromata, 268
Cystectomy
    partial, 586
    total, 587
Cystic hygroma, 242
Cystitis, 525
Cysto-urethroscopy, 516
Cystograms, 505, 509
Cystoscopy, 521–2
Cystostomy, suprapubic, 575
Cystourethroscopy, 592
Cysts
    bone, 113, 116
    branchial, 240
    breast, 277
    dermoid, 7, 152, 224
    epididymal, 632
    hydatid, of liver, 377
    lymph, 242
    mucous, 149
    ovarian, 639–40
    pancreas, 404, 405
    parovarian, 643
    popliteal, 103
    ranulas, 225
    renal, 554
    sebaceous, 6
    superficial tissues, 5–8
    thyroglossal
        mouth, 226
        neck, 241

Dehydration, 310
Deltopectoral flap, 14, 246–7
Denham pin, 118, 119
Dental infections, 223
DeQuervain's syndrome, 24
Dermoids, 7
    facial, 224
    implantation, 152
Diabetes, amputations in, 166
    foot, 182
    Syme's, 186
Diaphragm
    congenital malformation, 305
    herniae, 305
        traumatic, 307
    ruptured, 285, 307
Diarrhoea, post-operative, 353, 354
Digital arteries, palmar, 173
Disarticulation
    elbow, 178
    hip, 194
    knee, 190
    metacarpophalangeal joint, 175
    shoulder joint, 179
    toes, 181, 182
    wrist, 177
Dislocation
    hip
        congenital, 98
        surgical, 94
    mandible, 226
    patella, 103
    shoulder, 88

Diverticulectomy
    bladder, 577
    Meckel's, 447
Diverticulitis, 451
Drainage
    bile ducts, 394
    gall-bladder, 389
    intestines, 421
    perforated appendix, 412, 413
    peritoneal cavity, 321
    stomach, 345
    suction, 2, 237, 261, 275, 321, 394,
        421, 496, 531
    wound see Wounds, drainage
Drop
    foot, 108
    wrist, 77
Ductus arteriosus, patent, 298
Dumping after gastric surgery, 353
Duodenum
    anatomy, 334
        arteries, 335
        lymphatics, 336
        nerves, 337
        veins, 335
    congenital abnormalities, 364
    disease, investigation, 339
    division of, 349
    injuries, 332
    ulcers, 340
        bleeding, 356–8
        operations for, 340, 342–52, 355–8
        perforated, 345, 354
        recurrent (anastomotic), 341, 342,
            353
Dupuytren's contracture, 10, 133, 147–9
Dura mater
    incision of, 208
    treatment, 200

Ears
    external
        haematoma, 224
        tumours, 232
    protruding, 223
Echo-encephalography, 203
Eggert's operation, 105
Elastic stockings, 48, 50, 51
Elbow
    arthroplasty, 91
    disarticulation at, 178
    exposure, 90
    intra-articular fracture, 121
    arthrodesis, 91
Electrolyte balance, 310
    in intestinal obstruction, 421
Ellik evacuator, 602
Embolectomy, 45
Empyema
    pleural, 286
        tuberculous, 290
    subdural, 211
Encephalography, air, 207
Endo-aneurysmorrhaphy, obliterative,
    41
Endometriosis, 643
Endoscopy

Endoscopy (*cont'd*)
  gastric, 340, 357
  urological
    equipment, 516–21
    photographs, 525–6
    technique, 521–2
Enterogastric reflux, 353
Epididymectomy, 630
Epididymostomy, 634
Epithelioma, 8
Erythrocyanosis, 80
Evacuator, Ellik, 602
Exomphalos, 497
Extracorporeal circulation, 295
Extradural haemorrhage, 202–3

Face
  congenital abnormalities, 232
  dermoid cysts, 224
  fractures, 221–3
  incisions, 1
  suture methods, 220
  tumours, 226
    malignant, 226–32
  wounds, 220, 222
  see also specific parts of face
Facial
  artery, 263
  nerve, 263
    paralysis, 266
    repair, 79
  vein, 263
Factor VIII, concentrates, 62
Factor IX, concentrates, 62
Faecalith, 428
Fasciectomy, 148
Femoral
  arteries, 191, 194
    anatomy, 32
    embolectomy, 45
    exposure, 33
  canal, 490
    closure of, 492, 493
  hernia, 491
    operations for, 491–4
    strangulated, 502
  nerve, 191, 194
  vein, 191, 194
Femur
  excision of head and neck, 98
  exposure, 95
  fractures, 118, 122
    complications, 124
    internal fixation, 122, 124
    midshaft, 125
    subtrochanteric, 124
    supracondylar, 126
    transcervical, 122
    trochanteric, 124
  head, replacement, 123
  tumours, 194, 195
Fibrinogen, replacement, 61
Fibroadenoma, breast, 278
Fibrosarcomas, 114, 116
Fingers
  amputations, 172
    disarticulation, 175

    indications for,173
    middle or proximal phalanx,
      175
    terminal phalanx, 174
  anatomy, 172
  arthritis, 149–52
  arthrodesis, 141, 149
  extensor tendon repair, 22
  flexor tendon repair, 21
  fractures, 139
  infections, 141
  injuries, 137
    ring avulsion, 137
  mallet, 22
  nails
    infections, 142
    injuries, 137
    splinters under, 138
    tumours at, 153
  replantation, 139
  swan-neck deformity, 151
  tips, injuries, 137
  tourniquets, 131
  traction, 138
  trigger, 25
  ulnar deviation, 151
Finney gastroduodenostomy, 346
Fistula
  anal, 472–4
  branchial, 240
  colo-vesical, 452, 589
  thyroglossal, 241
  tracheo-oesophageal, 303
  urethral, 613
  vesical, 589
Flaps
  latissimus dorsi, 15, 281
  osteoplastic, 208
  pectoralis major, 14, 229, 245–6
  skin
    local, 9
    pedicle, 14, 137
    rotation-advancement,10
    transposition, 10
Fluid
  balance, 310
    daily, 310
  intravenous infusions, 310
    intestinal obstruction, 421
Foot
  amputations in, 182
  claw, 107, 108
  club, 107, 108
  drop, 108
  flat, 108
  forefoot
    arthroplasty, 112
    operations on, 108–12
  hindfoot
    arthrodesis, 107, 108
    calcaneal osteotomy, 107
    operations on, 107–9
Forearm *see* Arm
Forehead, lined flap, 228
Foreign bodies
  brain, 201
  hand, 138

  spine, 215
  wounds, 157
Fossa ovalis defect, 296
Fournier's gangrene, 635
Fractures
  Bennett's, 140
  compound
    hand, 141
    management, 117
    in elderly, 117, 122
  hand, 139–41
  internal fixation, 118–28
    compression, 119, 121
    hand, 140
    intramedullary nailing, 122, 125,
      127
    plates, 124–7
    screws, 119, 120, 124–8
    tension band wiring, 120, 126
  intra-articular, 120
  management, 116–18
  Monteggia, 122
  non-union, 128
  skeletal traction, 118
  see also under specific sites of fracture
Frey's syndrome, 266
Fundoplication, 306

Gall-bladder
  anastomosis to gastro-intestinal tract,
    398
  anatomy, 381
  carcinoma, 378, 379, 384, 392
  injuries, 332
  operations on, 389–92, 398–9
    choice of, 388
    general technique, 385–8
    indications for, 383–5
    surgical diagnosis, 387
  stones, 383, 384
    ileus, 420
    impacted, 428
    removal, 389
Ganglia
  hand, 149, 152
  joints and tendons, 92
Ganglionectomy, 92
  fingers, 149, 152
  lumbar, 83
Gangrene
  diabetic, 166
  dry, 165, 183
  Fournier's, 635
  gas, 161, 163, 165
Gardner tongs, 215
Garrod's pads, 147
Gas gangrene, 161, 163, 165
Gastrectomy
  partial, 342, 347
    Billroth I, 351
    effect on gastric motility, 339
    Polya, 252, 348, 352
    radical, 360
Gastrin, 338, 340
Gastroduodenostomy, Finney, 346
Gastrojejunocolic fistula, 354
Gastrojejunostomy, 323, 346

Gastroschisis, 497
Gastrostomy, 362
  in children, 362
Gastrotomy, 362
Gauze packing, 158
Genu
  valgum, 105
  varum, 105
Girdlestone pseudarthrosis, 98
Girdlestone's operation, 109
Gliomas, 209
Glomus tumour, 153
Glossectomy, 229
Goitre, 257–8
  lymphadenoid see Thyroiditis,
    autoimmune
  removal, 259–61
  retrosternal, 261
Grafts
  arteries, 36, 37
    aneurysms, 43
  bone, 115, 128
    cancellous strip, 129
    onlay, 92
    tumour cases, 230
  bypass, vascular, 37
  nerve, 71, 266
  skin, 9–15
    failure, 13
    full thickness, 13
    infection and, 11, 13
    mesh, 13
    pinch, 14
    split, 10–13
    strip, 13
  tendon, 20
  Thiersch, 10
  Wolfe, 9
Granuloma, pyogenic, hand, 145
Grease gun injury, 139
Gritti-Stokes amputation, 194
Gunshot wounds, 194
  brain, 201
  face, 222
  rectum, 460
  spine, 215
  treatment, 156, 157
Gut see Intestines
Gynaecological operations in general
    surgery, 636
Gynaecomastia, 278

Haemangioma
  capillary, 7
  cavernous, 7
Haematoceles, 631
Haematoma
  extradural, 204
  subdural, 205
    chronic, 211
Haemophilia
  joint disorders and, 101
  treatment, 62
Haemorrhage
  arrest of
    arterial wounds, 27, 34
    dural vessels, 200

femoral vein, 49
  limbs, 34
  oesophagus, 370
  peptic ulcer, 357
  scalp, 197
  skin incisions, 1
blood transfusions in, 59–61
extradural, 202
  diagnosis, 202–3
  treatment, 203
gastrointestinal, 356, 370, 447, 452
haemolytic transfusion reactions, 62
post-operative, peptic ulcer surgery,
    352
secondary, soft tissue injuries, 161
subarachnoid, 211
subdural, 202
  chronic haematoma, 211
  diagnosis, 202–3
  treatment, 205
Haemorrhoids, 461, 468–71
Haemothorax, 284, 285
Hallux
  clawing, 111
  rigidus, 111
  valgus, 110
Hamilton Russell traction, 98, 125
Hamstrings, division, 23
Hand
  amputations in, 172–7
    indications, 173
    optimum levels, 165
  anaesthesia, 131
  anatomy, 172
  congenital anomalies, 146
  Dupuytren's contracture, 10, 133,
    147–9
  fractures, 139
    compound, 141
  immobilization, 133
  incisions, 133
    fasciectomy, 148
  infections, 141–6
    palmar spaces, 145
    septic arthritis, 144
    subcutaneous, 142
    subcuticular, 142
    tendon sheaths, 143
  injuries, 136–41
    aftercare, 135
    management, 136
    traumatic amputation, 139
  osteoarthritis, 149
  position of function, 134
  preparation for surgery, 131–3, 136
  replantation, 139
  rheumatoid arthritis, 150
  skin grafts, 137
  swelling, treatment, 135
  tendon repair, 20–2, 24
  tenosynovitis, 24
  tourniquets, 131
  tumours, 152
  see also Fingers; Thumb
Hartmann's procedure, 428, 444, 462, 467
Hashimoto's disease see Thyroiditis,
    autoimmune

Hauser's operation, 103
Head see Brain; Scalp; Skull
Healing, skin wounds, 2
Heart
  arrest, 293
  compression of, 294
  congenital defects, 296, 298
  disease, 298
    ischaemic, 297
  open surgery, 295–8
  surgical approach, 292
  valve replacement, 297
  wounds, 294
Heel, inversion, correction of, 107,
    108
Heineke-Mikulicz pyloroplasty, 345
Heller's operation, 305
Heparin, 39, 43
  in abdominal surgery, 312, 326
Hepatitis, neonatal, 399
Hepatitis A, prophylaxis, 62
Hepatitis B
  prophylaxis, 62
  transmission by transfusion, 63
Hernia
  diaphragmatic, 305
  direct inguinal, 488
    operation for, 489–90
  epigastric, 498
  femoral, 490
    strangulated, 502
  hiatus, 305
  incisional, 498
  oblique inguinal, 480
    in children, 482
    operations for, 481–8
    reconstructive procedures, 485
    strangulated, 502
  obturator, 499
  Richter's, 500, 501
    strangulated, 502
  sliding, 490
  strangulated, 500–2
  traumatic, 307
  umbilical
    adults, 494–6
    children, 496–8
    operations for, 494–8
Hiccough, post-operative, 326
Hip joint
  adduction deformities, 23
  amputations at, 194
  anatomy, 194
  arthrodesis, 96
  arthroplasty, 98
  aspiration, 93
  dislocation
    congenital, 98
    surgical, 94
  exposure, 93
  open reduction, 99
  replacement, 95
Hirschsprung's disease, 452–4
Hodgkin's disease, 367, 369
Horner's syndrome, 79, 80, 81
Human normal immunoglobulin (HNI),
    62

Human specific immunoglobulin (HSI),
  62
Humerus
  amputation through, 180
  exposure, 85
  intra-articular fracture, 120
Hydatid disease of liver, 377
Hydroceles, 630
Hydrocephalus, 214
Hydronephrosis, 549
Hygroma, cystic, 242
Hyperaldosteronism, 557
Hyperhidrosis, 80, 81
Hpernephroma *see* Renal cell carcinoma
Hyperparathyroidism, 262
Hypersplenism, 367, 368
Hypertension, portal, 369–73
Hypoalbuminaemia, treatment, 61
Hypoparathyroidism, 262
Hypopharynx, 246
  operations on, 246–8
Hypoproteinaemia, treatment, 61
Hypospadias, 622
Hypothermia in open heart surgery, 295
Hypothyroidism, 262
Hypovolaemia, fluid replacement, 61
Hysterectomy, 641–2, 643

Ileal conduit, 569
Ileitis, regional, 448
Ileocolitis, regional, 448
Ileostomy, 432, 449
  in children, 450
  complications, 450
  with ileorectal anastomosis, 451
  technique, 449
Ileum
  anatomy, 417
  diverticulum, 447
  kinking, 411
  tuberculosis, 448
Ileus
  gall-stone, 420
  paralytic, 419
    indications for operation, 423
    post-operative, 429
    treatment, 420, 422
Iliac arteries
  anatomy, 31
  aneurysm, 43
  embolectomy, 45
  exposure, 32
Ilium
  crest, cancellous grafting, 129
  osteotomy, 99
Immunoglobulins, transfusion
    preparations, 62
Incisions
  abdomen, 314–17
    in children, 317–19
  hand, 133
    fasciectomy, 148
  hockey stick, 387
  kidney, 529–34
  Kocher's, 317, 387
  Lanz, 316, 355, 409
  McFee, 253

Mayo-Robson, 387
Nagamatsu, 532
neck, 236, 253
Pfannenstiel's, 317
Rutherford Morison, 316, 411
Schechter, 253
skin, 1
  closure, 2–5
Weber Fergusson, 231
see also under specific operations
Infection
  abdominal surgery, 319, 320, 322,
    386, 413, 437
    appendicectomy, 413
  amputations and, 164
  dental, 223
  neck, 237
  prostatectomy, 604
  see also Wound infection
Infusions
  blood, 56
  intravenous, 55
Inguinal
  canal, 480
  hernia
    direct, 488–90
    oblique, 480–8
    strangulated, 502
  lymph nodes
    anatomy, 620
    dissection, 620
    treatment in penile carcinoma, 620
Injection injuries, 139
Interosseus nerve, posterior, 76, 77
Interphalangeal joints, 173, 180
  arthritis in, 149
  arthrodesis, 141, 149
Intervertebral discs
  compression of, 216
  protrusion of, 216
Intestines
  in abdominal surgery
    handling, 319
    repositioning, 321
  anastomoses, 322
  drainage, 421
    external (stoma), 432–5
  hernia
    external, 420
    internal, 428
  indications for operation, 422
  intussusception, 420, 425, 447
  large *see* Colon
  malrotation, 426
  obstruction, 418
    adhesive, 420, 422, 424–7
    assessment, 418
    differential diagnosis, 420
    exploratory laparotomy, 423,
      424
    level of, 421
    mechanical, 419
    post-operative, 429
    pseudo-, 420
  operations on, 423–54
    short-circuiting, 431
  plication procedure, 424

pre-operative treatment, 420
  irrigation, 445
resection, 501
small
  anatomy, 417
  atresia, 427
  injuries, 331
  obstruction, 418, 422, 424
  resection, 331, 429
  short-circuiting, 431
  strangulated hernia, 501
  volvulus, 426
strangulation, 419, 500
  internal, 425
sutures of, 320
volvulus, 427
*see also under specific conditions of
  intestines*
Intravenous infusion
  technique, 55
  see also Fluid, intravenous infusion
Intussusception, 425
  in infancy, 420, 425
  retrograde jejunogastric, 354
Ischaemia, traumatic, muscles, 17
Ischio-rectal abscess, 471
Isotope scanning
  bone, 272
  cerebral, 206
  kidney, 511
  Meckel's diverticulum, 447
  spinal, 214
  stomach, 353
  subphrenic, 375
  thyroid, 257

Jaboulay procedure for hydrocele, 631
Jaundice
  obstructive, 384, 399
  surgery in patients with, 385, 387
Jaw
  clicking, 226
  fractures, 221
  osteomyelitis, 223
Jejunogastric retrograde
    intussusception, 354
Jejunum, anatomy, 417
Joints
  aspiration, 85
  hand, surface marking, 172
  replacement, antibiotic cover, 85
  surgery, 84–130
    operative techniques, 84
  see also specific joints
Jones' operation, 111

Kasai's operation, 400
Kidneys
  anatomy, 528
  congenital anomalies, 550–2
  cysts, 554
  ectopic, 551
  failure, post-operative, 327
  hydronephrotic, 538
  injuries, 332, 552
  investigation of, 504–12

see also specific investigative
techniques
operations on, 534–55
  percutaneous, 555
removal, 534–8
  partial, 539, 541
stones, 540
  indications for operation, 541
  removal, 541–5
surgical approaches to, 529–34
transplantation, 555
tumours, 538, 539
  angiograms, 507
transitional cell, 539
  see also Renal cell carcinoma
see also Renal . . .
Knee
  arthrodesis, 103
  arthroplasty, 100
  arthroscopy, 99
  aspiration, 99
  disarticulation at, 190
  exposure, 100
  flexion deformities, 104–5
  genu valgum, 105
  genu varum, 105
  loose body removal, 102
  meniscectomy, 101
  osteochondritis dissecans, 102
  patellectomy, 103
  synovectomy, 100
Knife wounds, 154
Knots
  tying with left hand, 2
  types, 2
Kocher's incision, 317, 387
Krukenberg amputation, 178
Küntscher nail, 119, 125

Ladd's bands, 426, 427
Laminectomy, 215, 216
Langer's lines, 236
Lanz incision, 316, 355, 409
Laparoscopy, 333, 384, 638
Laparotomy, 329, 638
  intestinal obstruction, 423
  intraperitoneal injuries, 329
  peritonitis, 332
  technique, 330
Laryngeal nerves, 257
  paralysis, 262
Laryngectomy, 248–50
Laryngo-pharyngo-oesophagectomy,
  247
Laryngocoele, 243
Laryngopharyngectomy, 246
Laryngotomy, 248
Larynx, tumours of, 248–50
Latissimus dorsi flap, 28
Lawnmower injuries, 155, 158
Leg
  amputation through
    below knee, 186–90
    in upper third, 190
    in vascular disease, 188
  anatomy, 186
Lembert sutures, 319, 320, 322, 323

Leukoplakia, 225
Limbs
  amputation *see* Amputations
  congenital deficiency, 165
  reattachment, 163
Lipoma, 7
Lips
  cleft, 232
  leukoplakia, 225
  tumours, 227
Litholapaxy, 580
Lithotriptor, ultrasonic, 581
Lithotrites, 580, 581
Liver
  abscesses
    amoebic, 377
    pyogenic, 376
  anatomy, 374
  hydatid disease, 377
  injuries, 330
  needle biopsy, 380, 384
  resection, 378
    wedge, 379
  tumours, 378, 379
Lobectomy, 291
Lord's procedure for hydrocele, 631
Ludwig's angina, 239
Lumbar
  block, 80
  puncture, 213
Lungs
  abscess, 290
  cancer, 290, 292
  infections, post-operative, 326
  resection, 289, 291
    indications for, 290
  tuberculosis, 289
  wet, 283
Lymph glands
  anal canal, 458
  axillary, 270
    examination of, 271
  carcinoma, 8, 252, 267, 620
  cervical
    malignant disease, 252–6
    tuberculosis, 256
  colon, 417
  Hodgkin's disease, 367, 369
  rectum, 457
  stomach, 336
Lymph nodes, inguinal *see* Inguinal
  lymph nodes
Lymphangiography, pedal, 509, 620
Lymphangioma, 242
Lymphangitis, hand, 145

McBurney's point, 316, 408
McEvedy's operation for femoral
  hernia, 494, 502
Macewen's triangle, 206
McFee incision, 253
Magnesium deficiency, 311
Mallet finger, 22
Mandible
  bone graft, 230
  excision, 230, 245, 268
  fractures, 221

Mandibular joint, affections of, 226
Mastectomy
  modified radical, 276
  operative staging, 274
  radical, 277
  reconstruction following, 281
  simple (total), 275
    indications for, 273
Mastoiditis, 206
Maxilla
  excision, 231
  fractures, 222
Mayo-Robson incision, 387
Mayo's operation for umbilical hernia,
  494
Meatomes, 561
Meatotomy, 610, 622
Meckel's diverticulum, 447
Median nerve
  anatomy, 72, 177, 179
  compression, 73
  forearm, 177
  injury, 72
  repair, 73
  upper arm, 178
Melanoma
  amelanotic, 7
  malignant, 8
    hand, 153
Meningiomas, 209, 218
Meningocoele, 214
Meniscectomy
  knee, 101
  mandibular joint, 226
Menisci of knee, 101
Meralgia paraesthetica, 79
Mesentery
  anatomy, 417
  haematoma, 331
  injuries, 331
  vascular occlusion, 420, 428
Mesotenon, 18
Metacarpal bones
  fracture, 139
  osteotomy, 150
Metacarpophalangeal joint, 173
  arthritis, 152
  arthrodesis, 141, 150
  bites at, 138
  disarticulation at, 175
  subluxation, 151
Metatarsophalangeal joint, 180
  arthrodesis, 111
  disarticulation at, 181, 182
Metatarsus
  head resection, 112
  osteotomy, 110
Microsurgery
  fibula transplant, 113
  and limb reattachment, 163
  see also Replantation
Microvascular surgery, 15, 38, 71, 113,
  139, 163
Midtarsal joint, arthrodesis, 107, 108
Mikulicz operation, 429
Miller-Abbott tube, 421
Milnes Walker operation, 372

Minnesota tube, 370
Mitral valve disease, 297, 298
Monteggia fracture, 122
Moore's hip prosthesis, 123
Morton's neuroma, 79
Motor cycle injuries, brachial plexus, 71
Mousseau-Barbin tube, 301
Mouth
  congenital abnormalities, 232
  cysts, 224, 225, 226
  floor
    cysts, 225
    tumours, 230
  leukoplakia, 225
  tumours, 227–32
Muscles
  abscesses, 17
  contracture, 17
  hernia, 16
  management at amputation, 169
  rupture, 16
  transfer, 79
  traumatic ischaemia, 17
Musculocutaneous nerve, arm, 178, 179
Myelography, 214
Myelomenigocoele, 214
Myodesis, 167
Myoplasty, 167
  at amputation, 169

Naevi, 7
Nagamatsu incision, 532
Nails see Finger nails; Toe nails
Nasal bones, fracture, 223
Nasopharynx, 244
  operations on, 244
Neck
  congenital abnormalities, 239–44
  incisions, 1
  infections, 237
  operations, 236–62
    general techniques, 236
    incisions, 236, 253
    radical dissection, 253–6
    see also specific parts of neck
  tumours, 244–7
    lymph glands, 252–6
  wounds, 237
Needles
  arteries, 27
  gut, 320
  infusion, 54
  liver biopsy, 380
  skin, 5
Nephrectomy, 534–6
  indications for, 534
  partial, 539–40, 541
  for renal carcinoma, 536–8
  for stones, 541
  subcapsular, 536
Nephro-ureterectomy, 538
Nephrolithotomy, 541, 543–5
Nephropexy, 554
Nephrostomy, 547
Nerves
  anatomy, 68
  compression, 79

fibres, 68
grafting, 71, 266
injuries
  assessment, 69
  classification, 68
  hand, 137
  management, 70
  recovery from, 69
  see also individual nerves
management at amputation, 169
repair, 70
Wallerian degeneration, 69, 70
see also Sympathetic nervous system;
    individual nerves
Neuralgia, trigeminal, 211
Neurapraxia, 68
Neuromas, 218
  acoustic, 209
Neurotmesis, 68
Nipples, indrawn, 280
No-touch technique
  colon, 439
  orthopaedic, 84
Nose
  rhinophyma, 224
  see also Nasal . . .
Nuclear medicine, 510
Nutrition, parenteral, 312
Nylon darn, 487, 490, 499

Oesophagectomy, 247
Oesophagogastrectomy, 373
Oesophagus
  achalasia, 305
  arrest of haemorrhage, 370
  atresia, 303
  carcinoma, 300–303
  congenital malformation, 306
  excision, 299
  hiatus hernia, 305
  resection, 300, 301
  stricture of, 304
  transection, 370, 372
Ogilvie's syndrome, 420
Olecranon, fractures, 120
Omentum, 334
  strangulated, 502
Onychogryphosis, 109
Oophorectomy, 639–40, 643
Orchidectomy, 629
  direct inguinal hernia, 490
  subcapsular, 630
Orchidopexy, 625, 626–8
Oropharynx, 244
  operations on, 244–6
Orthopaedic surgery, 84–130
  see also Bones; Joints; and specific sites
Osteoarthritis, hand, 149
Osteochondritis dissecans, 102, 111
Osteochondromas, 114
Osteomas, oesteoid, 114
Osteomyelitis, 112
  jaws, 223
Osteoplastic flaps, 208
Osteoplasty, 169
Osteosarcoma, 114, 116

Osteotomy, 85
  with arthrodesis, 97
  calcaneus, 107
  femur, 99
  iliac, 99
  intertrochanteric, 97
  metatarsus, 110
  -osteoclasis, 85
  subtrochanteric, 97
  supracondylar, 105
  tibial, 105
  Wilson, 110
Ostium primum defect, 296
Ostium secundum defect, 296
Otoplasty, 223
Ovarian
  artery, 637
  cysts, 639–40
  vein, 637
Ovaries
  anatomy, 636
  removal, 639–40, 643
  tumours, 640

Pain, intractable, analgesic surgery, 218
Palate
  cleft, 233
  tumours, 231
Palm, repair with skin from finger, 174
Palmar spaces, infections, 145
Paloma operation for varicocele, 633
Pancreas
  abscess, 404
  anatomy, 382
  inflammatory conditions, 403–6
  injury, 406
  operations on, 400–3
    surgical diagnosis, 387
  pseudocyst, 404, 405
  tumours, 400–3
    carcinoma, 384, 388, 400–3
Pancreatectomy, 402, 406
  distal, 405
Pancreaticoduodenectomy, 401
Pancreatitis
  acute, 403–5
  chronic, 405
Papillomata
  breast, 278
  colon, 452
  face and mouth, 226
  rectum, 460
  skin, 7
Papillotomy, endoscopic, 396
Paracolic abscess, 451
Paranasal sinuses, fractures involving,
    201
Parapharyngeal abscess, 238
Paraphimosis, 617
Paratenon, 19
Parathyroid glands
  anatomy, 257, 262
  removal, 262
  tumours, 262
Paravertebral block, 80
Parenteral nutrition, 312
Paronychia, 142

Parotid gland
  anatomy, 263
  calculi, 264
  operations on, 264–7
    complications, 266
    indications for, 263
  sialectasis, 264
  tumours, 263, 264, 266
Parotidectomy
  conservative, 263, 264
  superficial, 264
  total, 266
Parotitis
  acute suppurative, 263
  chronic, 264
  post-operative, 328
Patella
  dislocation, 103
  removal of, 103
Pauchet manoeuvre, 352
Pectoralis major flaps, 14, 229, 245–6
Pedicle flaps, 14
  hand surgery, 137
Pelvis
  abscess, 143
  drainage, 322
    perforated appendix, 412, 413
  tumours, 195
Penis
  amputation, 618–20
  anatomy, 615
  balanitis, 616
  circumcision, 616–18
  congenital anomalies, 621–3
  curvature, 621
  paraphimosis, 617
  phimosis, 616
  straightening, 622
  tumours, 618–22
Pepsin secretion, 338
Peptic ulcers
  bleeding, 356–8
  investigation, 339
  perforated, 354–6
  post-operative management, 352
  recurrent, 341, 342, 353
  surgery, 434–52, 355–8
    choice of operation, 342, 356, 358
    complications, 352
    indications for, 340
Pericarditis
  acute suppurative, 299
  constrictive, 299
Pericardium, drainage, 299
Perinephric abscess, 548
Perineum, dissection, 464
Peripheral vascular disease, 80
Peritoneal cavity
  drainage, 321
    suction, 321
  exploratory laparotomy, 329
  lavage, 321, 333, 355, 405, 413, 437, 452
  prevention of soiling, 319
Peritoneum
  closing of, 321
  opening of, 319

Peritonitis
  appendix, 412
  due to salpingitis, 333
  laparotomy for, 332
  pneumococcal, 333
  post-operative, 327
  streptococcal, 333
  tuberculous, 333
Peroneal artery, 187
Pes cavus, 107, 108
Pes planus, 108
Peyronie's disease, 621
Pfannenstiel's incision, 317
Phaeochromocytomata, 557
Phalanges, hand
  amputation, 174
  fracture, 139
Pharyngeal pouch, removal, 247
Pharynx
  operations on, 244–50
  tumours, 244–7
Phimosis, 616
Phlebothrombosis, post-operative, 326
Phlegmasia caerulea dolens, 52
Pilonidal sinus, 477
Pirogoff's amputation, 186
Pituitary gland, tumours, 209
Plasma
  freeze dried, 61
  fresh dried, 61
  fresh frozen, 61
Plasma Protein Fraction (PPF), 61
Platelet concentrates, 61
Pleural
  aspiration, 286
  decortication, 289
  drainage, 286
  empyema, 286
Pleurectomy, 285
Pneumonectomy, 291
Pheumothorax
  in chest injuries, 283
  chronic (recurrent), 285
  open, 284
  spontaneous, 285
  tension (valvular), 283
Politano-Leadbetter operation, 565, 566
Polya partial gastrectomy, 348, 352, 353
Polypi
  colon, 452
  rectum, 460
Popliteal
  arteries, 191
    anatomy, 33
    aneurysm, 43
    exposure, 33
  cysts, 103
  nerves, 191
Port-wine stains, 7
Portal hypertension, 369–73
Portal vein shunts, 371
Potassium deficiency, 311
Pott's disease, 217
Pott's multi-point clamps, 298
Pregnancy, ruptured ectopic, 637–9
Princeps pollicis artery, 173
Pringle's manoeuvre, 379

Proctocolectomy, total, 449, 452
Proctoscopy, 458
Proctotomy, internal, 461
Profundaplasty, 38
Prostate
  anatomy, 589
  cystoscopic photographs, 526
  hypertrophy, 590
    choice of operation, 593
    diagnosis, 592
  stones, 606
  tumours, 595
    carcinoma, 604–6
Prostatectomy
  complications, 604
  punch, 603
  retropubic, 595–8
  transurethral, 598–604
  transvesical, 594
Protein deficiency, 311
Pruritus ani, 475
Pseudocyst of pancreas, 404, 405
Pseudomyxoma peritonei, 640
Psoas hitch, 562
Pulmonary
  embolism, post-operative, 326
  valve, stenosis of, 296
  see also Lungs
Purpura, idiopathic thrombocytopenic, 367
Putti-Platt procedure, 89
Pyelo-ureterography, antegrade, 509
Pyelography, retrograde, 507
Pyelolithotomy, 541, 542, 544
  coagulum, 543
  extended, 542
  percutaneous, 542
Pyeloplasty, 549
Pyelostomy, 547
Pyloromyotomy, 363
  in gastrectomy, 302, 361
Pyloroplasty, 345
Pylorus, stenosis of, 358
  congenital hypertrophic, 363
Pyomyositis tropicans, 17

Quadricepsplasty, 105

Radial
  artery, 177
  bursa, infection, 144
  nerve, 177, 178
    anatomy, 76
    exposure, 77
    injury, 77
Radialis indicis artery, 173
Radical nerve, paralysis, 24
Radius
  exposure, 91
  fractures, 121
  head
    dislocation, 122
    fractures, 120
Ramstedt's operation, 363
Raney clamps, 197, 198
Ranula, 225
Raynaud's syndrome, 80

Rectosigmoidectomy, 461
Rectum
  anatomy, 457
  carcinoma, 459, 462, 641
    choice of operation, 463
    operative techniques, 463–7
    pre-operative treatment, 463
  congenital anomalies, 475
  examination, 458
  Hirschsprung's disease, 452
  injuries, 459
  operative techniques
    abdominal excision, 467
    abdominoperineal dissection, 463
    anterior resection, 466
    palliative, 467
  proctocolectomy, 449
  prolapse, 461
  strictures, benign, 461
  tumours
    benign, 460
    differential diagnosis, 459
    see also Rectum, carcinoma
Rectus sheath, 313
Red cells
  antigens/antibodies, 57
  concentrates, 60
  leucocyte-depleted, 61
Renal
  angiography, 506
  artery, embolization, 537, 540
  cell carcinoma (Hypernephroma), 510
    operations for, 533, 536–8, 539
  failure, acute, 545
    treatment, 545–8
  ischaemia, 555
  pedicle, haemorrhage from, 538
  scan, 511
  vein, thrombosis, 510
  see also Kidneys
Renography, 510
Replantation, fingers, 139
Resectoscopes, 519, 598
Retropharyngeal abscess, 238
Rhesus (Rh) blood group system, 57
Rheumatoid arthritis
  hand, 150
  hip, 95
  knee, 101
Rhinophyma, 224
Rhinorrhoea, cerebrospinal fluid, 201, 202
Rhizotomy, spinal cord, 218
Ribs
  cervical, 243
  resection, 287
Richter's hernia, 500, 501, 502
Riedel's struma, 261
Ring avulsion, 137
Road traffic accident injuries
  abdominal, 329
  bladder, 332, 576
  brachial plexus, 71
  bumper, 154
  facial, 222
  renal, 552
  spine, 214
  thoracic, 283
  tibia, 126

Rodent ulcer, 8
Rotation-advancement flaps, 10
Rotator cuff muscles, 89
Roux loop, 302, 307, 308, 309
Roux-Goldthwart procedure, 103
Rush pin, 119
Rutherford Morison incision, 316, 411

Salivary glands
  anatomy, 263
  operations on, 264–9
    indications for, 263
  tumours, 263, 264, 266, 267
    ectopic, 268
Salpingectomy, 638, 640
Salpingitis, 333, 639
Saphenous
  nerve, 191
  veins, 187, 191
Sarcoma
  bone, 114, 116
  Ewing's, 165
  femur, 194
  stomach, 361
Scalenectomy, 243
Scalp
  anaesthesia, 197, 199
  anatomy, 197
  arrest of haemorrhage, 197
  suture methods, 198
  wounds, 197
    large, 199
Schechter incision, 253
Sciatic nerve, 191, 194
  anatomy, 78
  exposure, 78
  injuries, 77
Scrotum, operations on, 635
Semimembranosus bursa, 103
Shaving, 84
  head, 198
Shearing injuries, 154
Shock, fluid replacement, 61
Shotgun injuries, 154
Shoulder
  amputation at, 179
  anatomy, 178
  arthrodesis, 90
  dislocation, 88
  exposure, 86–8
  frozen, 256
Shouldice repair of inguinal hernias, 487
Sigmoidoscopy, 458
Sinuses
  pilonidal, 477
  tuberculous, neck, 256
Skin
  flaps see Flaps, skin
  grafting, 9–15
    hand, 137
  incisions, 1
    closure, 2–5
  management at amputation, 168
  preparation for surgery, 84
    hand, 132, 136
    soft tissue injuries, 156
  tumours, 5–8
    malignant, 8–9

Skull
  Burr hole exploration, 203, 205, 212
  defects, 212
  fractures, 199, 200
    depressed, 200, 205
    involving paranasal sinuses, 201
  open wounds, 199
  traction, 215
Smillie pins, 103, 121
Sodium deficiency, 311
Soft tissues
  injuries, 154–61
    face, 222
  management at amputation, 168
Souttar's tube, 301
Spermatic cord, torsion of, 628
Spermatoceles, 632
Spherocytosis, congenital, 367
Sphincteroplasty, transduodenal, 395, 398, 405
Spina bifida, 214
Spine
  analgesic surgery, 218
  anterolateral decompression, 217
  diagnostic procedures, 213
  fusion, 218
  infections, 216
  injuries, 214
    fractures, 214, 215
  laminectomy, 215, 216
  neoplasms, 218
  tuberculosis, 217
    treatment, 217
Spinothalamic tract, sectioning of, 218
Spleen
  anatomy, 366
  enlarged
    and blood dyscrasia, 367
    portal hypertension, 369
    removal of, 369
  injuries, 330
  removal of
    indications for, 366
    portal hypertension, 373
    technique, 368
  rupture, 366, 368, 369
Splinters, 139
Sports injuries
  Achilles tendon rupture, 22
  kidneys, 552
  knee, 101
    arthroscopy, 99
  muscle/tendon, 16
  quadriceps tendon, 23
Stable Purified Protein Solution (SPPS), 61
Stapling of wounds
  intestines, 443
  oesophagus, 370
  rectum, 463, 466
  stomach and duodenum, 349, 351, 361
Steindler's operation, 108
Steinmann pin, 118
Stereotaxy, 212
Stitches
  types, skin wounds, 3–4
  see also Sutures

Stockings, elastic, 48, 50, 51
Stomach
  anatomy, 334
    arteries, 335
    lymphatics, 336
    nerves, 337
    veins, 335
  aspiration, 309
  congenital abnormalities, 363
  diseases, investigation, 339
  drainage, 345
  injuries, 332
  lavage, 309
  minor operations, 362
  motility, 339
  physiology, 338
    acid and pepsin secretion, 338
  transection, 350
  tumours
    benign, 362
    carcinoma, 358–61
    differentiation, 339
    post-operative, 354
    sarcomas, 361
  ulcers, 341
    bleeding, 356–8
    differentiation, 339
    formation, 338
    operations for, 341, 342–52,
      355–8
    perforated, 354
    recurrent (anastomatic), 341, 353
Stomata
  intestinal surgery, 432
    care of, 432, 434
    construction, 433, 450, 466
    in children, 434, 450
    siting, 450
    temporary, 446
  urinary tract, 569–71
Stones, 540
  biliary, 383, 384, 420, 428
  bladder, 540, 578
  diagnosis, 541
  dislodger, Dormia type, 561
  indications for operation, 541
  kidney, 541–5
  prostatic, 606
  ureter, 559
  urethra, male, 613
  see also Calculi
Strangulation
  colon, 422, 501
  intestines, 419, 500, 502
    small, 501
  omentum, 502
Stryker frame, 215
Stumps, amputation, 167
  post-operative management, 171
Sturge-Kalischer-Weber syndrome, 7
Subarachnoid haemorrhage, 211
Subclavian arteries
  anatomy, 29
  aneurysms, 43
  exposure, 29
Subdural haemorrhage, 202–3, 205
  chronic haematoma, 211

Submandibular
  calculus, 226
  gland
    anatomy, 263
    calculi, 267
    removal, 267–8
    tumours, 267, 268
  space, infections of, 239
Subphrenic
  abscess, 375
  space, 375
Subtalar joint, arthrodesis, 107
Supraspinatus muscles, tendonitis, 90
Suture(s)
  Connell, 320, 430
  fascial, 487
  gastrectomy, 351, 361
  inguinal hernia, 487
  intestines, 320, 437
    anastomosis, 322, 441
  laryngectomy, 250
  Lembert, 319, 320, 322, 323
  materials
    abdomen, 321, 437
    arteries, 27, 35
    face wounds, 224, 225, 232, 233,
      234
    gastrectomy, 349, 351–2, 361
    hernia repairs, 486, 490, 495, 499
    intestines, 321, 431, 437, 441, 442, 446
    kidney operations, 534
    larynx, 250
    neck wounds, 237
    nerves, 70, 137
    perforated ulcer, 355
    pharynx, 245, 247
    pyloroplasty, 346
    skin wounds, 4, 220
    tendon repair, 19, 138
    vas deferens, 633, 634
    vascular, 27, 35
  nerve, 70, 71
  nylon darn, 487, 499
  Pulvertaft, 20
  pyloroplasty, 346
    in gastrectomy, 361
  skin, 5
    facial, 220
  skin ribbon, 487
  stapling device for, see Stapling of
      wounds
  tendon, 20
  unbilical hernia, 495
Swabs, safeguards against retention, 320
Syme's amputation, 166, 167, 183–5
  in diabetes, 186
  modified, 186
Sympathectomy, 79–83
  cervicothoracic, 81
  lumbar, 82
    chemical, 80
  transaxillary (transpleural), 82
Sympathetic nervous system
  disorders, 79–83
  paravertebral block, 80
Synovectomy, 101
Synovitis, pigmented villonodular, 152

Talipes equinovarus, 108
Telescopes, urinary tract endoscopy, 518
Tendo Achilles
  in club foot, 107
  lengthening, 23
  rupture, 22
Tendons
  anatomy, 18
  extensor, repair, 22
  fingers, 172
  flexor, repair, 19, 20–2, 25, 138
  hamstring, division, 23
  injuries, hand, 138
  quadriceps, repair, 23
  repair, 19–23
    grafting, 20,21
    hand, 20–2, 24
    silastic rods, 21
    suture, 19
  rupture, 16
  sheaths
    giant cell tumour, 152
    infection, 143
  tenotomy, 25
  transplantation, 24
Tenosynovitis, stenosing, 24
Tenotomy, 23
Testes
  anatomy, 623
  imperfect descent, 624
    management, 625–8
  removal, 629
  torsion, 628
  tumours, 625, 629
Tetanus, prophylaxis, 62
Tetany, 262
Tetralogy of Fallot, 296
Thiersch operation, 462, 475
Thigh
  amputation through, 191–4
  anatomy, 191
Thomson hip prosthesis, 123
Thoracoplasty, 289
Thorax
  injuries, 283–5
    see also Pneumothorax
  operations on, 286–307
Throat, cut, 237
Thrombo-angeitis obliterans, 80
Thrombo-endarterectomy, 37
Thrombocytopaenia, 61
Thrombolysis, 39
Thrombosis
  arterial, 44
  venous, 52
  see also Phlebothrombosis
Thumb
  amputations, 176
  anatomy, 172
  arthritis, 152
  arthrodesis, 150
  fractures, 139
  immobilization, 134
  malignant melanoma, 153
  tendon repair, 22, 24, 25
  trapeziometacarpal joint, 150
  Z-deformity, 151

Thymus, 299
Thyroglossal
    cysts
        lingual, 226
        neck, 241
    fistulae, 241
Thyroid
    arteries, 256
    glands
        anatomy, 256
        carcinoma, 257, 261
        isthmus, excision, 261
        operations on, 257–62
    scan
        isotope, 257
        ultrasound, 257
    veins, 256
Thyroidectomy
    hemi-, 261
    indications for, 257
    post-operative complications, 261
    pre-operative treatment, 258
    subtotal, 259
    total, 261
Thyroiditis
    autoimmune, 258, 261, 262
    chronic, 261
Thyrotoxicosis, 258
    recurrent, 262
Tibia
    fractures, 126
        non-union, 128
    osteotomy, 105
Tibial
    arteries, 187
    nerve, 187
Tinel sign, 68
Toes
    amputation, 181
    anatomy, 180
    arthrodesis, 11, 109, 110
    clawing, 108, 109, 182
    fifth, overlapping, 111
    hammer, 109
    mallet, 110
    nails, ingrowing, 109
    see also Hallux
Tongue
    excision, 229
    leukoplakia, 225
    stitch, 221
    tumours, 228–30
Tonsillectomy, 244
Torticollis, 23, 239
Tourniquets, 84
    hand, 131
Trachea, anatomy, 250
Tracheostomy, 250–2
    aftercare, 251
    in laryngectomy, 250
Traction
    after amputation, 172
    Hamilton Russell, 98, 125
    skeletal, 118
Tractotomy, spinothalamic, 218
Transplantation
    kidneys, 555

tendons, 24
Transposition flaps, 10
Trapeziometacarpal joint, osteoarthritis,
    150
Trendelenburg operation, 48
Trendelenburg position, 312
Trigeminal nerve, neuralgia, 211
Trigger finger, 25
Trigonectomy, 595
Trochanter, fracture of, 124
Tuberculosis
    anal canal, 472, 474
    cervical lymph glands, 256
    ileocaecal, 448
    pulmonary, 289
    spinal, 217
Tubes
    Cantor's, 421
    Miller-Abbott, 421
    Minnesota, 370
    Mousseau-Barbin, 301
    Souttar's, 301
Tumours
    amputation for, 165, 166
    Buschke-Loewenstein, 618
    Ewing's, 114, 115, 116, 165
    fulguration, 467, 584
    giant cell
        bone, 114, 116
        joints, 114, 116
        tendon sheath, 152
    superficial tissues, 5–8
    see also specific sites and types of tumour

Ulcers
    peptic see Peptic ulcers
    rodent, 8
    venous, 51
Ulna
    exposure, 92
    fractures, 121
Ulnar
    bursa, infection, 144
    nerve
        anatomy, 74
        compression, 75
        exposure, 75
        forearm, 177
        shoulder, 179
        transposition, 75
        upper arm, 178
Ultrasound, 257, 375, 385, 401, 505,
    549, 555, 557
Umbilicus, congenital anomalies,
    496–8, 502
Urachus, patent, 498
Ureter
    anatomy, 558
    catheterization, 526, 545
    exposure, 558
    implantation, 564
    injuries, 562
    orifice, 525
    repair, 562
    stones, 559–62
    transplantation
        into colon, 568

        to skin surface, 571
Ureterectomy with nephrectomy, 538
Ureterocystostomy, 564
Ureterolithotomy, 559–62
Ureterolysis, 571
Ureterosigmoidostomy, 568
Ureterostomy, 547, 562
    cutaneous, 571
Urethra
    catherization, 512
    male
        anatomy, 607
        catheterization, 608
        dilatation, 610
        fistulae, 613
        injuries, 607–9
        operations on, 610–15
        reconstruction, 612, 622
        stones, 613
        strictures, 609, 612
        tumours, 609
    prostatic, anatomy, 601
Urethrectomy, 587
Urethrocystography, 509
Urethroplasty, 612, 622
Urethroscopy, 517
Urethrostomy, 611
    perineal, 613, 620
Urethrotomes, 611
Urethrotomy, internal, 611–12
Urinary diversion operations, 568–71
Urinary tract
    investigative techniques, 504–27
        see also individual techniques
    see also individual parts of urinary tract
Urine
    residual, measurement of, 592
    retention
        post-operative, 326
        prostatic, 591–4
        urethral stricture and, 611
Urodynamics, 511, 593
Urography, intravenous (excretory), 504
Uterine
    artery, 637
    tube
        anatomy, 637
        infection, 639
        removal, 638, 640
        rupture, 637–9
    vein, 637
Uterus
    anatomy, 636
    broad ligament, 637
    cysts, 643
    removal, 641–2, 643

V–Y advancement, 10
Vagina, 636
Vagotomy, 342, 343–5
    effect on gastric motility, 339
Vagus nerves, 337, 338
VanderMeulen's operation for
    hypospadias, 622
Vanwelkenhuyzen's operation, 589
Varicoceles, 632
Varicose veins see Veins, varicose

Vas deferens, ligation/division *see*
        Vasectomy
Vascular
    anastomoses, 27, 35
    clamps, 26
    disease
        amputation for, 163, 166
        amputation in, 166, 188, 190
        obliterative, 36, 38
        peripheral, 80
Vasectomy, 633
    along with prostatectomy, 594
    reversal, 634
Vaso-epididymostomy, 634
Veins
    anatomy, 26
    cannulation, 55
    femoral
        arrest of haemmorhage, 49
        ligation, 53
    internal jugular, percutaneous
        puncture, 56
    pulmonary, embolism, 52
    saphenous
        anatomy, 46
        operations on, 48–51
    subclavian, percutaneous puncture,
        56
    thrombosis, 52
    ulcers, 51
    varicose, 46
        assessment, 47
        ligation, 50
        operations on, 48–51
        sclerotherapy, 48
        stripping, 49
Vena cava, inferior, interruption of, 53
Ventriculography, cerebral, 207

Verner Morison syndrome, 403
Vesical fistulae, 589
Vesico-vaginal fistulae, 589
Vesicolithotomy, 581
Viscera, repositioning after surgery, 321
Vitello-intestinal duct, patent, 498
Volkmann's ischaemic contracture, 17
Vomiting, post-operative, 326, 327

Waltman-Walters syndrome, 392
Warfarin, 39
Warts
    infective, 7
    pigmented, 7
    venereal, 618
Weber Fergusson incision, 231
Whipple's procedure, 401
Whitaker's test, 549
Wounds
    closed irrigation, 160
    closure
        hand, 136
        neck, 237
        skin, 2–5
        soft tissue injuries, 157
    debridement
        infected wounds, 160
        scalp, 198
        soft tissue injuries, 157, 160
    drainage
        abdomen, 322, 413
        neck, 237
        skin, 2
    excision
        hand injuries, 136
        scalp, 198
        soft tissue injuries, 156
    gunshot *see* Gunshot wounds

healing, 2
heart, 295
immobilization, soft tissue injuries,
        158
infection, 154
    appendicectomy, 413
    debridement and, 160
    gas gangrene, 161
    prevention, 155–6
    and skin grafting, 11, 13
    soft tissue injuries, 154, 155, 159–62
lacerated, repair, 10, 11
neck, 237
penetrating
    abdomen, 329, 330, 332
    arterial injury, 43
    brain, 201
    thorax, 283, 284
soft tissue, 154
    infected, 159–61
    treatment, 155–61
    types of, 154
thorax, 283, 284
see also Incisions
Wrist
    arthritis, 152
    arthrodesis, 92
    disarticulation of, 177
    drop, 77
    exposure, 92
    ganglionectomy, 92

Zadek's operation, 109
Z-plasty, 10
    hand surgery, 133, 148
Zollinger-Ellison syndrome, 340,
        403
Zygomatic bone, fractures, 223